Neuroimaging

Neuroimaging

William W. Orrison, Jr., M.D.

Professor and Chairman
Department of Radiology
University of Utah School of Medicine
Salt Lake City, Utah

W.B. SAUNDERS COMPANY
A Division of Harcourt Brace & Company
Philadelphia   London   Toronto   Montreal   Sydney   Tokyo

W.B. SAUNDERS COMPANY
A Division of Harcourt Brace & Company

The Curtis Center
Independence Square West
Philadelphia, Pennsylvania 19106

Library of Congress Cataloging-in-Publication Data

Neuroimaging / [edited by] William W. Orrison, Jr.

p.   cm.

Includes bibliographical references and index.

ISBN 0–7216–6799–6

1. Nervous system—Imaging.   2. Head—Imaging.   3. Neck—Imaging.
I. Orrison, William W.
[DNLM: 1. Central Nervous System Diseases—diagnosis.   2. Central Nervous
System—anatomy & histology.   3. Central Nervous System—pathology.
4. Head—pathology.   5. Diagnostic Imaging.   WL 300   N4938155 1998]
RC349.D52N476 1998

616.8′04754—dc21   97-39761

The editor gratefully acknowledges the contribution of the Society of Nuclear Medicine in allowing the reproduction of numerous figures and tables from *The Journal of Nuclear Medicine.*

NEUROIMAGING   ISBN 0–7216–6799–6
                                                      Volume 1 0–7216–6800–3
                                                      Volume 2 0–7216–6801–1

Last digit is the print number: 9   8   7   6   5   4   3   2   1

This text is dedicated to the memory of Wayman R. Spence, M.D.,
who was my relative, friend, mentor, confidant, and guide.

AND

To the women and men who have contributed of their time,
experience, and knowledge in order to make this text possible.
To each of you I am eternally grateful.

WILLIAM W. ORRISON, JR., M.D.

Contributors

ANDREW L. ALEXANDER, Ph.D.
Assistant Research Professor, University of Utah,
Salt Lake City, Utah
  *Neurovascular Magnetic Resonance and Computed
  Tomographic Angiography*

ROSEANNE ASTURI, R.D.M.S.
Ultrasound Technologist, Supervisor, Allegheny General
Hospital, Pittsburgh, Pennsylvania
  Transcranial Doppler Sonography

IRWIN BECKMAN, D.O., F.A.C.R., A.B.
Assistant Professor of Radiologic Sciences, Senior
Attending Radiologist, Allegheny General Hospital,
Allegheny University of the Health Sciences,
Pittsburgh, Pennsylvania
  Transcranial Doppler Sonography

FRANÇOIS BENARD, M.D.
Senior Fellow, Nuclear Medicine, University of
Pennsylvania; Senior Research Fellow, Nuclear
Medicine, University of Pennsylvania Medical Center,
Philadelphia, Pennsylvania
  Thyroid and Parathyroid

EDWARD C. BENZEL, M.D.
Professor, Department of Neurosurgery, Cleveland
Clinic Foundation, Cleveland, Ohio
  Spine Trauma

ROBERT DOWNEY BOUTIN, M.D.
Assistant Professor of Radiology, University of California,
San Diego; Musculoskeletal Radiologist, University of
California, San Diego Medical Center, and Veterans
Affairs Medical Center, San Diego, California
  Myelography; Degenerative Diseases of the Spine

BRIAN C. BOWEN, Ph.D., M.D.
Associate Professor of Radiology and Neurological
Surgery, Neuroradiology Section, Department of
Radiology, University of Miami School of Medicine;
Attending Radiologist, Jackson Memorial Medical
Center, Miami, Florida
  Salivary Glands and Lymph Nodes

WILLIAM G. BRADLEY, M.D, Ph.D.
Professor of Radiological Sciences, University of
California, Irvine; Director, MRI and Radiology
Research, Long Beach Memorial Medical Center,
Long Beach, California
  Hydrocephalus and Cerebrospinal Fluid Flow

JOHN A. BUTMAN, M.D., Ph.D.
Fellow, Neuroradiology, University of New Mexico,
Alburquerque, New Mexico
  Spine Trauma

SHARON E. BYRD, M.D.
Associate Professor, Department of Radiology,
Northwestern Medical School and Hospital; Head,
Division of Neuroimaging, Department of Radiology,
Children's Memorial Hospital, Chicago, Illinois
  *Normal Development of the Neonate's, Infant's, and
  Young Child's Brain*

RAYMOND F. CARMODY, M.D.
Professor of Radiology, Neuroradiology Section,
Department of Radiology, University of Arizona,
Tucson, Arizona
  The Orbit and Visual System

LINDA R. CASEY, M.D.
Staff Radiologist, Lovelace Hospital,
Albuquerque, New Mexico
  Cerebral Angiography

MAURICIO CASTILLO, M.D.
Associate Professor, Chief of Neuroradiology, University
of North Carolina School of Medicine, Chapel Hill,
North Carolina
  *The Larynx; Imaging of Congenital Malformations of
  the Brain; Imaging of Congenital Abnormalities of the
  Spine and Spinal Cord; Imaging of Congenital
  Abnormalities of the Face*

BRIAN W. CHONG, M.D., F.R.C.P.(C.)
Associate Professor, University of Utah, School of
Medicine; Medical Director, Center for Advanced
Medical Technologies and Functional Brain Imaging
Program, Department of Radiology, University of Utah,
Salt Lake City, Utah
  *Functional Magnetic Resonance Imaging; Magnetic
  Source Imaging; The Normal Brain*

EDWIN L. CHRISTIANSEN, D.D.S., Ph.D.
Professor and Director, Oral Medicine/TMJ Clinic;
Associate Professor, Department of Radiation Sciences,
Loma Linda University Schools of Dentistry and
Medicine, Loma Linda, California
  *Essential and Advanced Temporomandibular Joint
  Imaging: A Study of Cases*

VIJAYA V. CHUNDI, M.D.
Neuroradiologist, North Florida Regional Hospital;
North Florida Radiology, Gainesville, Florida
  Extra-Axial Tumors Including Pituitary and Parasellar

CAROL L. CLERICUZIO, M.D.
Associate Professor of Pediatrics and Chief, Division of
Clinical Genetics/Dysmorphology, University of New
Mexico School of Medicine, Albuquerque, New Mexico
Neurocutaneous Syndromes

CRYSTAL F. DARLING, M.D.
Assistant Professor, Department of Radiology, Division
of Neuroimaging, Children's Memorial Hospital,
Northwestern University School of Medicine;
Department of Radiology, Northwestern Memorial
Hospital, Chicago, Illinois
*Normal Development of the Neonate's, Infant's, and
Young Child's Brain*

NILIMA DASH, M.D.
Associate Professor of Radiologic Sciences, Allegheny
University of the Health Sciences, MCP, Hahnemann
School of Medicine, Allegheny Campus; Senior
Attending Staff Radiologist, Allegheny General Hospital,
Pittsburgh, Pennsylvania
Transcranial Doppler Sonography

H. CHRISTIAN DAVIDSON, M.D.
Assistant Professor of Radiology, The University of Utah;
Chief of Imaging Service, Veterans Affairs Medical
Center, Salt Lake City, Utah
The Temporal Bone; The Skull Base

DONALEE A. DAVIS, R.N., C.N.R.N.
Technical Director, Neurovascular Laboratory,
Department of Radiology, Cleveland Clinic Foundation,
Cleveland, Ohio
Transcranial Doppler Sonography

MARK H. DEPPER, M.D.
Chief, Neuroradiology, Walter Reed Army Medical
Center, Washington, District of Columbia
Pediatric Brain Tumors; Neurocutaneous Syndromes

PEDRO J. DIAZ-MARCHAN, M.D.
Assistant Professor, Department of Radiology, Baylor
College of Medicine; Chief of Neuroradiology, Ben Taub
General Hospital, Houston, Texas
Intracranial Hemorrhage

ROSALIND B. DIETRICH, M.B., Ch.B.
Professor of Radiological Sciences, Vice Chair of
Research, and Director of MRI, University of California,
Irvine, Orange, California
Anoxic Ischemic Injury in Children

MARY K. EDWARDS-BROWN, M.D.
Professor of Radiology and Neurology,
Indiana University School of Medicine,
Indianapolis, Indiana
*Metabolic and Endocrine Diseases; Traumatic Brain
Injury in Children*

REGINA GANDOUR-EDWARDS, M.D.
Assistant Clinical Professor of Pathology, Department of
Pathology, University of California, Davis Medical
Center, Sacramento, California
The Nasal Cavity and Paranasal Sinuses

CHRISTINE M. GLASTONBURY, M.B.B.S.
Clinical Instructor, Department of Radiology,
Neuroradiology Section, The University of Utah,
Salt Lake City, Utah
Adult White Matter Disease; The Skull Base

KENT GLEDHILL, M.D.
Director of Medical Imaging, Timpanogas Regional
Hospital, Orem; Staff Radiologist, Mountain View
Hospital, Payson; Adjunct Clinical Professor,
Department of Radiology, The University of Utah, Salt
Lake City, Utah
Cerebrovascular Disease

H. RIC HARNSBERGER, M.D.
Professor of Radiology, The University of Utah,
Salt Lake City, Utah
The Temporal Bone

BLAINE L. HART, M.D.
Associate Professor, Department of Radiology, University
of New Mexico, Albuquerque, New Mexico
*Intra-Axial Brain Tumors; Spine Trauma; Pediatric
Brain Tumors; Neurocutaneous Syndromes; Traumatic
Brain Injury in Children*

MICHAEL F. HARTSHORNE, B.A., B.S., M.D.
Professor of Radiology, University of New Mexico;
Chief, Joint Imaging Service, Veterans Affairs Medical
Center, Albuquerque, New Mexico
*Positron Emission Tomography in the Central Nervous
System; Single-Photon Emission Computed
Tomography of the Central Nervous System*

L. ANNE HAYMAN, M.D.
Professor, Department of Radiology; Professor,
Department of Psychiatry and Behavioral Sciences;
Director, Herbert J. Frensley Center for Imaging
Research, Baylor College of Medicine, Houston, Texas
Intracranial Hemorrhage

JOHN M. JACOBS, M.D.
Adjunct Clinical Professor of Radiology, The University
of Utah, Salt Lake City, Utah
Neurointervention; Cerebrovascular Disease

BLAKE A. JOHNSON, M.D.
Director of CNS Imaging, Center for Diagnostic
Imaging, St. Louis Park, Minnesota
Intracranial Infections

GREGORY M. JONES, Ph.D.
Medical Health Physicist, Center for Advanced Medical
Technologies, University of Utah, Salt Lake City, Utah
Functional Magnetic Resonance Imaging

EMANUEL KANAL, M.D., F.A.C.R.
Associate Professor of Radiology and Director, Clinical
and Educational Magnetic Resonance, University of
Pittsburgh Medical Center, Pittsburgh, PA
Magnetic Resonance: Bioeffects and Safety

JOHN P. KARIS, M.D.
Staff Neuroradiologist, The Barrow Neurological
Institute, St. Joseph's Hospital and Medical Center,
Phoenix, Arizona
*Magnetic Resonance Imaging Artifacts: A Practical
Approach; The Aging Brain and Neurodegenerative
Disorders*

RONALD L. KORN, M.D., Ph.D.
Staff Radiologist, Scottsdale Memorial Hospital,
Scottsdale, Arizona
Thyroid and Parathyroid

ROLAND R. LEE, M.D.
Associate Professor of Radiology, University of New
Mexico School of Medicine; Director of Neuroimaging,
Veterans Affairs Medical Center, Albuquerque, New
Mexico
Neoplasms of the Spine

JONATHAN S. LEWIN, M.D.
Associate Professor, and Vice Chairman for Research
and Academics, Case Western Reserve University School
of Medicine; Director of Magnetic Resonance Imaging,
University Hospitals of Cleveland, Cleveland, Ohio
Imaging of the Parapharyngeal and Masticator Spaces

JEFFREY DAVID LEWINE, Ph.D.
Scientific Director, Center for Advanced Medical
Technologies; Director, Functional Brain Imaging
Program and Magnetic Source Imaging Facility;
Associate Professor of Radiology, The University of
Utah, Salt Lake City, Utah
Magnetic Source Imaging; The Normal Brain

VIRGINIA A. LIVOLSI, M.D.
Professor, Pathology and Laboratory Medicine,
University of Pennsylvania; Vice Chairman, Anatomic
Services, Department Pathology and Laboratory
Medicine, University of Pennsylvania Medical Center,
Philadelphia, Pennsylvania
Thyroid and Parathyroid

ANTHONY R. LUPETIN, M.D., F.A.C.R.
Professor of Radiology, Allegheny University of the
Health Sciences, MCP, Hahnemann School of Medicine,
Allegheny Campus; Director, Division of Body Imaging;
Senior Attending Radiologist, Allegheny General
Hospital, Pittsburgh, Pennsylvania
Transcranial Doppler Sonography

ALEXANDER S. MARK, M.D.
Director of MRI, Washington Hospital Center; Associate
Clinical Professor of Radiology and Neurosurgery,
George Washington University Hospital, Washington,
District of Columbia
Infections and Inflammatory Diseases of the Spine

VINCENT P. MATHEWS, M.D.
Associate Professor of Radiology, Indiana University
School of Medicine, Indianapolis, Indiana
Metabolic and Endocrine Diseases

ELIAS MELHEM, M.D.
Assistant Professor of Radiology, Boston University
School of Medicine; Section Head, Neuroradiology,
Boston Medical Center, Boston, Massachusetts
Neoplasms of the Spine

KEVIN R. MOORE, M.D.
Clinical Instructor, Department of Radiology,
Neuroradiology Section, The University of Utah,
Salt Lake City, Utah
*Cerebrovascular Disease; Neuroimaging and Head
Trauma; The Skull Base*

SURESH K. MUKHERJI, M.D.
Assistant Professor of Radiology and Surgery; Chief,
Head and Neck Radiology, University of North Carolina
School of Medicine; Adjunct Assistant Professor of
Diagnostic Sciences, University of North Carolina
School of Dentistry, Chapel Hill, North Carolina
*The Pharynx and Oral Cavity; The Larynx; Imaging
of Congenital Malformations of the Brain; Imaging of
Congenital Abnormalities of the Spine and Spinal
Cord; Imaging of Congenital Abnormalities of
the Face*

GERARD J. MURO, M.D.
The Barrow Neurological Institute, St. Joseph's Hospital
and Medical Center, Phoenix, AZ
The Aging Brain and Neurodegenerative Disorders

SANDY NAPEL, Ph.D.
Associate Professor of Radiology, Department of
Radiology, Radiological Sciences Laboratory, Stanford
University School of Medicine, Stanford, CA
*Neurovascular Magnetic Resonance and Computed
Tomographic Angiography*

WILLIAM R. NEMZEK, M.D.
Assistant Clinical Professor of Radiology, Department of
Radiology, University of California, Davis Medical
Center, Sacramento, California
The Nasal Cavity and Paranasal Sinuses

WILLIAM W. ORRISON, JR., M.D.
Professor and Chairman, Department of Radiology,
University of Utah, Salt Lake City, Utah
*The History of Neuroradiology; Magnetic Source
Imaging; Neurointervention; Intra-Axial Brain
Tumors; Cerebrovascular Disease; Adult White Matter
Disease; Neuroimaging and Head Trauma; The Skull
Base; Hydrocephalus and Cerebrospinal Fluid Flow*

JUNG K. PARK, M.D.
Director of Neuroradiology, Arrowhead Community
Hospital; Radiologist, Arizona Medical Imaging,
Phoenix, Arizona
Imaging of the Parapharyngeal and Masticator Spaces

DENNIS L. PARKER, Ph.D.
Professor, Department of Radiology, Medical Imaging
Research Laboratory, University of Utah, Salt Lake City,
Utah
*Neurovascular Magnetic Resonance and Computed
Tomographic Angiography*

JESSE R. RAEL, M.D.
Assistant Professor, Department of Radiology, University of New Mexico, Albuquerque, New Mexico
Cerebral Angiography; Neurointervention

DONALD RESNICK, M.D.
Professor of Radiology, University of California, San Diego School of Medicine; Chief, Osteoradiology Section, Veterans Affairs Medical Center, San Diego, California
Degenerative Diseases of the Spine

FREDERICK WILLIAM RUPP, JR., M.D.
Assistant Professor of Neuroradiology, University of New Mexico Health Sciences Center/School of Medicine, Albuquerque, New Mexico
Myelography

JOHN A. SANDERS, Ph.D.
Research Assistant Professor, Department of Radiology, University of New Mexico School of Medicine; Health Scientist, Albuquerque Veterans Affairs Medical Center, Albuquerque, New Mexico
Computed Tomography and Magnetic Resonance Imaging; Functional Magnetic Resonance Imaging

WILLIAM P. SANDERS, M.D.
Senior Staff Neuroradiologist, Department of Radiology, Henry Ford Hospital, Detroit, Michigan
Extra-Axial Tumors Including Pituitary and Parasellar

ALICE M. SCHEFF, M.D.
Staff Radiologist, Santa Clara Valley Medical Center, San Jose, California
Thyroid and Parathyroid

JOACHIM F. SEEGER, M.D., F.A.C.R.
Professor and Head of Neuroradiology, Department of Radiology, University of Arizona Health Sciences Center, Tucson, Arizona
Normal Variations of the Head

JAMES J. SELL, M.D.
Associate Professor, Department of Radiology, University of New Mexico School of Medicine, Albuquerque, New Mexico
Contrast Agents in Neuroradiology

FRANK J. SHELLOCK, Ph.D.
Clinical Professor of Radiology, University of Southern California School of Medicine, Los Angeles, CA
Magnetic Resonance: Bioeffects and Safety

H. JOSEPH SPAETH, M.D.
Staff Radiologist, Suburban Radiologic Consultants, Minneapolis, Minnesota
Degenerative Diseases of the Spine

LISA M. SULLIVAN, M.D.
Private Practice, Lincoln, Nebraska
Fetal Neurosonography; Neonatal, Spinal, and Intraoperative Neurosonography

JAMES N. SUOJANEN, M.D.
Instructor in Radiology, Harvard Medical School; Neuroradiologist, Beth Israel Deaconess Medical Center, Boston, Massachusetts
The Hypopharynx

KATHERINE H. TABER, Ph.D.
Assistant Professor, Department of Radiology, Baylor College of Medicine, Houston, Texas
Intracranial Hemorrhage

LAWRENCE N. TANENBAUM, M.D.
Assistant Professor, Department of Neuroscience, Seton Hall School of Graduate Medical Education, Newark; Section Chief, Neuroradiology, MRI, and CT, New Jersey Neuroscience Institute, JFK Medical Center, Edison, New Jersey
Seizure Imaging

MICHAEL R. THEOBALD, M.D.
The Barrow Neurological Institute, St. Joseph's Hospital and Medical Center, Phoenix, AZ
The Aging Brain and Neurodegenerative Disorders

JOSEPH R. THOMPSON, M.D.
Neuroradiology Section, Loma Linda University Medical Center, Loma Linda, California
Essential and Advanced Temporomandibular Joint Imaging: A Study of Cases

SHEILA MULLIGAN WEBB, B.S., M.F.A.
Department Editor, Department of Radiology, University of Utah, Salt Lake City, Utah
The History of Neuroradiology

JANE WEISSMAN, M.D.
Associate Professor of Radiology and Otolaryngology; Director, Head and Neck Imaging, University of Pittsburgh School of Medicine, Pittsburgh, Pennsylvania
The Pharynx and Oral Cavity

DAVID G. WESTMAN, M.D., F.R.C.P.(C.)
Staff Radiologist, Stratford General Hospital, Stratford, Ontario, Canada
The Nasal Cavity and Paranasal Sinuses

MICHELLE L. WHITEMAN, M.D.
Assistant Professor of Clinical Radiology, Otolaryngology and Neurological Surgery, Department of Radiology, Section of Neuroradiology, University of Miami School of Medicine; Attending Radiologist, Jackson Memorial Medical Center, Miami, Florida
Salivary Glands and Lymph Nodes

PHILIP W. WIEST, M.D.
Associate Professor of Radiology, Vice-Chairman for Clinical Affairs, Department of Radiology, University of New Mexico, Health Sciences Center, School of Medicine, Albuquerque, New Mexico
Fetal Neurosonography; Neonatal, Spinal, and Intraoperative Neurosonography

Foreword

"Good grief!" Charlie Brown exclaimed to Lucy as he rolled his eyeballs. "Not *another* neuroradiology book!" He complained about his overloaded sagging bookshelves and stretched budget. "Hey," continued Charlie, "Wonderful teaching texts are already available. Highly detailed tomes that serve as excellent references in single modalities (such as MR) sit on our shelves. There are superb texts that focus on specific age groups, e.g., pediatrics. And there are still more that address subspecialty areas such as head and neck, spine and cord. We've got handbooks. Case Books. Self-evaluation quiz books. We even have some very fine books on specific disease entities such as head trauma and myelin disorders. So what's the big deal?"

Well, to the "Charlie Browns" among us, there's a mighty good reason to have another book on your shelf. When Bill Orrison and I discussed the already crowded field of neuroimaging texts several years ago, what became readily apparent is what we *don't* have. There really isn't an up-to-date multimodality, multisubspecialty, comprehensive reference text that includes hot new imaging techniques such as functional magnetic resonance imaging (fMRI), advanced magnetic resonance angiography (MRA), magnetoencephalography (MEG), and other emerging tools for imaging the central nervous system and its disorders. Bill Orrison's landmark new text, *Neuroimaging*, is designed to fill this need. It even includes (thank you, Bill!) modalities such as transcranial Doppler sonography (TCD) that are usually outside the domain of traditional neuroradiology.

Intended as a comprehensive reference for radiologists, clinicians, and allied neuroscience professionals, *Neuroimaging* isn't a book one sits down and reads cover to cover. It *is* the one you want to have handy when you need to look up "stuff." When you're puzzled about a difficult diagnosis. When you wonder what additional studies might be useful in elucidating an unusually puzzling problem. The illustrations are beautiful, the hefty references provide further suggested reading, and the hot new modalities are dazzling. Bill and his coauthors have done a monumental job in collating a huge amount of information on a spectrum of diseases (both major, "usual suspects," and minor but important pathology).

I hope you'll enjoy having such an invaluable resource right at your fingertips. I will!

ANNE G. OSBORN, M.D.

Preface

This text has been created to serve as a master reference file on the field of neuroimaging. The goal was to catalog and include all aspects of the practice of neuroimaging. It is hoped that this text will serve as a resource for physicians and neuroscientists in the fields of diagnostic radiology, neuroradiology, neurosurgery, neurology, psychiatry, psychology, neurophysiology, and neurobiology. Such an undertaking was by its very nature far more than any one individual could attempt, and therefore experts were sought in each of the subspecialty areas of neuroimaging to supply the most comprehensive information available. Omissions that may be present are not intentional and, if noted, are solely my responsibility.

The first section of this work deals with the history and technology that have made the field of neuroimaging possible. It includes sections on computed tomography (CT) and magnetic resonance (MR) technology, CT and MR angiography, functional MR, positron emission tomography, single-photon emission computed tomography, magnetic source imaging, cerebral angiography, neurointervention, neurosonography, transcranial Doppler sonography, myelography, contrast agents, and the safety issues and artifacts encountered in MR. There appears to be a real need for this type of information. This seems to be particularly true for physicians in training or those who work around, but not necessarily directly with, a given modality.

The second section focuses on the brain. Chapters here discuss the normal brain, normal variations encountered in neuroimaging, intra- and extra-axial neoplasms, vascular disease, infections, adult white matter disorders, the aging brain and neurodegenerative disorders, intracranial hemorrhage, brain trauma, and seizure imaging. A comprehensive review of all of the modalities that are currently used to evaluate the brain as well as the diseases encountered should make this a valuable reference tool for both the practicing clinician and the active neuroscientist.

The third section is dedicated to the head, neck, and spine. Included in this section are chapters on the temporal bone and skull base, the orbit and visual system, the nasal cavity and paranasal sinuses, the pharynx and oral cavity, the larynx, the hypopharynx, the parapharyngeal and masticator spaces, the thyroid and parathyroid, the salivary glands and lymph nodes, the temporomandibular joint, degenerative diseases of the spine, neoplasms of the spine, infectious and inflammatory diseases of the spine, and spinal trauma. This is perhaps the most complicated area in neuroimaging, especially when the head and neck are emphasized. Therefore, a comprehensive reference guide should be of benefit to those who work and study in this field.

The fourth section covers pediatric neuroimaging. This section includes chapters on the normal development of the neonatal, infant, and young child's brain, the imaging of congenital malformations of the brain, the imaging of congenital spine and spinal cord abnormalities, pediatric brain tumors, metabolic and endocrine diseases, the imaging of congenital abnormalities of the face, anoxic ischemic injury, hydrocephalus and cerebrospinal fluid flow, neurocutaneous syndromes, and traumatic brain injury in children. Pediatric neuroimaging is complex, and reference material is frequently needed. In the words of the late Dr. Derek Harwood-Nash, and true to spirit of what he has taught us, "Children are not small adults."

This exhaustive work would not have been accomplished without the dedication and effort of many people. Primary among them are the authors whose work we are privileged to present here. I would also like to acknowledge the assistance of Beth Hatter and Judy Spahr from the W.B. Saunders Company who prodded us through the publishing process. I would particularly like to thank Lisette Bralow for her patience and understanding during the final months of the editing of this text. There are no words to express my appreciation for the work performed by Sheila Mulligan Webb. For your countless hours of editing and your dedication to perfection—I sincerely thank you. Finally, I would like to thank my children, Bill, Jenny, and Mike, for their patience as they would ask every day, "Dad, how many more chapters do you have left?" The answer, kids, for once, is none! And to my wife, Becky, your support, your love, and your acceptance sometimes defy understanding.

This comprehensive textbook of neuroimaging is being published in the last year of the second millennium. It will at the very least serve as a marker of the advancements made in this field as of this point in time. The field of neuroradiology or neuroimaging came into existence in the latter part of this century. As we approach the next century, neuroimaging has become a cornerstone in medical care and a symbol of excellence in scientific accomplishment. Based on the successes we have witnessed thus far, the future appears unimaginable. In the words of my mentor and friend, Dr. Wayman R. Spence, "The best is yet to come!"

WILLIAM W. ORRISON, JR., M.D.
Salt Lake City, Utah

Contents

PEDIATRICS 1473

43. Normal Development of the Neonate's, Infant's, and Young Child's Brain 1475

    Sharon E. Byrd, M.D., and
    Crystal F. Darling, M.D.

44. Imaging of Congenital Malformations of the Brain 1516

    Mauricio Castillo, M.D., and
    Suresh K. Mukherji, M.D.

45. Imaging of Congenital Abnormalities of the Spine and Spinal Cord 1536

    Mauricio Castillo, M.D., and
    Suresh K. Mukherji, M.D.

46. Pediatric Brain Tumors 1550

    Mark H. Depper, M.D., and
    Blaine L. Hart, M.D.

47. Metabolic and Endocrine Diseases 1643

    Mary K. Edwards-Brown, M.D., and
    Vincent P. Mathews, M.D.

48. Imaging of Congenital Abnormalities of the Face 1670

    Mauricio Castillo, M.D., and
    Suresh K. Mukherji, M.D.

49. Anoxic Ischemic Injury in Children 1685

    Rosalind B. Dietrich, M.B.B.S.

50. Hydrocephalus and Cerebrospinal Fluid Flow 1704

    William G. Bradley, Jr., M.D., Ph.D., and
    William W. Orrison, Jr., M.D.

51. Neurocutaneous Syndromes 1717

    Blaine L. Hart, M.D.,
    Mark H. Depper, M.D., and
    Carol L. Clericuzio, M.D.

52. Traumatic Brain Injury in Children 1760

    Mary K. Edwards-Brown, M.D., and
    Blaine L. Hart, M.D.

Index i

Head, Neck, and Spine

28

The Temporal Bone*

H. CHRISTIAN DAVIDSON, M.D.
H. RIC HARNSBERGER, M.D.

NORMAL ANATOMY
Osseous Components

Classic descriptions of the temporal bone are based on its five embryologically distinct osseous components: the petrous, mastoid, tympanic, squamous, and styloid portions.

Petrous Portion

The petrous portion is a pyramid-shaped wedge of bone that forms the medial aspect of the temporal bone. The apex of the pyramid points medially and rests adjacent to the clivus, and this relationship defines the petro-occipital fissure. The "sides" of the pyramid are made up of three surfaces: an anterior surface, a posterior surface, and an inferior surface. The dense bone of the otic capsule lies within the center of the petrous bone and contains the structures of the inner ear. The tympanic cavity is a complex space that lies laterally within the petrous bone and constitutes the middle ear.

Mastoid Portion

The mastoid portion comprises the bulbous posterolateral portion of the temporal bone and the inferiorly projecting mastoid process. The medial margin of the mastoid is intracranial and forms part of the border of transverse sinus. The mastoid contains multiple aerated cells, which communicate with the middle ear. The mastoid process is not ossified at birth.

Tympanic Portion

The tympanic portion is a U-shaped bony plate that forms the bulk of the bony external auditory canal (EAC) and the posterior (nonarticular) part of the mandibular fossa. The fissures that are formed by the junctions of the tympanic and other portions of the temporal bone are of anatomic interest and are discussed at length in other works dedicated to the study of the temporal bone.[1]

Squamous Portion

The squamous portion is composed of a flat bony plate that forms the lateral wall of the middle cranial fossa and medial wall of the high masticator space. This portion contributes the posterior segment of the zygomatic arch and also forms the anterior (articular) part of the mandibular fossa.

Styloid Portion

The styloid portion is a thin, finger-like bony projection that extends inferiorly from the posterolateral aspect of the inferior surface of the petrous bone. The base of the styloid process is located at the anterior margin of the external aperture of the stylomastoid foramen. Like the mastoid process, the styloid process is not ossified at birth.

Functional Anatomic Classification

The anatomic classification used in this chapter defines six functional regions of the temporal bone (Table 28–1). This organization groups together lesions that share common clinical, diagnostic imaging, and therapeutic considerations.

Internal Auditory Canal

The internal auditory canal (IAC) traverses the petrous bone in a roughly horizontal plane extending anterolaterally from the porus acusticus to the fundus. The facial nerve (cranial nerve VII) and the nervus intermedius travel in the anterosuperior aspect of the canal. The cochlear branch of the vestibulocochlear nerve (cranial nerve VIII) is found in the anteroinferior aspect of the canal, and the superior and inferior vestibular branches travel in the posterior half of the canal. Vascular structures found in the IAC include the intracanalicular loop of the anterior inferior cerebellar artery and internal auditory artery.

At the fundus of the IAC, the nerves pass two bony septa before entering the labyrinth through thin perforate bone. The crista falciformis is a horizontal septum that separates the facial nerve and superior vestibular nerve above from the cochlear nerve and inferior vestibular nerve below. Bill's bar is a vertical bony septum in the upper half of the fundus that separates the facial nerve in front from the superior vestibular nerve behind. The cochlear nerve traverses the base of the cochlea to give rise to spiral ganglia in the modiolus. The vestibular

---

*The text and figures in this chapter are from Davidson HC. The Temporal Bone. Salt Lake City, Electronic Medical Education Research Group, 1999.

TABLE 28–1 Temporal Bone Functional Anatomic Regions

Region	Contents
Internal auditory canal	Intracanalicular cistern; cerebellopontine angle cistern Cranial nerves VII and VIII
Inner ear (labyrinth)	Cochlea; vestibule; semicircular canals Endolymphatic duct and sac
Intratemporal facial nerve	Labyrinthine, geniculate, tympanic, and mastoid segments Excludes intracanalicular and intraparotid segments
Petrous bone	Petrous apex, pneumatized cells; carotid canal Petrous bone proper except for otic capsule and tympanic cavity
Middle ear and mastoid	Epitympanum; mesotympanum; hypotympanum Tympanic membrane; ossicular chain; round and oval windows Mastoid bone; mastoid antrum and additus
External ear	Bony, cartilaginous, and soft tissue external canal Pinna and associated cutis

Used with permission from Davidson HC. The Temporal Bone. Salt Lake City, Electronic Medical Education Research Group, 1999.

nerves traverse the area cribrosa at the medial wall of the vestibule and give rise to ganglia that serve the vestibular sense organs.

Lesions of the IAC typically result in seventh and eighth cranial nerve dysfunction, particularly hearing loss. Lesions of the cerebellopontine angle (CPA) cistern are considered together with lesions of the IAC. Such lesions are usually best evaluated with dedicated high-resolution contrast-enhanced and fast spin echo (FSE) magnetic resonance (MR).

Inner Ear

The inner ear consists of the components of the membranous and bony labyrinth. The intratemporal facial nerve is considered separately.

The cochlea is a gently tapered tubular structure wound in a spiral with 2½ turns located anteroinferiorly in the otic capsule. The cochlear spiral has the shape of a flat cone, the apex of which points anterolaterally and just slightly downward. The membranous cochlea is divided along its length into two roughly equal perilymphatic chambers, the scala vestibuli (anterior) and scala tympani (posterior), which are separated by the osseous spiral lamina. The scala media, or cochlear duct, is a small endolymphatic chamber anterior to the spiral lamina that contains the organ of Corti; it is not reliably distinguishable on MR or computed tomographic (CT) imaging. The modiolus, the tissue core at the central axis of the cochlear spiral, is composed of the nervous tissue of the

spiral ganglia as well as the supporting bone and soft tissue of the spiral lamina. The round window, a small opening at the posterolateral aspect of the basal turn of the cochlea, is covered by a membrane that separates the cochlea from the middle ear.

The cochlear aqueduct is a small bony channel that extends from the basal turn of the cochlea to the lateral margin of the jugular foramen. This perilymphatic channel runs just below and roughly parallel to the IAC, for which it is sometimes mistaken by inexperienced radiologists.

The vestibule is an ovoid chamber located posterosuperiorly relative to the cochlea. The membranous vestibule contains two endolymphatic subunits, the saccule and utricle, which are surrounded by perilymph. Both subunits are in contiguity with each other, with the endolymphatic duct, and with the cochlear duct. These distinct endolymphatic components and their connecting ducts are not reliably visible on MR or CT imaging.

The three semicircular canals arise from the vestibule, each with an arc of two thirds to three fourths of a full circle, oriented at right angles to each other. The superior semicircular canal is in an oblique sagittal plane, roughly perpendicular to the long axis of the petrous bone. The bony roof of the superior semicircular canal forms the arcuate eminence, a landmark on the superior surface of the petrous bone. The posterior semicircular canal is in an oblique coronal plane, roughly parallel to the long axis of the petrous bone. The lateral semicircular canal is in a nearly transverse plane that slopes downward anteriorly, perpendicular to the other two semicircular canals. Each canal is contiguous at both ends with the vestibule; the medial limbs of the posterior and superior semicircular canals join together into the crus communis, which in turn is contiguous with the vestibule. The endolymphatic ducts of the semicircular canals and the ampullae that occur at the junctions of these ducts and the utricle are not distinguishable from the surrounding perilymphatic fluid on MR or CT imaging.

The endolymphatic duct is a small duct that arises from the saccule and utricle. The endolymphatic duct is contained in the bony vestibular aqueduct, which courses posterolaterally just behind and medial to the posterior semicircular canal, terminating in a small dimple on the posterior surface of the petrous bone. The endolymphatic sac is the flared terminus of the endolymphatic duct; its proximal portion is in the distal vestibular aqueduct, and its distal portion is between leaves of dura mater. These structures are small but reliably visible on MR and CT.

Lesions of the inner ear typically give rise to sensorineural hearing loss or vestibular symptoms. Such lesions are usually best evaluated with dedicated high-resolution contrast-enhanced and FSE MR, with use of CT as an adjunct to define associated bony abnormalities.

Intratemporal Facial Nerve

The course of the facial nerve (cranial nerve VII) in the temporal bone is complex. The first intratemporal segment is the labyrinthine segment, which courses laterally from the fundus of the IAC and curves anteriorly to the geniculate fossa, a small depression that houses the geniculate ganglion. This ganglion also marks the takeoff of the greater superficial petrosal nerve. The nerve makes a U-turn at the geniculate fossa, forming the anterior genu, and courses posteriorly and laterally to become the tympanic, or horizontal, segment. The horizontal facial canal courses just above the oval window and immediately below the lateral semicircular canal. The horizontal segment has a bony covering that is visible as a prominence in the upper medial aspect of the mesotympanum. At its posterior extent, the tympanic segment of the nerve segment takes a 90-degree turn downward to form the posterior genu and becomes the mastoid segment. The nerve exits the temporal bone at the stylomastoid foramen and enters the parotid space.

Lesions of the intratemporal facial nerve typically give rise to facial paresis or hemifacial spasm. Secondary vestibulocochlear symptoms may also be present, particularly hearing loss due to compression of the cochlear nerve in the IAC or due to ossicular compromise in the middle ear. Facial nerve lesions are usually best evaluated with dedicated high-resolution MR, with use of CT as an adjunct to define associated bony abnormalities.

Petrous Bone

The petrous bone has a pyramidal shape with three surfaces and a medially directed apex. The anterior, or superior, surface forms the posterior margin of the middle cranial fossa floor and serves as the bony roof of the middle and internal ear apparatus. The posterior surface is oriented more vertically and forms the anterior margin of the posterior cranial fossa; it is perforated by the porus acusticus as well as the apertures of the vestibular and cochlear aqueducts. The inferior surface forms part of the external topography of the bony skull base; it forms the anterolateral border of the jugular foramen and contains the proximal aperture to the petrous carotid canal. The bone of the petrous apex often shows penumatization, which has a wide range of variation among individuals. These pneumatized cells are subject to the same processes that affect other aerated cavities in the skull.

The jugular foramen is an anatomically complex structure located between the petrous bone anterolaterally and the occipital bone posteromedially. The pars vascularis, the larger posterolateral part of the foramen, contains cranial nerve X, cranial nerve XI, and the jugular vein. The smaller pars nervosa, the anteromedial part of the foramen, contains cranial nerve IX and the inferior petrosal sinus. Lesions of the jugular foramen can be grouped with other lesions that affect the central and posterior skull base. As such, this chapter addresses only those lesions that affect the temporal bone directly, and a complete description of jugular foramen lesions is given in Chapter 29.

Several neoplastic, infectious, and inflammatory conditions account for the majority of lesions affecting the petrous bone. Many such lesions have characteristic soft tissue appearance but also affect the osseous structures directly, and therefore both CT and MR play a role in their evaluation.

Middle Ear and Mastoid

The middle ear, or tympanic cavity, is a complex space with six walls formed from the surrounding petrous bone.

The medial wall of the middle ear is formed by the bony labyrinth. The prominence of the lateral semicircular canal forms an overhang at the upper aspect of the medial wall, below which is found the prominence of the tympanic facial canal. The oval window niche is just below the facial canal prominence and contains the oval window, which is covered by the footplate of the stapes. Just below the oval window is the cochlear promontory, which is the portion of the otic capsule that covers the lateral aspect of the basal turn of the cochlea. The round window niche is at the posteroinferior margin of the cochlear promontory and contains the round window, which is covered by the secondary tympanic membrane. Two small bony projections at the posteromedial wall help to define the sinus tympani: the subiculum at the superolateral margin of the round window niche, and the ponticulus at the inferolateral margin of the oval window.

The posterior wall of the tympanic cavity is formed by the mastoid bone and has three important landmarks: the sinus tympani, the pyramidal eminence, and the facial nerve recess. The sinus tympani is a deep depression located medially in the low posterior wall, just lateral to and above the round window niche. The bony ridge of the subiculum partially separates the concave contours of the round window and sinus tympani. The facial nerve recess is a shallower depression lateral to the sinus tympani and marks the location of the bony canal of the descending facial nerve. Between the two depressions of the sinus tympani and facial nerve recess is the bony prominence of the pyramidal eminence. The upper part of the posterior wall of the mesotympanum communicates with the mastoid through the additus ad antrum.

The lateral wall of the middle ear is formed by the tympanic membrane and the squamous bone above the level of the tympanic membrane. The inferior margin of the squamous bone is a pointed bony spicule called the scutum. The tympanic membrane is attached superiorly at the tip of the scutum and inferiorly at the tympanic anulus.

The superior wall, or roof, of the middle ear is the tegmen tympani, which forms part of the superior surface of the petrous bone. The inferior wall, or floor, is formed by the bony covering of the petrous carotid canal anteriorly and the roof of the jugular bulb posteriorly.

The middle ear is subdivided into three subregions: the epitympanum, the mesotympanum, and the hypotympanum. The epitympanum, or attic, is that portion of the middle ear that extends above a line drawn from the top of the tympanic membrane to the horizontal facial canal. The lateral space between the scutum and the ossicles is known as Prussak's space. The mesotympanum, or middle ear proper, is that portion of the tympanic cavity between the levels of the upper and lower margins of the tympanic membrane. The hypotympanum is that portion of the middle ear below the level of the tympanic membrane.

The ossicular chain is composed of three bones: the malleus, the incus, and the stapes. The manubrium of the malleus is attached to the tympanic membrane. The head of the malleus articulates with the body of the incus in the epitympanum. The long process of the incus articulates with the head of the stapes in the mesotympanum. The footplate of the stapes covers the oval window.

The mastoid bone contains multiple pneumatized spaces, the largest of which is the mastoid antrum. The antrum communicates with the mesotympanum through a channel that opens into the upper posterior wall of the middle ear, known as the additus ad antrum. The descending or mastoid segment of the facial nerve traverses the mastoid bone in a vertical trajectory, just deep to the facial recess in the posterior wall of the middle ear.

Lesions of the middle ear and mastoid are manifest primarily as changes of bony structures or soft tissue density in aerated spaces, and these lesions are best evaluated with thin-section CT. MR is a useful adjunct, particularly in lesions that are large or have intracranial complications.

External Ear

The external ear is composed of the EAC and pinna. The EAC is a tubular cavity formed of cartilage and bone, lined by dermis. The walls of the lateral segment of the EAC are made up of fibrocartilage that is contiguous with cartilage of the pinna. The walls of the medial segment of the EAC are formed by the temporal bone. The U-shaped tympanic portion of the temporal bone forms the floor and most of the anterior and posterior margins of the medial EAC. The roof of the medial EAC is formed by the squamous portion of the temporal bone. The medial margin of the EAC is delineated by the tympanic membrane.

IMAGING TECHNIQUES

CT and MR are the primary techniques used in temporal bone imaging. Most temporal bone lesions are adequately visualized for diagnosis and therapeutic planning by one or both of these techniques. On occasion, angiographic, plain radiographic, and radioisotopic imaging provide additional correlative imaging or therapeutic options.

Computed Tomography

The strength of CT in imaging the temporal bone is its superior capability for defining osseous structures. Modern CT imaging provides exquisite visualization of submillimeter structures in the temporal bone, including the bony labyrinth, IAC, petrous apex, ossicles and middle ear cavity, EAC, and mastoid.

The standard technique for CT imaging of the temporal bone consists of thin-section axial and coronal acquisitions, described in Table 28–2. Contiguous slices are obtained, with slice thickness set as thin as possible, ideally at 1 mm and no more than 2 mm. Conventional axial acquisition is preferred, although helical scanning can also be used provided that adequate technique is achieved. Administration of contrast material is not necessary in most cases, because CT is used primarily for evaluation of osseous structures, and enhanced imaging is better achieved with MR. The exception is in patients who are unable to undergo MR imaging, in which case contrast-enhanced CT can replace MR. Temporal bone CT should always be read with use of a window width of 4000; lesser widths may conceal significant osseous detail. Examples

TABLE 28–2 Technique for Routine Temporal Bone Computed Tomography

	Axial	Coronal
Setup		
Localization	From top of petrous apex to inferior tip of mastoid (36–40 slices)	From anterior margin of petrous apex to posterior margin of mastoid (32–36 slices)
Position	Supine	Prone, or "hanging head" supine

	Sequential	Spiral
Acquisition		
Collimation	1 mm	1 mm
Spacing	1 mm (contiguous)	1 mm, pitch 1:1
Technique	400 mAs, 2 sec, 120 kVp	300–400 mAs, 120 kVp
Post Processing		
Reconstruction	Bone algorithm, 12-cm FOV, each ear separately	
Display	Window/level = 4000/400	

Used with permission from Davidson HC. MR Protocol Advisor. Salt Lake City, Electronic Medical Education Research Group, 1999. *Abbreviation:* FOV, field of view.

of these images are shown in the subsequent section on normal anatomy.

Magnetic Resonance Imaging

The strength of MR in temporal bone imaging is its superior tissue contrast for defining lesions within the cranial vault, IAC and labyrinth, osseous structures of the temporal bone itself, and adjacent deep soft tissues. The standard technique for MR imaging of the temporal bone consists of multiplanar thin-section T1-weighted image (T1WI) acquisitions without and with contrast enhancement, described in Table 28–3. Examples of these images are shown in the subsequent section on normal anatomy.

High-resolution T2 FSE imaging is a non–contrast-enhanced T2-weighted imaging (T2WI) technique that provides a valuable adjunct to conventional enhanced imaging. This technique takes advantage of the intrinsic tissue contrast of the fluid-filled IAC and membranous labyrinth and is particularly useful in the evaluation of the inner ear and IAC. The protocol for T2 FSE acoustic MR is described in Table 28–4. Examples of these images are shown in the subsequent section on normal anatomy.

IMAGING ANATOMY
Normal Anatomy on Computed Tomography

Normal anatomic structures of the temporal bone as seen on axial and coronal thin-section CT are demonstrated in Figures 28–1 and 28–2.

TABLE 28–3 Technique for Contrast-Enhanced Temporal Bone Magnetic Resonance Imaging

Setup	Axial Sequences		Coronal Sequences			Whole Brain Screen
Localization	From petrous apex superiorly to mastoid tip inferiorly (12–14 3-mm slices)		From petrous apex anteriorly to aerated mastoid posteriorly (12–14 3-mm slices)			Routine brain (as indicated)

Sequence	AX T2 FSE	AX T1	COR T1	AX T1 +	COR T1 +	Whole Brain
Plane	Axial	Axial	Coronal	Axial	Coronal	Routine FLAIR, T2-weighted FSE, or post–contrast-enhanced as indicated
Fat saturation	✓					
Contrast				✓	✓	
Parameters						
TR/TE	FSE 4000/100	Spin echo 500/min–full	Spin echo 500/min–full	Spin echo 667/min–full	Spin echo 667/min–full	
Acquisition						
Slice/skip	FOV 16 cm 3–4 mm/0 mm	FOV 16 cm 3 mm/0 mm	FOV 16 cm 3 mm/0 mm	FOV 16 cm 3 mm/0 mm	FOV 16 cm 3 mm/0 mm	
Matrix	256 × 256	256 × 192	256 × 192	256 × 192	256 × 192	
Frequency	A-P	A-P	S-I	A-P	S-I	
Number of excitations	3–4	2	2	2	2	

Used with permission from Davidson HC. MR Protocol Advisor. Salt Lake City, Electronic Medical Education Research Group, 1999.
Abbreviations: AX, axial; COR, coronal; FLAIR, fluid attenuated inversion recovery; FOV, field of view; FSE, fast spin echo.

Normal Anatomy on Magnetic Resonance Imaging

Normal anatomic structures of the temporal bone as seen on enhanced T1WI are shown in Figure 28–3. Corresponding anatomy as seen on thin-section T2 FSE MR is shown in Figure 28–4.

INTERNAL AUDITORY CANAL AND CEREBELLOPONTINE ANGLE LESIONS

Lesions that arise within or involve the IAC can be considered together with lesions affecting the CPA cis-

TABLE 28–4 Technique for High-Resolution Fast Spin Echo Acoustic Magnetic Resonance Imaging

	Axial		Coronal		Oblique Sagittal
Setup					
Localization	From superior semicircular canal to bottom of cochlea inferiorly		From apex of cochlea anteriorly to posterior semicircular canal		From CPA cistern medially to cochlear modiolus laterally
Coil	Dual phased-array surface coil (TMJ coil or other dual phased-array specialty coil)				

Sequence	AX 3-D	COR 3-D	AX 2-D°	COR 2-D°	O-SAG 2-D
Plane	Axial	Axial	Axial	Coronal	Oblique sagittal
Parameters	3-D FSE	3-D FSE	2-D FSE	2-D FSE	2-D FSE
TR/TE	~4000/~130	~4000/~130	~4500/~110	~4500/~110	~4500/~110
Echo train	64	64	32	32	16
Acquisition	FOV 14 cm	FOV 14 cm	FOV 20 × 10 cm	FOV 20 × 15 cm	FOV 10 cm
Slice/skip	0.8 mm/0 mm	0.8 mm/0 mm	2 mm/0 mm†	2 mm/0 mm†	2 mm/0 mm
Matrix	256 × 256	256 × 256	512 × 512	512 × 384	256 × 256
Phase FOV	Full	Full	One half	Three fourths	Full
Frequency	R-L	S-I	R-L	S-I	S-I
Flow comp	Yes	Yes			
Number of excitations	1	1	6	4	4

Used with permission from Davidson HC. MR Protocol Advisor. Salt Lake City, Electronic Medical Education Research Group, 1999.
Abbreviations: AX, axial; COR, coronal; CPA, cerebellopontine angle; FSE, fast spin echo; FOV, field of view; TMJ, temporomandibular joint.
°Axial and coronal two-dimensional (2-D) sequences are alternatives to axial and coronal three-dimensional (3-D) sequences if 3-D FSE is not available.
†Slices can be overlapped (2-mm-thick slices at 1-mm spacing) by performing two separate acquisitions that are offset 1 mm. Thinner slices can also be obtained by use of zero-filled interpolation.

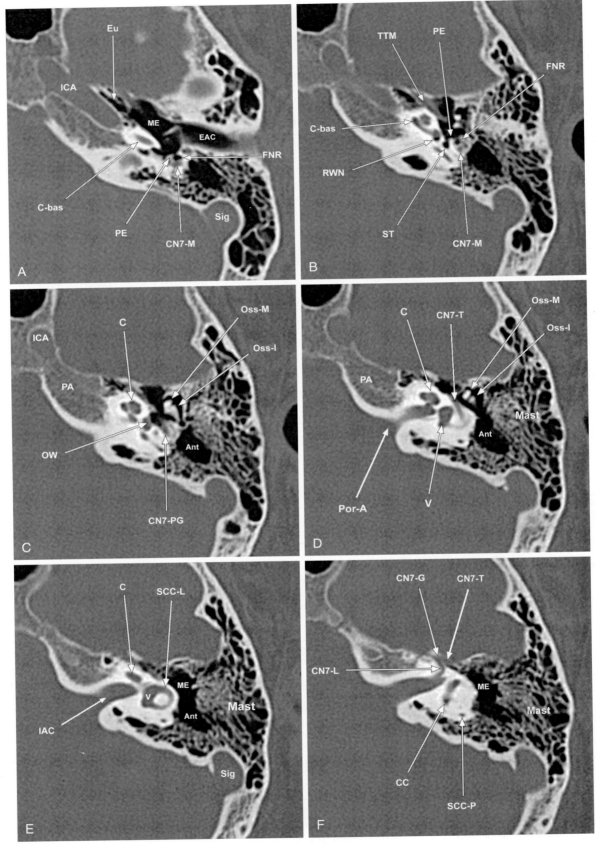

FIGURE 28–1 *See legend on opposite page*

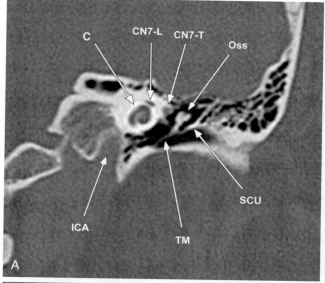

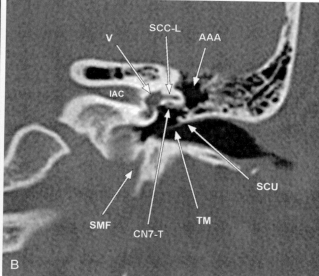

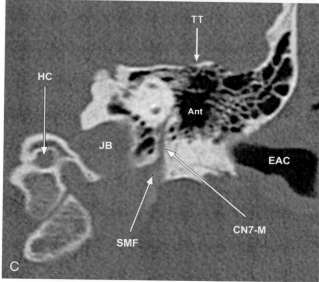

FIGURE 28–2 Normal CT. *A–C,* Coronal thin-section CT scans of the temporal bone. See Figure 28–1 legend for key. (*A–C,* Used with permission from Davidson HC. Digital Teaching File. Salt Lake City, Electronic Medical Education Research Group, 1999.)

FIGURE 28–1 Normal computed tomography (CT). *A–F,* Axial thin-section CT scans of the temporal bone. AAA, additus ad antrum; Ant, antrum; C, cochlea; C-bas, cochlear basal turn; CC, common crus; CN7, cranial nerve VII (facial nerve); CN7-G, geniculate fossa of cranial nerve VII; CN7-L, labyrinthine segment of cranial nerve VII; CN7-M, mastoid segment of cranial nerve VII; CN7-PG, posterior genu of cranial nerve VII; CN7-T, tympanic segment of cranial nerve VII; CN8, cranial nerve VIII (vestibulocochlear nerve); CN8-C, cochlear branch of cranial nerve VIII; CN8-Vs, superior vestibular branch of cranial nerve VIII; CN8-Vi, inferior vestibular branch of cranial nerve VIII; CPA, cerebellopontine angle; EAC, external auditory canal; ELD, endolymphatic duct; ET, epitympanum; Eu, eustachian tube; FNR, facial nerve recess; GSP, greater superficial petrosal nerve; HC, hypoglossal canal; IAC, internal auditory canal; ICA, internal carotid artery; ISS, interscalar septum; IV, fourth ventricle; JB, jugular bulb; Mast, mastoid; ME, middle ear cavity; MOD, modiolus; Oss, ossicles; Oss-I, incus; Oss-M, malleus; OW, oval window; P, parotid gland; PA, petrous apex; PE, pyramidal eminence; Por-A, porus acusticus; RWN, round window niche; SCC-L, lateral semicircular canal; SCC-P, posterior semicircular canal; SCC-S, superior semicircular canal; SCU, scutum; Sig, sigmoid sinus; SMF, stylomastoid foramen; SS, sphenoid sinus; ST, sinus tympani; Teg. Tymp., tegmen tympani; TM, tympanic membrane; TTM, tensor tympani muscle; V, vestibule. (*A–F,* Used with permission from Davidson HC. Digital Teaching File. Salt Lake City, Electronic Medical Education Research Group, 1999.)

tern. This group of lesions consists of neoplastic and cystic masses arising from normal or ectopic structures in the CPA region as well as inflammatory and vascular processes that affect the CPA and IAC cisterns and the cranial nerves located there. In addition to lesions specific to this region, any intra-axial or extra-axial process that involves subarachnoid cisternal spaces in general can also be seen here.

Vestibulocochlear Schwannoma

Vestibulocochlear schwannoma (VCS) is a benign, slowly growing neoplasm that arises from Schwann cells in the nerve sheath of the vestibulocochlear nerve. This tumor can affect other cranial nerves as well but has a predilection for the eighth nerve, in particular the vestibular portion of the nerve, which has led to the preferred use of the designation VCS rather than *acoustic neuroma,* the well-known synonym.[2] The majority of intracranial schwannomas affect the vestibular portion of the eighth nerve, and only a small minority affect the cochlear portion. Two histologic subtypes of schwannoma have been described: Antoni's type A, more common in VCS, which shows a compact tissue organization; and type B, which

shows a looser tissue texture, often with areas of cyst formation.

VCS is a relatively common tumor that accounts for about three fourths of all CPA masses and about one tenth of all intracranial tumors.[3, 4] Patients with VCS usually present in the fourth to sixth decades. The most common symptom is progressive unilateral sensorineural hearing loss, often accompanied by tinnitus.[5] Vestibular symptoms of vertigo and dizziness are less common, which is curious given that most of these tumors arise from the vestibular portion of the nerve. This phenomenon may be due to a lesser susceptibility of the nerve to the effects of compression or to the central nervous system's better ability to compensate for unilateral vestibular denervation.[6] Large tumors in the CPA may also present with symptoms of cerebellar dysfunction or neuropathy of the lower cranial nerves.

VCS is associated with neurofibromatosis type 2 (NF-2),[7] and this condition should be suspected when VCS is bilateral or is discovered in a child or young adult. The presence of NF-2 should also heighten the radiologist's awareness of possible associated lesions, including meningiomas and ependymomas. Malignant degeneration of VCS is rare and associated with NF-1.[8] *Melanotic*

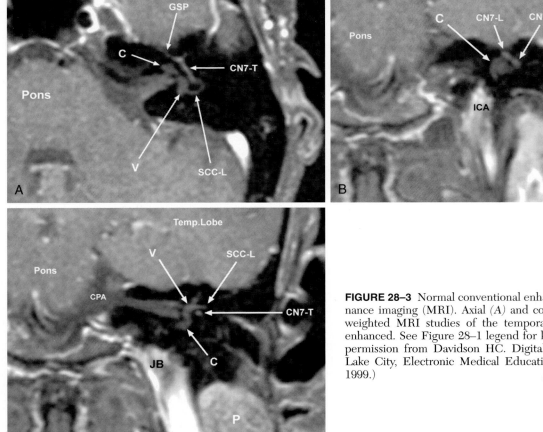

FIGURE 28–3 Normal conventional enhanced magnetic resonance imaging (MRI). Axial *(A)* and coronal *(B* and *C)* T1-weighted MRI studies of the temporal bone, gadolinium-enhanced. See Figure 28–1 legend for key. (*A–C,* Used with permission from Davidson HC. Digital Teaching File. Salt Lake City, Electronic Medical Education Research Group, 1999.)

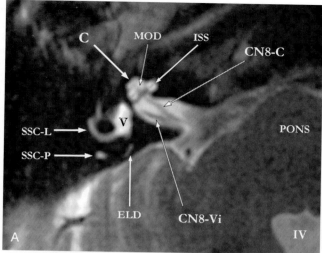

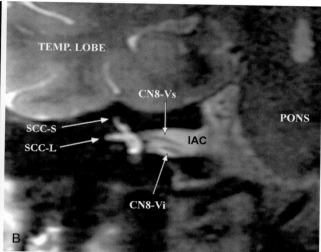

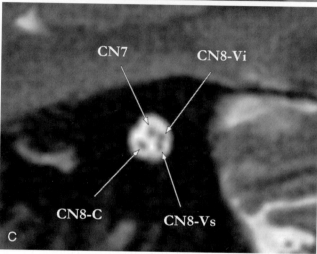

FIGURE 28–4 Normal acoustic high-resolution T2-weighted MRI. Axial (A), coronal (B), and oblique sagittal (C) T2-weighted fast spin echo (FSE) MRI studies of the temporal bone. See Figure 28–1 legend for key. (A–C, Used with permission from Davidson HC. Digital Teaching File. Salt Lake City, Electronic Medical Education Research Group, 1999.)

schwannoma is another malignant variant of VCS that may arise from melanocytes that share their neural crest origin with Schwann cells.[9]

Facial schwannoma is a related lesion of the seventh cranial nerve. The majority of these lesions occur in the intratemporal segments of the facial nerve and are discussed in a subsequent section of this chapter. A facial schwannoma may occasionally involve the intracanalicular facial nerve, in which case it may be radiographically and clinically indistinguishable from a VCS, unless the tumor can be seen extending along the expected course of the nerve into the labyrinthine facial canal.[10, 11]

MR is the preferred imaging modality for detecting and describing VCS, unless MR is contraindicated.[12] On unenhanced T1WI, schwannomas appear isointense to brain and can usually be detected as masses that displace the normal cerebrospinal fluid (CSF) signal. After administration of contrast material, schwannomas typically show uniform enhancement, although heterogeneity may be seen when areas of internal cystic or hemorrhagic change are present.[13]

VCSs are typically centered near the porus acusticus and are classically described as having an elongated intra-canalicular component and bulbous CPA cisternal component that results in an "ice cream cone" configuration. Small lesions that are 15 mm or less may be contained entirely within the IAC and have a tubular shape (Fig. 28–5).[14] Large lesions that are 30 mm or greater typically have a dominant CPA component. VCSs are usually solid but may show cystic or hemorrhagic change, particularly in large or rapidly growing tumors (Fig. 28–6).[15]

Contrast-enhanced MR is widely considered to be the first-line imaging technique for VCS evaluation because of the sensitivity afforded by the intense enhancement that these tumors typically manifest, in even small lesions.[16] However, high-resolution T2 FSE imaging is a supplemental non–contrast-enhanced technique that can provide exquisite imaging of the CSF and nerves in the CPA and IAC. On T2 FSE imaging, VCSs appear as nodules or filling defects against the background of bright CSF. This technique allows detection of tumors as small as a few millimeters and can provide adjunctive information that is useful in surgical planning, such as identifying from which nerve component the tumor arises, defining the exact extent of the tumor boundaries, and determining whether there is a CSF cap at the fundus of the IAC

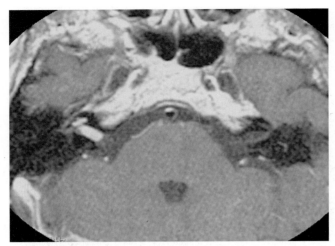

FIGURE 28–5 Vestibulocochlear schwannoma. Axial T1-weighted MRI study with contrast enhancement in a patient with progressive sensorineural hearing loss. The intensely enhancing schwannoma nearly fills the internal auditory canal, with only a small amount of cerebrospinal fluid (CSF) at the fundus. The tumor extends through the modiolus into the basal turn of the cochlea and probably originates from the cochlear branch of the eighth cranial nerve. (Used with permission from Davidson HC. Digital Teaching File. Salt Lake City, Electronic Medical Education Research Group, 1999.)

(Fig. 28–7). In the proper clinical setting, T2 FSE imaging can serve as an inexpensive screening technique for patients with uncomplicated sensorineural hearing loss.[17]

Facial schwannoma that is limited to the IAC may be indistinguishable from a VCS on contrast-enhanced imaging. If the tumor is small, the origin of the tumor at the facial nerve may be demonstrable on T2 FSE imaging.

Meningioma

Meningiomas are neoplasms that arise from arachnoid cap cells, dural fibroblasts, or arachnoid membrane.[18] The last accounts for lesions in the CPA region. These tumors are typically benign and well circumscribed, and they are epidemiologically and histologically similar to meningiomas that occur elsewhere in the cranial vault.

The incidence of meningioma in the CPA region is a distant second to VCS, accounting for about 5% to 10% of CPA masses.[19, 20] Depending on their location, CPA meningiomas may present with cranial neuropathy, cerebellar dysfunction, or other symptoms due to local mass effect. Rarely, a meningioma that is limited to the IAC may mimic a VCS clinically.[21]

On non–contrast-enhanced CT, meningiomas may be isointense or hyperintense, and unlike schwannomas, they may show calcification in up to one fourth of lesions.[22] The presence of hyperostosis on CT also suggests a diagnosis of meningioma. On MR, meningiomas show T1 signal that is roughly similar to brain; they may be hyperintense or hypointense on T2WI. The hallmark imaging features of meningioma include extra-axial dura-based location, intense enhancement, hyperostosis, and calcification (Fig. 28–8). The dural origin of these tumors typically results in a hemispherical mass with a broad dural margin that forms an obtuse angle against the adjacent bone, compared with the spheroid or nodular mass with acute angle typically seen in VCS.[22–24] The presence of a "dural tail" also favors the diagnosis of meningioma, although this sign is not totally specific.[25]

Epidermoid and Other Cystic and Congenital Masses

Another group of lesions that can affect the CPA and IAC is an assortment of cystic and congenital masses that includes epidermoid cysts, arachnoid cysts, dermoid cysts, lipomas, and hamartomas. Of these, the most common is epidermoid, which is the third most common CPA region mass after VCS and meningioma.

Because these lesions develop slowly, they may become large before causing symptoms. Symptoms, when

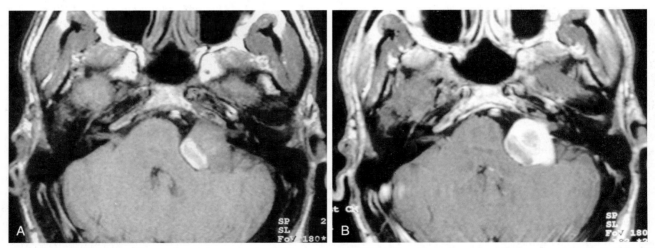

FIGURE 28–6 Vestibulocochlear schwannoma. *A*, Axial T1-weighted MRI study without contrast enhancement. Intrinsic high T1-weighted signal in the posteromedial portion of the cerebellopontine angle tumor represents subacute blood products due to hemorrhage in this schwannoma. *B*, Post–contrast-enhanced image demonstrates typical intense enhancement in the remainder of the tumor. (*A* and *B*, Used with permission from Davidson HC. Digital Teaching File. Salt Lake City, Electronic Medical Education Research Group, 1999.)

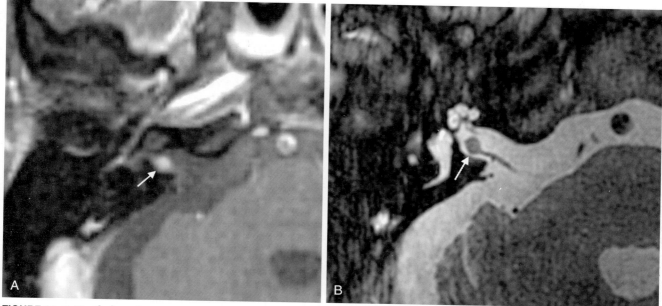

FIGURE 28–7 Vestibular schwannoma. *A*, Axial T1-weighted post–contrast-enhanced image of the internal auditory canal. Enhanced image demonstrates a nodule of intense enhancement *(arrow)*, corresponding to a small intracanalicular schwannoma. *B*, Axial high-resolution T2-weighted FSE MRI study clearly demonstrates the tumor nodule *(arrow)*, which originates from the inferior vestibular branch of the eighth cranial nerve. (*A* and *B*, Used with permission from Davidson HC. Digital Teaching File. Salt Lake City, Electronic Medical Education Research Group, 1999.)

they develop, are the result of local mass effect and include sensorineural hearing loss, vertigo, dizziness, and cerebellar dysfunction. Larger lesions can also cause other cranial neuropathies as well as seizures related to involvement of the mesial temporal lobe.

Epidermoid cyst, also known as *congenital cholestea-* *toma* or *epidermoid tumor*, is caused by congenital rests of ectoderm in the CPA cistern. Epidermoid cyst can also occur in the ventricles, petrous bone, tympanic cavity, skull base, and calvarium.[26, 27] The squamous epithelium in these rests of ectoderm gives rise to accumulations of desquamated keratin debris. This keratinaceous material

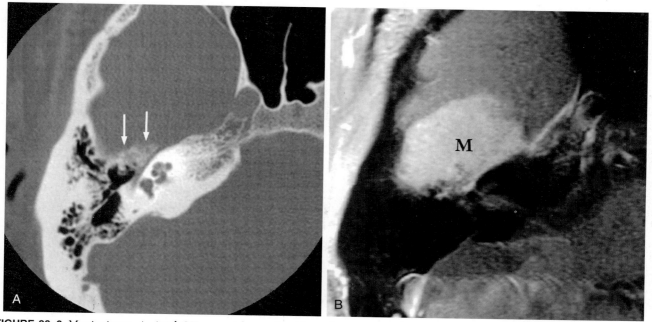

FIGURE 28–8 Meningioma. *A*, Axial CT scan at bone algorithm of a patient with a temporal bone meningioma centered over the petrous bone at the posterior floor of the middle cranial fossa. The hyperostotic bony changes are characteristic for meningioma. *B*, Post–contrast-enhanced T1-weighted MRI study shows characteristic enhancement of the meningioma (M). (*A* and *B*, Used with permission from Davidson HC. Digital Teaching File. Salt Lake City, Electronic Medical Education Research Group, 1999.)

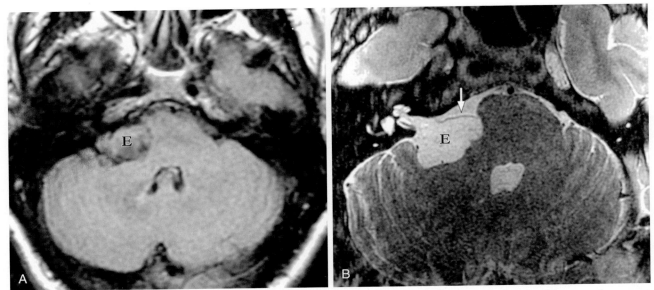

FIGURE 28–9 Epidermoid. *A*, Axial T1-weighted image of the cerebellopontine angle region in a 35-year-old man with worsening vertigo. An epidermoid cyst is present (E), displacing the adjacent pons and cerebellum. The mass appears hyperintense relative to CSF. *B*, Axial high-resolution T2-weighted FSE MRI study allows identification of the vestibulocochlear nerves and demonstrates anterior displacement of the cochlear branch (*arrow*) by the epidermoid cyst. The mass shows T2-weighted signal identical to CSF. (*A* and *B*, Used with permission from Davidson HC. Digital Teaching File. Salt Lake City, Electronic Medical Education Research Group, 1999.)

has a glistening, pearly gross appearance that has led to this lesion's being called "the beautiful tumor."[28] Patients with epidermoid typically present with symptoms in young or middle adulthood.

Epidermoid cyst shows CT density that is similar to or slightly greater than that of CSF. On MR, epidermoid cyst appears fairly homogeneous, with signal characteristics that are similar to CSF. On T1WI, epidermoid cyst is hypointense but usually slightly brighter than CSF, giving rise to the term "dirty CSF." In contrast to other CPA region tumors, epidermoid cyst does not enhance. Epidermoid cyst is characteristically hyperintense on T2WI and in some cases may be indistinguishable from CSF. When conventional MR sequences are indeterminate, diffusion-weighted imaging can be useful and will greatly increase the conspicuity of the lesion (Fig. 28–9).

Arachnoid cysts are simple loculated CSF collections that form as a result of a congenital focal defect or duplication of the arachnoid membrane.[29] Arachnoid cysts can be seen in any location where the arachnoid membrane is found, but some of the more common locations include the middle cranial fossae, sylvian cisterns, and hemispherical convexities. Less common locations include the CPA cisterns, suprasellar cistern, and cisterna magna.

The imaging features of arachnoid cyst are those of a large uniform CSF collection with smooth, rounded margins. Arachnoid cyst appears isodense to CSF on CT and isointense to CSF on T1WI and T2WI, showing no contrast enhancement. Arachnoid cyst may appear similar to epidermoid cyst. Mass effect on adjacent brain or mild remodeling of adjacent bone is often present (Fig. 28–10). When the cyst wall cannot be seen, differentiation between a simple enlarged CSF space and a small arachnoid cyst can be difficult.

Dermoid cyst is similar to epidermoid cyst in that it is the result of a congenital ectodermal inclusion but differs in that it includes tissues from all three ectodermal layers. Dermoid cysts may contain fat, dermal appendages (including hair and teeth), and calcification. Dermoid cysts

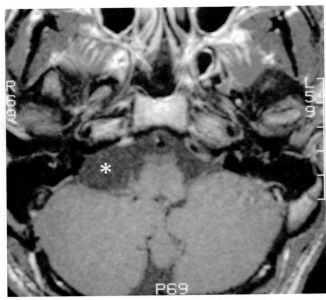

FIGURE 28–10 Arachnoid cyst. Axial T1-weighted MRI study through the cerebellopontine angle cistern demonstrates a homogeneous CSF signal collection (*asterisk*) that causes mild mass effect on the adjacent brain structures. The cyst wall is incompletely perceptible. (Used with permission from Davidson HC. Digital Teaching File. Salt Lake City, Electronic Medical Education Research Group, 1999.)

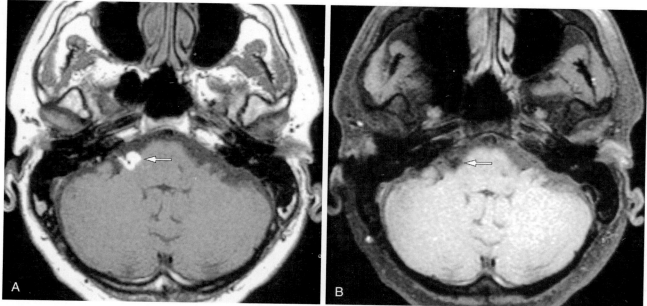

FIGURE 28–11 Lipoma. *A*, Axial T1-weighted MRI study shows a cerebellopontine angle mass *(arrow)* with intrinsic T1-weighted hyperintensity that is characteristic of lipoma. *B*, Axial T1-weighted MRI study with fat suppression confirms the fatty nature of the mass *(arrow)*. (*A* and *B*, Used with permission from Davidson HC. Digital Teaching File. Salt Lake City, Electronic Medical Education Research Group, 1999.)

may rupture, resulting in spread of contents in the subarachnoid space and causing a chemical meningitis. *Lipomas* are congenital hamartomatous lesions that are distinct from dermoid cysts. Lipomas are masses of ectopic fat that probably form as a result of fatty maldevelopment of primitive meningeal mesodermal tissues.[30] Intracranial lipomas are most commonly seen at the midline, often in association with callosal or other midline anomalies, but they can also occur in the CPA region.[31] Lipomas within the IAC have been described.[32] Both dermoid cysts and lipomas on MR show characteristic hyperintense fat signal on T1WI. Lipomas tend to be smaller and more homogeneous (Fig. 28–11). Dermoid cysts often contain heterogeneous elements, including calcification, which is best appreciated on CT. Dermoid cysts typically have greater mass effect and may rupture, producing a characteristic appearance of scattered fat droplets in the CSF space.

Malignant, Inflammatory, and Infectious Meningitides

Any process that affects the meninges and subarachnoid spaces generally can affect the CPA and IAC cisterns. Spread of a malignant process to the subarachnoid space and CSF results in *carcinomatosis*, which may be seen in patients with primary central nervous system malignant neoplasia, adenocarcinoma (especially breast and lung), lymphoma, melanoma, leukemia, or other metastatic malignant disease.[33, 34] Infectious meningitis, particularly tuberculous and fungal meningitis, results in focal meningeal disease that is most prominent in the basilar cisterns. Noninfectious inflammatory conditions also cause localized meningeal changes, including sarcoidosis, histiocytosis, idiopathic hypertrophic pachymeningitis, and postoperative meningeal reaction.[35–38]

Meningeal disease is best evaluated with contrast-enhanced MR. Abnormal enhancement may appear as multiple nodular deposits or as focal or diffuse leptomeningeal or pachymeningeal thickening (Fig. 28–12).[39–41] A solitary meningeal deposit may mimic meningioma.[42] In

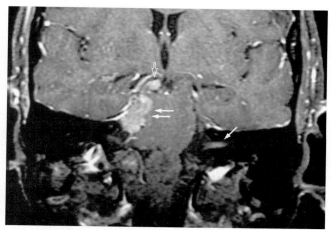

FIGURE 28–12 Lymphoma. Coronal T1-weighted MRI study with gadolinium enhancement and fat suppression in an elderly patient with a prior history of non-Hodgkin's lymphoma and new onset of multiple cranial neuropathies. Extensive leptomeningeal enhancement is present, including enhancement filling the left internal auditory canal affecting the left seventh and eighth nerves *(single solid arrow)*, bulky tumor in the lateral recess of the upper prepontine cistern affecting the right fifth nerve *(double solid arrows)*, and nodular enhancement in the interpeduncular cistern along the right third nerve *(open arrow)*. (Used with permission from Davidson HC. Digital Teaching File. Salt Lake City, Electronic Medical Education Research Group, 1999.)

general, when a focal meningeal process is discovered in the CPA or IAC, the remainder of the intracranial contents and spinal axis should be examined to evaluate for possible disseminated meningeal disease.

INNER EAR LESIONS

Lesions of the inner ear consist of conditions that affect the membranous and bony labyrinth, including the cochlea, vestibule, and associated endolymphatic and perilymphatic structures. A wide variety of congenital, neoplastic, and inflammatory lesions affect the inner ear, most of which present as disturbance of cochlear or vestibular function.

Large Endolymphatic Duct and Sac

Large endolymphatic duct and sac (LEDS) is a congenital enlargement of the intracranial extension of the inner ear endolymphatic system. The defining feature of this condition is enlargement of the endolymphatic sac and duct and corresponding enlargement of the bony vestibular aqueduct. The original synonym for this condition, large vestibular aqueduct syndrome, comes from the hallmark finding of vestibular aqueduct enlargement seen on CT and plain tomographic studies.[43]

LEDS was first described in the late 1970s, but has since come to be recognized as one of the most common causes of congenital sensorineural hearing loss. LEDS is the most commonly identified radiographic anomaly of the inner ear.[43–45] Patients typically present with progressive, severe sensorineural hearing loss in childhood or early adulthood, often exacerbated by minor trauma.[44]

The hallmark imaging characteristic of LEDS on CT is enlargement of the bony vestibular aqueduct, defined as a diameter greater than 1.5 mm at a point halfway between the crus communis and the intracranial aperture of the aqueduct. On T2 FSE MR, the underlying endolymphatic structure abnormalities are readily demonstrated, consisting of enlargement of the endolymphatic sac and duct (Fig. 28–13). In some cases, enlargement of the sac is more conspicuous than that of the duct, and T2 FSE MR is the preferred modality for making this diagnosis.

Inner Ear Dysplasias

The inner ear dysplasias are a heterogeneous group of congenital lesions that result from malformation of the vestibulocochlear structures at various stages of inner ear embryologic development, which occurs from the third to the eighth week of gestation.[46] These lesions are addressed collectively here; for a more detailed description of specific entities in this group and associated embryologic considerations, the reader is referred to works dedicated to this topic.[47, 48]

The *cochlear dysplasias* can be differentiated by the stage of maturation at which developmental insult occurs.[46, 49] Arrested development at the earliest stage results in complete aplasia, known as Michel's aplasia, a rare condition with total failure of inner ear development.[50] Developmental arrest in the fourth gestational week results in a single labyrinthine cystic structure, called a common cavity. Arrest of cochlear development during the fifth and sixth weeks results in cochlear aplasia and hypoplasia. In these conditions, the cochlea is present as an amorphous cavity showing little or no development of internal cochlear architecture.

Developmental arrest in the seventh week gives rise

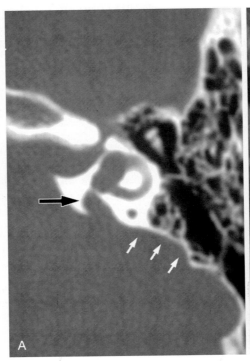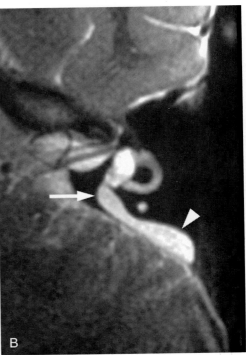

FIGURE 28–13 Large endolymphatic duct and sac. *A,* Axial bone CT image in a middle-school student who experienced sensorineural hearing loss after a minor head injury. Enlargement of the bony vestibular aqueduct *(black arrow)* is present, as is bony remodeling of the posterior margin of the petrous bone secondary to the enlarged endolymphatic sac *(white arrows). B,* Axial T2-weighted FSE MRI study demonstrates the enlarged fluid signal endolymphatic duct *(arrow),* corresponding to the enlarged bony aqueduct. MRI also clearly demonstrates the enlarged endolymphatic sac in its entirety *(arrowhead). (A* and *B,* Used with permission from Davidson HC. Digital Teaching File. Salt Lake City, Electronic Medical Education Research Group, 1999.)

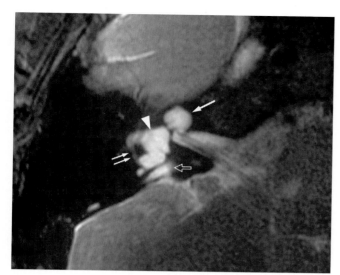

FIGURE 28–14 Severe inner ear dysplasia. Axial T2-weighted FSE MRI study in a child with bilateral sensorineural hearing loss. Severe cochlear dysplasia is present, and the cochlea appears as a common cavity with little internal architecture *(single solid arrow)*. The vestibule is also dysplastic and appears grossly enlarged *(arrowhead)*. The lateral semicircular canal is hypoplastic *(double solid arrows)*. A large endolymphatic duct is also apparent *(open arrow)*. (Used with permission from Davidson HC. Digital Teaching File. Salt Lake City, Electronic Medical Education Research Group, 1999.)

to a number of specific conditions that manifest partial internal cochlear maturation. Incomplete partition is a condition in which the individual cochlear turns and interscalar septa are only partially formed. Classic Mondini's dysplasia features incomplete partition as a typical manifestation.[47, 51] Other anomalies involving the vestibule and semicircular canals are frequently associated with this type of cochlear dysplasia. *Mondini's dysplasia* is a term that has been applied to a range of morphologic anomalies resulting from late-stage arrest and does not describe a single entity. Another specific type of late-stage cochlear arrest is cochleosaccular dysplasia, also known as Scheibe's dysplasia, which results from incomplete development of the cochlear duct and saccule.

Vestibular dysplasias are almost always seen in association with other anomalies of the inner ear. Dysplastic changes include maldevelopment of the endolymphatic compartments and ducts in the vestibule and semicircular canals, with associated enlargement or obliteration of the corresponding bony labyrinthine structures.

There are a large number of developmental conditions that result in sensorineural hearing loss but that do not have specific radiologic manifestations. This group of conditions includes a host of genetic, metabolic, toxic, infectious, and idiopathic factors that affect the vestibulocochlear apparatus, many of which have distinct clinical and histologic manifestations.[48] Patients with these conditions may present with congenital or progressive hearing loss and therefore may be referred for imaging studies of the temporal bone.

The inner ear dysplasias are best evaluated with a combination of thin-section non–contrast-enhanced CT

to evaluate the bony labyrinth and T2 FSE MR to evaluate the membranous labyrinth. Common labyrinthine cavity is seen as a simple fluid-filled space in the bony otic capsule without internal cochlear or vestibular differentiation. Cochlear aplasia and hypoplasia show a dysmorphic cochlear cavity without discrete internal cochlear architecture, often with coexistent vestibular anomalies (Fig. 28–14).

The milder dysplastic changes of incomplete partition are manifest as a distortion of the normal contours of the middle and apical cochlear turns. Other features of mild dysplasia include a deficient modiolus and incomplete interscalar septum with asymmetric or undivided scalar chambers (Fig. 28–15).[52] Classic late-stage Mondini-type dysplasia shows a flat cochlea with an incomplete number of turns (1 1/2 instead of 2 1/2). Dysplastic changes of the vestibule may be seen as bulbous enlargement. The semicircular canals may be small or enlarged, or they may appear to be assimilated into an enlarged vestibule (see Fig. 28–14). The endolymphatic changes of late-stage anomalies, such as cochleosaccular dysplasia, as well as many developmental causes of hearing loss are frequently not visible, even with high-resolution MR imaging.

Labyrinthitis

Labyrinthitis is a nonspecific inflammation of the membranous labyrinth.[53, 54] A commonly used classification scheme subdivides the causes of labyrinthitis into hematogenic, tympanogenic, meningogenic, traumatic, and spontaneous categories. Most commonly, labyrinthitis is the

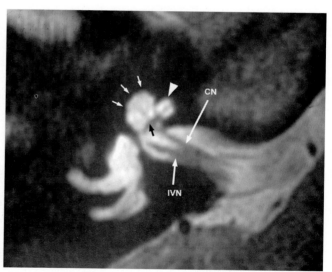

FIGURE 28–15 Mild inner ear dysplasia. Axial T2 FSE MRI study in a teenager with sensorineural hearing loss. Mild cochlear dysplasia is present, manifest as modiolar deficiency *(black arrow)*, abnormal cochlear apex with incomplete scalar partition and distorted contour *(white arrows)*, and enlargement of the anterior scalar chamber relative to the posterior chamber in the basal turn *(arrowhead)*. This patient also had an enlarged endolymphatic sac and duct (not shown). CN, cochlear nerve; IVN, inferior vestibular nerve. (Used with permission from Davidson HC. Digital Teaching File. Salt Lake City, Electronic Medical Education Research Group, 1999.)

result of viral infection. A host of other conditions can lead to labyrinthitis, including otomastoid disease, demyelinating disease, granulomatous disease, and metastatic malignant disease. Syphilis was a common cause of labyrinthitis in the preantibiotic era and has become more frequent again in recent years. Autoimmune labyrinthitis has also recently been recognized as a distinct entity.[55]

The clinical presentation of labyrinthitis typically includes vertigo, dizziness, and sensorineural hearing loss. These symptoms can be extremely debilitating, often with acute onset but occasionally becoming chronically recurrent or persistent. In the chronic phase, labyrinthitis may progress to labyrinthine ossificans, which is described in the next section.

In the era before high-resolution cross-sectional imaging, there were few direct radiographic findings of labyrinthitis. Contrast-enhanced MR of the temporal bone is the most sensitive technique for detecting labyrinthine inflammation. Labyrinthitis is usually manifest as diffuse mild or moderate enhancement that involves the entire membranous labyrinth (Fig. 28–16). Enhancement is occasionally limited to a subportion of the labyrinth, and such segmental involvement has been shown to correlate with clinical symptoms.[54] Enhancement may be unilateral or bilateral and may persist for months after the onset of

symptoms.[56] Meningogenic labyrinthitis is typically bilateral, whereas labyrinthitis due to tympanogenic and traumatic causes is unilateral. When labyrinthitis is tympanogenic, associated findings of otomastoiditis should be apparent, and evaluation with CT is warranted.

Labyrinthine Ossificans

Labyrinthine ossificans is a postinflammatory process of the inner ear that causes fibro-osseous obliteration of the labyrinth.[57] Labyrinthine ossificans occurs as a sequela of long-standing labyrinthitis[58, 59] and is due to a proliferation of fibroblasts and osteoblasts in the membranous labyrinth.[60] The clinical presentation of labyrinthine ossificans is one of chronic profound deafness and loss of vestibular function.

The imaging hallmark of labyrinthine ossificans is osseous obliteration of the labyrinth (Fig. 28–17). This obliteration is best appreciated on thin-section CT[61] but can also be readily appreciated on thin-section T2 FSE images.[57, 62] The imaging changes of labyrinthine ossificans develop during several months to years. Imaging findings in the acute phase of labyrinthitis are described in the preceding section. In the early stages of labyrinthine ossificans, the membranous labyrinth begins to fill with ill-

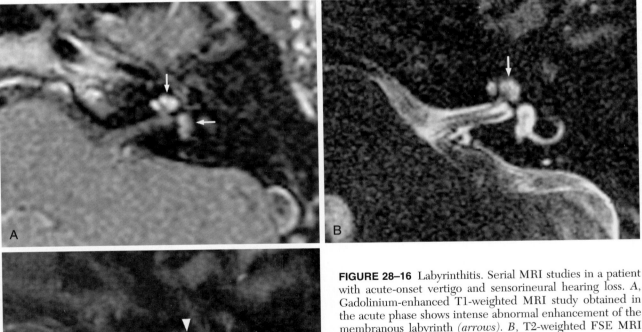

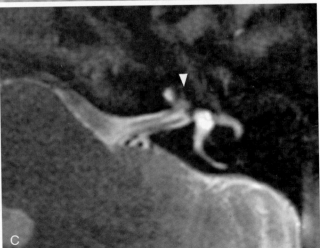

FIGURE 28–16 Labyrinthitis. Serial MRI studies in a patient with acute-onset vertigo and sensorineural hearing loss. *A,* Gadolinium-enhanced T1-weighted MRI study obtained in the acute phase shows intense abnormal enhancement of the membranous labyrinth *(arrows)*. *B,* T2-weighted FSE MRI study in the acute phase shows partial obscuration of the fluid signal in the cochlea due to inflammatory debris *(arrow),* but without discrete filling defect. The patient subsequently had regression of vertigo but progression of hearing loss. *C,* T2-weighted FSE MRI study obtained 1 year later shows osseous obliteration of the cochlea *(arrowhead),* representing labyrinthine ossificans secondary to labyrinthitis. (*A–C,* Used with permission from Davidson HC. Digital Teaching File. Salt Lake City, Electronic Medical Education Research Group, 1999.)

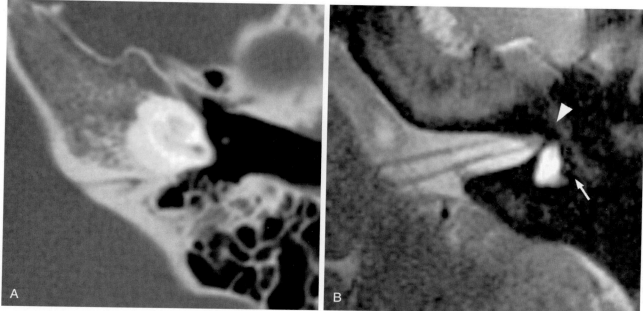

FIGURE 28–17 Labyrinthine ossificans. *A,* Axial bone CT scan of the inner ear in a patient with a history of childhood meningitis and subsequent progressive profound sensorineural hearing loss. Nearly complete osseous obliteration of the cochlea is apparent, with only a ghost of the cochlear contour remaining. *B,* T2-weighted FSE MRI study shows complete absence of fluid signal in the expected location of the cochlea *(arrowhead).* The lateral semicircular canal is also obliterated *(arrow).* (*A* and *B,* Used with permission from Davidson HC. Digital Teaching File. Salt Lake City, Electronic Medical Education Research Group, 1999.)

defined fibrous inflammatory debris. These early changes are more difficult to detect on CT, and T2 FSE imaging is a useful adjunct to CT at this stage. As osseous proliferation continues, portions of the labyrinth become filled in by bone and may progress to complete obliteration in severe cases. In the absence of appropriate clinical history, end-stage labyrinthine ossificans may be mistaken for congenital labyrinthine hypoplasia.

Labyrinthine Schwannoma

Labyrinthine schwannoma (LS) is a rare variation of VCS that arises within or secondarily involves the membranous labyrinth.[63, 64] LSs are histologically similar to other intracranial schwannomas but arise from the termini of the fibers of the vestibular and cochlear nerves. Like VCS, LS typically presents with symptoms of sensorineural hearing loss or vestibular symptoms, depending on tumor location. These tumors tend to grow slowly, and patients often present with gradual onset of symptoms that may last for decades.[55, 65] Because of the typically nonaggressive nature of these lesions and the morbidity of labyrinthine surgery, the diagnosis of LS is often made presumptively, particularly when the tumor is small.

Before the advent of MR, the diagnosis of LS was not made without surgical exploration of the labyrinth. LS is demonstrable on enhanced thin-section T1WI, where it is readily seen as focal intense enhancement within the membranous labyrinth.[62–64] A corresponding filling defect can be demonstrated on thin-section T2 FSE imaging (Figs. 28–18 and 28–19). The vestibule is cited to be a frequent location of LS, although LS may be intracochlear and, when large, may involve all labyrinthine segments.[66, 67]

Endolymphatic Sac Tumor

Endolymphatic sac tumor, also referred to as *papillary adenomatous tumor of the temporal bone,* is a rare neoplasm that occurs as a locally invasive mass at the posteromedial petrous bone.[68–70] This tumor has been mistaken for a variety of other adenomatous tumors before it was described relatively recently.[71] Endolymphatic sac tumor occurs most commonly in patients with von Hippel–Lindau disease and may be bilateral,[72] but it may also occur sporadically. Patients with endolymphatic sac tumor typically present with sensorineural hearing loss and vestibular symptoms, which may be complicated by facial nerve dysfunction if fistulization with the facial canal occurs.

Both CT and MR are valuable in the imaging evaluation of endolymphatic sac tumor. On CT, the tumor is seen as a locally erosive or destructive process at the posteromedial margin of the temporal bone, often with a stippled or irregular margin. On MR, non–contrast-enhanced T1WI shows heterogeneity including foci of high signal from blood products. The tumor is relatively vascular and will show contrast enhancement (Fig. 28–20).

Otosclerosis

Otosclerosis is an idiopathic process that causes replacement of the normal dense endochondral bone of the otic capsule with abnormal spongy vascular bone.[73, 74] Although the foci of abnormal new bone may recalcify, the underlying process of hypodense spongy bone formation has led many to consider the term otosclerosis a misnomer, preferring rather the more descriptive term *otospon-*

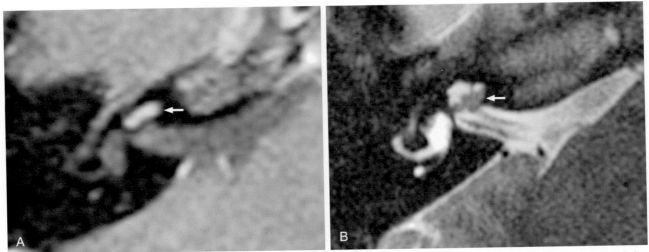

FIGURE 28–18 Labyrinthine schwannoma. *A*, Axial T1-weighted gadolinium-enhanced image of the inner ear in a patient with long-standing unilateral right sensorineural hearing loss. A small cochlear schwannoma *(arrow)* fills the basal turn of the cochlea, showing characteristic intense enhancement. *B*, Axial T2-weighted FSE MRI study shows a filling defect *(arrow)* that is complementary to the nodule of enhancement. The schwannoma just traverses the cochlear modiolus. (*A* and *B*, Used with permission from Davidson HC. Digital Teaching File. Salt Lake City, Electronic Medical Education Research Group, 1999.)

giosis.[75] Two major forms of otosclerosis occur, fenestral and cochlear.[61] *Fenestral otosclerosis* involves the region of the oval window at the medial wall of the tympanic cavity and to a lesser extent the round window as well.[76] *Cochlear otosclerosis,* also called retrofenestral otosclerosis, involves the bone surrounding the cochlea but is almost always accompanied by fenestral otosclerosis, which suggests that cochlear otosclerosis represents a more advanced stage of the disease.[77] Patients with fenestral disease present with progressive conductive hearing loss, whereas patients with combined cochlear and fenestral disease present with mixed elements of conductive and sensorineural hearing loss. Otosclerosis usually ap-

pears in the second and third decades, has a 2:1 female predominance, and is bilateral in approximately 80% of patients.[78–80]

Evaluation of otosclerosis is best accomplished with thin-section multiplanar CT. It is also useful to be familiar with the appearance of otosclerosis on MR inasmuch as changes may be noted incidentally on routine brain scanning or screening acoustic examinations. The most common CT finding is fenestral otosclerosis of the oval window, which appears as an osseous plaque in the space immediately lateral to the oval window (the fissula ante fenestram), with resultant narrowing or obliteration of the oval window. In more advanced disease, manifestations of

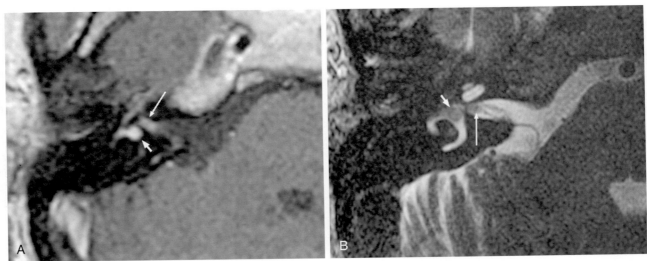

FIGURE 28–19 Labyrinthine schwannoma. *A*, Axial T1-weighted gadolinium-enhanced image of the inner ear in a patient with chronic vertigo. A small schwannoma is seen as nodular enhancement in the vestibule *(short arrow)*, extending into the fundus of the internal auditory canal *(long arrow)*. *B*, T2-weighted FSE MRI study shows corresponding filling defects in the vestibule and internal auditory canal. (*A* and *B*, Used with permission from Davidson HC. Digital Teaching File. Salt Lake City, Electronic Medical Education Research Group, 1999.)

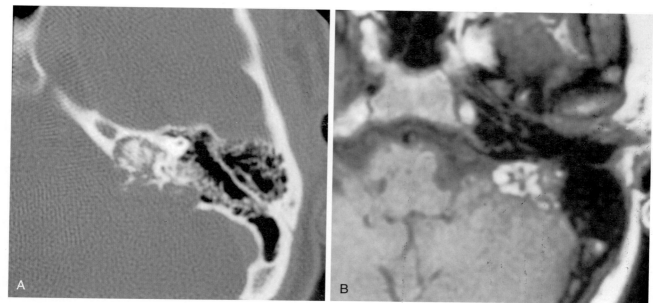

FIGURE 28–20 Endolypmhatic sac tumor. *A,* Axial bone CT scan in a 24-year-old woman with left-sided sensorineural hearing loss. A destructive mass is centered at the upper petrous bone, with stippled calcifications and irregular margins. *B,* Axial T1-weighted MRI study shows heterogeneous enhancement. (*A* and *B,* Used with permission from Davidson HC. Digital Teaching File. Salt Lake City, Electronic Medical Education Research Group, 1999.)

cochlear otosclerosis are apparent, with multiple foci of demineralization in the otic capsule surrounding the cochlea (Fig. 28–21). In contrast to labyrinthine ossificans, the lesions of otosclerosis show decreased mineralization, not osseous obliteration.

INTRATEMPORAL FACIAL NERVE LESIONS

A variety of neoplastic and inflammatory conditions affect the intratemporal segments of the facial nerve. These lesions cause a peripheral type of facial nerve palsy. The number of disease states that have been associated with peripheral facial nerve palsy is large, but only those conditions that affect the intratemporal facial nerve primarily are discussed in this section. The preferred imaging technique for evaluating facial nerve lesions is enhanced thin-section MR to identify enhancing tumor or inflamed nerve, supplemented by thin-section CT to assess for bony changes of the facial canal.

Viral Facial Neuritis

Facial neuritis is a nonspecific inflammation of the seventh cranial nerve. *Bell's palsy* is perhaps the most well recognized facial neuritis. Long considered idiopathic, Bell's palsy has now been associated with herpes simplex infection, possibly involving reactivation of latent virus.[81, 82] Bell's palsy presents with acute onset of lower motor neuron facial paralysis, often preceded by a viral prodrome and frequently accompanied by disturbance of taste due to involvement of gustatory fibers of the chorda tympani.

Ramsay Hunt syndrome, or *herpes zoster oticus,* is another type of herpetic facial neuritis caused by herpes

zoster infection of the external ear as well as of the facial nerve. Patients with Ramsay Hunt syndrome present with facial palsy and painful vesicles involving the pinna, external canal, and tympanic membrane. Involvement of the

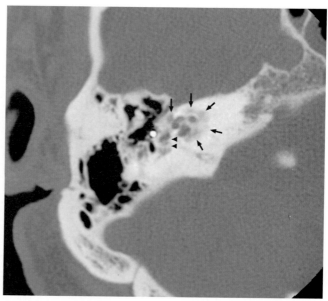

FIGURE 28–21 Otosclerosis. Axial thin-section CT scan of the temporal bone in a patient with mixed conductive and sensorineural hearing loss. The bone of the otic capsule surrounding the cochlea is markedly abnormal, with multiple foci of otospongiotic demineralization *(arrows).* Abnormal osseous plaque is also present at the medial wall of the tympanic cavity *(arrowheads).* Note the presence of a cochlear implant lead. (Used with permission from Davidson HC. Digital Teaching File. Salt Lake City, Electronic Medical Education Research Group, 1999.)

vestibulocochlear nerve may also result in hearing and balance disturbance.[83]

In cases of viral neuritis with classic clinical presentation, imaging is often unnecessary, particularly when the condition is self-limited. The need for diagnostic imaging arises when the clinical course is atypical with unresolving or progressive symptoms, which raises suspicion of a tumor or other nonneuritic etiology. Enhanced MR is the study of choice, demonstrating uniform enhancement of the intratemporal facial nerve, with little or no enlargement and no focal nodularity (Fig. 28–22).[84, 85] Facial nerve enhancement in Bell's Palsy has been reported between 60% and 100%.[86–88] The entire intratemporal length of the nerve may enhance, with the distal segments (mastoid and distal tympanic segments) enhancing less frequently. Enhancement of the nerve characteristically extends to the fundus of the IAC.[87–89] Because mild enhancement of the geniculate ganglion and tympanic segment can be normal, comparison with the uninvolved contralateral nerve provides an important internal control. The pattern of enhancement does not correlate with prognosis and may persist for months after resolution of symptoms.[85–89]

In Ramsay Hunt syndrome, intratemporal facial nerve enhancement may be seen in a manner identical to Bell's palsy, although half of MR scans of Ramsay Hunt syndrome fail to show enhancement. Intracanalicular and even vestibular enhancement may be seen, particularly when there is concomitant involvement of the vestibulocochlear nerve.[90, 91]

Facial Nerve Schwannoma

Facial schwannoma is an uncommon benign nerve sheath tumor that is similar to other cranial nerve schwannomas.

Facial schwannoma may involve any segment of the facial nerve, with a predilection for the geniculate ganglion as well as a tendency to involve multiple segments of the nerve.[92–98] Clinical presentation of facial schwannoma depends on tumor location. Facial nerve palsy is a common symptom, usually with gradual onset but occasionally occurring acutely and mimicking viral facial neuritis.[98] Sensorineural hearing loss is also a common symptom with facial schwannoma, particularly when the tumor is located in the IAC. Because the heavily myelinated motor axons of the facial nerve are less sensitive to mechanical compression, hearing loss may be present while facial motor function is simultaneously preserved.[95, 99] Facial schwannoma in the IAC may be clinically indistinguishable from acoustic schwannoma.[98]

Imaging of facial nerve tumors is best accomplished by a combination of enhanced MR to show enhancing tumor followed by bone CT to show associated bony changes and to illuminate relevant surgical anatomy. Detailed description of tumor extent and location is critical for preoperative evaluation, in terms of both surgical planning and anticipation of the potential risk of nerve injury.[94, 95, 98, 100]

Like other schwannomas, facial schwannomas are seen as homogeneously enhancing masses on post–contrast-enhanced temporal bone MR; larger lesions appear more heterogeneous owing to cystic or hemorrhagic change.[101] Nodular or tubular tumor is characteristically seen in the region of the geniculate ganglion and adjacent intratemporal nerve segments but may be seen anywhere along the length of the nerve (Fig. 28–23).[92, 95–97] CT shows enlargement or focal expansion of the facial canal due to slowly growing tumor. These bony changes, particularly when they are seen in the region of the geniculate fossa

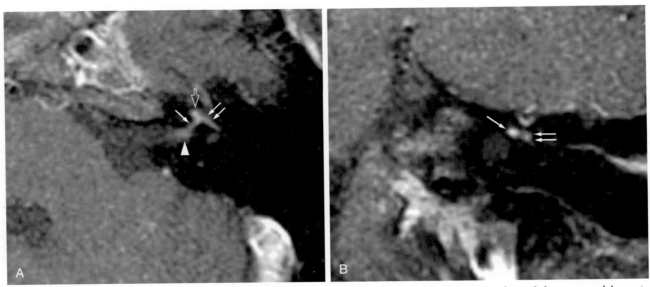

FIGURE 28–22 Facial neuritis. Axial *(A)* and coronal *(B)* contrast-enhanced T1-weighted MRI studies of the temporal bone in a patient with acute onset of left facial paralysis and a clinical diagnosis of Bell's palsy. Abnormal enhancement of the facial nerve is apparent in the labyrinthine portion *(single solid arrow)*, geniculate portion *(open arrow* in *A)*, and tympanic portion *(double arrows)* of the facial nerve. A small amount of abnormal enhancement is also seen in the fundus of the internal auditory canal *(arrowhead* in *A)*. The two side-by-side dots of enhancement of the labyrinthine and proximal tympanic segments of the nerve on coronal section *(B)* have been referred to as "snake eyes." *(A* and *B,* Used with permission from Davidson HC. Digital Teaching File. Salt Lake City, Electronic Medical Education Research Group, 1999.)

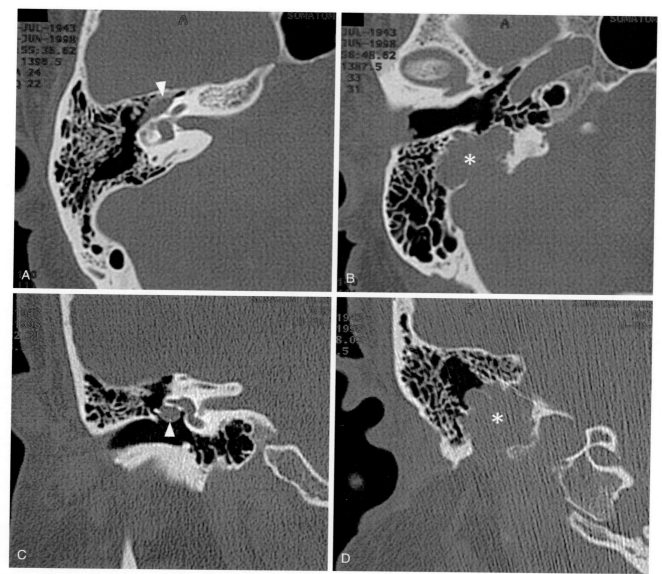

FIGURE 28–23 Facial nerve schwannoma. Axial *(A and B)* and coronal *(C and D)* 1-mm CT sections through the temporal bone in a patient with a 5-year history of right facial nerve paralysis. Images through the tympanic segment of the facial nerve show enlargement of the horizontal facial canal *(arrowhead)*. Schwannoma is seen extending distally, involving the mastoid segment of the nerve, with bulky soft tissue that markedly enlarges the descending facial canal *(asterisk)*. *(A–D, Used with permission from Davidson HC. Digital Teaching File. Salt Lake City, Electronic Medical Education Research Group, 1999.)*

and labyrinthine facial canal, are extremely useful in differentiating facial schwannoma from other petrous bone lesions.[98, 100]

Facial Nerve Hemangioma

Hemangioma of the facial nerve is a benign vascular malformation that has also come to be known as *benign vascular tumor.*[102, 103] Hemangiomas are composed of multiple vascular channels of varying size; cavernous and capillary subtypes are defined on the basis of channel size.[104, 105] Hemangiomas were previously considered rare but have recently come to be recognized as frequently as facial nerve schwannomas.[104–107] Hemangiomas present with symptoms of facial palsy and hemifacial spasm, often

at an earlier stage than their schwannomatous counterparts because they invade the nerve rather than simply compress it. Early detection of hemangioma is crucial to preservation of facial nerve function.

Complete characterization of hemangiomas usually requires both CT and contrast-enhanced MR. Hemangiomas most commonly occur in the region of the geniculate ganglion, to a lesser extent in the labyrinthine facial nerve and distal IAC. On CT, hemangiomas produce widening of the geniculate fossa and affected portion of the facial canal as well as characteristic intratumoral bony spicules and "honeycomb" changes in the adjacent bone.[103, 107] This feature has led to the synonymous term *ossifying hemangioma.* Because of their vascular nature, hemangiomas appear hyperintense on T2WI and manifest intense

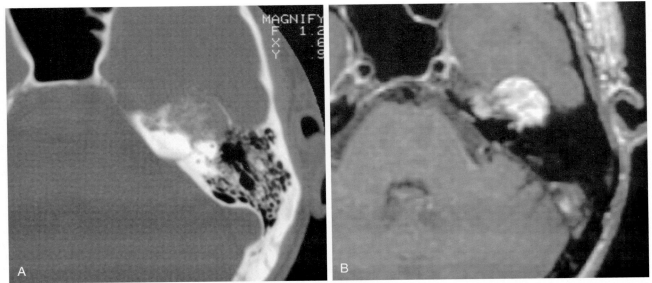

FIGURE 28–24 Facial nerve hemangioma. *A*, Axial bone CT of the temporal bone in a patient with left facial palsy. A mass is centered at the geniculate fossa in the anterior petrous bone with characteristic intratumoral calcific spicules. *B*, T1-weighted MRI study after gadolinium administration shows intense enhancement of the mass. (*A* and *B*, Used with permission from Davidson HC. Digital Teaching File. Salt Lake City, Electronic Medical Education Research Group, 1999.)

enhancement on post–contrast-enhanced T1WI (Fig. 28–24).[105, 108, 109] Heterogeneity on MR may reflect the presence of bony spicules in the soft tissue mass.

GENERALIZED OSSEOUS LESIONS

Processes that affect osseous structures generically elsewhere in the body may also affect the temporal bone. Lesions in this group include bony dysplasias, osseous neoplasms, trauma, and idiopathic conditions.

Otodystrophies and Bone Dysplasias

The otodystrophies and bone dysplasias are a group of idiopathic, dysplastic, and inherited conditions that result in abnormal bone formation in the petrous temporal bone as well as in other bones in the body. These include Paget's disease, fibrous dysplasia, osteogenesis inperfecta, and osteopetrosis. A related condition, otosclerosis, affects primarily the bony labyrinth and is discussed in a previous section.

Evaluation of the otodystrophies is best accomplished with thin-section CT. It is also useful to be familiar with the appearance of the otodystrophies on MR inasmuch as changes may be noted incidentally on routine scanning in patients with mild or asymptomatic disease.

Paget's disease, also called *osteitis deformans,* is a progressive idiopathic process that is characterized by abnormal turnover of bone, particularly the axial skeleton (Fig. 28–25). The condition manifests both lytic and sclerotic phases. In the lytic phase, accelerated osteoclastic activity results in increased bone resorption and increased vascularity. Subsequently, increased new bone is formed in the sclerotic phase that is denser and less vascular than normal bone. Paget's disease is relatively common; it is found in up to 3% of patients older than 40 years, and it occurs

four times more often in men than in women. Malignant degeneration to osteosarcoma occurs in approximately 1% of cases.[110, 111] When the temporal bone is involved by Paget's disease, lytic changes predominate, often in association with the classic changes of osteoporosis circumscripta of the skull. Sclerotic lesions, as well as the mixed lytic and sclerotic "cotton-wool" lesions characteristic of the disease elsewhere in the skull can be seen.[112]

Fibrous dysplasia is an inherited abnormality in which

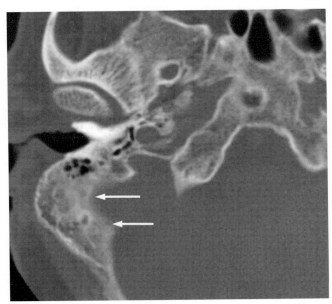

FIGURE 28–25 Paget's disease. Axial bone CT scan in an elderly man with polyostotic Paget's disease. Typical expansile changes of the right mastoid bone are present (*arrow*). (Used with permission from Davidson HC. Digital Teaching File. Salt Lake City, Electronic Medical Education Research Group, 1999.)

normal bone is replaced by fibrous tissue and irregular trabeculae formed of woven bone. The monostotic form is more common than the polyostotic form, occuring in approximately three fourths of patients. The skull and face are the sites of involvement in approximately one fourth of patients with monostotic disease and in one half of patients with polyostotic disease. When fibrous dysplasia involves the temporal bone, the clinical presentation typically consists of hearing loss that is most often conductive in nature but that may also have a sensorineural component. Tinnitus, awareness of a bony mass, and facial nerve dysfunction may also be presenting symptoms. Fibrous dysplasia may also be complicated by cholesteatoma. Symptoms usually present in the second decade, typically becoming quiescent after puberty or progressing into young adulthood. Females are affected two to three times as often as are males.[113–115] The imaging appearance of fibrous dysplasia in the temporal bone is similar to that elsewhere in the skull base and is discussed in more detail in Chapter 29.

Osteogenesis imperfecta is a group of inherited conditions that are characterized by faulty production of type I collagen. Four subtypes of osteogenesis imperfecta have been described.[116] Type I, the most common type, represents the classic *tarda* form of osteogenesis imperfecta. Clinical features of type I include autosomal dominant inheritance, pale blue sclerae, fractures in early childhood but with preserved stature, and abnormal dentition. Type II represents the classic *congenita* form of osteogenesis imperfecta. Features of type II include autosomal recessive inheritance, marked skeletal deformity, and stillbirth or death in infancy. Type III, or progressive deforming osteogenesis imperfecta, is a recessive form that is somewhat less severe. Features of type III include multiple fractures, progressive skeletal deformity, and abnormal dentition. Type IV is a dominant form of osteogenesis imperfecta that is similar to type I except that the sclerae appear normal. Hearing loss due to temporal bone involvement with osteogenesis imperfecta is most commonly seen in type I disease.

Osteopetrosis is a group of rare inherited conditions that are characterized by abnormal bone remodeling due to osteoclast dysfunction, resulting in overproduction of thick, dense, immature bone.[117, 118] Two forms exist, a severe form that manifests recessive inheritance and a more benign form with dominant inheritance.[119, 120] Patients with the recessive form suffer from anemia and hematopoietic deficiency due to marrow replacement as well as multiple fractures of dense but fragile bones.[119] Recessive osteopetrosis usually leads to death in infancy or childhood. Foraminal stenosis in the skull may lead to cranial neuropathy, and temporal bone involvement in particular can lead to conductive hearing loss and facial nerve dysfunction. Recessive disease has also been associated with renal tubular acidosis and resultant intracranial calcifications.[121] Patients with the dominant form of osteopetrosis present later with less extreme manifestations of fractures and cranial neuropathies and may be asymptomatic.[120]

Benign and Malignant Osseous Neoplasm

Like any other bone, the petrous bone is subject to osseous neoplasm of primary or secondary origin. Primary hematopoietic malignant neoplasms that involve the temporal bone include lymphoma and myeloma. Metastatic tumor that spreads to the temporal bone hematogenously most frequently originates from breast, lung, prostate, gastrointestinal tract, and genitourinary tract. In pediatric patients, additional considerations include Langerhans cell histiocytosis and rhabdomyosarcoma.[122] Squamous cell carcinoma and adenocarcinoma primarily involve the middle and external ear but may extend into the petrous bone proper. Because many of these lesions have a similar appearance, the specific diagnosis of a malignant petrous lesion often requires biopsy or is made presumptively on the basis of clinical history.

Primary tumors of osteocartilaginous origin are rare in the skull base. Giant cell tumor and aneurysmal bone cyst have been described in the temporal bone.[122–125] Osteoblastoma can occur in the temporal bone and is usually seen in younger patients.[126] Osteosarcoma is rare in the temporal bone and may be seen secondarily in the setting of prior irradiation or Paget's disease.[127] One lesion that has a predilection for the skull base is chondrosarcoma, which is typically centered in the petrosphenoid and petro-occipital synchondroses and frequently extends into the petrous apex.[126] A more complete description of chondrosarcoma and other regional tumors is given in Chapter 29.

The imaging features of primary hematopoietic and metastatic malignant tumors of the temporal bone are generally nonspecific. CT is often more helpful than MR in distinguishing malignant from benign lesions because malignant lesions show more permeative bone destruction and greater loss of cortical margins (Fig. 28–26). On CT, most malignant lesions appear lytic with a varying amount of associated soft tissue mass. Metastatic prostate cancer is primarily blastic but may be lytic, particularly in older patients. Breast cancer may be primarily lytic, blastic, or mixed. Other metastatic types that may be blastic include lung (carcinoid), stomach, bladder, and some central nervous system malignant neoplasms. Enhanced MR with fat suppression shows the soft tissue extent of malignant tumors to greater advantage and is of particular value in assessing the extent of intracranial disease.

Primary osseous tumors in the temporal bone appear as in other bones of endochondral origin. Giant cell tumors appear as expansile, often large, variably destructive tumors. Aneurysmal bone cysts appear as expansile multiloculated lesions with fluid levels.[125] Tumors with osteocartilaginous tissues will show characteristic matrix on CT.

Trauma

Trauma to the temporal bone is usually the result of severe blunt head injury. The number and complexity of structures in the temporal bone means that clinical signs of trauma can vary widely. Direct signs of injury include otorrhea, hemotympanum, and mastoid ecchymosis (Battle's sign). Disruption of the ossicles or middle ear may cause conductive hearing, whereas fracture involving the labyrinth may cause sensorineural hearing loss, vertigo, or facial nerve palsy.[127–129] Related complications may also develop, including CSF leak and meningitis. In the setting of severe trauma, temporal bone fractures may be over-

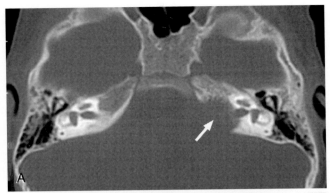

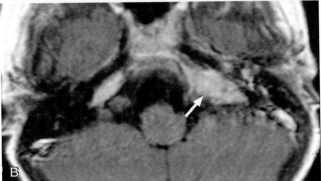

FIGURE 28–26 Eosinophilic granuloma. *A,* Axial bone CT scan of the temporal bone in a pediatric patient. A destructive mass is present at the posteromedial petrous temporal bone and involves the internal auditory canal *(arrow).* The appearance of the lesion is malignant but nonspecific. *B,* Post–contrast-enhanced T1-weighted MRI study shows diffuse, slightly irregular enhancement *(arrow).* Pathologic examination revealed Langerhans cell histiocytes. (*A* and *B,* Used with permission from Davidson HC. Digital Teaching File. Salt Lake City, Electronic Medical Education Research Group, 1999.)

looked initially while other more acute injuries are managed.

Temporal bone fractures are described according to the orientation of the fracture relative to the long axis of the temporal bone and are classically classified as *longitudinal* or *transverse.*[130–132] Longitudinal fractures are more common, seen in 79% to 90% of cases, and result from temporoparietal impact. Longitudinal fractures typically involve the middle ear, with resultant conductive hearing loss. Facial nerve injury is uncommon in longitudinal fractures, seen in 10% to 20% of cases, and is often incomplete with delayed presentation.[133–136] By comparison, transverse fractures are less common, seen in 10% to 30% of cases, and result from frontal or occipital impact. Transverse fractures more frequently violate the labyrinth, resulting in sensorineural hearing loss and vertigo. Transverse fractures have a higher incidence of facial nerve injury, seen in up to 50% of cases, with palsy that is more often acute and complete.[133–136]

High-resolution temporal bone CT is essential in the evaluation of temporal bone trauma, although in many cases the opportunity to perform a dedicated scan does not present itself until after the patient is stabilized. Longitudinal fractures are oriented along the long axis

of the temporal bone, with the fracture line frequently extending into the otic capsule and labyrinth. Transverse fractures are oriented in a perpendicular direction and tend to involve the tympanic cavity; middle ear and mastoid fluid is typical, and ossicular disruption may be apparent. Although the distinction between transverse and longitudinal fractures is a useful tool for discussion, in practice many fractures have features that suggest both types or that do not clearly fit either type and are best described as oblique, mixed, or complex (Fig. 28–27).[137–139]

Other portions of the temporal bone may be fractured with trauma. Styloid process fracture may be seen in combination with other fractures or as an isolated fracture. Mandible and temporomandibular joint injuries may result in fracture of the tympanic portion. The squamous portion may also be fractured in association with other calvarial or skull base injuries.

PETROUS BONE LESIONS

Lesions that affect the petrous bone proper include congenital vascular anomalies and infectious and inflammatory conditions that involve petrous apex air cells. Lesions of the jugular foramen, such as glomus jugulare paraganglioma, are discussed in the section on poster skull base lesions in Chapter 29. Imaging evaluation of lesions of the petrous bone usually includes thin-section bone CT. MR is useful in evaluating the soft tissue components and

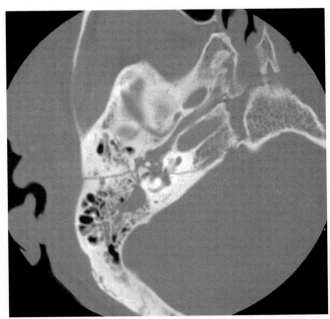

FIGURE 28–27 Temporal bone fracture. Axial thin-section CT image of the temporal bone in a motor vehicle accident victim. A fracture line traverses the temporal bone obliquely, with features of both transverse and longitudinal type fractures. Both the middle ear and the bony labyrinth are breached. The middle ear and mastoid are opacified with fluid and blood, although the ossicles in the epitympanum appear grossly aligned. (Used with permission from Davidson HC. Digital Teaching File. Salt Lake City, Electronic Medical Education Research Group, 1999.)

complications of inflammatory conditions and in demonstrating anomalous vessels.

Anomalous Internal Carotid Artery

The normal internal carotid artery (ICA) follows a tortuous course through the petrous carotid canal. Anomalies of the intratemporal ICA arise as a result of disturbed development of the primitive hyoid artery and proximal dorsal aortic arches.[140] The most common of these anomalies is *aberrant ICA*, also called *intratympanic ICA*, which results from regression of the cervical ICA during embryogenesis. Intratympanic ICA develops from the anastomosis of an enlarged ascending pharyngeal branch (the inferior tympanic artery) and an enlarged derivative of the primitive hyostapedial trunk (the caroticotympanic artery).[140, 141] This uncommon lesion is often asymptomatic, although patients may experience conductive hearing loss or subjective or objective pulsatile tinnitus.[141, 142] In the clinical setting of a vascular retrotympanic mass, differentiation of aberrant ICA from surgical lesions, such as paraganglioma, is critical.[143, 145]

Intratympanic ICA is most easily recognized on CT, where the appearance of the aberrant bony canal is characteristic.[141, 146] The aberrant ICA enters the tympanic cavity posteriorly through an enlarged tympanic canaliculus, coursing anteriorly at the cochlear promontory, and reentering the posterior aspect of the normal horizontal petrous canal through a bony dehiscence (Fig. 28–28).[147] Aberrant ICA is also recognizable on angiographic images and MR angiography three-dimensional projections by the abnormally lateral and posterior position of the vertical petrous ICA.

Benign Petrous Apex Fluid

Benign sterile fluid in the petrous apex is a postinflammatory process that occurs as a sequela of prior otomastoid disease. This chronic accumulation of "trapped" fluid presupposes the presence of air cells, which are present in about one-third of normal individuals.[148] This process is benign and is discovered incidentally, but it is probably the most common radiographically identified lesion of the petrous apex.[149] The asymmetry of petrous apex pneuma-

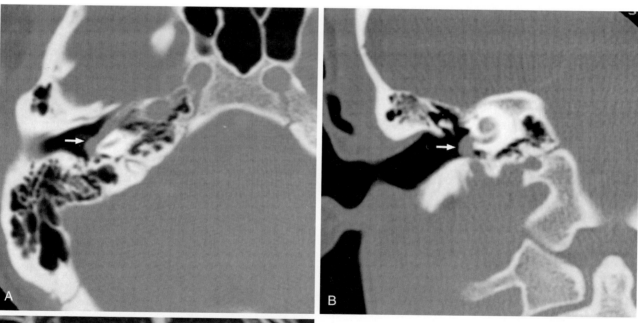

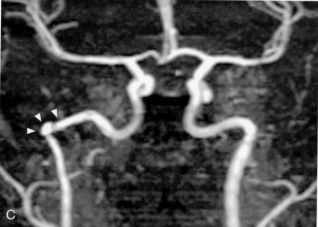

FIGURE 28–28 Aberrant internal carotid artery. Axial *(A)* and coronal *(B)* thin-section bone CT images in a patient with a right ear vascular retrotympanic mass. The aberrant internal carotid artery is clearly seen entering the posterior tympanic cavity medially and coursing anteriorly past the cochlear promontory *(arrows)*. *C,* Maximal intensity projection from three-dimensional time-of-flight magnetic resonance angiogram shows the characteristic lateral course of the aberrant internal carotid artery *(arrowheads)*. (A–C, Used with permission from Davidson HC. Digital Teaching File. Salt Lake City, Electronic Medical Education Research Group, 1999.)

tization and fluid may be striking, particularly on MR, leading to a diagnostic dilemma when petrous apex fluid is noted incidentally on scans done for unrelated clinical conditions but not recognized as a "leave me alone" lesion.[149]

The appearance of benign petrous apex fluid on CT is characteristic, showing nonexpansile opacification of pneumatized cells in the petrous apex without bony erosion. The appearance on MR is more complicated, appearing consistently hyperintense on T2WI but with signal on T1WI that may be hypointense, isointense, or hyperintense, depending on the proteinaceous nature of the fluid (Fig. 28–29). When both T2WI and T1WI appear hyperintense, the signal characteristics of benign fluid mimic those of cholesterol granuloma. If there is uncertainty about the diagnosis in this situation, comparison with CT to exclude an expansile lesion and long-term imaging follow-up are prudent to rule out early cholesterol granuloma.[149]

A related normal variant is the presence of asymmetric fatty marrow in the petrous apex. The degree of marrow signal asymmetry in the petrous apex can be striking on MR, particularly with the widespread use of neuroimaging protocols that employ T2WI techniques such as FSE and fluid attenuated inversion recovery that show much higher signal from fat than earlier conventional T2WI techniques do. As with benign petrous apex fluid, CT can be used to exclude an underlying expansile or destructive lesion when uncertainty exists.

Cholesterol Granuloma of the Petrous Apex

Cholesterol granuloma is a complication of chronic otomastoid inflammation that is characterized pathologically by specialized granulation tissue, blood products, and cholesterol crystals.[150] The most common location for cholesterol granuloma is the middle ear, although classic descriptions often focus on petrous apex lesions. Cholesterol granuloma that is localized in the petrous apex may present with hearing loss, tinnitus, or multiple cranial nerve deficits, depending on size and position.[151–153] Rarely, cholesterol granuloma of the petrous apex occurs in the absence of a history of chronic otomastoid disease, in which case the lesion is referred to as a cholesterol cyst.[153]

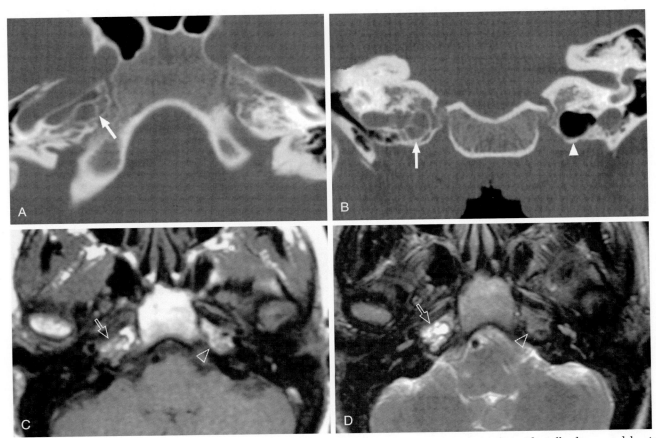

FIGURE 28–29 Benign petrous apex fluid. Axial *(A)* and coronal *(B)* CT images in a patient with incidentally discovered benign petrous apex fluid. Opacified air cells are visible in the right petrous apex *(arrows)*. There is no evidence of expansion, trabecular disruption, or body destruction. Note that a single large aerated cell is visible on the left on coronal scan *(arrowhead in B)*. Axial T1-weighted *(C)* and FSE T2-weighted *(D)* MRI studies show the fluid in the right apex cells *(arrows)* to have hyperintense T2- and mixed T1-weighted signal, consistent with complex fluid that is probably postinflammatory in nature. Note the presence of fatty marrow in the contralateral left petrous apex *(arrowheads)*. *(A–D, Used with permission from Davidson HC. Digital Teaching File. Salt Lake City, Electronic Medical Education Research Group, 1999.)*

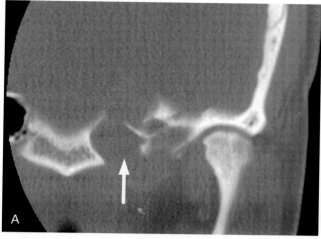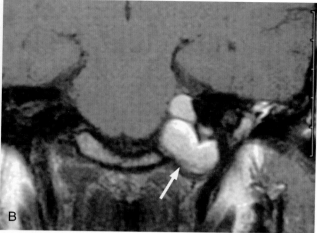

FIGURE 28–30 Petrous apex cholesterol granuloma. *A,* Coronal CT image demonstrates an expansile mass *(arrow)* centered in the petrous apex. The bony margins are smooth and scalloped. *B,* T1-weighted non–contrast-enhanced MRI signal shows intrinsic T1 shortening *(arrow)*, consistent with blood products, which is typical for cholesterol granuloma. (*A* and *B,* Used with permission from Davidson HC. Digital Teaching File. Salt Lake City, Electronic Medical Education Research Group, 1999.)

A related lesion is mucocele of the petrous apex, which develops as a postobstructive sequela to inflammatory insult, similar to that seen in the sinonasal cavities.[154] The petrous apex is an uncommon place for mucocele, but when large, it can present clinically similar to cholesterol granuloma.

Cholesterol granuloma in the petrous apex is seen as an expansile mass with smooth bony margins on CT. On MR, the presence of chronic blood products and fluid debris give rise to hyperintense signal on both T1WI and T2WI. Post–contrast-enhanced images show nonenhancement centrally, with enhancement of granulation tissue at the periphery of the lesion (Fig. 28–30).[152] Large lesions may compromise the inner ear, IAC, or sphenoid sinus.[155]

Mucocele of the petrous apex is indistinguishable from cholesterol granuloma on CT, appearing as an expansile mass with smooth bony margins. MR of petrous apex mucocele typically shows hypointensity on T1WI and hyperintensity on T2WI, distinguishing mucocele from cholesterol granuloma. However, signal on T1WI is variable, depending on the protein composition of the fluid contents, and may appear hyperintense, in which case differentiation from cholesterol granuloma is more difficult.

Apical Petrositis and Osteomyelitis

Apical petrositis is an acute infection of the pneumatized air cells of the petrous apex. Infection presumably spreads from nearby otomastoid disease, which presupposes the presence of petrous apex pneumatization[155] (see earlier discussion of trapped petrous apex fluid). If untreated, apical petrositis progresses to osteomyelitis in the surrounding bone. Patients with apical petrositis present with signs and symptoms of acute infection and usually manifest some or all of the classic symptoms of *Gradenigo's syndrome,* which consists of purulent otomastoiditis, abducens palsy due to compromise of the sixth nerve as it passes through Dorello's canal, and deep facial and retro-orbital pain along the trigeminal nerve distribution.[156]

In the early stages of acute apical petrositis without osteomyelitis, CT and MR show simple opacification or air-fluid levels in petrous apex cells with enhancement as well as evidence of otomastoid disease. As the infection progresses to osteomyelitis, bony changes of trabecular breakdown and cortical destruction become apparent on CT (Fig. 28–31).[154] Advanced intracranial disease is best evaluated on MR, which may show involvement of the adjacent cisterns or IAC as well as possible complications of abscess or venous sinus thrombosis.

MIDDLE EAR AND MASTOID LESIONS

Lesions that affect the middle ear and mastoid include congenital anomalies, congenital and acquired inflammatory conditions, and infectious processes. Complex dysplasias that involve the middle and external ear are discussed together in this section.

Middle and External Ear Dysplasia

Middle and external ear dysplasia represents a spectrum of congenital anomalies resulting from abnormal embryogenesis of the first and second branchial arches and tympanic ring.[157–159] The middle and external ear develop in concert from these structures, which explains the usual association of these anomalies. By contrast, the inner ear is usually preserved in cases of middle and external ear dysplasia, except in complex syndromic conditions such as craniofacial dysplasias and trisomies.[160, 161] Although it is possible to classify specific lesions according to the specific embryonic anlage from which the defects arise, in practice complex middle and external ear dysplasias can be addressed together. Patients with middle and external ear dysplasia present with congenital conductive hearing loss and obvious external deformity due to coexistent aural atresia. Males are affected more than females

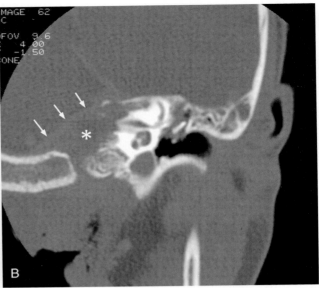

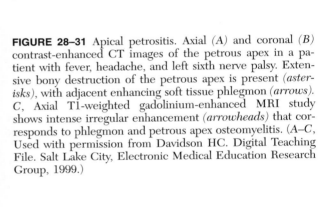

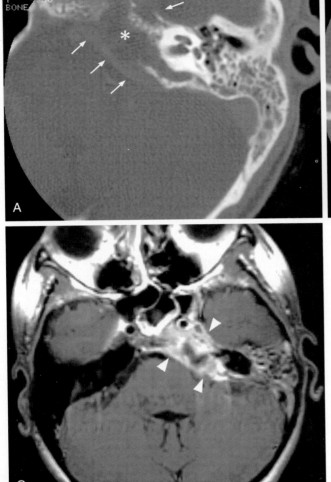

FIGURE 28–31 Apical petrositis. Axial (*A*) and coronal (*B*) contrast-enhanced CT images of the petrous apex in a patient with fever, headache, and left sixth nerve palsy. Extensive bony destruction of the petrous apex is present (*asterisks*), with adjacent enhancing soft tissue phlegmon (*arrows*). *C*, Axial T1-weighted gadolinium-enhanced MRI study shows intense irregular enhancement (*arrowheads*) that corresponds to phlegmon and petrous apex osteomyelitis. (*A–C*, Used with permission from Davidson HC. Digital Teaching File. Salt Lake City, Electronic Medical Education Research Group, 1999.)

at a 3:2 ratio. Bilateral disease is present in 30% of cases, and a family history is present in 15%.

The imaging evaluation of middle and external ear dysplasia is performed with thin-section CT. The main goals of imaging are to provide a presurgical assessment of temporal bone structures, evaluate for associated anomalies, and determine whether any complications are present (Fig. 28–32). To this end, a checklist of specific features should be assessed and explicitly reported for every ear with dysplasia (Table 28–5).[160, 162, 163]

The classification of external ear atresia depends on the degree of canal narrowing and whether the canal is obstructed by bone or soft tissue.[164] The size of the tympanic cavity is an important presurgical observation, because a coarcted (small and underdeveloped) middle ear significantly complicates surgery. A coarcted tympanic cavity that measures less than 3 mm in the lateral dimension may be inadequate for ossicular reconstruction.[163]

Anomalies of the ossicular chain include rotation, fusion, and absence of the ossicles as well as abnormalities of the associated suspensory ligaments. Fusion of the incus and malleus in the epitympanum is a commonly seen pattern. The status of the stapes has the greatest significance relative to surgical prognosis.[163] The stapes is best evaluated in the coronal plane, with its footplate located in the oval window at the medial wall of the

TABLE 28–5 Middle and External Ear Dysplasia Imaging Checklist

Type and thickness of external atresia
Degree of middle ear and mastoid coarctation
Morphology and position of ossicular chain
Status of the oval and round windows
Course of the intratemporal facial nerve
Coexistence of congenital cholesteatoma
Anomalies of the inner ear

Used with permission from Davidson HC. The Temporal Bone. Salt Lake City, Electronic Medical Education Research Group, 1999.

tympanic cavity, just medial to and below the lateral semicircular canal and facial canal. The oval window should measure 2 mm on the coronal image. The round window is best evaluated in the axial plane and should be visible as an air-filled pocket adjacent to the lateral margin of the basal turn of the cochlea.

An anomalous course of the intratemporal facial nerve is usual in middle ear dysplasia. In the absence of normal development of the second branchial arch middle ear structures, the posterior genu and vertical segment migrate anteriorly away from their normal position. This anterior displacement places the nerve at risk for injury

during surgical reconstruction, and precise description of nerve position is critical for presurgical planning. The tympanic segment may also take an anomalous course overlying the oval window, but this is less common.

Congenital cholesteatoma is seen in a small minority of dysplasia cases, but its presence will affect the approach and timing of surgical therapy.

Congenital Cholesteatoma

Congenital cholesteatoma is caused by the presence of an ectopic rest of epithelial tissue. Congenital cholesteatoma

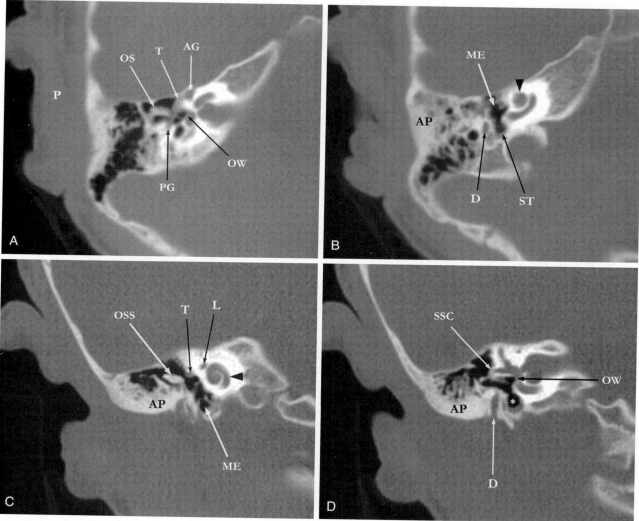

FIGURE 28–32 Middle and external ear dysplasia. *A,* Axial scan at the level of the epitympanum demonstrates ossicular fusion (OS). The anterior genu (AG) and proximal tympanic (T) segments of the facial nerve are normally positioned, but the posterior genu (PG) is located too far anteriorly. The oval window (OW) is clear. The pinna (P) is deformed. *B,* Axial scan at the level of the cochlear promontory shows absence of the external canal with a thick bony atresia plate (AP) and attenuated size of the middle ear (ME). The descending facial nerve (D) is located abnormally anterior relative to the sinus tympani (ST). The cochlea *(arrowhead)* is normal. *C,* Coronal scan at the level of the cochlea also shows the fused ossicles (OSS) in the epitympanum and the attenuated middle ear. The atresia plate has a horizontal orientation, and the tympanic portion of the temporal bone is aplastic. The cochlea *(arrowhead),* tympanic segment of facial nerve (T), and labyrinthine segment of facial nerve (L) appear normal. *D,* Coronal scan at the level of the oval window shows the abnormally anterior position of the descending facial nerve. A small amount of soft tissue or fluid is dependent in the attenuated hypotympanum *(asterisk)* but without evidence of cholesteatoma. The ossicles are partially annealed to the bony covering of the lateral semicircular canal (SCC). The oval window is clear. (*A–D,* Used with permission from Davidson HC. Digital Teaching File. Salt Lake City, Electronic Medical Education Research Group, 1999.)

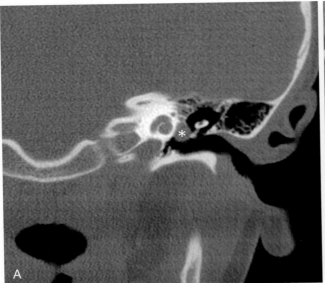 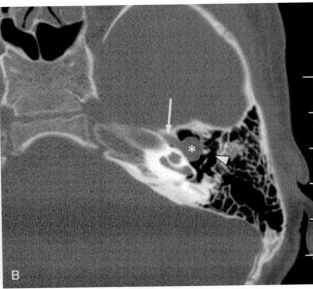

FIGURE 28–33 Congenital cholesteatoma. *A,* Coronal CT scan in a child with progressive conductive hearing loss who did not give a history of otitis media. A rounded soft tissue mass is present in the middle ear *(asterisk),* located between the wall over the cochlea medially and the ossicles laterally. Prussak's space and the rest of the epitympanum are clear. Note the proximity of the cholesteatoma to the tympanic segment of the facial nerve. *B,* Axial CT scan shows a soft tissue mass anteriorly in the middle ear at the entrance to the eustachian tube *(arrow).* This is the classic location for congenital cholesteatoma. In contrast to acquired cholesteatoma, Prussak's space is clear *(arrowhead).* (A and B, Used with permission from Davidson HC. Digital Teaching File. Salt Lake City, Electronic Medical Education Research Group, 1999.)

is histologically identical to epidermoid tumor. By convention, these lesions are referred to as epidermoid when they occur intracranially and as cholesteatoma when they occur in the temporal bone or intradiploic space. Although classically described in the petrous apex, congenital cholesteatoma is more commonly found in the middle ear and may also occur in the mastoid and external canal. Congenital cholesteatomas are much less likely than their acquired counterparts. Clinical presentation usually consists of progressive conductive hearing loss, although other symptoms may be present depending on the location and degree of osseous destruction. Cholesteatoma is presumed to be congenital if there is no history of inflammatory middle ear disease and may be present for years before becoming symptomatic. Congenital cholesteatoma should be sought in any patient who is being evaluated for external or middle ear dysplasia.

The radiographic features of congenital cholesteatoma on CT consist of characteristic bony erosion associated with a nonenhancing soft tissue mass (Fig. 28–33). Congenital cholesteatoma in the middle ear is seen as an irregular nonenhancing soft tissue mass that has a propensity to occur anteriorly in the tympanic cavity near the eustachian tube. This location has embryologic significance in that a rest of squamous cells, called the epidermoid formation, occurs here at the epithelial transition between the eustachian tube and middle ear.[165] Congenital cholesteatoma also has a tendency to occur near the stapes but may occur anywhere in the middle ear or temporal bone. Large lesions show bony erosive changes similar to those seen in acquired cholesteatoma, described next. MR signal of congenital cholesteatoma is variable but is similar to that seen with intracranial epidermoid tumors. T1WI images show a mildly hypointense mass that is variably hyperintense on T2WI. Post–contrast-enhanced scans show little enhancement except for a thin line at the periphery. Labyrinthine enhancement is seen when fistulization is present.

Congenital cholesteatoma occurs less commonly in the petrous apex, where it presents as a nonenhancing mass with localized osseous changes, including scalloped enlargement of pneumatized air cells and erosion of bony margins.

Acquired Cholesteatoma

Acquired cholesteatoma is a complication of chronic otomastoiditis that consists of a collection of keratinaceous debris contained within a sac lined by stratified squamous epithelium.[166] Because this lesion may not contain cholesterol crystals, some consider the term *cholesteatoma* a misnomer, preferring the term *keratoma.*[167] Acquired cholesteatoma arises as a result of disruption of the normal physiologic maintenance of the tympanic squamous epithelium, although some disagreement exists as to the exact mechanism of acquired cholesteatoma formation. The most widely accepted theory suggests that retraction pockets form in the tympanic membrane as a result of inflammatory insult, which in turn disrupts the normal migration and turnover of squamous epithelial layers.[168, 169] Another theory suggests that acquired cholesteatoma is due to invasion of stratified epithelium from the outer surface of the tympanic membrane into the middle ear through a perforation in the membrane.[170] Other theories suggest that acquired cholesteatoma may occur as the result of basal cell hyperplasia in the tympanic membrane or as a sequela of squamous metaplasia in the middle ear.[171]

The clinical setting of acquired cholesteatoma includes a history of repeated episodes of otitis media, with associated tympanic membrane rupture or tympanostomy tube placement. Patients with acquired cholesteatoma suffer from progressive conductive hearing loss and may experience symptoms of facial nerve and vestibulocochlear dysfunction as osseous erosion progresses to involve adjacent temporal bone structures. Cholesteatoma is an acquired lesion in most cases; less than 5% are congenital in origin.

Acquired cholesteatoma is divided into two subtypes based on the part of the tympanic membrane from which it arises. *Pars flaccida* cholesteatomas originate superiorly in Prussak's space. Pars flaccida lesions displace the ossicles medially as they expand and also extend posteriorly in the attic along ossicular ligaments into the additus ad antrum.[172, 173] In contrast, *pars tensa* cholesteatomas arise posteriorly and are referred to as *sinus cholesteatomas* because they involve the posterior depressions of the facial recess and sinus tympani. Pars tensa lesions are more medial than pars flaccida lesions and displace the ossicles laterally instead of medially as they expand, but they also extend posteriorly into the additus ad antrum similar to the pars flaccida type.[168, 174]

The hallmark feature of cholesteatoma is bony erosion associated with nonenhancing soft tissue mass, best demonstrated on CT (Fig. 28–34). Ossicular erosion is common, with full preservation of the ossicular chain in only 30% of pars flaccida and 10% of pars tensa cholesteatomas.[175, 176] Erosion of the scutum is a classic finding in attic cholesteatoma, as is remodeling of the lateral attic wall. As cholesteatomas become large, local osseous erosion may be extensive and involve any portion of the middle ear. Complications of cholesteatoma are due to

erosion into adjacent vital structures and include facial canal dehiscence, labyrinthine fistula (particularly at the lateral semicircular canal), dehiscence of the tympanic tegmen, and extension into the dural venous sinuses.[172, 177, 178] Evidence of these potential complications should be sought on all studies in which cholesteatoma is suspected. MR signal of acquired cholesteatomas is similar to that described for congenital lesions, consisting of hypointensity on T1WI, variable hyperintensity on T2WI, and mild peripheral enhancement.

Noncholesteatomatous Chronic Inflammatory Change

Patients with chronic otomastoiditis may develop postinflammatory changes in the middle ear and mastoid without overt cholesteatoma formation. In the wake of repeated inflammatory insults, the development of ossicular erosion, ossicular disruption, ossicular fixation, tympanosclerosis, and other postinflammatory debris can lead to conductive hearing loss. These patients have clinical presentations similar to those of patients with cholesteatoma, but with lesser severity of complications.

As with cholesteatoma, other postinflammatory changes of the middle ear are best appreciated on CT. Focal erosion can affect any of the ossicles, but the incus appears to be the most vulnerable in the ossicular chain.[179] Erosions may be present even if the middle ear is normally aerated, and in fact the absence of inflammatory debris improves detection of underlying ossicular defects. Injury to the interossicular articulations leads to subluxation or frank disruption of the ossicular chain. Ossicular fixation is manifest as soft tissue density fibrous and granulation debris that encases the ossicular chain. Simple granulation tissue without hemorrhage or cholesterol

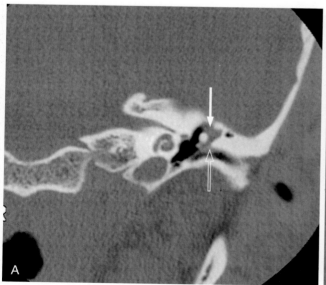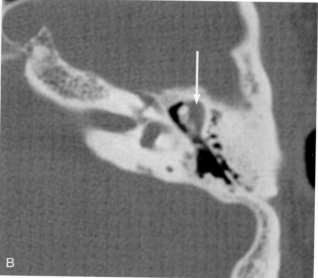

FIGURE 28–34 Acquired cholesteatoma. *A,* Coronal CT scan in a child with a history of multiple episodes of otitis media and previous placement of tympanostomy tubes. Soft tissue is present in the lateral epitympanum, extending into Prussak's space (*solid arrow*). Thickening of the pars flaccida of the tympanic membrane is present, as is early erosion of the scutum (*open arrow*). *B,* Axial CT scan shows classic location of cholesteatoma in Prussak's space (*arrow*). (*A* and *B,* Used with permission from Davidson HC. Digital Teaching File. Salt Lake City, Electronic Medical Education Research Group, 1999.)

crystals is probably more common than true cholesterol granuloma.[180]

Tympanosclerosis is a manifestation of inflammation and appears as multifocal punctate calcifications scattered within soft tissue debris in the middle ear cavity.[181] Postinflammatory thickening and adhesions of the tympanic membrane itself may also be visible on high-resolution CT.

Cholesterol Granuloma and Other Granulation Tissue

Granulation tissue in the middle ear results from chronic otomastoid inflammation. When uncomplicated, this process results in the accumulation of *simple granulation.* *Cholesterol granuloma* is a more complicated response to chronic inflammation that is characterized by the production of specialized granulation tissue.[182, 183] Cholesterol granuloma is prone to hemorrhage, resulting in the presence of chronic blood products and the development of cholesterol crystals, which in turn incite further aggravation of inflammatory response and perpetuate the process.[184] Cholesterol granuloma can occur anywhere along the tympanic cleft but is most commonly found in the middle ear proper. The terms *blue dome cyst* and *chocolate cyst* are used to describe a histologically identical lesion that occurs in a mastoidectomy cavity.[185] The distinctive features of cholesterol granuloma of the petrous apex are discussed in a previous section.

Simple granulation tissue and cholesterol granuloma of the middle ear are essentially always seen in the setting of chronic otomastoiditis. Chronic effusion is common, and hearing loss is variably present. These granulomatous lesions may coexist with other sequelae of chronic otomastoid inflammation, such as cholesteatoma.[156, 186] Because of its hemorrhagic nature, cholesterol granuloma may appear as a vascular retrotympanic mass on otologic inspection.

Both simple granulation tissue and cholesterol granuloma appear on CT to show accumulation of soft tissue debris in the middle ear. Simple granulation shows little bony change, whereas cholesterol granuloma may cause bony expansion and erosion. Interestingly, the degree of mass effect of these lesions is minimal, and the absence of a bulging tympanic membrane is a helpful diagnostic feature.[182, 187] MR is useful in differentiating cholesterol granuloma because the presence of chronic blood products and fluid debris gives rise to characteristic hyperintense signal on both T1WI and T2WI. Granulation tissue is often vascular and shows enhancement after administration of contrast material. Cholesterol granuloma will typically show peripheral enhancement that surrounds the chronic hemorrhagic fluid.[187, 188]

Acute Otomastoiditis

Acute otomastoiditis, a common infectious process, stems from upper respiratory infection and usually affects children. Bacterial etiology is the rule, with *Streptococcus pneumoniae* and *Haemophilus influenzae* accounting for the majority of cases.[189] Tuberculous otitis is uncommon but occurs more often in immunocompromised patients. Classically, tuberculous otitis presents with painless otorrhea, although a variety of presentations is possible.[152]

Acute otomastoiditis is readily managed with a course of antibiotics in most patients. The condition becomes complicated when secondary osseous infection develops that involves the ossicles, tympanic cavity, or mastoid. Coalescent mastoiditis, abscess formation, and fistula development are part of the spectrum of untreated disease. In advanced cases, intracranial extension of infection may result in meningitis, cerebritis, empyema, or dural venous thrombosis.[190]

In the setting of acute uncomplicated disease, imaging is not necessary; if imaging is done, nonspecific fluid and debris will be apparent in the middle ear and mastoid without evidence of bony erosion. In more advanced disease, evidence of osseous destruction is present, with loss of middle ear and mastoid bony landmarks and dehiscence into the inner ear and intracranial compartment (Fig. 28–35). Intracranial complications are best appreciated on contrast-enhanced MR.

Glomus Tympanicum Paraganglioma

Glomus tympanicum paraganglioma is tumor of glomus cells, or paraganglia, that reside in the inferior temporal bone. Glomus tympanicum paraganglioma is a subtype of paraganglioma that is localized to the glomus formations of the glossopharyngeal nerve (Jacobson's nerve) found near the cochlear promontory. Paragangliomas in the jugular foramen, the proximal carotid sheath, and the carotid bifurcation are referred to as *glomus jugulare, glomus vagale,* and *carotid body tumor,* respectively; the unique

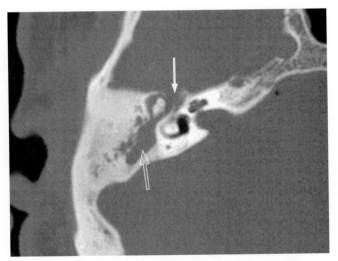

FIGURE 28–35 Acute otomastoiditis. Axial CT scan in a 40-year-old man with purulent otorrhea, facial weakness, hearing loss, and vertigo. Opacification of the middle ear is present, with dehiscence of the anterior tympanic wall and facial canal *(solid arrow).* Coalescence of air cells is seen in the mastoid antrum *(open arrow).* The presence of pneumolabyrinth in the cochlea and vestibule indicates a fistula. (Used with permission from Davidson HC. Digital Teaching File. Salt Lake City, Electronic Medical Education Research Group, 1999.)

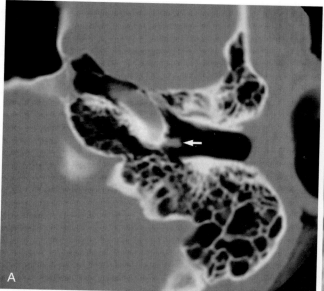
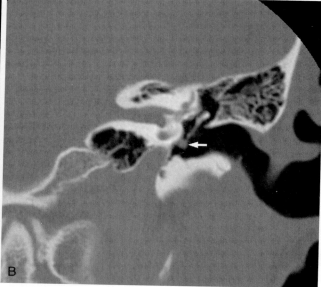

FIGURE 28–36 Glomus tympanicum paraganglioma. Axial (A) and coronal (B) CT scans in a 36-year-old woman with pulsatile tinnitus and retrotympanic mass on otoscopic examination. A small soft tissue mass is present at the medial wall of the middle ear overlying the lower portion of the cochlear promontory (arrows). (A and B, Used with permission from Davidson HC. Digital Teaching File. Salt Lake City, Electronic Medical Education Research Group, 1999.)

features of these lesions are discussed elsewhere. When a large glomus jugulare extends into the middle ear, the term *glomus jugulotympanicum* is used.

Glomus tympanicum paraganglioma is three times more common in women than in men, usually presenting in middle age.[191] Patients typically present with pulsatile tinnitus, conductive hearing loss, or inner ear symptoms. Large jugulotympanicum tumors may also present with multiple lower cranial neuropathies. On otologic examination, glomus tympanicum paraganglioma appears as a vascular retrotympanic mass.[192]

Small glomus tympanicum paraganglioma tumors are readily seen on thin-section CT. The lesion appears as a nodule of soft tissue at the medial wall of the middle ear, classically located at the cochlear promontory (Fig. 28–36). Larger tumors fill the middle ear but typically do not cause bone erosion and tend to spare the ossicles. Glomus tumors show intense enhancement on MR imaging because of their vascular nature. MR plays a critical role in defining the extension of glomus tympanicum paraganglioma intracranially and into the skull base, inasmuch as the surgeon can appreciate the tympanic part of the tumor only on otoscopy.

EXTERNAL EAR LESIONS

Lesions of the external ear include congenital anomalies, infectious and inflammatory processes that exhibit unique behavior in the external canal, and benign and malignant neoplasms of the soft tissue and bone of the external canal. Complex middle and external ear dysplasias are discussed in the previous section.

External Auditory Canal Atresia and Hypoplasia

EAC atresia and hypoplasia are part of the spectrum of congenital anomalies that result from abnormal embryogenesis of the first and second branchial arches. Because the middle and external ear develop together, EAC atresia is typically associated with middle ear anomalies, which are discussed in detail in a previous section. Anomaly of the auricle, or microtia, is occasionally isolated but is usually seen in association with EAC stenosis or atresia.

Evaluation of external ear anomalies is done as part of the overall assessment of middle and external ear dysplasia. Axial and coronal CT reveal the degree of canal narrowing and whether the canal is obstructed by bone or soft tissue.[164] Milder anomalies show stenosis or membranous atresia, whereas more severe anomalies show complete atresia with a bony plate and no identifiable canal (see Fig. 28–32).

Malignant Otitis Externa

Malignant otitis externa is an aggressive, potentially life-threatening infection of the external ear. Malignant otitis externa is typically seen in diabetic, elderly, or otherwise immunocompromised patients, whereas simple otitis externa in an immunocompetent patient is usually benign and self-limited. The offending organism in most cases is *Pseudomonas aeruginosa*, which thrives in the setting of hyperglycemia, moisture, and osteochondral infection.[193, 194]

Imaging evaluation of malignant otitis externa includes multiple modalities. CT is most useful in demonstrating destructive bony changes of the EAC and secondary mid-

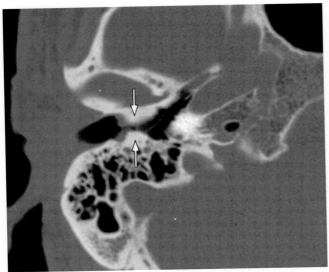

FIGURE 28–37 Surfer's ear. Axial CT scan in a young male competitive swimmer with external canal stenosis. Broad-based bony excrescence is present circumferentially at the medial external canal (*arrows*), resulting in severe stenosis. (Used with permission from Davidson HC. Digital Teaching File. Salt Lake City, Electronic Medical Education Research Group, 1999.)

dle ear and mastoid complications. MR provides excellent evaluation of the extent of soft tissue involvement as well as intracranial complications. Radionuclide studies have been advocated as a means of early diagnosis in symptomatic patients who are at risk.[195, 196]

External Auditory Canal Exostosis and Osteoma

Exostosis is a benign bony mass of the EAC and is the most common solid tumor of this region. Exostoses are found deep in the EAC and usually occur in patients with a history of chronic EAC irritation. "Surfer's ear" refers to exostosis due to prolonged exposure to cold seawater. The condition is bilateral in most cases, although presenting symptoms may be unilateral. Exostoses are best appreciated on CT, where they are seen as broad-based sessile bony masses located medially in the EAC (Fig. 28–37). Stenosis, but not occlusion, of the EAC is typical.[197, 198]

Osteoma is a benign bony mass that is distinct from exostosis. Osteomas are sporadic and typically unilateral and solitary. On CT, osteomas appear pedunculated and are found farther laterally in the EAC compared with exostoses.[197]

External Ear Cutaneous Malignant Neoplasms

Cutaneous malignant neoplasms that may affect the external ear include squamous cell, basal cell, ceruminous gland, and adenoid cystic carcinomas as well as melanoma. These lesions are most often found in elderly patients. Lesions may originate in the EAC or auricle. Basal cell carcinoma and melanoma are typically the re-

sult of solar exposure; they usually originate in the auricle and affect the EAC only secondarily.[199–202]

The purpose of imaging evaluation of these malignant neoplasms is to assess the degree of deep extension and regional spread of disease. Bone abnormalities may be subtle on CT, but any changes are suspicious if a known malignant process exists. MR is useful in determining soft tissue extent and degree of skull base invasion in more advanced lesions. Local spread to the parotid gland and regional lymphatic spread to parotid lymph nodes are also important features of radiologic staging.

References

1. Curtin HD, Som PM, Bergeron RT. Temporal bone embryology and anatomy. In Som PM, Curtin HD (eds). Head and Neck Imaging, Vol. 2, 3rd ed., pp. 1300–1318. St. Louis, Mosby–Year Book, 1996.
2. National Institutes of Health Consensus Development Conference Statement on Acoustic Neuroma, December 11–13, 1991. The Consensus Development Panel. Arch Neurol 1994;51:201–207.
3. Lo WWM, Solti-Bohman LG. Tumors of the temporal bone and the cerebellopontine angle. In Som PM, Curtin HD (eds). Head and Neck Imaging, Vol. 2, 3rd ed., p. 1450. St. Louis, Mosby–Year Book, 1996.
4. Swartz JD, Harnsberger HR. Imaging of the Temporal Bone, p. 420. New York, Thieme Medical, 1998.
5. Kasantikul V, Netsky MG, Glassock ME 3rd, Hayes JW. Acoustic neurilemmoma. Clinicoanatomical study of 103 patients. J Neurosurg 1980;52:28–35.
6. Weissman JL. Hearing loss. Radiology 1996;199:593–611.
7. Lo WWM, Solti-Bohman LG. Tumors of the temporal bone and the cerebellopontine angle. In Som PM, Curtin HD (eds). Head and Neck Imaging, Vol. 2, 3rd ed., p. 1451. St. Louis, Mosby–Year Book, 1996.
8. Gruskin P, Carberry JN. Pathology of acoustic tumors. In House WF, Luetze CM (eds). Acoustic Tumors, Vol. 1, pp. 85–148. Baltimore, University Park Press, 1979.
9. Earls JP, Robles HA, McAdams HP, Rao KC. General case of the day. Malignant melanotic schwannoma of the eighth cranial nerve. Radiographics 1994;14:1425–1427.
10. Latack JT, Gabrielsen TO, Knake JE, et al. Facial nerve neuromas: Radiologic evaluation. Radiology 1983;149:731–739.
11. McMenomey SO, Glassock ME 3rd, Minor LB, et al. Facial nerve neuromas presenting as acoustic tumors. Am J Otol 1994;15:307–312.
12. Curtin HD. CT of acoustic neuroma and other tumors of the ear. Radiol Clin North Am 1984;22:77–105.
13. Tali ET, Yuh WT, Nguyen HD, et al. Cystic acoustic schwannomas: MR characteristics. AJNR 1993;14:1241–1247.
14. Harnsberger HR. The lower cranial nerves. In Handbook of Head and Neck Imaging, 2nd ed., pp. 488–521. Chicago, Mosby–Year Book, 1995.
15. Charabi S, Mantoni M, Tos M, Thomson J. Cystic vestibular schwannomas: Neuroimaging and growth rate. J Laryngol Otol 1994;108:375–379.
16. Curati WL, Graif M, Kingsley DP, et al. Acoustic neuromas: Gd-DTPA enhancement in MR imaging. Radiology 1986;158:447–451.
17. Allen RW, Harnsberger HR, Shelton C, et al. Low-cost high-resolution fast spin-echo MR of acoustic schwannoma: An alternative to enhanced conventional spin-echo MR? [see comments] AJNR 1996;17:1205–1210.
18. Black PM. Meningiomas. Neurosurgery 1993;32:643–657.
19. Hasso AN, Smith DS. The cerebellopontine angle. Semin Ultrasound CT MR 1989;10:280–301.
20. Lo WWM. Cerebellopontine angle tumors. Categorical Course on Neoplasms of the Central Nervous System, American Society of Neuroradiology, 1990.
21. Langman AW, Jackler RK, Althaus SR. Meningioma of the internal auditory canal. Am J Otol 1990;11:201–204.
22. Valavanis A, Schubiger O, Hayek J, Pouliadis G. CT of meningiomas on the posterior surface of the petrous bone. Neuroradiology 1981;22:111–121.
23. Lalwani AK, Jackler RK. Preoperative differentiation between

meningioma of the cerebellopontine angle and acoustic neuroma using MRI. Otolaryngol Head Neck Surg 1993;109:88–95.

24. Mikhael MA, Ciric IS, Wolff AP. Differentiation of cerebellopontine angle neuromas and meningiomas with MR imaging. J Comput Assist Tomogr 1985;9:852–856.

25. Goldsher D, Litt AW, Pinto RS, et al. Dural "tail" associated with meningiomas on Gd-DTPA–enhanced MR images: Characteristics, differential diagnostic value, and possible implications for treatment. Radiology 1990;176:447–450.

26. Zimmerman RA, Bilaniuk LT, Dolinskas C. Cranial computed tomography of epidermoid and congenital fatty tumors of maldevelopmental origin. J Comput Tomogr 1979;3:40–50.

27. Swartz JD, Harnsberger HR. Imaging of the Temporal Bone, p. 411. New York, Thieme Medical, 1998.

28. Osborn AG. Diagnostic Neuroradiology, p. 631. St. Louis, CV Mosby, 1994.

29. Rock JP, Zimmerman R, Bell WO, Fraser RA. Arachnoid cysts of the posterior fossa. Neurosurgery 1986;18:176–179.

30. Smirniotopoulos JG, Yue NC, Rushing EJ. Cerebellopontine angle masses: Radiologic-pathologic correlation. Radiographics 1993;13:1131–1147.

31. Dalley RW, Robertson WD, Lapointe JS, Durity FA. Computed tomography of a cerebellopontine angle lipoma. J Comput Assist Tomogr 1986;10:704–706.

32. Cohen TI, Powers SK, Williams DW 3rd. MR appearance of intracanalicular eighth nerve lipoma. AJNR 1992;13:1188–1190.

33. Russell DS, Rubinstein LJ. Pathology of Tumors of the Nervous System. Baltimore, Williams & Wilkins, 1989.

34. Henson RA, Urich H. Cancer and the Nervous System. The Neurological Manifestations of Systemic Malignant Disease. Oxford, Blackwell Scientific, 1982.

35. Song SK, Schwartz IS, Strauchen JA, et al. Meningeal nodules with features of extranodal sinus histiocytosis with massive lymphadenopathy. Am J Surg Pathol 1989;13:406–412.

36. Ranoux D, Devaux B, Lamy C, et al. Meningeal sarcoidosis, pseudo-meningioma, and pachymeningitis of the convexity. J Neurol Neurosurg Psychiatry 1992;55:300–303.

37. Mayer SA, Yim GK, Onesti ST, et al. Biopsy-proven isolated sarcoid meningitis. Case report. J Neurosurg 1993;78:994–996.

38. Martin N, Masson C, Henin D, et al. Hypertrophic cranial pachymeningitis: Assessment with CT and MR imaging. AJNR 1989;10:477–484.

39. Sze G. Diseases of the intracranial meninges: MR imaging features. AJR 1993;160:727–733.

40. Sze G, Soletsky S, Bronen R, Krol G. MR imaging of the cranial meninges with emphasis on contrast enhancement and meningeal carcinomatosis. AJNR 1989;10:965–975.

41. Tyrrell RL 2nd, Bundschuh CV, Modic MT. Dural carcinomatosis: MR demonstration. J Comput Assist Tomogr 1987;11:329–332.

42. Buff BL Jr, Schick RM, Norregaard T. Meningeal metastasis of leiomyosarcoma mimicking meningioma: CT and MR findings. J Comput Assist Tomogr 1991;15:166–167.

43. Valvassori GE, Clemis JD. The large vestibular aqueduct syndrome. Laryngoscope 1978;88:723–728.

44. Jackler RK, De La Cruz A. The large vestibular aqueduct syndrome. Laryngoscope 1989;99:1238–1242; discussion 1242–1243.

45. Mafee MF, Charletta D, Kumar A, Belmont H. Large vestibular aqueduct and congenital sensorineural hearing loss. AJNR 1992;13:805–819.

46. Jackler RK, Luxford WM, House WF. Congenital malformations of the inner ear: A classification based on embryogenesis. Laryngoscope 1987;97(pt 2, Suppl 40):2–14.

47. Schuknecht HF. Pathology of the Ear, p. 177. Philadelphia, Lea & Febiger, 1993.

48. Schuknecht HF. Pathology of the Ear, pp. 115–189. Philadelphia, Lea & Febiger, 1993.

49. Hasso AN, Casselman JW, Schmalbrock P. Temporal bone congenital anomalies. In Som PM, Curtin HD (eds). Head and Neck Imaging, Vol. 2, 3rd ed., pp. 1361–1367. St. Louis, Mosby–Year Book, 1996.

50. Michel EM. Memoire sur les anomalies congenitales de l'oreille interne, avec la premiere observation authentique d'absence complete d'oreille moyenne chez un sourd et muet de naissance, mort a l'age de onze ans. Gaz Med Strasb 1863;23:55–58.

51. Mondini C. Anatomia surdi nati sectio. De Bononiensi Scientiarum et Artium Instituto atzue Academia Commentarii. Bononiae 1791;7:28–29, 419–431.

52. Lemmerling MM, Mancuso AA, Antonelli PJ, Kubilis PS. Normal modiolus: CT appearance in patients with a large vestibular aqueduct. Radiology 1997;204:213–219.

53. Seltzer S, Mark AS. Contrast enhancement of the labyrinth on MR scans in patients with sudden hearing loss and vertigo: Evidence of labyrinthine disease [see comments]. AJNR 1991;12:13–16.

54. Mark AS, Seltzer S, Nelson-Drake J, et al. Labyrinthine enhancement on gadolinium-enhanced magnetic resonance imaging in sudden deafness and vertigo: Correlation with audiologic and electronystagmographic studies. Ann Otol Rhinol Laryngol 1992;101:459–464.

55. Mark AS. Contrast-enhanced magnetic resonance imaging of the temporal bone. Neuroimaging Clin N Am 1994;4:117–131.

56. Downie AC, Howlett DC, Koefman RJ, et al. Case report: Prolonged contrast enhancement of the inner ear on magnetic resonance imaging in Ramsay Hunt syndrome. Br J Radiol 1994;67:819–821.

57. Swartz JD, Harnsberger HR. Imaging of the Temporal Bone, pp. 272–282. New York, Thieme Medical Publishers, 1998.

58. Suga F, Lindsay JR. Labyrinthitis ossificans. Ann Otol Rhinol Laryngol 1977;86(pt 1):17–29.

59. Weissman JL, Kamerer DB. Labyrinthitis ossificans. Am J Otolaryngol 1993;14:363–365.

60. Paparella MM. Labyrinthitis. In Paparella MM, Shumrick DA (eds). Otolaryngology: The Ear, Vol. 2, pp. 1735–1756. Philadelphia, WB Saunders, 1980.

61. Swartz JD, Mandell DW, Wolfson RJ, et al. Fenestral and cochlear otosclerosis: Computed tomographic evaluation. Am J Otol 1985;6:476–481.

62. Casselman JW, Kuhweide R, Ampe W, et al. Pathology of the membranous labyrinth: Comparison of T1- and T2-weighted and gadolinium-enhanced spin-echo and 3DFT-CISS imaging. AJNR 1993;14:59–69.

63. Brogan M, Chakeres DW. Gd-DTPA–enhanced MR imaging of cochlear schwannoma. AJNR 1990;11:407–408.

64. Saeed SR, Birzgalis AR, Ramsden RT. Intralabyrinthine schwannoma shown by magnetic resonance imaging. Neuroradiology 1994;36:63–64.

65. Davidson HC, Krejei CS, Harnsberger HR. MR evaluation of labyrinthine schwannomas. Scientific paper presentation, American Society of Neuroradiology Annual Meeting, Philadelphia, April 1998.

66. Forton GE, Somers T, Hermans R, et al. Preoperatively diagnosed utricular neuroma treated by selective partial labyrinthectomy. Ann Otol Rhinol Laryngol 1994;103:885–888.

67. Swartz JD. Temporal bone inflammatory disease. In Som PM, Curtin HD (eds). Head and Neck Imaging, Vol. 2, 3rd ed., pp. 1415–1418. New York, Mosby–Year Book, 1996.

68. Hassard AD, Boudreau SF, Cron CC. Adenoma of the endolymphatic sac. J Otolaryngol 1984;13:213–216.

69. Batsakis JG, el-Naggar AK. Papillary neoplasms (Heffner's tumors) of the endolymphatic sac [see comments]. Ann Otol Rhinol Laryngol 1993;102(pt 1):648–651.

70. Heffner DK. Low-grade adenocarcinoma of probable endolymphatic sac origin: A clinicopathologic study of 20 cases. Cancer 1989;64:2292–2302.

71. MacDougall AD, Sangalang VE. A previously unrecognized papillary endolymphatic sac tumor presenting as a cerebellopontine angle lesion. Can J Neurol Sci 1985;189:203–204.

72. Palmer JM, Coker NJ, Harper RL. Papillary adenoma of the temporal bone in von Hippel–Lindau disease. Otolaryngol Head Neck Surg 1989;100:64–68.

73. Valvassori GE. Otodystrophies. In Berrett A, Brunner S, Valvassori GE (eds). Modern Thin Section Tomography, pp. 109–117. Springfield, IL, Charles C Thomas, 1973.

74. Valvassori GE. Otosclerosis. Otolaryngol Clin North Am 1973;6:379–389.

75. Goodhill V. Ear: Diseases, Deafness and Dizziness, pp. 388–457. New York, Harper & Row, 1979.

76. Swartz JD, Faerber EN, Wolfson RJ, Marlowe FI. Fenestral otosclerosis: Significance of preoperative CT evaluation. Radiology 1984;151:703–707.

77. Swartz JD, Mandell DW, Berman SE, et al. Cochlear otosclerosis (otospongiosis): CT analysis with audiometric correlation. Radiology 1985;155:147–150.

78. Carhart R. Labyrinthine otosclerosis. Arch Otolaryngol 1963;78:477–508.

79. Lindsay JR. Otosclerosis. In Paparella MM, Shumrick DA (eds). Otolaryngology: The Ear, Vol. 2, pp. 1617–1644. Philadelphia, WB Saunders, 1980.

80. Ruedi L. Pathogenesis of otosclerosis. Arch Otolaryngol 1963;78:469–477.

81. Baringer JR. Herpes simplex virus and Bell palsy. [Editorial; comment] Ann Intern Med 1996;124(pt 1):63–65.

82. Murakami S, Mizobuchi M, Nakashiro Y, et al. Bell palsy and herpes simplex virus: Identification of viral DNA in endoneurial fluid and muscle [see comments]. Ann Intern Med 1996;124(pt 1):27–30.

83. Osumi A, Tien RD. MR findings in a patient with Ramsay-Hunt syndrome. J Comput Assist Tomogr 1990;14:991–993.

84. Daniels DL, Czervionke LF, Millen SJ, et al. MR imaging of facial nerve enhancement in Bell palsy or after temporal bone surgery. Radiology 1989;171:807–809.

85. Tien R, Dillon WP, Jackler RK. Contrast-enhanced MR imaging of the facial nerve in 11 patients with Bell's palsy. AJNR 1990;11:735–741.

86. Engstrom M, Thuomas KA, Naeser P, et al. Facial nerve enhancement in Bell's palsy demonstrated by different gadolinium-enhanced magnetic resonance imaging techniques. Arch Otolaryngol Head Neck Surg 1993;119:221–225.

87. Murphy TP, Teller DC. Magnetic resonance imaging of the facial nerve during Bell's palsy. Otolaryngol Head Neck Surg 1991;105:667–674.

88. Schwaber MK, Larson TC 3rd, Zealear DL, Creasy J. Gadolinium-enhanced magnetic resonance imaging in Bell's palsy. Laryngoscope 1990;100:1264–1269.

89. Murphy TP. MRI of the facial nerve during paralysis. Otolaryngol Head Neck Surg 1991;104:47–51.

90. Anderson RE, Laskoff JM. Ramsay Hunt syndrome mimicking intracanalicular acoustic neuroma on contrast-enhanced MR. AJNR 1990;11:409.

91. Korzec K, Sobol SM, Kubal W, et al. Gadolinium-enhanced magnetic resonance imaging of the facial nerve in herpes zoster oticus and Bell's palsy: Clinical implications. Am J Otol 1991;12:163–168.

92. O'Donoghue GM, Brackmann DE, House JW, Jackler RK. Neuromas of the facial nerve. Am J Otol 1989;10:49–54.

93. Conley J, Janecka I. Schwann cell tumors of the facial nerve. Laryngoscope 1974;84:958–962.

94. Jackson CG, Glasscock ME 3rd, Sismanis A. Facial paralysis of neoplastic origin: Diagnosis and management. Laryngoscope 1980;90(pt 1):1581–1595.

95. Latack JT, Gabrielsen TO, Knake JE, et al. Facial nerve neuromas: Radiologic evaluation. Radiology 1983;149:731–739.

96. Lin SR, Go EB. Neurilemmoma of the facial nerve. Neuroradiology 1973;6:185–187.

97. Pulec JL. Facial nerve neuroma. Laryngoscope 1972;82:1160–1176.

98. Dort JC, Fisch U. Facial nerve schwannomas. Skull Base Surg 1991;1:51–57.

99. Pillsbury HC, Price HC, Gardiner LJ. Primary tumors of the facial nerve: Diagnosis and management. Laryngoscope 1983;93:1045–1048.

100. Nelson RA, House WF. Facial nerve neuroma in the posterior fossa: Surgical considerations. In Graham MD, House WF (eds). Proceedings of the Fourth International Symposium on Facial Nerve Surgery, pp. 403–406. New York, Raven, 1982.

101. Lidov M, Som PM, Stacy C, Catalano P. Eccentric cystic facial schwannoma: CT and MR features. J Comput Assist Tomogr 1991;15:1065–1067.

102. Glasscock ME 3rd, Smith PG, Schwaber MK, Nissen AJ. Clinical aspects of osseous hemangiomas of the skull base. Laryngoscope 1984;94:869–873.

103. Curtin HD, Jensen JE, Barnes L Jr, May M. "Ossifying" hemangiomas of the temporal bone: Evaluation with CT. Radiology 1987;164:831–835.

104. Fisch U, Ruttner J. Pathology of intratemporal tumors involving the facial nerve. In Fisch U (ed). Facial Nerve Surgery, pp. 448–456. Birmingham, Aesculapius, 1977.

105. Lo WW, Shelton C, Waluch V, et al. Intratemporal vascular tumors: Detection with CT and MR imaging. Radiology 1989;171:445–448.

106. Glasscock ME 3rd, Smith PG, Schwaber MK, Nissen AJ. Clinical aspects of osseous hemangiomas of the skull base. Laryngoscope 1984;94:869–873.

107. Lo WW, Horn KL, Carberry JN, et al. Intratemporal vascular tumors: Evaluation with CT. Radiology 1986;159:181–185.

108. Martin N, Sterkers O, Nahum H. Haemangioma of the petrous bone: MRI. Neuroradiology 1992;34:420–422.

109. Lo WW, Brackmann DE, Shelton C. Facial nerve hemangioma. Ann Otol Rhinol Laryngol 1989;98:160–161.

110. Hasso AN, Opp RL. Paget's diseases and other rare otodystrophies. Riv Neuroradiol 1995;8:889–898.

111. Hasso AN, Opp RL, Swartz JD. Otosclerosis and dysplasias of the temporal bone. In Som PM, Curtin HD (eds). Head and Neck Imaging, Vol. 2, 3rd ed., pp. 1432–1448. Chicago, Mosby–Year Book, 1996.

112. Ginsberg LE, Elster AD, Moody DM. MRI of Paget disease with temporal bone involvement presenting with sensorineural hearing loss. J Comput Assist Tomogr 1992;16:314–316.

113. Megerian CA, Sofferman RA, McKenna MJ, et al. Fibrous dysplasia of the temporal bone: Ten new cases demonstrating the spectrum of otologic sequelae. Am J Otol 1995;16:408–419.

114. Pouwels AB, Cremers CW. Fibrous dysplasia of the temporal bone. J Laryngol Otol 1988;102:171–172.

115. Younus M, Haleem A. Monostotic fibrous dysplasia of the temporal bone. J Laryngol Otol 1987;101:1070–1074.

116. Herman TE, McAlister WH. Inherited diseases of bone density in children. Radiol Clin North Am 1991;29:149–164.

117. Felix R, Hofstetter W, Cecchini MG. Recent developments in the understanding of the pathophysiology of osteopetrosis. Eur J Endocrinol 1996;134:143–156.

118. Milroy CM, Michaels L. Temporal bone pathology of adult-type osteopetrosis. Arch Otolaryngol Head Neck Surg 1990;116:79–84.

119. Bartynski WS, Barnes PD, Wallman JK. Cranial CT of autosomal recessive osteopetrosis. AJNR 1989;10:543–550.

120. Bollerslev J, Grontved A, Andersen PE Jr. Autosomal dominant osteopetrosis: An otoneurological investigation of the two radiological types. Laryngoscope 1988;98:411–413.

121. Demirci A, Sze G. Cranial osteopetrosis: MR findings. AJNR 1991;12:781–782.

122. Swartz JD, Harnsberger HR. Imaging of the Temporal Bone, pp. 149–152. New York, Thieme Medical, 1998.

123. Livingston PA. Differential diagnosis of radiolucent lesions of the temporal bone. Radiol Clin North Am 1974;12:571–583.

124. McCluggage WG, McBride GB, Primrose WJ, et al. Giant cell tumour of the temporal bone presenting as vertigo. J Laryngol Otol 1995;109:538–541.

125. Shah GV, Doctor MR, Shah PS. Aneurysmal bone cyst of the temporal bone: MR findings. AJNR 1995;16:763–766.

126. Meyers SP, Hirsch WL Jr, Curtin HD, et al. Chondrosarcomas of the skull base: MR imaging features. Radiology 1992;184:103–108.

127. Zimmerman RA, Bilaniuk LT, Hackney DB, et al. Magnetic resonance imaging in temporal bone fracture. Neuroradiology 1987;29:246–251.

128. Holland BA, Brant-Zawadski M. High resolution CT of temporal bone trauma. AJNR 1984;5:391–395.

129. Schubiger O, Valavanis A, Stuckmann G, Antonucci F. Temporal bone fractures and their complications. Examination with high resolution CT. Neuroradiology 1986;28:93–99.

130. Wright JW Jr. Trauma of the ear. Radiol Clin North Am 1974;12:527–532.

131. Goodwin WJ Jr. Temporal bone fractures. Otolaryngol Clin North Am 1983;16:651–659.

132. Bellucci RJ. Traumatic injuries of the middle ear. Otolaryngol Clin North Am 1983;16:633–650.

133. Swartz JD, Harnsberger HR. Imaging of the Temporal Bone, p. 318. New York, Thieme Medical, 1998.

134. Lindeman RC. Temporal bone trauma and facial paralysis. Otolaryngol Clin North Am 1979;12:403–413.

135. Hough JVD. Otologic trauma. In Paparella MM, Shumrick DA (eds). Otolaryngology: The Ear, Vol. 2, pp. 1656–1679. Philadelphia, WB Saunders, 1980.

136. McCabe BF. Injuries to the facial nerve. Laryngoscope 1972;82:1891–1896.

137. Ghorayeb BY, Yeakley JW, Hall JW 3rd, Jones BE. Unusual complications of temporal bone fractures. Arch Otolaryngol Head Neck Surg 1987;113:749–753.

138. Gentry LR. Temporal bone trauma: Current perspective for diagnostic evaluation. Neuroimaging Clin N Am 1991;1:319–340.
139. Ghorayeb BY, Yeakley JW. Temporal bone fractures: Longitudinal or oblique? The case for oblique temporal bone fractures. Laryngoscope 1992;102:129–134.
140. Berenstein A, Lasjuanias P. Surgical Neuroangiography, Vol. 1, pp. 1–11. New York, Springer-Verlag, 1987.
141. Lo WW, Solti-Bohman LG, McElveen JT Jr. Aberrant carotid artery: Radiologic diagnosis with emphasis on high-resolution computed tomography. Radiographics 1985;5:985–993.
142. Lo WWM, Solti-Bohman LG. Vascular tinnitus. In Som PM, Curtin H (eds). Head and Neck Imaging, Vol. 2, 3rd ed., pp. 1535–1548. St. Louis, CV Mosby, 1996.
143. Lapayowker MS, Liebman EP, Ronis ML, Safer JN. Presentation of the internal carotid artery as a tumor of the middle ear. Radiology 1971;98:293–297.
144. Reilly JJ Jr, Caparosa RJ, Latchaw RE, Sheptak PE. Aberrant carotid artery injured at myringotomy. Control of hemorrhage by a balloon catheter. JAMA 1983;249:1473–1475.
145. Remley KB, Coit WE, Harnsberger HR, et al. Pulsatile tinnitus and the vascular tympanic membrane: CT, MR, and angiographic findings. Radiology 1990;174:383–389.
146. Swartz JD, Bazarnic ML, Naidich TP, et al. Aberrant internal carotid artery lying within the middle ear. High resolution CT diagnosis and differential diagnosis. Neuroradiology 1985;27:322–326.
147. Swartz JD, Harnsberger HR. Imaging of the Temporal Bone, p. 196. New York, Thieme Medical, 1998.
148. Swartz JD, Harnsberger HR. Imaging of the Temporal Bone, p. 450. New York, Thieme Medical, 1998.
149. Moore KR, Harnsberger HR, Shelton C, Davidson HC. 'Leave me alone' lesions of the petrous apex. AJNR 1998;19:733–738.
150. Plester D, Steinbach E. Cholesterol granuloma. Otolaryngol Clin North Am 1982;15:655–672.
151. Greenberg JJ, Oot RF, Wismer GL, et al. Cholesterol granuloma of the petrous apex: MR and CT evaluation. AJNR 1988;9:1205–1214.
152. Griffin C, DeLaPaz R, Enzmann D. MR and CT correlation of cholesterol cysts of the petrous bone. AJNR 1987;8:825–829.
153. Latack JT, Graham MD, Kemink JL, Knake JE. Giant cholesterol cysts of the petrous apex: Radiologic features. AJNR 1985;6:409–413.
154. Atlas MD, Moffat DA, Hardy DG. Petrous apex cholesteatoma: Diagnostic and treatment dilemmas. Laryngoscope 1992;102(pt 1):1363–1368.
155. Swartz JD. Temporal bone inflammatory disease. In Swartz JD, Harnsberger HR (eds). Imaging of the Temporal Bone, p. 1393. New York, Thieme Medical, 1998.
156. Mafee MF, Aimi K, Kahen HL, et al. Chronic otomastoiditis: A conceptual understanding of CT findings. Radiology 1986;160:193–200.
157. Anson BJ, David J. Developmental anatomy of the ear. In Paparella MM, Shumrick DA (eds). Otolaryngology: Basic Sciences and Related Disciplines, Vol. 1, pp. 3–25. Philadelphia, WB Saunders, 1980.
158. Pearson AA. Developmental anatomy of the ear. In English GM (ed). Otolaryngology, Vol. 1. Hagerstown, MD, Harper & Row, 1983.
159. Hasso AN, Casselman JW, Schmalbrock P. Temporal bone congenital anomalies. In Swartz JD, Harnsberger HR (eds). Imaging of the Temporal Bone, pp. 1355–1361. New York, Thieme Medical, 1998.
160. Swartz JD, Faerber EN. Congenital malformations of the external and middle ear: High-resolution CT findings of surgical import. AJR 1985;144:501–506.
161. Swartz JD, Wolfson RJ, Marlowe FI, et al. External auditory canal dysplasia: CT evaluation. Laryngoscope 1985;95(pt 1):841–845.
162. Swartz JD, Harnsberger HR. Imaging of the Temporal Bone. p. 21. New York, Thieme Medical, 1998.
163. Yeakley JW, Jahrsdoerfer RA. CT evaluation of congenital aural atresia: What the radiologist and surgeon need to know. J Comput Assist Tomogr 1996;20:724–731.
164. Jahrsdoerfer RA, Yeakley JW, Aguilar EA, et al. Grading system for the selection of patients with congenital aural atresia. Am J Otol 1992;13:6–12.
165. Michaels L. Origin of congenital cholesteatoma from a normally occurring epidermoid rest in the developing middle ear. Int J Pediatr Otorhinolaryngol 1988;15:51–65.
166. Moran WBJ. Cholesteatoma. New York, Harper & Row, 1980.
167. Cody DTR. The definition of cholesteatoma. In McCabe BF, Sade J, Abramson M (eds). Cholesteatoma. First International Conference, pp. 6–9. Birmingham, AL, Aesculapius, 1977.
168. Nager GT. Cholesteatoma of the middle ear: Pathogenesis and surgical indication. In McCabe BF, Sade J, Abramson M (eds). Cholesteatoma. First international conference, pp. 191–203. Birmingham, AL, Aesculapius, 1977.
169. Ruedi L. Acquired cholesteatoma. Arch Otolaryngol 1983;78:252.
170. Nager GT. Theories on the origin of attic retraction cholesteatoma. In Proceedings of the Shambaugh Fifth International Workshop on Middle Ear Microsurgery and Fluctuant Hearing Loss. Huntsville, AL, Strode, 1977.
171. Sade J. Pathogenesis of attic cholesteatoma: The metaplasia theory. In McCabe BF, Sade J, Abramson M (eds). Cholesteatoma. First International Conference, pp. 212–232. Birmingham, AL, Aesculapius, 1977.
172. Swartz JD. Cholesteatomas of the middle ear. Diagnosis, etiology, and complications. Radiol Clin North Am 1984;22:15–35.
173. Swartz JD, Varghese S. Pars flaccida cholesteatoma as demonstrated by computed tomography. Arch Otolaryngol 1984;110:515–517.
174. Phelps PD, Lloyd GA. The radiology of cholesteatoma. Clin Radiol 1980;31:501–512.
175. Tos M. Can cholesteatoma be prevented? In Sade J (ed). Cholesteatoma and Mastoid Surgery, pp. 591–598. Amsterdam, Kugler, 1982.
176. Sade J, Berco E, Buyanover D. Ossicular damage in chronic middle ear inflammation. In Sade J (ed). Cholesteatoma and Mastoid Surgery, pp. 347–358. Amsterdam, Kugler, 1982.
177. Johnson DW, Hinshaw DB Jr, Hasso AN, et al. Computed tomography of local complications of temporal bone cholesteatomas. J Comput Assist Tomogr 1985;9:519–523.
178. Silver AJ, Janecka I, Wazen J, et al. Complicated cholesteatomas: CT findings in inner ear complications of middle ear cholesteatomas. Radiology 1987;164:47–51.
179. Swartz JD, Harnsberger HR. Imaging of the Temporal Bone, p. 108. New York, Thieme Medical, 1998.
180. Martin N, Sterkers O, Nahum H. Chronic inflammatory disease of the middle ear cavities: Gd-DTPA–enhanced MR imaging. Radiology 1990;176:399–405.
181. Swartz JD, Wolfson RJ, Marlowe FI, Popky GL. Postinflammatory ossicular fixation: CT analysis with surgical correlation. Radiology 1985;154:697–700.
182. Plester D, Steinbach E. Cholesterol granuloma. Otolaryngol Clin North Am 1982;15:655–672.
183. Greenberg JJ, Oot RF, Wismer GL, et al. Cholesterol granuloma of the petrous apex: MR and CT evaluation. AJNR 1988;9:1205–1214.
184. Lo WW, Solti-Bohman LG, Brackman DE. Cholesterol granuloma of the petrous apex: CT diagnosis. Radiology 1984;153:705–711.
185. Swartz JD, Harnsberger HR. Imaging of the Temporal Bone, p. 80. New York, Thieme Medical, 1998.
186. Paparella MM, Meyerhoff WC. Clinical significance of granulation tissue of chronic otitis media. In Sade J (ed). Cholesteatoma and Mastoid Surgery, pp. 387–395. Amsterdam, Kugler, 1982.
187. Martin N, Sterkers O, Mompoint D, et al. Cholesterol granulomas of the middle ear cavities: MR imaging. Radiology 1989;172:521–525.
188. Greenfield BJ, Selesnick SH, Fisher L, et al. Aural tuberculosis. Am J Otol 1995;16:175–182.
189. Van Cauwenberge P. Definition and character of acute and secretory otitis media. Adv Otorhinolaryngol 1988;40:38–46.
190. Shanley DJ, Murphy TF. Intracranial and extracranial complications of acute mastoiditis: Evaluation with computed tomography. J Am Osteopath Assoc 1992;92:131–134.
191. Larson TC, Reese DF, Baker HL, McDonald TJ. Glomus tympanicum chemodectomas: Radiographic and clinical characteristics. Radiology 1987;163:801–806.
192. Lo WWM, Solti-Bohman LG. Tumors of the temporal bone and the cerebellopontine angle. In Som PM, Curtin H (eds). Head and Neck Imaging, Vol. 2, 3rd ed., pp. 1484–1499. St. Louis, CV Mosby, 1996.
193. Mendelson DS, Som PM, Mendelson MH, Parisier SC. Malignant external otitis: The role of computed tomography and radionuclides in evaluation. Radiology 1983;149:745–749.

194. Meyerhoff WL, Gates GA, Montalbo PJ. Pseudomonas mastoiditis. Laryngoscope 1977;87(pt 1):483–492.

195. Stokkel MP, Boot CN, van Eck–Smit BL. SPECT gallium scintigraphy in malignant external otitis: Initial staging and follow-up. Case reports. Laryngoscope 1996;106(pt 1):338–340.

196. Weber PC, Seabold JE, Graham SM, et al. Evaluation of temporal and facial osteomyelitis by simultaneous In-WBC/Tc-99m-MDP bone SPECT scintigraphy and computed tomography scan. Otolaryngol Head Neck Surg 1995;113:36–41.

197. Di Bartolomeo JR. Exostoses of the external auditory canal. Ann Otol 1979;88(Suppl 61):1–20.

198. Sheehy JL. Diffuse exostoses and osteomata of the external auditory canal: A report of 100 operations. Otolaryngol Head Neck Surg 1982;90(pt 1):337–342.

199. Crabtree JA, Britton BH, Pierce MK. Carcinoma of the external auditory canal. Laryngoscope 1976;86:405–415.

200. Goodwin WJ, Jesse RH. Malignant neoplasms of the external auditory canal and temporal bone. Arch Otolaryngol 1980;106:675–679.

201. Hicks GW. Tumors arising from the glandular structures of the external auditory canal. Laryngoscope 1983;93:326–340.

202. Langman A, Yarington T, Patterson SD. Malignant melanoma of the external auditory canal. Otolaryngol Head Neck Surg 1996;114:645–648.

203. Davidson HC. The Temporal Bone. Salt Lake City, Electronic Medical Education Resource Group, 1999.

204. Davidson HC. Digital Teaching File. Salt Lake City, Electronic Medical Education Resource Group, 1999.

205. Davidson HC. MR Protocol Advisor. Salt Lake City, Electronic Medical Education Resource Group, 1999.

29

The Skull Base

H. CHRISTIAN DAVIDSON, M.D.

WILLIAM W. ORRISON, Jr., M.D.

CHRISTINE M. GLASTONBURY, M.B.B.S.

KEVIN R. MOORE, M.D.

The availability of computed tomography (CT) and magnetic resonance (MR) imaging has permitted dramatic advances in the diagnosis and treatment of skull base abnormalities. Whereas MR has replaced CT for the primary evaluation of many head, neck, and spine disorders, CT remains of utmost importance in the evaluation of skull base abnormalities. The complex nature of the osseous skull base anatomy is exquisitely evaluated by CT, and CT and MR in combination provide more information than has previously been imaginable in the evaluation of this region. Such a remarkable definition of skull base disease has facilitated equally dramatic advances in skull base surgery. Although many neoplasms and other skull base disorders have traditionally been regarded as inoperable, the combination of these advanced imaging methods with the development of new microsurgical techniques has enabled growth of the field of skull base surgery. This field requires an interdisciplinary approach by physicians from multiple subspecialties including neuroradiology, otolaryngology, neurosurgery, ophthalmology, plastic surgery, and interventional neuroradiology to diagnose and treat skull base disease effectively. The accurate and complete diagnosis of skull base disorders is central to the effectiveness of the treatment of these conditions.[1]

NORMAL SKULL BASE ANATOMY

The skull base is composed of five distinct bones: (1) sphenoid bone, (2) ethmoid bone, (3) occipital bone, (4) paired frontal bones, and (5) paired temporal bones (Fig. 29–1). An extensive review of the normal and abnormal temporal bone is included in Chapter 28.

The *sphenoid bone* is made up of a body (basisphenoid), the greater and lesser wings, and the pterygoid processes. The body of the sphenoid consists of the dorsum sella, posterior clinoid processes, sella turcica, tuberculum sella, and sphenoid sinus. The greater wing of the sphenoid bone makes up part of the floor of the middle cranial fossa as does the lesser wing, which also includes the anterior clinoid processes. The *ethmoid bone* consists of the crista galli and the cribriform plate and forms part of the floor of the anterior cranial fossa. The *occipital bone* is made up of three parts: (1) the basiocciput composed of the clivus and the jugular tubercles, (2) the condylar part, and (3) the squamous part. The *frontal bone* forms a major portion of the anterior cranial fossa (see Fig. 29–1). The normal skull base contains multiple foramina and apertures through which various nerves, arteries, and veins pass. These can be appreciated on the normal CT images presented in Figure 29–2.

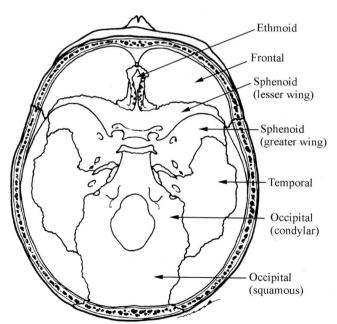

FIGURE 29–1 The normal skull base is composed of five bones: an unpaired ethmoid bone, paired frontal bones, the unpaired sphenoid bone (with paired lesser and greater wings), the paired temporal bones, and the unpaired occipital bone (squamous and condylar portions). (With permission from Davidson HC. Head and Neck Digital Teaching File. Salt Lake City, Electronic Medical Education Resource Group, 1999.)

Labels in figure: Ethmoid; Frontal; Sphenoid (lesser wing); Sphenoid (greater wing); Temporal; Occipital (condylar); Occipital (squamous)

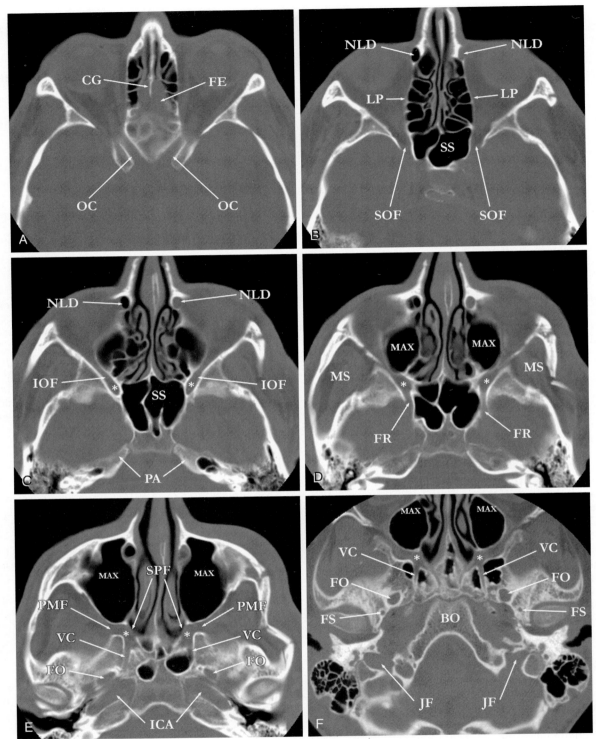

FIGURE 29–2 Normal skull base anatomy. Axial (*A–F*) and coronal (*G–L*) CT images through the skull base. AC, anterior clinoid; BO, basiocciput; C, cochlea; C1, C1 vertebral body; CG, crista galli; DPC, descending palatine canal; FE, fovea ethmoidalis; FL, foramen lacerum; FO, foramen ovale; FR, foramen rotundum; FS, foramen spinosum; HC, hypoglossal canal; IAC, internal auditory canal; ICA, internal carotid artery canal; IOF, inferior orbital fossa; JB, jugular bulb; JF, jugular foramen; M, mastoid bone; MAX, maxillary sinus; MS, masticator space; LP, lamina papyracea; LSCC, lateral semicircular canal; NLD, nasolacrimal duct; OC, optic canal; OCC, occipital condyle; OP, orbital process of frontal bone, OSS, ossicles; P, pterygoid fossa (bounded by pterygoid plates); PA, petrous apex; PC, posterior clinoid; PMF, pterygomaxillary fissure; SOF, superior orbital fissure; SPF, sphenopalatine foramen; SS, sphenoid sinus; SSCC, superior semicircular canal; Tymp, tympanic portion of temporal bone; V, vestibule, VC, vidian canal; *asterisk*, pterygopalatine fossa. (*A–L*, With permission from Davidson HC. Head and Neck Digital Teaching File. Salt Lake City, Electronic Medical Education Resource Group, 1999.)

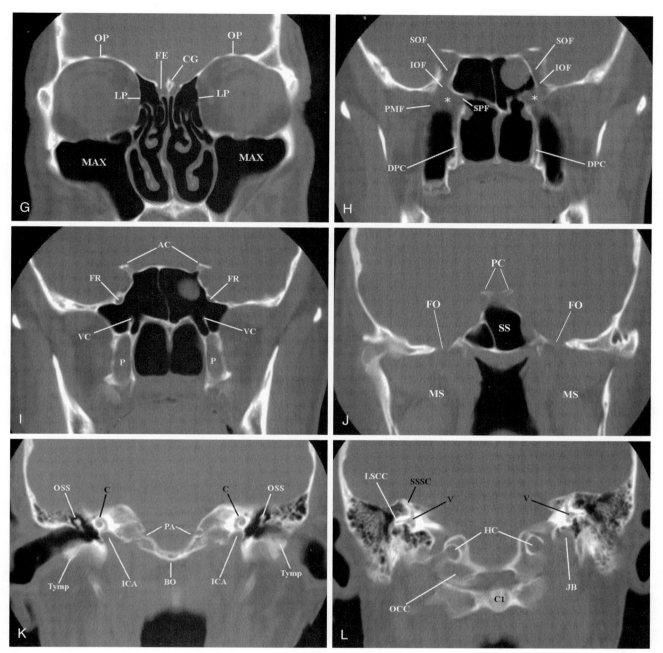

FIGURE 29–2 *Continued*

IMAGING THE SKULL BASE

In general, it is necessary to perform both skull base CT and MR for the complete neuroimaging evaluation of skull base lesions. On MR, it is important to perform T1, T2, and fat-suppressed contrast-enhanced imaging. Table 29–1 lists examples of CT and MR examinations that provide a good basis for the evaluation of skull base lesions.

SKULL BASE REGIONS

It is convenient to divide the skull base into regions in discussing the differential diagnosis of pathologic entities and the avenues of disease spread. The four major regions of the skull base are the anterior skull base, the central skull base, the posterior skull base, and the temporal bone (Fig. 29–3). Although it is technically part of the skull base, the temporal bone is traditionally discussed separately (see Chapter 28).

The anterior skull base consists of the frontal bones, the ethmoid bones, and the lesser wings of the sphenoid bones. Important anatomic contents include cranial nerve I (olfactory nerve) and the ethmoidal arteries. The major routes of contiguous spread of disease from the anterior skull base include the sinonasal passages, the orbits, the olfactory nerves, the meninges, and the inferior frontal lobes of the brain.

TABLE 29–1 Technique for Skull Base Imaging

	Axial	Coronal
Setup		
Localization		
Anterior	Orbital roof to hard palate	Frontal sinus to sella
Central	Orbit to hyoid	Orbit to basiocciput
Posterior	Sella to hyoid	Sella through foramen magnum
CT position	Supine	Prone or "hanging head"
MR coil	Head coil	Head coil

	Sequential	Spiral
CT Acquisition		
Collimation	3 mm	3 mm
Spacing	3 mm (contiguous)	3 mm, pitch 1:1
Technique	240–320 mAs; 120 kVp	240–320 mAs; 120 kVp
Contrast	No	No
Post processing	Bone reconstruction algorithm, 16 cm FOV Window/level = 2000–4000/150–400	

	AX T2 FSE	AX T1	COR T1	AX T1+	COR T1 +	SAG T1+
MR Acquisition						
Plane	Axial	Axial	Coronal	Axial	Coronal	Sagittal
Fat suppression	✓			✓	✓	✓
Contrast				✓	✓	✓
Parameters	FSE	SE	SE	SE	SE	SE
TR/TE	4000/100	500/min–full	500/min–full	667/min–full	667/min–full	667/min–full
Acquisition	FOV 16–18 cm	FOV 16–18 cm	FOV 16–18 cm	FOV 16–18 cm	FOV 16–18 cm	FOV 16–18 cm
Slice/skip	4/0 mm	3–4/0 mm	3–4/0 mm	3–4/0 mm	3–4/0 mm	3–4/0 mm
Matrix	256 × 256	256 × 192	256 × 192	256 × 192	256 × 192	256 × 192
Frequency	A-P	A-P	S-I	A-P	S-I	S-I
Number of excitations	2–3	2	2	2	2	2

From Electronic Medical Education Research Group, The University of Utah Department of Radiology, Salt Lake City, 1999.
Abbreviations: FOV, field of view; Ax, axial; Cor, coronal; FSE, fast spin echo; SE, spin echo; A-P, anterior to posterior; S-I, superior to inferior.
°Optional sequence.

The region of the central skull base consists of the greater wings of the sphenoid bones, the sella turcica, and the basisphenoid. This region contains cranial nerves II (optic nerve), III (oculomotor nerve), IV (trochlear nerve), V (trigeminal nerve), and VI (abducens nerve). Important foramina in the central skull base include the inferior and superior orbital fissures, the foramen rotundum, the vidian canal, the sphenopalatine foramen, the pterygomaxillary fissure, the palatine foramen, the foramen ovale, and the foramen spinosum. Disease spread within the central skull base is through the pterygopalatine fossa, the deep face perineural pathways, the pharyngeal mucosal space, the masticator space, the parapharyngeal space, the orbital apex, and the cavernous sinuses.

The posterior skull base consists of the foramen magnum, the jugular foramen, the hypoglossal canal, the occipital bone, the occipital synchondroses, and the jugular foramen. This region contains cranial nerves IX (glossopharyngeal), X (vagus), XI (spinal accessory), and XII (hypoglossal). Disease spread within the posterior skull base is through the jugular foramen; the temporal bone; the posterior fossa; and the posterior deep fascial spaces, namely, the retropharyngeal space, the perivertebral space, and the carotid space.

DISORDERS OF THE SKULL BASE

For purposes of this discussion, disorders of the skull base are divided into four categories (Table 29–2): (1) general disease of the skull base, (2) disorders of the anterior skull base, (3) disorders of the central skull base, and (4) disorders of the posterior skull base. The diseases of the temporal bone are discussed separately in Chapter 28.

GENERALIZED SKULL BASE LESIONS

Osteodystrophies

The skull base develops through endochondral bone formation and therefore is subject to any generalized disease process that affects cartilaginous bone. The basicranium can also be affected by any metabolic or hematologic disease that involves the entire bony skeleton. The features of bone softening and bone enlargement that may accompany bony disorders of the skull base can lead to compression of the brain stem, the spinal cord, or the cranial nerves. When generalized softening of the skull base occurs, either basilar invagination or platybasia may be seen. Platybasia represents a flattening of the skull

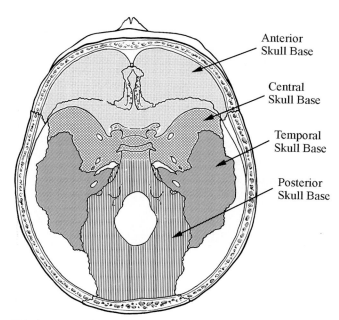

FIGURE 29–3 Skull base regions. For the purposes of this discussion, the skull base is divided into four regions: the anterior skull base, the central skull base, the temporal bone, and the posterior skull base. Although physically part of the skull base, the temporal bone is traditionally addressed separately from the remainder of the skull base. (With permission from Davidson HC. Head and Neck Digital Teaching File. Salt Lake City, Electronic Medical Education Resource Group, 1999.)

TABLE 29–2 Disorders of the Skull Base

Generalized Skull Base Lesions

Osteodystrophies
Trauma
Primary benign neoplasms
Primary malignant neoplasms
Diffuse hematopoietic osseous malignant neoplasms
Metastatic malignant disease

Anterior Skull Base Lesions

Congenital anomalies
Sinonasal inflammatory disease
Sinonasal neoplasms
Intracranial neoplasms

Central Skull Base Lesions

Congenital and genetic diseases
Inflammatory and infectious disease
Head and neck cancer
Sellar region neoplasm
Midbrain and cranial nerves

Posterior Skull Base Lesions

Vascular lesions
Jugular foramen region neoplasms
Osteocartilaginous neoplasms

From Electronic Medical Education Research Group, The University of Utah Department of Radiology, Salt Lake City, 1999.

base with an increase in the basal angle (Fig. 29–4). The *basal angle of Weneke* is formed between a line drawn from the nasion to the center of the sella turcica and from this point along the posterior margin of the clivus. This is normally noted to be approximately 140 degrees. This flattening of the skull base should not be confused with basilar invagination, which occurs when the softening of the skull base results in encroachment of the upper cervical spine into the base of the skull. *Chamberlain's line* is a line extending from the posterior margin of the hard palate to the posterior margin of the foramen magnum. Basilar invagination is present when the tip of the odontoid process projects 5 mm or more above Chamberlain's line. *McGregor's line* extends from the posterior margin of the hard palate to the most inferior aspect of the occipital bone posterior to the foramen magnum. If the tip of the ondontoid process is 7 mm above this line or if more than one-third of the odontoid process is above McGregor's line, basilar invagination is present (Fig. 29–5).[2]

General features of the osteodystrophies include dystrophic and fibrous changes, abnormal bone matrix, variable sclerotic bony changes, lytic regions, and often expansile or deformed areas of bone. Examples of the osteodystrophies include Paget's disease, fibrous dysplasia, metabolic osteodystrophies, osteogenesis imperfecta, and other dysostoses.

Paget's Disease

Paget's disease, or osteitis deformans, is an osseous lesion of unknown etiology that may be of viral origin. This disease is relatively common, affecting approximately 3% of the population older than 40 years and up to 10% older than 80 years. Paget's disease may be monostotic or polyostotic and can be focal or diffuse. The disease is a chronic and sometimes progressive disorder that most frequently affects the pelvis.

On histologic examination, Paget's disease demon-

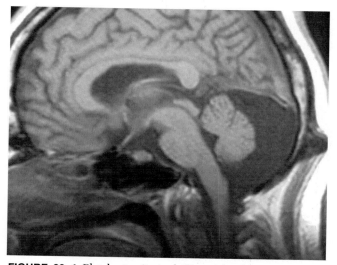

FIGURE 29–4 Platybasia. Sagittal T1-weighted magnetic resonance (MR) image shows flattening of the clival angle (platybasia) without basilar invagination. Note posterior fossa cyst and enlargement of the suprasellar cistern. (With permission from Glastonbury CM. Head and Neck Digital Teaching File. Salt Lake City, Electronic Medical Education Resource Group, 1999.)

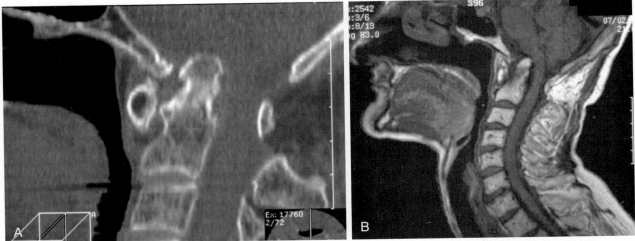

FIGURE 29–5 Basilar invagination. A 74-year-old woman with a history of rheumatoid arthritis. *A,* Sagittal computed tomography (CT) reconstruction (from 1-mm contiguous axial slices, bone algorithm) demonstrates irregularity with partial erosion of the dens and basilar invagination. *B,* The sagittal T1-weighted MR image clearly shows kinking of the cervicomedullary junction. (*A* and *B,* With permission from Glastonbury CM. Head and Neck Digital Teaching File. Salt Lake City, Electronic Medical Education Resource Group, 1999.)

strates osteoclastic resorption of trabeculae of the walls of the haversian canals of the compacta. This provides for the osteolytic phase characterized by early bone involvement. This imbalance between bone resorption and formation leads to the characterstic osseous deformities. There are three well-defined phases of the disease: (1) early destructive phase, (2) intermediate combined destructive and healing phase, and (3) late sclerotic or quiescent phase. Paget's disease may involve any bone and may be discovered as an incidental finding in many patients. Both CT and MR demonstrate bony expansion in the skull base. Because of softening of the bone, basilar invagination and platybasia may be present, which are more easily appreciated on MR than on CT because of the availability of multiplanar techniques. MR typically demonstrates high signal foci from fat on T1-weighted sequences as well as increased signal on T2-weighted imaging secondary to fibrovascular marrow (Fig. 29–6).[3–8]

Fibrous Dysplasia

Fibrous dysplasia is among the most common benign osseous skeletal disorders. Fibrous dysplasia is seen primarily in adolescents and young adults. Approximately 70% of patients have monostotic disease. Albright's syndrome is a rare unilateral polyostotic form of fibrous dysplasia with ipsilateral café au lait spots and endocrine dysfunction producing female precocious puberty.

Fibrous dysplasia is characterized by abnormal development of the fibroblasts as well as abnormal osseous mineralization. The bone is enlarged but usually follows the normal position or contour. CT reveals enlargement of the medullary space, but the normal cortex is usually maintained. The CT appearance varies, depending on how much fibrous and osteoid matrix is present. CT may show variations ranging from a lucent to a densely calcified medullary space. When a mixture of dense and sclerotic bony changes is present, the disease is referred to as *pagetoid.* The classic description of fibrous dysplasia

is that of a "ground-glass" appearance to the medullary space surrounded by an intact cortex (Fig. 29–7). MR imaging typically demonstrates expanded and thickened bone of low to intermediate signal on both T1- and T2-weighted sequences that may contain cystic or hemorrhagic foci (Fig. 29–8). Enhancement is variable but usually better appreciated on MR than on CT.[2–4, 9–13]

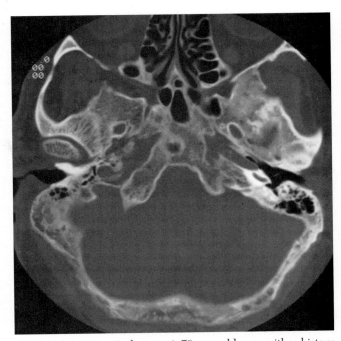

FIGURE 29–6 Paget's disease. A 78-year-old man with a history of Paget's disease and recent onset of sensorineural hearing loss. The axial CT scan demonstrates the lytic phase of Paget's disease involving the right temporal bone and occipital bones. (With permission from Glastonbury CM. Head and Neck Digital Teaching File. Salt Lake City, Electronic Medical Education Resource Group, 1999.)

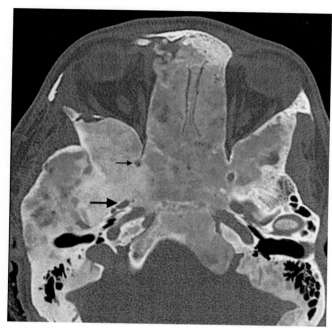

FIGURE 29–7 CT of fibrous dysplasia. A 15-year-old girl with a diagnosis of Albright's syndrome. Axial CT scan at 1-mm sections with bone algorithm shows marked expansion of the skull base with a heterogeneous mixed-density matrix. Note distortion of the right foramen ovale *(large arrow)* and foramen rotundum *(small arrow).* (With permission from Glastonbury CM. Head and Neck Digital Teaching File. Salt Lake City, Electronic Medical Education Resource Group, 1999.)

Osteogenesis Imperfecta

Osteogenesis imperfecta is a group of inherited conditions characterized by faulty collagen production that results in a weakened bone structure. Several types are known, with more severe manifestations in infants and young children in the congenital forms. The severity of this disorder is variable in the tarda forms, which are manifested by painless fractures after relatively minor trauma. Wormian bones and narrowing of the foramen magnum may be present. Osteogenesis imperfecta is characterized clinically by blue sclerae and frequent fractures. Additional abnormalities may include dental anomalies and deafness. Basilar invagination may occur secondary to skull base involvement. Osteogenesis imperfecta tarda and otosclerosis may share a common genetic abnormality. When osteogenesis imperfecta, otosclerosis, and blue sclerae are seen in combination, the disorder is referred to as *van der Hoeve's syndrome.* Imaging demonstrates diffuse osteoporosis, basilar invagination or platybasia, and temporal bone otosclerosis.[2, 5, 14]

Dysostoses

Multiple other bone dysplasias result in abnormalities of the skull base. Although the terminology used to describe these disorders varies considerably, the group includes dysostoses, osteopetroses, and osteochondrodysplasias.

Achondroplasia affects the skull base, and failure of growth at the spheno-occipital synchondrosis produces a short clivus and sphenoid bone that is reduced in size.

There may also be a decrease in the size of the foramen magnum and platybasia. The mucopolysaccharidoses are lysosomal storage disorders in which the skull base may show abnormal growth with thickening and basilar invagination. These disorders include Morquio's, Hurler's, Hunter's, and Maroteaux-Lamy. They may be associated with other craniovertebral anomalies as well as with atlantoaxial instability. Metabolic disorders, such as hyperparathyroidism, may also be associated with osteodystrophic changes of the skull base (Fig. 29–9).[2, 15, 16]

Trauma

The skull base provides part of the support for the facial skeleton as well as the floor of the cranial fossa. Skull base fractures are present in approximately one fourth of cases in which facial fractures are identified.[17–19] Skull base fractures are best identified by use of high-resolution thin-section CT with bone algorithm reconstruction and wide window filming. Trauma that involves the skull base invariably encompasses additional regional structures in the brain and face, and CT of the skull base should be performed in conjunction with evaluation of the facial skeleton, facial soft tissues, and brain to assess for concomitant injury. Both axial and coronal CT scans are beneficial for the evaluation of complex facial, skull base, and cranial injuries. In the event that direct coronal scanning is not possible because of the condition of the patient, re-formatted images derived from the axial scan may provide limited additional information. MR imaging can be of benefit in differentiating hemorrhage from other processes, such as infection or neoplasm, if necessary; for the most part, however, high-resolution CT is the modality of choice for the evaluation of skull base injury.[17, 20–24]

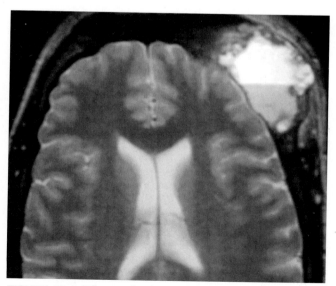

FIGURE 29–8 Fibrous dysplasia. Axial T2-weighted fast spin echo (FSE) MR image in a patient with monostotic fibrous dysplasia. The frontal bone shows marked osseous expansion. High T2-weighted signal centrally shows a fluid-fluid layer secondary to hemorrhage. (With permission from Davidson HC. Head and Neck Digital Teaching File. Salt Lake City, Electronic Medical Education Resource Group, 1999.)

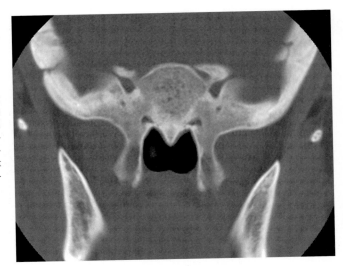

FIGURE 29–9 Hyperparathyroidism. Coronal CT scan in a patient with chronic renal failure and progressive vision loss. Diffuse sclerosis of the skull base is present as a manifestation of renal osteodystrophy due to secondary hyperparathyroidism. Encroachment of the optic canal in this patient required surgical decompression. (With permission from Davidson HC. Head and Neck Digital Teaching File. Salt Lake City, Electronic Medical Education Resource Group, 1999.)

Fractures of the skull base may result in cranial neuropathy, intracranial infection, cerebrospinal fluid leakage secondary to a dural tear, and damage to the internal carotid artery including thrombosis or pseudoaneurysm formation. Fractures of the sphenoid bone, although uncommon, are often accompanied by more extensive skull base fractures (Fig. 29–10). Sphenoid sinus opacification or a sphenoid sinus air-fluid level may indicate the presence of cerebrospinal fluid, hemorrhage, or in some cases poor sinus drainage. Injury of the sphenoid sinus may be life-threatening when the fracture extends to the adjacent cavernous sinus or carotid artery.[17, 20, 25]

A suspected dural tear can be evaluated initially by thin-section directed CT; however, the actual cerebrospinal fluid leak will be best demonstrated after the injection of intrathecal contrast material or by thin-section coronal MR. The most common locations for cerebrospinal fluid leaks are the cribriform plate and the tegmen of the temporal bone (Fig. 29–11).[17, 20, 25, 26]

Primary Benign Neoplasms

Benign neoplasms may originate within the cranial base or from any of its affiliated tissues, including those structures that pass through or are adjacent to the skull base. Meningiomas are a relatively frequently encountered, benign neoplasm associated with the skull base, particularly the greater wing of the sphenoid. These neoplasms are discussed in detail in Chapters 20, 22, and 25. Other benign neoplasms include paragangliomas, chordomas, neural sheath neoplasms, and primary bone tumors. Paragangliomas and nerve sheath tumors of the jugular foramen are discussed in the subsequent section on posterior skull base diseases.

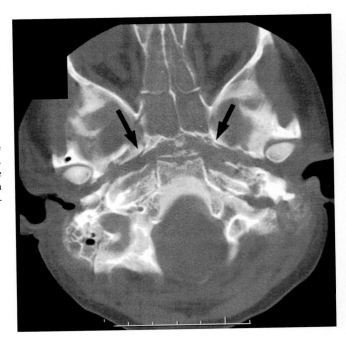

FIGURE 29–10 Sphenoid sinus fracture. Bone window axial image from a CT scan performed in a young male patient after trauma. The *arrows* indicate a fracture through the central skull base extending to the sphenoid sinus. (With permission from Davidson HC. Head and Neck Digital Teaching File. Salt Lake City, Electronic Medical Education Resource Group, 1999.)

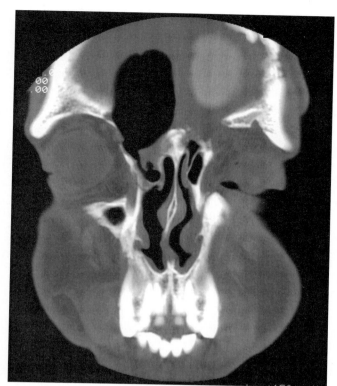

FIGURE 29–11 Cerebrospinal fluid leak on CT. A 29-year-old man who had sustained multiple facial injuries 3 months earlier in a motor vehicle accident re-presented with rhinorrhea. The coronal CT image (without intrathecal or intravenous administration of contrast material) demonstrates pneumocephalus secondary to a right anterior ethmoid leak with anterior skull base disruption. (With permission from Glastonbury CM. Head and Neck Digital Teaching File. Salt Lake City, Electronic Medical Education Resource Group, 1999.)

Of the primary benign bone neoplasms that may affect the skull base, the two most commonly seen are osteomas and giant cell tumors. Osteomas represent a form of benign bone tumor made up of mature cortical bone. Osteomas may involve the skull or facial bones and are seen as densely calcified, well marginated, smooth protuberances of bone. The osteoma may project externally or internally and typically spares the diploic space and inner table of the skull. An osteoma can occasionally be expansile or erosive. The frontal sinuses are the most commonly involved location in the head and neck. Osteomas of the skull base and paranasal sinuses are rarely of clinical significance and are most often seen as incidental findings (Fig. 29–12).[30–32] Osteochondromas (chondromas) may also rarely affect the skull base and are sometimes referred to as osteocartilaginous exostoses. These exostoses are histologically similar to normal bone and form a bony excrescence that has a cartilaginous covered cortex.[32–34]

Giant cell tumors may involve any region of the skull base, when seen in the jugular fossa. These tumors are grossly lytic, expansile lesions that tend to demonstrate locally aggressive behavior without crossing the periosteum. Giant cell tumors contain sinusoidal vessels with hypervascular stroma. Hemorrhagic change is frequent

and matrix mineralization is rare histologically. CT shows a lytic, expansile, destructive lesion. MR demonstrates a cystic mass of mixed signal intensity that may show evidence of hemorrhage in various stages.[33, 35–38]

Primary Malignant Neoplasms

Accurate evaluation of local tumor involvement and regional extension or systemic metastasis is crucial for the treatment planning of head and neck cancer. Primary cancers of the head and neck may be too small to be clinically detected before evidence of metastatic disease. CT and MR are often the most effective methods of locating the primary tumor in such cases, particularly when they are located within the skull base.[39]

Primary malignant neoplasms that affect the skull base include nasopharyngeal carcinomas, rhabdomyosarcomas, osteosarcomas, and chondrosarcomas. Primary malignant bone neoplasms are rare in the skull base region. Osteosarcomas arise spontaneously or occur in association with Paget's disease or previous radiation therapy. Osteosarcoma is characterized by mineralization of the tumor matrix and extensive bone destruction. These neoplasms often occur in the body or wing of the sphenoid when they involve the skull base, and the imaging diagnosis rests on the identification of an osteoid matrix best seen on high-resolution CT.[4, 40, 41]

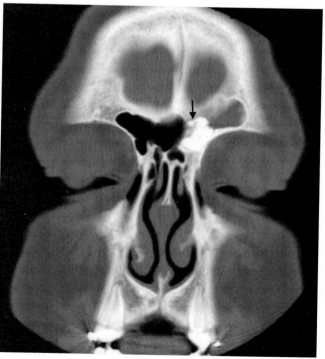

FIGURE 29–12 Osteoma of frontal sinus. Coronal CT image in an 11-year-old boy with left frontal sinus obstructive symptoms (fluid density in sinus) secondary to an osteoid osteoma (arrow). (With permission from Davidson HC. Head and Neck Digital Teaching File. Salt Lake City, Electronic Medical Education Resource Group, 1999.)

Diffuse Hematopoietic Osseous Malignant Neoplasms

Lymphoma

Lymphoma can be seen anywhere throughout the extracranial head and neck. Lymphomatous masses may be focal or multifocal and may demonstrate perineural spread. CT and MR are both characterized by discrete or infiltrative skull base lesions. MR scans demonstrate replacement of normal high-signal marrow, and fat-suppressed contrast-enhanced images are particularly effective for showing the extent of tumor involvement. The imaging appearance is nonspecific, however, and lymphoma of the skull base may be difficult to differentiate from other malignant skull base neoplasms (Fig. 29–13).[3, 31, 42, 43]

Myeloma

Multiple myeloma disease may present as either medullary or extramedullary tumor. On histologic examination, myeloma is characterized by sheets of plasma cells on a delicate reticular stroma. Specific histologic features are not necessarily related to tumor aggressiveness, and prognosis appears to be related more to tumor location and degree of marrow involvement. Although myeloma almost always begins in the bone marrow, it may manifest as a solitary bone neoplasm or extramedullary soft tissue mass. In the solitary form, it is referred to as a plasmacytoma. Some patients will succumb to generalized disease, whereas others may die of local invasion by a single lesion. There is an increased incidence of extramedullary myeloma in men with a male to female sex ratio of 3 to 1. The male to female ratio is equal for multiple myeloma. Although rare, 85% or more of plasmacytomas occur in the region of the head and neck. A solitary plasmacytoma is indistinguishable from a single lytic metastatic lesion (Fig. 29–14). Multiple myeloma may involve any of the bones of the skull base with diffuse permeative osseous changes. Neither CT nor MR reliably differentiates multiple myeloma from osteolytic metastatic disease.[3, 31, 44]

Langerhans Cell Histiocytosis

Langerhans cell histiocytosis, also known as histiocytosis X, most commonly presents as a solitary or monostotic eosinophilic granuloma. This disorder is probably a clonal neoplastic disorder that is seen primarily in the pediatric age group, but a less severe form of the disease also occurs in adults. Langerhans cell histiocytosis includes a spectrum of diseases with the common pathologic denominator being the presence of histiocytic proliferation that may involve bone or soft tissue. The disorders include (1) eosinophilic granuloma, which by definition is confined to bone; (2) Hand-Schüller-Christian disease, which includes soft tissue involvement but carries an intermediate prognosis; and (3) Letterer-Siwe disease, which includes visceral involvement and has the most severe prognosis. The disease may range from focal skull lesions to diffuse osteolytic skull base abnormalities and variably demonstrates a significant soft tissue component. On CT, a single "punched-out" lytic lesion with well-defined borders and

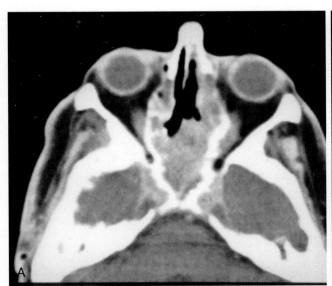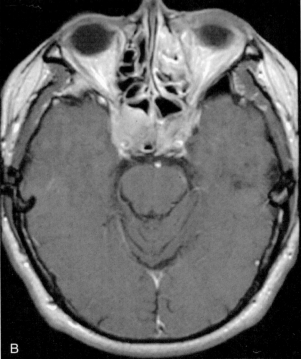

FIGURE 29–13 Skull base lymphoma. A 50-year-old man with bilateral proptosis, headaches, and a several-month history of general malaise. *A,* Post–contrast-enhanced axial CT at the level of the orbits demonstrates a predominantly expansile mass in the nasal cavity and sphenoid sinus, with enhancing but enlarged cavernous sinuses. *B,* MR axial post–contrast-enhanced T1-weighted image demonstrates intense enhancement of this mass. Pathologic examination revealed histiocytic lymphoma. (*A* and *B,* With permission from Davidson HC. Head and Neck Digital Teaching File. Salt Lake City, Electronic Medical Education Resource Group, 1999.)

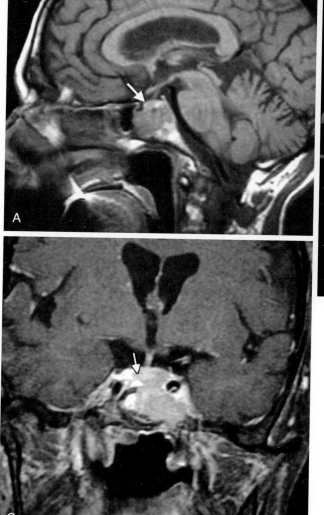

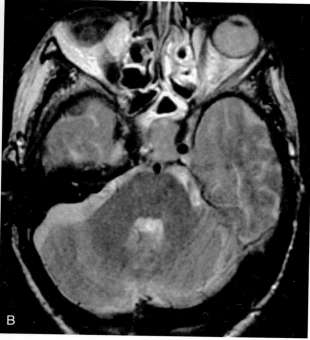

FIGURE 29–14 Plasmacytoma. An 80-year-old woman who presented with diplopia. Sagittal T1-weighted (A), axial T2-weighted (B), and post–contrast-enhanced coronal T1-weighted (C) images demonstrate a mass arising in the sphenoid centrally and extending anteriorly to the sinus and superiorly to surround and displace the pituitary gland (arrows in A and B). The dorsal margin of the clivus is intact. Plasmacytoma was diagnosed at biopsy. There was no evidence of systemic multiple myeloma at diagnosis or at 9-month follow-up. (A–C, With permission from Glastonbury CM. Head and Neck Digital Teaching File. Salt Lake City, Electronic Medical Education Resource Group, 1999.)

beveled edges is characteristic of simple cases of eosinophilic granuloma. Contrast enhancement is typical and is best evaluated on MR (Fig. 29–15).[3, 4, 45–54]

Metastatic Malignant Disease

Metastatic disease is the most common malignant neoplasm involving the skull base. Metastases may spread to the skull base either by direct invasion or by hematogenous spread and may be focal or diffusely lytic and destructive. The primary tumors that most frequently give rise to metastases to the skull base are lung, breast, and prostate cancer. When prostate or breast carcinoma metastasizes to the skull base, the lesions may be hyperostotic, destructive, or mixed. Perineural spread may occur with any form of metastatic disease and is best illustrated by MR. On CT, metastatic lesions appear nonspecific and

demonstrate lytic bony infiltration and destruction. On T1-weighted MR, displacement of the normal high-intensity marrow signal by lower intensity tumor is characteristic. Fat-suppressed contrast-enhanced images help to reveal the full extent of neoplastic involvement, which may extend well beyond the cortical margins (Fig. 29–16).[3, 31, 55]

ANTERIOR SKULL BASE LESIONS

Congenital Lesions

Congenital lesions of the anterior skull base include the anterior neuropore anomalies (anterior cephaloceles, nasal gliomas, and nasal dermoid). These lesions present clinically with a nasal mass, dermal sinus, or meningitis. The imaging features of these abnormalities include osse-

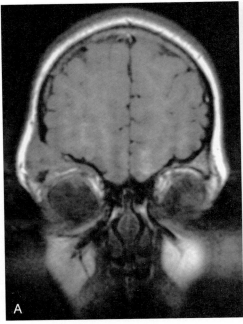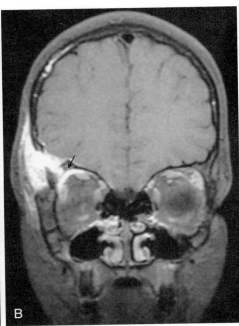

FIGURE 29–15 Eosinophilic granuloma. Pathologically confirmed eosinophilic granuloma of the anterior skull base in a young male patient. Coronal T1-weighted *(A)* and post–contrast-enhanced *(B)* images show the avid enhancement of this bone lesion and its extension infero-medially to the orbit *(arrow)*. (*A* and *B*, With permission from Chong BW. Head and Neck Digital Teaching File. Salt Lake City, Electronic Medical Education Resource Group, 1999.)

ous defects on CT and herniation of brain or meninges on MR (Fig. 29–17). These lesions are discussed in more detail in Chapter 44.

Sinonasal Inflammatory Disease

Skull base involvement by sinonasal inflammation occurs secondary to chronic underlying infectious or granulomatous disease, leading to meningitis, encephalitis, or abscess. The differential diagnosis of anterior skull base inflammatory disease includes Wegener's granulomatosis, sarcoidosis, polyposis, and fungal sinusitis. Imaging changes seen on both CT and MR include aggressive osseous changes, soft tissue masses, granulomas, polyps, inspissation, phlegmon, nasal septal destruction (granulomatous diseases), and secondary intracranial complications.

Sinonasal Neoplasms

Sinonasal neoplasms frequently present clinically with nasal obstruction or epistaxis. The differential diagnosis of these tumors includes squamous cell carcinoma, lymphoma, minor salivary gland tumors, olfactory neuroblastoma (esthesioneuroblastoma), melanoma, and sinonasal undifferentiated carcinoma. Imaging of sinonasal

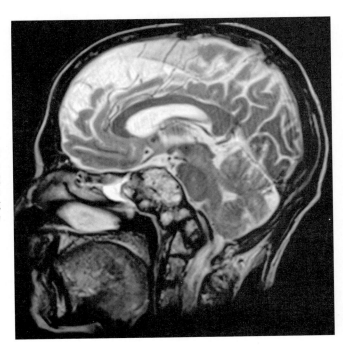

FIGURE 29–16 Metastatic disease. A 50-year-old man with widely metastatic renal cell carcinoma. The parasagittal T2-weighted image demonstrates a large heterogeneous hyperintense mass replacing the marrow of the clivus and basisphenoid, extending through the posterior cortex and compressing the pons. (With permission from Davidson HC. Head and Neck Digital Teaching File. Salt Lake City, Electronic Medical Education Resource Group, 1999.)

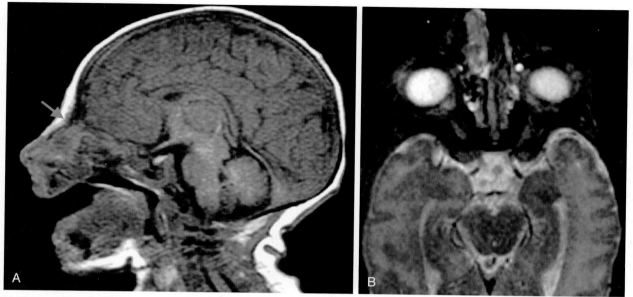

FIGURE 29–17 Nasal Glioma. A neonate with respiratory distress and noted to have a nasal mass. *A,* Sagittal T1-weighted image shows an isointense nasal mass extending posteriorly and superiorly toward the anterior cranial fossa *(arrow)*. *B,* Axial T2-weighted MR shows the right-sided mass to be hyperintense. This proved to be a nasal glioma. (*A* and *B,* With permission from Glastonbury CM. Head and Neck Digital Teaching File. Salt Lake City, Electronic Medical Education Resource Group, 1999.)

neoplasms with CT or MR typically demonstrates an enhancing mass high in the nasal cavity with variable bone destruction (Fig. 29–18). Aggressive tumors may demonstrate direct invasion of the cribriform plate, the anterior fossa dura, and the sphenoid bone as well as demonstrate perineural tumor spread.

CENTRAL SKULL BASE LESIONS

Congenital and Genetic Disease

Neurofibromatosis Type 1

The skull base changes typically associated with type 1 neurofibromatosis include bony dysplasia involving the

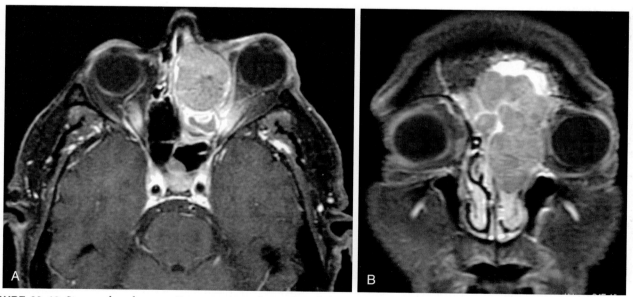

FIGURE 29–18 Sinonasal melanoma. Post–contrast-enhanced axial *(A)* and coronal *(B)* T1-weighted images with fat suppression. The bulky mass is centered high in the nasal cavity, with extension through the cribriform plate into the anterior cranial fossa and through the lamina papyracea into the left orbit with resulting proptosis. The mass shows moderate enhancement. (*A* and *B,* With permission from Davidson HC. Head and Neck Digital Teaching File. Salt Lake City, Electronic Medical Education Resource Group, 1999.)

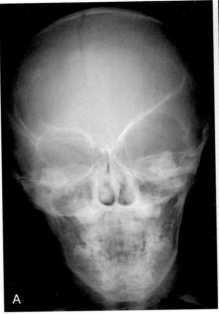

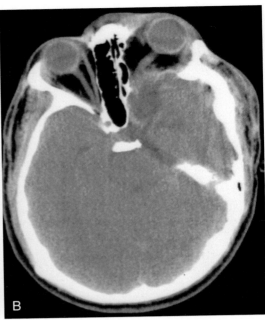

FIGURE 29–19 Neurofibromatosis type 1. Plain anteroposterior skull radiograph (A) and CT scan (B) in a child with neurofibromatosis type 1. Left sphenoid wing dysplasia with absence of the orbital roof is apparent on both plain film and CT. Herniation of right middle cranial fossa contents into the orbit with resultant proptosis is apparent on CT, as is periorbital soft tissue thickening due to cutaneous neurofibroma. (A and B, With permission from Orrison WW. Head and Neck Digital Teaching File. Salt Lake City, Electronic Medical Education Resource Group, 1999.)

sphenoid wing and orbit, with associated herniation of intracranial contents and clinical exophthalmos. Patients with type 1 neurofibromatosis also develop soft tissue neurofibromas and orbital and central nervous system neoplasms (Fig. 29–19). Neurofibromatosis is discussed in detail in Chapter 51.

Basal Cephalocele

The congenital basal cephalocele represents a defect in the fusion of the ossification centers and is typically

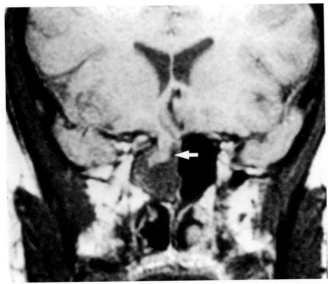

FIGURE 29–20 Transsphenoidal encephalocele. Coronal T1-weighted image at the level of the sphenoid sinus. The right sphenoid sinus is filled with cerebrospinal fluid signal. There is herniation of a portion of the frontal lobe into the sinus (arrow). (With permission from Davidson HC. Head and Neck Digital Teaching File. Salt Lake City, Electronic Medical Education Resource Group, 1999.)

named according to the area of passage, such as the transethmoidal, sphenoethmoidal, sphenorbital, transsphenoidal, and sphenomaxillary types. Imaging demonstrates an osseous defect on CT and soft tissue herniation on MR (Fig. 29–20).

Inflammatory and Infectious Disease

Sinonasal disease in the sphenoid sinus may spread to the central skull base secondarily with contiguous intracranial extension. In immunocompromised patients, invasive fungal infections such as rhinocerebral mucormycosis or aspergillosis can rapidly develop osteomyelitis and contiguous intracranial extension. The imaging findings demonstrate destructive bony changes and secondary intracranial complications. Although CT is excellent for demonstrating osseous destruction, MR imaging with contrast enhancement and fat saturation is preferred for delineation of soft tissue extension and intracranial complication.

Head and Neck Cancer

Primary neoplasms may spread to the central skull base from and through the central deep head and neck spaces, namely, the pharyngeal mucosal space, the masticator space, and the parapharyngeal space. Primary neoplasms that may spread in this way include squamous cell carcinoma, minor salivary carcinomas (adenoid cystic mucoepidermoid carcinoma), lymphoma, and sarcoma. CT and MR both typically show direct invasion of adjacent osseous structures with associated soft tissue mass. Perineural tumor spread may occur with any primary malignant neoplasm and may manifest skip lesions or even intracranial tumor extension (Fig. 29–21).

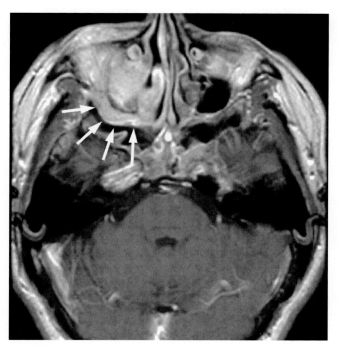

FIGURE 29–21 Perineural tumor spread. Post–contrast-enhanced axial T1-weighted image in a patient with non-Hodgkin's lymphoma involving the central skull base. Perineural spread of disease is manifest as marked thickening of a branch of the maxillary division of the trigeminal nerve *(arrows)* in the inferior orbital fissure and inferior orbital groove. (With permission from Davidson HC. Head and Neck Digital Teaching File. Salt Lake City, Electronic Medical Education Resource Group, 1999.)

POSTERIOR SKULL BASE LESIONS

Vascular Lesions

Jugular Bulb Anomalies

Some of the more common lesions of the posterior skull base are the jugular bulb anomalies. Normal developmental variants of the jugular bulb are common and include asymmetric enlargement, high position, and diverticulum. Although asymmetric enlargement and high jugular bulb are benign conditions that are virtually asymptomatic, the degree of asymmetry may be striking, confronting the radiologist with the dilemma of deciding whether a more worrisome process is present. When an enlarged bulb is present, the right side is the larger twice as often as the left side. A jugular bulb is considered high when the apex of the bulb rises above the level of the floor of the internal auditory canal. A diverticulum of the jugular bulb is seen as a superior projection from a normal, enlarged, or high bulb. A jugular bulb diverticulum projects more medially than the more common high jugular bulb and is not associated with dehiscence. On CT, the bony margins of a diverticulum or enlarged or high jugular bulb should show no irregularity or demineralization (Fig. 29–22 and 29–23). The MR appearance of an anomalous jugular bulb can be more of a problem because the turbulent flow signal may simulate a lesion. MR venography and bone CT are useful adjuncts when MR imaging is indeterminate.

Dural Sinus Thrombosis and Arteriovenous Fistula

Dural sinus thrombosis and associated dural arteriovenous fistula are included in the differential diagnosis of lesions found in the posterior skull base. These conditions are discussed in more detail in Chapter 21.

Venous sinus thrombosis is the cause of approximately 1% of strokes. The superior sagittal sinus is most frequently affected, followed by the transverse, sigmoid, and cavernous sinuses (Fig. 29–24). Patients with cerebral venous thrombosis present with a variety of symptoms including altered mental status, blurred vision, diplopia, personality change, focal neurologic findings, convulsions, and even coma. The clinical course tends to be slowly progressive but in the setting of acute thrombosis can proceed rapidly to coma and death. A variety of disorders can result in dural sinus thrombosis, although one-fourth of cases that are encountered clinically remain of unknown cause.

Jugular Foramen Region Neoplasms

Paraganglioma

The most common neoplasm of the jugular foramen is the paraganglioma, which accounts for approximately 90% of the tumors at this level. Paragangliomas, also referred to as glomus tumors, are neoplasms found in a variety of relatively predictable regions of the body, characterized by clusters of cells called *Zellballen*.[56, 57] The term *chemodectoma* was first used by Mulligan to describe tumors originating in the chemoreceptor system of the carotid body.[58, 59] When this type of neoplasm is found within the region of the jugular foramen arising from the paragangli-

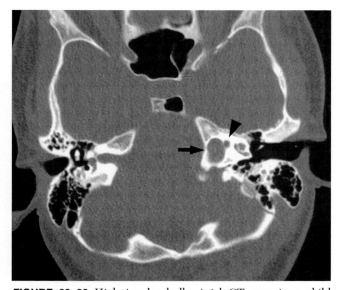

FIGURE 29–22 High jugular bulb. Axial CT scan in a child who was being evaluted for headache. An enlarged, medially positioned high jugular bulb is present *(arrow)*. A small laterally directed diverticulum is noted *(arrowhead)*. No dehiscence of the tympanic floor is present. (With permission from Davidson HC. Head and Neck Digital Teaching File. Salt Lake City, Electronic Medical Education Resource Group, 1999.)

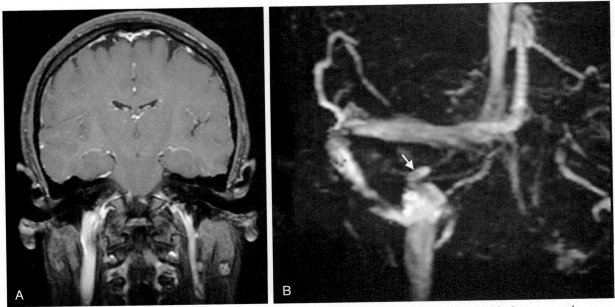

FIGURE 29–23 Jugular bulb diverticulum. Young female patient with pulsatile tinnitus that she could eliminate with pressure on the right side of her neck. Coronal post–contrast-enhanced T1-weighted image (A) shows normal position of the bulb but irregularity of its apex, which is clarified by the MR venogram performed the same day (B). The diverticulum of the jugular bulb is clearly demonstrated (arrow). (A and B, With permission from Glastonbury CM. Head and Neck Digital Teaching File. Salt Lake City, Electronic Medical Education Resource Group, 1999.)

onic cells around the jugular ganglion, it is referred to as a *glomus jugulare* tumor. Other paragangliomas of the head and neck include glomus tympanicum tumors, glomus vagale tumors, and carotid body tumors. The glomus jugulare tumor is typically found within the adventitia of the jugular bulb along the tympanic branch of the glossopharyneal nerve (Jacobson's nerve). Patients present with a variety of symptoms related primarily to cranial nerve IX (glossopharyngeal), X (vagus), and XI (spinal accessory) involvement. Glomus jugulare and glomus tympanicum tumors may present with pulsatile tinnitus.

Extension of the glomus jugulare tumor into the intracranial and extracranial spaces is common, with equal amounts of neoplasm occurring above and below the skull base centered about the jugular foramen. When this tumor extends laterally into the temporal bone and middle ear cavity, resulting in pulsatile tinnitus, it is referred to as a *glomus jugulotympanicum* tumor.[20, 58, 60]

Paragangliomas may be seen either as part of an autosomal dominant genetic pattern or spontaneously. Multiple tumors are more common in the familial types, and bilateral carotid body tumors may be seen in nearly one

FIGURE 29–24 Dural sinus thrombosis. A 40-year-old woman with a history of chronic mastoiditis and recent severe headaches. *A*, The MR venogram demonstrates absence of normal signal within the right transverse and sigmoid sinuses and the internal jugular vein. *B*, The axial T2-weighted MR image shows early venous infarct in the middle temporal gyrus *(arrow)*. (A and B, With permission from Glastonbury CM. Head and Neck Digital Teaching File. Salt Lake City, Electronic Medical Education Resource Group, 1999.)

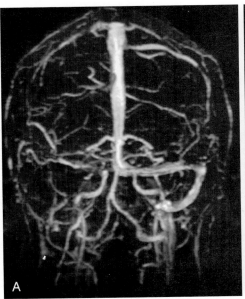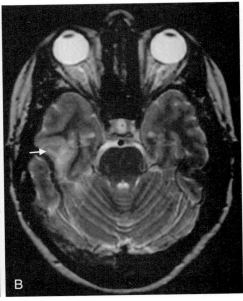

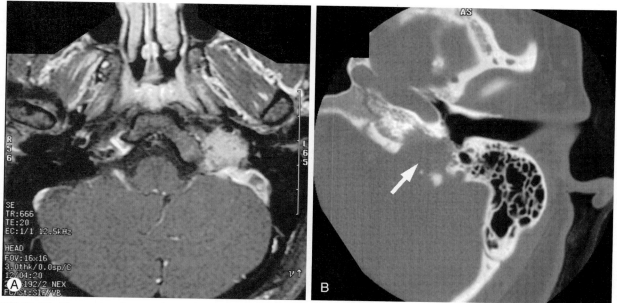

FIGURE 29–25 Glomus jugulare. Enhanced T1-weighted fat-suppressed MR image (A) and axial CT scan (B) of the posterior skull base in a middle-aged woman with pulsatile tinnitus. The MR shows an intensely enhancing jugular foramen mass with punctate foci of signal void corresponding to small blood vessels (arrow). The CT shows enlargement of the left jugular foramen with classic permeative bony margins. (A and B, With permission from Davidson HC. Head and Neck Digital Teaching File. Salt Lake City, Electronic Medical Education Resource Group, 1999.)

third of familial cases. However, presentation of multiple paragangliomas may be separated in time by months or even up to decades in some cases. Therefore, it is important to examine the carotid arteries bilaterally when any paraganglioma is identified.[58, 60]

Paragangliomas are highly vascular neoplasms that tend to have dramatic contrast enhancement on both CT and MR. Owing to the rapidity of blood flow within these hypervascular neoplasms, dynamic scanning may be required to demonstrate the full extent of contrast enhancement. As these neoplasms enlarge, tumor necrosis may occur, resulting in regions that lack contrast enhancement. Hemorrhage may also be present, with resulting focal areas of increased density on CT or hyperintensity on T1-weighted MR. In addition to focal areas of hemorrhage, sporadic regions of slow flow within the multiple vessels composing this neoplasm may also contribute focal areas of high signal. Small foci of signal void may also be seen because of flow voids within these highly vascular neoplasms. These multiple high- and low-intensity foci have been referred to as the *salt-and-pepper* appearance that is classically used to describe paragangliomas. The lesions appear hyperintense on T2-weighted imaging and show intense contrast enhancement. Paragangliomas demonstrate a characteristic permeative infiltration of bone on CT (Fig. 29–25).

Smaller tumors may not demonstrate these classic imaging features, and angiography may be required for diagnosis when imaging is indeterminate.[46, 47, 58, 61, 62] Selective external carotid arteriography typically demonstrates a dense reticular tumor stain that may show arteriovenous shunting. As the tumor enlarges, it may receive supply from branches of the internal carotid or vertebral arteries. Some neoplasms may be of sufficient vascularity to re-

ceive blood supply from the opposite carotid artery (Fig. 29–26).

Schwannoma

Schwannomas of the posterior skull base may arise from the glossopharyngeal (IX), vagus (X), or spinal accessory (XI) nerves at the level of the jugular foramen; the hypoglossal (XII) nerve may be affected at the level of the hypoglossal canal. Schwannomas of the jugular foramen have been classified into three types (A, B, and C) on the basis of location. Type A schwannomas are primarily intracranial and frequently result in acoustic or cerebellar symptoms. The type B tumors tend to be centered at the jugular foramen, and type C extends predominantly extracranially. The type B and type C schwannomas are most likely to cause jugular foramen syndromes. Distinguishing the parent nerve of origin in this area may be difficult.[35, 61, 63, 64]

Hypoglossal schwannomas may be intracranial, extracranial, or both, having a "dumbbell" shape. Schwannomas arising at the level of the hypoglossal canal may also extend into the spinal canal. Although the most classic symptom of hypoglossal nerve (XII) involvement is hemiatrophy of the tongue with fat replacement on CT and MR, other forms of neurologic compromise may be observed, such as those secondary to brain stem, cerebellar, and other cranial nerve compression. When a hypoglossal neoplasm is present, there is typically erosion of the hypoglossal canal, but this change is not universally seen. Neoplasms arising within the hypoglossal canal may extend to the jugular tubercle and clivus, which can make differentiating them from primary jugular foramen masses extremely difficult.[35, 61, 63, 65–67]

On CT, schwannomas of the jugular foramen typically

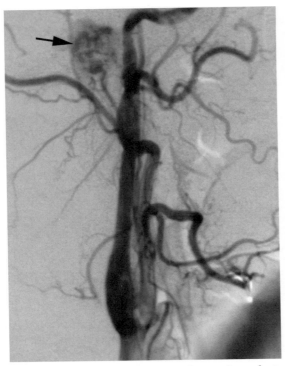

FIGURE 29–26 Angiogram of paraganglioma. Lateral view of digital subtraction angiography with carotid artery injection shows marked vascularity that is characteristic of paraganglioma (*arrow*). (With permission from Orrison WW. Head and Neck Digital Teaching File. Salt Lake City, Electronic Medical Education Resource Group, 1999.)

cause symmetric bony expansion; but in contrast to paragangliomas, they maintain a sharp osseous margin. CT often shows foraminal changes that aid in differentiating schwannoma from paraganglioma and a hypoglossal from a jugular lesion. The extent of the tumor is often best defined on MR, where coronal and sagittal imaging play a key role in demonstrating the full tumor extent (Fig. 29–27).

Other Jugular Foramen Region Neoplasms

Additional neoplasms that may be found at the level of the jugular foramen include meningiomas, neurofibromas, chondrosarcomas, and other primary or metastatic malignant neoplasms. Meningiomas are a relatively frequent benign neoplasm that may be encountered in the skull base and the jugular foramen, and these neoplasms are discussed in detail in Chapter 20. Neurofibromas of the skull base are frequently associated with neurofibromatosis type 1 and are discussed in Chapter 51. Metastatic disease or primary malignant neoplasia of the posterior skull base should always be included in the differential diagnosis of patients with a lower cranial neuropathy (Fig. 29–28).

Osteocartilaginous Neoplasms

Chondrosarcoma

Chondrosarcomas may originate from bone, from cartilage, or even from tissues without a cartilaginous component. Approximately 7% of these neoplasms arise in the

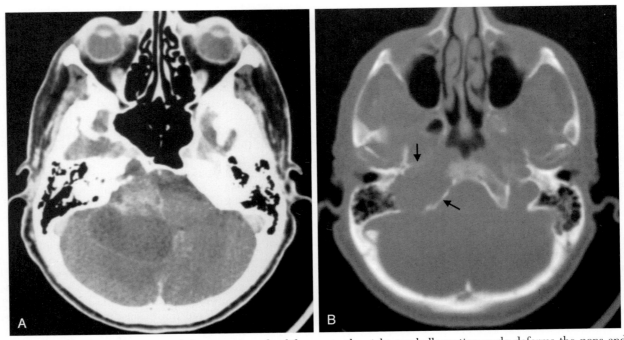

FIGURE 29–27 Jugular schwannoma. A large cystic and solid mass in the right cerebellopontine angle deforms the pons and the right cerebellum (*A*, post–contrast-enhanced axial CT) and appears to arise from the right jugular foramen (*B*, CT bone windows). Pathologically shown to be a giant schwannoma. Note the scalloped bone margins (*arrows* in *B*). (*A* and *B*, With permission from Orrison WW. Head and Neck Digital Teaching File. Salt Lake City, Electronic Medical Education Resource Group, 1999.)

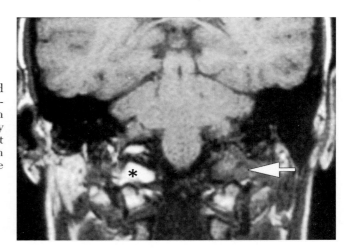

FIGURE 29–28 Ewing's sarcoma. Coronal non–contrast-enhanced T1-weighted MR image in a patient with left hypoglossal neuropathy. Tumor infiltration is seen in the left occipital condyle with extension into the hypoglossal canal. Note that the normal fatty marrow has been replaced *(arrow)*. Compare the normal bright T1 marrow signal on the right *(asterisk)*. (With permission from Davidson HC. Head and Neck Digital Teaching File. Salt Lake City, Electronic Medical Education Resource Group, 1999.)

head and neck and are particularly prone to arise from the petro-occipital synchondrosis, although they may also originate from the junction of the nasal septum and the rostrum of the sphenoid.

Chondrosarcomas are relatively slow growing, locally invasive tumors. Chondrosarcomas tend to be centered off-midline, which is an important feature in differentiating this lesion from midline chordoma. Chondrosarcomas rarely metastasize.[27, 68–71]

The CT appearance of chondrosarcoma varies according to the amount of chondroid matrix present. There is typically a generous soft tissue component that appears dense on CT before administration of contrast material, with at least partial enhancement. Calcification of the tumor in a ringlike pattern is characteristic but not invariably present. The margin between normal bone and neoplasm may be well defined but generally lacks a sclerotic rim. On MR imaging, the signal of a chondrosarcoma is relatively isointense on T1 but hyperintense on T2-weighted sequences. There is usually some degree of enhancement after gadolinium administration (Fig. 29–29).[3, 27, 72–74]

Chordomas

Chordomas are rare neoplasms arising from embryonic notochord remnants. The majority (50%) occur in the sacrococcygeal area; another 15% occur within a vertebral body, and approximately one-third originate in the skull base region of the clivus. The most frequent skull base location is the spheno-occipital synchondrosis, but these tumors may also arise from the basisphenoid and basiocciput.[3, 27, 75–77] Chordomas can occur at any age but have a peak incidence between the ages of 40 and 60 years for the sacrococcygeal region and between 30 and 50 years in the skull base. Chordomas are more common in men than in women.

On gross examination, a chordoma has a translucent gray appearance with a soft tissue component that is usually significantly larger than the amount of bone destruction present. The neoplasm is composed of nests or cords of vacuolar tumor cells containing glycogen and mucin. Dystrophic calcification and hemorrhage may be present. When cartilaginous matrix is noted, the tumor is referred to as a *chondroid chordoma*.[3, 27, 75–77]

Chordomas may involve the trigeminal nerve initially

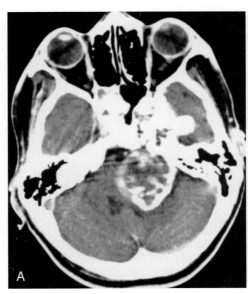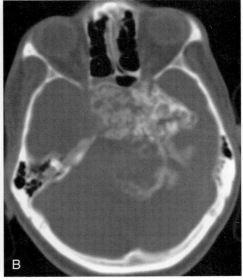

FIGURE 29–29 Chondrosarcoma. A 28-year-old man presented with dizziness, dysphagia, and cerebellar signs. *A*, Post–contrast-enhanced CT scan shows a large heterogeneous mass arising from the region of the apex of the petrous temporal bone and extending to the sphenoid bone and to the middle and posterior cranial fossae. *B*, The bone windows show a calcified matrix. (*A* and *B*, With permission from Davidson HC. Head and Neck Digital Teaching File. Salt Lake City, Electronic Medical Education Resource Group, 1999.)

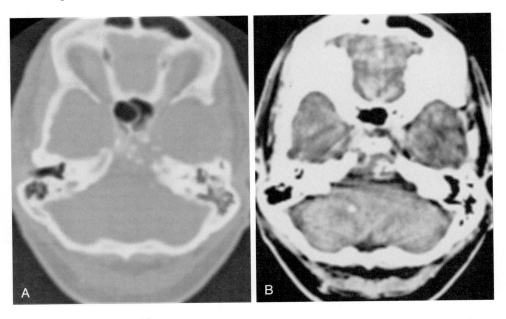

FIGURE 29–30 Clivus chordoma. *A*, Axial CT scan at bone windows demonstrates destruction and expansion of the clivus. *B*, Axial CT scan at soft tissue windows demonstrates soft tissue density replacing the normal bone density of the clivus. (*A* and *B*, With permission from Orrison WW. Head and Neck Digital Teaching File. Salt Lake City, Electronic Medical Education Resource Group, 1999.)

but may also extend to involve the facial and the vestibulocochlear nerves as they enter the internal auditory canal. Anterior tumor extension may encroach on the oculomotor, trochlear, and abducens nerves as well as the optic nerve, resulting in visual disturbance and ophthalmoplegia. Patients may also present with headaches or symptoms related to pituitary dysfunction as the neoplasm extends into the sella turcica. As the tumor increases in size, there may ultimately be brain stem compression. Although rare, it is also possible for chordomas to occur intracranially or within the nasopharynx. Chordomas tend to be relatively slow growing, but their location makes complete resection extremely difficult and therefore local recurrence is common. Chordomas also tend to be resistant to radiation therapy.[1, 27, 75–78]

As with most skull base disorders, both CT and MR are beneficial for the evaluation of a patient thought to have a clivus mass. It is not uncommon for chordomas to be first identified incidentally on CT or MR imaging. The CT examination typically reveals a midline clival mass with a prominent soft tissue component. Bone destruction is present in 95% of cases. The margin between normal bone and tumor is usually poorly defined and lacks a sclerotic margin. Soft tissue calcifications are visualized

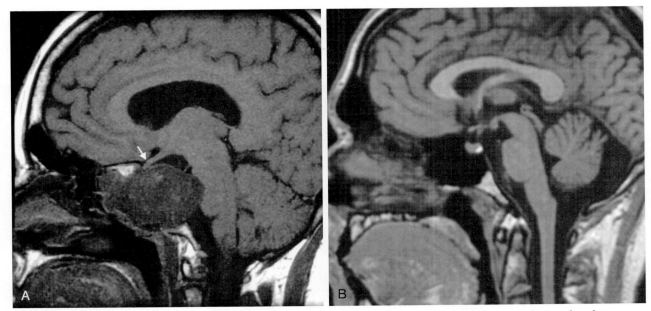

FIGURE 29–31 Chordoma. *A*, Sagittal T1-weighted image demonstrates a large low-intensity mass replacing the clivus marrow, disrupting its dorsal cortex, and compressing the pons. There is also anterior extension to the sphenoid sinus and superior extension elevating the optic chiasm *(arrow)*. Compare with the normal fatty marrow signal in the clivus from a normal scan in *B*. (*A* and *B*, With permission from Orrison WW. Head and Neck Digital Teaching File. Salt Lake City, Electronic Medical Education Resource Group, 1999.)

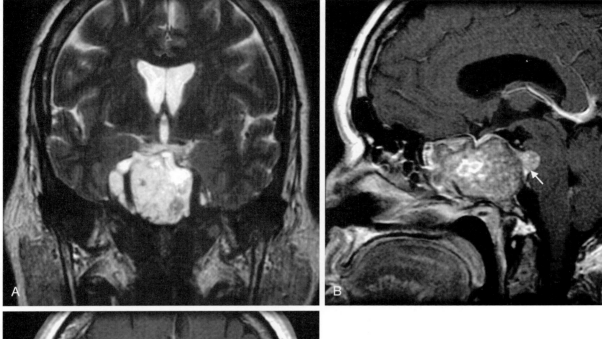

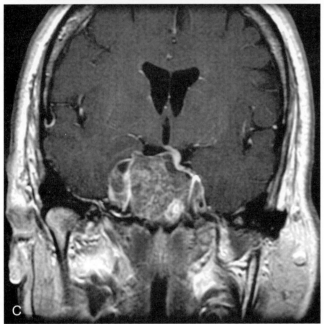

FIGURE 29–32 Chordoma. *A*, Coronal T2-weighted MR image of the same patient as in Figure 29–31. The high T2-weighted signal intensity of chordoma is well appreciated. Note the insinuation around the right cavernous internal carotid artery. Sagittal *(B)* and coronal *(C)* post–contrast-enhanced T1-weighted images. Heterogeneous but intense enhancement of the chordoma is demonstrated. A nodular component of the tumor is compressing the pons *(arrow* in *B)*, and the intimate relation of the chordoma to critical structures is apparent. *(A–C,* With permission from Glastonbury CM. Head and Neck Digital Teaching File. Salt Lake City, Electronic Medical Education Resource Group, 1999.)

on CT in half of these neoplasms and are generally considered remnants of bony destruction rather than tumor matrix (Fig. 29–30). Contrast enhancement is variable. MR usually shows T1 hypointensity within the clivus relative to the normally high fat signal intensity on T1-weighted sequences. Indeed, it is imperative that the reader be alert to the signal change within the clivus, because T1 isointensity may be the only clue that the clivus is abnormal in some cases. The sagittal T1-weighted scan that is standard in most MR cranial studies is ideal for making this distinction (Fig. 29–31). Because hemorrhagic change is frequent and mucinoid material abundant, focal regions of high signal may also be present on T1-weighed MR sequences. Increased signal is anticipated on long TR/TE sequences; however, focal regions

of low signal may be seen secondary to hemorrhage or residual bone. The tumor margins are often better visualized on MR than on CT, and the size of the soft tissue mass identified on MR is usually disproportionately larger than the degree of osseous destruction noted on CT. MR contrast enhancement is typically intense but heterogeneous (Fig. 29–32).[14, 27, 79–84]

SUMMARY

The pathologic spectrum of skull base lesions and their imaging presentations are myriad. As the field of head and neck imaging continues to develop, it is increasingly important for both the diagnosing and the treating physician to have a practical working understanding of skull base anatomy, which encompasses some of the most complex anatomy in the human body. The skull base in the past was considered virtually unapproachable surgically, but it is now routinely accessible to multidisciplinary surgical teams in large part owing to improvements in advanced imaging techniques. The combined application of advanced high-resolution CT and MR imaging techniques for osseous and soft tissue disease, respectively, provides the precise anatomic localization required for tailored preoperative planning of these complex lesions. Early diagnosis combined with aggressive surgical resection has translated into substantially improved prognosis for patients. The tailored use of contemporary imaging techniques usually permits a short differential list and sometimes permits the reader to suggest a specific tissue diagnosis as well.

References

1. Samii M, Cheatham ML, Becker DP. Atlas of Cranial Base Surgery. Philadelphia, WB Saunders, 1995.
2. Som PM, Curtin HD. Neck; orbit and visual pathways; skull base and temporal bone. In Head and Neck Imaging, Vol. 2, 3rd ed., pp. 1292–1293. St. Louis, Mosby–Year Book, 1996.
3. Harnsberger HR. Handbook of Head and Neck Imaging, 2nd ed., pp. 417–420. St. Louis, Mosby–Year Book, 1995.
4. Osborn AG. Diagnostic Neuroradiology, pp. 509–510. St. Louis, Mosby–Year Book, 1994.
5. Som PM, Curtin HD. Neck; orbit and visual pathways; skull base and temporal bone. In Head and Neck Imaging, Vol. 2, 3rd ed., pp. 1441–1446. St. Louis, Mosby–Year Book, 1996.
6. Isselbacher KJ, et al. Harrison's Principals of Internal Medicine, 13th ed., pp. 2105–2195. New York, McGraw-Hill, 1994.
7. Nager GT. Paget's disease of the temporal bone. Ann Otol Rhinol Laryngol 1975;84(Suppl 22):1–32.
8. Kelly JK, Denier JE, Wilner HI, et al. MR imaging of lytic changes in Paget disease of the calvarium. J Comput Assist Tomogr 1989;13:27–29.
9. Resnick D, Niwayama G. Diagnosis of Bone and Joint Disorders, Vol. 6, pp. 4057–4103. Philadelphia, WB Saunders, 1988.
10. Daffner RH, Kirks DR, Gehweiler JA Jr, et al. Computed tomography of fibrous dysplasia. AJR 1982;139:943–946.
11. Fries JW. The roentgen features of fibrous dysplasia of the skull and facial bones. AJR 1957;77:71–75.
12. Leeds NE, Seaman WB. Fibrous dysplasia of the skull and its differential diagnosis. Radiology 1962;78:570–578.
13. Casselman JW, DeJonge I, Neyt L, et al. MRI in craniofacial fibrous dysplasia. Neuroradiology 1993;35:234–237.
14. Harnsberger HR. Handbook of Head and Neck Imaging, 2nd ed. St. Louis, Mosby–Year Book, 1995.
15. Beighton P, Durr L, Hamersma H. Clinical features of sclerosteosis: A review of the manifestations in 25 affected individuals. Ann Intern Med 1976;84:393–397.
16. Beighton P, Hamersma H, Horan F. Craniometaphyseal dysplasia: Variability of expression within a large family. Clin Genet 1979;15:252–258.
17. Som PM, Curtin HD. Midface and sinonasal cavities; mandible and temporomandibular joints; upper aerodigestive tract. In Head and Neck Imaging, Vol. 1, 3rd ed., pp. 263–286. St. Louis, Mosby–Year Book, 1996.
18. Stanley RB Jr. Maxillofacial trauma. In Cummings CW, Fredrickson JM, Harker LA, et al. (eds). Otolaryngology–Head and Neck Surgery, 2nd ed., pp. 374–402. St. Louis, Mosby–Year Book, 1993.
19. Schwenzer N, Kruger E. Midface fracture. In Kruger E, Schilli W, Worthington P (eds). Oral and Maxillofacial Traumatology, Vol. 2, pp. 107–136. Chicago, Quintessence, 1986.
20. Harnsberger HR. Handbook of Head and Neck Imaging, 2nd ed., pp. 415–416. St. Louis, Mosby–Year Book, 1995.
21. Brant-Zawadzki MN, Minagi H, Federle MP, et al. High-resolution CT with image reformation in maxillofacial pathology. AJR 1982;138:477–483.
22. Zilkha A. Computed tomography in facial trauma. Radiology 1982;144:545–548.
23. Zimmerman RA, Bilaniuk LT, Hackney DB, et al. Paranasal sinus hemorrhage: Evaluation with MR imaging. Radiology 1987;162:499–503.
24. Manson PN, Markowitz B, Mirvis S, et al. Toward CT-based facial fracture treatment. Plast Reconstr Surg 1990;85:202–212.
25. Valvassori GE, Hord GE. Traumatic sinus disease. Semin Roentgenol 1968;3:160–171.
26. Sibbitt R, Orrison WW Jr, Wicks JD, Moradian G. Precise localization of CSF leaks by MRI. J Magn Reson Imaging 1987;5:120.
27. Som PM, Curtin HD. Neck; orbit and visual pathways; skull base and temporal bone. In Head and Neck Imaging, Vol. 2, 3rd ed., pp. 1260–1265. St. Louis, Mosby–Year Book, 1996.
28. Barnes L, Kapadia SB. The biology and pathology of selected skull base tumors. J Neurooncol 1994;20:213–240.
29. Batsakis JG. Vasoformative tumors. In Tumors of the Head and Neck: Clinical and Pathological Considerations, 2nd ed., pp. 297–327. Baltimore, Williams & Wilkins, 1979.
30. Orrison WW Jr. Introduction to Neuroimaging, p. 48. Boston, Little, Brown, 1989.
31. Osborn AG. Diagnostic Neuroradiology, p. 491. St. Louis, Mosby–Year Book, 1994.
32. Som PM, Curtin HD. Neck; orbit and visual pathways; skull base and temporal bone. In Head and Neck Imaging, Vol. 2, 3rd ed., p. 945. St. Louis, Mosby–Year Book, 1996.
33. Osborn AG. Diagnostic Neuroradiology, p. 883. St. Louis, Mosby–Year Book, 1994.
34. Albrecht S, Crutchfield JS, Segall GK. On spinal osteochondromas. J Neurosurg 1992;77:247–252.
35. Som PM, Curtin HD. Neck; orbit and visual pathways; skull base and temporal bone. In Head and Neck Imaging, Vol. 2, 3rd ed., pp. 1491–1492. St. Louis, Mosby–Year Book, 1996.
36. Dorwart RH, LaMasters DL, Watanabe TJ. Tumors. In Newton TH, Potts DG (eds). Computed Tomography of the Spine and Spinal Cord, pp. 115–147. San Anselmo, CA, Clavadel, 1983.
37. Aoki J, Moriya K, Yamashita K, et al. Giant cell tumors of bone containing large amounts of hemosiderin: MR-pathologic correlation. J Comput Assist Tomogr 1991;15:1024–1027.
38. Post MJD. Primary spine and cord neoplasms. In Categorical Course on Spine and Cord Imaging, pp. 58–70. American Society of Neuroradiology, 1988.
39. Myers EN, Suen JY. Cancer of the Head and Neck, 3rd ed., p. 35. Philadelphia, WB Saunders, 1996.
40. Som PM, Curtin HD. Neck; orbit and visual pathways; skull base and temporal bone. In Head and Neck Imaging, Vol. 2, 3rd ed., pp. 1276–1277. St. Louis, Mosby–Year Book, 1996.
41. Lee YY, Van Tassel P, Navert C, et al. Craniofacial osteosarcomas: Plain film, CT, and MR findings: 46 cases. AJNR 1988;9:379–385.
42. DePena CA, Lee YY, Van Tassel P. Lymphomatous involvement of the trigeminal nerve and Meckel's cave: CT and MR appearance. AJNR 1989;10:515–517.
43. Parker GD, Harnsberger HR. Clinical-radiologic issues in perineural tumor spread of malignant diseases of the extracranial head and neck. Radiographics 1991;11:383–399.
44. Myers EN, Suen JY. Cancer of the Head and Neck, 3rd ed., pp. 664–665. Philadelphia, WB Saunders, 1996.
45. Som PM, Curtin HD. Neck; orbit and visual pathways; skull base and temporal bone. In Head and Neck Imaging, Vol. 2, 3rd ed., pp. 1517–1518. St. Louis, Mosby–Year Book, 1996.
46. Willman CL, Busque L, Griffith BB, et al. Langerhans'-cell histiocytosis (histiocytosis X): A clonal proliferative disease. N Engl J Med 1994;331:154–160.
47. Stool SE, Goodman ML. A 13-year-old boy with a destructive lesion of the left mastoid bone. N Engl J Med 1991;324:1489–1495.
48. Shelby JH, Sweet RM. Eosinophilic granuloma of the temporal bone: Medical and surgical management in the pediatric patient. South Med J 1983;76:65–70.
49. Nezelof C, Frederique FH, Cronier-Sachot J. Disseminated histiocytosis X: Analysis of prognostic factors based on a retrospective study of 50 cases. Cancer 1979;44:1824–1838.
50. Cunningham MJ, Curtin HD, Butkiewicz BL. Histiocytosis X of the temporal bone: CT findings. J Comput Assist Tomogr 1988;12:70–74.
51. Bonafe A, Joomye H, Jaeger P, et al. Histiocytosis X of the petrous bone in the adult: MRI. Neuroradiology 1994;36:330–333.

52. Sampson JH, Rossitch E Jr, Young JN, et al. Solitary eosinophilic granuloma invading the clivus of an adult. Neurosurgery 1992;31:755–758.
53. Caresio JF, McMillan H, Batnitzky S. Coexistent intra- and extracranial mass lesions: An unusual manifestation of histiocytosis X. AJNR 1991;12:80–81.
54. De Schepper AMA, Ramon F, Van Marck E. MR imaging of eosinophilic granuloma: Report of 11 cases. Skeletal Radiol 1993;22:163–166.
55. Laine FJ, Nadel L, Braun IF. CT and MR imaging of the central skull base. Radiographics 1990;10:797–821.
56. Som PM, Curtin HD. Head and Neck Imaging, Vol. 2, 3rd ed., pp. 808–809. St. Louis, Mosby–Year Book, 1996.
57. Barnes L, Peel RL, Verbin RS. Tumors of the nervous system. In Barnes L (ed). Surgical Pathology of the Head and Neck, pp. 659–724. New York, Marcel Dekker, 1985.
58. Som PM, Curtin HD. Head and Neck Imaging, Vol. 2, 3rd ed., pp. 932–936. St. Louis, Mosby–Year Book, 1996.
59. Mulligan RM. Chemodectoma in the dog. [Abstract] Am J Pathol 1950;26:690.
60. Zak FG, Lawson W. The Paraganglionic Chemoreceptor System: Physiology, Pathology, and Clinical Medicine, pp. 287–411. New York, Springer-Verlag, 1982.
61. Valavanis A, Schubiger O, Naidich TP. Clinical Imaging of the Cerebellopontine Angle, pp. 30–172. New York, Springer-Verlag, 1986.
62. Kaye AH, Hahn JF, Kinney SE, et al. Jugular foramen schwannomas. J Neurosurg 1984;60:1045–1053.
63. Dolan EJ, Tucker WS, Rotenberg D, et al. Intracranial hypoglossal schwannoma on an unusual cause of facial nerve palsy. J Neurosurg 1982;56:420–423.
64. Fugiwara S, Hachisuga S, Numaguchi Y. Intracranial hypoglossal neurinoma: Report of a case. Neuroradiology 1980;20:87–90.
65. Horn KL, House WF, Hitselberger WE. Schwannomas of the jugular foramen. Laryngoscope 1985;95:761–765.
66. Di Chiro G, Fisher RL, Nelson KB. The jugular foramen. J Neurosurg 1964;21:447–460.
67. Valvassori GE, Kirdani HA. The abnormal hypoglossal canal. AJR 1967;99:705–711.
68. Pritchard DJ, Lunke RJ, Taylor WF, et al. Chondrosarcoma: A clinicopathologic and statistical analysis. Cancer 1980;45:149–152.
69. Jones HM. Cartilaginous tumors of the head and neck. J Laryngol Otol 1973;87:135–138.
70. Lee YY, Van Tassel P. Craniofacial chondrosarcomas: Imaging findings in 15 untreated cases. AJNR 1989;10:165–171.
71. Guccion JG, Font RL, Enziger FM, et al. Extraskeletal mesenchymal chondrosarcoma. Arch Pathol 1973;95:336–337.
72. Brown E, Hug EB, Weber AL. Chondrosarcoma of the skull base. Neuroimaging Clin N Am 1994;4:529–541.
73. Osborn AG. Diagnostic Neuroradiology, p. 505. St. Louis, Mosby–Year Book, 1994.
74. Meyers SP, Hirsch WL Jr, Curtin HD, et al. Chondrosarcomas of the skull base: MR imaging features. Radiology 1992;184:103–108.
75. Burger PC, Scheihauer BW. Atlas of Tumor Pathology. Tumors of the Central Nervous System. Washington, DC, Armed Forces Institute of Pathology, 1994.
76. Mabrey RE. Chordoma: A study of 150 cases. Am J Cancer 1935;25:501–506.
77. Batsakis JG, Kittleson AC. Chordomas: Otorhinolaryngologic presentation and diagnosis. Arch Otolaryngol 1963;78:168–172.
78. Batsakis JG. Soft tissue tumors of the head and neck: Unusual forms. In Tumors of the Head and Neck: Clinical Considerations, 2nd ed., pp. 353–385. Baltimore, Williams & Wilkins, 1979.
79. Krol G, Sundaresan N, Deck M. Computed tomography of axial chordomas. J Comput Assist Tomogr 1983;7:286–290.
80. Weber AL, Liebsch NJ, Sanchez R, et al. Chordomas of the skull base: Radiologic and clinical evaluation. Neuroimaging Clin N Am 1994;4:515–527.
81. Firooznia H, Pinto RS, Lin JP, et al. Chordoma: Radiologic evaluation of 20 cases. AJR 1976;127:797–799.
82. Sze G, Uichanco LS III, Brant-Zawadzki MN, et al. Chordomas: MR imaging. Radiology 1988;166:187–191.
83. Meyers SP, Hirsch WL Jr, Curtin HD, et al. Chordomas of the skull base: MR features. AJNR 1992;13:1627–1636.
84. Oot RF, Melville GE, New PFJ, et al. The role of MR and CT in evaluating clival chordomas and chondrosarcomas. AJNR 1988;9:715–723.
85. Davidson HC. Head and Neck Digital Teaching File. Salt Lake City, Electronic Medical Education Resource Group, 1999.
86. Glastonbury CM. Head and Neck Digital Teaching File. Salt Lake City, Electronic Medical Education Resource Group, 1999.
87. Chong BW. Head and Neck Digital Teaching File. Salt Lake City, Electronic Medical Education Resource Group, 1999.
88. Orrison WW. Head and Neck Digital Teaching File. Salt Lake City, Electronic Medical Education Resource Group, 1999.

C H A P T E R

30

The Orbit and Visual System

RAYMOND F. CARMODY, M.D.

The visual apparatus represents a complex and highly specialized portion of the central nervous system with its own unique anatomy and physiology. The disease processes affecting the orbit and visual system are numerous and present a formidable challenge to the neuroradiologist. Whereas the globe, conjunctiva, and optic disk can be inspected by direct vision, the remainder of the orbit and visual pathways is much more amenable to neuroimaging techniques. In this chapter, we review the anatomy of the visual system and the radiologic manifestations of diseases affecting this area. Since computed tomography (CT) and magnetic resonance imaging (MRI) are the mainstays of orbital radiology, most of the discussion focuses on these modalities.

IMAGING TECHNIQUES

Although MRI is clearly superior to CT for imaging most of the central nervous system, both modalities are well suited for use in the orbit. CT is capable of producing excellent images because of the natural contrast provided by retrobulbar fat, bone, and air in the adjacent paranasal sinuses. Conversely, MRI offers multiplanar capabilities, no ionizing radiation to the lens, and better soft tissue discrimination than CT. Moreover, MRI is far better than CT for depicting the intracanalicular optic nerves, chiasm, and posterior visual pathways.

Computed Tomography

In most cases, both axial and coronal slices should be obtained. Axial slices are done parallel to the anthropologic baseline (inferior orbital rim to external auditory meatus), since this line is roughly parallel to the long axis of the orbit (Fig. 30–1). Contiguous 3-mm slices are ideal for screening purposes. Thinner (1 to 2 mm) slices can be obtained through the optic canal when fine detail is needed. Coronal images are obtained as close to perpendicular to the baseline as possible, but they are angled to avoid spray artifact from dental fillings (Fig. 30–2). In patients who cannot tolerate the coronal position, thin-section helical CT is a suitable alternative, since excellent coronal re-formations are possible. Iodinated contrast material is not always necessary but is used when evaluating orbital masses, vascular lesions, or intracranial extension

of orbital disease processes. Because of the wider range of densities present, soft tissue images of the orbit are filmed at wider windows than those used for brain. Window widths of 300 to 400 Hounsfield units work well. The images are also filmed at bone window settings.

Magnetic Resonance Imaging

Coil Selection

The choice of receiver coil depends in part on what the primary area of interest is. For high anatomic detail of the orbit or globe, a 7.5-cm surface coil provides excellent resolution, on the order of 0.3-mm pixel size if a 256 × 256 matrix and 8-cm field of view are used.[1, 2] With phased-array coils, both orbits can be imaged simultaneously without compromising signal-to-noise. The strong signal from these coils allows short imaging times, which helps to reduce eye motion artifact. Using dual 12.7-cm phased-array coils and a 14- to 16-cm field of view, Breslau and coworkers were able to obtain excellent, high signal-to-noise images of the entire anterior visual pathway, including the chiasm.[3] Disadvantages of surface coils are their high sensitivity to eye motion and the dropoff in signal posterior to the orbital apex and chiasm. Moreover, structures close to the receiver coil may appear excessively bright owing to the high signal, sometimes obscuring detail.

With some loss of resolution, the quadrature head coil can image the entire visual pathway on the same sequence. Pixel size is in the range of 0.9 mm,[4] which is usually adequate for screening purposes for retrobulbar, chiasmal, and posterior visual pathway lesions. Since the field of view is larger and the signal is weaker, more excitations must be done to obtain a satisfactory signal-to-noise ratio. Hence, imaging times are longer, increasing the potential problem of patient motion.

MRI Sequences

T1-weighted spin-echo images provide the best anatomic detail of the orbit and should be obtained in at least two planes (Table 30–1 and Figs. 30–3 and 30–4).[5] If the head coil is used, we typically perform axial and coronal T1-weighted images with 3- to 4-mm slice thickness, interleaved or 1-mm interslice gap. The TR and TE used depend on the type and field strength of the scanner; two

Text continued on page 1015

1009

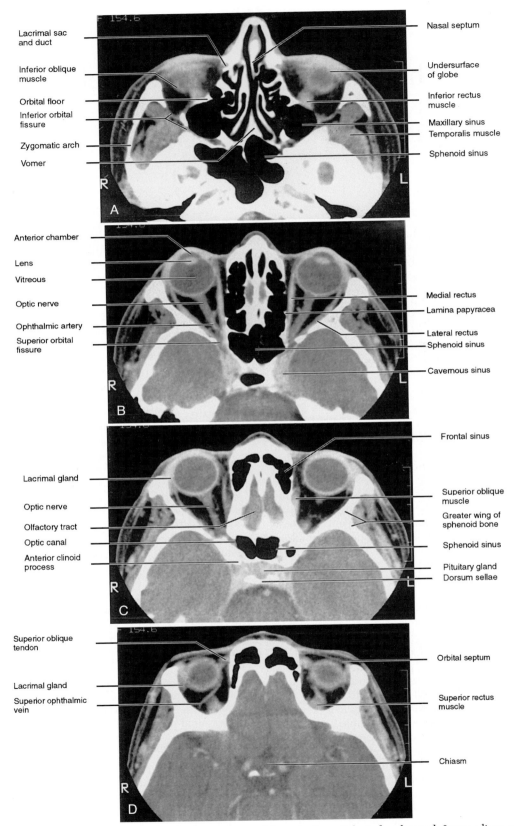

Lacrimal sac and duct
Inferior oblique muscle
Orbital floor
Inferior orbital fissure
Zygomatic arch
Vomer

Nasal septum
Undersurface of globe
Inferior rectus muscle
Maxillary sinus
Temporalis muscle
Sphenoid sinus

R   L   A

Anterior chamber
Lens
Vitreous
Optic nerve
Ophthalmic artery
Superior orbital fissure

Medial rectus
Lamina papyracea
Lateral rectus
Sphenoid sinus
Cavernous sinus

R   L   B

Lacrimal gland
Optic nerve
Olfactory tract
Optic canal
Anterior clinoid process

Frontal sinus
Superior oblique muscle
Greater wing of sphenoid bone
Sphenoid sinus
Pituitary gland
Dorsum sellae

R   L   C

Superior oblique tendon
Lacrimal gland
Superior ophthalmic vein

Orbital septum
Superior rectus muscle
Chiasm

R   L   D

FIGURE 30–1 Normal computed tomography (CT) anatomy, axial projection. Selected enhanced 2-mm slices progressing from inferior (*A*) to superior (*D*).

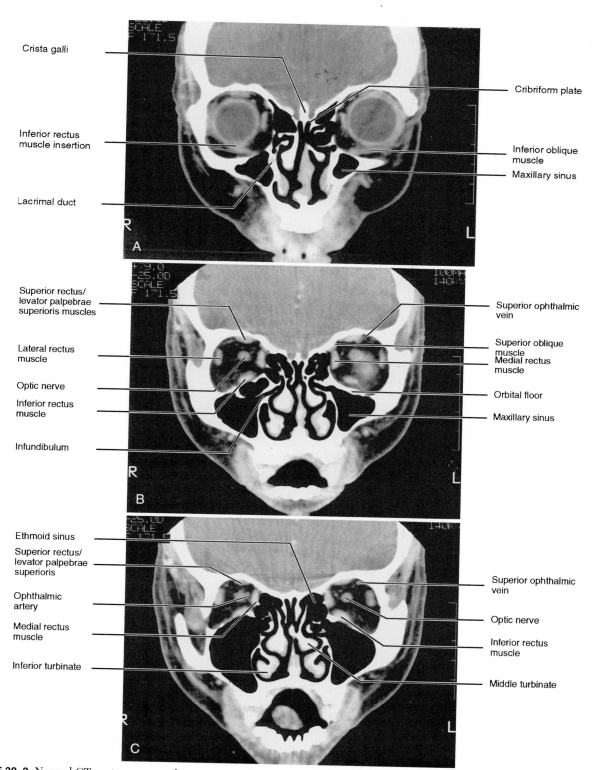

FIGURE 30–2 Normal CT anatomy, coronal projection. Selected enhanced 2-mm slices progressing from anterior (*A*) to posterior (*C*).

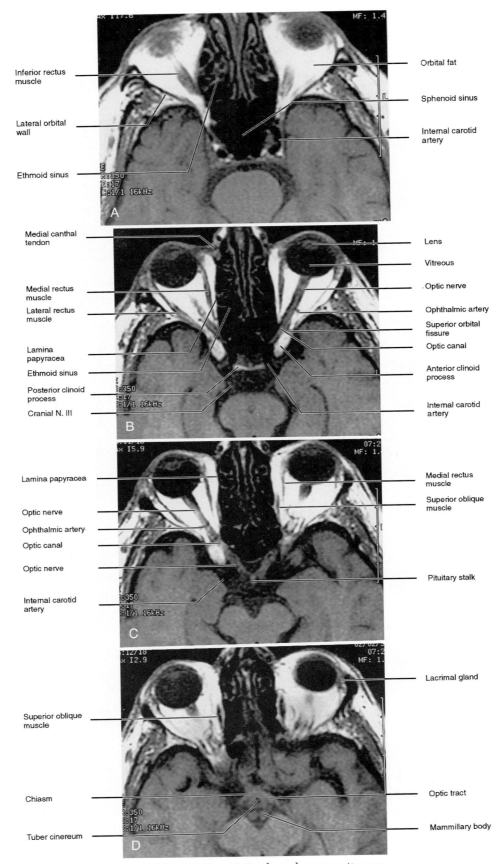

Inferior rectus muscle

Lateral orbital wall

Ethmoid sinus

Orbital fat

Sphenoid sinus

Internal carotid artery

Medial canthal tendon

Medial rectus muscle

Lateral rectus muscle

Lamina papyracea

Ethmoid sinus

Posterior clinoid process

Cranial N. III

Lens

Vitreous

Optic nerve

Ophthalmic artery

Superior orbital fissure

Optic canal

Anterior clinoid process

Internal carotid artery

Lamina papyracea

Optic nerve

Ophthalmic artery

Optic canal

Optic nerve

Internal carotid artery

Medial rectus muscle

Superior oblique muscle

Pituitary stalk

Lacrimal gland

Superior oblique muscle

Chiasm

Tuber cinereum

Optic tract

Mammillary body

FIGURE 30–3 *A–D. See legend on opposite page*

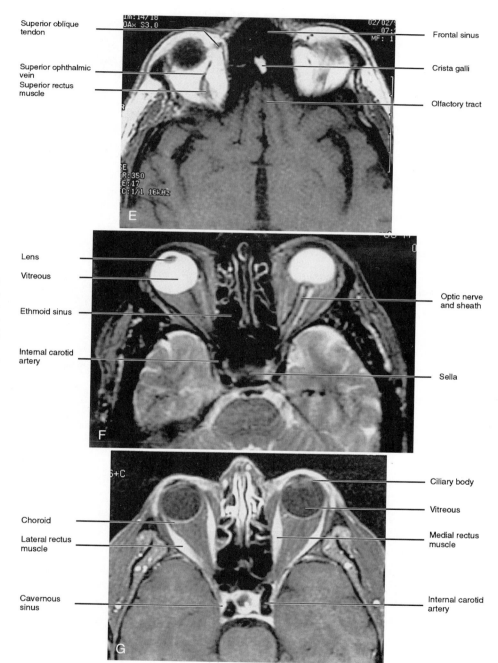

FIGURE 30–3 Normal magnetic resonance imaging (MRI) anatomy, axial projection. *A–E,* Selected 3-mm T1-weighted spin-echo (SE) images progressing from anterior *(A)* to posterior *(E)*. *F,* T2-weighted image at the level of the optic nerves. *G,* Gadolinium-enhanced, fat-suppressed T1-weighted image.

Superior oblique tendon

Superior ophthalmic vein

Superior rectus muscle

Frontal sinus

Crista galli

Olfactory tract

Lens

Vitreous

Ethmoid sinus

Internal carotid artery

Optic nerve and sheath

Sella

Choroid

Lateral rectus muscle

Cavernous sinus

Ciliary body

Vitreous

Medial rectus muscle

Internal carotid artery

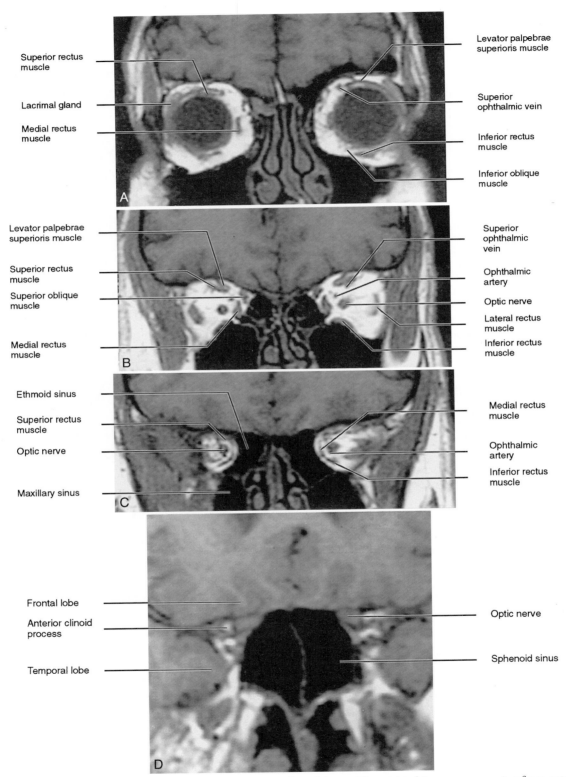

Superior rectus muscle

Lacrimal gland

Medial rectus muscle

Levator palpebrae superioris muscle

Superior ophthalmic vein

Inferior rectus muscle

Inferior oblique muscle

A

Levator palpebrae superioris muscle

Superior rectus muscle

Superior oblique muscle

Medial rectus muscle

Superior ophthalmic vein

Ophthalmic artery

Optic nerve

Lateral rectus muscle

Inferior rectus muscle

B

Ethmoid sinus

Superior rectus muscle

Optic nerve

Maxillary sinus

Medial rectus muscle

Ophthalmic artery

Inferior rectus muscle

C

Frontal lobe

Anterior clinoid process

Temporal lobe

Optic nerve

Sphenoid sinus

D

FIGURE 30–4 Normal MRI anatomy, coronal projection. *A–D*, Selected 3-mm T1-weighted images progressing from anterior *(A)* to posterior *(D)*.

TABLE 30–1 Orbital Magnetic Resonance Imaging Technique: Head Coil

T1-weighted image sagittal
    TR 500, TE minimum
    256 × 192 matrix, 5-mm slice thickness, skip 2
    22 cm FOV, 1 NEX, 2 min
T1-weighted image axial
    TR 450, TE minimum
    256 × 192 matrix, 3-mm thick, interleaved
    22 cm FOV, 2 NEX, 4.5 min
PD (or FLAIR), T2-weighted image axial
    TR 2400, TE 17/102
    256 × 192 matrix, 5-mm thick, interleaved
    22 cm FOV, 3 NEX, 4 min
    Include brain
T1-weighted image axial and coronal fat-suppressed,
        gadolinium-enhanced
    TR 400, TE minimum
    256 × 192 matrix, 3-mm thick, interleaved
    18 cm FOV, 2 NEX, 4.5 min

Abbreviations: FOV, field of view; NEX, number of excitations; PD, proton density; FLAIR, fluid attenuated inversion recovery.

to four excitations are done, with 265 × 192 matrix. A sagittal T1-weighted sequence of the entire head is also performed. A long-TR/long-TE axial sequence is obtained, usually fast spin echo with fat suppression. The T2-weighted images are also used to screen the entire brain for additional lesions, such as tumor or demyelinating disease. In most cases, these sequences are followed by gadolinium–diethylenetriaminepenta-acetic acid (DTPA)–enhanced, fat-suppressed axial and coronal images. During the scan acquisition, the patient is asked to fixate gaze at a particular point, preferably straight ahead, with the eyes open.

If surface or paired phased-array coils are used, finer matrices (256 × 256 or 256 × 512) can be used with a smaller field of view without inordinately lengthy acquisition times. Additional sequences are obtained, such as oblique sagittal T1-weighted images, along the axis of the optic nerve.

ANATOMY

Bony Orbit

The orbit is a cone-shaped structure with somewhat flattened sides. The orbital apices are directed medially, with the lateral walls forming an angle of approximately 90 degrees with each other. The thin medial wall is formed by the lesser wing of the sphenoid posteriorly, the lamina papyracea of the ethmoid in the midportion, the lacrimal bone anteriorly, and the frontal process of the maxilla in its most anterior portion. The roof consists of the orbital plate of the frontal bone. The greater wing of the sphenoid and the superior portion of the zygoma form the lateral wall. Most of the orbital floor is made up of the maxillary bone, and the anterolateral portion is formed by the zygomatic bone. The palatine bone forms a tiny portion of the floor near the apex.

Superior Orbital Fissure

The superior orbital fissure is bounded by the lesser wing of the sphenoid medially and the greater wing laterally, and it connects the orbit with the middle cranial fossa. Through it pass a number of important nerves and vessels: the oculomotor, trochlear, and abducens nerves; the lacrimal, frontal, and nasociliary branches of the ophthalmic division of cranial nerve V; and the superior ophthalmic vein.

Optic Canal

The optic canal lies medial to the superior orbital fissure and is separated from it by a short plate of bone known as the *optic strut* (Fig. 30–5). The canal is typically 8 to 10 mm in length and 4.5 to 6 mm in diameter. Through it pass the optic nerve with its three meningeal coverings, the ophthalmic artery, and some sympathetic nerves.

Inferior Orbital Fissure

The inferior orbital fissure separates the lateral wall of the orbit from the floor posteriorly, and it connects the orbit with the pterygopalatine and infratemporal fossae. Through it course the infraorbital nerve and artery and some venous connections between the inferior ophthalmic vein and the pterygoid plexus.

Periosteum

The bony orbit has a periosteal lining referred to as the *periorbita*. In the posterior aspect of the orbit, the periorbita is connected with the dura through the fissures and optic canal. Anteriorly it blends in with the periosteum of the facial bones at the orbital rim to form the *arcus marginalis*. From the arcus marginalis arises a vertical band of fibrous tissue, the *orbital septum*. The septum extends from the arcus marginalis to insert into the levator aponeurosis of the upper lid and into the tarsal plate of the lower lid. The compartment anterior to the septum is called the *preseptal space*, and posterior to it is the *postseptal space*. Although it is difficult to visualize by CT, the orbital septum can be seen on sagittal T1-weighted MRI with appropriate windows (Fig. 30–6).

The Extraocular Muscles

Six muscles control eye movement. The four rectus muscles take origin from a tendinous ring surrounding the optic nerve in the posterior orbit, the *annulus of Zinn*.[6] They insert into the sclera anterior to the equator of the globe (Figs. 30–7 and 30–8). Connecting the four rectus muscles is an incomplete intermuscular membrane, combining to form the *muscle cone* (Fig. 30–8). The fat-filled space inside the muscle cone is designated the *intraconal compartment,* and outside it is the smaller *extraconal compartment.*

The superior oblique muscle arises from the orbital apex where it is attached both to the sphenoid bone and to the tendinous origin of the medial rectus. It courses anteriorly along the medial orbital wall superior to the medial rectus, and its tendon passes through a cartilaginous ring, the *trochlea.* The superior oblique tendon then turns posterolaterally and inferiorly to insert on the sclera

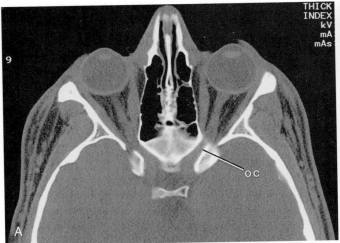

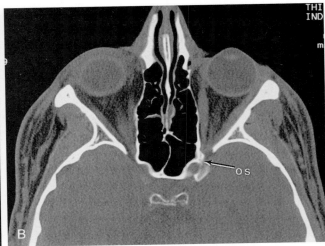

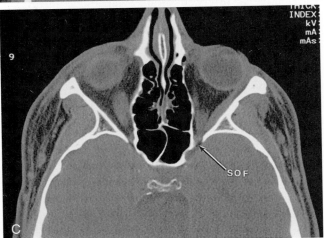

FIGURE 30–5 Normal axial thin-section CT to illustrate the bony anatomy of the orbital apex. *A–C,* Slices progressing from inferior *(A)* to superior *(C)*. OC, optic canal; OS, optic strut; SOF, superior orbital fissure.

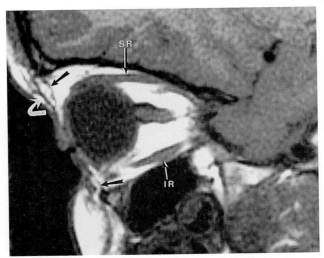

FIGURE 30–6 Normal MRI of the orbit, T1-weighted image, sagittal view. *Black arrows* indicate the orbital septum. *White arrow* indicates the orbicularis oculi muscle. SR, superior rectus/levator palpebrae superioris muscles; IR, inferior rectus muscle.

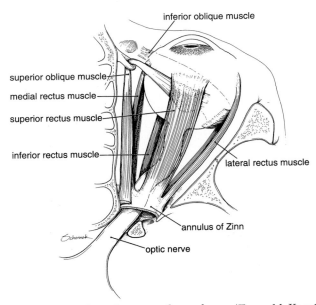

FIGURE 30–7 The orbit, seen from above. (From McKenzie JD, Drayer BP. Computed tomography and magnetic resonance imaging of the orbits. BNI Q 1993;9:35–45.)

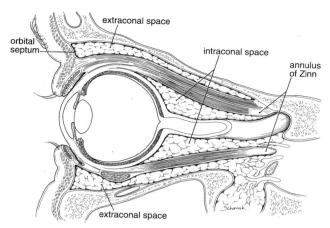

FIGURE 30–8 Sagittal view of the orbit. Note the intraconal and extraconal spaces and the position of the orbital septum. (From McKenzie JD, Drayer BP. Computed tomography and magnetic resonance imaging of the orbits. BNI Q 1993;9:35–45.)

under the superior rectus tendon. The inferior oblique muscle has its origin in the anteromedial aspect of the orbit, lateral to the nasolacrimal canal in the upper maxilla. It courses laterally, posteriorly, and superiorly between the inferior rectus tendon and the floor of the orbit to insert on the sclera behind the equator of the globe.

The levator palpebrae superioris muscle originates from the lesser wing of the sphenoid and runs anteriorly under the orbital roof to insert into the tarsal plate of the upper lid. Its function is to elevate the eyelid. Immediately beneath the levator muscle is the superior rectus, and below the superior rectus is the superior ophthalmic vein (see Fig. 30–4).

Innervation of the Extraocular Muscles

The superior, medial, and inferior recti and the inferior oblique and the levator palpebrae superioris muscles are innervated by the oculomotor nerve (cranial nerve III). This nerve also sends parasympathetic fibers to the constrictor pupillae and ciliary muscles. The sole function of the trochlear nerve (cranial nerve IV) is to supply the superior oblique muscle. The abducens nerve (cranial nerve VI) innervates the lateral rectus muscle.

Imaging Features

The extraocular muscles are readily depicted by both CT and MRI. With CT, the superior and inferior recti are not optimally seen on axial sections, and they are better defined on coronal sections (see Fig. 30–2). Coronal T1-weighted MRI nicely demonstrates all six muscles, which appear as intermediate signal intensity, surrounded by hyperintense fat (see Fig. 30–4). On gadolinium-enhanced, fat-suppressed T1-weighted images, the extraocular muscles enhance intensely (see Figs. 30–3 and 30–6). Without fat suppression, the enhancing muscles tend to be obscured by the fat.

The Globe

The globe is approximately 25 mm in diameter and is constructed of three primary layers. The outermost layer,

the *sclera*, is composed of collagenous tissue (Fig. 30–9). It extends from the margin (limbus) of the cornea anteriorly to the optic nerve posteriorly, where it is continuous with the dura. The middle layer is the *choroid*, which is predominantly vascular tissue; its main function is vascular supply to the globe and temperature regulation. The choroid, iris, and ciliary body form the *uveal tract*. Melanocytes are found throughout the uveal tract. The innermost layer of the eye can be subdivided into two main parts: the inner sensory retina, where the photoreceptor cells and other neural elements are found, and the outer retinal pigment epithelium.[7] The choroid forms the basement membrane for the retinal pigment epithelium. The retina extends from the ora serrata anteriorly to the optic nerve head posteriorly. Another connective tissue layer, *Tenon's capsule,* is present external to the sclera. This fibroelastic membrane envelopes the posterior four-fifths of the globe and also reflects back over the insertions of the rectus muscles and optic nerve. A potential space exists between the sclera and Tenon's capsule, called either the *episcleral space* or *Tenon's space*.

The lens and its attachments (zonular fibers and ciliary body) separate the anteriorly located aqueous humor from the much larger and posteriorly located vitreous body. Anterior to the lens is the iris. The space between the iris and the cornea is the *anterior chamber,* and the smaller space between the iris and the lens is the *posterior chamber* (see Fig. 30–9).

Imaging Features

The vitreous body, being about 98% water, is water density on CT. On MRI, it is isointense to cerebrospinal fluid on all sequences. The lens is only 66% water, the rest of it being protein. It is dense on CT, relatively hyperintense on T1-weighted images, and hypointense on T2-weighted images (Fig. 30–10). The dark signal on T2-weighted images results from the highly ordered nature of the lens protein, which restricts water mobility and accelerates dephasing of protons.[8]

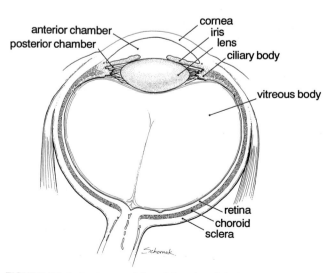

FIGURE 30–9 Anatomy of the globe. (Modified from McKenzie JD, Drayer BP. Computed tomography and magnetic resonance imaging of the orbits. BNI Q 1993;9:35–45.)

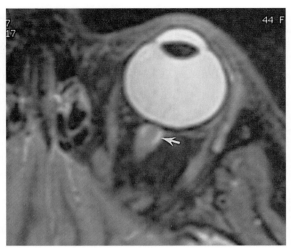

FIGURE 30–10 Normal MRI of the globe. Fast short-tau inversion recovery (STIR) sequence, 6-inch phased-array coil. The aqueous and vitreous humor have high signal owing to their high water content. The lens has low signal. Note cerebrospinal fluid in the optic nerve sheath *(arrow)*. (Courtesy of Kenneth Maravilla, M.D., University of Washington.)

The Optic Nerve

In its course from the posterior globe to the chiasm, the optic nerve has an intraorbital segment, about 25 mm in length, a 4- to 9-mm intracanalicular segment, and an intracranial segment about 10 mm long. The optic nerve is composed mainly of axons of secondary sensory neurons whose cell bodies reside in the retina. Hence, its MRI signal intensity parallels that of white matter. The intraorbital segment of the optic nerve has an undulating course to facilitate eye motion[9] (see Fig. 30–7). All three meningeal layers invest the nerve, and the subarachnoid space surrounding it is in direct connection with the intracranial subarachnoid space.[10] The clinical significance of this is that disease processes that affect the intracranial subarachnoid compartment, such as meningitis or leptomeningeal carcinomatosis, can also spread to the optic nerve sheath. On MRI, cerebrospinal fluid can usually be seen surrounding the nerve, particularly on coronal images. The diameter of the optic nerve is variable, but typically it is about 3 to 4 mm.

The dura investing the nerve blends in with the periosteal lining of the optic canal. Since the nerve is rather tightly confined by its bony covering while it traverses the optic canal, it is especially vulnerable to trauma in this area. Medially the intracanalicular optic nerve is in close proximity to the posterior ethmoid air cells and sphenoid sinus,[11] and compression from sinus disease is possible. Moreover, great potential exists for optic nerve injury during endoscopic sinus surgery because of these anatomic relationships.

The ophthalmic artery, which originates from the supraclinoid portion of the internal carotid, passes through the optic canal along the undersurface of the nerve. Once inside the orbit, the ophthalmic artery loops over the nerve from lateral to medial in roughly 85% of the cases, and under it in the remainder. From here, it divides into its various branches, after giving off the central retinal artery.

TABLE 30–2 Extraconal Lesions

Extraorbital Origin

Sinus tumors
Mucocele
Metastasis, myeloma
Histiocytosis
Fibrous dysplasia
Middle fossa meningioma
Capillary hemangioma
Wegener's granulomatosis

Intraorbital Origin

Infection (cellulitis, abscess)
Inflammatory pseudotumor
Sarcoid
Dermoid
Metastasis
Lymphoma, leukemia
Lymphangioma
Lacrimal gland lesions (see Table 30–10)
Epithelial cyst
Hematoma, hematic cyst
Rhabdomyosarcoma
Lacrimal sac lesions
Lipoma

The Lacrimal Gland

The lacrimal gland is located in the superolateral anterior orbit in the lacrimal gland fossa. The aponeurosis of the levator palpebrae superioris divides the gland into two parts: a larger orbital portion and a smaller palpebral portion. The superior surface of the gland is in contact with the periorbitum. On CT scans, the gland is readily seen as a moderate-density structure bordered by hypodense fat. On MRI, the lacrimal gland is clearly demonstrated on T1-weighted images as an area of intermediate signal intensity. The gland enhances prominently on contrast-enhanced CT and MRI.

IMAGING OF THE EYE AND ORBIT

In order to optimize the radiologic examination of the orbit, it is necessary to first obtain adequate clinical information. Having reliable clinical data is key to planning the appropriate imaging strategy and for developing a relevant differential diagnosis once the imaging findings are known. Regardless of whether plain radiographs, CT,

TABLE 30–3 Intraconal Lesions

Cavernous hemangioma
Optic nerve lesions (see Table 30–9)
Inflammatory pseudotumor
Metastasis
Lymphoma, leukemia
Cellulitis, abscess
Varix
Schwannoma, neurofibroma
Lymphangioma
Hematoma
Increased fat deposition (from exogenous obesity, corticosteroid therapy, Cushing's disease, Graves' disease)

or MRI is used, the examination should be tailored to the problem at hand in order that the appropriate views, slice thickness, imaging planes, and pulse sequences are selected. The decision to use intravenous contrast material is also based on the clinical situation.

Once an abnormality is recognized on an imaging study, the radiologist can use an algorithmic approach. The location is an important consideration, since certain disease processes are likely to be found in specific areas. For example, extraconal lesions have certain possibilities, as do intraconal masses (Table 30–2). When the lesion is extraconal, it is important to look for bone or periosteal involvement and to examine the adjacent paranasal sinuses as a possible source of disease. Intraconal masses lead to a different list of diagnostic possibilities, although considerable overlap exists (Table 30–3). With intraconal lesions, one should try to determine whether the optic nerve or globe is involved, either primarily or secondarily.

In addition to considering lesion location, the CT and MRI characteristics are of critical importance. Factors such as a lesion in the globe containing calcium, degrees and patterns of enhancement, T1 and T2 signal characteristics, and whether the disease process is unilateral or bilateral must all be considered. Once these questions are answered, the clinical data are again reviewed in order to

formulate a differential diagnosis. Even with a decision tree approach, the orbit is still a difficult area for the radiologist because many diseases have similar imaging findings.

In this chapter, the disease processes are grouped along anatomic lines in three broad categories: (1) abnormalities of the globe, (2) lesions of the orbit proper, and (3) disease processes affecting the optic pathways. As a general principle, most workups for a visual abnormality should image the entire visual system, from the globe to the occipital poles. This is easily and rapidly accomplished with today's technology.

LESIONS OF THE GLOBE

Abnormalities in Size or Shape

Coloboma

A coloboma is a defect, such as a notch or cleft, in the retina, choroid, iris, lens, or optic nerve due to failure of closure of the fetal optic fissure.[12] A posterior coloboma involving the globe or optic nerve is seen on CT or MRI as a funnel-shaped defect or cyst centered at the optic disk (Fig. 30–11). An associated extraocular cyst may be

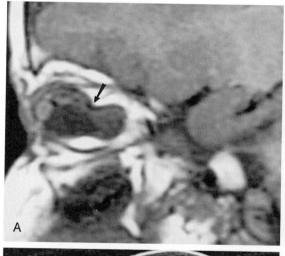
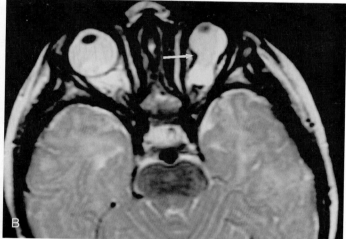
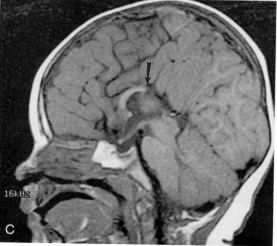

FIGURE 30–11 Coloboma with microphthalmia in an 11-month-old boy. Sagittal T1-weighted (A) and axial T2-weighted (B) images show a small right globe with a posterior defect (arrows). An associated cyst is seen posterior to the globe. C, Sagittal T1-weighted image shows dysgenesis of the corpus callosum, with absence of the posterior body (arrow).

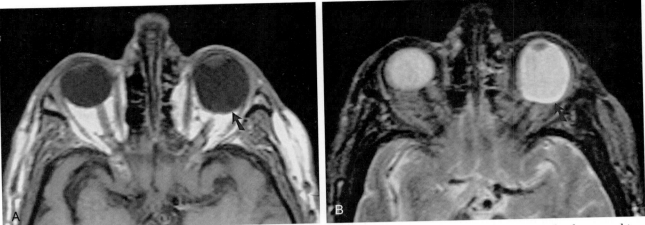

FIGURE 30–12 Staphyloma in a 65-year-old man. Axial T1-weighted (A) and T2-weighted (B) images show a focal outpouching of the posterolateral wall of the left globe (arrow in A). Axial myopia is also present, owing to the markedly elongated eye.

present. The cyst is caused by an abnormal proliferation of the neurosensory retina, which everts through the defect. Microphthalmia is often an associated feature, especially when a large extraocular cyst is present.[13] Other congenital anomalies may occur, such as encephalocele, agenesis of the corpus callosum, and olfactory dysplasia.[12] Clinically, a visual field scotoma is found, sometimes with profound visual loss.

Staphyloma

A staphyloma is a focal outpouching of the sclera or cornea. A typical location is along the posterior surface of the globe on the temporal side of the optic disk (Fig. 30–12). Staphylomas are composed of both sclera and choroid and are usually acquired defects resulting from weakening and thinning of the sclera. Scleral inflammation may be the cause (Fig. 30–13), and some are post-traumatic. Peripapillary staphylomas may be confused with colobomas. Posterior staphylomas are associated with severe myopia.[14] Choroidal and retinal detachments are common with staphylomas, and poor vision and blindness are frequent sequelae.

Macrophthalmia

An enlarged globe presents with proptosis, usually in a child. Since retinoblastoma and other intraocular masses may produce globe enlargement, it is important to exclude tumor as a cause. The most common cause of eye enlargement is axial myopia, which is an elongation of the long axis of the globe. This condition is usually idiopathic, but it has also been associated with Graves' disease and infection.[15] It may be unilateral or bilateral. Imaging studies show the globe to be elongated in the long axis and to have an oval shape (Fig. 30–14). The sclera may be thinned.

Buphthalmos refers to an enlarged eye resulting from congenital glaucoma. This form of globe enlargement is seen in childhood when the sclera is soft and pliable,[16] and rarely in adults. Buphthalmos is also seen with neurofibromatosis type 1 and Sturge-Weber syndrome.[17]

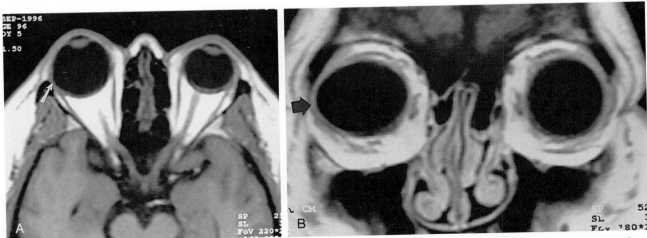

FIGURE 30–13 Staphyloma and macrophthalmia due to scleral inflammation (polyarteritis nodosa) in 56-year-old woman. A, On the axial T1-weighted image note the enlargement of the right globe with outward bulging of the sclera on the temporal side (arrow). B, Coronal T1-weighted image. Staphyloma is more apparent (arrow). (A and B, Courtesy of Norman Komar, M.D., Tucson, AZ.)

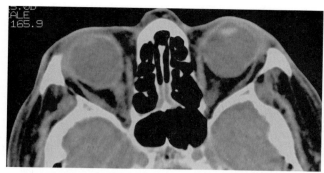

FIGURE 30–14 Bilateral axial myopia in a 72-year-old man. Axial CT demonstrates enlarged, elongated globes.

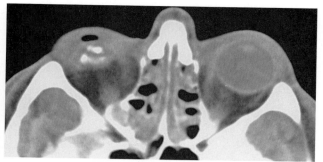

FIGURE 30–16 Phthisis bulbi in a 39-year-old man, cause unknown. CT shows a small, calcified right globe.

Connective tissue disorders such as Marfan's syndrome, Ehler-Danlos syndrome, and homocystinuria are also associated with macrophthalmia. With Marfan's syndrome, the lenses are frequently dislocated owing to weakened zonular fibers.[18]

Microphthalmia

A small globe may occur as an isolated congenital abnormality, or it may be associated with other craniofacial anomalies, such as hemifacial microsomia. Intrauterine infections, especially rubella, sometimes produce microphthalmia (Fig. 30–15). Other causes include persistent hyperplastic primary vitreous (PHPV), retinopathy of prematurity (ROP), and posterior colobomas.[19]

Phthisis Bulbi

Phthisis bulbi refers to a scarred, retracted, shrunken globe, usually with dystrophic calcification. It may be the end result of infection, trauma, noninfectious inflammation, or some other insult (Figs. 30–16 and 30–17).

Globe Trauma

Neuroimaging studies, mainly CT, can be very helpful to the ophthalmologist in the setting of acute trauma to the

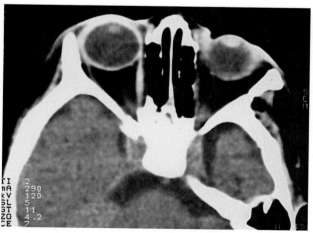

FIGURE 30–15 Microphthalmia with aniridia. CT shows a small left globe with a malformed anterior chamber. (Courtesy of Norman Komar, M.D., Tucson, AZ; From Zimmerman RA, Gibby WG, Carmody RF [eds]. Neuroimaging: Clinical and Physical Principles. New York, Springer-Verlag, 1999.)

eye. Intraocular hemorrhage into the anterior chamber (hyphema) may preclude adequate direct inspection of the globe. Penetrating foreign bodies need to be accurately localized, so that appropriate treatment can be initiated. CT is the procedure of choice for localization of metallic foreign bodies (Fig. 30–18); MRI is contraindicated in this setting because the magnetic field may induce movement of the particle and cause intraocular hemorrhage. Thin-section axial and coronal CT is the best means of determining whether the fragment is still inside the globe or whether it has passed into the retrobulbar tissues. If available, helical CT may be substituted for coronal slices. Although some metallic foreign bodies are well tolerated, copper may cause purulent inflammation and iron may induce retinal siderosis.[20] Organic foreign objects, such as wood or other plant material, are likely to cause endophthalmitis.

Loss of normal globe contour on imaging studies is usually an indication of globe rupture or laceration ("flat-tire" sign) (Figs. 30–19 and 30–20). Dislocation of the lens is demonstrable by both CT and MRI (Fig. 30–21). With blunt trauma to the anterior orbit, the transverse diameter of the globe is suddenly increased, which results in rupture of the zonular fibers that hold the lens in place.[21]

Detachments

Retinal or choroidal detachment may result from blunt ocular trauma. These detachments can be difficult to diagnose by funduscopy in the presence of intraocular hemorrhage. Retinal detachment occurs between the sensory retina and the underlying retinal pigmented epithelium.[22] The retina is tightly adherent to the other layers of the globe in only two locations: anteriorly it is attached at the ora serrata and posteriorly at the optic disk. On CT and MRI, therefore, retinal detachments have a V-shaped configururation, with the apex of the V at the optic nerve head. The MRI signal characteristics of the subretinal fluid depend on its chemical composition. If the fluid has a high protein content, it will be hyperintense to vitreous on T1-weighted images (Figs. 30–22 and 30–23). Hemorrhagic detachments follow the predictable course of MRI signal changes for hematomas elsewhere.

Choroidal detachments are caused by the accumulation of fluid or hemorrhage between the choroid and the sclera. On CT or MRI, they may extend anteriorly to the ciliary body, but they seldom extend to the optic nerve

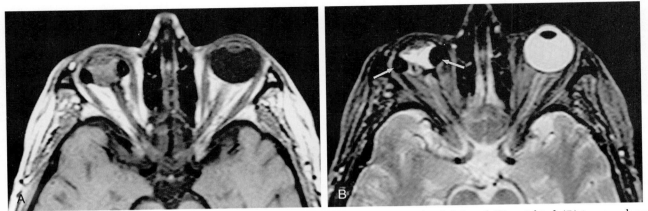

FIGURE 30–17 Phthisis bulbi in a 63-year-old man, cause unknown. Axial T1-weighted *(A)* and T2-weighted *(B)* images show a shrunken right globe with high T1 signal intensity. *Arrows* in *B* indicate a scleral band for treatment of retinal detachment.

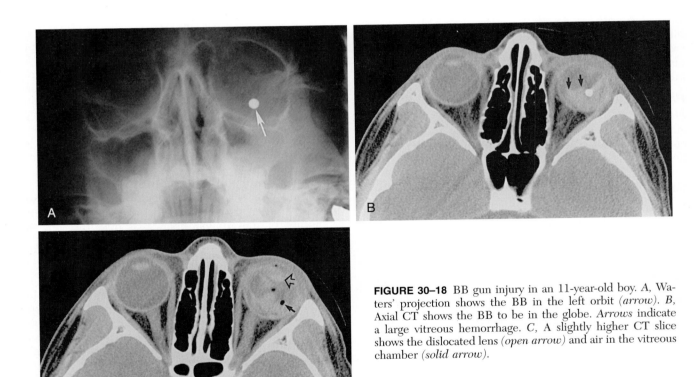

FIGURE 30–18 BB gun injury in an 11-year-old boy. *A,* Waters' projection shows the BB in the left orbit *(arrow). B,* Axial CT shows the BB to be in the globe. *Arrows* indicate a large vitreous hemorrhage. *C,* A slightly higher CT slice shows the dislocated lens *(open arrow)* and air in the vitreous chamber *(solid arrow).*

CHAPTER 30 The Orbit and Visual System   **1023**

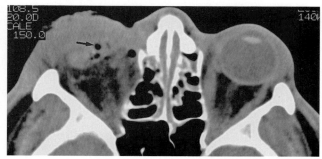

FIGURE 30–19 Ruptured globe due to a gunshot wound in a 23-year-old man. CT shows loss of the normal contour of the right eye with intraocular air bubbles *(arrow).*

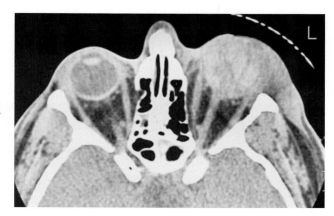

FIGURE 30–20 Ruptured globe with severe intraocular hemorrhage in a 30-year-old man who was kicked in eye. CT shows high-density material (blood) filling the left globe.

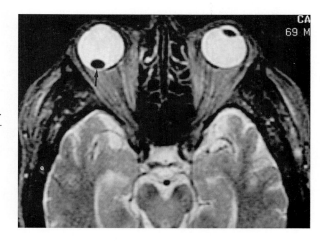

FIGURE 30–21 Traumatic dislocation of the lens in a 69-year-old man. Axial T2-weighted image shows the lens lying posteriorly in the vitreous chamber of the right eye *(arrow).*

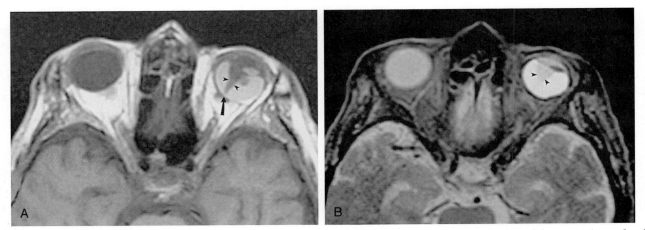

FIGURE 30–22 Retinal detachment in a 78-year-old man. *A,* T1-weighted image. Note the detached leaves of the retina *(arrowheads)* forming a V with the apex at the optic nerve head *(arrow).* Proteinaceous subretinal fluid is hyperintense to vitreous. *B,* On the T2-weighted image, the subretinal fluid remains hyperintense.

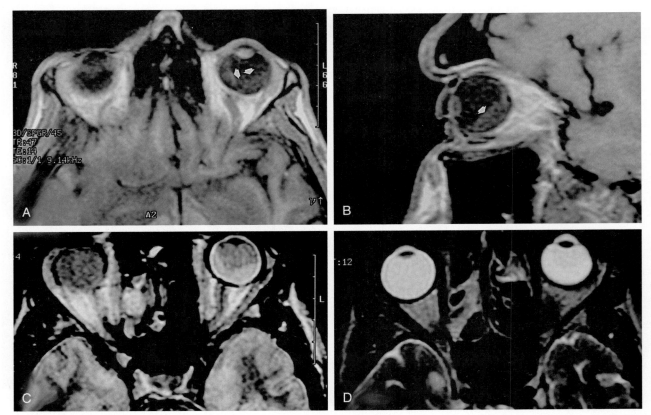

FIGURE 30–23 Retinal detachment in 40-year-old man with human immunodeficiency virus (HIV) chorioretinitis. Axial *(A)* and sagittal *(B)* T1-weighted images demonstrate detached leaves of the retina *(arrow)* of the left eye. Subretinal fluid is slightly hyperintense to vitreous. *C,* Subretinal fluid remains slightly hyperintense on proton density–weighted image. *D,* On the T2-weighted image, the subretinal fluid is nearly isointense to vitreous.

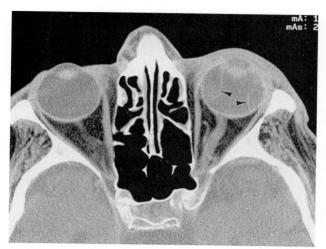

FIGURE 30–24 Choroidal detachment in a 72-year-old man with sporotrichal endophthalmitis. On axial enhanced CT, *arrowheads* indicate detached leaves of the choroid. Note that the leaves do not extend posteriorly to the optic nerve head, as is frequently seen with retinal detachments.

head because of the tethering effect of the vortex veins[23] (Fig. 30–24).

Detachments have many other causes besides trauma, including intraocular surgery (Fig. 30–25), inflammation (Fig. 30–26), tumor, severe axial myopia, staphyloma, and diabetic retinopathy.

Intraocular Tumors and Tumor-Like Conditions

Retinoblastoma

Retinoblastoma is a rare, congenital, highly malignant primitive neuroectodermal tumor with an incidence of 1 in every 18,000 to 30,000 live births.[24] It arises from the nuclear layer of the retina, from the cells destined to become the photoreceptors.[25] About 40% of retinoblastoma cases are inherited as an autosomal dominant trait, and the rest represent spontaneous mutations. Twenty-five percent to 33% of retinoblastomas are bilateral, and these cases are always hereditary. On occasion, a third, histologically similar tumor arises simultaneously in the pineal gland ("trilateral retinoblastoma").[26, 27]

Most retinoblastomas present clinically with *leukokoria*, a whitish or pinkish-white pupillary light reflex. In the developed countries, the average age at presentation is 13 months.[25] The diagnosis is confirmed by ophthalmoscopy. With early detection and treatment, the 5-year survival rate is 92%, with a good chance of preservation of useful vision in the affected eye.[7, 28] However, extraocular spread carries a poor prognosis for survival.

Imaging Findings. Imaging of the retinoblastoma patient has several intended functions: (1) to confirm the clinical and ophthalmoscopic suspicion of tumor, (2) to evaluate for retrobulbar spread, (3) to search for intracranial metastases, and (4) to exclude a second intraocular tumor, in both the affected eye and the contralateral eye. CT, with its high sensitivity to calcifications, is the procedure of choice for tumor detection, since 95% of retinoblastomas calcify.[7] CT typically shows a mass containing calcium arising from the retina and projecting into the vitreous chamber (Fig. 30–27). Large tumors may fill the entire globe.

On MRI, retinoblastomas tend to have mildly to moderately increased signal on T1-weighted images and are hypointense to vitreous on T2-weighted images (Fig. 30–28). The calcifications within the lesions appear as low signal on all sequences.[7, 29] Prominent enhancement is seen after Gd-DTPA administration. MRI is more sensitive than CT for detecting early spread along the optic nerve and into the intracranial compartment.

Other Causes of Leukokoria

Whereas retinoblastoma accounts for about half of all cases of childhood leukokoria,[30] many other intraocular diseases may present with this finding (Table 30–4). Fortunately these are all rare, and only a few of them are discussed here.

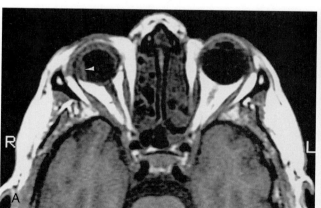
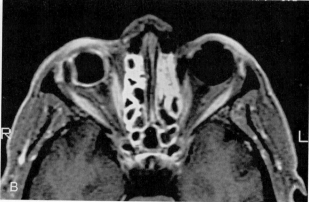

FIGURE 30–25 Small lateral choroidal detachment after corneal transplant in a 60-year-old woman. *A,* Axial T1-weighted image demonstrates a small area of increased signal intensity in the lateral aspect of the right globe *(arrow)*. The location and curvilinear configuration are consistent with choroidal detachment with proteinaceous material in suprachoroidal space. *B,* On the gadolinium-enhanced, fat-suppressed T1-weighted image, the entire choroid enhances, indicating an inflammatory process. (*A* and *B,* Courtesy of Rick Park, M.D., Owensboro, KY.)

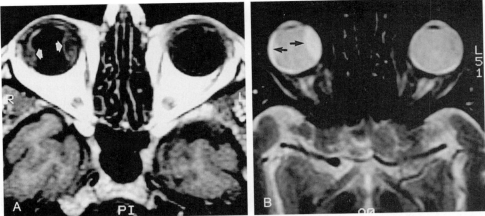

FIGURE 30–26 Bilateral choroidal detachments in a 63-year-old woman with choroidal effusions due to rheumatoid arthritis. A, T1-weighted MRI shows slightly hyperintense fluid between the choroid and the sclera (*arrows*). Detachment does not extend to the optic nerve head because of the tethering effect of the vortex veins. B, T2-weighted image shows the effusions (*arrows*) to be slightly hyperintense to vitreous. (*A* and *B*, From Zimmerman RA, Gibby WG, Carmody RF [eds]. Neuroimaging: Clinical and Physical Principles. New York, Springer-Verlag, 1999.)

Persistent Hyperplastic Primary Vitreous

PHPV is caused by failure of the embryonic hyaloid vasculature to regress normally.[31] Most often unilateral, it accounts for about 10% of all cases of leukokoria.[30] Additional clinical features include profound vision loss, microphthalmia, vitreous hemorrhage, retinal detachment, and cataract.[25, 32]

On CT, PHPV appears as increased density of the vitreous chamber (Fig. 30–29). If intravenous contrast agent is administered, the vitreous material may enhance. The globe is typically small, although buphthalmos is occasionally seen. A fluid-fluid level due to hemorrhage may be found in the posterior globe. Discrete tubular or triangular densities may be seen, owing to persistence of fetal tissue.[33] A deformed, anteriorly displaced lens may be present.[34]

MRI typically demonstrates increased signal intensity in the vitreous on all pulse sequences, owing to blood breakdown products from multiple hemorrhages. Fluid-fluid levels may be found, and retinal detachment may be seen.[33]

Retinopathy of Prematurity

ROP, previously called retrolental fibroplasia, develops in premature infants with prolonged exposure to supplemental oxygen. Leukokoria, usually bilateral, is often the presenting clinical finding. This is due to a fibrovascular mass behind a clear lens, and sometimes there is also persistence of the fetal hyaloid vasculature.

CT and MRI in ROP show features practically identical to those of PHPV; without a history, these two diseases may be indistinguishable. ROP is most often bilateral, but it is frequently asymmetric. Microphthalmia is common, but calcification is unusual, except in far-advanced cases (Fig. 30–30).[7, 35]

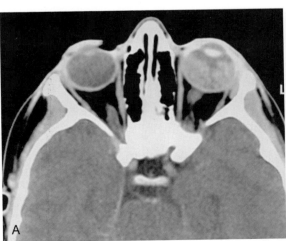
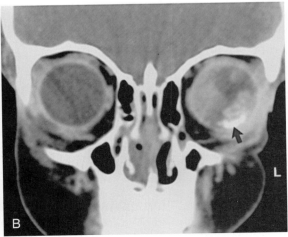

FIGURE 30–27 Retinoblastoma of the left eye in a 2-year-old girl. *A*, Axial CT shows a large mass arising from the retina and filling most of the vitreous chamber. *B*, Coronal CT. Note calcification (*arrow*) along the inferior surface of the tumor. (*A* and *B*, Courtesy of Boyd Ashdown, M.D., Tucson, AZ.)

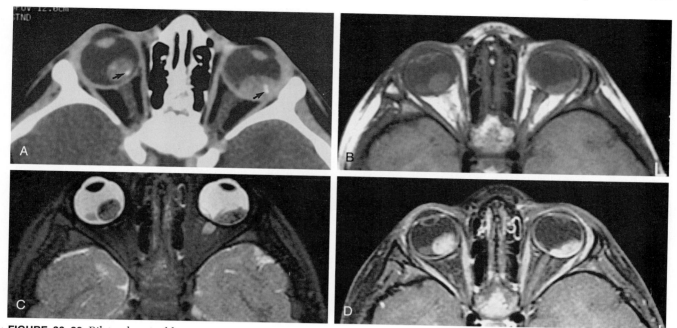

FIGURE 30–28 Bilateral retinoblastoma in a 3-year-old boy. *A,* Axial enhanced CT demonstrates ovoid masses arising from the retinas of both globes. Note calcifications *(arrows)* within the masses. *B,* On T1-weighted image, the lesions are slightly hyperintense to vitreous. *C,* On T2-weighted image, the tumors are markedly hypointense. *D,* After gadolinium administration, the masses enhance prominently. (*A–D,* Courtesy of James Schnur, M.D., Phoenix, AZ.)

Coats' Disease

Coats' disease is characterized by retinal telangiectasia and exudative retinal detachment. Almost always unilateral, it usually occurs in young boys (4 to 8 years). On ophthalmoscopic examination, Coats' disease may be indistinguishable from retinoblastoma, which has often led to an unnecessary enucleation.

Both CT and MRI can be helpful in distinguishing between Coats' disease and retinoblastoma. Calcification is not a feature of Coats' disease, but it is seen in the vast majority of retinoblastomas.[24, 36] With retinoblastoma a hypointense mass is seen on T2-weighted images, whereas with Coats' disease the subretinal exudate is hyperintense on T2-weighted images. Because of the retinal telangiectasia, the detached leaves of the retina enhance after gadolinium administration.[25]

Other Causes of Ocular Calcifications

In older individuals, small foci of calcifications are commonly seen on CT at the insertions of the medial and lateral rectus muscles (Fig. 30–31). These are known as

TABLE 30–4 Causes of Childhood Leukokoria

Retinoblastoma
Persistent hyperplastic primary vitreous
Retinopathy of prematurity
Coats' disease
Toxocaral endophthalmitis
Total retinal detachment
Retinal astrocytoma

Modified from Smirniotopolos JG, Bargallo N, Mafee MF. Differential diagnosis of leukokoria: Radiologic-pathologic correlation. Radiographics 1994;14:1059–1079.

focal scleral translucencies, and they are of no clinical significance. Scleral calcifications are also seen in disorders of calcium metabolism, as in chronic renal insufficiency (Fig. 30–32). Optic nerve head *drusen* (hyaline bodies) are caused by deposition of hyaline-like material on or under the surface of the optic disk. They are often bilateral and commonly calcify (Fig. 30–33). Drusen may produce visual field defects. Other causes of ocular calcification are listed in Table 30–5.

Ocular Melanoma

Malignant melanoma, which arises from the uveal tract, is the most common intraocular malignancy in adults. It

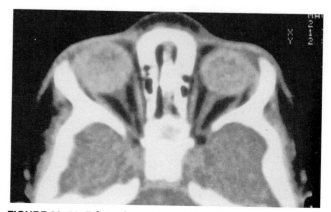

FIGURE 30–29 Bilateral persistent hyperplastic primary vitreous in an 8-month-old boy. CT demonstrates high-density material in both vitreous chambers. (Courtesy of Mahmood Mafee, M.D., Chicago, IL; from Zimmerman RA, Gibby WG, Carmody RF [eds]. Neuroimaging: Clinical and Physical Principles. New York, Springer-Verlag, 1999.)

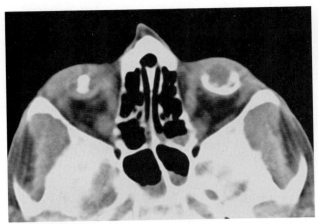

FIGURE 30-30 Phthisis bulbi due to retinopathy of prematurity in a 45-year-old man. Unenhanced CT shows small, shrunken, calcified globes bilaterally.

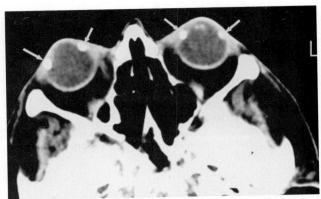

FIGURE 30-31 Focal scleral translucencies in an 81-year-old woman. Axial CT demonstrates calcifications at the insertions of the medial and lateral rectus muscles (*arrows*).

TABLE 30-5 Ocular Calcifications

Neoplastic	Infectious	Metabolic and Degenerative
Retinoblastoma	Cytomegalovirus	Optic nerve head drusen
Choroidal osteoma	Rubella	Cataracts
Astrocytic hamartoma	Toxoplasmosis	Phthisis bulbi
(with phakomatoses)	Herpes simplex	Retinopathy of prematurity
	Larval granulomatosis (rarely)	Retinal detachment
		Hypercalcemic states

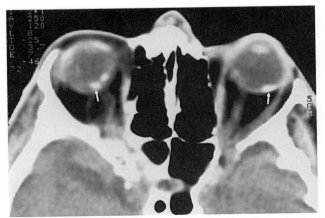

FIGURE 30-32 Scleral calcifications (*arrows*) in a 42-year-old man with chronic renal disease and secondary hyperparathyroidism. (Courtesy of Norman Komar, M.D., Tucson, AZ.)

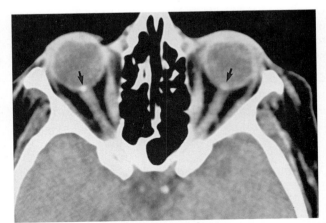

FIGURE 30-33 Optic nerve head drusen in a 56-year-old woman. *Arrows* indicate calcifications at both optic papillae.

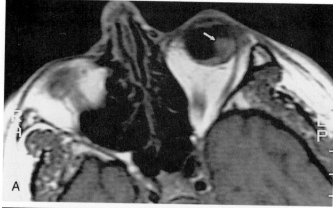

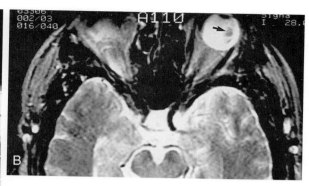

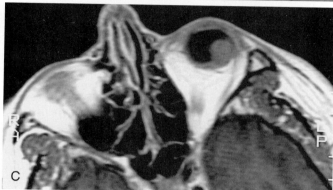

FIGURE 30–34 Ocular melanoma in a 45-year-old man. *A,* Axial T1-weighted image demonstrates a mildly hyperintense mass in the left globe *(arrow)*. *B,* On T2-weighted image, the mass *(arrow)* is hypointense to vitreous. *C,* After gadolinium administration, the tumor shows mild enhancement. (*A–C,* Courtesy of Rick Park, M.D., Owensboro, KY.)

is almost always unilateral and is rare in blacks (15:1 white to black ratio).[25] Because it occurs in older individuals, it is unlikely to be confused with retinoblastoma. The typical melanoma arises from the choroid, produces a retinal detachment, and presents as a mushroom-shaped mass projecting into the vitreous. Although melanoma is a funduscopic diagnosis, imaging studies are helpful in detecting extraocular extension and also aid in the differential diagnosis.

Imaging Findings. Although the CT appearance of melanoma will vary depending on the morphology of the tumor, the most common finding is that of a well-defined elevated mass of increased density that projects into the vitreous chamber.[37, 38] Moderate contrast enhancement is usually seen. One should search carefully for extension of

the tumor into the optic disk and Tenon's space. An occasional melanoma is discoid or ring-shaped.

Melanotic ocular melanomas have a characteristic appearance on MRI, which helps to confirm the clinical diagnosis. The tumor is hyperintense to vitreous on T1-weighted and proton-density–weighted images and hypointense on T2-weighted images (Figs. 30–34 and 30–35).[18, 39–43] These signal characteristics are thought to be caused by the presence of paramagnetic stable free radicals in the melanin pigment, which produce T1 and T2 shortening.[44] Lesions with cystic or necrotic components are more heterogeneous in appearance. Amelanotic melanomas produce less T1 and T2 shortening, but they are still hyperintense to vitreous on T1-weighted images. Moderate enhancement after gadolinium administration

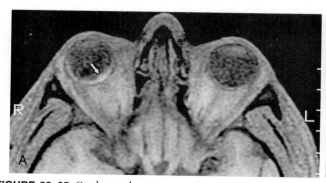

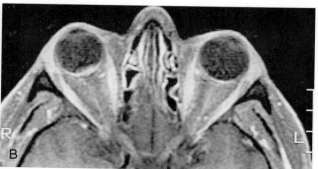

FIGURE 30–35 Ocular melanoma in a 46-year-old man. *A,* Fat-suppressed T1-weighted image shows a hyperintense mass in the posterior right globe *(arrow)*. *B,* After gadolinium administration, the tumor enhances. (*A* and *B,* Courtesy of Rick Park, M.D., Owensboro, KY.)

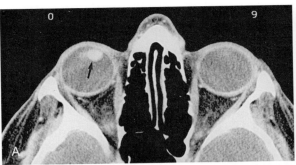
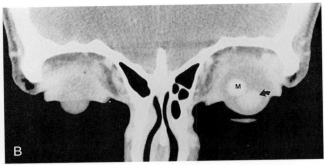

FIGURE 30–36 Metastatic carcinoid to the ciliary body in a 40-year-old woman. *A,* Axial enhanced CT shows a dense lesion *(arrow)* that superficially resembles the lens. *B,* On the coronal slice, the lens *(arrow)* can be seen separate from the metastasis (M).

is the rule. Choroidal metastases from mucin-producing adenocarcinomas may have a similar MRI appearance because of the T1 and T2 shortening effect of protein.[45] Many other lesions may simulate uveal melanoma, either clinically or on imaging studies (Table 30–6).

Ocular Metastases

The choroid, being a highly vascular tissue, is the occasional site of a metastatic deposit, particularly from lung or breast carcinoma. Although melanoma is rarely bilateral, about a third of ocular metastases occur bilaterally.[25] On CT, choroidal metastases tend to be flatter and less protuberant than melanomas, although they may be round or ovoid (Figs. 30–36 and 30–37).[7, 37] Retinal detachment is common. On MRI, uveal metastases tend to be diffusely infiltrative; they are usually isointense or hyperintense on T1-weighted images and hyperintense on T2-weighted images, and they enhance with gadolinium.[25]

LESIONS OF THE ORBIT PROPER

Trauma

By a marvelous design of nature, the orbital contents are deeply recessed in the skull and are surrounded by bone. Although this provides excellent protection against mild or moderate trauma, high-energy forces may nevertheless fracture the bony structures and cause soft tissue damage. In addition to blunt trauma, penetration of the orbit by foreign objects may damage the globe, extraocular muscles, nerves, and vascular structures. Not uncommonly, the clinical examination of the traumatized orbit is made difficult by marked swelling or hematoma to the extent that the patient is unable to open the eye. Moreover, the victim may be obtunded and unable to cooperate for an assessment of vision.

CT is the procedure of choice for evaluating orbital trauma.[46] Conventional radiography is less informative and used mainly as a screening examination for minor trauma. Now almost universally available, CT can be performed rapidly, often in conjunction with examination of the head for intracranial injury. This adds little time to the radiologic examination and provides a wealth of information. Three-mm axial and coronal images of the entire orbit can be obtained, with thinner cuts through the apex if fracture of the optic canal is suspected. Direct coronal slices are preferred, but these should not be attempted until the cervical spine has been "cleared." Coronal and sagittal re-formations of axial images are less desirable, but they may suffice in these cases. The new helical scanners allow for very rapid examination of the orbit. It is important to view the images at both soft tissue and bone window settings.

MRI is seldom necessary in the acute setting, but it may be helpful in certain situations, such as in assessing the intracanalicular portion of the optic nerve, the optic chiasm, or the posterior visual pathways. MRI should not be attempted until an intraocular metallic foreign body has been excluded.

Orbital Fractures
Zygomaticomaxillary Fractures

These are also called zygomatic complex fractures, tripod fractures, or trimalar fractures. This common injury re-

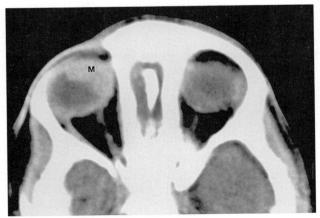

FIGURE 30–37 Metastatic sarcoma to the choroid in a 2-year-old girl. Axial enhanced CT scan shows a diffusely infiltrating, lobulated mass (M) in the superomedial portion of the globe.

**TABLE 30–6 Malignant Uveal Melanoma:
Differential Diagnosis**

Metastasis
Choroidal nevus
Choroidal hemangioma
Choroidal detachment
Choroidal cyst
Granulomatous lesions (e.g., sarcoid)
Hemorrhage

sults from a blow to the cheek, such as from a closed fist. Typically, the lateral wall of the orbit is fractured near or at the zygomaticofrontal suture, the floor is fractured near the infraorbital canal, and the lateral wall of the maxillary sinus is fractured (Figs. 30–38 and 30–39). The zygomatic arch is fractured in one or more places. A mobile fragment is created, which is usually displaced inferiorly, laterally, and posteriorly. The lateral canthus is pulled downward, and the globe may also be displaced. If not properly treated, significant permanent cosmetic deformity results.[47]

CT helps in the preoperative planning of the reduction and fixation of zygomatic complex fractures by demonstrating the position and degree of comminution of the bony fragments. It is also important to search for intraorbital hematomas, since these have the potential for optic nerve compression and may need decompression if large.

LeFort Fractures

In 1901, Rene LeFort, a French surgeon, reported on a number of symmetric midface fractures he had produced experimentally in cadavers.[48] Three types of fractures were described, having the following features in common: (1) all are bilateral; (2) all are associated with a mobile facial fragment; and (3) all have fracture lines exiting posteriorly through the pterygoid plates. The LeFort I fracture, the least common of the three, involves the nasal cavity and the maxillary sinuses bilaterally, creating a "floating palate." Since it does not involve the orbit, it will not be considered further here. The LeFort II fracture is a bilateral infrazygomatic fracture extending from the nasofrontal suture across the medial wall of the orbit, orbital floor, anterior and posterior walls of the maxillary sinus, and pterygoid plates[49] (Fig. 30–40). A pyramid-shaped central facial fragment results, with various degrees of comminution and posterior displacement.

The LeFort III injury is an extensive bilateral suprazygomatic fracture. The fracture lines extend from the region of the nasofrontal suture through the medial wall of the orbit, across the floor and the lateral wall of the orbit, the zygomatic arch, the posterolateral maxillary antrum, and the pterygoid plates[21] (Fig. 30–41). The sphenoid sinus and cribriform plate may also be involved. This spectrum of fractures produces a "craniofacial separation," with a mobile face. The involvement of the zygomatic arches is the simplest way to distinguish between a LeFort II and a LeFort III fracture. Pure LeFort III fractures are uncommon, and it is often the case that a LeFort II fracture will be present on one side and a LeFort III on the other.

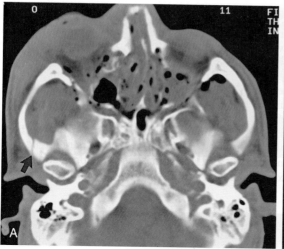

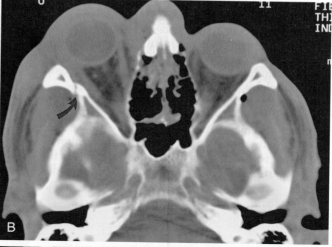

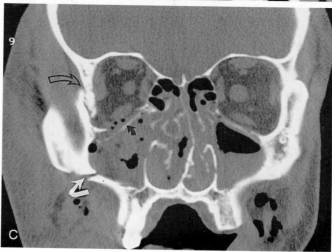

FIGURE 30–38 Zygomatic complex fracture in a 31-year-old man. *A,* CT at the level of the zygomatic arches shows a nondisplaced fracture of the posterior right arch *(arrow)*. *B,* Higher slice demonstrates a fracture of the right lateral orbital wall *(arrow)*. *C,* Coronal CT slice shows fractures of the right lateral maxillary antrum *(white arrow)*, lateral orbital wall *(open arrow)*, and orbital floor *(black arrow)*. Additional fractures of the medial maxillary walls, nasal septum, and alveolar ridges are also present.

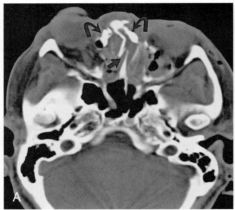
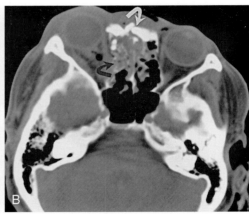

present in the antrum. Coronal CT is the best procedure for determining the size of the floor defect, the degree of displacement of the bony fragment, and whether or not the inferior rectus is entrapped.[60, 61] MRI has also been shown to be effective for demonstrating blowout fractures.[62]

Small orbital floor fractures usually do not require surgical repair, unless muscle entrapment is present.[63] Larger fractures, where a major portion of the floor is involved, may result in enophthalmos, inferior displacement of the globe, or permanent diplopia if not corrected.[49] The optimal time for surgical repair of a blowout fracture is about 10 to 14 days after injury.[56, 64]

Medial wall blowout fractures occur about half as frequently as floor fractures, and the two occur concurrently in 20% to 40% of the cases.[65] Even though the lamina papyracea is thinner than the orbital floor, it is buttressed by the ethmoid septae. Medial blowout fractures are much more likely to cause orbital emphysema, which may be made markedly worse by sneezing or nose blowing. Plain radiographs are less sensitive for diagnosing these fractures, and CT is preferred. Both axial and coronal images demonstrate a soft tissue mass projecting through a defect in the medial wall (Fig. 30–46). Medial rectus muscle entrapment is distinctly uncommon. Unless they are extensive, most medial blowout fractures do not need surgical repair.[66]

Orbital Roof Fractures

Fractures of the roof of the orbit are less common than floor or medial wall fractures and are usually caused by a blow to the superior orbital rim. The most common part of the roof to fracture is the area where it is weakened by the superior orbital fissure and optic canal.[67–69] When the fracture extends into the optic canal, injury to the optic nerve may result. Associated frontal bone fracture and frontal lobe contusion are common.[68] If the fracture involves the posterior wall of the frontal sinus, an epidural abscess may develop. Orbital hematoma may interfere with the superior rectus function and cause vertical diplopia as well as inferior displacement of the globe. Orbital roof fracture is slightly more common in children, and large defects may produce encephaloceles. Coronal CT is the best means of demonstrating the fracture and its sequelae; in equivocal cases of encephalocele, MRI may be confirmatory.

Penetrating Injuries

In addition to injury to the globe, foreign object penetration of the orbit may also damage the extraocular muscles, nerves, vascular structures, and lacrimal apparatus. With orbital trauma, it is not always possible to deduce the presence of an intraorbital foreign body by clinical examination alone. Retained foreign material, especially dirt, wood, or other vegetable material, commonly results in

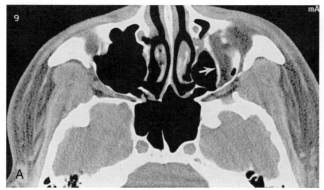
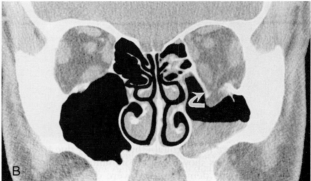

FIGURE 30–44 Orbital floor blowout fracture in a 23-year-old man. *A,* Axial CT demonstrates a bone fragment *(arrow)* projecting into the left maxillary antrum from the orbital floor. *B,* Coronal CT more clearly depicts the fragment *(arrow)* as well as the orbital fat herniated into the sinus.

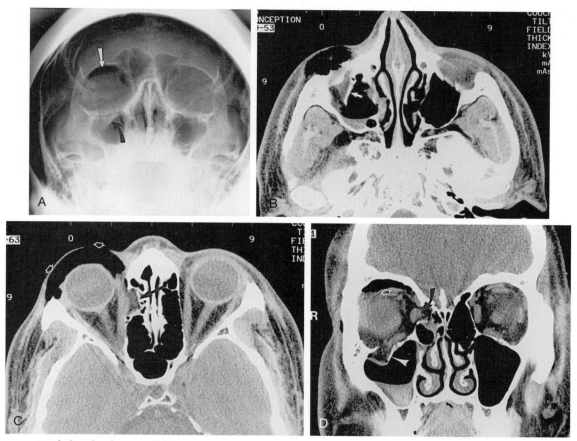

FIGURE 30–45 Medial and inferior wall blowout fractures in a 21-year-old man. *A,* Waters' projection demonstrates the "trapdoor" fragment of the orbital floor displaced inferiorly into the maxillary sinus *(black arrow).* Orbital emphysema is also present *(white arrow). B,* Axial CT slice demonstrates the orbital floor fragment in the antrum *(arrow). C,* Higher slice demonstrates a fracture of the lamina papyracea *(solid arrow)* and prominent orbital emphysema *(open arrows).* Medial rectus muscle contusion is also evident. *D,* Coronal slice depicts the medial wall fracture and medial rectus muscle hematoma *(curved arrow),* orbital emphysema *(open arrow),* and orbital floor fracture *(arrowhead).* The orbital emphysema is probably due to the medial fracture.

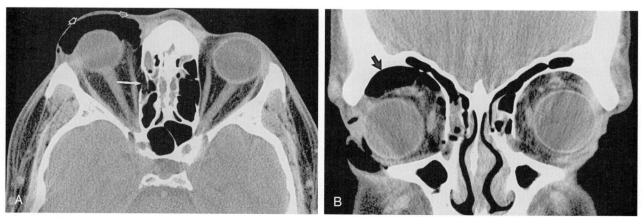

FIGURE 30–46 Pure medial blowout fracture in a 27-year-old man. *A,* Axial CT shows a small fracture of the lamina papyracea *(solid arrow)* and orbital emphysema *(open arrows). B,* Coronal CT shows a large amount of air in the superior orbit *(arrow).*

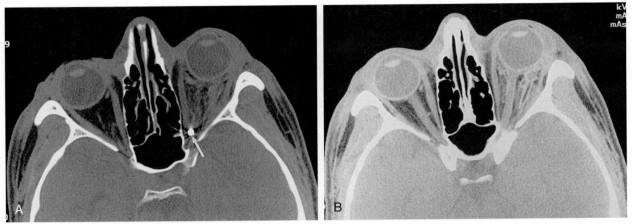

FIGURE 30–47 Penetrating injury to the left orbit (shotgun wound) in a 28-year-old man. *A,* Axial CT shows the pellet *(arrow)* in the orbital apex. *B,* Slightly higher slice depicts the intact optic nerve and hemorrhage into the intraconal compartment.

orbital cellulitis, abscess, and even draining fistulas. Metal and glass fragments are better tolerated. CT is very accurate for detecting metal, glass, and bone fragments (Fig. 30–47), but wood fragments may present a problem. Wood may be hyperdense, isodense, or hypodense to orbital soft tissues,[70–72] and it may simulate air. MRI has also been used to detect and localize intraorbital wood.[72]

Penetrating trauma may also cause an intraorbital hematoma, which can present as proptosis, impaired ocular motility, or visual loss (Fig. 30–48). In most cases, the hemorrhage can be treated conservatively, unless vision is compromised. One should also search carefully for evidence of intracranial penetration, which has the potential for causing meningitis, brain abscess, or carotid-cavernous sinus fistula.

Inflammatory Diseases of the Orbit

Infection

Most infections of the orbit originate in the paranasal sinuses, usually the ethmoid.[73] The lamina papyracea is perforated by valveless veins, and perivascular spaces surround the ethmoid arteries. These channels allow the spread of infection from the ethmoid sinus into the medial subperiosteal space of the orbit. This periostitis may progress to a subperiosteal abscess, with lifting of the periosteum off the bone. Gas may accumulate in the subperiosteal space in the event of infection with a gas-forming organism, or if there is direct communication with the ethmoid. Frontal and maxillary sinusitis are less common causes of orbital infection.

Penetrating trauma and bacteremia are other causes of orbital infection. Orbital cellulitis may involve the preseptal space (Fig. 30–49), in which case it is apparent by clinical examination. However, if the inflammatory process is located posterior to the orbital septum (postseptal cellulitis), the situation is more serious and should be investigated by cross-sectional imaging.[74, 75] Postseptal cellulitis is typically found in the extraconal space.

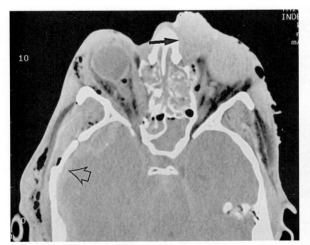

FIGURE 30–48 This 26-year-old man was shot in the left eye while making a withdrawal at an automated teller machine. Axial CT demonstrates hemorrhage into the left globe and the adjacent medial orbital hematoma *(solid arrow)*. Both the right and the left ethmoid sinuses have comminuted fractures. The right optic nerve was also damaged. Subdural hematoma *(open arrow)* and subarachnoid hemorrhage are present. Follow-up: Blind, both eyes.

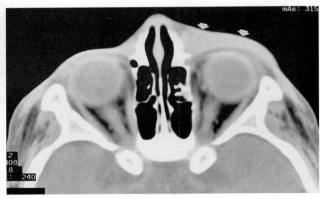

FIGURE 30–49 Preseptal cellulitis in a 5-year-old boy. Enhanced axial CT demonstrates soft tissue edema of the left ocular adnexa *(arrows)*. The orbital fat is "clean."

With postseptal cellulitis, CT shows loss of definition of and increased density to the orbital fat. Subperiosteal abscesses are identified as areas of fluid density with rim enhancement, typically medial to the medial rectus muscle (Fig. 30–50). Some degree of proptosis is usually present. On MRI, there is loss of the normal high signal intensity of the orbital fat on T1-weighted images and increased T2 signal owing to edema.

Unrecognized or improperly treated orbital cellulitis or abscess may lead to serious or life-threatening complications. The infection may spread through the valveless veins of the orbit into the cavernous sinus to produce cavernous sinus thrombosis and septic thrombophlebitis. Cerebritis and brain abscess may develop. Scarring, adhesions, and permanent blindness in the involved eye may be late sequelae.

Idiopathic Orbital Inflammation (Pseudotumor)

Orbital pseudotumor is a nongranulomatous inflammatory process with no known cause that may involve virtually any structure in the orbit. Clinically and radiologically, it may present in a number of ways: (1) extraocular muscle infiltration (myositis), (2) episcleritis, (3) lacrimal gland enlargement (dacryoadenitis), (4) optic nerve sheath thickening, and (5) diffuse infiltration of the orbit ("dirty orbit").[76] The acute variety of pseudotumor often presents clinically with pain, proptosis, and impaired ocular motility. In some cases, there may also be decreased visual acuity, uveitis, and even retinal detachment.[73] The chronic form often presents as a slowly developing mass that causes proptosis or impaired motility. Pseudotumor is most common in middle age but can occur in children. It is more likely to be unilateral, although occasionally it may be bilateral, especially in children.

The histology of pseudotumor is variable, depending on its chronicity. Acute forms demonstrate infiltration with lymphocytes, plasma cells, neutrophils, eosinophils, and macrophages. In the chronic form, a dense fibrotic response may be seen.[73, 77] These variable histologic features are thought to account for the inconsistent signal intensities observed on MRI.

When pseudotumor involves the orbital apex, superior orbital fissure, and cavernous sinus, a clinical symptom complex known as the *Tolosa-Hunt syndrome* results. The clinical features are painful ophthalmoplegia, minimal proptosis, and hypesthesia of the periorbital skin. The ophthalmoplegia reflects involvement of the third, fourth, and sixth cranial nerves, and the hypesthesia is due to involvement of the first division of the fifth nerve.[73]

Imaging Findings. The CT and MRI findings in orbital pseudotumor reflect the degree, duration, and location of involvement. In the myositic form of the disease, the extraocular muscles are enlarged. The enlargement may involve only the muscle belly, as in Graves' disease, but more often it has a tubular shape owing to thickening of the tendinous insertions of the muscles[78, 79] (Fig. 30–51). Prominent enhancement of the affected muscles is seen. With lacrimal gland involvement, the gland is enlarged but retains its normal shape, although its margins may be somewhat indistinct.[73] Contrast enhancement is prominent. When the globe is affected, it is usually in the form of thickening and enhancement of the posterior wall (episcleritis). With optic nerve sheath pseudotumor, the nerve is thickened and its meningeal coverings enhance, often in a "tram-track" pattern[80] (Fig. 30–52). With diffuse involvement, the orbital fat may have increased density on CT ("dirty fat"). In the tumefactive variety, a solid-appearing mass may fill the entire orbital cavity, closely resembling primary tumor or lymphoma (Fig. 30–53).

MRI can be helpful in differentiating pseudotumor from other orbital masses. On T1-weighted spin-echo images, pseudotumor tends to be isointense to muscle; on T2-weighted images, its signal is close to that of orbital fat—that is, darker than most other lesions (Figs. 30–54 and 30–55).[81] In more chronic cases, where there is a predominance of fibrous tissue, low signal on T2-weighted images is typical. T2 signal may be higher in acute cases, where inflammatory cells and edema predominate.

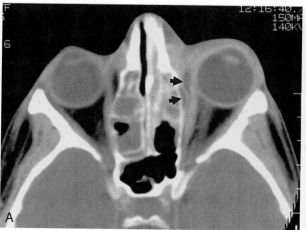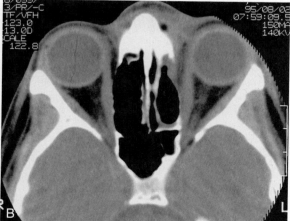

FIGURE 30–50 Pre- and postseptal cellulitis in a 14-year-old boy. *A,* Enhanced axial CT demonstrates bilateral ethmoid sinusitis and elevation of the periorbitum from the lamina papyracea on the left *(arrows).* A fluid collection is seen medial to the medial rectus muscle. Periorbital edema is also present. *B,* Follow-up CT 2 weeks later, after decompression and ethmoidectomy. The lamina papyracea has been resected, and the phlegmon is no longer seen.

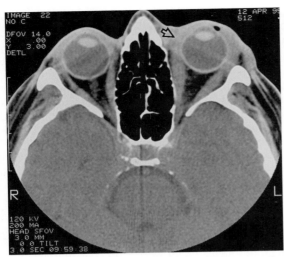

FIGURE 30–51 Inflammatory pseudotumor of the left orbit in a 65-year-old woman. The medial rectus muscle is enlarged, including its tendinous insertion on the globe *(arrow)*. The periorbital soft tissues are infiltrated, and slight enlargement of the lateral rectus muscle is seen. (Courtesy of Mark Yoshino, M.D., Tucson, AZ.)

Several other diseases may closely resemble orbital pseudotumor. The myositic form can be similar in appearance to Graves' disease. Lymphoma is almost always in the differential diagnosis of tumefactive pseudotumor, as is metastatic carcinoma. A helpful distinguishing feature is that pseudotumor rarely causes bone destruction, which is common with metastases. Sarcoidosis may involve the lacrimal gland, the optic nerve sheath or the posterior globe, or it may cause Tolosa-Hunt syndrome.[82] Since pseudotumor, especially the acute form, responds dramatically to corticosteroids, a short course of steroids may be confirmative.

Graves' Ophthalmopathy

Graves' disease (thyroid ophthalmopathy) is the most common cause of both bilateral and unilateral proptosis.

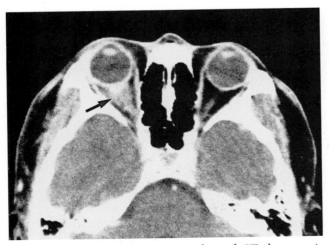

FIGURE 30–52 Optic perineuritis. Enhanced CT shows an irregular mass surrounding the right optic nerve *(arrow)* as well as some thickening of the posterior sclera. (Courtesy of Mahmood Mafee, M.D., Chicago, IL.)

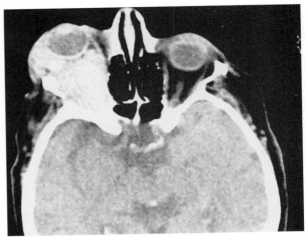

FIGURE 30–53 Tumefactive pseudotumor in an 83-year-old woman. Axial CT demonstrates a large, dense mass filling the right orbit and causing marked proptosis. (Courtesy of Mahmood Mafee, M.D., Chicago, IL.)

This autoimmune disorder, which affects 1 out of every 200 individuals, occurs in both hyperthyroid and euthyroid states. It has a female to male predominance of 4 to 1 and is most common in the fifth and sixth decades of life. Physical findings include eyelid retraction, exophthalmos, and vascular congestion of the eyes in the acute stage. The thyroid gland is usually enlarged.

The pathologic changes include enlargement of the extraocular muscles owing to infiltration with lymphocytes, plasma cells, and mast cells.[77] In later stages, the muscles may undergo fibrosis and fatty infiltration. Some patients have an increase in the orbital fat, which can also show inflammatory or fibrotic change.

Imaging Findings. Although both CT and MRI are well suited for demonstrating the abnormalities in this disease, CT is certainly adequate in most cases, providing that both axial and coronal slices are obtained. If only axial images are performed, an enlarged inferior rectus muscle may be mistaken for an orbital tumor, especially by the neophyte (Fig. 30–56). Graves' disease is bilateral in 90% of the cases, although it is often asymmetric.[83] Many cases that are thought to be unilateral on clinical grounds will have bilateral findings on imaging studies. The inferior rectus is often the first muscle to enlarge, followed by the medial rectus (Fig. 30–57). The superior rectus is the next most commonly involved. Lateral rectus involvement occurs later and may be minimal. In some cases, all six muscles are swollen. The enlarged muscles typically have a spindle shape, owing to infiltration of the muscle belly and sparing of the tendons. Occasionally, the tendon is affected, as with pseudotumor. On MRI, the muscles may demonstrate fatty infiltration in some patients, which is another differential feature between Graves' and pseudotumor.[84] Marked gadolinium enhancement is characteristic. Infrequently, the muscles may appear normal and the orbital fat is increased, with anterior bulging of the orbital septum[85] (Fig. 30–58). Mild to moderate lacrimal gland enlargement may occur.

In cases of severe extraocular muscle enlargement, crowding of the orbital apex may cause compressive optic

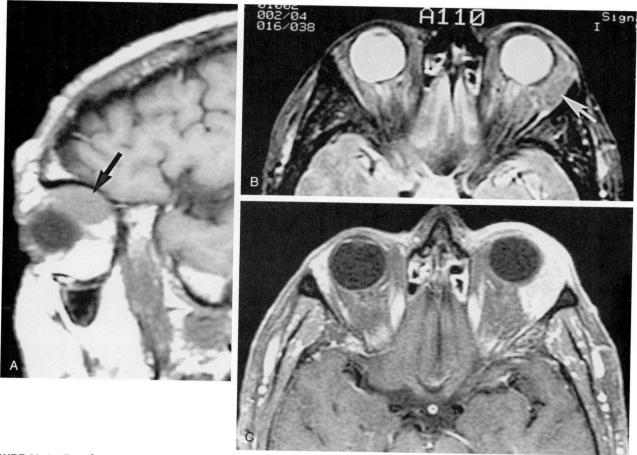

FIGURE 30–54 Pseudotumor involving the lacrimal gland in a 65-year-old man. *A*, T1-weighted sagittal image shows a superolateral orbital mass *(arrow)* that is isointense to muscle. *B*, On T2-weighted image, the mass *(arrow)* is isointense to orbital fat. *C*, Gadolinium-enhanced T1-weighted image shows prominent enhancement of the mass. *(A–C,* Courtesy of James Johnson, M.D., Bend, OR; From Zimmerman RA, Gibby W, Carmody RF [eds]. Neuroimaging: Clinical and Physical Principles. New York, Springer-Verlag, 1999.)

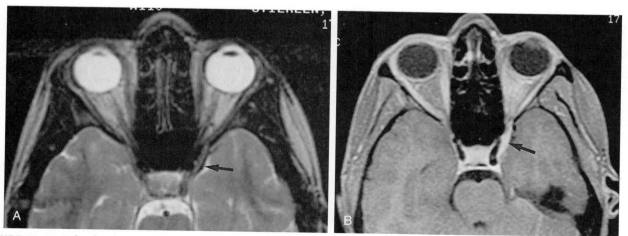

FIGURE 30–55 Orbital apex pseudotumor presenting as Tolosa-Hunt syndrome in a 17-year-old girl. *A*, T2-weighted MRI shows a subtle low-signal-intensity mass *(arrow)* adjacent to the left cavernous sinus. *B*, Gadolinium-enhanced image demonstrates prominent homogeneous enhancement of the lesion *(arrow)*, which is extending anteriorly into the superior orbital fissure. Diffuse enhancement of intraconal fat is also seen. *(A* and *B*, Courtesy of Jordan Cohen, M.D., Phoenix, AZ.)

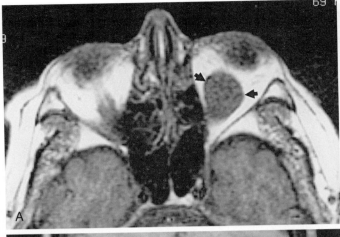

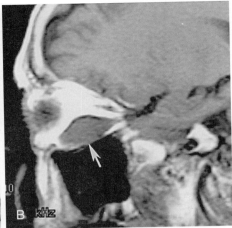

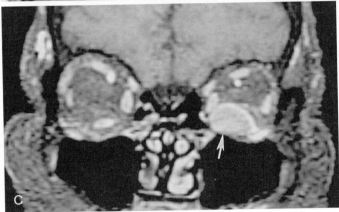

FIGURE 30–56 Graves' disease limited to the left inferior rectus muscle in a 69-year-old woman. *A,* Axial T1-weighted image demonstrates a masslike lesion *(arrows)* in the left orbit. *B,* Sagittal T1-weighted image shows that the "mass" is an enlarged inferior rectus muscle belly *(arrow). C,* Coronal Gd-DTPA–enhanced, fat-suppressed MRI demonstrates the enlarged muscle belly *(arrow),* which enhances prominently.

neuropathy[86, 87] (Fig. 30–59). Another sign of compressive optic neuropathy that has been recently described is protrusion of orbital fat through the superior orbital fissure into the intracranial compartment.[88]

The main differential diagnostic consideration for Graves' disease is pseudotumor, which has already been discussed. However, a number of other diseases can cause extraocular muscle enlargement, and these are listed in Table 30–7.

Optic Neuritis

Optic neuritis is usually caused by an immune-related inflammatory reaction in the optic nerve. Clinical manifestations include pain behind the globe, decreased visual

TABLE 30–7 Causes of Extraocular Muscle Enlargement

Graves' disease
Inflammatory pseudotumor (myositic form)
Metastasis
Lymphoma, leukemia
Hematoma
Carotid-cavernous or dural arteriovenous fistula
Infection, parasitic diseases
Acromegaly
Rhabdomyosarcoma
Amyloidosis

acuity, and impaired color vision (dyschromatopsia). In acute cases, visual loss may progress rapidly in a few days. The condition is bilateral in 30% of patients.[89] Although many cases are idiopathic, about half of all patients presenting with optic neuritis will develop multiple sclerosis. Young adults have an even greater chance of developing multiple sclerosis. Of all cases of multiple sclerosis, optic neuritis is the initial presenting symptom in 15% to 20%, and 35% to 40% of multiple sclerosis patients will have optic neuritis sometime in the course of their disease.[89] Other causes of optic neuritis include radiation, sarcoidosis, and neurosyphilis.[82, 90, 91]

Imaging Findings. MRI is the preferred modality for radiologic evaluation of the optic neuritis patient. Three- or 4-mm axial and coronal images are standard, and parasagittal oblique slices along the course of the nerve are helpful. T2-weighted images and short-tau inversion recovery (STIR) sequences show increased signal intensity in the substance of the nerve, sometimes in multiple segments. The nerve is frequently enlarged. Gadolinium-enhanced fat-suppressed T1-weighted images show areas of focal enhancement[92, 93] (Fig. 30–60). Another advantage of MRI over CT is that the entire brain can be examined at the same time to look for multiple sclerosis (Fig. 30–61). The sensitivity of MRI for optic neuritis is relatively low; in one study of 13 patients, Gd-DTPA–enhanced MRI was able to confirm the clinical diagnosis in 7 cases.[93] However, the main function of imaging is not to make the diagnosis but to rule out other causes of optic

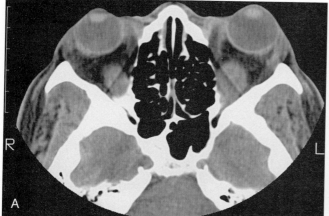

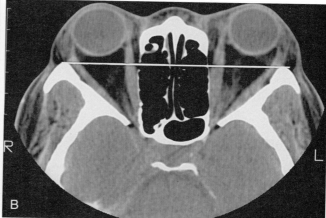

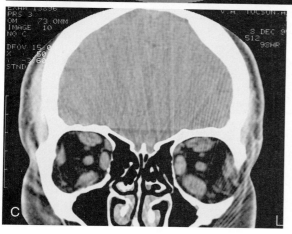

FIGURE 30–57 Moderate bilateral Graves' disease in a 42-year-old woman. *A,* Axial CT demonstrates bilateral inferior rectus muscle enlargement. *B,* Higher slice shows enlargement of both medial rectus muscles, as well as proptosis. Normally, about one-third of the globe should be behind the *white line* connecting the two zygomatic bones. *C,* Coronal CT shows enlargement of the rectus muscles bilaterally.

nerve compromise, such as an orbital tumor. Additionally, patients with no evidence of multiple sclerosis on their initial MRI are less likely to ultimately develop the disease.

In some patients, the pattern of gadolinium enhancement is different, with enhancement of only the optic nerve sheath. This condition is commonly referred to as *optic perineuritis* or *perioptic neuritis.* This is usually an infectious or granulomatous optic neuropathy.[94] The tram-track enhancement pattern is nonspecific and is seen in several other conditions (Table 30–8).

Sarcoidosis

Sarcoidosis is a multiple system granulomatous disease of unknown cause, but it may represent an exaggerated immune response to an antigenic stimulus. Approximately 25% of the patients have ophthalmic involvement, most commonly uveitis.[95, 96] Structures affected include the globe, lacrimal gland, conjunctiva, extraocular muscles, retrobulbar fatty reticulum, optic nerve, chiasm, and optic radiations. Ocular disease may be the first manifestation of sarcoid.[97]

Imaging Findings. MRI is the procedure of choice for evaluating orbital sarcoidosis, since its superior tissue characterization may add specificity to the findings. Infil-

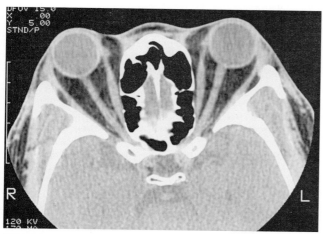

FIGURE 30–58 Graves' disease manifested as increased orbital fat in a 45-year-old man. Axial CT demonstrates bilateral proptosis, but the extraocular muscles are not enlarged.

TABLE 30–8 Causes of the "Tram-Track" Sign

Optic nerve sheath meningioma
Metastasis
Lymphoma, leukemia
Optic neuritis/perineuritis
Inflammatory pseudotumor
Sarcoid

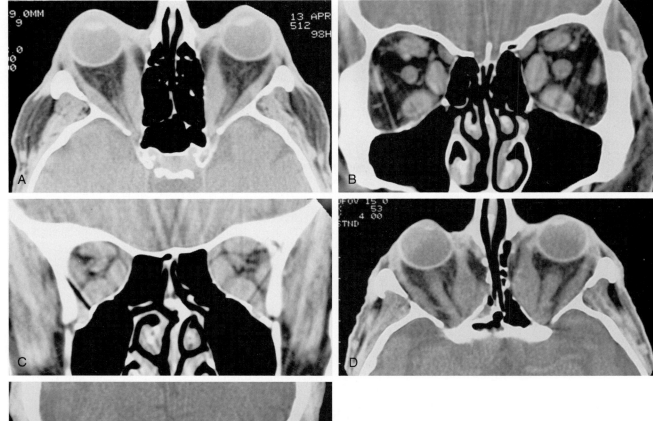

FIGURE 30–59 Advanced Graves' disease in a 63-year-old man. *A,* Axial CT demonstrates marked medial and moderate lateral rectus muscle enlargement. *B,* Coronal CT demonstrates enlargement of all the muscle bellies. *C,* Coronal CT slice through the posterior orbit shows orbital apex "crowding." *D* and *E,* Follow-up scans 18 months later, after orbital decompression. Note absence of the ethmoid sinuses. Proptosis is much improved, even though the muscle enlargement has progressed.

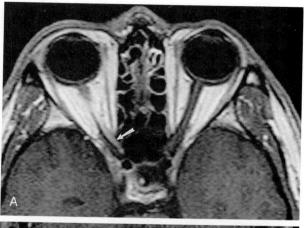
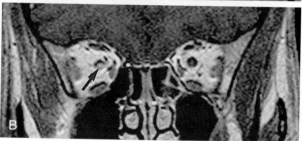

FIGURE 30–60 Optic neuritis in 33-year-old man. Axial *(A)* and coronal *(B)* T1-weighted gadolinium-enhanced images demonstrate enhancement along the medial aspect of the right optic nerve *(arrows)*.

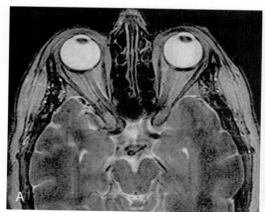
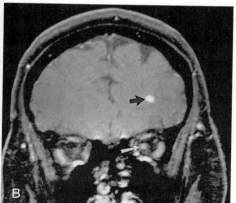

FIGURE 30–61 Optic neuritis in a 55-year-old woman. *A,* Axial T2-weighted image shows no abnormality. *B,* Gadolinium-enhanced fat-suppressed coronal image demonstrates left optic nerve enhancement *(white arrow)* as well as enhancing multiple sclerosis plaque *(black arrow)*.

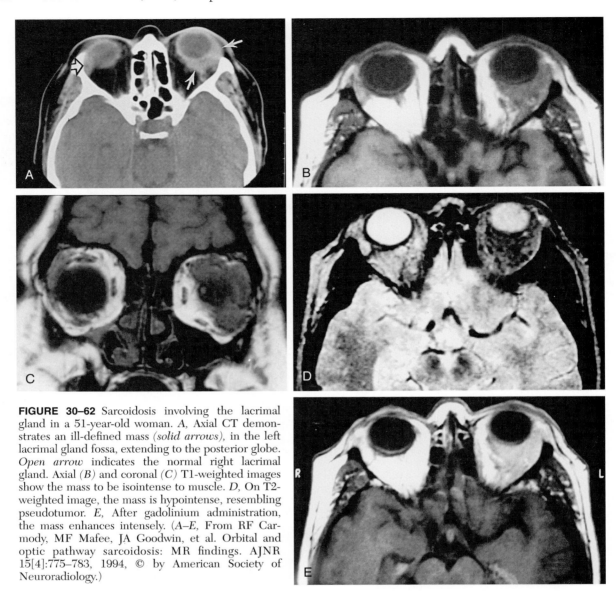

FIGURE 30–62 Sarcoidosis involving the lacrimal gland in a 51-year-old woman. *A,* Axial CT demonstrates an ill-defined mass *(solid arrows),* in the left lacrimal gland fossa, extending to the posterior globe. *Open arrow* indicates the normal right lacrimal gland. Axial *(B)* and coronal *(C)* T1-weighted images show the mass to be isointense to muscle. *D,* On T2-weighted image, the mass is hypointense, resembling pseudotumor. *E,* After gadolinium administration, the mass enhances intensely. *(A–E,* From RF Carmody, MF Mafee, JA Goodwin, et al. Orbital and optic pathway sarcoidosis: MR findings. AJNR 15[4]:775–783, 1994, © by American Society of Neuroradiology.)

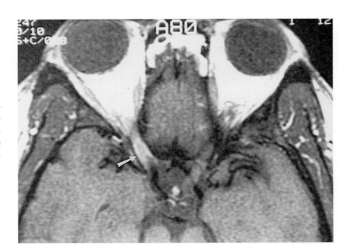

FIGURE 30–63 Optic neuritis due to sarcoidosis in a 26-year-old woman. Axial gadolinium-enhanced T1-weighted image shows perineural enhancement of the right optic nerve *(arrow).* (From RF Carmody, MF Mafee, JA Goodwin, et al. Orbital and optic pathway sarcoidosis: MR findings. AJNR 15[4]:775–783, 1994, © by American Society of Neuroradiology.)

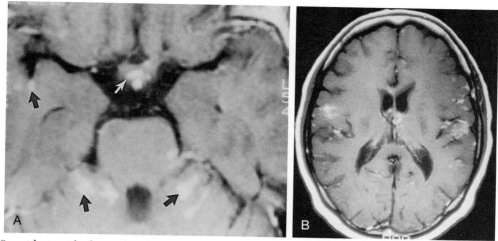

FIGURE 30–64 Sarcoidosis with chiasmal and meningeal enhancement in a 50-year-old woman. *A,* Axial gadolinium-enhanced T1-weighted image at the level of the suprasellar cistern demonstrates perichiasmal enhancement *(white arrow)* as well as basal meningeal enhancement *(black arrows)*. *B,* Higher slice shows prominent meningeal enhancement.

tration of the lacrimal gland causes glandular enlargement and prominent enhancement (Fig. 30–62). On T2-weighted images, the abnormal tissue is usually hypointense.[82] Optic nerve involvement causes nerve enlargement with enhancement, in either a solid or a tram-track pattern (Fig. 30–63). Perichiasmal enhancement is not uncommon, along with enhancement of the basal meninges (Fig. 30–64). Periventricular white matter abnormalities similar to those seen with multiple sclerosis are sometimes observed (Fig. 30–65). Orbital apex and superior orbital fissure involvement may cause Tolosa-Hunt syndrome[82] (Fig. 30–66). Since many of the imaging features of orbital sarcoid overlap those of pseudotumor, it is important to search for evidence of systemic disease to confirm the diagnosis.

Orbital Tumors and Tumor-Like Conditions

Tumors of the Optic Nerve and Nerve Sheath

Optic Glioma

Optic nerve gliomas are almost always low-grade astrocytomas. These uncommon neoplasms occur during the first decade of life in 75% of the cases, with 90% occurring during the first 2 decades.[89] About half of all optic nerve gliomas occur in patients with neurofibromatosis type 1, and 10% to 15% of individuals with neurofibromatosis type 1 develop optic gliomas.[98] Clinical signs and symp-

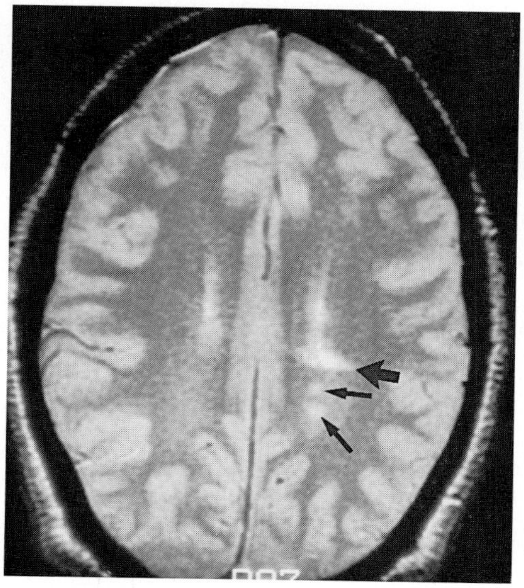

FIGURE 30–65 Periventricular lesions in an 18-year-old man with chiasmal sarcoidosis. Proton density–weighted (2900/30) image shows linear periventricular lesions resembling multiple sclerosis *(arrows)*.

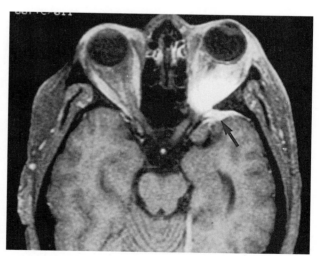

FIGURE 30–66 Orbital apex sarcoidosis presenting as Tolosa-Hunt syndrome. Gadolinium-enhanced fat-suppressed T1-weighted image demonstrates a markedly enhancing left orbital apex mass that has extended through the superior orbital fissure into the middle cranial fossa *(arrow)*. (From RF Carmody, MF Mafee, JA Goodwin, et al. Orbital and optic pathway sarcoidosis: MR findings. AJNR 15[4]:775–783, 1994, © by American Society of Neuroradiology.)

toms include proptosis, decreased visual acuity, dyschromatopsia, scotomata, and afferent pupillary defect. On ophthalmoscopic examination, papilledema or optic atrophy may be seen.

Imaging Findings. Although both CT and MRI can satisfactorily demonstrate these tumors, MRI is better for showing intracranial extension of disease. The typical case shows fusiform enlargement of the nerve, although eccentric or nodular lesions are also seen[94, 99–101] (Figs. 30–67 and 30–68). On T1-weighted images the tumor is hypointense to isointense to white matter, and on T2-weighted images it is isointense to hyperintense.[89] Mild to moderate contrast enhancement is usually seen. Bilateral optic nerve gliomas are virtually pathognomonic of neurofibromatosis type 1 (Fig. 30–69).

The clinical course of optic gliomas is unpredictable, which makes therapeutic decisions difficult. Some tumors remain stable for many years, whereas others behave more aggressively.[102] For this reason, regular follow-up with MRI is advisable.

Meningioma

Optic nerve sheath meningiomas are uncommon tumors that tend to occur in middle age, with a 3 to 1 female predominance. They can occur in younger individuals, especially those with neurofibromatosis type 2. Whereas nerve sheath meningiomas develop from the arachnoid surrounding the optic nerve,[103] meningiomas may also arise from arachnoid rests elsewhere in the orbit or from the meningeal coverings or periosteum lining the optic canal, superior orbital fissure, and bony orbit.[93] Nerve sheath meningiomas present clinically with gradual loss of vision, dyschromatopsia, scotomata, and proptosis. Funduscopic examination may show disk edema, pallor, or optic atrophy.

Imaging Findings. Both CT and MRI have a role in imaging orbital meningiomas. CT is much better at detecting the calcifications found in many of these tumors, and MRI is superior for demonstrating extension into the optic canal and intracranial compartment.[104] The imaging findings reflect the pattern of growth of the lesion. In the classic nerve sheath meningioma, the tumor surrounds the nerve in a tubular fashion, producing a tram-track appearance on axial CT or MRI and the "doughnut sign" on coronal images (Fig. 30–70). This is most apparent on enhanced studies, since these neoplasms demonstrate prominent enhancement. With MRI, the enhancement is best appreciated on fat-suppressed sequences[101] (Fig. 30–71). Growth of the tumor may be eccentric, with the nerve off to one side of the mass. On T1-weighted images, meningiomas tend to be isointense to muscle, and they are usually (although not always) low signal intensity on

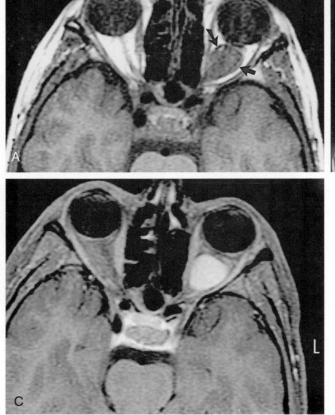
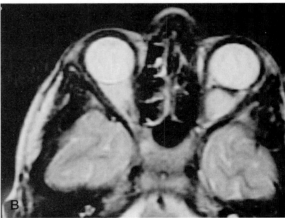

FIGURE 30–67 Optic nerve glioma in a 12-year-old boy. *A,* Axial T1-weighted image demonstrates a fusiform mass *(arrows)* replacing the normal left optic nerve. *B,* On T2-weighted fast spin echo (FSE) image, the mass is hyperintense to brain. *C,* Axial gadolinium-enhanced T1-weighted image. The tumor enhances prominently. (*A–C,* From Zimmerman RA, Gibby W, Carmody RF [eds]. Neuroimaging: Clinical and Physical Principles. New York, Springer-Verlag, 1999.)

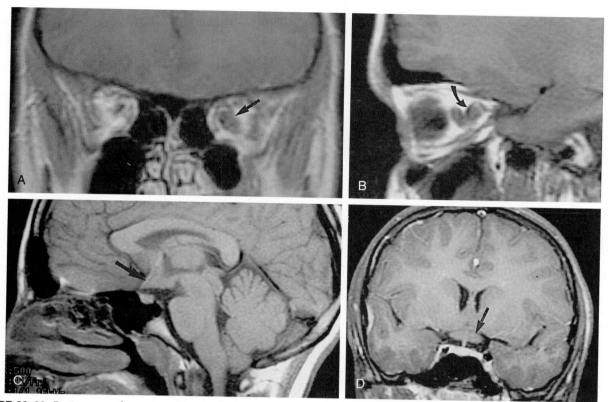

FIGURE 30–68 Optic nerve glioma in a 10-year-old boy with neurofibromatosis 1. Coronal (*A*) and sagittal (*B*) T1-weighted images demonstrate fusiform enlargement of the optic nerve (*arrows*), which is also elongated. Sagittal unenhanced (*C*) and coronal enhanced (*D*) T1-weighted images show involvement of the chiasm (*arrows*). The tumor did not enhance.

FIGURE 30–69 Bilateral optic nerve and chiasmal gliomas in a 10-year-old girl with neurofibromatosis 1. *A*, Axial enhanced CT demonstrates a suprasellar mass (*arrows*) that does not enhance appreciably. *B*, Axial T1-weighted MRI shows enlargement of the chiasm (arrow), both intracranial optic nerves, and both optic tracts. The tumor is isointense to white matter. (*A* and *B*, From Carmody RF, Van Dalen J. Magnetic resonance imaging. In Lessell S, Van Dalen J [eds]. Yearbook of Neuroophthalmology. St. Louis, Mosby–Year Book, 1991.)

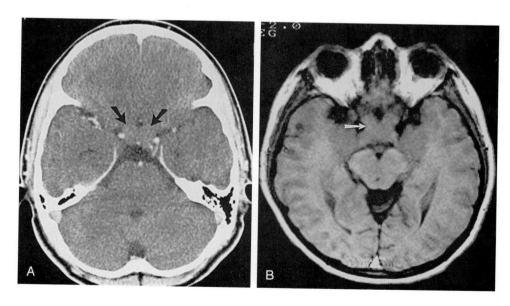

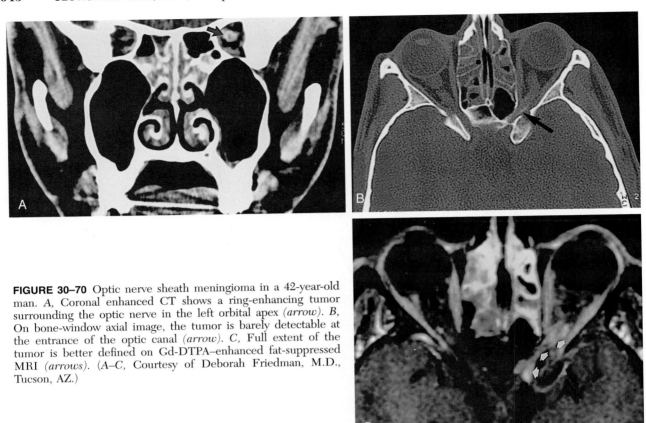

FIGURE 30–70 Optic nerve sheath meningioma in a 42-year-old man. *A,* Coronal enhanced CT shows a ring-enhancing tumor surrounding the optic nerve in the left orbital apex *(arrow). B,* On bone-window axial image, the tumor is barely detectable at the entrance of the optic canal *(arrow). C,* Full extent of the tumor is better defined on Gd-DTPA–enhanced fat-suppressed MRI *(arrows). (A–C,* Courtesy of Deborah Friedman, M.D., Tucson, AZ.)

T2-weighted images, similar to intracranial meningiomas.[105] Other conditions that may cause enlargement of the optic nerve are listed in Table 30–9.

Vascular Lesions of the Orbit

Hemangioma

Cavernous hemangiomas are hamartomatous malformations composed of large vascular channels lined by epithelial cells. They are the most common benign orbital neoplasm and are most likely to occur in females in their second to fourth decade of life.[106] Often large and bulky tumors, they are most likely to occur in the intraconal space, but they may extend into the extraconal compartment.[106] They have a tendency to spare the orbital apex

TABLE 30–9 Causes of Optic Nerve Enlargement

Optic nerve glioma
Nerve sheath meningioma
Metastasis
Inflammatory pseudotumor
Compressive optic neuropathy
Papilledema
Perineural hematoma
Graves' disease
Granulomatous disease (e.g., sarcoid)
Perineural hematoma
Normal variant

but may extend through the superior orbital fissure. Clinically, they present with proptosis and diplopia. Visual loss is uncommon, since they seldom cause optic nerve compression. Another interesting feature is stress proptosis, which can be elicited by a Valsalva maneuver or jugular compression.[107]

Imaging Findings. Because hemangiomas are filled with blood, they are hyperdense on unenhanced CT scans[108] (Fig. 30–72). Marked homogeneous contrast enhancement is seen on both CT and MRI studies. The lesions have distinct margins and do not deform the globe when they abut against it—a reflection of their soft consistency. Bone destruction is not a feature, although large hemangiomas may induce bone remodeling. Phleboliths are occasionally demonstrated at CT. On T1-weighted images, cavernous hemangiomas have been variously reported as having low to isointense to mixed signal intensity.[34, 107] On T2-weighted images, they are usually isointense or slightly hyperintense. Areas of high signal on T1-weighted images most likely represent intravascular thrombosis.[34] Hemorrhage into a cavernous hemangioma is rare.

Capillary hemangiomas are congenital malformations that present in the pediatric age group and may grow rapidly during infancy.[109] They occur on the eyelids and surrounding skin, which shows a port-wine discoloration. An unsuspected intraorbital component may be demonstrated by imaging studies. CT demonstrates an irregularly lobulated mass that enhances intensely. On MRI,

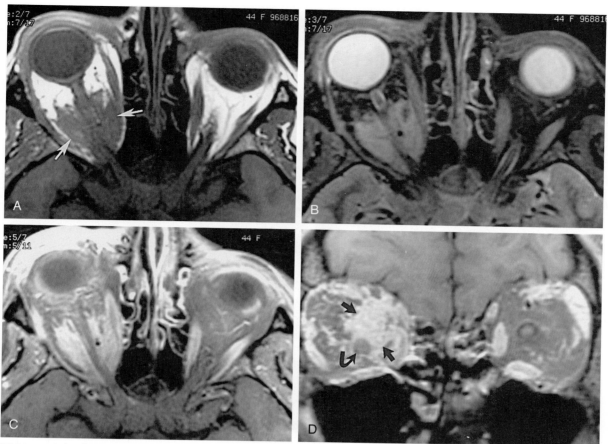

FIGURE 30–71 Orbital apex meningioma in a 44-year-old woman. *A,* T1-weighted image demonstrates a bulky mass *(arrows)* that is isointense to gray matter surrounding the right optic nerve. *B,* On fast STIR image, the tumor remains isointense to gray matter. *C,* Gadolinium-enhanced FSE T1-weighted image. The tumor enhances prominently. Notice that the optic nerve can be seen coursing through the tumor, which would not be the case if it were an optic glioma. *D,* Coronal enhanced image shows the eccentric location of the tumor *(straight arrows)* to the optic nerve *(curved arrow)*. (*A–D,* Courtesy of Kenneth Maravilla, M.D., University of Washington.)

they have variable signal characteristics, with low to isointense signal on T1-weighted images and hyperintense signal on T2-weighted images[107] (Fig. 30–73). Capillary hemangiomas usually regress spontaneously during later childhood, and those that do not will often respond to steroids.

Lymphangiomas

Lymphangiomas are soft, bulky, nonencapsulated infiltrative lesions composed of clear fluid channels.[110] They occur in a younger age group than cavernous hemangiomas, often in children or young adults. They are more likely to be extraconal than intraconal, but frequently they involve both compartments. Lymphangiomas have a tendency for spontaneous hemorrhage, which often results in sudden onset of proptosis.[106]

Imaging Findings. CT may show an irregular mass of mixed attenuation (Fig. 30–74). On MRI, lymphangiomas have a characteristic appearance (Fig. 30–75). Heterogeneous signal intensity is found on both T1- and T2-weighted images, owing to the repeated episodes of hemorrhage.[111] High signal on T1-weighted images represents

methemoglobin. Areas of low signal on T2-weighted images reflect the presence of deoxyhemoglobin or hemosiderin. High signal on T2-weighted images is due to cystic fluid-filled spaces. Contrast enhancement is variable and not as intense as with hemangiomas; some lymphangiomas do not enhance.

Lymphangiomas are difficult management problems, since complete surgical extirpation is often impossible and repeat partial excisions are commonly performed. Some investigators recommend conservative management in lieu of resection.[112]

Orbital Varix

A varix is a rare malformation consisting of a focally dilated vein. It causes proptosis with a Valsalva maneuver, with bending over, or with certain changes in head position. They are often undetectable on routine CT, but they become apparent with a Valsalva maneuver, with jugular venous compression, or with scanning in the prone position.[113, 114] Since it is a lot easier to scan during a Valsalva maneuver with CT, this is the preferred procedure for

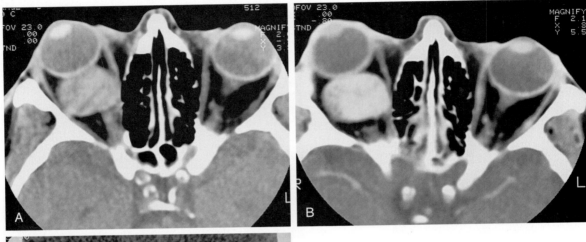

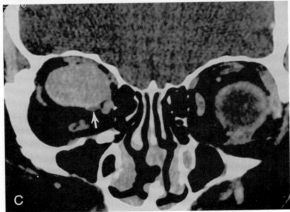

FIGURE 30–72 Cavernous hemangioma in a 65-year-old woman. *A*, Unenhanced axial CT demonstrates a large intraconal mass posterior to the right globe. The tumor is denser than muscle or brain tissue. *B*, After intravenous injection of contrast material, the lesion enhances intensely. *C*, On coronal scan, the optic nerve *(arrow)* can be identified inferior to the tumor. The sharp margins are typical for this neoplasm. (*A–C*, Courtesy of Boyd Ashdown, M.D., Tucson, AZ.)

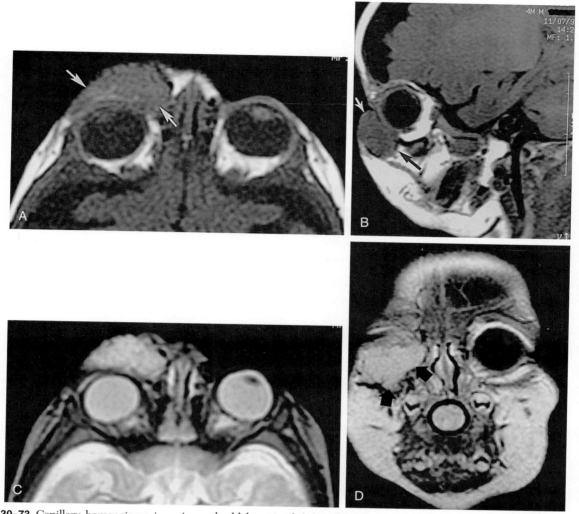

FIGURE 30–73 Capillary hemangioma in a 4-month-old boy. Axial *(A)* and sagittal *(B)* T1-weighted images demonstrate a bulky mass involving the right lower eyelid *(arrows). C,* The lesion is hyperintense to brain on the T2-weighted image. *D,* Coronal gadolinium-enhanced T1-weighted image. The lesion enhances homogeneously *(arrows).*

FIGURE 30–74 Orbital lymphangioma in a 14-year-old girl. *A,* Axial enhanced CT demonstrates a poorly circumscribed mass filling the left orbit and causing marked proptosis. *B,* Coronal CT. Owing to the infiltrative nature of the lesion, it is difficult to identify the normal orbital structures.

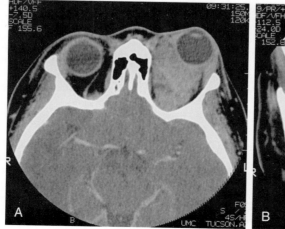
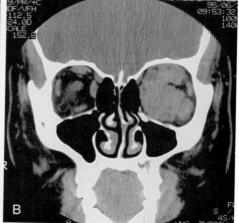

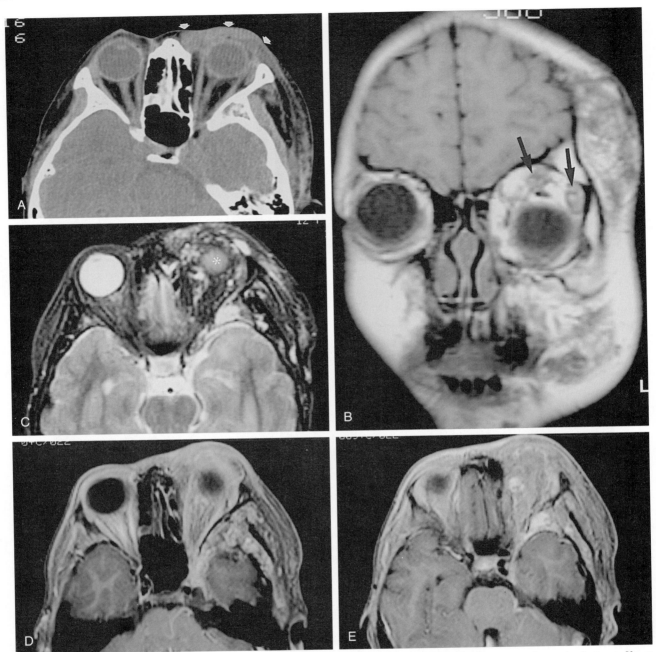

FIGURE 30–75 Extensive facial and orbital lymphangioma in a 12-year-old girl. *A,* Unenhanced CT scan shows the lesion infiltrating the eyelids and conjunctiva *(arrows). B,* Coronal T1-weighted MRI shows inferior displacement of the left globe and infiltration of the extraocular muscles *(arrows).* Note the extensive involvement of the face and scalp on the left side. *C,* Axial T2-weighted image demonstrates an ill-defined, inhomogeneous mass of mixed signal intensity in both intra- and extraconal compartments. Mixed signal is due to hemoglobin breakdown products of varying age. The top of the left globe *(asterisk)* is barely visible. *D* and *E,* T1-weighted gadolinium-enhanced, fat-suppressed images show mild, inhomogeneous enhancement of the lesion.

demonstrating a varix. On MRI, a flow void may be seen in the dilated vein.

Carotid-Cavernous Fistula

Fistulous communications between the external carotid artery and the cavernous sinus (dural arteriovenous fistula) or between the internal carotid artery and the cavernous sinus may result from head trauma, rupture of an

internal carotid aneurysm, or atherosclerotic disease (Fig. 30–76). The increased flow through the cavernous sinus results in increased venous pressure, which in turn is transmitted to the valveless orbital veins. The result is marked orbital venous distention and chemosis.[7] CT or MRI shows dilatation of the superior ophthalmic vein on the side of involvement, and there may also be engorgement of the extraocular muscles. Other causes of supe-

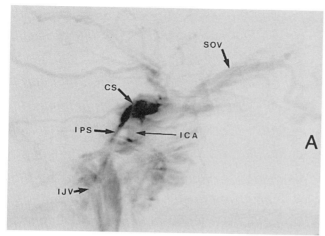

FIGURE 30–76 Carotid-cavernous sinus fistula in a 33-year-old woman who had sustained closed head trauma 3 days earlier. Left internal carotid arteriogram, lateral projection, anterior (A) to the viewer's right. With early arterial injection, there is opacification of the cavernous sinus (CS) by the fistula. Retrograde flow into a dilated superior ophthalmic vein (SOV) is seen. IPS, inferior petrosal sinus; ICA, internal carotid artery; IJV, internal jugular vein.

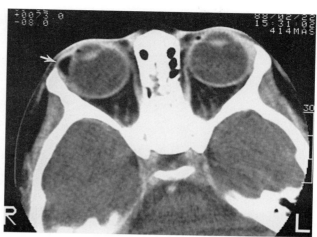

FIGURE 30–77 Orbital dermoid in a 3-year-old girl. Enhanced CT shows a fat-density mass (*arrow*) lateral to the right globe. (From Zimmerman RA, Gibby W, Carmody RF [eds]. Neuroimaging: Clinical and Physical Principles. New York, Springer-Verlag, 1999.)

rior ophthalmic vein distention include cavernous sinus thrombosis, Graves' disease, and orbital apex masses.

Dermoids and Epidermoids

Dermoids and epidermoids arise from ectodermal inclusions in the intraorbital suture lines.[115] They are the most common congenital lesions of the orbit. They often are located superficial and lateral to the globe, arising from the zygomaticofrontal suture. Since they are slow-growing benign masses, they remodel rather than invade bone. Some may also occur in a subconjunctival location. Dermoids have a well-defined capsule that contains skin appendages. Their contents vary from fat to fluid to keratinaceous material. Epidermoids contain keratin but not fat.

Imaging Findings. On CT, a well-defined mass of variable density is seen. Those that contain fat are hypodense (Fig. 30–77), and those that contain fluid vary from hypodense to isodense with muscle. A capsule that may contain calcium is identifiable (Fig. 30–78). The rim usually enhances, but the central portion does not.[115] Fat-fluid levels are not uncommon.[116] On MRI, fat-filled dermoids are hyperintense on T1-weighted images. In other cases, they may have intermediate T1 signal and hyperintense T2 signal.

Lipomas

Lipomas are rare in the orbit. When they do occur, it is usually in the fifth or sixth decade of life, and they present with gradually worsening proptosis.[117] CT shows a fat-density mass with little or no capsule (Fig. 30–79). Enhancement is uncommon. MRI confirms the presence of fatty material, with its characteristic bright signal on T1-weighted images.

Liposarcomas are aggressive, infiltrative tumors that

present with rapidly progressive proptosis. CT and MRI experience with this lesion is limited, but some have been reported as being cystic or diffusely infiltrating on CT and to have some fat density within them.[118]

Nerve Sheath Tumors

Neurofibromas and schwannomas (neurilemmomas) can arise from any of the numerous nerves in the orbit, except for the optic nerve. The optic nerve is not involved, since it is covered by meninges and not Schwann cells. The ophthalmic division of the fifth cranial nerve is the most likely source of nerve sheath tumors. Histologically, neurofibromas are a mixture of Schwann cells, axons, fibroblasts, and perineural cells.[119] Schwannomas are composed of Schwann cells arranged in the familiar Antoni A and B patterns. *Plexiform neurofibromas* occur in children with neurofibromatosis type 1; these are diffusely infiltrating, nonencapsulated, highly vascular lesions that may involve the eyelids, orbital fat, extraocular muscles, or lacrimal gland fossa.[120] Concomitant facial deformity is

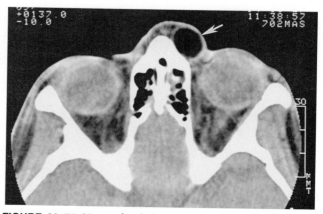

FIGURE 30–78 Naso-orbital dermoid in a 27-year-old woman. Axial CT demonstrates an encapsulated fat-density mass (*arrow*) anterior to the medial canthal tendon.

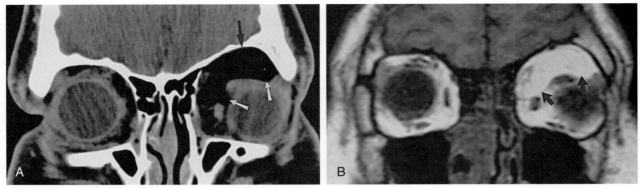

FIGURE 30–79 Orbital lipoma in a 19-year-old boy. *A,* On coronal CT, a large low-density mass is seen in the superior left orbit *(white arrows).* The globe is displaced inferolaterally. The orbital roof is elevated *(black arrow),* indicating chronicity of the lesion. *B,* On coronal T1-weighted MRI, the lesion *(arrows)* is isointense and indistinguishable from the normal orbital fat. *(A* and *B,* Courtesy of Jeffrey Popp, M.D., Omaha, NE.)

common. Additional symptoms include proptosis, decreased visual acuity, and a palpable mass. MRI demonstrates an ill-defined mass with low to moderate signal intensity on T1-weighted images and high T2 signal intensity.[120] Contrast enhancement is found on both CT and MRI.

Solitary neurofibromas are usually spherical or ovoid, well-circumscribed masses that typically occur in the superior orbit or lacrimal gland fossa. They are more common in the third to fifth decades of life.[121] On CT, they are isodense to muscle and show uniform contrast en-

hancement (Fig. 30–80). On MRI, solitary neurofibromas are hypointense or isointense to muscle on T1-weighted images and hyperintense on T2-weighted images. Enhancement with gadolinium is the rule.

Schwannomas occur in adults and present with slowly progressive proptosis and, not uncommonly, diplopia. These well-encapsulated tumors usually cannot be distinguished from solitary neurofibromas by imaging studies, since they have similar CT and MRI features. Occasionally, schwannomas are partially cystic or may contain intratumoral hemorrhage, which helps to distinguish them

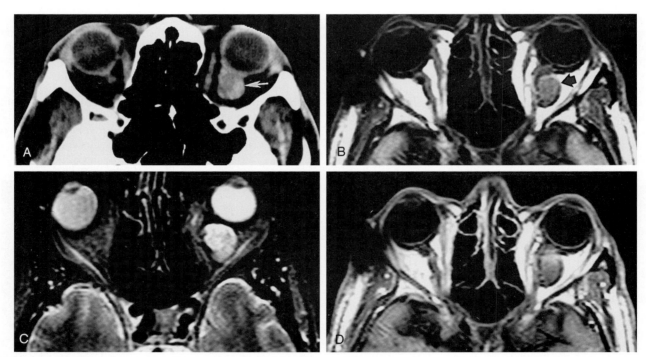

FIGURE 30–80 Neurofibroma in a 57-year-old man with known neurofibromatosis 1. *A,* Axial unenhanced CT demonstrates a well-circumscribed intraconal lesion *(arrow). B,* On T1-weighted MRI, the mass *(arrow)* is isointense to muscle. *C,* The tumor is hyperintense on T2-weighted image. *D,* On gadolinium-enhanced image, the neurofibroma shows only mild enhancement, which is atypical for nerve sheath tumors. *(A–D,* From Zimmerman RA, Gibby W, Carmody RF [eds]. Neuroimaging: Clinical and Physical Principles. New York, Springer-Verlag, 1999.)

from neurofibromas.[34] Schwannomas and solitary neurofibromas may closely resemble cavernous hemangiomas on imaging studies.

Lacrimal Gland Masses

About half of all lacrimal gland masses are epithelial in origin, and the rest are either lymphoid or inflammatory in nature (Table 30–10).[122] Of the epithelial tumors, half are benign mixed tumors (pleomorphic adenomas) and the remainder are carcinomas. Cell types of the carcinomas include adenoid cystic carcinoma, malignant mixed tumor, mucoepidermoid carcinoma, adenocarcinoma, squamous cell carcinoma, and anaplastic carcinoma.[7, 123] Lacrimal gland tumors present with a palpable mass in the lacrimal gland fossa or with proptosis. Although pain may indicate an active inflammatory process, it can also be present with adenoid cystic carcinoma, which has a propensity for perineural spread.[119]

On imaging studies, pleomorphic adenomas appear as well-marginated heterogeneous lesions causing lacrimal gland enlargement (Fig. 30–81). Scalloping of adjacent bone may be present, but bone destruction is absent. Some degree of contrast enhancement is usually seen. The carcinomas tend to have more irregular margins and early bony invasion. Spread to the paranasal sinuses, cavernous sinus, and intracranial compartment occurs early, and the prognosis is poor. On MRI, the carcinomas tend to be hypointense on T1-weighted images and hyperintense on T2-weighted images.[119] High signal intensity on T1-weighted images may be seen with mucoepidermoid carcinoma. It is generally not possible on the basis of imaging studies to distinguish between the various cell types of carcinomas, since the imaging features are nonspecific.

A number of lymphoid and inflammatory diseases may occur in the lacrimal gland. In the lymphoid group, the

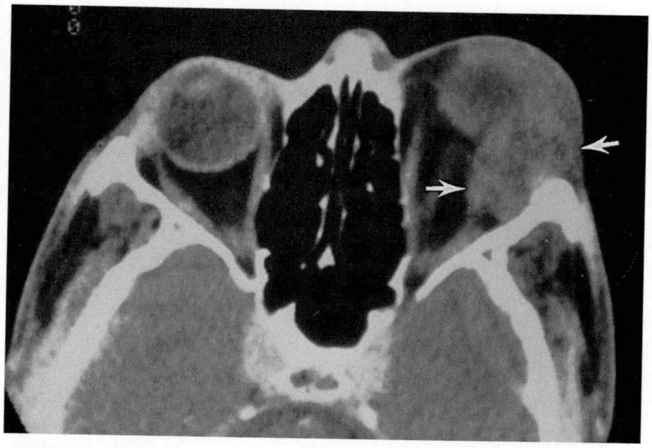

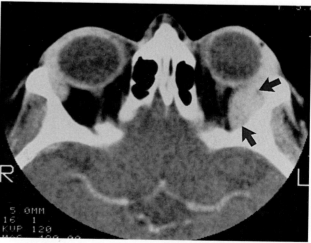

FIGURE 30–81 Pleomorphic adenoma of the left lacrimal gland. Enhanced axial CT shows a poorly enhancing, somewhat heterogeneous mass (arrow) in the left lacrimal gland fossa. (Courtesy of Mahmood Mafee, M.D., Chicago, IL.)

spectrum ranges from lymphoid hyperplasia to malignant lymphoma. Lymphomas tend to cause diffuse enlargement of the gland with homogeneous contrast enhancement (Fig. 30–82). Bone destruction seldom occurs, and the tumor tends to mold itself to the surrounding structures, such as the globe. Most lymphomas are hypointense on T1-weighted images and hypointense to hyperintense on T2-weighted images, depending on the cellularity of the lesion (Fig. 30–83). Sarcoidosis and pseudotumor are more likely to be hypointense on T2-weighted images.[82] Other inflammatory conditions to affect the lacrimal gland in addition to sarcoid and pseudotumor include Sjögren's and Mikulicz's syndromes (Fig. 30–84), and Wegener's granulomatosis. None of these diseases has distinctive

TABLE 30–10 Lacrimal Gland Masses

Epithelial Neoplasms

Pleomorphic adenoma (benign mixed tumor)
Adenoid cystic carcinoma
Mucoepidermoid carcinoma
Adenocarcinoma
Malignant mixed tumor
Undifferentiated carcinoma
Squamous cell carcinoma
Sebaceous carcinoma

Nonepithelial Lesions

Lymphoid hyperplasia
Lymphoma
Inflammatory pseudotumor
Sarcoid
Cyst
Dermoid
Sjögren's syndrome
Mikulicz' syndrome
Wegener's granulomatosis
Metastasis
Dacryoadenitis

FIGURE 30–82 Lacrimal gland and conjunctival lymphoma in a 63-year-old woman. Axial enhanced CT shows a homogeneously enhancing mass replacing the left lacrimal gland (arrows), conjunctival infiltration, and slight enlargement of the right lacrimal gland. (From Carmody RF, Yang PJ. Computed tomography of orbital tumors. Contemp Diagn Radiol 1988;11[3]:1–6.)

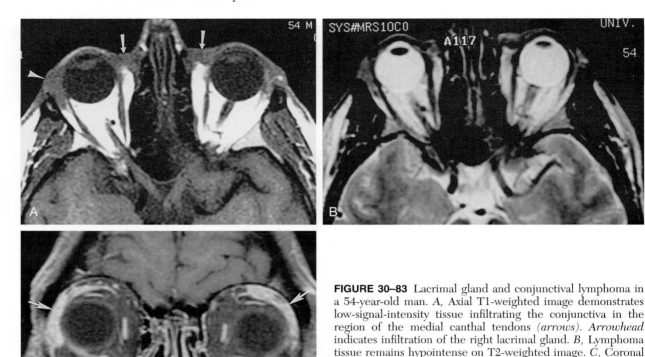

FIGURE 30–83 Lacrimal gland and conjunctival lymphoma in a 54-year-old man. *A,* Axial T1-weighted image demonstrates low-signal-intensity tissue infiltrating the conjunctiva in the region of the medial canthal tendons *(arrows)*. *Arrowhead* indicates infiltration of the right lacrimal gland. *B,* Lymphoma tissue remains hypointense on T2-weighted image. *C,* Coronal Gd-DTPA–enhanced, fat-suppressed image shows intense enhancement of the lymphoma *(arrows)*.

imaging features, although all of them cause gland enlargement.

Lymphoproliferative Disease

Lymphoid masses in the orbit and adnexa are classified according to their histologic aggressiveness as reactive lymphoid hyperplasia (pseudolymphoma), atypical lymphoid hyperplasia (borderline lesions), and malignant lymphoma.[124] Whereas reactive lymphoid hyperplasia is mixed T-cell and B-cell type, the malignant lymphomas consist primarily of B-cell lymphocytes. About 30% to 35% of orbital lymphomas are associated with systemic lymphoma, and most are of the non-Hodgkin type.[125] The higher the grade of orbital lymphoma, the more likely the patient has systemic disease.[124] After a biopsy has determined that lymphoma is present in the orbit, the patient needs to have a workup for systemic disease.

Orbital lymphoid tumors present clinically with

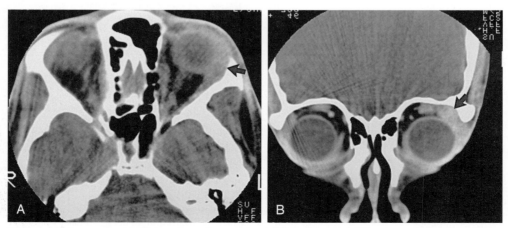

FIGURE 30–84 A 24-year-old woman with Sjögren's syndrome. Axial *(A)* and coronal *(B)* enhanced CT demonstrate enlargement of the left lacrimal gland *(arrows)* with mild enhancement. (*A* and *B,* From Zimmerman RA, Gibby W, and Carmody RF [eds]. Neuroimaging: Clinical and Physical Principles. New York, Springer-Verlag, 1999.)

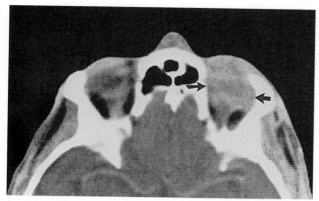

FIGURE 30–85 Non-Hodgkin's lymphoma in a 69-year-old man. Axial CT demonstrates an enhancing mass (*arrows*) filling the superior aspect of the left orbit. The lacrimal gland is also involved.

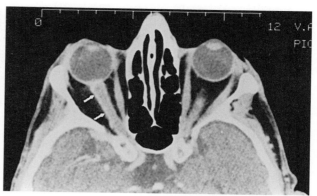

FIGURE 30–87 Lymphoma infiltrating the right optic nerve sheath. Axial enhanced CT demonstrates the "tram track" pattern of enhancement (*arrows*), similar to that seen with optic perineuritis or nerve sheath meningioma. (From Carmody RF, Yang PJ. Computed tomography of orbital tumors. Contemp Diagn Radiol 1988;11[3]:1–6.)

proptosis, globe displacement, visual impairment, ptosis, diplopia, and mild motility disorders.[124] Unlike pseudotumor, they are more likely to be painless. Females have a higher incidence, and the most common age at presentation is 50 to 70 years.[124] Although virtually any structure in the orbit can be involved, the extraocular muscles are usually spared.

Imaging Findings. Some of the imaging features of lymphoma have been discussed in the section on lacrimal gland tumors. CT is usually adequate for evaluating orbital lymphoid lesions, with MRI occasionally providing additional helpful information. Lymphoma commonly occurs in the extraconal compartment, often in the superior orbit, where it may obscure the superior rectus and levator palpebrae superioris muscles and cause inferior displacement of the globe (Fig. 30–85). Molding of the tumor around the globe is characteristic (Fig. 30–86). Infiltration of the anterior orbital structures, such as the lids and conjunctivae, may be seen. Involvement of Tenon's space causes apparent thickening of the posterior wall of the globe. The optic nerve sheath may be infiltrated, creating an appearance indistinguishable from perioptic neuritis or pseudotumor[126] (Fig. 30–87). Although bone destruction is uncommon except in cases of the most malignant cell types, lymphoma not infrequently

extends out of the orbit via the superior and inferior orbital fissures and various foramina. Lymphoid masses tend to be hyperdense and homogeneous on CT and show mild to moderate enhancement (Fig. 30–88). As discussed previously, they are hypointense on T1-weighted images and hypointense to hyperintense on T2-weighted images, with prominent gadolinium enhancement.

Leukemia also occurs in the orbit and has a predilection for the choroid of the globe (Fig. 30–89),[127] although any structure may be involved. Optic nerve sheath infiltration is not uncommon.

Langerhans Cell Histiocytosis

Formerly known as histiocytosis X, this reticuloendothelial disorder of unknown cause may involve the orbits in pediatric patients. Extensive lytic bone destruction is the rule, especially of the lateral orbital wall and middle

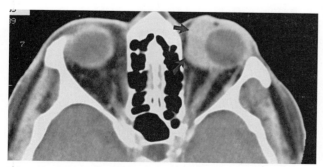

FIGURE 30–86 Orbital lymphoma in a 63-year-old man. Axial enhanced CT shows a homogeneously enhancing mass in the medial orbit (*arrows*). Note how the tumor is molding itself to the adjacent globe, a characteristic feature of lymphoma.

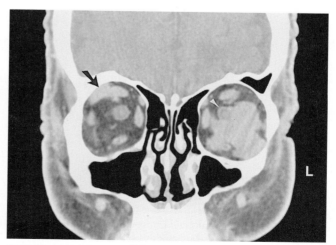

FIGURE 30–88 Large cell lymphoma in a 73-year-old man. Coronal enhanced CT shows a large intraconal mass (*arrowhead*) in the left orbit, partially surrounding the optic nerve. A smaller tumor deposit (*arrow*) is seen in the right orbit.

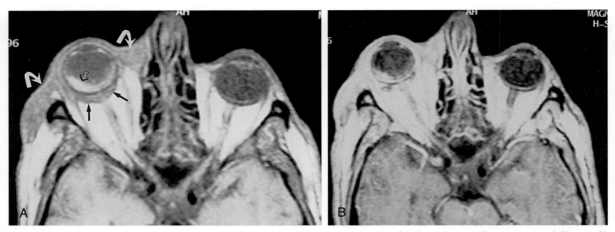

FIGURE 30–89 Leukemic infiltration of the orbit of a 35-year-old man. *A,* T1-weighted axial MRI demonstrates diffuse infiltration of the ocular adnexa *(curved arrows)* and Tenon's space *(black arrows)*. Choroidal hemorrhage is present *(open arrow)*. *B,* After Gd-DTPA administration, the leukemic infiltrate enhances prominently. (*A* and *B,* Courtesy of Thomas Spera, M.D., Tucson, AZ.)

cranial fossa. Associated soft tissue masses are seen in the orbit, typically in the lateral extraconal compartment. On CT, the masses are isodense to hyperdense with prominent contrast enhancement (Fig. 30–90). MRI discloses hypointense to isointense T1 signal and hypointense to occasionally hyperintense T2 signal.[128]

Rhabdomyosarcoma

Rhabdomyosarcoma is the most common primary malignant soft tissue tumor of the head and neck in childhood. The orbit and the paranasal sinus are the usual sites of involvement. The tumor arises from primitive mesenchymal elements in the orbit, or it may invade the orbit secondarily from adjacent structures. The neoplasm is uncommon in adults, with 90% of patients being under age 16 years.[129, 130] The embryonal cell type is the most common in the orbit.[129, 131] Clinical findings include rapidly progressive proptosis, dystopia, eyelid ecchymosis, and ophthalmoplegia[132] (Fig. 30–91).

Imaging Findings. On CT, rhabdomyosarcomas appear as well-defined masses that are isodense with the extraocular muscles and enhance after contrast administration.[132] Bone remodeling or destruction may be seen. Invasion into the paranasal sinuses, nasopharynx, or intracranial compartment frequently occurs. On MRI, rhabdomyosarcoma is of intermediate signal intensity on all pulse sequences and enhances after gadolinium administration.[133]

Metastatic Disease to the Orbit

The orbit is occasionally the site of metastatic deposits, most commonly from carcinoma of the breast and lung.[134]

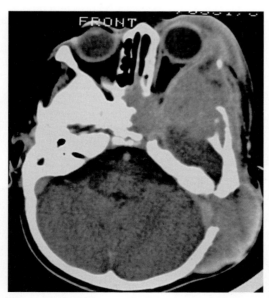

FIGURE 30–90 Langerhans cell histiocytosis in a 2-year-old girl. Enhanced CT shows extensive destruction of the left lateral orbital wall, sphenoid bone, and temporo-occipital region by the enhancing mass. (From WK Erly, RF Carmody, RM Dryden. Orbital histiocytosis X. AJNR 16[6]:1258–1261, 1995, © by American Society of Neuroradiology.)

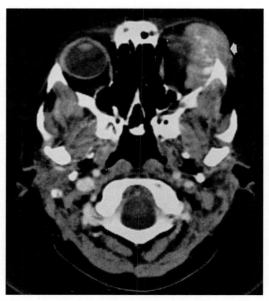

FIGURE 30–91 Rhabdomyosarcoma in a 58-year-old woman. Enhanced axial CT demonstrates a heterogeneous enhancing mass *(arrow)* in the lateral left orbit.

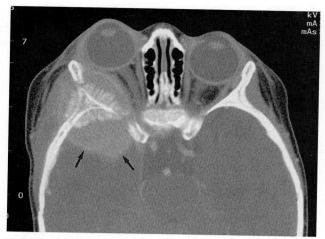

FIGURE 30–92 Metastatic neuroblastoma in a 9-year-old girl. Axial CT demonstrates a mass originating from the greater wing of the sphenoid on the right, with invasion of the lateral orbit and medial displacement of the lateral rectus muscle. The tumor extends into the middle cranial fossa *(arrows)*. Note the characteristic starburst pattern of the bone spicules in neuroblastoma bone involvement.

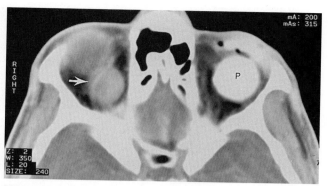

FIGURE 30–94 Metastatic melanoma to the right orbit in a 57-year-old man. Axial enhanced CT shows an intraconal mass *(arrow)* posterior to the globe. A hydroxyapatite prosthesis (P) is seen in the left orbit.

In children, neuroblastoma frequently metastasizes to the orbit. Any structure in the orbit may be affected, including the globe. Most metastases are located in the extraconal space, but eventually the entire orbit may be diffusely infiltrated. Bone destruction is common. Although most patients with orbital metastasis present with proptosis, metastatic scirrhous carcinoma of the breast or stomach may cause enophthalmos.[135]

Imaging Findings. The CT and MRI findings in metastatic disease are quite variable, depending on the primary tumor of origin and the location of disease in the orbit. Typically, an infiltrating, rather poorly marginated mass is seen in the extraconal space, often with invasion of the adjacent bone (Figs. 30–92 through 30–94). Slight to moderate contrast enhancement is usually found. MRI findings are nonspecific, with decreased signal on T1-weighted images and increased signal on T2-weighted images[136] (Fig. 30–95).

Paranasal Sinus Diseases That May Involve the Orbit

Mucocele

Mucoceles are expansile, mucus-filled lesions that result from obstruction of a sinus ostium or a compartment of a septated sinus.[133] They are most common in the frontal sinuses, followed in decreasing order by the ethmoids, maxillary sinuses, and sphenoid sinus. The affected sinus is completely airless and undergoes slow remodeling and expansion. Frontal sinus mucoceles may expand inferiorly into the orbit and cause downward displacement of the globe. Anterior ethmoid mucoceles expand the lamina papyracea and cause lateral displacement of the globe and diplopia. Rarely, a large maxillary antral mucocele may elevate the floor of the orbit. Sphenoid sinus involvement may eventually compromise the orbital apex and optic nerve. Mucoceles may also occur as a complication of facial fractures (Fig. 30–96).

Imaging Findings. On plain radiographs, the frontal sinus mucocele causes clouding of the sinus, with smooth expansion and obliteration of the normal septations. On CT, the sinus cavity is filled with fluid-density material and the walls are bowed outward. In some cases, the bony sinus walls become markedly thinned or even invisible (Figs. 30–97 and 30–98). The MRI appearance of mucoceles is quite variable, depending on the protein content and the degree of inspissation of the secretions within the sinus. If the secretions have a high water content, the T1-weighted images have hypointense signal and the T2-weighted images hyperintense signal. Partially inspissated mucoceles are hyperintense on all sequences, and completely inspissated lesions may be hypointense on all sequences.[137]

Mucormycosis

Rhinocerebral mucormycosis occurs in certain predisposed individuals, especially uncontrolled diabetics and

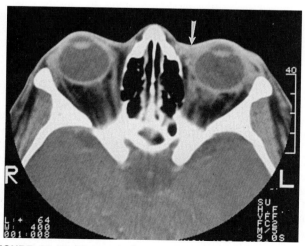

FIGURE 30–93 Metastatic breast carcinoma in a 49-year-old woman. Enhanced axial CT shows infiltration of the medial canthal area *(arrow)*, conjunctiva, medial rectus muscle, and Tenon's capsule.

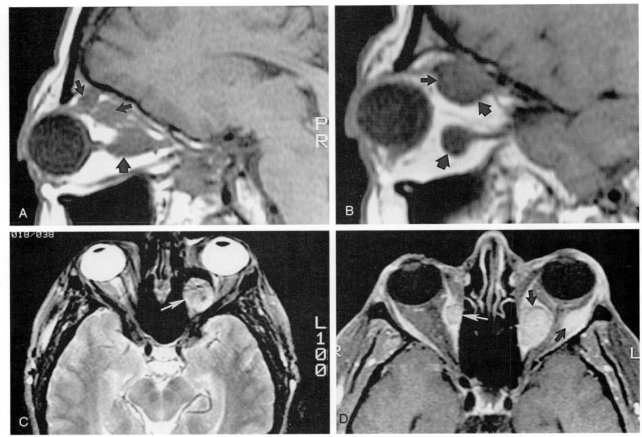

FIGURE 30–95 Melanoma metastatic to both orbits in a 48-year-old woman. *A* and *B,* Sagittal T1-weighted images of the right and left orbits show multiple masses *(arrows)*. *C,* Axial T2-weighted image demonstrates a heterogeneous mass *(arrow)* in the medial left orbit. *D,* Axial fat-suppressed, gadolinium-enhanced T1-weighted image demonstrates enhancing masses *(arrows)* within the bellies of the rectus muscles. *(A–D,* Courtesy of Rick Park, M.D., Owensboro, KY.)

immunocompromised patients. The disease is caused by several genera of fungi of the family Mucoraceae, most commonly *Rhizopus, Mucor,* and *Absidia*.[133] The infection typically starts in the nasal cavity, then spreads to the paranasal sinuses and next to the orbit (Fig. 30–99). The fungus invades blood vessel walls, causing thrombosis and tissue necrosis. Bony destruction is extensive. Orbital involvement may lead to proptosis, ptosis, ophthalmoplegia, and eventually blindness. If uncontrolled, the infection spreads to the cavernous sinus via the orbital veins to cause widespread cerebral infarction.

Carcinoma

Paranasal sinus tumors not uncommonly invade the orbit by direct extension through the orbital walls. Most paranasal sinus malignancies are squamous cell carcinomas, with the maxillary antrum being the sinus most frequently affected. However, ethmoid sinus carcinoma is more likely to invade the orbit. Multiplanar imaging studies are critically important to the management of paranasal sinus neoplasms, and demonstration of orbital invasion significantly alters treatment.

Imaging Findings. CT or MRI demonstrates a soft tissue mass within the affected sinus, often with associated bone destruction, particularly with squamous cell carcinoma (Fig. 30–100). Whereas bone destruction is the hallmark of sinus carcinoma, some neoplasms such as mucoepidermoid carcinoma and lymphoma may cause bony remodeling.[133] MRI is superior to CT for distinguishing solid tumor within the sinus from sinus obstruction with retained secretions. Tumors tend to have intermediate signal intensity on T2-weighted images, whereas retained secretions have increased T2 signal. CT is helpful for confirming subtle areas of bone destruction.

The necrotizing vasculitides may produce a clinical and radiographic picture similar to that of carcinoma and can involve both the paranasal sinuses and the orbit. Wegener's granulomatosis commonly involves the upper and lower respiratory tract and affects the orbit in 18% to 22% of cases.[7] Pulmonary and renal disease are part of the syndrome. Imaging findings in the orbit may be indistinguishable from pseudotumor. Similar to Wegener's granulomatosis is polymorphic reticulosis, formerly known as lethal midline granuloma. This entity causes extensive destructive lesions in the nose, paranasal sinuses, facial bones, and frequently, the orbit.

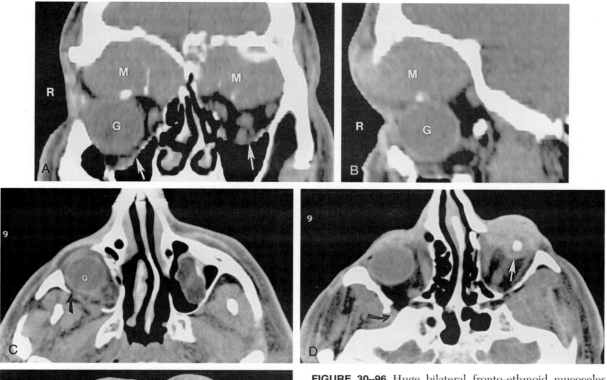

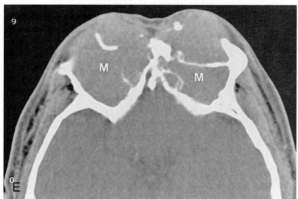

FIGURE 30–96 Huge bilateral fronto-ethmoid mucoceles in a 40-year-old man with an old, untreated LeFort III fracture. *A,* Coronal re-formatted CT demonstrates mucoceles (M) filling the superior portions of the orbits. The right globe (G) is displaced inferiorly into the maxillary sinus. The bilateral orbital floor fractures *(arrows)* have healed in poor positions. R, right. *B,* Sagittal re-formations through the right orbit. *C,* Axial CT through the maxillary sinuses shows the right globe in the antrum and an un-united lateral maxillary sinus wall fracture *(arrow)*. *D,* Higher axial slice shows the small, calcified (phthisic) left globe *(white arrow)*. The displaced fracture of the right lateral orbital wall is seen *(black arrow)*. *E,* Axial slice through the superior orbits shows mucoceles.

FIGURE 30–97 Frontal sinus mucocele in a 40-year-old man. *A,* Axial enhanced CT shows a mass *(arrows)* anterior to the right globe. The periphery of the mass enhances, but the central part does not. *B,* Coronal CT shows a soft tissue mass filling the right frontal sinus, with erosion of the orbital roof *(solid arrows)*. The globe *(open arrow)* is displaced inferiorly. Extensive chronic sinusitis is present.

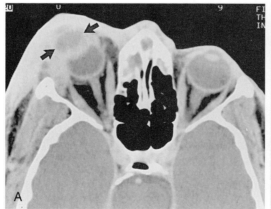

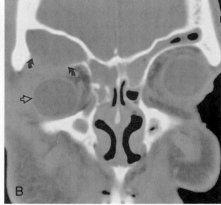

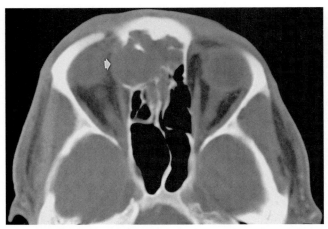

FIGURE 30–98 Ethmoid sinus mucocele in a 53-year-old man. Axial CT shows a soft tissue density mass in the anterior ethmoid region on the right. The mucocele *(arrow)* has eroded through the lamina papyracea and protrudes into the orbit.

THE POSTERIOR VISUAL PATHWAYS

Anatomic Considerations

At the optic chiasm, nerve fibers from the nasal side of each retina decussate to the contralateral optic tract. Axons from the temporal side of the retina do not cross at the chiasm; thus, the left optic tract contains axons from both the left temporal and the left nasal hemiretinas. Light rays from the right side of the visual field fall on the left side of both retinas, so that the left optic tract conducts visual impulses from the right visual field. From the chiasm, the optic tracts course posterolaterally around the hypothalamus in the ambient cistern to the lateral geniculate nuclei, where most of the fibers terminate. A small number of fibers bypass the lateral geniculate nu-

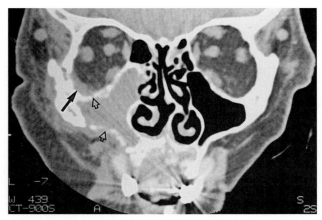

FIGURE 30–99 Mucormycosis in a 76-year-old diabetic woman. On coronal CT scan, the right maxillary antrum is opacified, with destruction of the lateral and superior walls *(open arrows)*. The infection has broken through into the inferolateral orbit *(solid arrow)*. (From Zimmerman RA, Gibby W, Carmody RF [eds]. Neuroimaging: Clinical and Physical Principles. New York, Springer-Verlag, 1999.)

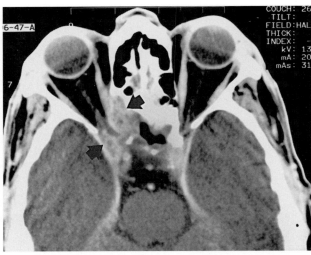

FIGURE 30–100 Sphenoethmoid squamous cell carcinoma with orbital involvement in a 53-year-old woman. Axial enhanced CT shows destruction of the posterior ethmoid cells on right, with the tumor *(arrows)* filling the orbital apex.

cleus and terminate in the superior colliculus and pretectal region of the midbrain. These are afferent pupillary fibers and are involved in the pupillary light reflex.[138]

After synapsing in the lateral geniculate nuclei, the visual fibers proceed to the visual cortex as the optic radiations. After fanning out from the lateral geniculate body, the optic radiations pass through the retrolenticular portion of the internal capsule and divide into two groups:

1. The more anterior fibers sweep forward around the temporal horn of the lateral ventricle (Meyer's loop) and then course posteriorly to the inferior calcarine cortex. This fiber group represents the superior position of the visual field.
2. The posterior fibers course posteriorly along the lateral surface of the occipital horn of the lateral ventricle, terminating in a more superior portion of the calcarine cortex. These fibers represent the inferior portion of the visual field.

In the visual cortex, the fibers representing macular vision project to the posterior third of the occipital lobe. The peripheral visual fields are mapped topographically in the more anterior portion of the medial surface of the occipital lobe. The superior portion of the calcarine cortex represents the inferior portion of the visual field, and the superior fields are mapped on the inferior visual cortex.

Visual Pathway Pathology

A complete discourse on all the various types of lesions affecting the visual pathways is well beyond the scope of this chapter; only the basic principles are discussed, since these have great relevance to planning an imaging strategy. In general, MRI is the procedure of choice for imaging the visual pathways. A diagrammatic overview of the effects of optic pathway lesions is presented in Figure 30–101.

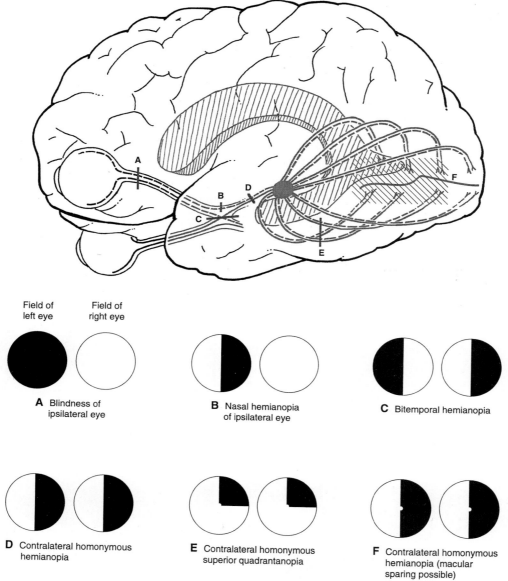

Field of left eye   Field of right eye

A Blindness of ipsilateral eye

B Nasal hemianopia of ipsilateral eye

C Bitemporal hemianopia

D Contralateral homonymous hemianopia

E Contralateral homonymous superior quadrantanopia

F Contralateral homonymous hemianopia (macular sparing possible)

FIGURE 30–101 Visual defects produced by interruption of the optic pathways at various sites (labeled *A–F* on *top figure* to correspond to *bottom figures*). *A,* Destruction of one optic nerve causes ipsilateral monocular blindness. *B,* Damage to one side of the optic chiasm destroys the noncrossing fibers from the ipsilateral eye. These fibers arise in the temporal retina, so a nasal hemianopia of the ipsilateral eye results. *C,* Pressure on the center of the optic chiasm, typically from a pituitary tumor, destroys the crossing fibers from both eyes, causing a bitemporal hemianopia. *D,* Destruction of one optic tract causes contralateral homonymous hemianopia. *E,* Damage to one temporal lobe could destroy part of the optic radiation, specifically the fibers representing the contralateral superior quadrant of each visual field. Since the optic radiation is rather spread out at this point, some fibers are likely to be spared (e.g., in this case, the macular fibers remain intact). *F,* Massive damage to one occipital lobe *(shaded area),* such as might be caused by occlusion of one posterior cerebral artery, causes contralateral homonymous hemianopia. The macular representation is quite large, and some of it is likely to survive, resulting in macular sparing. (*A–F,* From Nolte J. The Human Brain, 3rd ed. St. Louis, Mosby–Year Book, 1993.)

Optic Nerve

Injury to the optic nerve causes monocular visual loss and an *afferent pupillary defect*. The ipsilateral pupil constricts poorly or not at all in response to light stimulation owing to interruption of the afferent pupillary fibers in the optic nerve. However, it will constrict if a light is shone in the contralateral eye (consensual reflex), since pupil constriction is mediated by parasympathetic fibers from the Edinger-Westphal nucleus, which receives bilateral innervation from the pretectal region. The pupillomotor fibers reach the eye via the oculomotor nerve. Many of the conditions that cause optic neuropathy have already been discussed. Others include vascular lesions, such as ischemia and aneurysm; bony lesions compromising the optic canal, such as fibrous dysplasia and metastatic disease; and paranasal sinus lesions, such as tumor or infection of the posterior ethmoid or sphenoid sinuses.

Chiasm

The chiasm may be primarily affected by inflammatory lesions (e.g., demyelinating disease, sarcoid), tumors (e.g., chiasmatic glioma, lymphoma), vascular lesions (e.g., cavernous angiomas, arteriovenous malformations, ischemia), radiation injury, or trauma. More often, however, the chiasm is secondarily involved by a wide array of lesions that can occur in the suprasellar cistern. The most common of these is the pituitary adenoma, which compresses the chiasm and causes a bitemporal hemianopia. The decussating fibers from the nasal hemiretinas are the ones compromised by these large tumors. Sagittal and coronal MRI with gadolinium enhancement is the optimal way of assessing chiasmal compression (Figs. 30–102 and 30–103). Radiation injury to the chiasm appears as thickening and enhancement on MRI.[139]

Optic Tract

Complete transection of the optic tract produces a homonymous hemianopia and a subtle contralateral afferent pupillary defect.[140] More often, an incomplete lesion is present, which causes an incongruous hemianopia. Lesions of the optic tract are distinctly uncommon. Chiasmal gliomas may grow posteriorly along the optic tract. Others include aneurysm (Fig. 30–104), demyelinating disease, craniopharyngioma, ischemia, and radiation injury.

Lateral Geniculate Nucleus

Lesions of the lateral geniculate body produce a congruous contralateral hemianopia. Unlike optic tract lesions,

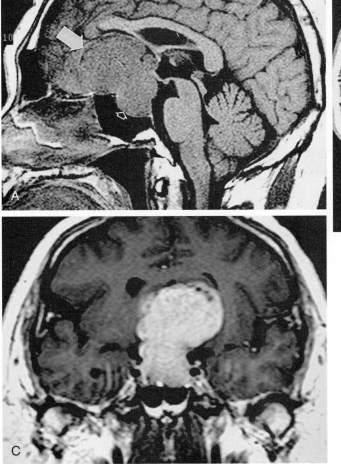
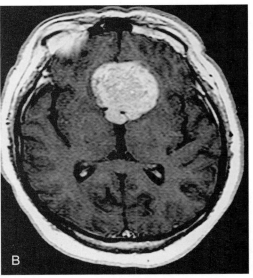

FIGURE 30–102 Pituitary adenoma. A, Sagittal T1-weighted MRI shows a mass filling the sella turcica *(open arrow)*, with massive suprasellar extension *(solid arrow)*. The optic tracts and chiasm are not identifiable with certainty. Axial *(B)* and coronal *(C)* Gd-DTPA–enhanced T1-weighted images show a homogeneously enhancing tumor with marked suprasellar extension. The patient had severe bilateral visual loss due to chiasmal compression.

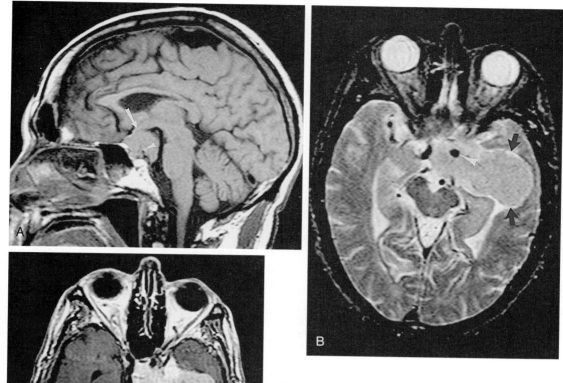

FIGURE 30–103 Suprasellar meningioma in a 74-year-old man. *A,* Sagittal T1-weighted MRI shows a mass in the suprasellar cistern with elevation of the chiasm and optic tracts *(arrow).* The dorsum sellae is eroded *(arrowhead).* *B,* Axial T2-weighted image shows the tumor to extend into the right middle cranial fossa *(arrows)* and to encase the left internal carotid artery *(arrowhead).* *C,* Axial T1-weighted image after Gd-DTPA administration demonstrates homogeneous enhancement, typical of meningioma.

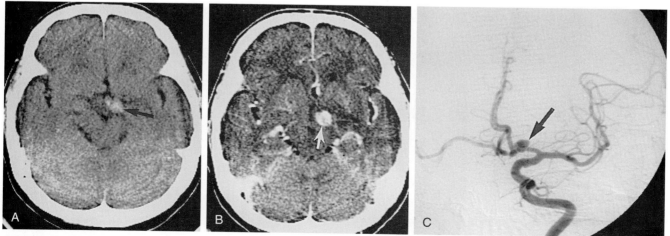

FIGURE 30–104 Optic tract compression from an anterior cerebral artery aneurysm. *A,* Unenhanced CT shows a high-density lesion in the region of the left optic tract, most likely representing the aneurysm and surrounding hemorrhage *(arrow).* *B,* Enhanced scan depicts the lumen of the aneurysm *(arrow).* *C,* Left internal carotid angiogram shows the aneurysm *(arrow)* arising from the horizontal segment of the anterior cerebral artery. The patient had a right visual field defect. (*A–C,* From Zimmerman RA, Gibby W, Carmody RF [eds]. Neuroimaging: Clinical and Physical Principles. New York, Springer-Verlag, 1999.)

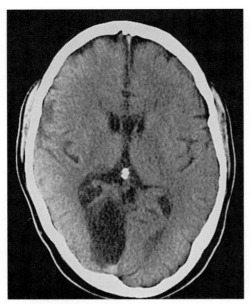

FIGURE 30–105 A 68-year-old male developed left homonymous hemianopia after chiropractic manipulation a few months earlier. Unenhanced CT scan demonstrates a hypodense area in the right occipital lobe due to infarction. Stroke was caused by vertebral artery dissection.

the pupillary responses are preserved. Infarction, tumor, vascular malformation, and trauma are some causative possibilities that may be demonstrated on imaging studies. It would be unusual for an infarct to involve only the lateral geniculate body, and other ipsilateral thalamic findings are usually present.

Optic Radiations

As discussed earlier, part of the optic radiations loop through the temporal lobes (anterior bundles) and part pass through the parietal lobes (posterior bundles). Hence, a lesion in the temporal lobe may produce a homonymous superior quadrantanopia and a parietal lobe lesion causes a homonymous inferior quadrantanopia. Infarction, tumor, infection, and vascular malformation are a few of the many conditions that can damage the optic radiations.

Visual Cortex

The macular fibers, which travel through the central portion of the optic radiations, are disproportionally represented in a large area of the occipital poles, extending out laterally over the occipital lobes. Lesions occurring in the tips of the occipital poles cause homonymous paracentral scotomata (half of each macular region),[141, 142] with preservation of peripheral vision. More-anterior occipital lobe lesions cause a contralateral homonymous hemianopia with macular sparing. If only the superior aspect of the occipital lobe (cuneus) is involved, a homonymous inferior quadrantanopia may result. Conversely, damage to the inferior occipital lobe (lingual gyrus) may cause a superior quadrant field defect. Bilateral occipital lobe destruction causes cortical blindness.

Infarctions are the most common lesions to affect the visual cortex (Figs. 30–105 and 30–106); fortunately, many of them spare the occipital pole, probably because of the dual blood supply to this area (posterior and middle cerebral arteries). Other lesions include trauma, neoplasm, infection, and hypertensive encephalopathy.

CONCLUSION

The complex anatomy and pathology of the visual system makes this area a formidable but fascinating challenge to the clinician and to the radiologist. As is the case with any organ system, a thorough knowledge of the anatomy and physiology as well as the pathologic processes that affect this region will enable one to formulate a reasonable differential diagnosis for most radiologic findings. CT and MRI are both important modalities for orbital imaging. CT is better at detecting calcifications and provides superior bone detail. MRI provides better soft tissue discrimination and offers readily obtainable multiplanar

FIGURE 30–106 Subacute occipital lobe infarction. *A,* T2-weighted MRI shows a region of increased signal intensity *(arrows)* in the right occipital lobe. *B,* T1-weighted image after gadolinium administration shows marked enhancement of the infarct. In this case, no macular sparing was found, owing to involvement of the occipital pole.

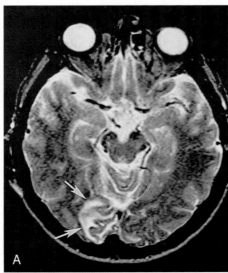
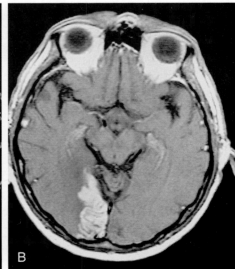

capabilities. MRI is superior for imaging the visual pathways. Although these modalities can, at times, provide a precise diagnosis, on other occasions they cannot because many orbital lesions look alike. Fortunately, when all the relevant clinical information is added in to the equation, the list of reasonable possibilities is usually short.

References

1. Schenck JF, Hart HR, Foster TH, et al. Improved MR imaging of the orbit at 1.5 T with surface coils. AJR 1985;144:1033–1036.
2. Sullivan JA, Harms SE. Surface coil MR imaging of orbital neoplasms. AJNR 1986;7:29–34.
3. Breslau J, Dalley RW, Tsruda JS, et al. Phased array surface coil MR of the orbits and optic nerves. AJNR 1995;16:1247–1251.
4. De Marco JK, Bilaniuk LT. Magnetic resonance imaging: Technical aspects. In Newton TH, Bilaniuk LT (eds). Radiology of the Eye and Orbit, pp. 1.1–1.14. New York, Raven, 1990.
5. Edwards JH, Hyman RA, Vacirca SJ. 0.6 T magnetic resonance imaging of the orbit. AJR 1985;144:1015–1020.
6. Daniels DA, Pech P, Kay MC, et al. Orbital apex: Correlative anatomic and CT study. AJR 1985;145:1141–1146.
7. Mafee MF. Eye and orbit. In Som PM, Curtin HD (eds). Head and Neck Imaging, pp. 1009–1128. St. Louis, Mosby–Year Book, 1996.
8. Gomori JM, Grossman RI, Shields JA, et al. Ocular MR imaging and spectroscopy: An ex vivo study. Radiology 1986;160:201–205.
9. Smiddy WE, Michels RG, Kumar AJ. Magnetic resonance imaging of retrobulbar changes in optic nerve position with eye movement. Am J Ophthalmol 1989;107:82–83.
10. Manelfe C, Pasquini U, Bank WO. Metrizamide demonstration of the subarachnoid space surrounding the optic nerves. J Comput Assist Tomogr 1978;2:545–547.
11. DeLano MC, Yun FY, Zinreich SJ. Relationship of the optic nerve to the posterior paranasal sinuses: A CT anatomic study. AJNR 1996;17:669–675.
12. Simmons JD, LaMasters D, Char D. Computed tomography of ocular colobomas. AJR 1983;141:1223–1226.
13. Hopper KD, Sherman JL, Boal DKB. Abnormalities of the orbit and its contents in children: CT and MR imaging findings. AJR 1991;156:1219–1224.
14. Anderson RL, Epstein GA, Dauer EA. Computed tomographic diagnosis of posterior ocular staphyloma. AJNR 1983;21:90–91.
15. Brodey PA, Randel S, Lane B, et al. Computed tomography of axial myopia. J Comput Assist Tomogr 1983;7:484–485.
16. Smith M, Castillo M. Imaging and differential diagnosis of the large eye. Radiographics 1994;14:721–728.
17. Castillo M, Quencer RM, Glaser J, Altman N. Congenital glaucoma and buphthalmos in a child with neurofibromatosis. J Clin Neuroophthalmol 1988;8:69–71.
18. Char DH, Unsold R, Sobel DF, et al. Ocular and orbital pathology. In Newton TH, Hasso AN, Dillon WP (eds). Computed Tomography of the Head and Neck, pp. 9–15. New York, Raven, 1988.
19. Osborne DR, Foulks GN. Computed tomographic analysis of deformity and dimensional changes in the eyeball. Radiology 1984;153:669–674.
20. Gerkowicz K, Prost M, Wawrzyniak M. Experimental ocular siderosis after extrabulbar administration of iron. Br J Ophthalmol 1985;69:149–153.
21. Lustrin ES, Brown JH, Novelline R, Weber AL. Radiologic assessment of trauma and foreign bodies of the eye and orbit. Neuroimaging Clin N Am 1996;6:219–237.
22. Mafee MF, Peyman GA. Retinal and choroidal detachments: Role of magnetic resonance imaging and computed tomography. Radiol Clin North Am 1987;25:487–507.
23. Mafee MF, Peyman GA. Choroidal detachment and ocular hypotony: CT evaluation. Radiology 1984;153:697–670.
24. Mafee MF, Goldberg MF, Greenwald MJ, et al. Retinoblastoma and simulating lesions: Role of CT and MR imaging. Radiol Clin North Am 1987;25:667–682.
25. Mafee MF, Ainbinder D, Afshani E, Mafee RF. The eye. Neuroimaging Clin N Am 1996;6:29–59.
26. Jakobiec FA, Tso MOM, Zimmerman LE, et al. Retinoblastoma and intracranial malignancy. Cancer 1977;39:2048–2058.
27. Bader JL, Miller RW, Meadows AT, et al. Trilateral retinoblastoma. Lancet 1980;2:582–583.
28. Abramson DH, Ellsworth RM, Tretter P, et al. Treatment of bilateral groups I through III retinoblastoma with bilateral radiation. Arch Ophthalmol 1981;99:1761–1762.
29. Peyster RG, Augsburger JJ, Shields JA, et al. Intraocular tumors: Evaluation with MR imaging. Radiology 1988;168:773–779.
30. Howard GM, Ellsworth RM. Differential diagnosis of retinoblastoma. Am J Ophthalmol 1965;60:610–618.
31. Mafee MF, Goldberg MF, Valvassori GE, et al. Computed tomography in the evaluation of patients with persistent hyperplastic primary vitreous (PHPV). Radiology 1982;145:713–717.
32. Magill HL, Sobeil LH, Brooks MT, et al. Case of the day. Pediatric. Persistent hyperplastic primary vitreous (PHPV). Radiographics 1990;10:515–518.
33. Mafee MF, Goldberg MF. CT and MR imaging for diagnosis of persistent hyperplastic primary vitreous. Radiol Clin North Am 1987;25:683–692.
34. Atlas SW, Galetta SL. The orbit and visual system. In Atlas SW (ed). Magnetic Resonance Imaging of the Brain and Spine, pp. 709–791. New York, Raven, 1991.
35. Hopper KD, Katz NNK, Dorwart RH, et al. Childhood leukokoria: Computed tomographic appearance and differential diagnosis with histopathologic correlation. Radiographics 1985;5:377–394.
36. Sherman JL, McLean IW, Brallier DR. Coats' disease: CT-pathologic correlation in two cases. Radiology 1983;146:77–78.
37. Mafee MF, Peyman GA, McKusick MA. Malignant uveal melanoma and similar lesions studied by computed tomography. Radiology 1985;156:403–408.
38. Peyster RG, Augsburger JJ, Shields JA, et al. Choroidal melanoma: Comparison of CT, fundoscopy, and US. Radiology 1985;156:675–680.
39. Bilaniuk LT, Schenck JF, Zimmerman RA, et al. Ocular and orbital lesions: Surface coil MR imaging. Radiology 1985;156:669–674.
40. Gomori JM, Grossman RI, Shields JA, et al. Choroidal melanomas: Correlation of NMR spectroscopy and MR imaging. Radiology 1986;158:443–445.
41. Mafee MF, Peyman GA, Grisolano JE, et al. Malignant uveal melanoma and simulating lesions: MR imaging evaluation. Radiology 1986;160:773–780.
42. Zimmerman RA, Bilaniuk LT. Ocular MR imaging. Radiology 1988;168:875–876.
43. Marx HF, Colletti PM, Raval JK. Magnetic resonance imaging features in melanoma. Magn Reson Imaging 1990;8:223–229.
44. Damadian R, Zaner K, Hor D, et al. Human tumors by NMR. Physiol Chem Phys 1973;5:381–402.
45. Mafee MF. MRI and in vivo proton spectroscopy of lesions of the globe. Semin Ultrasound CT MR 1988;9:59–71.
46. Manson PN, Markowitz B, Mirvis S, et al. Toward CT-based facial fracture treatment. Plast Reconstr Surg 1990;85:202–214.
47. Zingg M, Chowdhury K, Ladrach K, et al. Treatment of 813 zygoma-lateral orbital complex fractures. Arch Otolaryngol Head Neck Surg 1991;117:611–622.
48. LeFort R. Etude experimentale sur les fractures de la machoire superieure. Rev Chir 1901;23:208–227, 360–379, 479–507.
49. Pathria MN, Blaser SI. Diagnostic imaging of craniofacial fractures. Radiol Clin North Am 1989;27:839–853.
50. Harris JH, Ray RD, Rauschkolb EN. An approach to mid-facial fractures. Crit Rev Diagn Imaging 1984;21:105–132.
51. Guyon JJ, Brant-Zawadzki M, Seiff SR. CT demonstration of optic canal fractures. AJR 1984;143:1031–1034.
52. Unger JM. Orbital apex fractures: The contribution of computed tomography. Radiology 1984;150:713–717.
53. Russell EJ, Czervionke L, Huckman M. CT of the inferomedial orbit and the lacrimal drainage apparatus: Normal and pathologic anatomy. AJR 1985;145:1147–1154.
54. Gentry LR, Manor WF, Turski PA, et al. High-resolution CT analysis of facial struts in trauma: 1. Normal anatomy. AJR 1983;140:523–532.
55. Gentry LR, Manor WF, Turski PA, et al. High-resolution CT analysis of facial struts in trauma: 2. Osseous and soft tissue complications. AJR 1983;140:533–541.
56. Hammerschlag SB, Hughes S, O'Reilly GV, et al. Another look at blow-out fractures of the orbit. AJR 1982;139:133–137.
57. Koorneef L. Orbital septa: Anatomy and function. In Symposium: Tumors of the lids and orbit. Ophthalmology 1979;86:876–880.
58. Koorneef L, Zonneveld FW. The role of direct multiplanar high

resolution CT in the assessment and management of orbital trauma. Radiol Clin North Am 1987;25:753–766.

59. Weinstein JM, Lissnar GS. Trauma to the orbit, neurovisual system and oculomotor apparatus. Neuroimaging Clin N Am 1991;1:357–377.
60. Lyon DB, Newman SA. Evidence of direct damage to extraocular muscles as a cause of diplopia following orbital trauma. Ophthal Plast Reconstr Surg 1989;5:81–91.
61. Gilbard SM, Mafee MF, Lagouros PA, et al. Orbital blowout fractures: The prognostic significance of computed tomography. Ophthalmology 1985;92:1523–1528.
62. Tonami H, Yamamoto I, Matsuda M, et al. Orbital fracture: Surface coil MR imaging. Radiology 1991;179:789–794.
63. Putterman AM, Stevens T, Urist MJ. Nonsurgical management of blow-out fractures of the orbital floor. Am J Ophthalmol 1974;77:232–239.
64. Dutton JJ, Manson PM, Iliff N, Putterman AM. Management of blow-out fractures of the orbital floor. Surv Ophthalmol 1990;35:279–298.
65. Coker NJ, Brooks BS, El Gammel T. Computed tomography of orbital medial wall fractures. Head Neck Surg 1983;5:383.
66. Segrest DR, Dortzbach RK. Medial orbital wall fractures: Complications and management. Ophthal Plast Reconstr Surg 1989;5:75–80.
67. Curtin HD, Wolfe P, Schramm V. Orbital roof blow-out fractures. AJR 1982;139:969–972.
68. Chirico PA, Mirvis SE, Kelman SE, et al. Orbital "blow-in" fractures: Clinical and CT features. J Comput Assist Tomogr 1989;13:1017–1022.
69. Sullivan WG. Displaced orbital roof fractures: Presentation and treatment. Plast Reconstr Surg 1991;87:657–661.
70. Bhimani S, Virapongse C, Sarwar M. Computed tomography in penetrating injury to the eye. Am J Ophthalmol 1984;97:583–586.
71. Etherington RJ, Hourihan MD. Localisation of intraocular and intraorbital foreign bodies using computed tomography. Clin Radiol 1989;40:610–614.
72. Green BF, Kraft SP, Carter KD, et al. Intraorbital wood: Detection by magnetic resonance imaging. Ophthalmology 1990;97:608–611.
73. Weber AL, Jakobiec FA, Sabates NR. Pseudotumor of the orbit. Neuroimaging Clin N Am 1996;6:73–92.
74. Towbin R, Bokyung KH, Kaufman RA, et al. Postseptal cellulitis: CT in diagnosis and management. Radiology 1986;158:735–737.
75. Handler LC, Davey IC, Hill JC, et al. The acute orbit: Differentiation of orbital cellulitis from subperiosteal abscess by computerized tomography. Neuroradiology 1991;33:15–18.
76. McNicholas MMJ, Power WJ, Griffin JF. Idiopathic inflammatory pseudotumour of the orbit: CT features correlated with clinical outcome. Clin Radiol 1991;44:3–7.
77. Jones IS, Jakobiec FA. Diseases of the Orbit. Hagerstown, MD, Harper & Row, 1979.
78. Harr DL, Quencer RM, Abrams GW. Computed tomography and ultrasound in the evaluation of orbital infection and pseudotumor. Radiology 1982;142:395–401.
79. Dresner SC, Rothfus WE, Slamovits TL, et al. Computed tomography of orbital myositis. AJR 1984;143:671–674.
80. Flanders AE, Mafee MF, Rao VM, et al. CT characteristics of orbital pseudotumors and other orbital inflammatory processes. J Comput Assist Tomogr 1989;13:40–47.
81. Atlas SW, Grossman RI, Savino PJ, et al. Surface-coil MR of orbital pseudotumor. AJR 1987;148:803–808.
82. Carmody RF, Mafee MF, Goodwin JA, et al. Orbital and optic pathway sarcoidosis: MR findings. AJNR 1994;15:775–783.
83. Rothfus WE, Curtin HD. Extraocular muscle enlargement: A CT review. Radiology 1984;151:677–681.
84. Hosten N, Sander B, Cordes M, et al. Graves ophthalmopathy: MR imaging of the orbits. Radiology 1989;172:759–762.
85. Weber AL, Dallow RL, Sabates NR. Graves' disease of the orbit. Neuroimaging Clin N Am 1996;6:61–72.
86. Barrett L, Glatt HJ, Burde RM. Optic nerve dysfunction in thyroid eye disease: CT. Radiology 1988;167:503–507.
87. Neigel JM, Rootman J, Belkin RI, et al. Dysthyroid optic neuropathy: The crowded orbital apex syndrome. Ophthalmology 1988;95:1515–1521.
88. Birchall D, Goodall KL, Noble JL, Jackson A. Graves ophthalmopathy: Intracranial fat prolapse on CT images as an indicator of optic nerve compression. Radiology 1996;200:123–127.
89. Weber AL, Klufas R, Pless M. Imaging evaluation of the optic nerve and visual pathway. Neuroimaging Clin N Am 1996;6:143–177.
90. Beardsley TL, Brown SV, Sydnor CF, et al. Eleven cases of sarcoidosis of the optic nerve. Am J Ophthalmol 1984;97:62–77.
91. Adams R, Victor M. Principles of Neurology, 4th ed. Companion Handbook. New York, McGraw-Hill, 1991.
92. Miller DH, Newton MR, Van Der Poel JC, et al. Magnetic resonance imaging of the optic nerve in optic neuritis. Neurology 1988;38:175–179.
93. Guy J, Mancuso A, Quisling RG, et al. Gadolinium-DTPA–enhanced magnetic resonance imaging in optic neuropathies. Ophthalmology 1990;97:592–600.
94. Rothfus WE, Curtin HD, Slamovits TL, et al. Optic nerve/sheath enlargement. Radiology 1984;150:409–415.
95. Jabs DA, Johns CJ. Ocular involvement in chronic sarcoidosis. Am J Ophthalmol 1986;102:297–301.
96. James DG. Ocular sarcoidosis. Ann N Y Acad Sci 1986;465:551–563.
97. Obenauf CD, Shaw HE, Sydnor CF, Klintworth GK. Sarcoidosis and its ophthalmic manifestations. Am J Ophthalmol 1988;23:232–237.
98. DiMario FJ, Ramsby G, Grennastein R, et al. Neurofibromatosis type I: Resonance imaging findings. J Child Neurol 1993;8:32–39.
99. Peyster RG, Hoover ED, Hershey BL, Haskin ME. High-resolution CT of lesions of the optic nerve. AJR 1983;140:869–874.
100. Daniels DL, Herfkins R, Gager WE, et al. Magnetic resonance imaging of the optic nerves and chiasm. Radiology 1984;152:79–83.
101. Hendrix LE, Kneeland JB, Haughton VM, et al. MR imaging of optic nerve lesions: Value of gadopentetate dimeglumine and fat-suppression technique. AJNR 1990;11:749–754.
102. Wright JE, McNab AA, McDonald WI. Optic nerve glioma and the management of optic nerve tumours in the young. Br J Ophthalmol 1989;73:967–974.
103. Azar-Kia B, Mafee MF, Horowitz SW, et al. CT and MRI of the optic nerve and sheath. Semin Ultrasound CT MR 1988;9:443–454.
104. Zimmerman CF, Schatz NJ, Glaser JS. Magnetic resonance imaging of optic nerve meningiomas. Ophthalmology 1990;97:585–591.
105. Atlas SW, Bilaniuk LT, Zimmerman RA, et al. Orbit: Initial experience with surface coil spin-echo imaging at 1.5T. Radiology 1987;164:501–509.
106. Mafee MF, Putterman A, Valvassori GE, et al. Orbital space-occupying lesions: Role of computed tomography and magnetic resonance imaging. Radiol Clin North Am 1987;25:529–559.
107. Forbes GS. Vascular lesions in the orbit. Neuroimaging Clin N Am 1996;6:113–122.
108. Forbes GS, Earnest F, Waller RR. Computed tomography of orbital tumors, including late-generation scanning techniques. Radiology 1982;142:387–394.
109. Shields JA, Bakewell B, Augsburger JJ. Classification and incidence of space-occupying lesions of the orbit: A survey of 645 biopsies. Arch Ophthalmol 1984;102:1606–1611.
110. Graeb DA, Rootman J, Robertson WD. Orbital lymphangiomas: Clinical, radiologic, and pathologic characteristics. Radiology 1990;175:417–421.
111. Bilaniuk LT, Atlas SW, Zimmerman RA. The orbit. In Lee SH, Rao KC, Zimmerman RA (eds). Cranial MRI and CT, pp. 119–191. New York, McGraw-Hill, 1992.
112. Wilson ME, Parker PL, Chavis RM. Conservative management of childhood orbital lymphangioma. Ophthalmology 1989;96:484–489.
113. Ball WS, Towbin RB, Kaufman RA. Pediatric case of the day. Radiographics 1987;7:1181–1182.
114. Shnier R, Parker G, Hallinan JM, et al. Orbital varices: New technique for noninvasive diagnosis. AJNR 1991;12:717–718.
115. Nugent RA, Lapointe JS, Rootman J, et al. Orbital dermoids: Features on CT. Radiology 1987;165:475–478.
116. Barnes PD, Robson CD, Robertson RL, Young-Pouissant T. Pediatric orbital and visual pathway lesions. Neuroimaging Clin N Am 1996;6:179–198.
117. Brown HH, Kersten RC, Kulwin DR. Lipomatous hamartoma of the orbit. Arch Ophthalmol 1991;109:240–243.
118. Jakobiec FA, Rini F, Char D, et al. Primary liposarcoma of the orbit: Problems in the diagnosis and management in five cases. Ophthalmology 1989;96:180–191.

119. Warner MA, Weber AL, Jakobiec FA. Benign and malignant tumors of the orbital cavity including the lacrimal gland. Neuroimaging Clin N Am 1996;6:123–142.
120. Aoki S, Barkovich AJ, Nishimura K. Neurofibromatosis types 1 and 2: Cranial MR findings. Radiology 1989;172:527–534.
121. Krohel GB, Rosenberg PN, Wright JE, et al. Localized orbital neurofibromatosis. Am J Ophthalmol 1985;100:458–464.
122. Hesselink JR, Davis KR, Dallow RL, et al. Computed tomography of masses in the lacrimal gland region. Radiology 1979;131:143–147.
123. Balchunas WR, Quencer RM, Byrne SF. Lacrimal gland and fossa masses: Evaluation by computed tomography and A-mode echography. Radiology 1983;149:751–758.
124. Weber AL, Jakobiec FA, Sabates NR. Lymphoproliferative diseases of the orbit. Neuroimaging Clin N Am 1996;6:93–111.
125. Knowles DM, Jakobiec FA, McNally L, et al. Lymphoid hyperplasia and malignant lymphoma occurring in the ocular adnexa (orbit, conjunctiva, and eyelids): A prospective multiparametric analysis of 108 cases during 1977 to 1987. Hum Pathol 1990;21:959–973.
126. Kattah JC, Suski ET, Killen JY. Optic neuritis and systemic lymphoma. Am J Ophthalmol 1980;89:431–436.
127. Kincaid MC, Green WZ. Ocular and orbital involvement in leukemia. Surv Ophthalmol 1983;27:211–232.
128. Erly WK, Carmody RF, Dryden RM. Orbital histiocytosis X. AJNR 1995;16:1258–1261.
129. Jones IS, Reese AB, Krout J. Orbital rhabdomyosarcoma: An analysis of 62 cases. Trans Am Ophthalmol Soc 1965;63:223–255.
130. Spaeth EB, Cleveland AF. Rhabdomyosarcoma in infancy and childhood. Am J Ophthalmol 1952;53:463–466.
131. Porterfield JT, Zimmerman LE. Rhabdomyosarcoma of the orbit: A clinicopathologic study of 55 cases. Virchows Arch Pathol [Anat] 1962;335:329.
132. Lallemand DP, Brasch RC, Char DH, et al. Orbital tumors in children: Characterization by computed tomography. Radiology 1984;151:85–88.
133. Som PM, Brandwein M. Sinonasal cavities: Inflammatory diseases, tumors, fractures, and postoperative findings. In Som PM, Curtin HD (eds). Head and Neck Imaging, pp. 126–315. St. Louis, Mosby–Year Book, 1996.
134. Hesselink JR, Davis KR, Weber AL, et al. Radiological evaluation of orbital metastases with emphasis on computed tomography. Radiology 1980;137:363–366.
135. Cline RA, Rootman J. Enophthalmos: A clinical review. Ophthalmology 1984;91:229–237.
136. Peyster RG, Shapiro MD, Haik BG. Orbital metastasis: Role of magnetic resonance imaging and computed tomography. Radiol Clin North Am 1987;25:647.
137. Som PM, Dillon WP, Fullerton GD, et al. Chronically obstructed sinonasal secretions: Observations on T_1 and T_2 shortening. Radiology 1989;172:515–520.
138. Langer BG, Charlotta DA, Mafee MF, et al. MRI of the normal optic pathway. Semin Ultrasound CT MR 1988;9:401–412.
139. Zimmerman CF, Schatz NJ, Glaser JS. Magnetic resonance imaging of radiation optic neuropathy. Am J Ophthalmol 1990;110:389–394.
140. Levin LA. Clinical signs and symptoms requiring computed tomography and magnetic resonance imaging evaluation. Neuroimaging Clin N Am 1996;6:1–14.
141. Bilaniuk LT, Zimmerman RA, Savino PJ. Visual pathways. Neuroimaging Clin N Am 1993;3:71–83.
142. Armington WG, Zimmerman RA, Bilaniuk LT. Visual pathways. In Som PM, Curtin HD (eds). Head and Neck Imaging, pp. 1184–1229. St. Louis, Mosby–Year Book, 1996.

31

The Nasal Cavity and Paranasal Sinuses

WILLIAM R. NEMZEK, M.D.

REGINA GANDOUR-EDWARDS, M.D.

DAVID G. WESTMAN, M.D.

The key to understanding sinonasal disease is a thorough grasp of the anatomy. The sinuses are the result of a mysterious process in which solid skeletal facial elements are invaded by respiratory mucosa and become pneumatized.[1] The paranasal sinuses are named for the bones they pneumatize and consist of the maxillary, frontal, ethmoid, and sphenoid sinuses. The sinuses drain into ostia on the lateral wall of the nose.[1, 2]

Throughout this chapter, cross-sectional imaging is emphasized. The reader may refer to Som and Brandwein's or Mafee and Carter's work for an excellent discussion of plain film anatomy.[3, 4]

PNEUMATIZATION AND DEVELOPMENT OF THE PARANASAL SINUSES

Sinus Development

The paranasal sinuses arise as evaginations from the primitive nasal fossa in the third month of fetal life and are not fully developed until 18 years of age (Figs. 31–1 to 31–3).[2, 5]

The *maxillary sinus* is the first paranasal sinus to develop. At birth the rudimentary maxillary sinus has a volume of 6 to 8 cm³. Pneumatization continues laterally under the orbit until 15 years of age. After the maxillary adult teeth have erupted, pneumatization is completed by extending into the alveolar ridge.[6]

Ethmoid air cells are present at birth and continue to grow until late puberty. Opacification of the maxillary and ethmoid sinuses is normal in the first few years of life.[1]

At birth the *sphenoid* bone contains only red marrow and is not pneumatized. Conversion of red marrow to fatty marrow precedes pneumatization.[7] Fatty marrow conversion occurs first in the presphenoid between 7 months and 2 years of age and then proceeds posteriorly into the basisphenoid. Pneumatization begins at 2 years and is completed by 14 years of age.

The *frontal sinus* is the last to develop. The frontal sinus is considered an extension of the anterior ethmoid sinus. Pneumatization begins shortly after 2 years and continues until after puberty. It is not fully developed until 16 to 18 years of age in males and 12 to 14 years in females.[8]

Normal Anatomy and Anatomic Variants

The *maxillary sinus* contains complete or incomplete septations in 1% to 2.5% of cases (see Fig. 31–2). Maxillary sinus septa are usually found anteriorly and are usually unilateral.[2] Asymmetry in size and shape is common. Unilateral hypoplasia occurs in 7% and bilateral hypoplasia in 2% of adults. Hypoplasia of the maxillary sinus is caused by failure of embryologic development or arrest of pneumatization secondary to trauma or infection (Table 31–1).[9]

The infraorbital nerve (V2) crosses the roof of the maxillary sinus to exit the infraorbital foramen (see Fig. 31–3). The medial wall of the sinus forms the inferior aspect of the lateral wall of the nose. The ostium of the maxillary sinus empties into the hiatus semilunaris beneath the middle turbinate (Figs. 31–4 and 31–5). Accessory ostia are found inferior to the major opening in 28% of cases.[10] These are small holes in thin membranes that cover natural bony dehiscences in the middle meatus

TABLE 31–1 Maxillary Sinus Hypoplasia

Primary
   Failure of development
Secondary
   Trauma
   Infection
Miscellaneous
   First branchial arch anomalies
     (e.g., Treacher Collins syndrome)
   Cretinism
   Thalassemia
   Osteopetrosis

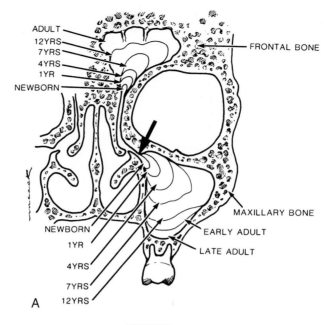

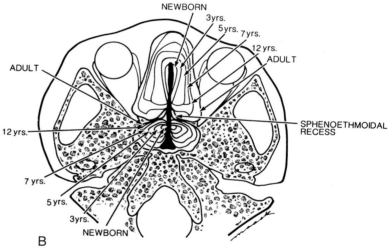

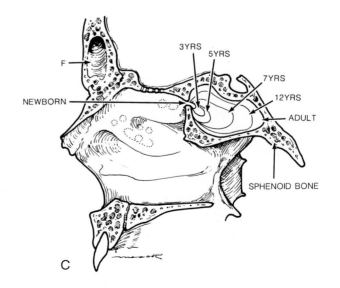

FIGURE 31–1 Composite drawings show development of the sinuses from birth to maturity. *A,* The maxillary sinus develops from the ethmoid infundibulum *(wide arrow)* in an inferolateral direction. Pneumatization is complete when the permanent teeth erupt, allowing the sinus floor to extend below the level of the hard palate. The frontal sinus is a superior extension of the anterior ethmoid sinus into the frontal bone. *B,* The lateral walls of the ethmoid sinuses expand laterally, becoming parallel in early childhood and convex in early adulthood. The sphenoid sinuses expand inferolaterally and may extend into the pterygoid plates and the anterior clinoid processes. The perpendicular plate of the ethmoid bone and vertical sphenoid septum are blackened, illustrating fusion of the ethmoid air cells and the sphenoid sinus. *C,* Development of the sphenoid sinus. F, frontal sinus. (*A–C,* From Scuderi AJ, Harnsberger HR, Boyer RS. Pneumatization of the paranasal sinuses: Normal features of importance to the accurate interpretation of CT and MR images. AJR 1993; 160:1101–1104. Reprinted with permission from AJR, Reston, VA.)

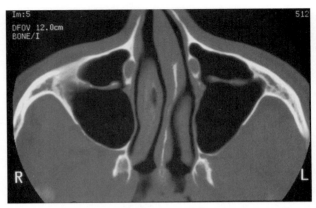

FIGURE 31–2 Congenital septation of the anterior maxillary sinuses.

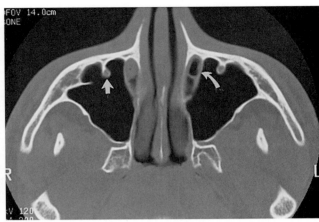

FIGURE 31–3 Infraorbital nerve *(straight arrow)* in the roof of the maxillary sinus. Note that the left nasolacrimal duct is filled with air *(curved arrow)* and the right contains tears.

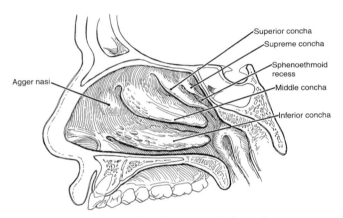

FIGURE 31–4 Lateral wall of the nose with the turbinates intact. (From Donald PJ. Anatomy and histology. In Donald PJ, Gluckman JL, Rice DH [eds]. The Sinuses, pp. 25–48. Philadelphia, Lippincott-Raven, 1995.)

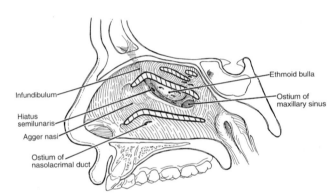

FIGURE 31–5 Lateral wall of the nose with the turbinates removed. (From Donald PJ. Anatomy and histology. In Donald PJ, Gluckman JL, Rice DH [eds]. The Sinuses, pp. 25–48. Philadelphia, Lippincott-Raven, 1995.)

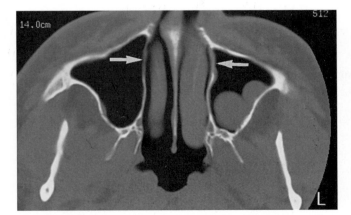

FIGURE 31–6 Fontanelles in the medial wall of the maxillary sinuses *(arrows)*, a normal variant. The mucosal surfaces are in apposition with no intervening bone. Note the retention cysts in the left maxillary sinus.

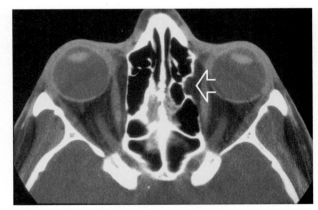

FIGURE 31–7 Congenital dehiscence in the lamina papyracea of the ethmoid sinus *(arrow)*.

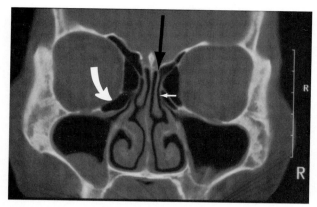

FIGURE 31–8 Computed tomography (CT) scan in the coronal plane. Note the vertical attachment *(straight black arrow)* of the middle turbinate to the junction of the fovea ethmoidalis and the lateral cribriform plate; the frontal recess *(straight white arrow)* opens into the middle meatus. Haller's cells *(curved white arrow)* are infraorbital ethmoid air cells. U, uncinate process.

called *fontanelles*.[1] The fontanelle is formed by a double layer of mucosa with no intervening bone, located inferior to the uncinate process (Fig. 31–6).[11, 12]

The *ethmoids* are divided into anterior and posterior air cells by the grand or basal lamella of the middle turbinate.[13] (The anterior ethmoids may be further subdivided into the anterior and the posterior group.) Air cells that are entirely within the ethmoid are *intramural,* and those developing outside the ethmoid are referred to as

extramural (Table 31–2).[14] Haphazard growth of air cells gives each individual an ethmoid labyrinth that is as unique as a fingerprint. Fortunately the basic anatomic landmarks are similar.[15] The anterior ethmoids arise inferior to the attachment of the middle turbinate, and the posterior develop superior to the middle turbinate.[5] The anterior group drains into the middle meatus and the posterior into the superior meatus. There are between 7 and 11 air cells on each side.[1] There is also dehiscence in the lamina papyracea of the ethmoid that may be congenital or acquired secondary to trauma (Fig. 31–7).[16] Defects in the lamina papyracea place the orbital contents in jeopardy during surgery.

Three groups of ethmoid cells deserve mention. *Haller's cells* are ethmoid cells that extend beneath the floor of the orbit between the orbit and the maxillary infundibulum (Fig. 31–8). They are found in 10% of the population.[2, 17] They arise from the attachment of the middle turbinate to the lateral nasal wall. Haller's cells may obstruct the maxillary sinus ostium or the infundibulum.[10] *Onodi's* cells are the most posterior ethmoid air cells that extend into the anterior superior sphenoid sinus. These cells may surround the optic nerve and optic canal and extend to the anterior wall of the sella turcica (Fig. 31–9). This anomaly may place the optic nerve at greater risk of accidental surgical trauma.[18] They are found in about 25% of the population.[1, 2, 17] The *agger nasi cells* are the most anterior ethmoid cells that are located anterior to the frontal recess and represent pneumatization of the lacrimal bone (Fig. 31–10).[1, 2, 17] Because of the proximity of the agger (Latin, mound) nasi cell to the lacrimal sac, sinus disease involving these cells may produce ocular

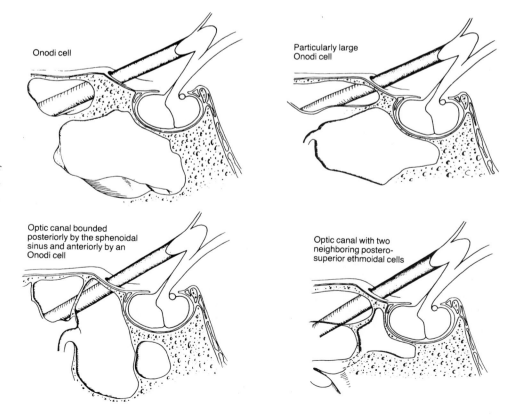

FIGURE 31–9 Various types of Onodi's cells surround the optic nerve. (From Lang J. Clinical Anatomy of the Nose, Nasal Cavity and Paranasal Sinuses. New York, Thieme Medical, 1989.)

TABLE 31–2 Ethmoid Sinus

Anterior Ethmoid Air Cells

Anterior group
    Infundibular and frontal: give rise to frontal recess,
        portion of frontal sinus, ethmoid infundibula, anterior
        air cells, and agger nasi cells
Middle group
    Ethmoid bullae, Haller's cells

Posterior Ethmoid Air Cells

    Posterior air cells, Onodi's cells

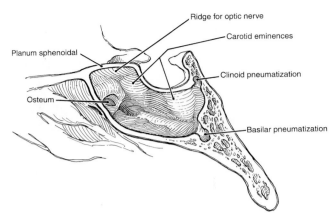

FIGURE 31–11 Lateral wall of the sphenoid sinus. (From Donald PJ. Anatomy and histology. In Donald PJ, Gluckman JL, Rice DH [eds]. The Sinuses, pp. 25–48. Philadelphia, Lippincott-Raven, 1995.)

symptoms. These cells may also provide surgical access to the frontal sinus and frontal recess.

The *sphenoid sinus* is usually paired but asymmetrically developed. The intersinus septum is usually off midline and deviates from the vertical plane. The wall of the sphenoid sinus is intimately related to important structures, including the internal carotid artery, the optic nerve, the pituitary gland, and the vidian and maxillary nerves (Figs. 31–11 through 31–13).[1, 18] Extension of pneumatization to the greater sphenoid wing and base of the pterygoid process is common (Fig. 31–14A). Pneumatization of the lesser sphenoid wing and anterior and posterior clinoid processes occurs less frequently (Figs 31–14B).[18] The sphenoid sinus drains via the sphenoethmoid recess into the superior meatus (Figs. 31–15 and 31–16).[5]

Unilateral aplasia of the frontal sinus occurs in 15% and bilateral aplasia in 5% of adults.[8] Aplasia of the frontal sinus occurs in 12% to 17% of Europeans and 52% of Eskimos.[19] The communication between the frontal sinus and the anterior middle meatus in the nasal cavity is the *frontal recess* (see Fig. 31–8).[12] Lang found that 77% of frontal sinuses have a defined nasofrontal duct and 23% possess only an ostium.[19]

The *nasal septum* divides the nasal cavity into halves. The septum is predominately cartilage anteriorly, with the posterior aspect formed by the vomer inferiorly and the perpendicular plate of the ethmoid superiorly (Fig. 31–17).[20] The septum attaches to the body of the sphenoid bone posteriorly and the nasal bone and spine of the

frontal bone anteriorly.[12] The palate forms the floor of the nose, with the palatine bone posteriorly and the maxilla anteriorly. The cribriform plate and the olfactory region form the roof of the nasal vault.[20]

At birth, the nasal septum is straight and thick. *Septal deviation* is acquired because the nasal septum grows more rapidly than the lateral walls of the nasal fossa and because of asymmetric eruption of the medial central incisor teeth.[21]

Septal deviation is more common toward the right at the junction of the ethmoid bone and vomer (Fig. 31–18).[21] Septal deviation is found in about half the population.[2]

Lateral Nasal Wall

There are three *turbinates* suspended from the lateral side of the nose: the inferior, middle, and superior. Uncommonly a fourth turbinate, the supreme turbinate, is located superior to the superior turbinate.[17] Each turbinate is composed of a scroll of thin bone, called a *concha*, which is covered by mucosa. The superior and middle conchae are part of the ethmoid bone. The inferior concha is a separate bone.[22] The superior, middle, and inferior meati are located beneath their respective turbinates (see Figs. 31–4 and 31–5).[1, 12]

The *inferior turbinate* is the largest. The nasolacrimal duct is the only structure to drain beneath the inferior turbinate. The nasolacrimal duct connects superiorly with the lacrimal sac and courses along the anterior wall of the maxillary sinus. The nasolacrimal duct is normally filled either with tears or with air and is seen best on axial images (see Fig. 31–3).

The *middle turbinate* arises from the medial ethmoid labyrinth. It attaches to two areas of delicate bone. Superiorly, there is vertical attachment to the roof of the ethmoid at the junction of the fovea ethmoidalis (ethmoid roof) and the lateral aspect of the cribriform plate (Fig. 31–19A).[12] There is also a lateral attachment to the ethmoid sinus (Fig. 31–19B). Anteriorly, the middle turbinate attaches to the agger nasi cell and the superior edge of the uncinate process.[22] Posteriorly, the attachment of

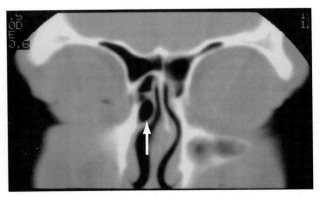

FIGURE 31–10 Coronal CT scan. Agger nasi cell (*arrow*), which is the most anterior ethmoid air cell, located anterior to the frontal recess.

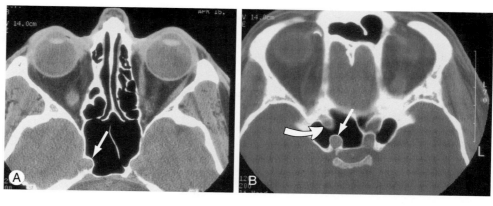

FIGURE 31–12 Axial CT scan through the sphenoid sinuses. *A,* Groove for the internal carotid artery on the posterior aspect of the sphenoid sinus *(arrow). B,* More superior axial CT scan shows the internal carotid artery within the sphenoid sinus *(straight arrow)* surrounded by a thin layer of bone and the optic nerve *(curved arrow).*

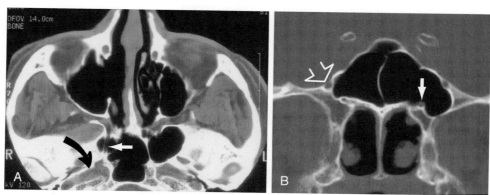

FIGURE 31–13 Axial *(A)* and coronal *(B)* CT scans. Vidian nerve canal is nearly completely surrounded by air *(white straight arrow)* in the sphenoid sinus. Note the canal for the horizontal petrous internal carotid artery *(curved black arrow)* near the posterior opening of the vidian canal. *White open arrow* indicates the foramen rotundum.

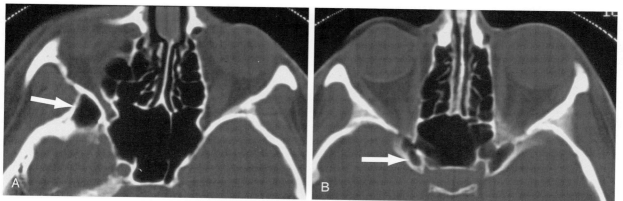

FIGURE 31–14 Variants of normal sphenoid sinus pneumatization. *A,* Pneumatization of the greater wing of the sphenoid *(arrow).* *B,* Pneumatization of the anterior clinoids *(arrow).*

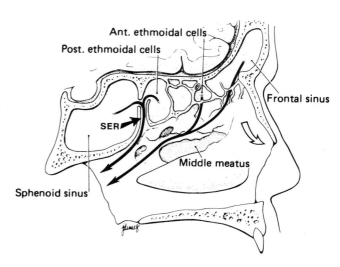

FIGURE 31–15 Diagram of the lateral nasal wall shows the mucociliary drainage from the frontal, anterior ethmoid, and maxillary sinuses into the middle meatus and then into the nasopharynx. The sphenoid and posterior ethmoid sinuses drain into the sphenoethmoid recess (SER). Drainage anterior to the middle meatus is forward. (From Zinrich SJ, Kennedy DW, Rosenbaum AE, et al. Paranasal sinuses: CT imaging requirements for endoscopic surgery. Radiology 1987;163:769–775.)

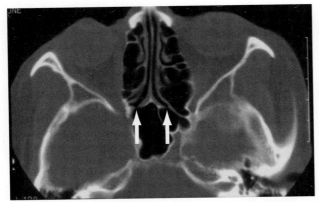

FIGURE 31–16 Axial CT scan shows the opening of the sphenoid sinus (*arrows*) into the sphenoethmoid recess bilaterally.

the middle turbinate curves superiorly and laterally, assuming a coronal orientation posterior to the ethmoid bulla and attaching the middle turbinate to the lamina papyracea. This coronal extension of the basal lamella is

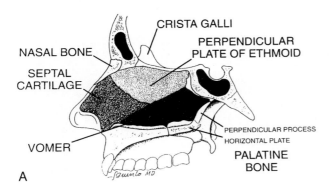

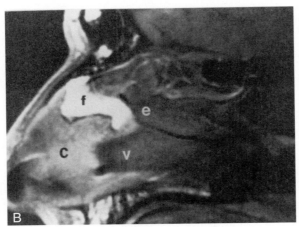

FIGURE 31–17 *A*, Diagram of the nasal septum. *B*, Sagittal T1-weighted image of the nasal septum. e, perpendicular plate of the ethmoid; v, vomer; c, quadrangular cartilage; f, fat in the nasal septum, which is a normal variant. (*A* and *B*, From Allbery SM, Chaljub G, Cho NL, et al. MR imaging of nasal masses. Radiographics 1995;15:1311–1327.)

called the *basal* or *ground lamella*. The basal lamella divides the anterior from the posterior ethmoid air cells and is the posterior landmark for an anterior ethmoidectomy.[12, 14, 15, 17] The *lateral sinus* is the space between the ethmoid bulla and the coronal extension of the basal lamella (Fig. 31–20).[11, 22]

A *concha bullosa* is a pneumatized middle turbinate and is an anatomic variation of ethmoid air cell development with a prevalence of about 34% (Fig. 31–21).[8, 17] Pneumatization extends from the ethmoid air cells to the middle turbinate. The concha bullosa drains into the frontal recess or into the lateral sinus. This large air cell may cause nasal obstruction or impair drainage of the osteomeatal complex.[2, 17] A massively enlarged concha bullosa may be confused with an intranasal mass such as a juvenile nasopharyngeal angiofibroma (Fig. 31–22).[21] The concha bullosa may fill with secretions and fail to drain, becoming infected (Fig. 31–23).

The convexity of the normal middle turbinate is directed medially toward the nasal septum, the same as the inferior turbinate. A *paradoxically curved middle turbinate* bone is curved laterally. This anomaly has a prevalence of about 25%.[2]

The *superior turbinate* bone is the smallest of the three. The superior meatus drains the posterior ethmoid air cells through multiple ostia.[17] The sphenoid sinus drains into the sphenoethmoid recess, which lies postero-superior to the superior turbinate between the posterior wall of the ethmoid and anterior wall of the sphenoid sinus (see Fig. 31–16).[17]

With the middle turbinate removed, three prominent underlying structures are apparent: the *uncinate process* anteriorly, the ethmoid bulla posteriorly, and the *hiatus semilunaris* in between (see Figs. 31–5 and 31–15).[17] The *uncinate process* is a thin curved bony plate arising from the lateral aspect of the ethmoid labyrinth and forms a portion of the lateral nasal wall (Fig. 31–24; see also Figs. 31–8 and 31–19A). The *semilunar hiatus* is a crescentic semicircular groove between the free margin of the uncinate process and the ethmoid bulla.[11, 12] The ostia for the frontal sinus (*frontal recess* anteriorly), the anterior ethmoids, and the maxillary sinus drain beneath the *middle turbinate* into the *semilunar hiatus* (see Fig. 31–15). Superior to the semilunar hiatus is a bubble-shaped piece of bone, the *ethmoid bulla*, the largest anterior ethmoid air cell, which is pierced by the exiting foramina for the ethmoid air cells (see Figs. 31–19A and 31–24).[1]

The *infundibulum* is the channel connecting the maxillary sinus with the middle meatus. It is bordered by the uncinate process medially and the inferomedial wall of the orbit laterally (see Fig. 31–24).[11]

Osteomeatal Complex

The critical anatomy for understanding chronic sinus disease is the *osteomeatal complex* (OMC). The OMC includes the maxillary sinus ostium and infundibulum; uncinate process; hiatus semilunaris; ethmoid bulla; middle turbinate; and frontal recess (Table 31–3) (see Fig. 31–24). This functional importance of the sinuses and OMC is discussed in the section on functional endoscopic sinus surgery.

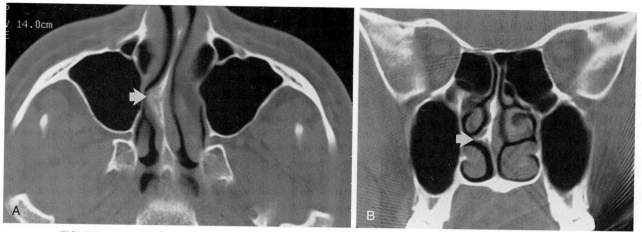

FIGURE 31–18 Axial *(A)* and coronal *(B)* CT scans show the nasal septal deviation with a spur *(arrow)*.

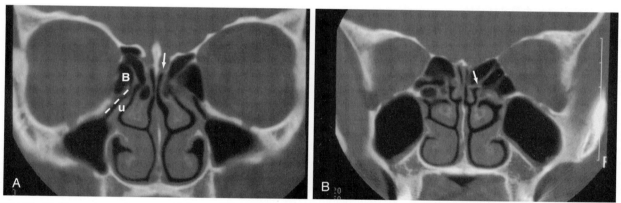

FIGURE 31–19 Normal attachments of the middle turbinate. *A,* Coronal CT scan shows the vertical attachment of the middle turbinate to the junction of the roof of the ethmoid sinus with the lateral cribriform plate *(arrow)*. U, uncinate process; B, ethmoid bulla; *dashed line,* maxillary infundibulum. *B,* Coronal CT scan slightly posterior to *A.* Note the lateral attachment of the middle turbinate to the ethmoid sinus *(arrow)*.

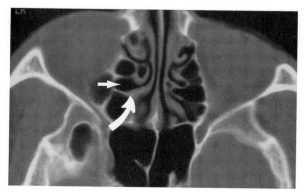

FIGURE 31–20 Axial CT scan shows the lateral sinus (sinus lateralis) *(straight arrow)* between the grand lamella of the middle turbinate *(curved arrow)* and the posterior wall of the anterior ethmoid sinus.

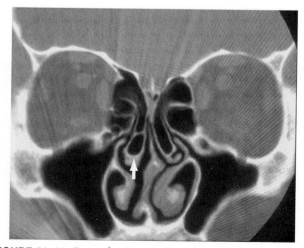

FIGURE 31–21 Coronal CT scan shows bilateral concha bullosa *(arrow)*, which is pneumatization of the middle turbinate.

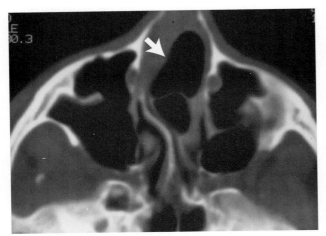

FIGURE 31–22 Massive concha bullosa *(arrow)*, which can simulate a nasal mass.

CONGENITAL LESIONS

Choanal Atresia

The nasal cavity begins as an ectodermal thickening, the *nasal placode*, on the surface of the fetus. The primitive nasal sac is separated from the anterior oral cavity by the thin *oronasal membrane*, which disappears during the seventh week to establish the primitive posterior choanae (Fig. 31–25).[23, 24] The *oropharyngeal membrane* separates the ectodermally lined stomodeum (primitive mouth) from the endoderm of the pharyngeal gut.[23] A mesodermal plate separates the stomodeum from the ectoderm that forms the cranium and brain. Bony choanal atresia is caused by failure of resorption of this mesodermal plate. Membranous choanal atresia is caused by failure of perforation of the oronasal membrane. Most cases (90%) of choanal atresia occur at the posterior nasal choanae.[23]

Early studies, before computed tomography (CT), described choanal atresia as being partially or completely osseous in 90% and membranous in 10%.[21] Recent work finds that nearly all patients with choanal atresia have bony abnormalities, with narrowing of the posterior nasal cavity. About 30% have purely osseous atresia, and 70%

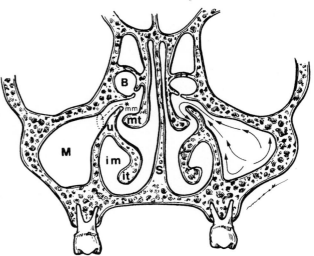

FIGURE 31–24 Coronal diagram of the normal osteomeatal unit. Normal flow of mucociliary drainage of the maxillary sinus *(arrows)*. *Dotted oval,* maxillary osteum; *dashed line,* maxillary infundibulum; *asterisk,* hiatus semilunaris; B, ethmoid bulla; M, maxillary sinus; U, uncinate process; mt, middle turbinate; im, inferior meatus; it, inferior turbinate; S, nasal septum; mm, middle meatus. (From Pollei SR, Harnsberger HR. The radiologic evaluation of the sinonasal region. Postgrad Radiol 1989;8:242–265.)

have a mixed bony and membranous atresia.[25, 26] Completely membranous atresia is very rare.

Choanal atresia occurs once in every 8000 births. From 50% to 60% of cases are unilateral.[25] Choanal atresia is two times more common in girls.[21] Bilateral choanal atresia produces respiratory distress in the neonate because infants are obligatory nose breathers.

The diagnosis may be made by instilling contrast material into the nasal cavity under fluoroscopy. The contrast material fails to reach the nasal cavity. Thin-section CT is now the diagnostic method of choice. CT scans should be performed with the gantry angled 5 degrees cephalic to a line perpendicular to the hard palate.[5] In the neonate, the normal choana should measure 8 mm in height and 6 mm in width.[19] Narrowing of the posterior nasal airway is caused by thickening and medial bowing of the lateral

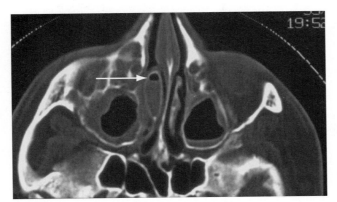

FIGURE 31–23 Concha bullosa with trapped secretions *(arrow)* and an air-fluid level ("concha bullitis").

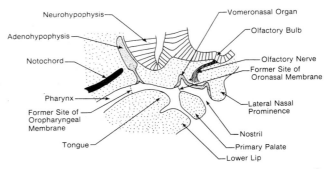

FIGURE 31–25 Sagittal diagram through the anterior craniofacial region of a fetus of 7 weeks' gestation. (From Sperber GH. Craniofacial Embryology, 4th ed., pp. 31–57. London, Butterworth Heinemann, 1989.)

TABLE 31–3 Ostiomeatal Complex (Common Drainage for Anterior Ethmoid, Maxillary, and Frontal Sinuses)

Maxillary sinus ostium and infundibulum
Uncinate process
Ethmoid bullae
Frontal recess
Hiatus semilunaris
Middle turbinate

walls of the nasal cavity, expansion of the medial pterygoid plate, and enlargement of the vomer (Fig. 31–26A).[21, 26] The vomer is fused with the lateral nasal walls in bony atresia. With combined bony and membranous atresia, the lateral walls approach the vomer and narrow the nasal cavity; there is also a central membrane connecting the vomer and the medial pterygoid.[26]

Other associated anomalies have been described, with the most frequent anomalies linked with the acronym CHARGE. This includes *c*olobomas, *h*eart disease, *a*tresia of the choanae, *r*etarded growth, *g*enital hypoplasia, and *e*ar anomalies.[21, 23, 27]

Bony stenosis of the anterior nares (nasal piriform aperture) also occurs (10%) and is easily differentiated by CT scanning (see Fig. 31–26B).[21, 23]

Mucocele of the Nasolacrimal Duct (Endonasal Dacryocystocele)

A mucocele of the nasolacrimal duct (endonasal dacryocystocele) should be considered in a child with a submucosal nasal mass arising under the inferior turbinate. It often presents in association with inner canthal swelling and epiphora (excessive tearing) (Fig. 31–27). If the mucocele becomes infected, dacryocystitis (inflammation of the lacrimal sac), periorbital cellulitis, or sepsis may result.[28]

The lesion may be considered to result from maldevelopment of the nasolacrimal drainage system. There is usually distal nasolacrimal duct obstruction at the valve of Hasner, where the epithelial lining of the nasolacrimal duct meets the nasal mucosa, and a proximal obstruction

at the entrance to the lacrimal sac at the valve of Rosenmüller (Fig. 31–28).[28–31]

Kallmann's Syndrome

Kallmann's syndrome is congenital anosmia associated with hypogonadism.[32] In this genetic disorder, olfactory cells and cells that secrete luteinizing hormone–releasing factor fail to migrate from the olfactory placode into the hypothalamus and septal area and remain in the nasal cavity. The anterior lobe of the pituitary is unable to synthesize follicle-stimulating and luteinizing hormone. The clinical result is hypogonadotropic hypogonadism.[33]

Magnetic resonance imaging (MRI) demonstrates hypoplasia or absence of the olfactory sulcus and olfactory bulbs (Fig. 31–29). If pituitary hypofunction is severe, the pituitary appears small on sagittal MRI images.[34]

Congenital Nasal Masses

Congenital midline nasal masses are unusual lesions (Table 31–4). The differential diagnosis includes dermoid and epidermoid tumors (usually seen with an associated dermal sinus tract), nasal cerebral heterotopias (also called nasal gliomas), and nasal cephaloceles. Other even more unusual midline masses are inclusion cysts, hemangiomas, and anomalies of the ethmoid sinuses.

During development of the nasofrontal region, two spaces are temporarily formed. The first is the *fonticulus nasofrontalis*, which is a small midline fontanelle between the paired frontal and nasal bones. The second is the *prenasal space* between the nasal bones anteriorly and the developing nasal cartilage posteriorly.[34, 35]

Between 7 and 8 weeks' gestation, a dural diverticulum extends from the anterior skull base through the embryologic foramen cecum into the prenasal space to come in contact with the superficial ectoderm of the nose (Fig. 31–30). As the fetus develops, the nasal processes of the frontal bone grow to surround the dural diverticulum. The dura process involutes, leaving the *foramen cecum*, which is filled with a fibrous cord representing the obliterated dural projection.[35]

If the dural diverticulum fails to involute, an epithelial sinus tract persists. A small dimple may be seen on the

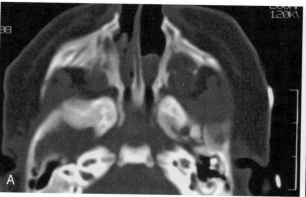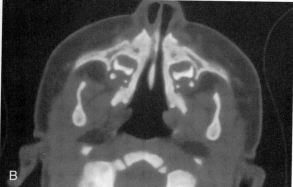

FIGURE 31–26 Congenital nasal obstruction. *A,* Choanal atresia in a newborn. Note the thickening and medial bowing of the lateral nasal wall, causing narrowing of the posterior nasal cavity. There was a membrane, completing the choanal atresia. *B,* Piriform aperture stenosis in a neonate. (*B,* Courtesy of Suresh Mukherji, M.D., Chapel Hill, NC.)

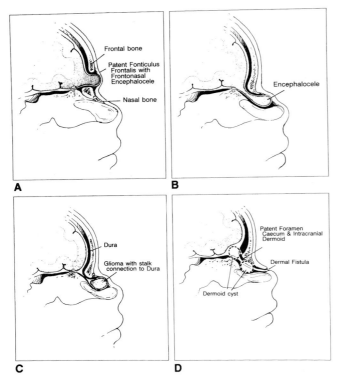

FIGURE 31–31 Diagrams show abnormal development of the anterior skull base. *A,* The fonticulus frontalis fails to close, resulting in a frontonasal encephalocele. *B,* The foramen cecum fails to close, resulting in a frontoethmoid encephalocele. *C,* If the dural projection through the foramen cecum fails to involute, a nasal glioma may develop with a fibrous stalk connecting to the foramen cecum or the intracranial contents. *D,* If the dural projection fails to involute, a dermal sinus will result that may contain a dermoid or epidermoid cyst. (*A–D,* From Barkovich AJ, Vandermarck P, Edwards MB, et al. Congenital nasal masses: CT and MR features in 16 cases. AJNR 1991;12:105–116; adapted from Hughes GB, Sharpino G, Hunt W, Tucker HM. Management of the congenital midline nasal mass: a review. Head Neck Surg 1980;2:222–233. Copyright © 1980. Reprinted by permission of John Wiley & Sons, Inc.)

The cause may be enlargement of arachnoid villi or draining veins. Imperfect fusion of presphenoid and postsphenoid ossification centers has also been implicated.[39]

PHYSIOLOGY

The nose and paranasal sinuses are lined with pseudostratified columnar ciliated epithelium. This epithelium contains goblet cells. *Seromucinous* glands are found submucosally under the basement membrane. Although seromucinous glands are found throughout the nasal septum and the turbinates, they are located almost exclusively around the sinus ostia and are rare in the sinus walls.[1]

Nasal Cycle

There is a rich submucosal network of blood vessels whose histology is similar to that of the corpora cavernosa of the penis.[1] There is normal intermittent congestion of the mucosa of the nasal septum, turbinates, and ethmoid air cells called the *nasal cycle.* These cyclical changes alternate sides every 50 minutes to 6 hours.[10, 40, 41]

Normal Secretions

The primary physiologic role of the nasal passages is to humidify, warm, and remove particulate matter from the inspired air.[40] About 2 liters of serous watery secretions is produced daily by the sinonasal mucosa. The largest deposits of inhaled particulate debris are trapped in the thin layer of mucus covering the inner surface of the sinuses.[40]

In the sinuses the cilia of the upper respiratory mucosa propel the mucous blanket toward the sinus ostia at the rate of about 1 cm/min. The mucous layer in the normal maxillary sinus is renewed on the average every 20 to 30 minutes.[12] In the maxillary sinus, mucociliary movement begins at the sinus floor and then extends superiorly along the walls of the sinus to the ostium (see Fig. 31–24).[40] In the frontal sinus, the mucus blanket moves in a circular pattern from the medial wall up to the sinus roof, then laterally along the sinus roof, down along the lateral wall, and medially to the sinus ostium. Mucus is swept from the nares to the choanae in the nasal cavity, then into the nasopharynx, where it is swallowed.[1, 10, 14, 42]

It is important to remember that even though a surgical defect is created in the wall of the sinus for drainage, the cilia will continue to transport the mucus blanket toward the natural sinus ostium.[42]

Normal sinus secretions are 95% water and 5% macromolecular proteins (predominately mucous glycoprotein). The normal watery secretions have long T1 and T2 relaxation times and are dark on T1-weighted and bright on T2-weighted images.[43]

Obstructed Secretions

When the sinuses are obstructed, the amount of protein increases and the amount of free water decreases. The secretions change from a primarily serous composition into a loose mucous collection, and finally into a stonelike mucous plug. Protein acts as a catalyst to shorten both the T1 and T2 relaxation times.[41] As the protein content rises from 5% to 25% the T1-weighted signal intensity brightens. At 25% to 40% protein concentration, secretions have the consistency of syrup or paste. T1- and T2-weighted signal intensity decreases. Above 40% protein content, secretions have a solid consistency and are depicted as signal voids on both T1- and T2-weighted images (Figs. 31–35 and 31–36). Extremely dessicated secretions are soft tissue density on CT but produce a signal void on MRI, simulating a normal air-filled sinus.[43–45]

Secretions that become desiccated and semisolid may have a high attenuation on CT, similar to that of a cellular tumor. Dried, semisolid secretions almost always have a thin zone of lower attenuation between them and the sinus wall, which represents sinus mucosa and additional newer mucoid secretion (see Fig. 31–36). The differential diagnosis of an opacified sinus with a central zone of high attenuation and a peripheral zone of lower attenuation includes desiccated secretions, sinus fungal infection with a mycetoma, and intrasinus hemorrhage (Table 31–5).[43–45]

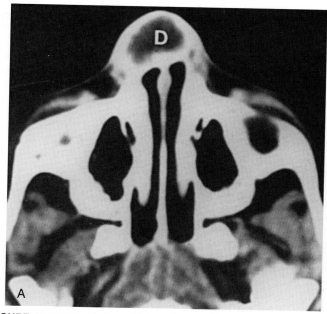
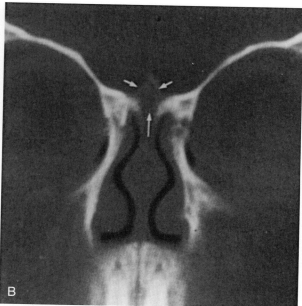

FIGURE 31–32 Nasal dermoid in a 5-year-old child with meningitis and presumed abscess at the tip of the nose. A, Axial CT scan shows a hypodense mass (D) that was found to be infected dermoid surrounded by thickened, inflamed skin. B, Coronal CT scan demonstrates a widely patent foramen cecum (long arrow) and widened crista galli (short arrows), suggesting intracranial communication. At surgery, a pedicle was found to extend from the dermoid to the meninges through a patent foramen cecum. (A and B, From Castillo M. Congenital abnormalities of the nose: CT and MR findings. AJR 1994;162:1211–1217. Reprinted with permission from AJR, Reston, VA.)

FIGURE 31–33 Basal encephalocele presenting as an intranasal mass. Sagittal T1-weighted (A) and coronal T1-weighted (B) images show a defect in the sphenoid and ethmoid bones with herniation of the intracranial contents, including the hypothalamus and third ventricle. Note agenesis of the corpus callosum. (A and B, Courtesy of Hugh Curtin, M.D., Boston, MA.)

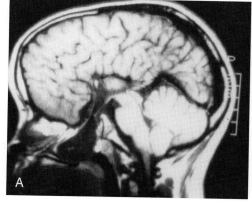
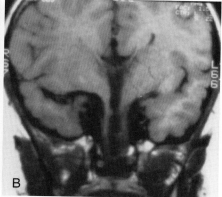

FIGURE 31–34 Intrasphenoid cephalocele. A and B, Mass seen on the superolateral aspect of the sphenoid sinus. No bony dehiscence is identified. (A and B, From Albernaz MS, Horton WD, Adkins WY, et al. Intrasphenoidal encephalocele. Otolaryngol Head Neck Surg 1991;104:279–281.)

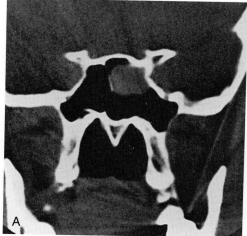
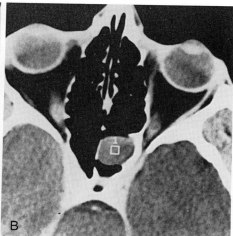

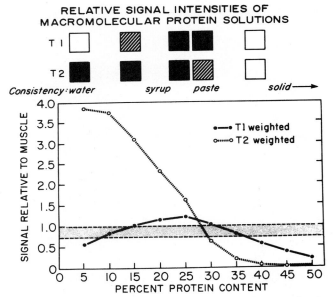

RELATIVE SIGNAL INTENSITIES OF MACROMOLECULAR PROTEIN SOLUTIONS

FIGURE 31–35 Observed signal intensities of macromolecular protein solutions versus protein content. (From Som PM, Curtin HD. Chronic inflammatory sinonasal diseases including fungal infections. The role of imaging. Radiol Clin North Am 1993;31:33–44.)

IMAGING INFLAMMATORY DISEASE

Plain radiographs are adequate to detect about 75% of significant disease.[46] However, overlap of structures obscures anatomy and causes either over- or underdiagnosis of disease. Minimal disease is usually missed. Evaluation with plain radiographs is insufficient to evaluate the OMC and to plan surgical procedures.

MRI renders excellent soft tissue detail but fails to depict the thin osseous sinus walls and ostia. If CT scanning has already been performed for inflammatory disease, a "limited" MRI examination with T2-weighted images for residual mucosal disease might prove to be a valuable follow-up screening examination that does not use ionizing radiation.

CT scanning yields both excellent soft tissue and bone detail and is the best technique for preoperative imaging of sinonasal inflammatory disease.[17] Limited axial CT is adequate for identification of disease. The limited examination includes a minimum of four slices, with at least one image to include the frontal, maxillary, ethmoid, and sphenoid sinuses. For detection of disease, the limited sinus CT scan is in agreement with a full coronal sinus CT scan about 88% of the time.[46] The coronal plane gives the best demonstration of the OMC and simulates the plane seen by the endoscopist.[17]

TABLE 31–5 Dense Sinus Secretions on Computed Tomography

Hemorrhage
Desiccated secretions
Fungal disease

Ideally sinus CT should be performed after treatment with antibiotics and decongestants, when the patient is least symptomatic. A sympathomimetic nasal spray and vigorous nose blowing have been recommended immediately before scanning. The goal is to identify disease that has not responded to conventional medical therapy and may require surgical intervention.[11, 20, 47] Patients are examined in the supine or prone position, with the neck extended. The gantry is angled perpendicular to the hard palate. The prone position is preferred because fluid accumulates in the most dependent portion of the maxillary sinus floor and does not obscure the OMC. To define the anatomy of critical regions, such as the OMC, 3-mm contiguous scans are necessary.[48] Data are acquired using a bone algorithm. Hard copy is photographed using a single intermediate window and level (window level 2500 HU and window width 250 HU). This provides adequate bone and soft tissue detail on a single set of images. Contrast material is only necessary to evaluate the complications of sinus disease. Patients who are acutely ill with suspected orbital or intracranial complications of sinusitis should be imaged in the coronal and axial planes with both bone and soft tissue windows after receiving intravenous contrast material.[49]

INFECTION AND INFLAMMATORY SINUS DISEASE

Acute Sinusitis

Acute sinusitis usually develops during a viral upper respiratory infection. The most common symptoms are cough, nasal discharge, fever, headache, facial pain over the infected sinus, and swelling.[50–52]

Acute sinusitis may result from colonization of bacteria from the nasal cavity, due to obstruction of the sinus ostia.[41] Common pathogens include *Streptococcus pneumoniae* and *Haemophilus influenzae* in about 50% of patients. Viruses may be isolated in about 20% of cases of acute sinusitis.[41] In patients positive for human immunodeficiency virus (HIV), as in the immunocompetent population, most sinonasal disease is inflammatory, rather than neoplastic. In addition to the common pathogens, other organisms such as *Pseudomonas aeruginosa, Cryptococcus neoformans, Legionella pneumophila, Pneumocystis carinii,* cytomegalovirus, and fungi have been described as a cause of sinusitis.[53, 54]

The radiographic findings of acute sinusitis include air-fluid levels, partial or complete opacification, and mucous membrane thickening of at least 4 mm (Fig. 31–37).[7, 41] Air-fluid levels do not always indicate acute sinusitis, but may represent retained secretions without infection (Table 31–6).[47] Transient mucosal thickening and air-fluid levels are frequent radiologic findings in adults with a common cold.[55] Even with radiographic abnormalities, plus the appropriate clinical symptoms, sampled sinus secretions yielded a positive culture for bacteria in only 75% of children.[56] Fluid levels in sinuses may result from hemorrhage secondary to trauma or sinus lavage and are common after nasal intubation that causes obstruction of sinus ostia.[51]

From 1 to 2 mm of mucosal thickening in the ethmoid

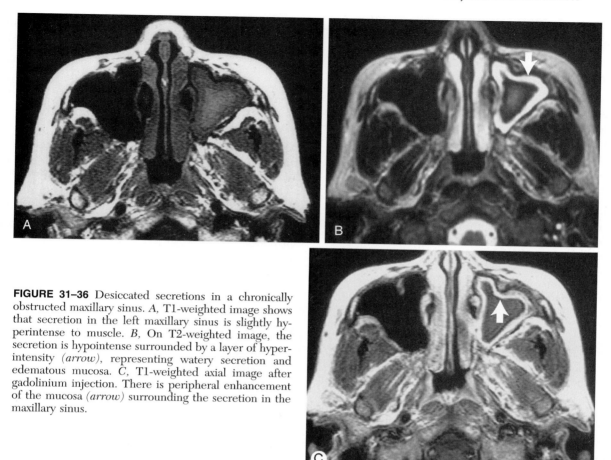

FIGURE 31–36 Desiccated secretions in a chronically obstructed maxillary sinus. *A,* T1-weighted image shows that secretion in the left maxillary sinus is slightly hyperintense to muscle. *B,* On T2-weighted image, the secretion is hypointense surrounded by a layer of hyperintensity *(arrow)*, representing watery secretion and edematous mucosa. *C,* T1-weighted axial image after gadolinium injection. There is peripheral enhancement of the mucosa *(arrow)* surrounding the secretion in the maxillary sinus.

sinuses and up to 3 mm of mucosal thickening in the other paranasal sinuses are an incidental finding in about 65% of asymptomatic adults.[57] Minimal ethmoid mucosal thickening is probably a physiologically normal variant related to the nasal cycle.[57, 58]

On MRI, inflamed edematous sinus mucosa has a low signal intensity on T1-weighted and high signal intensity on T2-weighted images. Retention cysts and sinus polyps have similar MRI signal characteristics.[41]

The radiographic diagnosis of sinusitis in children is controversial. Some authors find opaque sinuses in infants to be a normal condition due to "redundant" mucosa and accumulation of tears associated with crying.[21, 49, 51, 59–61] Incidental sinus opacification in apparently asymptomatic infants and children occurs in 30% to 50% of radiographs and CT scans.[59, 60] Asymptomatic sinus opacification is found in about 50% of children between the ages of 1 and 16 years with a history of uncomplicated upper respiratory tract infection in the past 2 weeks, but only in 7% of children with no recent history of recent respiratory tract infection.[62] Therefore, upper respiratory infection alone may account for much of the sinus abnormality in asymptomatic children.[61] The radiologist should be wary of making the diagnosis of acute sinusitis in children

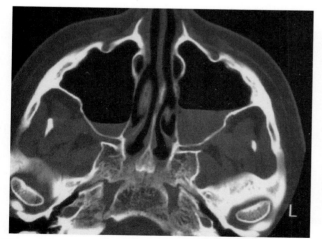

FIGURE 31–37 Axial CT scan. Bilateral maxillary sinusitis with air-fluid levels in both maxillary sinuses.

TABLE 31–6 Sinus Air-Fluid Level

Sinusitis
Upper respiratory infection
Blood (fracture)
Lavage
Intubation
Tears

younger than 5 years without compelling clinical and laboratory corroboration.[21]

Chronic Sinusitis

The persistence of sinus disease for more than 3 months constitutes chronic disease.[46] Chronic sinusitis is unusual in children younger than 16 years and should prompt a search for an underlying abnormality.[51] In children, systemic disease associated with chronic sinusitis includes asthma, allergic rhinitis, cystic fibrosis, immune deficiency, and immotile cilia syndrome (Kartagener's syndrome). Local factors predisposing to chronic sinus disease include nasal foreign bodies and polyps.[50]

About 25% of cases of chronic sinusitis are associated with dental disease.[41] Chronic sinusitis is manifest radiographically by mucosal thickening and sinus opacification, but the hallmark of chronic sinusitis is osseous thickening of the bony sinus wall (Fig. 31–38).[17] The bony changes represent remodeling and new bone formation in response to long-standing inflammation.[17]

Allergic Sinusitis

Symptoms of allergic sinusitis rarely occur before 2 years of age and reach a peak incidence in postadolescent teenagers.[51] CT reveals bilateral polypoid mucosal thickening involving the sinuses and turbinates. Air-fluid levels are usually absent unless there is superimposed acute bacterial infection.[17, 51]

Chronic Allergic Sinusitis

Chronic allergic sinusitis is discussed in the section on chronic allergic fungal sinusitis.

Fungal Sinusitis

Fungal sinusitis is unusual, and many pathogens that are part of the normal respiratory flora are also responsible for both indolent and aggressive fungal sinus disease.

Fungal sinonasal disease is classified into four distinct categories.[45, 63, 64]

1. Noninvasive
   A. Noninvasive mycotic colonization (mycetoma)
   B. Allergic fungal sinusitis
2. Invasive fungal sinus disease
   A. Acute fulminate invasive disease
   B. Chronic invasive disease

Mycetoma

Mycetoma, or "fungus ball," is a benign saprophytic colonization of the sinus, without mucosal invasion, in an immunocompetent patient.[45, 64] A mycetoma results from colonization of inadequately treated bacterial sinusitis. The mycetoma is most frequently found in the maxillary sinus.[51]

This type of fungal sinus disease produces dense sinus secretions on CT. MRI images show decreased signal on T1-weighted and markedly decreased signal intensity on T2-weighted images.[41] This abnormal MRI signal can be explained by the presence of calcium and magnesium within the mycetomas.

Chronic Allergic Fungal Sinusitis

Allergic fungal sinus disease occurs in immunocompetent adolescents and young adults with a history of atopy, sinonasal polyposis, and asthma. This is associated with elevated serum IgE levels, eosinophilia, and skin sensitivity to fungal antigens.[45, 64–66] Histologically there is thick mucus admixed with plasma cells, eosinophils, neutrophils, and scattered fungal hyphae that may be difficult to find. The fungus is most commonly *Aspergillus* or a dematiaceous species such as *Bipolaris*.[45, 67, 68] Multiple sinuses are involved. Typically the sinus is expanded with dense secretions on CT representing fungus and inspissated secretion. The dense secretions may have a serpiginous or an "onion-skin" laminated appearance. Areas of bone resorption are also seen in 19% to 64% of cases (Fig. 31–39).[64, 65]

Invasive Fungal Sinus Disease

Acute invasive fungal sinus disease usually occurs in an immunocompromised or diabetic patient.[17, 41] Two of the

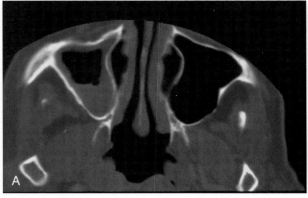
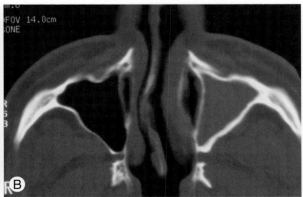

FIGURE 31–38 Chronic maxillary sinusitis. *A*, Acute and chronic right maxillary sinusitis with mucosal thickening, air-fluid level and thickening, and sclerosis of the bony sinus wall. *B*, Chronic left maxillary sinusitis. Left maxillary sinus is opaque with a thickened, sclerotic wall.

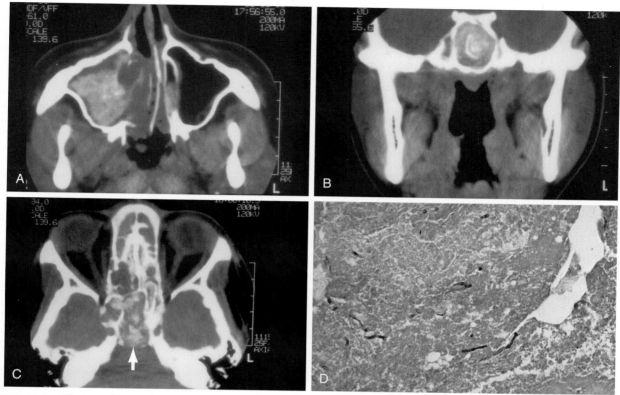

FIGURE 31–39 Chronic allergic fungal sinusitis—*Aspergillus* infection. Axial *(A)*, coronal *(B)*, and axial *(C)* CT scans. Dense, laminated secretions fill the right maxillary and both ethmoid and sphenoid sinuses. Note bone resorption of the posterior wall of the sphenoid sinus *(arrow in C)*. D, Scattered fungal hyphae are embedded in thick mucus (silver methenamine 100×).

most common pathogens are *Mucor* and *Aspergillus*. Both diseases have a predilection for vascular invasion, producing endothelial damage, thrombosis, and necrosis and progressing from the paranasal sinuses to involve the orbit and intracranial structures.[51]

Aspergillus

The most prevalent species are *Aspergillus fumigatus, A. flavus,* and *A. niger.* Histologically one sees uniform, septate hyphae, 3 to 6 μm in diameter, with dichotomous, forked branching (Fig. 31–40). When the condition is

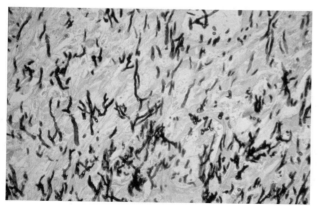

FIGURE 31–40 *Aspergillus* (silver methenamine 200×). Numerous uniform, septate hyphae with forked branching are seen.

noninvasive, the hyphae are typically seen as a tangled ball with little accompanying inflammation. When it is invasive, the hyphae are present within tissue and preferentially involve blood vessels with resulting ischemic necrosis. The typical mixed inflammation of neutrophils, lymphocytes, and macrophages may be less severe in immunosuppressed patients.

Mucormycosis

Mucormycosis is a generic term for disease caused by the *Zygomycetes* species of fungi such as *Rhizopus, Mucor,* and *Absidia* (in descending order of frequency).[45] Histologic examination reveals broad, nonseptate hyphae 6 to 50 μm in diameter with irregular branching (Fig. 31–41). Mucormycosis most commonly invades the lungs, skin, gastrointestinal tract, and blood vessels.[41] The ethmoid air cells are the most commonly involved paranasal sinus. Tissue invasion results in profound necrosis. Both vascular and neural invasion result in often-rapid spread to the orbit and brain. Clinically the nasal turbinates, nasal septum, and soft palate are necrotic and black. (Fig. 31–42).[41] Aggressive surgical débridement plus medical therapy may be lifesaving.[69]

Invasive fungal sinus disease is best imaged with a combination of CT and MRI. CT is best for evaluation of bone involvement, and MRI demonstrates leptomeningeal and intracranial spread (Fig. 31–43).[51] Invasive fungal disease produces mucosal thickening associated with bone destruction that can mimic a destructive tumor. Unlike

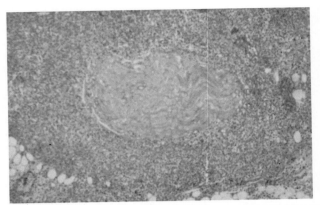

FIGURE 31–41 *Mucor* (hematoxylin and eosin [H&E] 200×). Broad, nonseptate hyphae surround the peripheral branches of the third division of the trigeminal nerve.

neoplasm, areas of bone thickening and sclerosis may also be found in the involved sinus.[17]

Fungal abscesses in the brain are ring-enhancing lesions with a hypointense rim on T2-weighted MRI images, due to the presence of methemoglobin or free radicals produced by macrophages in the capsule wall. Similar hypointense rings on T2-weighted images have been described in pyogenic abscesses, metastases, and subacute hematomas (Fig. 31–44).[70]

Chronic invasive fungal sinusitis is also seen in immunocompromised patients but has a slower course with sclerosis and bone destruction that simulates neoplasm (Fig. 31–45). Unlike acute bacterial sinusitis, which demonstrates hyperintense edematous mucosa on T2-weighted images, the mucosal disease is hypointense with fungal sinus involvement. MRI may direct the surgeon to biopsy the areas of greatest diagnostic yield (Fig. 31–46).[54, 71]

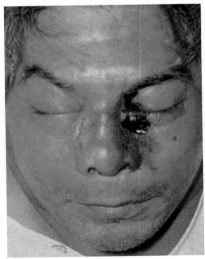

FIGURE 31–42 Mucormycosis. Infarction of the skin of the face, eyes, and nose. (From Donald PJ. Fungal infections of the sinuses. In Donald PJ, Gluckman JL, Rice DH [eds]. The Sinuses, pp. 271–285. Philadelphia, Lippincott-Raven, 1995.)

Functional Endoscopic Sinus Surgery

Functional endoscopic sinus surgery (FESS) has revolutionized the surgical therapy of sinus disease.[42] FESS is based on the premise that the OMC is the linchpin to the pathogenesis of chronic sinus disease.[12] The goal in treating chronic sinusitis with FESS is to relieve the obstruction of the OMC that is responsible for dysfunction of mucociliary drainage.[11, 12] Since the sinus ostia are frequently not gravity dependent, physiologic surgical therapy is necessary to enhance normal mucociliary drainage.[20] FESS has reduced the need for traditional, more extensive surgery, such as Caldwell-Luc or intranasal fenestration procedures.[11, 12]

There are two common pathways for mucociliary drainage that divide the sinuses into two functional and anatomic groups.

The first group includes the maxillary, anterior ethmoid, and frontal sinuses, which drain into the middle meatus (see Figs. 31–15 and 31–24). OMC is the critical connecting channel through which these sinuses drain. The OMC includes the maxillary sinus ostium, infundibulum, frontal recess, ethmoid bulla, uncinate process, hiatus semilunaris, and middle meatus.[10, 11, 17, 20, 47] This region is frequently involved by inflammatory disease processes.[17]

The second group includes the posterior ethmoid and sphenoid sinuses, which drain into a common area called the *sphenoethmoidal recess*, and the superior meatus (see Fig. 31–15).[17]

Five recurring patterns of sinonasal inflammatory disease have been indentified (Table 31–7). These are infundibular, OMC, sphenoethmoid recess, sinonasal polyposis, and unclassified.[47]

The infundibular pattern results in isolated maxillary sinusitis secondary to obstruction of the maxillary ostium and infundibulum. Obstruction of the OMC by mucosal swelling, enlarged turbinates, or polyps leads to inflammatory disease in the ipsilateral maxillary, frontal, and anterior ethmoid sinuses. Obstruction of the sinus ostia posteriorly, in the sphenoethmoid recess, results in posterior ethmoid and sphenoid sinus disease. Isolated sphenoid or posterior ethmoid disease may also occur with this pattern because of the separation of the ostia of these sinuses. The sphenoid sinus drains into the sphenoethmoid recess, whereas the posterior ethmoids drain both into the sphenoethmoid recess and more anteriorly into the superior meatus.

With sinonasal polyposis, polyps fill the nasal cavity and paranasal sinuses, producing obstruction of all the sinus ostia and pansinusitis. The diffuse polyposis produces infundibular enlargement and convex bulging of the ethmoid sinuses, with thinning of the bony nasal septum and ethmoid trabeculae. Finally, about 24% defy classification.

Imaging and Functional Endoscopic Sinus Surgery

Coronal sinus CT is indispensable for planning FESS, and radiologists should be familiar with the anatomy, anatomic variants, and pathology of the lateral nasal wall.[11, 47, 72–74] Recognition of anatomic variants helps avoid

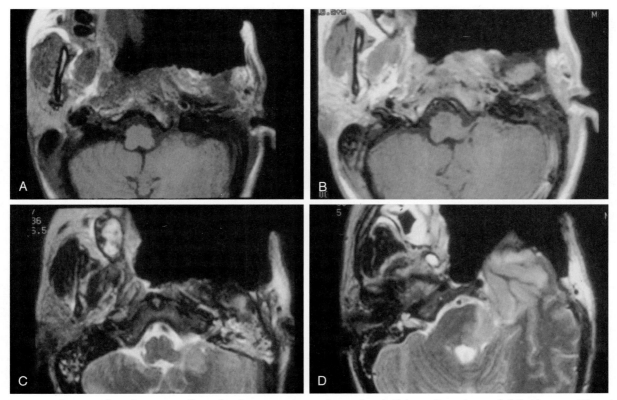

FIGURE 31–43 Invasive fungal sinusitis after orbital exenteration and anterior skull base dissection and débridement. T1-weighted images before *(A)* and after *(B)* gadolinium injection. Note the contrast enhancement in the surgical bed. *C* and *D*, T2-weighted images. Increased signal in the pons, cerebellum, and left temporal lobe is due to involvement by fungal infection.

TABLE 31–7 Recurring Patterns of Sinonasal Inflammatory Disease

Pattern	Percentage	Involved Sinuses
Infundibular	26	Maxillary
Ostiomeatal complex	25	Maxillary, frontal, anterior ethmoid
Sphenoethmoid recess	6	Posterior ethmoid, sphenoid
Sinonasal polyposis	10	Pansinusitis
Unclassified	25	

Adapted from Babbel RW, Harnsberger HR, Sonkens J, et al. Recurring patterns of sinonasal inflammatory disease demonstrated on screening sinus CT. AJNR 1992;13:903–912.

FIGURE 31–44 *Aspergillus* abscess of the left frontal lobe in an immuno-compromised patient. *A,* T1-weighted image after gadolinium injection shows a faint ring-enhancing lesion in the left frontal lobe. *B,* T2-weighted image. The left frontal lobe mass has a low-intensity rim and marked surrounding edema.

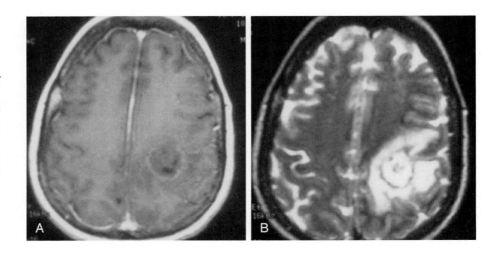

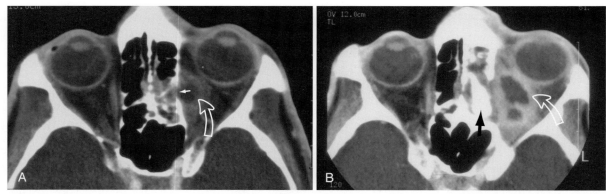

FIGURE 31–45 Chronic invasive aspergillosis in a patient with acquired immunodeficiency syndrome (AIDS). *A,* Axial CT scan. There is ethmoid sinus disease with dehiscence in the lamina papyracea *(straight arrow)* and an adjacent subperiosteal abscess *(curved arrow).* Note sclerosis of the lamina papyracea. *B,* Axial CT scan 4 months after drainage. There is a larger subperiosteal abscess *(curved arrow)* with greater involvement of the left ethmoid air cells and a sequestrum *(straight arrow).*

potentially disastrous complications of FESS. Crucial anatomic relationships between the paranasal sinuses and the orbit, optic nerve, internal carotid artery, cavernous sinuses, cribriform plate, and fovea ethmoidalis are optimally assessed on coronal CT scans.[11, 75] A systematic approach to the radiographic report is helpful (Table 31–8). One should begin anteriorly and proceed posteriorly noting normal anatomy and anatomic variants that

may affect surgery. Then one should evaluate mucosal disease and the two common pathways for sinus damage. Finally, note the character and integrity of the bony sinus walls.[76]

Anatomic variants may obstruct sinus ostia and impair mucociliary drainage resulting in recurrent sinusitis. These include concha bullosa, large ethmoid bulla; paradoxically bent middle turbinate; large or laterally deviated

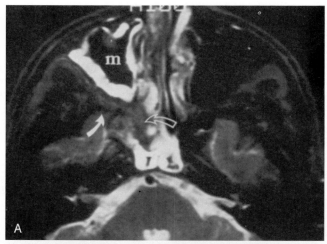

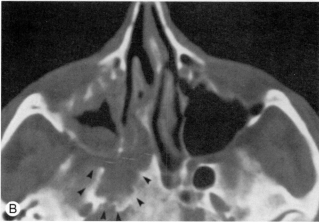

FIGURE 31–46 Chronic invasive aspergillosis in a 36-year-old AIDS patient who noted numbness of the right cheek after shaving. Neurologic examination confirmed decreased sensation in the second division of the trigeminal nerve. *A,* Axial T2-weighted image demonstrates the mass *(open arrow)* in the posterior nasal cavity with extension into the pterygopalatine fossa *(closed arrow).* Note that the mass is hypointense relative to the typical bright signal of inflammatory mucosal disease in the right maxillary sinus (m). *B,* Axial CT scan shows irregular destruction of the right skull base *(arrowheads).* (*A* and *B,* From Holliday RA. Manifestations of AIDS in the oromaxillofacial region: The role of imaging. Radiol Clin North Am 1993;31:45–73.)

TABLE 31–8 Functional Endoscopic Sinus Surgery Radiology Report Should Include

Extent of mucosal disease
Evaluation of the two common pathways of sinus
    drainage
    Osteomeatal complex
    Sphenoethmoidal recess
Anatomic variants
    Dehiscent bone surrounding
        Optic nerve
        Internal carotid artery
    Lamina papyracea, dehiscence
    Fovea ethmoidalis
        Low, asymmetric, dehiscent
    Pneumatization anterior clinoid
    Haller's cells
    Onodi's cells
    Prominent ethmoid bulla
    Uncinate process
        Pneumatized, lateral deviation
    Septal deviation and spurs
    Concha bullosa
    Paradoxic middle turbinate (convex laterally)
Postsurgical changes
    Resection of vertical insertion of middle turbinate

uncinate process (Fig. 31–47); nasal septal deviation with spur; and Haller's cells.[11, 77] Other authors have found that these anatomic variants play no significant role in recurrent sinusitis and are found with equal frequency in normal patients.[72]

Other anatomic variants that may lead to surgical complication should be reported by the radiologist. These include Onodi's cells, dehiscence of the bony canal for the internal carotid artery in the sphenoid sinus, and incidental dehiscence of the lamina papyracea. Aeration of the anterior clinoid places the canalicular portion of the optic nerve at increased risk. An abnormally low or asymmetric position of the roof of the ethmoid sinus, known as the *fovea ethmoidalis*, may lead to accidental surgical penetration.[49]

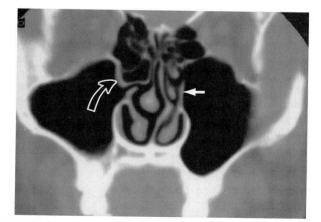

FIGURE 31–47 Coronal CT scan. There is anomalous vertical orientation of the left uncinate process *(straight arrow)*. Note the Haller cell on the right *(curved arrow)*, with lateral deviation of the uncinate process.

After sinus surgery, the integrity of the vertical attachment of the middle turbinate to the cribriform plate should be noted. This is an important landmark for the surgeon, who tries to remain lateral to it to avoid intracranial entry through the cribriform plate.[42, 49]

Complications of Endoscopic Sinus Surgery

The proximity of the paranasal sinuses to key anatomic structures provides potential for disaster (Table 31–9). Because of the small confined space and the lack of depth perception when a monocular endoscope is used, even the most experienced surgeon may encounter problems.

Complications include minor sequelae, such as recurrent inflammatory disease (7% to 18%). Major complications are rare, but blindness, dysfunction of the extraocular muscles, vascular injury with hemorrhage, cerebrospinal fluid leak, meningitis, brain abscess, pneumocephalus, carotid-cavernous fistula, and death have been reported.[12, 78]

Accidental violation of the lateral wall of the ethmoid sinuses may lead to orbital hemorrhage and emphysema, extraocular muscle injury, damage to the lacrimal drainage system, and optic nerve injury.[79] The optic canal often bulges into the posterior ethmoid and sphenoid sinuses and is nearly surrounded by air (see Fig. 31–12B). There is usually only thin bone separating the optic canal from the sinus, and in about 4% of cases, there is complete bony dehiscence of the optic canal.[17, 78] The canalicular portion of the optic nerve is medial to the anterior clinoid process. Extensive pneumatization of the anterior clinoid places the optic nerve at risk with posterior sphenoid surgery. Blindness may result from direct injury to the optic nerve or an acute intraorbital hemorrhage producing pressure on the optic nerve, with ischemia and loss of vision.[78] Breach of the fovea ethmoidalis and dura may cause a cerebrospinal fluid fistula and meningitis (Fig. 31–48).

The internal carotid artery may be injured as it passes adjacent to the sphenoid sinus. The internal carotid artery often bulges into the sphenoid sinus (see Fig. 31–14). In two-thirds of patients there is less than 1 mm of bone separating the internal carotid artery from the sphenoid sinus. This thin bony partition is less than 0.5 mm in 8.8%, and absent in 4% to 8% of cases.[17] Carotid-cavernous fistula and severe intraoperative hemorrhage have been reported.

Complications of Sinusitis

Undiagnosed or inadequately treated sinus disease may result in intraorbital and intracranial complications (Table

TABLE 31–9 Complications of Functional Endoscopic Sinus Surgery

Minor
    Subcutaneous or orbital emphysema
    Nasal synechiae
    Small orbital hematoma
    Tooth pain
Major
    Cerebrospinal fluid leak
    Meningitis
    Hemorrhage, subarachnoid or intranasal
    Blindness

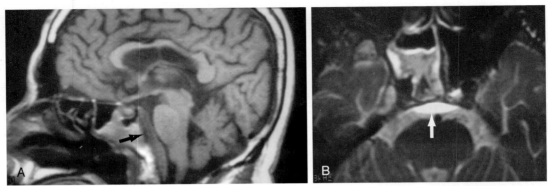

FIGURE 31–51 Sphenoid sinusitis causing right sixth-nerve palsy in a 68-year-old man with a 1-month history of headache and diplopia. *A*, Unenhanced sagittal T1-weighted scan shows a dural mass *(arrow)* adjacent to the clivus. *B*, Axial T2-weighted scan reveals an air-fluid level in the sphenoid sinus and hyperintense inflammatory dural thickening (pachymeningitis) posterior to the clivus *(arrow)*. (*A* and *B*, From Nemzek W, Postma G, Poirier V, et al. MR features of pachymeningitis presenting with sixth-nerve palsy secondary to sphenoid sinusitis. AJNR 1995;16:960–963.)

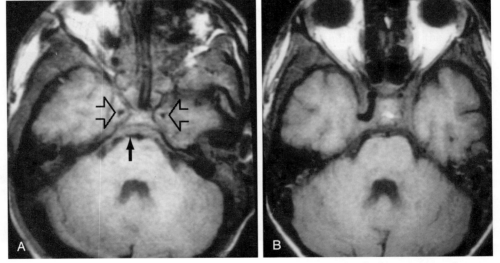

FIGURE 31–52 Sphenoid sinusitis in 17-year-old boy with a 1-week history of fever, headache, nausea, and vomiting. He developed bilateral sixth-nerve palsies and rapid deterioration of vision. *A*, Unenhanced axial T1-weighted image shows inflammatory dural thickening overlying the clivus *(arrow)*, which would explain the sixth-nerve palsies. Note the narrowing of both internal carotid arteries *(open arrows)* in the cavernous sinus. There is fluid in the mastoids and ethmoid and sphenoid sinusitis. *B*, Unenhanced axial T1-weighted image 1 month later shows lack of a flow void in the cavernous portion of the left internal carotid artery compatible with carotid occlusion. (*A* and *B*, From Nemzek W, Postma G, Poirier V, et al. MR features of pachymeningitis presenting with sixth-nerve palsy secondary to sphenoid sinusitis. AJNR 1995;16:960–963.)

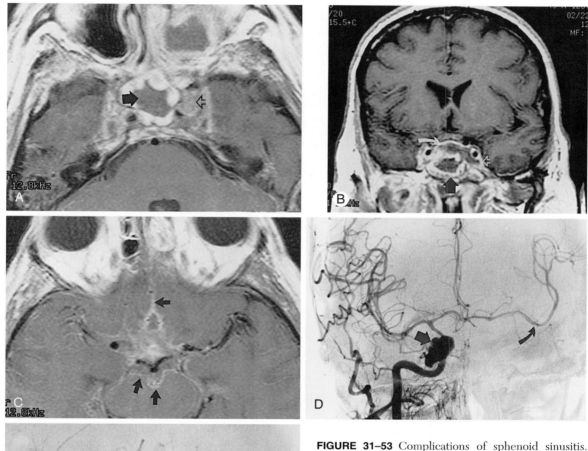

FIGURE 31–53 Complications of sphenoid sinusitis. Enhanced axial (A) and coronal (B) T1-weighted images show mucosal thickening and a fluid-filled sphenoid sinus (black arrow). A pituitary abscess (curved arrow in B) extends into the left cavernous sinus (open arrows). C, Axial T1-weighted scan after gadolinium injection demonstrates diffuse meningeal enhancement (arrows) compatible with meningitis. Anteroposterior (D) and lateral (E) right carotid arteriograms 1 week later show pseudoaneurysm of the right internal carotid artery (straight arrows) and flow to the contralateral anterior cerebral and middle cerebral arteries (curved arrow in D) owing to occlusion of the left internal carotid artery.

through thin or dehiscent sphenoid walls. Transverse sinus thrombosis is a complication of mastoiditis.

A contrast-enhanced CT scan shows a filling defect or no opacification of a bulging (outwardly convex) cavernous sinus. Another clue is dilatation of the superior ophthalmic vein (Fig. 31–54).

Thrombosis of the transverse sinus may extend to the superior sagittal sinus. Superior sagittal thrombosis is also caused by frontal sinusitis. Frontal sinus infection may spread into the anterior cranial fossa via emissary veins with no evidence of bone erosion.[51] Contrast-enhanced CT shows a hypodense venous sinus containing thrombus, surrounded by enhancing dura (the "empty delta sign" in the case of the occluded superior sagittal sinus).

MR venography also demonstrates an absent flow in an occluded venous sinus. The occluded sinus may contain methemoglobin, which is of high signal intensity on both T1- and T2-weighted images. Flow and methemoglobin both have increased signal on time-of-flight magnetic resonance arteriography (MRA) that uses gradient-echo images. Phase contrast angiography provides suppression of high signal intensity from hemorrhage so only flow is imaged as a bright signal. Phase contrast MRA is more accurate for the assessment of venous thrombosis.

Venous infarction and intracranial hemorrhage are complications of venous thrombosis. Bilateral (or unilateral) subcortical hemorrhage occurs.

NONNEOPLASTIC SINONASAL LESIONS

Sinonasal Retention Cysts and Polyps

Retention Cysts

Mucous retention cysts are found in 10% to 35% of patients.[45] They are common after inflammatory sinusitis and are due to obstruction of minor seromucinous glands, which become filled with mucus (Fig. 31–55; see also Fig. 31–6).[41, 57]

Sinonasal polyps are inflammatory swellings of the submucosa rather than true neoplastic growths. The majority occur in the ethmoid recesses and upper lateral nasal wall near the middle turbinate and may be single, multiple, and bilateral.

Grossly, polyps are soft, polypoid, translucent masses up to several centimeters in diameter. Polyps increase in size by accumulating water in the lamina propria.[41, 45] Polyps are associated with allergy, atopy, infection, and vasomotor impairment.[45]

Histologically the surface mucosa is typically intact and covered by respiratory epithelium with increased mucous cells or areas of squamous metaplasia or both. The stroma is edematous and myxomatous with scattered fibroblasts and variable vascularity and a mixed inflammatory cell infiltrate of eosinophils, lymphocytes, plasma cells, and tissue mast cells (Fig. 31–56). Chronic polyps may have a fibrotic stroma.

Antrochoanal Polyp and Sinonasal Polyposis

Occasionally a polyp originating in the maxillary sinus enlarges and protrudes through the sinus ostium, through the middle meatus, and into the nasal cavity. It may then extend to the choana (junction of the nasal cavity and nasopharynx). The term *antrochoanal polyp* is applied to these lesions, which represent 4% to 6% of all nasal polyps.

The antrochoanal polyp is the most common benign sinus tumor in children.[51] A large polyp may present as a nasopharyngeal or oropharyngeal mass.[87] Most antrochoanal polyps occur in teenage and young adults.[45] Rarely a choanal polyp may arise from the sphenoid sinus.[87] These are typically solitary, unilateral lesions, and the gross appearance is similar to that of common sinonasal polyps.[88] Histologically, although generally similar to standard polyps, the antrochoanal polyps tend to have a more fibrous and vascular appearance.

Polyps are the most common mass lesion of the nasal

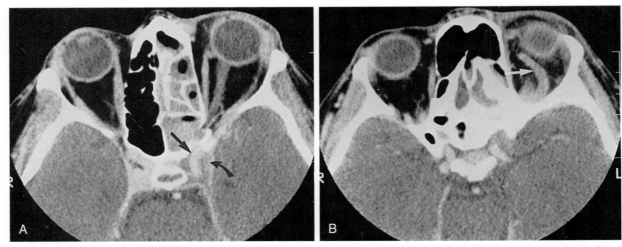

FIGURE 31–54 Ethmoid and sphenoid sinusitis causing partial cavernous sinus thrombosis. *A* and *B,* Contrast-enhanced axial CT scans show left ethmoid and sphenoid sinusitis. Note the patent enhanced left cavernous internal carotid artery (*straight black arrow*) surrounded by unenhanced thrombus (*curved black arrow*) in the cavernous sinus. The left superior ophthalmic vein is enlarged (*straight white arrow*).

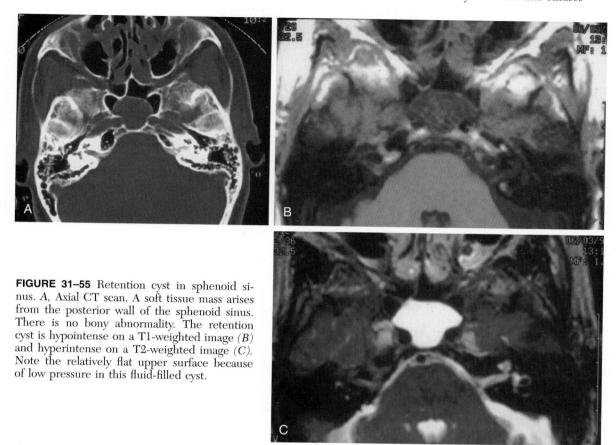

FIGURE 31–55 Retention cyst in sphenoid sinus. *A,* Axial CT scan. A soft tissue mass arises from the posterior wall of the sphenoid sinus. There is no bony abnormality. The retention cyst is hypointense on a T1-weighted image *(B)* and hyperintense on a T2-weighted image *(C).* Note the relatively flat upper surface because of low pressure in this fluid-filled cyst.

cavity.[45] Nasal polyps have increased incidence in patients with diabetes mellitus, allergies, vasomotor rhinitis, infectious rhinosinusitis, aspirin intolerance, and asthma. In children, chronic sinusitis and nasal polyps are associated with cystic fibrosis.[51, 89]

Polyps and retention cysts are indistinguishable by imaging. Both are of low attenuation on CT. Since polyps and cysts are predominately water, they have low T1-weighted and high T2-weighted signal intensities. Minimal enhancement is seen at the mucosal surface (Fig. 31–57).[51] With time, or after infection, retention cysts

may have increased T1-weighted signal intensity, due to elevated protein content in the cyst fluid.[45]

Large retention cysts, because of relatively low internal pressure, have a relatively flat upper surface, resembling a flat tire. This appearance may be mistaken for an air-fluid level (see Fig. 31–55).[45]

Sinonasal Polyposis

Multiple extensive polyps are seen in patients with a history of allergic or nonallergic atopic rhinitis, asthma, and aspirin sensitivity.[90–92] Many patients with cystic fibrosis develop sinonasal polyposis.

The polypoid masses are usually bilateral and are present in the nasal cavity in the region of the middle turbinate. The maxillary infundibulum is usually widened. The sinuses are opaque and filled with polyps and obstructed inflammatory secretions. Multiple conglomerate polyps may trap secretions and may contain mucoceles. MRI reveals a mixture of signal intensities ranging from high to intermediate to signal void. The polyps may remodel bone with intracranial and intradural extension. The nasal septum may be eroded.

On MRI, the extensive form of sinonasal polyposis has variable signal intensities and may simulate neoplasm.[45] Squamous cell carcinoma typically has a monotonous intermediate signal intensity. On CT, the signature of ethmoid polyposis is expansion of the sinus wall, yet the delicate sinus septations are spared (Fig. 31–58).[45]

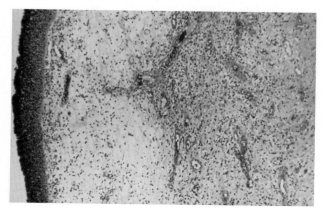

FIGURE 31–56 Sinonasal polyp (H&E 100×). Intact respiratory-type epithelium and edematous stroma.

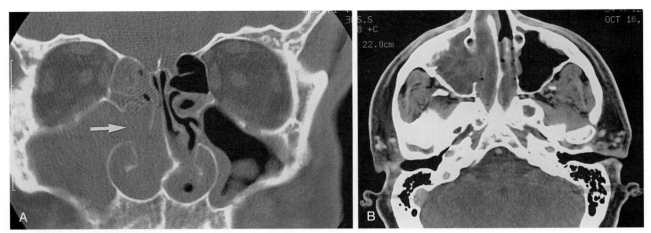

FIGURE 31–57 Antrochoanal polyp. *A,* Coronal CT scan. The mass fills the maxillary sinus and spills into the nasal cavity. The polyp reached the nasal choana (not shown). Note widening of the ostium of the maxillary sinus *(arrow)* and erosion of the uncinate process. *B,* Axial CT scan after contrast medium injection. There is minimal peripheral enhancement of the polyp.

Mucocele

A mucocele is an obstructed, airless sinus, filled with secretion with expansion and remodeling of its bony walls. (Figs. 31–59 through 31–61).[31, 41] Mucoceles are the most common expansile lesions of the paranasal sinuses.[51] Mucoceles are most common in the *f*rontal sinus (60%),

followed by the *e*thmoid (25%), *m*axillary (10%), and *s*phenoid (5%) sinuses[51] (mnemonic FEMS). In children, the ethmoid sinus is the most common site for mucocele. Ethmoid mucoceles usually arise in the anterior ethmoid cells, because the anterior ostia are the smallest of any of the paranasal sinuses.[31]

Patients present with proptosis and nasal obstruction.

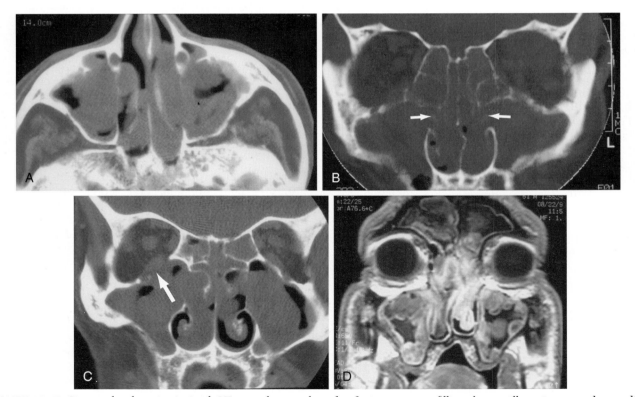

FIGURE 31–58 Sinonasal polyposis. *A,* Axial CT scan shows polypoid soft tissue masses filling the maxillary sinuses and extending into the nasal cavity. *B,* Coronal CT scan. There is expansion of the ethmoid sinuses with intact trabeculae. The maxillary sinus ostia are widened *(arrows). C,* Coronal CT posterior to *B.* Note erosion of the floor of the right orbit *(arrow). D,* Coronal T1-weighted image enhanced with gadolinium of a different patient shows multiple polyps with peripheral enhancement filling the sinuses and nasal cavity and pansinus disease. The polyps were of increased intensity on unenhanced T1-weighted images (not shown).

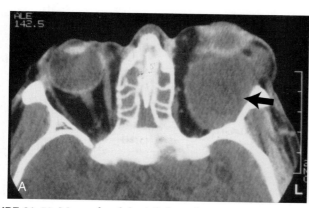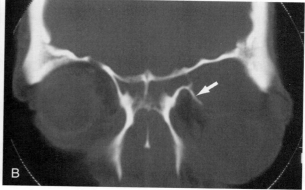

FIGURE 31-59 Mucocele of the left frontal sinus causing proptosis in a 52-year-old man with sinonasal polyposis. *A,* Axial CT scan shows a mass *(arrow)* in the left orbit displacing the globe anteriorly. The mass is the same attenuation as the vitreous. *B,* Coronal CT scan shows the mass arising from the left frontal sinus with displacement and remodeling of the inferior medial wall of the frontal sinus *(arrow).*

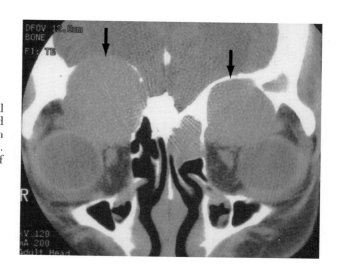

FIGURE 31-60 Bilateral frontal mucoceles in a woman with bilateral proptosis and a remote history of a frontal lobotomy performed through the frontal sinuses. There is inferior displacement of both globes by the airless, expanded, remodeled frontal sinuses *(arrows).* Note that the density of the mucoceles is greater than that of the vitreous.

FIGURE 31-61 Bilateral maxillary mucoceles in a 10-year-old child with cystic fibrosis. Axial *(A)* and coronal *(B)* CT scans. The maxillary sinuses are airless and expanded with marked pressure erosion and thinning remodeling of the medial walls. Note the mucoceles encroaching on the nasal cavity, which could simulate an intranasal mass.

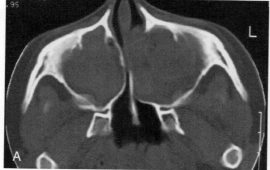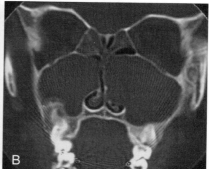

The MRI appearance of a mucocele may be confusing. The signal intensity depends on the hydration of the obstructed sinus secretions. Watery secretions are dark on T1-weighted and bright on T2-weighted images. Markedly inspissated secretion is hypointense on T1- and T2-weighted sequences and may be mistaken for a normally aerated sinus on MRI. CT demonstrates an opaque sinus, however.[41]

Gadolinium shows rim enhancement of the mucosa, which is typical for a mucocele, thereby excluding tumor.[41]

Granulomatous Sinus Disease

Wegener's Granulomatosis

Wegener's granulomatosis is a chronic idiopathic systemic necrotizing vasculitis characterized by focal, granulomatous arteritis involving the upper and lower respiratory tract, kidneys, and other organs. Histologic examination reveals a variable mixture of three elements: vasculitis, granulomatous inflammation, and necrosis (Fig. 31–62). The vasculitis affects small to medium-sized arteries with transmural fibrinoid necrosis and neutrophils. The granulomas are often ill defined and composed of multinucleate giant cells admixed with macrophages and lymphocytes. The necrosis is typically irregular and geographic in pattern with admixed neutrophilic abscesses.

Mucosal disease is present in the nasal cavity and paranasal sinuses. Bone destruction occurs in the nasal septum (Table 31–11) and in the medial wall of the maxillary sinuses in advanced cases.[93] Imaging demonstrates nodular mucosal thickening, but the hallmark of the disease is extensive bone destruction without an associated soft tissue mass (Fig. 31–63).

Small infarcts occur in the brain in about 25% of patients.[93]

Midline Granuloma

The terms *lethal midline granuloma, polymorphic reticuloses,* and *lymphomatoid granulomatosis* are gone and have been replaced by the appreciation that most of these lesions are actually a precursor or a type of nasal

TABLE 31–11 Nasal Septum Destruction
Infectious
Syphilis
Rhinoscleroma
Leprosy
Noninfectious
Cocaine
Sarcoid
Postsurgical
Nasal lymphoma (lethal midline granuloma)
Wegener's granulomatosis
Polyposis

lymphoma.[94] Lymphoma is discussed with malignant neoplasm.

Cocaine Granuloma ("Cocaine Nose")

Cocaine abuse causes necrotizing vasculitis with granuloma formation that eventually produces destruction of the nasal septum (Fig. 31–64).[45]

Wegener's granulomatosis, midline granuloma, and cocaine nose may appear similar on sinonasal imaging. It is important to make the distinction because therapy is very different for each entity. Wegener's granulomatosis usually causes less bone destruction and also involves the respiratory tract and kidneys. Therapy includes steroid and cytotoxic drugs. Local radiation is the treatment for nasal lymphoma. Antibiotic therapy and abstinence are the treatment for cocaine nose.[95]

Rhinoscleroma

Rhinoscleroma is a chronic, progressive, granulomatous infection that affects upper and lower airways but has a predilection for the nose. The disease is caused by the bacterium *Klebsiella rhinoscleromatis*. Although most cases occur in rural areas of developing countries, sporadic cases are found in the United States because of immigration from endemic areas. This disease is associated with altered T-cell immunity and should be added to the list of opportunistic infections that can occur in

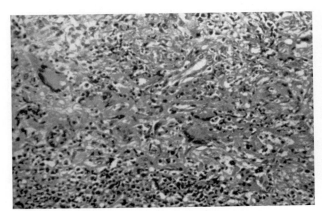

FIGURE 31–62 Wegener's granulomatosis (H&E 100×). Numerous multinucleated giant cells are admixed with lymphocytes, neutrophils, and areas of necrosis.

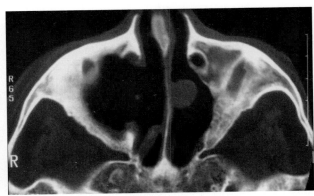

FIGURE 31–63 The patient had a 20-year history of Wegener's granulomatosis. Axial CT scan. There is destruction of the turbinates and medial wall of the maxillary sinuses with no associated soft tissue mass. The lateral walls of the maxillary sinuses are thickened and sclerotic.

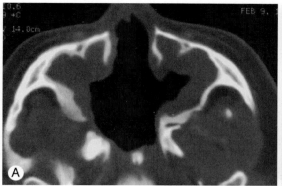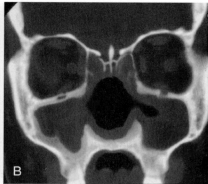

FIGURE 31–64 Long history of cocaine use in a 33-year-old woman with no history of previous surgery. Axial *(A)* and coronal *(B)* CT scans reveal destruction of the nasal septum, the medial wall of the maxillary sinuses, and the ethmoid sinuses. There is mucosal disease with reactive sclerosis of the lateral walls of the maxillary sinuses.

patients with acquired immunodeficiency syndrome (AIDS).

The nose is affected in 95% to 100% of cases, the pharynx in 18% to 43%, the paranasal sinuses in 26%, the trachea in 12%, and the bronchi in 2% to 7%.[96] On CT, one finds inflammatory soft tissue masses that may distort the midface producing a rhinoceros-like appearance. The nasal septum may be destroyed (see Table 31–11).[45, 97] The differential diagnosis includes leprosy and syphilis.

Inflammatory Pseudotumor

Inflammatory pseudotumor is an uncommon, idiopathic, benign, slow-growing lesion composed of inflammatory cells, fibroblasts, and histiocytes. The most common site is the lung, followed by the orbit. Paranasal sinus extension from the orbit is uncommon, and primary pseudotumor is rare.[98]

Radiographically, inflammatory pseudotumor may simulate an aggressive neoplasm. There is a soft tissue mass associated with bone destruction, but also thickened sclerotic bone (Fig. 31–65). The differential diagnosis includes carcinoma, lymphoma, and chronic fungal disease.[98]

SYNDROMES ASSOCIATED WITH SINUSITIS

Cystic Fibrosis

Abnormal secretions of the exocrine glands of the respiratory tract in cystic fibrosis lead to impaired mucociliary transport, which produces recurrent infections.[99] The most common abnormalities include nasal polyposis and mucocele or mucopyocele of the maxillary sinus in children with cystic fibrosis. Nasal polyposis is bilateral, with inflammatory polyps arising from the middle meatus. Some children have extreme narrowing of the nasal cavity due to a mucocele or pyomucocele with marked medial bowing of the medial wall of the maxillary antrum, which reaches the nasal septum (see Fig. 31–61). There may be pressure erosion of the medial wall of the maxillary sinus caused by polyps and the trapped secretions of the mucocele.[99]

Kartagener's Syndrome (Immotile Cilia Syndrome)

The immotile cilia syndrome (Kartagener's syndrome) is included in the differential diagnosis of chronic, recurrent sinobronchial disease in children and adults. Clinically the patient presents with obstructive lung disease, chronic otitis media, and sinusitis. Males are sterile, and situs inversus is present in 50% of patients.[100]

MISCELLANEOUS SYNDROMES INVOLVING THE SINUSES

Osteopetrosis

Osteopetrosis is characterized by defective osteoclastic function and failure of bone remodeling. The primary calcified spongiosa cannot be absorbed, and the result is the radiologic finding of dense "marble bone." The para-

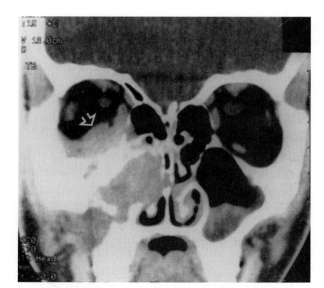

FIGURE 31–65 Inflammatory pseudotumor. Coronal CT scan. There is a soft tissue mass *(arrow)* in the right maxillary sinus, extending into the nasal fossa and the orbit. Note the associated bone destruction and sclerosis. (From Maldjian JA, Norton KI, Groisman GM, et al. Inflammatory pseudotumor of the maxillary sinus in a 15-year-old boy. AJNR 1994;15:784–786.)

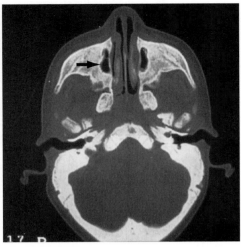

FIGURE 31–66 Osteopetrosis in a 9-year-old boy. Axial CT scan. There is thickening and sclerosis of the bone of the skull base and paranasal sinuses. Note only minimal aeration of the maxillary sinuses *(arrow)*.

nasal sinuses fail to develop and pneumatize, and the skull base foramina are narrowed (Fig..31–66).[101]

Camurati-Engelmann Disease

Camurati-Engelmann disease (progressive diaphyseal dysplasia) is a rare disorder of bone metabolism characterized by hyperostosis of the diaphysis of long bones, the skull, and other membranous bones. The bones are thickened and sclerotic. Skull base foramina are narrowed, causing cranial nerve deficits. Narrowing of the foramen magnum may produce brain stem compression and death.[102] The sinuses fail to pneumatize (Fig. 31–67).

Fibrous Dysplasia

Fibrous dysplasia is discussed in the section on fibro-osseous lesions.

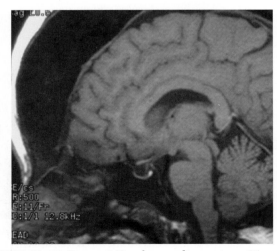

FIGURE 31–67 Camurati-Engelmann disease in a 25-year-old woman. Sagittal T1-weighted image. There is a markedly thickened diploic space with no pneumatization of the frontal or sphenoid sinuses.

SINONASAL NEOPLASM OVERVIEW AND IMAGING

The diverse tissues that constitute the nasal cavity and paranasal sinuses are some of the most complex in the human body. The lining includes squamous and respiratory mucosa as well as specialized olfactory epithelium. The submucosa includes numerous seromucinous or minor salivary glands, blood and lymphatic vessels, peripheral nerves, and connective tissue. These mucosae and soft tissues are adherent to underlying bone and hyaline cartilage. This complex array of tissue types gives rise to a number of benign and malignant tumors (Tables 31–12 and 31–13).[103]

Malignant sinonasal neoplasms account for less than 1% of all malignancies and 3% of all head and neck tumors. From 50% to 65% arise in the maxillary sinus, 15% to 30% in the nasal cavity, 10% to 25% in the ethmoid sinuses, and 0.1% to 4% in the frontal and sphenoid sinuses.[104–106] Sinonasal malignancies may be divided into tumors of epithelial or minor salivary gland origin.[106] Tumors of epithelial origin include papilloma, squamous cell carcinoma, undifferentiated carcinoma, malignant melanoma, and esthesioneuroblastoma. Squamous cell carcinoma represents 80% of sinonasal malignant tumors.[41] Glandular tumors account for 10% to 14% of sinonasal malignancies. This group of neoplasms includes adenoid cystic carcinoma; adenocarcinoma; mucoepidermoid carcinoma; and acinic cell carcinoma.[106, 107] Other malignancies include lymphoma, plasmacytoma, metastases, and sarcomas.[41, 105]

Neoplasms of the paranasal sinuses are unusual in children. Fibro-osseous lesions (especially fibrous dyspla-

TABLE 31–12 Benign Sinonasal Neoplasms

Benign epithelial lesions
  Papilloma
  Pleomorphic adenoma
Benign mesenchymal lesions
  Juvenile angiofibroma
  Hemangioma
  Neurogenic lesions
  Meningioma
Pituitary adenoma
Osseous lesions
  Fibro-osseous lesions
    Osteoma
    Osteoblastoma
    Fibrous dysplasia
    Ossifying fibroma
  Giant cell tumor (osteoclastoma)
  Giant cell reparative granuloma
  "Brown tumor" of hyperparathyroidism
Odontogenic lesions
  Radicular cyst
  Follicular cysts (primordial and dentigerous cysts)
  Keratocyst
  Ameloblastoma
Fissural cyst
  Globulomaxillary cyst
Aneurysmal bone cyst
Langerhans cell histiocytosis

TABLE 31–13 Malignant Sinonasal Neoplasms

Malignant epithelial neoplasms
  Squamous cell carcinoma
  Sinonasal undifferentiated carcinoma
  Minor salivary gland neoplasms
    Adenoid cystic carcinoma
    Sinonasal adenocarcinoma
    Mucoepidermoid carcinoma
  Malignant melanoma
  Esthesioneuroblastoma
Malignant mesenchymal neoplasms
  Sarcoma
    Rhabdomysarcoma
    Chondrosarcoma
    Osteosarcoma
    Dermatofibrosarcoma protuberans (malignant
      fibrous histiocytoma)
Hemangiopericytoma
Lymphoma
Plasmacytoma
Metastatic tumor

sia) and odontogenic tumors are the most common benign neoplasms. Rhabdomyosarcoma and undifferentiated carcinoma are the most frequent malignancies.[51]

Presenting clinical symptoms are those of chronic sinusitis, including nasal obstruction, nasal drainage, and epistaxis. A high degree of suspicion must be maintained when patients are unresponsive to medical therapy or have recurrent or unilateral symptoms.[106]

CT is the best modality to detect bone erosion. Key areas to scrutinize include the bony orbital walls, cribriform plate, fovea ethmoidalis, posterior wall of the maxillary sinus, pterygoid plates, and pterygopalatine fossa. Tumors of the sphenoid sinus extend laterally into the cavernous sinus and middle cranial fossa, or anteriorly into the nasopharynx. Frontal sinus tumors extend posteriorly into the anterior cranial fossa or inferiorly into the ethmoid sinuses.[106, 107]

CT imaging includes 5-mm-thick axial images from the top of the frontal sinus to the hyoid bone and 3-mm coronal scans from the nose to the back of the sphenoid sinus with iodinated contrast enhancement.[49] Metastatic nodes are unusual at presentation for squamous cell carcinoma. The most common nodes initially involved are the retropharyngeal, submandibular, and high internal jugular,[45] which are included in the imaging protocol. The entire neck should be scanned with recurrent tumor, because the chance of metastatic adenopathy increases in such cases.[49]

Absence of bone does not always indicate destruction by neoplasm. When bone involvement is evaluated, pressure erosion from a slow-growing lesion can be distinguished from the permeative bone destruction of an aggressive neoplasm. Absent bone in the center portions of a lesion may represent simple pressure erosion or invasive destruction.[44, 45] When evaluating bone destruction, one must carefully examine the margins of the lesion and not the central portions for appropriate clues (Table 31–14). The signature of an indolent process is bone expansion and remodeling. Slowly expanding processes cause pres-

sure erosion and deossification of adjacent bone, but the outer periosteum has the opportunity to rebuild bone at the margins of the lesion. Examples of this type of marginal bone remodeling include mucoceles (see Figs. 31–59 through 31–61), polyps, inverted papillomas, and low-grade sarcomas.[45] Rapidly growing lesions invade and destroy marginal bone leaving a permeative path of destruction. Aggressive bone destruction is typical of squamous cell carcinoma (see Fig. 31–107). Fungal infection may cause a combination of destruction and remodeling (see Fig. 31–45). These types of marginal bone response are found in the facial bones and nasal vault. Skull base lesions demonstrate a limited remodeling response.[44, 45]

It is important to realize that the bone-remodeling does not always correlate with the biologic aggressiveness of the tumor. Lesions such as melanoma, some sarcomas, and esthesioneuroblastoma may grow slowly enough to permit remodeling of bone, yet the prognosis and patient survival statistics may be abysmal (see Fig. 31–123).[44]

MRI is superior in differentiating inflammatory tissue and retained secretion from neoplasm.[41, 106] Inflammatory tissue contains predominately free water, which produces high signal intensity on T2-weighted images. *Most* sinonasal tumors are highly cellular and are of only intermediate signal intensity on T2-weighted scans.[41] Gadolinium enhancement shows that neoplasm enhances centrally and inflammatory tissue enhances peripherally (see Fig. 31–36C).[108] Exceptions with a high water content and increased T2-weighted signal intensity include polyps; papillomas; minor salivary gland tumors; schwannomas; and adenoid cystic carcinoma.[104, 109–111]

Even though the T2-weighted signal intensity of most sinonasal neoplasms is less than that of watery sinus secretions, the T2-weighted signal intensity of tumors exceeds the T1-weighted signal intensity. If the window width and level are constant, the observer sees a relative brightening of tumor between the T1- and T2-weighted MRI scans.[44] It also follows that if the T2-weighted signal

TABLE 31–14 Marginal Bone Response to Lesions of Nasal Vault and Face

Bone destruction
  Squamous cell carcinoma
  Undifferentiated carcinoma
  Metastases
Destruction and remodeling
  Aggressive chronic infection (e.g., fungal disease)
  Inflammatory pseudotumor
Bone remodeling
  Mucocele
  Polyps
  Angiofibroma
  Low-grade sarcoma
  Hemangiopericytoma
  Inverting papilloma
  Lymphoma
  Plasmacytoma
  Melanoma
  Esthesioneuroblastoma

Data from Som PM, Curtin HD. Inflammatory lesions and tumors of the nasal cavities and paranasal sinuses with skull base involvement. Neuroimaging Clin North Am 1994;4:499–513.

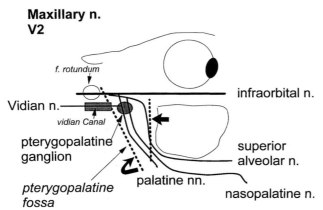

FIGURE 31–68 Lateral diagram of the maxillary nerve division (V2) and the branches arising in the pterygopalatine fossa. The pterygopalatine fossa lies between the posterior wall of the maxillary sinus *(straight arrow)* and the pterygoid process of the sphenoid *(curved arrow)*. (From Nemzek WR. The trigeminal nerve. Top Magn Reson Imaging 1996;8:132–154.)

intensity is less than that of the T1-weighted signal, the diagnosis is most likely to be inspissated secretion, a fungus ball, or fibrous dysplasia.[43, 44]

The MRI protocol includes the same areas covered by CT. Precontrast T1-weighted 3- to 4-mm axial images and conventional or fast spin echo coronal and axial images are obtained. If there is a question of violation of the skull base with intracranial extension, then gadolinium-enhanced coronal images with fat saturation are most useful.[44] In cases of brain invasion, T2-weighted images will show subtle areas of edema. After contrast administration, an irregular tumor-brain interface with distortion of normal anatomy indicates brain involvement (see Figs. 31–109 and 31–124). Dura involved by tumor or inflammation also enhances (see Figs. 31–82B and 31–108A).

When tumor has violated the posterior wall of the maxillary sinus, the malignancy reaches the pterygopalatine fossa (PPF). Any discussion of paranasal sinus malignancy must include the PPF and the potential for perineural spread along branches of the trigeminal nerve.[112–115] This space is found between the pterygoid process of the sphenoid and the posterior wall of the maxillary sinus (Figs. 31–68 and 31–69). The PPF is the crossroads of the head and neck and a junction for branches of V2. Branches arising here include the zygomatic, palatine, and superior alveolar nerves. Tumor may spread along V2 through the *foramen rotundum,* gaining access to the cavernous sinus, Meckel's cave, and the middle cranial

TABLE 31–15 Pterygopalatine Fossa

Connects with	By Way of
Orbit	Inferior orbital fissure
Middle fossa	Foramen rotundum
Foramen lacerum	Vidian canal
Nasal cavity	Sphenopalatine foramen
Infratemporal fossa	Pterygomaxillary fissure
Palate	Greater and lesser palatine foramen

fossa. The vidian nerve (formed by the greater superficial petrosal branch [parasympathetic] of cranial nerve VII [CN VII] and the deep petrosal nerve [sympathetic fibers traveling along the internal carotid artery]) passes through the *vidian canal.* The vidian canal provides communication between the PPF and the foramen lacerum. The palatine nerves run inferiorly through the *pterygopalatine canal* and *greater* and *lesser palatine foramen* to the mucosa of the hard palate. Once tumor has reached the PPF it may spread laterally through the wide *pterygomaxillary fissure* to the infratemporal fossa. Medially the *sphenopalatine foramen* communicates with the nasal cavity. Superiorly the PPF connects with the *inferior orbital fissure* and the apex of the orbit (Table 31–15).

The predominant constituent of the PPF is fat, which provides excellent radiographic contrast. Absence of fat in the PPF indicates abnormality (see Figs. 31–76, 31–107, and 31–115B).

BENIGN SINONASAL NEOPLASMS

Papilloma

Papillomas are of three histologic types: fungiform or septal (50%), inverted (47%), and cylindrical cell papilloma (3%). Papillomas arise from mucosa derived from ectoderm. This mucosa is called the *schneiderian membrane,* giving rise to the term *schneiderian papillomas.*[116] Sinonasal papillomas are derived from schneiderian epithelium and composed of columnar or ciliated respiratory epithelium with varied degrees of squamous differentiation. Fungiform papillomas occur almost exclusively on the nasal septum, where the inverted and cylindrical cell types occur along the lateral nasal wall and less frequently in the paranasal sinuses.

Septal (fungiform) papillomas have a characteristic exophytic, cauliflower-like appearance. Histologically, they are composed of papillary fronds of thick squamous, transitional, or respiratory epithelium with delicate fibrovascular cores (Fig. 31–70).

Inverted papillomas usually arise from the lateral nasal wall adjacent to the middle turbinate. They are unilateral and often secondarily extend into the ethmoid and maxillary sinuses. Inverted papillomas are typically large, polypoid masses that are composed of epithelial nests that grow in an endophytic or "inverted" pattern. The epithelium may be squamous or columnar or both admixed with goblet cells and mucin-containing microcysts (Fig. 31–71).

Inverted papillomas are three to five times more common in men and typically occur in patients between 40 and 60 years of age.[108] Inverted papillomas have a notorious propensity for recurrence.[106] From 5% to 27% harbor squamous cell carcinoma.[41, 106, 108] The nasal vault may be remodeled with expansion of the nasal fossa on CT.[44] Calcification may occasionally be found on CT. Bone destruction due to pressure necrosis has been reported in up to 30% of cases (Figs. 31–72 and 31–73). Inverted papillomas are isointense to slightly hyperintense to muscle on T1-weighted MRI and of intermediate to high signal intensity on T2-weighted MRI. There is heterogeneous enhancement after gadolinium administration.[108]

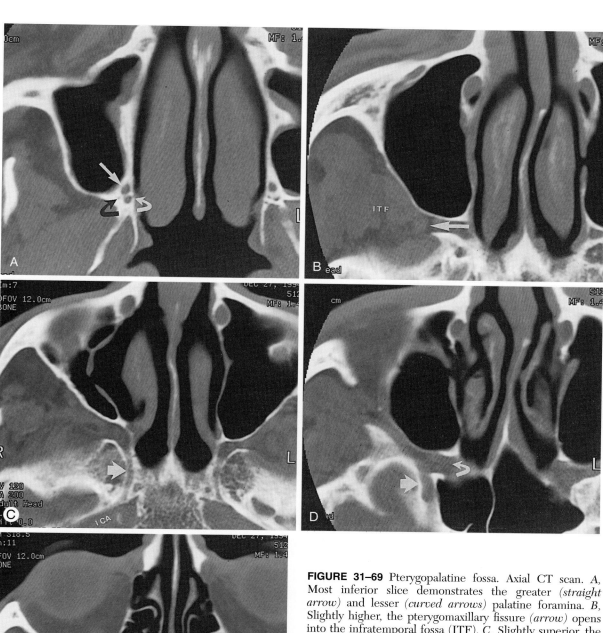

FIGURE 31–69 Pterygopalatine fossa. Axial CT scan. *A,* Most inferior slice demonstrates the greater *(straight arrow)* and lesser *(curved arrows)* palatine foramina. *B,* Slightly higher, the pterygomaxillary fissure *(arrow)* opens into the infratemporal fossa (ITF). *C,* Slightly superior, the vidian canal *(arrow)* connects the pterygopalatine fossa with the region of the foramen lacerum and canal for the petrous portion of the internal carotid artery (ICA). *D,* Slightly higher are the foramen rotundum *(straight arrow)* and the sphenopalatine foramen *(curved arrow)*, which opens into the nasal cavity. *E,* The most superior slice shows the inferior orbital fissure *(arrow)*, which communicates with the orbit. (*A–E,* From Nemzek WR. The trigeminal nerve. Top Magn Reson Imaging 1996;8:132–154.)

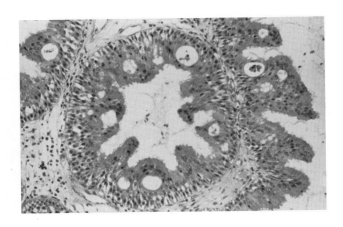

FIGURE 31–70 Septal papilloma (H&E 100×). Uniform squamous and mucous cells project in a papillary pattern.

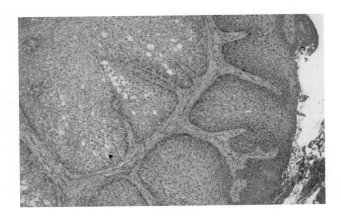

FIGURE 31–71 Inverted papilloma (H&E 100×). Uniform squamous cells with a smooth, "pushing" border proliferate along preformed ducts in the mucosa.

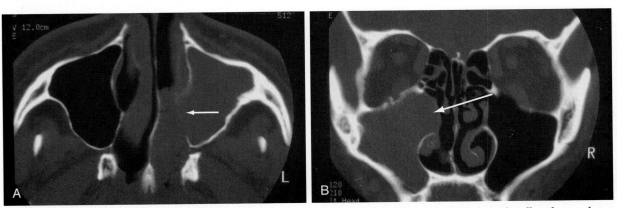

FIGURE 31–72 Inverted papilloma. Axial (A) and coronal (B) CT scans. Mass arises from the lateral nasal wall and extends into the left maxillary sinus. Note the widening of the maxillary sinus ostium (arrows).

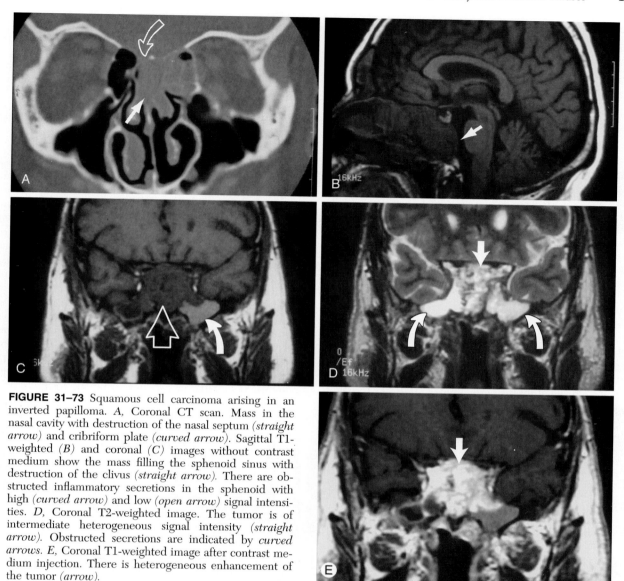

FIGURE 31–73 Squamous cell carcinoma arising in an inverted papilloma. *A*, Coronal CT scan. Mass in the nasal cavity with destruction of the nasal septum (*straight arrow*) and cribriform plate (*curved arrow*). Sagittal T1-weighted (*B*) and coronal (*C*) images without contrast medium show the mass filling the sphenoid sinus with destruction of the clivus (*straight arrow*). There are obstructed inflammatory secretions in the sphenoid with high (*curved arrow*) and low (*open arrow*) signal intensities. *D*, Coronal T2-weighted image. The tumor is of intermediate heterogeneous signal intensity (*straight arrow*). Obstructed secretions are indicated by *curved arrows*. *E*, Coronal T1-weighted image after contrast medium injection. There is heterogeneous enhancement of the tumor (*arrow*).

Cylindrical cell papillomas are characterized by dense pink, oncocytic epithelium and abundant mucin-filled cysts.

Pleomorphic Adenoma

These variegated tumors are of salivary duct origin. Variable-sized glands, ducts, and solid sheets of epithelial cells are surrounded by stellate and spindle-shaped myoepithelial cells. The myxoid stroma is characteristic, and islands of cartilage are commonly present (Fig. 31–74). Malignancy, most often an adenocarcinoma, occurs infrequently in tumors of long duration.

Benign Mesenchymal Neoplasms

Juvenile Angiofibroma

Juvenile angiofibroma is the most common benign tumor of the nasopharynx, occurring almost exclusively in ado-

lescent boys.[51, 117] Although benign, these are locally aggressive vascular tumors, representing less than 0.5% of all head and neck neoplasms.[117] The patient presents with recurrent epistaxis and nasal obstruction. The tumor typically arises in the nasopharynx and extends through the sphenopalatine foramen into the PPF.[41, 51] These tumors exit the PPF through the pterygomaxillary fissure into the infratemporal fossa. The PPF is expanded, and typically there is anterior displacement and remodeling of the posterior wall of the maxillary sinus ("antral bowing sign") (Fig. 31–75). Juvenile angiofibromas may extend into the nasopharynx, maxillary or ethmoid sinuses (30%), and intracranial cavity (5% to 10%) (Fig. 31–75).[51] Because the tumors are highly vascular (Fig. 31–75D), biopsy may be associated with significant hemorrhage.[51]

Histologically various-sized vascular channels are lined by plump, uniform, endothelial cells that are embedded in a stroma of spindle or stellate fibroblastic cells. The vascular spaces are irregular and "staghorn" in shape, and

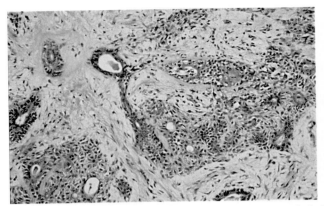

FIGURE 31–74 Pleomorphic adenoma (H&E 100×). Epithelial cells form ducts and small glands that are surrounded by spindle-shaped myoepithelial cells. A background myxoid stroma is characteristic.

their walls have no elastic tissue and little or no smooth muscle (Fig. 31–76D).

CT features include a solid enhancing mass centered in the sphenopalatine foramen with smooth bone remodeling ("antral bowing sign") (see Fig. 31–75). The angiofibroma has intermediate signal intensity on T1-weighted and variable signal intensity on T2-weighted MRI images. Flow void may be seen within the lesion, indicative of

large feeding vessels.[51] Preoperative embolization may reduce surgical blood loss and facilitate complete removal.[107] Major supply is from the internal maxillary and ascending pharyngeal arteries. Large tumors may parasitize blood supply from the internal carotid artery and the contralateral external carotid artery.[51]

Hemangioma

Hemangioma is a common soft tissue tumor and is the most common tumor of the head and neck in children.[118] Histologically hemangiomas are of two types: capillary and cavernous. Capillary hemangioma is more common, usually appearing in infancy or early childhood and involuting by the age of 5 or 6 years.[118] Cavernous hemangiomas are composed of large endothelial-lined vascular spaces. The endothelial lining cells are frequently prominent and tufted in appearance. The vessels are arranged in clusters or lobules with central slightly larger vessels surrounded by those of smaller caliber. Accompanying granulation tissue and inflammation is common.

Hemangioma of the nasal cavity presents with epistaxis, nasal stuffiness, and cosmetic deformity. Capillary hemangiomas commonly arise in the anterior portion of the nasal septum known as Little's area, or near Kiesselbach's triangle. The cause is unclear, but the lesions are associated with trauma and pregnancy.[119] Grossly, they are smooth, polypoid masses measuring up to 1.5 cm with surface ulceration.

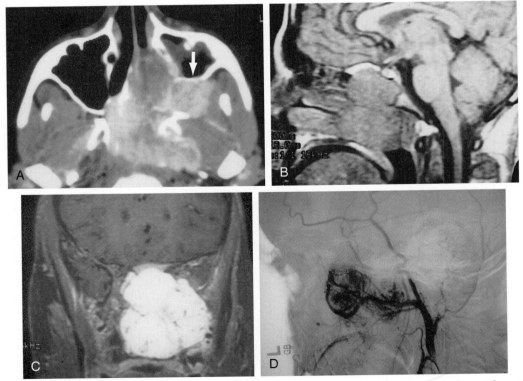

FIGURE 31–75 Juvenile nasopharyngeal angiofibroma in a 12-year-old boy. A, Axial CT with contrast medium. There is an enhancing mass in the nasopharynx, extending into the nasal cavity and pterygopalatine fossa and invading the infratemporal fossa. Note the widening of the pterygopalatine fossa, with anterior displacement and remodeling of the posterior wall of the maxillary sinus (arrow), the "antral bowing sign." Sagittal (B) and coronal (C) T1-weighted images after contrast medium with fat saturation. The angiofibroma is isointense with muscle and shows marked contrast enhancement. D, Lateral external carotid arteriogram. The hypervascular mass is supplied predominantly by branches of the internal maxillary artery.

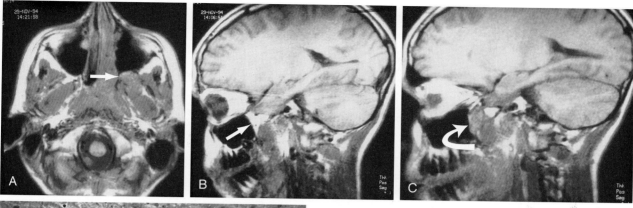

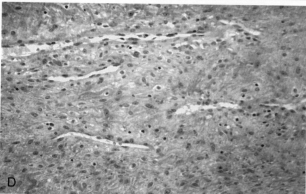

FIGURE 31–76 Juvenile angiofibroma in a 14-year-old boy. *A,* Axial T1-weighted image. Mass arises from the region of the left sphenopalatine foramen with extension into nasal cavity and nasopharynx. There is widening of the pterygopalatine fossa *(arrow)* and involvement of the infratemporal fossa. Sagittal T1-weighted image to the right *(B)* and the left *(C)* of midline. There is normal bright signal intensity of fat in the right pterygopalatine fossa *(straight arrow)* and intermediate signal of tumor filling and expanding the left pterygopalatine fossa *(curved arrow)*. *D,* Angiofibroma (H&E 100×). The irregular tumor vessels lack a smooth muscle wall and are embedded in a stroma of stellate fibroblasts and collage.

Cavernous hemangiomas are less common and are usually found in the lateral nasal wall.[120] These lesions are usually located within the inferior or middle turbinate and may extend into the maxillary sinus, with deviation of the contralateral nasal septum. There is usually expansion and remodeling of bone compatible with an indolent process. Extensive bone destruction has also been reported (Fig. 31–77).[120] On MRI, hemangiomas are usually isointense on T1-weighted and hyperintense on T2-weighted images with peripheral areas of hypointensity due to hemosiderin, calcification, or clotted blood.[41] Capillary hemangiomas enhance intensely, whereas cavernous hemangiomas demonstrate mild to moderate enhancement with gadolinium.[41] Arteriography may demonstrate pooling of contrast material with slow arteriovenous shunting.[118]

Neurogenic Tumors

Neurogenic tumors include *schwannoma* and *neurofibroma*. *Schwannomas* are encapsulated tumors arising from any nerve with a Schwann cell sheath. The olfactory nerve is thus excluded.[121, 122] From 25% to 45% of schwannomas occur in the head and neck, but sinonasal schwannomas are uncommon. They are usually found in the nasoethmoid region.[107] Schwannomas are characterized by sheets of spindle cells with serpentine nuclei arranged in wavy or whorled bundles. The classic pattern has areas of high cellularity (Antoni's A) and low cellularity (Antoni's B). The cellular areas often form palisaded groups called *Verocay's bodies* (Fig. 31–78).

Neurofibromas are unencapsulated tumors that contain the same constituents as normal nerves, that is, nerve fibers, perineural Schwann's cells, and connective tissue. They are characterized by haphazard sheets of spindle cells with serpentine nuclei and scant cytoplasm that are embedded in a loose matrix of short collagen fibers. There is some histologic overlap between these two benign entities.[123–125]

Patients with neurofibromatosis I (von Recklinghausen's disease) have an increased incidence of both neurofibroma and schwannoma. Neurofibromas almost always occur within the context of von Recklinghausen's disease.[123–125] Neurofibromas may undergo sarcomatous degeneration in 6% to 16% of cases (Fig. 31–79).[107]

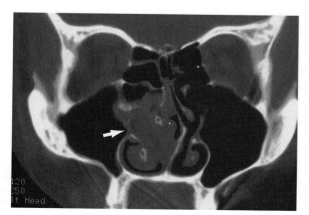

FIGURE 31–77 Hemangioma of the middle turbinate with pressure erosion of the medial wall of the maxillary sinus *(arrow)*.

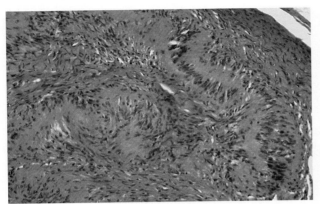

FIGURE 31–78 Schwannoma (H&E 100×). Sheets of spindle cells with serpentine nuclei form a pattern of densely cellular areas (Antoni's A) and acellular areas (Antoni's B). Focally, the nuclei are arranged in parallel or palisades that are called *Verocay's bodies.*

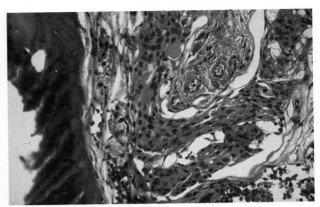

FIGURE 31–80 Meningioma (H&E 100×). These uniform, plump spindle cells are arranged in characteristic whorls.

Meningioma

Meningiomas may seldom extend into the sinonasal region from an intracranial origin. Rarely, a meningioma may arise primarily in an unexpected location, such as the sinuses, from an ectopic rest of arachnoid cells.[126]

Primary meningiomas are found most frequently in the frontal sinus (59%), followed by the ethmoid (23%), sphenoid (9%), and maxillary sinuses (9%).[127] Histologically there is a variable mixture of plump epithelium-like (meningoepithelial) cells, and spindle-shaped cells are arranged in characteristic whorls. Individual cells have uniform nuclei with rare intranuclear cytoplasmic inclusions, and pale pink cytoplasm with indistinct cell borders. Psammoma bodies, which are concentric calcified concretions, are a frequent component (Fig. 31–80).

Meningiomas are associated with both hyperostosis and bone destruction (Fig. 31–81). On CT, meningiomas are homogeneously hyperdense relative to muscle, with uniform contrast enhancement. Calcification is found in 20% to 25% of meningiomas. On MRI the lesion is usually isointense to gray matter with prominent contrast enhancement (Fig. 31–82). Over half of meningiomas exhibit a "dural tail" that represents either tumor infiltration or simply reactive change in the adjacent dura.[128]

Pituitary Adenoma

Extracranial extension of an intrasellar pituitary adenoma may involve the sphenoid sinus and nasopharynx. Ectopic pituitary tumors may arise from embryologic rests along the course of Rathke's pouch in the sphenoid bone and sinus (Fig. 31–83).[129, 130]

Fibro-Osseous Lesions (Table 31–16)

Osteoma

Osteomas are benign tumors consisting of thick lamellar bone. Osteomas are most commonly found in the frontal

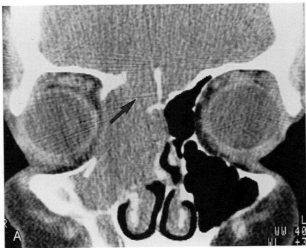
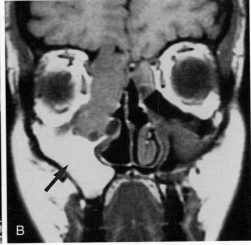

FIGURE 31–79 A 34-year-old woman with a neurofibrosarcoma arising in the ethmoid sinus. *A,* CT scan reveals erosion of the cribriform plate and the fovea ethmoidalis *(arrow)* and the medial wall of the right orbit and maxillary sinus. *B,* T1-weighted image reveals erosion of the cribriform plate and fovea ethmoidalis. The destruction of the thin bony septa of the medial orbit and maxillary sinus may be surmised, but it is more definitively evaluated on the CT scan. Note the high signal intensity of the secretions in the chronically obstructed maxillary sinus *(arrow).*

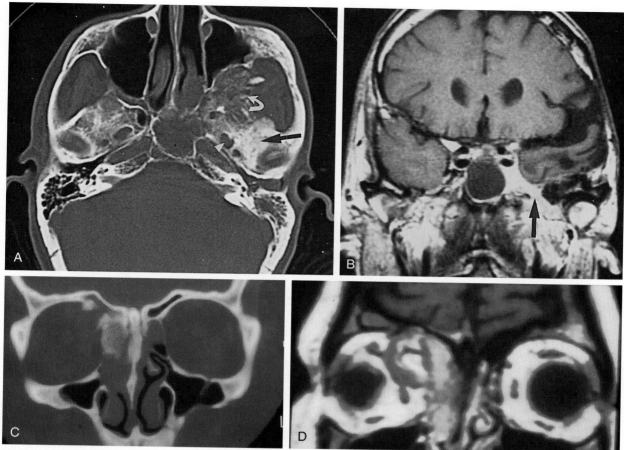

FIGURE 31–81 Meningioma. *A,* 47-year-old man with a skull base meningioma. There is sclerotic change in the sphenoid bone *(straight arrow)* associated with a meningioma that is difficult to appreciate on magnetic resonance imaging (MRI). The foramen ovale is normal in size *(arrowhead).* There is extension of calcified tumor into the infratemporal fossa with remodeling of the posterior wall of the maxillary sinus *(curved arrow). B,* MRI after gadolinium injection. There is contrast enhancement in the foramen ovale *(arrow)* on MRI compatible with perineural spread along the third division of the trigeminal nerve. Coronal CT *(C)* scan and MRI *(D)* with contrast media in a different patient show meningioma arising in the right ethmoid sinus with invasion of the orbit. There is sclerosis of the lamina papyracea on CT scan and heterogeneous enhancement of the tumor on MRI. *(C–D,* Courtesy of Suresh Mukherji, M.D., Chapel Hill, NC.)

and ethmoid sinuses. Less common sites include the mandible, maxilla, external auditory canal, mastoid, and petrous bone. Osteomas are usually incidental findings on plain films and CT scans in asymptomatic patients, with an incidence of 3% in the paranasal sinuses.[131] Rarely an osteoma becomes large enough to obstruct a sinus ostium, producing sinusitis or a mucocele. Osteomas are predominately cortical bone (Fig. 31–84) but may contain a fibrous component that enhances on MRI after gadolinium administration.[104]

Multiple osteomas and colonic polyposis constitute Gardner's syndrome. Associated lesions include desmoid tumors of the skin, epidermoid and sebaceous cysts, and impacted permanent and supernumerary teeth. The osteomas are detected before the development of polyposis. The colonic polyps invariably become malignant.[132]

Osteoblastoma

Osteoblastoma is related to osteoid osteoma of long bones but is by definition greater than 1 cm. Osteoblastoma may be transformed into osteosarcoma.[133] On histologic examination, one finds multiple irregular islands of miner-

alized bone and osteoid surrounded by osteoblasts and osteoclasts. The stroma is vascularized and highly cellular with spindle cells and individual osteoblasts (Fig. 31–85). Aggressive variants are characterized by plump, atypical osteoblasts often arranged in sheets.

Radiologically, there is a central area of less dense bone surrounded by a rim of sclerotic bone. There is moderate to marked contrast enhancement on MRI.[134] Osteoblastoma is associated with widespread inflammatory response that may lead to an incorrect diagnosis of lymphoma or Ewing's sarcoma (Fig. 31–86).[135]

TABLE 31–16 Fibro-Osseous Lesions

Osteoma	Osteogenic sarcoma
Osteoblastoma	Chondrosarcoma
Fibrous dysplasia	Chondroblastoma
Ossifying fibroma	Chondromyxoid fibroma
Giant cell tumor	Fibromyxoma
Aneurysmal bone cyst	Paget's disease

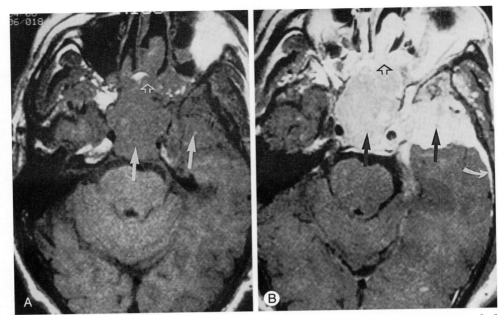

FIGURE 31–82 A 46-year-old man with an extensive skull base meningioma. T1-weighted images before (*A*) and after (*B*) gadolinium enhancement. After the infusion of gadolinium, both tumor (*straight arrows*) and dural enhancement (*curved arrow* in *B*) are evident. There is involvement of the anterior, middle, and posterior fossae, sphenoid sinus, and nasopharynx (*open arrows*).

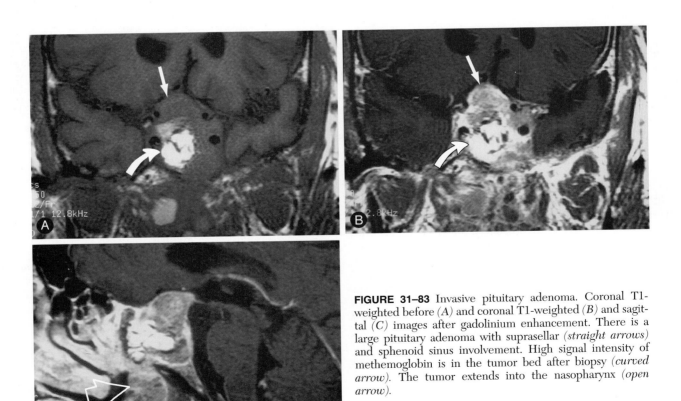

FIGURE 31–83 Invasive pituitary adenoma. Coronal T1-weighted before (*A*) and coronal T1-weighted (*B*) and sagittal (*C*) images after gadolinium enhancement. There is a large pituitary adenoma with suprasellar (*straight arrows*) and sphenoid sinus involvement. High signal intensity of methemoglobin is in the tumor bed after biopsy (*curved arrow*). The tumor extends into the nasopharynx (*open arrow*).

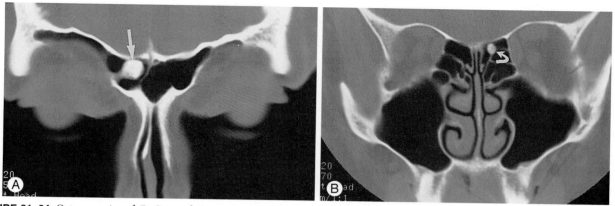

FIGURE 31–84 Osteoma. *A* and *B,* Coronal CT scans show osteomas in the frontal *(straight arrow* in *A)* and ethmoid *(curved arrow* in *B)* sinuses.

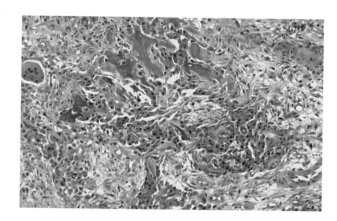

FIGURE 31–85 Osteoblastoma (H&E 100×). Sheets of osteoblasts surround several nests of osteoid as well as mineralized matrix. Numerous osteoclasts are also present.

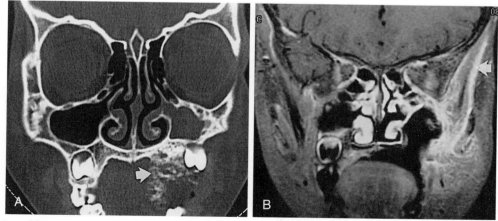

FIGURE 31–86 Osteoblastoma. *A,* Coronal CT scan. An expansile mass with a calcified matrix arises from the left maxillary alveolar ridge *(arrow).* Note the marked inflammatory disease in the adjacent left maxillary sinus. *B,* Coronal T1-weighted image after enhancement with fat saturation after excisional biopsy. There is swelling and enhancement of the temporalis muscle *(arrow).* Osteoblastoma is associated with a marked inflammatory response.

Fibrous Dysplasia

Fibrous dysplasia is the most common fibro-osseous lesion, followed by ossifying fibroma.[51]

Fibrous dysplasia may be monostotic (one bone) or polyostotic (several bones) and frequently involves the craniofacial complex. Monostotic disease accounts for 80% of cases, with 20% to 25% involvement of the head and neck. The polyostotic form accounts for 20% of all cases, with skull and facial bone involvement in 40% to 60%.[45]

Albright's syndrome consists of polyostotic fibrous dysplasia, sexual precocity in females, and irregularly marginated (coast of Maine) skin pigmentation.[45]

Fibrous dysplasia is a self-limited process that starts in childhood, but its slow growth may not cause symptoms until adulthood. In the craniofacial area, fibrous dysplasia occurs most commonly in the calvarium and maxilla.[136] Malignant transformation of fibrous dysplasia to sarcoma has been reported (0.5%), particularly after radiation.[45, 137] The sarcomas include osteosarcoma (65%), fibrosarcoma (18%), chondrosarcoma (10%), and giant cell sarcoma (7%).[138]

Histologically, fibrous dysplasia consists of multiple irregular, immature fibrillar or woven bony trabeculae surrounded by loose, uniform fibroblastic spindle cells. The trabeculae often have C or Y shapes and have been described as "Chinese characters." Osteoclasts are rarely observed and osteoblasts are seen infrequently (Fig. 31–87).

This lesion may replace and expand the sinus. A "ground glass" appearance is characteristic (Figs. 31–88 through 31–90). MRI reveals a lesion with low to intermediate signal on all pulse sequences with gadolinium enhancement. The T2-weighted signal intensity is less than that of the T1-weighted signal (Fig. 31–90). The MRI appearance may cause the lesion to be mistaken for an aggressive tumor.

Ossifying Fibroma

Ossifying fibroma is the second most common fibro-osseous lesion after fibrous dysplasia. It is a benign indolent fibro-osseous tumor of bone treatable by simple curet-

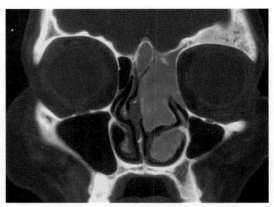

FIGURE 31–88 Fibrous dysplasia in a 17-year-old girl. Coronal CT scan. Expansion and sclerosis of the left middle and inferior turbinates, the left ethmoids, and the crista galli. (Courtesy of Deiter Enzmann, M.D., Palo Alto, CA.)

tage. Ossifying fibroma is more aggressive than fibrous dysplasia and has a tendency to recur after surgery. Ossifying fibroma occurs between the second and fourth decade and is more common in women, with male to female ratios between 1.8:1 and 5:1. Ossifying fibroma is almost always a monostotic lesion found in the cranial bones. Seventy-five percent of lesions occur in the mandible. Fibrous dysplasia is an arrest of bone maturation in the woven stage of development. Ossifying fibroma is a circumscribed lesion composed of a highly cellular fibrous stroma with various-sized islands of bone rimmed by osteoblasts, with the potential for destructive growth. It may originate from periodontal tissue or primitive mesenchymal cells. When it involves the midface and paranasal sinuses, it is a potentially aggressive, destructive lesion. Maxillary lesions in children can be very extensive, and wide local excision can be necessary for control.[139] On CT the lesion is expansile with areas of nonossified fibrous tissue (Fig. 31–91).

Giant Cell Tumor (Osteoclastoma)

Giant cell tumor is a benign tumor that constitutes 4% to 5% of bone neoplasms. Seventy-five percent are located

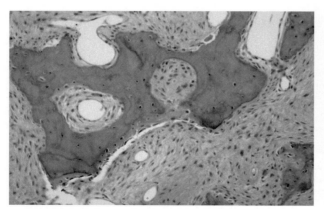

FIGURE 31–87 Fibrous dysplasia (H&E 100×). Irregular islands of bone are embedded in a densely cellular stroma of stellate fibroblasts. Only scant osteoblasts or osteoclasts are present.

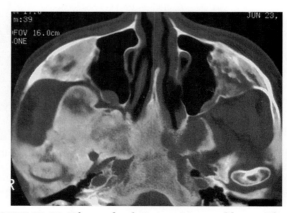

FIGURE 31–89 Fibrous dysplasia in a 34-year-old man. There is sclerosis and expansion on the lateral wall of the maxillary sinus and sphenoid bone.

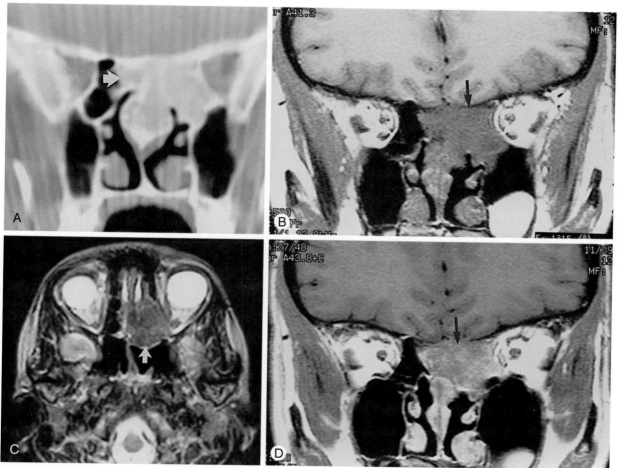

FIGURE 31–90 Fibrous dysplasia. *A*, Coronal CT scan. There is sclerosis and expansion of the left ethmoids and nasal septum, with extension into the right ethmoid air cells *(arrow)*. *B*, Coronal T1-weighted image without enhancement. The lesion *(arrow)* is isointense to muscle. *C*, Axial T2-weighted image. The mass is hypointense *(arrow)*. *D*, T1-weighted image after gadolinium injection. Note the slight homogeneous enhancement *(arrow)*.

in the epiphyses of long bones. Rarely they occur in the head and neck.

Giant cell tumors tend to destroy and remodel bone. On MRI there is low signal intensity of all pulse sequences. Contrast enhancement is noted.[45]

Giant Cell Reparative Granuloma

Giant cell reparative granuloma arises in the maxillary or mandibular alveolus. The lesion is more common in women older than 20 years and is associated with trauma such as tooth extraction or poorly fitting dentures.

This reactive lesion is composed of multinucleated giant cells surrounded by a fibrous stroma. Variable vascularity and areas of hemosiderin deposition are commonly seen (Fig. 31–92A).

Radiographically the lesion is multiloculated and may exhibit bone destruction (Fig. 31–92B and C).

Brown Tumor of Hyperparathyroidism

The brown tumor of hyperparathyroidism is an expansile lesion that remodels bone and may be indistinguishable

from giant cell reparative granuloma and giant cell tumor by biopsy. Clinical correlation is imperative. Parathyroid hormone and serum calcium levels are elevated with a brown tumor of hyperparathyroidism.[45]

Odontogenic Lesions

The most common cystic expansile mass arising in a paranasal sinus is a mucocele. Cystic lesions arising outside the maxillary antrum, from the maxillary alveolar process, demonstrate a bony partition between the lesion and the maxillary sinus. This bony plate represents the expanded, remodeled floor of the maxillary sinus. These extra-antral lesions include fissural cysts, odontogenic cystic lesions, and ameloblastoma (Table 31–17).[140]

Radicular Cyst (Periodontal or Periapical Cyst)

Radicular cysts are the most common jaw cysts, representing a granuloma at the root of an infected erupted tooth. The cyst may grow and break into the maxillary sinus. Histologically often disrupted, the cyst has a variable lining of hyperplastic nonkeratinizing squamous epi-

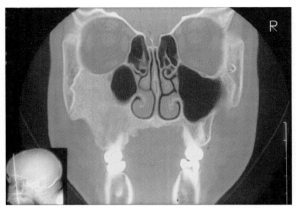

FIGURE 31–91 Ossifying fibroma. Coronal CT scan. An expansile bony mass that is partially ossified arises from the lateral wall of the right maxillary sinus. (Courtesy of Suresh Mukherji, M.D., Chapel Hill, NC.)

thelium surrounded by granulation tissue (Fig. 31–93). The fibrous stroma is frequently infiltrated by neutrophils, macrophages, and multinucleate giant cells. Hemosiderin and cholesterol clefts are frequent.

Follicular Cysts (Primordial and Dentigerous Cysts)

Dentigerous cysts are expansile unilocular lesions that incorporate the crown of an unerupted tooth (Fig. 31–94). Dentigerous cysts represent 35% of all odontogenic

TABLE 31–17 Maxilla Cystic Expansile Masses

Mucocele
Extra-antral
   Fissural cysts
   Odontogenic lesions
      Radicular (periapical) cyst
      Primordial cyst
      Dentigerous cyst
      Odontogenic keratocyst
      Ameloblastoma
   Giant cell reparative granuloma
   Giant cell tumor
   "Brown tumor" (hyperparathyroidism)
   Aneurysmal bone cyst
   Metastasis (renal, thyroid)

cysts.[45] The cyst is lined by a thin layer of nonkeratinizing squamous epithelium surrounded by a dense fibrous stroma (Fig. 31–95). A primordial cyst is a well-circumscribed unilocular lesion that results from degeneration of the enamel organ and contains no recognizable tooth structures.

Keratocyst

Odontogenic keratocysts are aggressive lesions that have a propensity for recurrence. There is an association with Marfan's syndrome and the basal cell nevus syndrome.[45] The basal cell nevus syndrome (Gorlin's syndrome) con-

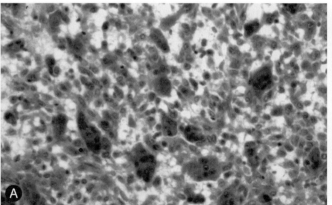

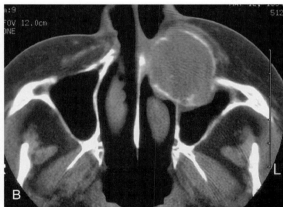

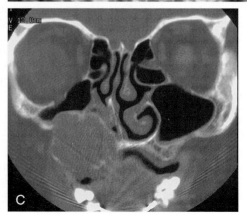

FIGURE 31–92 Giant cell reparative granuloma. *A,* Sheets of multinucleated giant cells are surrounded by stellate fibroblasts (H&E 200×). Axial *(B)* and coronal *(C)* CT scans. Expansile mass with remodeled and eroded bony margins extends into the hard palate and the floor of the maxillary sinus.

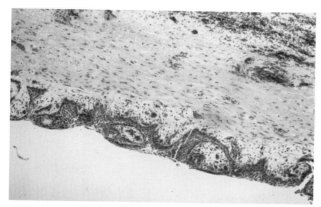

FIGURE 31–93 Radicular cyst (H&E 100×). A thin but irregular layer of nonkeratinizing squamous epithelium is surrounded by granulation tissue.

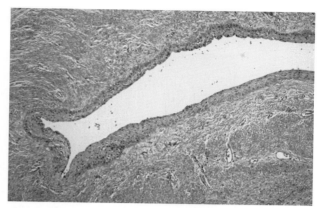

FIGURE 31–95 Dentigerous cyst (H&E 100×). A thin, uniform layer of nonkeratinizing squamous cells is surrounded by fibrous tissue.

sists of multiple keratocysts, cutaneous basal cell carcinomas, dural calcifications, and vertebral and rib anomalies.

Two histologic types are identified. The parakeratotic variant, which is most common, is lined by a layer of stratified squamous epithelium with an uneven corrugated surface of nucleated keratin cells and luminal keratin debris. The orthokeratotic type has a layer of stratified squamous epithelium with a prominent granular cell layer, a smooth surface, and multilayers of anucleate keratin (Fig. 31–96).

The lesions occur two to four times more frequently in the mandible. They may be destructive or have a thin scalloped sclerotic rim (Fig. 31–97).

Ameloblastoma

Ameloblastoma is a benign odontogenic tumor and the most common odontogenic tumor. It occurs most commonly in the third and fourth decades.

Histologic examination reveals basaloid epithelial cells arranged in sheets; cysts and cords surround an inner

core of stellate cells in a myxoid stroma (the stellate reticulum). The follicular pattern (Fig. 31–98) is most common.

Radiographically it is a multiloculated lytic lesion containing both cystic and solid components (Fig. 31–99). There is variable signal intensity on T2-weighted images.[45]

Fissural Cyst

Fissural cysts arise from epithelium entrapped in the fusion lines of the maxilla and palate during facial development (Fig. 31–100).[45] These masses are painless unless secondarily infected and are usually found in patients younger than 30 years. The *globulomaxillary cyst* occurs between the maxillary lateral incisor and canine teeth and may extend into the maxillary sinus (Fig. 31–101). The *central cysts* (incisive canal cysts, cysts of the papillatine papilla, and median palatal cysts) are confined to the hard palate and do not involve the maxillary sinus (Fig. 31–102). The nasoalveolar cyst is a soft tissue lesion.[45]

Histologically these simple cysts may be lined by stratified squamous, cuboidal, or columnar epithelium.

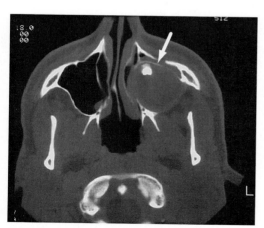

FIGURE 31–94 Dentigerous cyst. Axial CT scan. Expansile mass in the left maxillary sinus incorporates the crown of a tooth. There is erosion of the walls of the maxillary sinus. Note the thin bony partition (*arrow*), which is the remodeled alveolus, separating the lesion from the maxillary sinus. (Courtesy of Hugh Curtin, M.D., Boston, MA.)

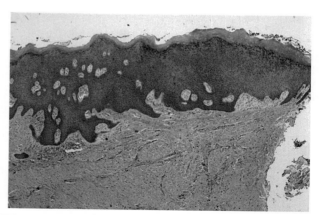

FIGURE 31–96 Odontogenic keratocyst (H&E 100×). A thick, irregular layer of squamous epithelium has a prominent granular cell layer and abundant surface keratin. This is an orthokeratotic type of odontogenic keratocyst.

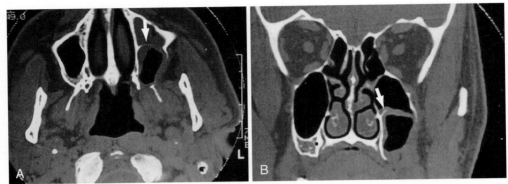

FIGURE 31–97 Axial *(A)* and coronal *(B)* CT scans. Odontogenic keratocyst arises in the alveolus of the maxilla. This expansile destructive lesion contains air. The patient presented with spontaneous foul-tasting and foul-smelling drainage. Note the thin bone of expanded alveolus *(arrow)* separating the cyst from the maxillary sinus.

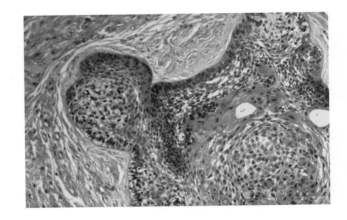

FIGURE 31–98 Ameloblastoma (H&E 100×). Sheets of tumor are composed of an outer edge of basaloid epithelial cells and an inner stroma of stellate mesenchymal cells (the stellate reticulum).

FIGURE 31–99 Axial CT scans through the mandible *(A)* and the maxilla *(B)*. Ameloblastoma arises as a multiloculated destructive mass in the mandible with extension to the maxilla and infratemporal fossa.

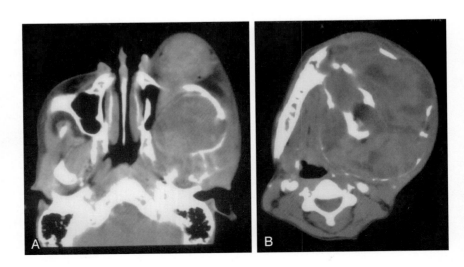

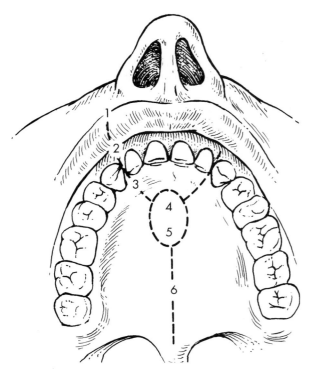

FIGURE 31–100 Location of fissural cysts: 1, nasolabial cyst; 2, nasoalveolar cyst; 3, globulomaxillary cyst; 4, nasopalatine cyst; 5, cyst of palatine papilla; and 6, median palatal cyst. (From Som PM, Brandwein M. Sinonasal cavities: Inflammatory diseases, tumors, fractures, and postoperative findings. In Som PM, Curtin HD [eds]. Head and Neck Imaging, pp. 126–315. St. Louis, Mosby–Year Book, 1996.)

Radiographically, the globulomaxillary cyst is a well-defined lucent lesion in the maxillary alveolus that separates the roots of adjoining teeth and assumes a pear shape as it increases in size (see Fig. 31–101).[132, 141]

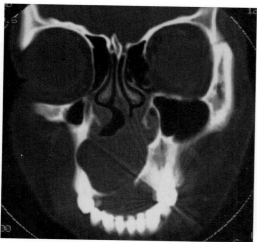

FIGURE 31–101 Coronal CT scan. Globulomaxillary cyst. Expansile cystic mass arises off the midline and extends into the nasal cavity.

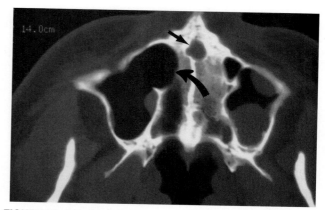

FIGURE 31–102 Axial CT scan. Nasopalatine cyst. Midline mass in the anterior hard palate expands the incisive canal *(straight arrow)*. Note the incidental pneumocele with expansion of the medial wall of the maxillary sinus *(curved arrow)*.

Aneurysmal Bone Cyst

Aneurysmal bone cyst is a nonneoplastic lesion occurring more commonly in women older than 20 years. Between 3% and 12% of these lesions occur in the head and neck. They are found in the maxilla, orbit, ethmoid, and frontal bone.[45]

Histologically, blood-filled cystic spaces are lined by fibroblasts admixed with multinucleated giant cells. Foci of immature bone or osteoid are present as well as foamy macrophages and hemosiderin (Fig. 31–103).

On MRI, the aneurysmal bone cyst is a multicystic lesion with fluid-fluid levels.

Langerhans Cell Histiocytosis (Eosinophilic Granuloma)

Langerhans cell histiocytosis encompasses a spectrum of disease from an isolated bone or soft tissue lesion to a fulminant fatal disseminated systemic illness.[142]

Letterer-Siwe disease is an acute disseminated process occurring in infants younger than 1 year. It is character-

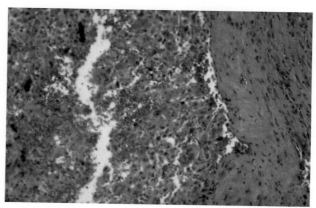

FIGURE 31–103 Aneurysmal bone cyst (H&E 100×). Collapsed, blood-filled cysts are lined by reactive fibrous tissue. Macrophages with hemosiderin are present as well as numerous osteoclasts.

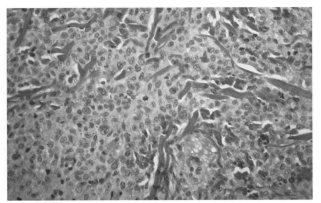

FIGURE 31–104 Eosinophilic granuloma (H&E 100×). Sheets of large, individual histiocytes have cleaved nuclei and abundant cytoplasm. Admixed eosinophils are a variable feature.

ized by hepatosplenomegaly, lymphadenopathy, anemia, and thrombocytopenia.[143] *Hand-Schüller-Christian* disease occurs in children 1 to 10 years of age and is more common in boys (male to female ratio of 2 to 1). The classic triad includes skull defects, exophthalmos, and diabetes insipidus. *Eosinophilic granuloma* is the mildest form of the disease and is more common in men between 20 and 30 years of age.[132]

Langerhans cell histiocytosis of bone most commonly involves the skull, ribs, femur, and pelvis. Lesions of the mastoid and external auditory canal are common. Langerhans cell histiocytosis of the sinonasal region is rare.[45, 143]

Histologically, the tumor cell is a large monocyte-like cell (Langerhans cell) with a characteristic reniform nucleus. These are present in sheets admixed with eosinophils, plasma cells, macrophages, and multinucleated giant cells. Areas of necrosis and fibrosis may be present. The tumor cells are reactive with S-100 protein; with electron microscopy, a characteristic cytoplasmic, tennis

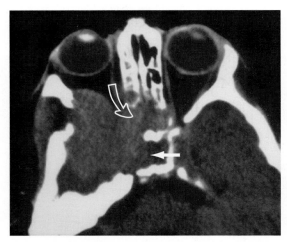

FIGURE 31–105 Axial CT scan. A. 1-year-old boy with eosinophilic granuloma. Soft tissue mass destroys the lateral wall of the orbit and the greater wing of the sphenoid with extension into the middle fossa, and the sphenoid (*straight arrow*) and ethmoid (*curved arrow*) sinuses.

TABLE 31–18 Staging of Maxillary Sinus Tumor

Tis	Carcinoma in situ
T1	Tumor limited to antral mucosa with no erosion or destruction of bone
T2	Tumor with erosion or destruction of infrastructure including hard palate or middle nasal meatus or both
T3	Tumor invading any of following: skin of cheek; posterior wall of maxillary sinus; floor or medial wall of orbit; anterior ethmoid sinus
T4	Tumor invading orbital contents or any of following or both: cribriform plate; posterior ethmoid or sphenoid sinuses; nasopharynx, soft palate; pterygomaxillary or temporal fossa; base of skull

Used with the permission of the American Joint Committee on Cancer, Chicago, Illinois. The original source for this material is the AJCC Manual for Staging of Cancer, 4th edition (1992) published by J. B. Lippincott Company, Philadelphia.

racket–shaped inclusion body (Birbeck's granules) can be demonstrated (Fig. 31–104).

Radiographically the lesions are moderately well defined, with "punched-out" borders and beveled edges. Contrast enhancement is noted with CT and MRI (Fig. 31–105).[144]

MALIGNANT SINONASAL NEOPLASMS

Staging

The American Joint Committee on Cancer staging system applies only to the maxillary sinus, which is the most common site (80%) for malignancy (Table 31–18).[107, 145] Anatomic boundaries are based on *Ohngren's line*; this is a theoretical plane extending from the medial canthus of the eye to the angle of the mandible. This line divides the maxillary sinus into an anteroinferior segment (infrastructure) and a posterosuperior portion (suprastructure). Anteromedial malignancies have a better prognosis than posterolateral cancers.[107]

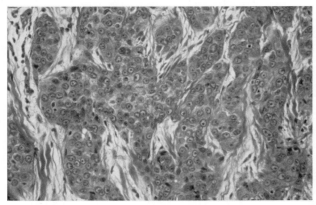

FIGURE 31–106 Squamous cell carcinoma (H&E 100×). Moderately differentiated tumor with moderate pink cytoplasm, intercellular bridges, and scant keratin.

Malignant Epithelial Lesions

Squamous Cell Carcinoma

Squamous cell carcinoma is the most common malignancy of the nasal cavity and paranasal sinuses. Squamous cell carcinoma is twice as common in men and usually occurs in the sixth and seventh decades of life.[106] In descending order of frequency the most common sites are the maxillary, ethmoid, frontal, and sphenoid sinuses, and the nasal cavity.

Squamous cell carcinoma is characterized by a disorganized, invasive growth of large epithelial cells with intercellular bridges and cytoplasmic keratin. Adjacent or over-

lying atypia of the surface mucosa is typically present. Squamous cell carcinoma is graded into well, moderate, and poorly differentiated types by the degree of resemblance to normal squamous tissue. Specific criteria include definition of intercellular bridges, amount of keratinization, nuclear pleomorphism, mitotic rate, and degree of cell cohesion (sheets versus small nests) (Fig. 31–106).

Squamous cell carcinoma is characterized by aggressive bone destruction. T2-weighted MRI images can differentiate the very bright signal of inflammatory changes from the intermediate signal intensity of squamous cell carcinoma.[41] There is moderate contrast enhancement with gadolinium (Figs. 31–107 through 31–109).[45] Lymph

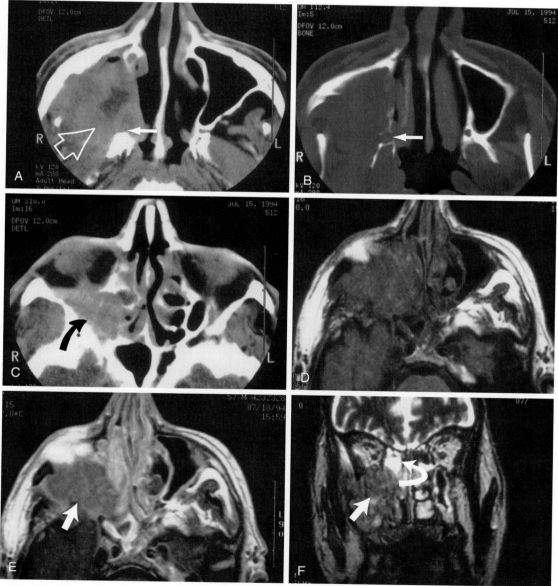

FIGURE 31–107 Squamous cell carcinoma. *A–C,* Axial CT scans with contrast enhancement. The mass destroys the medial and lateral walls of the right maxillary sinus. Marginal bone remodeling is lacking. The tumor extends into the pterygopalatine *(straight arrow)* and infratemporal fossa *(open arrow),* then cephalad through the inferior orbital fissure *(curved arrow)* into the orbital apex. Axial T1-weighted images before *(D)* and after *(E)* gadolinium enhancement. The tumor is isointense with muscle and shows only moderate contrast enhancement *(arrow). F,* Coronal T2-weighted image. The tumor is of moderate signal intensity *(straight arrow)* compared with hyperintense sinus secretions *(curved arrow).*

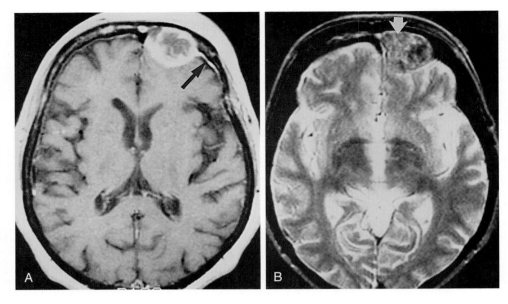

FIGURE 31–108 Squamous cell carcinoma, left frontal sinus in a 65-year-old woman. *A,* Axial T1-weighted image with contrast enhancement. There is enhancement of a necrotic mass destroying the left frontal sinus. Note the dural enhancement *(arrow).* At surgery, there was neoplastic invasion of the dura. *B,* Axial T2-weighted image shows a tumor *(arrow)* of moderate signal intensity. The adjacent frontal lobe is displaced but of normal signal intensity.

node metastases have been reported in about 10% of patients at presentation.

Mucoepidermoid Carcinoma

Mucoepidermoid carcinoma is common in the salivary glands, especially the parotid gland. Rarely mucoepidermoid carcinoma arises in the paranasal sinuses and shares similar imaging characteristics with squamous cell carcinoma.

These tumors of salivary origin are composed of a mixture of mucous and squamous cells. A third component, called *intermediate cells,* consists of epithelial cells that appear to be a transitional form between mucous and squamous. Three grades of mucoepidermoid carci-

noma are recognized, that is, low, intermediate, and high. Low-grade tumors are cystic with predominant mucous cells. Intermediate-grade lesions have a higher proportion of intermediate and squamous cells (Fig. 31–110). High-grade tumors are infiltrating nests and cords of predominately squamous and intermediate cells with mitoses, pleomorphism, and a desmoplastic stroma.

Sinonasal Undifferentiated Carcinoma

Sinonasal undifferentiated carcinoma is a relatively recently identified aggressive, undifferentiated carcinoma of the nasal cavity and paranasal sinuses. The tumor presents as a large, fungating mass in the nasal cavity with extension to multiple paranasal sinuses.[146, 147] Microscopically,

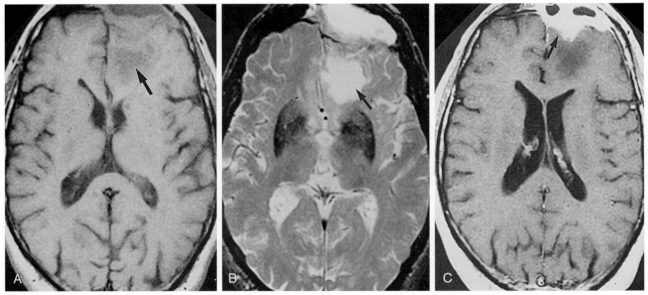

FIGURE 31–109 Squamous cell carcinoma, left frontal sinus, with brain invasion, in a 69-year-old man. Axial T1-weighted image before contrast enhancement *(A)* and T2-weighted axial image *(B).* A mass is destroying the left frontal sinus. There is edema of the adjacent frontal lobe *(arrow).* C, Axial T1-weighted image after contrast enhancement. Note the irregular enhancement at the tumor-brain interface *(arrow),* indicating invasion of the frontal lobe.

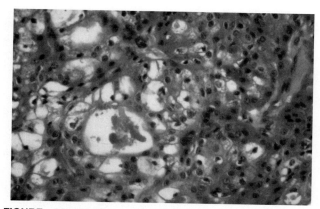

FIGURE 31-110 Mucoepidermoid carcinoma, intermediate grade (H&E 100×). Sheets of squamous and mucous cells are admixed with intermediate cells with transitional cell features.

medium-sized, pleomorphic cells are arranged in nests and sheets with large, irregular nuclei and a small to moderate amount of pink cytoplasm. Mitotic figures are abundant. Vascular channels distended with tumor that has central necrosis is commonly seen (Fig. 31–111).

Aggressive permeative bone destruction is similar to that of squamous cell carcinoma. On MRI, sinonasal undifferentiated carcinoma is of intermediate signal on T2-weighted images with moderate enhancement (Fig. 31–112).

Minor Salivary Gland

The minor salivary glands are ubiquitous in the upper aerodigestive system. Tumors of the minor salivary glands usually arise in the palate and then extend to the paranasal sinuses or nasal cavity.[106]

Adenoid Cystic Carcinoma

Adenoid cystic carcinoma (ACC) is a treacherous unpredictable neoplasm. This tumor is characterized by a slow, relentless malignant course with distant metastases occurring many (10 to 15) years after the primary diagnosis even with local control.[148] The task of the radiologist, to define the presence, location, and extent of the neoplasm,

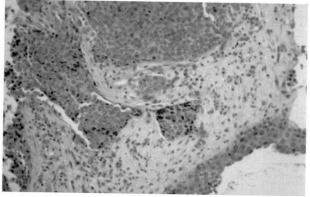

FIGURE 31-111 Sinonasal undifferentiated carcinoma (H&E 100×). Nests of large, undifferentiated tumor have significant necrosis and a brisk mitotic rate.

is even more difficult because ACC has a strong propensity for perineural spread, allowing this insidious neoplasm to "resurface" at distant locations.[149–151] ACC characteristically spreads along perineural spaces including those of the maxillary division of the trigeminal nerve and may traverse the foramen ovale to the gasserian ganglion.[152]

ACC accounts for less than 1% of all head and neck malignancies and about 10% of salivary gland neoplasms.[153] About 40% of cases arise in the major salivary glands (parotid, submandibular, and sublingual glands). ACC is the most common malignant tumor of minor salivary (seromucinous) glands. The majority of cases (60%) occur in the minor seromucinous glands found in the oral cavity, nasal cavity, paranasal sinuses, nasopharynx, and trachea.[148] In the paranasal sinuses, the maxillary sinus is most commonly involved.[41]

Three patterns are described: tubular, solid, and cribriform; tumors are classified by which pattern dominates (e.g., greater than 50% of the tumor). The cribriform type is the most common and is considered the "classic" pattern. Nests of cells demonstrate multiple circular spaces filled with bluish mucinous material or pink, hyalinized material (Figs. 31–113 and 31–114).

The tubular pattern consists of cells arranged in individual ducts or tubules, whereas the solid pattern, as expected from the name, has nests or sheets of basaloid cells with little cystic formation.

Prognosis correlates with the predominant histologic pattern (tubular, cribriform, or solid) and the degree of cellularity, which increases from tubular to the solid form. The greater the cellularity the worse the prognosis. Perzin and colleagues found a correlation between these histologic patterns and survival rates as follows: tubular 8 years, cribriform 9 years and solid 5 years.[154, 155] Recurrence rates were tubular 59%, cribriform 89%, and solid 100%.

ACC is isointense with muscle on T1-weighted MRI images. On T2-weighted images the signal intensity of the tumor depends on the water content and the degree of cellularity. Tumors with high signal intensity on T2-weighted images had low cellularity and were associated with the best prognosis. Tumors with low signal intensity on T2-weighted images had dense cellularity and a poorer prognosis (Figs. 31–115 through 31–117).[111]

Lymphatic spread in low regional nodal metastases occurs in approximately 10% of patients. Hematogenous metastasis is high (40%), with lung and bone representing the most common sites of distant spread.[155] Bone invasion by contiguous spread may be destructive or sclerotic, or ACC may invade marrow spaces leaving the involved bone with a relatively normal appearance on CT or plain films.[156] CT is necessary for imaging fine bone detail, but MRI is better for detection of marrow invasion.

Sinonasal Adenocarcinoma

Sinonasal adenocarcinomas are also called *mucinous, colonic type,* or *enteric* adenocarcinomas. The tumor occurs predominantly in 50- to 60-year-old men[41] and is associated with wood dust exposure. Sinonasal adenocarcinomas typically arise from the middle turbinate or ethmoid sinus and less commonly from the antrum. Only rare reports

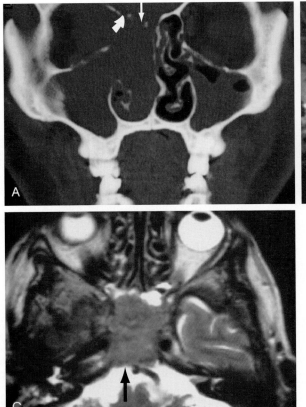

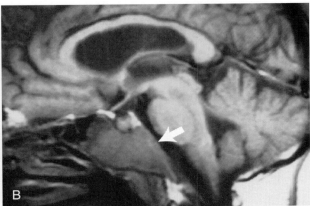

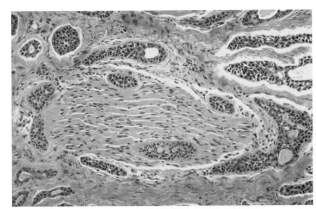

FIGURE 31–112 Sinonasal undifferentiated carcinoma. *A,* Coronal CT scan. Tumor arises in the right ethmoid sinus with destruction of the medial wall of the orbit and the maxillary sinus, with extension into the nasal cavity and erosion of the nasal septum, cribriform plate *(straight arrow),* and fovea ethmoidalis *(curved arrow).* Sagittal T1-weighted *(B)* and axial T2-weighted *(C)* images of a different patient. Tumor is of intermediate signal, fills the sphenoid sinus, and destroys the clivus *(arrow).*

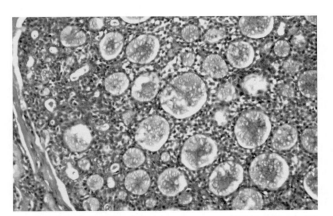

FIGURE 31–113 Adenoid cystic carcinoma (H&E 100×). The classic Swiss-cheese appearance of the cribriform pattern.

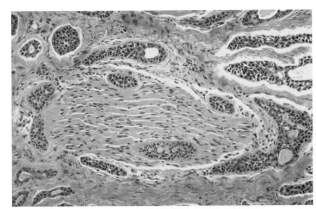

FIGURE 31–114 Adenoid cystic carcinoma (H&E 100×). Invasion of the perineural sheath of the trigeminal nerve.

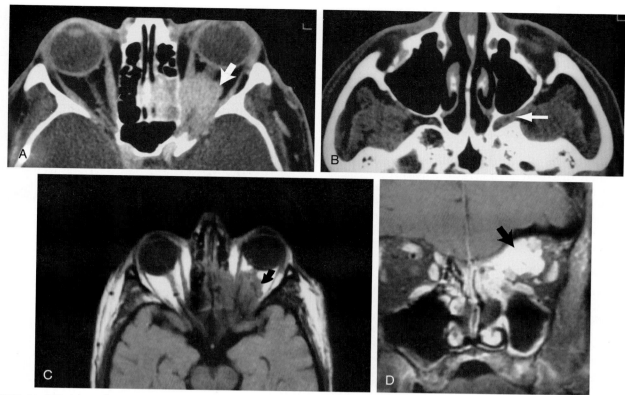

FIGURE 31–115 Adenoid cystic carcinoma arises in the left ethmoid sinus in a 49-year-old man. *A,* Axial CT scan with contrast enhancement. Tumor in the left ethmoid sinus involves the orbit *(arrow),* with little bony disruption of the lamina papyracea. *B,* Axial CT scan inferior to *A.* There is neoplasm in the pterygopalatine fossa *(arrow).* Note the normal fat in the normal contralateral side. Axial T1-weighted *(C)* and coronal T1-weighted *(D)* images with gadolinium enhancement and fat saturation. The tumor is isointense to muscle and enhances with contrast media *(arrows).*

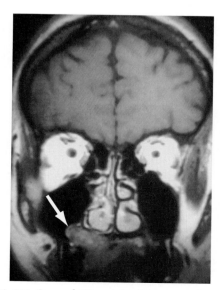

FIGURE 31–116 Coronal T1-weighted image with contrast enhancement. Moderately enhancing adenoid cystic carcinoma of the palate extends into the right maxillary sinus *(arrow).*

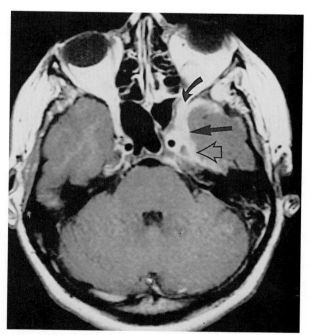

FIGURE 31–117 T1-weighted image with contrast enhancement. Adenoid cystic carcinoma arises in the nasopharynx in a 42-year-old woman. There is perineural invasion with enhancement of the superior orbital fissure *(curved arrow),* cavernous sinus *(straight arrow),* and Meckel's cave *(open arrow).*

of colonic adenocarcinoma metastatic to the sinonasal tract have been published. The clinical course is similar to that of adenoid cystic carcinoma with local invasion and low rate of nodal and systemic metastases.[157, 158]

The tumor forms papillae and various-sized irregular glands. The papillary type arises from surface mucosa and consists of multiple fronds of columnar epithelial cells with large, pleomorphic nuclei on fibrovascular cores. This histologic pattern is considered low grade and has the best prognosis of the group. The sessile type is felt to arise from minor salivary ducts and contains goblet cells and glands that bear a striking resemblance to colonic adenocarcinoma (Fig. 31–118). The alveolar-mucoid variant arises from seromucinous glands and remains within the lamina propria. It contains signet ring cells, numerous goblet cells, and nests of tumor cells suspended in mucinous pools reminiscent of a "colloid carcinoma" pattern.

Malignant Melanoma

Sinonasal mucosal melanomas constitute 0.6% to 2.5% of all malignant melanomas and arise from melanocytes that have migrated from the neural crest.[159] The majority of these tumors occur in the nasal cavity, especially along the nasal septum, lateral wall, and inferior and middle turbinates. The prognosis is dismal. Reported 5-year survival rates for nasal and paranasal sinus mucosal melanomas are 11% to 30% and generally worse than for cutaneous melanomas. Nasal cavity melanomas demonstrate a 50% recurrence rate. Factors such as size, location, pigmentation, and histologic type have not shown prognostic significance. Regional lymph node metastases and distant metastases occur in approximately 20% of patients.[160, 161]

Grossly, the tumors are sessile or polypoid and may be pink, brown, or black with mucosal ulceration. Microscopically, the tumor cells are typically large and pleomorphic with epithelioid or spindle morphology. The growth pattern may be papillary, solid, organoid and/or mixed. Dense brown cytoplasmic melanin granules may be seen and confirmed by a Fontana stain. A significant number (10% to 30%) of sinonasal melanomas are amelanotic and require immunohistochemistry with S-100 or HMB-45 antibodies to confirm the diagnosis (Figs. 31–119 and 31–120).

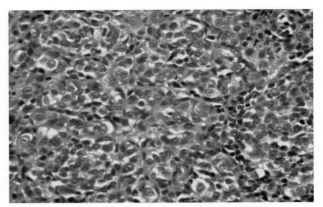

FIGURE 31–119 Sinonasal melanoma (H&E 100×). The individual cells have dark but otherwise uniform nuclei and no cytoplasmic melanin pigment.

Despite their poor prognosis, nasal melanomas may remodel bone, mimicking an indolent process. Melanomas are expected to be bright on T1-weighted and dark on T2-weighted images. The signal intensity is a function of the melanin pigment, which has a paramagnetic effect, shortening the T1 and T2 relaxation times. The fact that these lesions frequently hemorrhage also contributes to their MRI appearance. Amelanotic melanomas may be isointense to muscle on T1-weighted and bright on T2-weighted images.[162] On MRI melanomas have a variable pattern of signal intensity, and it is not possible to separate melanotic from amelanotic on the basis of the MRI signal (Fig. 31–121).[163]

Esthesioneuroblastoma

Esthesioneuroblastoma, or olfactory neuroblastoma, is an uncommon tumor of neuroectodermal origin that arises from the olfactory epithelium in the superior nasal cavity in the cribriform region in the upper third of the nasal septum, and along the superior and supreme turbinates.[164] The incidence of esthesioneuroblastoma ranges between 2% and 3% of all intranasal malignancies.[165] This slowly growing vascular neoplasm occurs in all ages but has a bimodal incidence, with peaks between 11 and 20 years

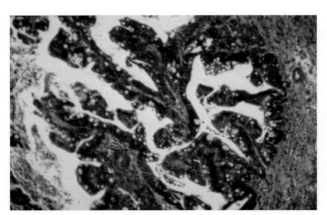

FIGURE 31–118 Sinonasal adenocarcinoma (H&E 100×). The tumor surface has goblet cells and resembles primary adenocarcinoma of the colon.

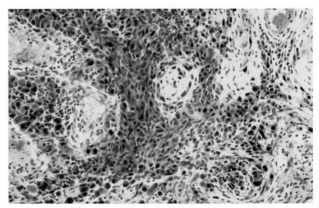

FIGURE 31–120 Melanoma (100×). Immunohistochemistry with anti–S-100 antibody decorates the melanoma cells.

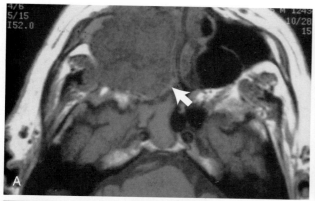

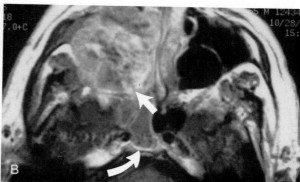

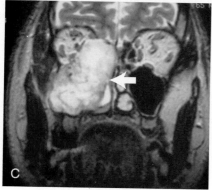

FIGURE 31–121 Sinonasal melanoma in a 65-year-old man. Axial T1-weighted image before *(A)* and after *(B)* contrast enhancement. *(C),* Coronal T2-weighted image. Necrotic mass *(straight arrow)* arises in the nasal cavity and extends to the ethmoid and maxillary sinuses. The lesion is isointense with muscle on T1-weighted and hyperintense on T2-weighted images with heterogeneous contrast enhancement. Note obstructed secretions in the sphenoid sinus with peripheral enhancing mucosa *(curved arrow in B).*

of age, and again in the 50- to 60-year-old group.[4, 164] The most common presenting symptoms are epistaxis and nasal obstruction. Metastases have been reported in 14% to 62%, with the most common site being the cervical lymph nodes. Local recurrences occur in about 50% of patients.[4, 164]

The tumor consists of clustered masses of small cells with round uniform nuclei representing the primitive neuroblasts (Fig. 31–122). A variable amount of pink, fibrillar tissue is admixed and represents neural fibrils that are felt to be cytoplasmic extensions from the neuroblasts.

This tumor is usually homogeneous on CT and MRI but may show areas of calcification (inverted papillomas and chondroid tumors also calcify) (Table 31–19)[165] and

cystic degeneration (Figs. 31–123 and 31–124). Esthesioneuroblastoma is hypointense to brain on T1-weighted and hyperintense on T2-weighted images.[4] This tumor is locally invasive and frequently involves the orbit (17%), olfactory bulbs and anterior cranial fossa (15%), and adjacent paranasal sinuses.[41, 164] Distant metastases to cervical nodes, lungs, and bone occur in 20% of cases.[41] Pathologically, esthesioneuroblastoma may be confused with other small cell malignancies, including lymphoma, amelanotic melanoma, undifferentiated squamous cell carcinoma, extramedullary plasmacytoma, and meningioma.[164]

Malignant Mesenchymal Neoplasms

Sarcoma

Rhabdomyosarcoma

The most common soft tissue sarcoma in infants and children is rhabdomysarcoma. This neoplasm ranks sev-

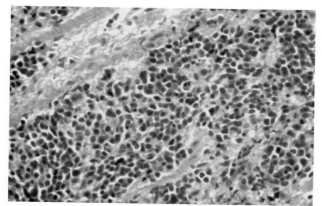

FIGURE 31–122 Olfactory neuroblastoma (H&E 100×). Uniform, small neuroblasts with pink neuronal extensions.

TABLE 31–19 Sinonasal Lesions with Calcification

Chronic inflammatory disease
Inverting papilloma
Dentigerous cyst
Esthesioneuroblastoma
Osteoblastoma
Osteosarcoma and chondrosarcoma
Chordoma
Fibro-osseous lesions
Meningioma

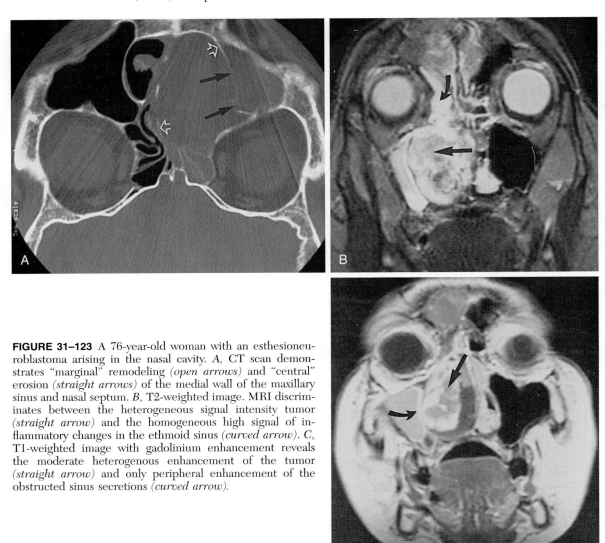

FIGURE 31–123 A 76-year-old woman with an esthesioneu-roblastoma arising in the nasal cavity. *A,* CT scan demonstrates "marginal" remodeling *(open arrows)* and "central" erosion *(straight arrows)* of the medial wall of the maxillary sinus and nasal septum. *B,* T2-weighted image. MRI discriminates between the heterogeneous signal intensity tumor *(straight arrow)* and the homogeneous high signal of inflammatory changes in the ethmoid sinus *(curved arrow). C,* T1-weighted image with gadolinium enhancement reveals the moderate heterogenous enhancement of the tumor *(straight arrow)* and only peripheral enhancement of the obstructed sinus secretions *(curved arrow).*

enth among the common malignancies in childhood. There is a bimodal peak age distribution, between 2 and 5 years and 15 and 19 years of age. The most common sites are the head and neck, genitourinary tract, extremities, trunk, and retroperitoneum.

Sinonasal rhabdomyosarcomas commonly present with a polypoid configuration that is described histologically as botryoid or grapelike in appearance. Four histologic subtypes are described: embryonal, alveolar, pleomorphic, and mixed. The embryonal variant is the most common, with sheets of large round and spindle cells with abundant eosinophilic cytoplasm called *rhabdomyoblasts.* Cross-striations resembling those found in skeletal muscle fibers are often present. The alveolar subtype consists of poorly defined groups of single, small, dense, round cells with irregular nuclei and scant cytoplasm. This histologic appearance is included in the poorly differentiated "small round blue cell tumors of childhood." An alveolar pattern with cell clusters resembling lung alveoli is variable, and the primitive cells may appear in solid sheets or trabecular nests. Mitoses and necrosis are common (Fig. 31–125).

The prognosis is strongly linked to the histologic type, with the alveolar variant having a less favorable course than the embryonal type at all stages. Rhabdomyosarcoma metastasizes to regional lymph nodes as well as hematogenously to bone, lung, and brain.

Rhabdomyosarcoma can both destroy and remodel bone.[4]

Chondroma and Chondrosarcoma

Chondrosarcoma is found in bone that has ossified from cartilage. Common sites include the nasal septum and the sphenoid and ethmoid. Chondrosarcoma may also arise in the maxillary sinus from cartilaginous cell rests.[107]

Histologically, conventional chondrosarcoma is characterized by increased cellularity and the presence of one or more cells that lie within clear spaces called *lacunae.* The nuclei vary from dense and hyperchromatic to vesicular with prominent nucleoli. Mitoses are sparse. The stroma is usually composed of a hyaline matrix but may be spindled and myxoid. The majority of sinonasal chondrosarcomas are well (grade I) to moderately (grade II)

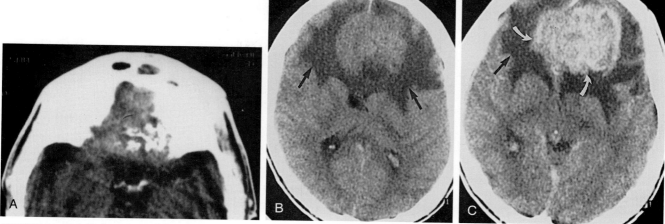

FIGURE 31–124 Esthesioneuroblastoma arises in the nasal cavity, with brain invasion, in a 23-year-old man. *A,* Axial CT scan before contrast enhancement. There is destruction of the cribriform plate and anterior skull base. The tumor contains calcifications. CT scans before *(B)* and after *(C)* contrast enhancement. Note the low-density edema of the frontal lobes *(straight arrows)* and the irregular enhancement at the tumor-brain interface *(curved arrows* in *C)* indicating brain invasion.

differentiated. Poorly differentiated (grade III) tumors are uncommon (Fig. 31–126).

On CT these are destructive lesions with dense nodular plaquelike calcification (Fig. 31–127). Other lesions with calcification include inverting papilloma and meningioma (see Table 31–19). These tumors induce sclerosis in adjacent bone. Osteosarcomas frequently produce bone formation that is diffuse and ill defined; however, the CT appearance may be indistinguishable from that of

chondrosarcoma. MRI features include increased signal intensity on T2-weighted images and contrast enhancement.[166]

Osteosarcoma

Osteosarcoma is the second most common malignant bone tumor after multiple myeloma. Osteosarcomas are twice as common as chondrosarcomas.[45] Only 6% of osteosarcomas occur in the head and neck region, with the

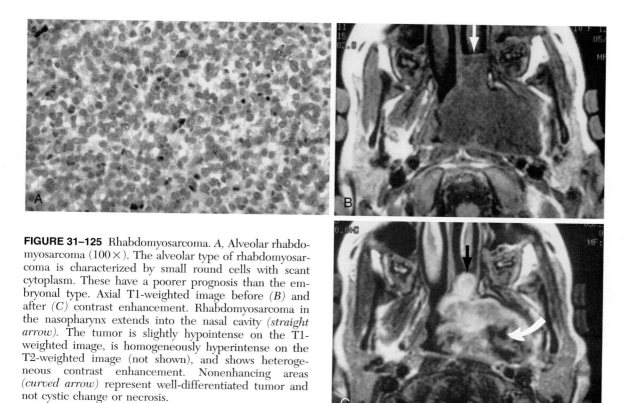

FIGURE 31–125 Rhabdomyosarcoma. *A,* Alveolar rhabdomyosarcoma (100×). The alveolar type of rhabdomyosarcoma is characterized by small round cells with scant cytoplasm. These have a poorer prognosis than the embryonal type. Axial T1-weighted image before *(B)* and after *(C)* contrast enhancement. Rhabdomyosarcoma in the nasopharynx extends into the nasal cavity *(straight arrow).* The tumor is slightly hypointense on the T1-weighted image, is homogeneously hyperintense on the T2-weighted image (not shown), and shows heterogeneous contrast enhancement. Nonenhancing areas *(curved arrow)* represent well-differentiated tumor and not cystic change or necrosis.

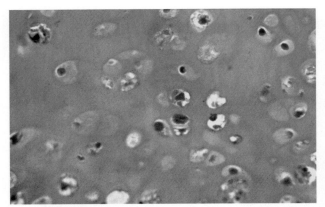

FIGURE 31–126 Chondrosarcoma, low grade (H&E 200×). Scattered plump chondrocytes are present with lacunar spaces within a chondroid matrix. No mitoses or densely cellular areas are present.

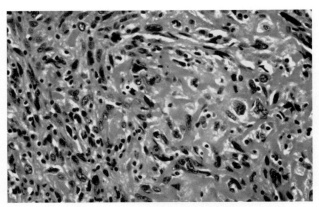

FIGURE 31–128 Osteosarcoma (H&E 200×). Large pleomorphic spindle cells are embedded in a dense pink matrix of osteoid.

majority occurring in the mandible.[167] The maxilla is the second most common head and neck site, however, and tumors in the maxillary and ethmoid sinuses have been reported. Head and neck osteosarcoma is most common in men in the third and fourth decades of life.[45] The tumors present as poorly defined, destructive masses and grossly may be firm, gritty, fleshy, or fibrous. The prognosis for sinonasal osteosarcomas is generally poor, with reported recurrence rates of 80% usually occurring within the first postoperative year. Metastases to lungs and brain typically occur within the first 2 years and reduce survival to zero.[168]

Microscopy shows cellular sheets of large spindle and pleomorphic cells admixed with osteoid. Osteoid has a dense, pink, and often lacelike appearance and is essential for diagnosis. Fibrous and chondroblastic elements may be present; however, the presence of osteoid classifies the sarcoma as osteosarcoma or osteogenic sarcoma (Fig. 31–128).

Radiographically, osteosarcoma varies from a purely lytic destructive mass to an osteoblastic lesion. Dense

bone, calcification, or a "sunburst" periosteal bone reaction is noted (Fig. 31–129). Signal intensity is variable on MRI. Ossified areas exhibit decreased signal intensity, and "nonossified" areas are brighter on all pulse sequences.[45]

Dermatofibrosarcoma Protuberans

Dermatofibrosarcoma protuberans is an uncommon low-grade cutaneous sarcoma, characterized by indolent infiltrative growth and a marked propensity for recurrence after simple excision. This tumor is of intermediate-grade malignancy, between benign and malignant fibrous histiocytoma. The most common site is the trunk, followed by the extremities and the head and neck. The lesion is found slightly more often in males, with a peak age distribution of 30 to 40 years.[169–171]

Dermatofibrosarcoma protuberans is a highly cellular tumor that invades the dermis and subcutis and is composed of dense sheets of mildly pleomorphic spindle cells with large mildly atypical spindle-shaped nuclei. The stroma has variable amounts of collagen and myxoid sub-

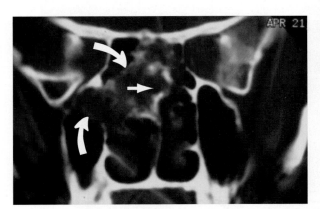

FIGURE 31–127 Chondrosarcoma arises in the nasal septum. Coronal CT scan. There is destruction of the nasal septum (*straight arrow*) by a calcified mass in the nasal cavity. There is involvement of the adjacent sphenoid and maxillary sinuses (*curved arrows*).

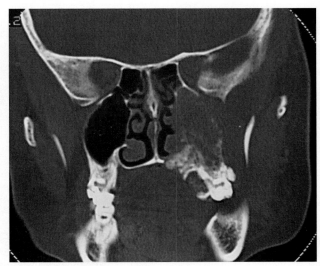

FIGURE 31–129 Osteosarcoma. Coronal CT scan. A soft tissue mass with calcification is associated with destruction of the walls of the left maxillary sinus.

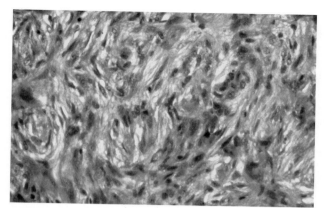

FIGURE 31–130 Dermatofibrosarcoma protuberans (H&E 200×). Sheets of plump, spindle-shaped cells are arranged in a cartwheel or storiform pattern.

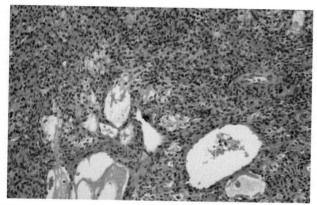

FIGURE 31–132 Sinonasal hemangiopericytoma (H&E 100×). Irregular, "staghorn" vessels are surrounded by densely packed spindle cells.

stance. The pattern can be storiform or cartwheel-like. Scattered mitoses are usually seen (Figs. 31–130 and 31–131).

Hemangiopericytoma

Hemangiopericytoma is an uncommon soft tissue tumor with a controversial etiology. Most investigators feel that the tumor arises from pericytes that are spindle cells that surround blood vessels and are thought to have smooth muscle and baroreceptor functions.[172, 173] From 15% to 20% of hemangiopericytomas occur in the head and neck, with greater than 50% of these occurring in the sinonasal tract. The majority appear to arise in the paranasal sinuses with secondary involvement of the nasal cavity.

Patients present with nasal obstruction and epistaxis.[174] The majority of sinonasal hemangiopericytomas behave indolently with a 60% recurrence if inadequately treated surgically. Malignant hemangiopericytomas are characterized by cellular anaplasia and increased mitoses. Only 10% have distant metastases to the lung. Lymph node metastases are rare. The tumors are considered to be radioresistant.[175] Grossly, they are red-tan to gray-tan polypoid masses high in the nasal cavity.

Densely cellular sheets of uniform spindle cells surround thin-walled, irregular endothelium-lined spaces. The vascular spaces are classically described as having a staghorn- or antler-like configuration. Reticulin fibers outline individual cells. (Fig. 31–132). Considerable histologic variation is reported such as a fibrosis, hyalinization, or a myxoid degeneration. Occasional mitoses are present, but significant mitotic activity and necrosis are not typical features.

Hemangiopericytoma is a highly vascular tumor, and

FIGURE 31–131 Dermatofibrosarcoma protuberans in a 74-year-old woman. *A*, Coronal CT scan shows a soft tissue mass in the nasal cavity with expansion and remodeling of the lamina papyracea of the left ethmoid sinus *(straight arrow)* and nasal septum *(curved arrow)*. There is erosion of the fovea ethmoidalis *(open arrow)*. Coronal T1-weighted *(B)* and T2-weighted *(C)* images. The tumor is isointense to muscle. *D*, T1-weighted image after gadolinium injection shows homogeneous enhancement.

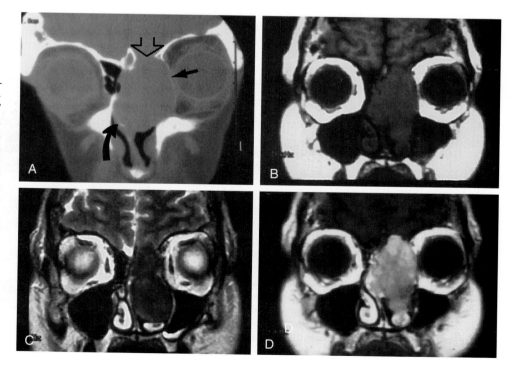

preoperative embolization may facilitate surgery and decrease intraoperative blood loss.[174]

These lesions expand and remodel bone. Hemangiopericytomas are low to intermediate signal intensity on T1-weighted images, bright signal intensity on T2-weighted images, and enhance.[45]

Lymphoma

After squamous cell carcinoma, non-Hodgkin's lymphoma is the second most frequent malignancy of the head and neck.[176] non-Hodgkin's lymphoma of the head and neck is the second most common type of extranodal lymphoma, following the lymphoma of the gastrointestinal tract, and accounts for 10% of paranasal sinus neoplasia.[31, 41, 176]

Malignant lymphomas are currently divided into Hodgkin's and Non-Hodgkin's types, although advancing molecular biology continues to shape our understanding and classification of these tumors. Non-Hodgkin's lymphoma is the most common type seen in the sinonasal tract, with Hodgkin's type occurring rarely. Non-Hodgkin's lymphomas are also currently classified by their B- or T-cell phenotype utilizing immunohistochemistry and flow cytometry for surface marker analysis.

Both B-cell and T-cell lymphomas, as well as a minority portion of nonclassifiable phenotypes, occur in the sinonasal tract. Studies report variable proportions of B- and T-cell lymphomas;[177, 178] however, it is clear that the T-cell phenotype is more common in the nasal cavity than other Waldeyer's ring sites or other extranodal sites. Both B- and T-cell lymphomas of the sinonasal tract have demonstrated associated Epstein-Barr virus antigens in Asian and non-Asian populations.[179]

Idiopathic midline destructive granuloma is a misnomer, and its diagnosis should be abandoned. Recent studies have found that a majority of lesions previously classified as midline granuloma and polymorphic reticulosis are indeed T-cell lymphoma.[180, 181] The T-cell sinonasal lymphomas have a propensity for angioinvasion with secondary "vasculitis" and necrosis of bone, cartilage, and soft tissues.[94] Neoplastic oral and sinonasal fistulas are more common with lymphoma than with Wegener's granulomatosis. Like paranasal sinus carcinomas, the B-cell lymphomas invade adjacent structures, such as the orbit, PPF, anterior cranial fossa, and cheek.[94] Histologically, sinonasal B-cell lymphomas tend to be diffuse, monomorphous infiltrates of large cleaved or immunoblastic, or both, cells that invade throughout the mucosa and soft tissues (Fig. 31–133). The T-cell lymphomas are diffuse, large pleomorphic cells with frequent necrosis and angioinvasion (Fig. 31–134).

Lymphoma is isointense to gray matter on T1-weighted MRI and iso- or slightly hypo- or hyperintense on T2-weighted images.[176] There is enhancement with gadolinium. Lymphoma may involve the sphenoid and cavernous sinuses and encase the internal carotid artery without narrowing the lumen. Meningioma has similar imaging characteristics but may cause hyperostosis with narrowing of the carotid artery.[176] Lymphoma exhibits a variable effect on bone. Lymphoma may cause bone remodeling with minimal destruction, or lymphoma may permeate bone, leaving an intact cortex with little evidence of bone

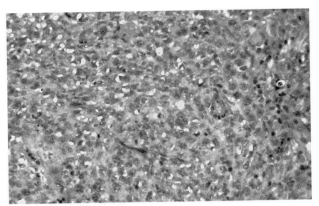

FIGURE 31–133 Nasal B-cell lymphoma (H&E 200×). Sheets of large, individual, pleomorphic cells have large nuclei and scant cytoplasm.

destruction. Lymphoma may also be associated with bone destruction (Fig. 31–135).[31, 41, 176]

The differential diagnosis of lymphoma involving the sphenoid sinus (Table 31–20) would include squamous cell carcinoma, meningioma, chordoma, chondrosarcoma, and invasive pituitary adenoma.[176, 182]

Plasmacytoma

Plasmacytoma accounts for 4% of all nonepithelial neoplasms of the head and neck. Extramedullary or solitary plasmacytomas are defined masses of atypical neoplastic plasma cells. Most patients are men in their sixth to seventh decades. The upper respiratory mucosa is a common site, with the majority of these neoplasms occurring in the sinonasal tract. Approximately 75% arise in the sinonasal region and nasopharynx, 10% in the oropharynx, and 15% in the larynx.[183]

It is unusual for patients to have increased serum or urine levels of immunoglobulins; however, immunohistochemical studies typically demonstrate monoclonal immunoglobulins in plasmacytoma. The lesions are usually treated with radiotherapy, and a 50% 10-year survival is

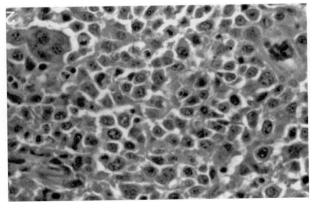

FIGURE 31–134 Sinonasal T-cell lymphoma (H&E 200×). Sheets of large, individual cells have significant pleomorphism and areas of vascularity.

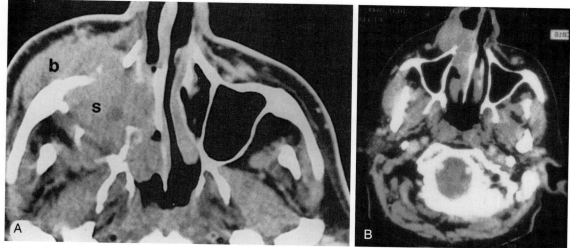

FIGURE 31–135 Lymphoma. *A,* Immunoblastic lymphoma in a 35-year-old man with a rapidly growing right cheek mass and low-grade fever. Axial contrast-enhanced CT scan shows a mass involving the right maxillary sinus (s), extending into the buccal space (b). There is destruction of the wall of the maxillary sinus. *B,* Lymphoma arises from the nasal cavity and extends through the piriform aperture. (*A,* From Holliday RA. Manifestations of AIDS in the oromaxillofacial region: The role of imaging. Radiol Clin North Am 1993;45–73. *B,* Courtesy of Suresh Mukherji, M.D., Chapel Hill, NC.)

reported. Some patients, however, have local recurrences, and others eventually develop multiple myeloma.[184]

Grossly, the lesions may be polypoid or submucosal masses. Microscopically, plasmacytoma consists of sheets of oval cells with basophilic cytoplasm and eccentrically placed nuclei. The nuclear chromatin pattern is distinctive with multiple dense chromatin masses arranged in a cart-wheel pattern. Varied numbers of less differentiated cells may be present with increased large, pleomorphic or binucleate nuclei, and mitotic figures (Fig. 31–136).

On CT, plasmacytoma is usually a localized, well-demarcated tumor, without infiltration. Occasionally it may be an aggressive lesion marked by bone destruction and involvement of adjacent structures. The lesions are isointense or slightly hyperintense with respect to muscle on T1-weighted images and of only moderate signal intensity on T2-weighted images. There is intense contrast enhancement with central inhomogeneity.[183, 185, 186]

Metastatic Tumor

Metastatic tumor to the sinonasal cavities is unusual. Most metastases are hematogenous to bone. The most common

metastasis is from renal cell carcinoma (Fig. 31–137).[4, 104] Other primary tumors include, in decreasing order of frequency, lung, breast, prostate, testis, and gastrointestinal malignancies.[4, 104]

MAXILLOFACIAL TRAUMA

Anatomy

Because of the complex nature of most midfacial fractures, radiologic evaluation requires a good understanding of the normal osseous anatomy. Before analyzing the facial skeleton, it is helpful to review the supporting buttresses that provide the basic framework for its structure. There are three main vertical and three horizontal buttresses.[187, 188]

Vertical Buttresses

The three paired vertical buttresses (Fig. 31–138) are

The nasomaxillary (nasofrontal) buttress
The zygomaticomaxillary buttress
The pterygomaxillary buttress

The nasomaxillary buttress extends from the anterior alveolus of the maxilla, along the lateral wall of the piriform (anterior nasal) aperture, and into the medial wall of the orbit. Important components of the nasomaxillary buttresses include (1) the lower maxilla, the medial walls of the maxillary sinuses, and the frontal process of the maxilla; (2) the nasal bones and the nasofrontal suture (nasion); and (3) the medial orbital walls including the lacrimal bone.

The more laterally situated zygomaticomaxillary buttress is formed by the body of the zygoma and its frontal process as well as the lateral portion of the maxilla. It transmits vertically directed forces from the midmaxilla to the frontal bone.

The pterygomaxillary buttress extends from the poste-

TABLE 31–20 Sphenoid Sinus (and Central Skull Base) Lesions

Squamous cell carcinoma
Lymphoma
Adenoid cystic carcinoma
Metastasis
Meningioma
Chordoma
Chondrosarcoma
Pituitary adenoma (invasive)
Aneurysm
Mucocele
Intrasphenoid encephalocele

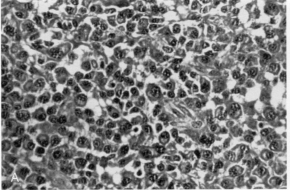
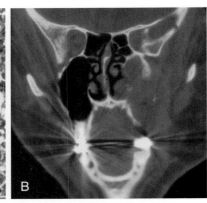

FIGURE 31–136 Plasmacytoma. *A*, Extramedullary plasmacytoma (H&E 200×). Sheets of pleomorphic and binucleate plasma cells are present in this nasal lesion. *B*, Plasmacytoma destroys the maxillary sinus and invades the nasal cavity. (*B*, Courtesy of Suresh Mukherji, M.D., Chapel Hill, NC.)

rior maxillary alveolus (tuberosity) cranially to the skull base and includes the pterygoid process and plates of the sphenoid and the posterolateral and posteromedial walls of the adjacent maxillary sinus. It transmits forces from the posterior aspect of the hard palate and the alveolar ridges to the skull base.

In addition to the three paired vertical buttresses, there is also a centrally located buttress, the nasoethmoid buttress. It is composed of the ethmoid and vomer and represents an important bony bridge between the cranium and the lower facial skeleton. These buttresses have evolved as mechanical adaptations of the skull and facial

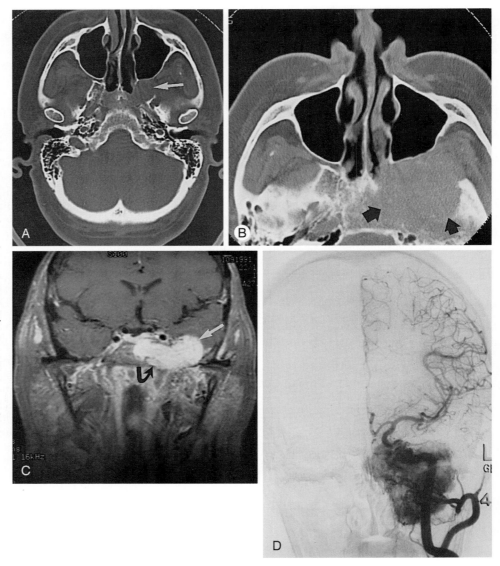

FIGURE 31–137 Metastatic renal cell carcinoma in a 56-year-old woman. *A*, Axial CT scan, performed for suspected transient ischemic attack, shows incidental widening of the pterygopalatine fossa (*arrow*) and erosion of the pterygoid plates and posterior wall of the left maxillary sinus. *B*, Axial CT scan. The patient initially refused further work-up and returned 6 months later with a large mass eroding the skull base (*arrows*). *C*, Coronal T1-weighted contrast-enhanced image. There is homogeneous enhancement of the tumor, which invades the middle cranial fossa (*straight arrow*) and the sphenoid sinus (*curved arrow*). *D*, Left common carotid angiogram (anteroposterior projection) shows a hypervascular mass fed predominantly by branches of the external carotid artery.

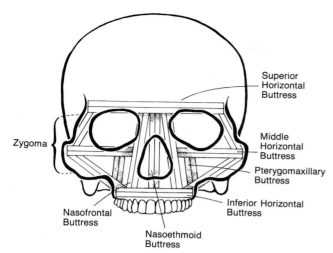

FIGURE 31–138 Schematic drawing of the facial buttresses. (From DelBalso AM, Hall RE, Margarone JE. Radiographic evaluation of maxillofacial trauma. In DelBalso AM [ed]. Maxillofacial Imaging, pp. 35–128. Philadelphia, WB Saunders, 1990.)

bones to masticatory forces. The zygomaticomaxillary buttress absorbs the majority of the occlusal forces as evidenced by the thick cortical bone present in the body of the zygoma.

Horizontal Buttresses

Overall the previously mentioned vertical buttresses tend to have a somewhat curved shape requiring reinforcement by axial struts for maximal strength. Thus the sagittally oriented buttresses are interconnected by three axially oriented struts. These three horizontal struts (see Fig. 31–138) are named

    The superior horizontal buttress
    The middle horizontal buttress
    The inferior horizontal buttress

The superior horizontal buttress is composed of the floor of the anterior cranial fossa including the orbital roofs (frontal bone), the roofs of the ethmoid air cells (frontal bone), and the cribriform plate of the ethmoid.

The middle horizontal buttress includes (1) the orbital surface of the maxilla and segments of the frontal process of the maxilla; (2) the body, temporal process, and infraorbital process of the zygoma; and (3) the zygomatic process of the temporal bone. It provides lateral stability to the facial skeleton and protects the central facial skeleton from horizontally directed forces.

The inferior horizontal buttress is composed of the alveolar ridge and the hard palate and acts as an important bony bridge between the two maxillary bones.

Imaging in Acute Facial Trauma

Although conventional radiographs (i.e., facial bone series) continue to be the first examination usually requested in patients presenting with suspected facial trauma, CT is the modality of choice for the complete evaluation of the facial skeleton, facial soft tissues, the brain, and so forth, and has become an essential study

for proper treatment planning. Patients who are clinically stable and have no clinical or radiographic evidence of cervical or thoracic spine trauma are best evaluated with both axial and direct coronal views. The axial images should extend from the mandible to the top of the frontal sinuses, and the coronal images should extend from the nasal arch anteriorly to the sphenoid sinus posteriorly. If both axial and coronal views can be obtained, an adequate study can be performed using 3-mm collimation and incrementation. If the patient has definite or possible cervical or thoracic spine injuries, however, axial 1-mm scans can be obtained and coronal (and if necessary oblique sagittal) two-dimensional reconstructions of the face and mandible may be performed.

In those patients who are clinically unstable, studies can be performed in the helical scanning mode using 3-mm collimation and a 1:1 or 1:2 pitch. Once again in these patients obtaining coronal and oblique sagittal two-dimensional reconstructions greatly increases the diagnostic value of the study.

Depending on the clinical situation, three-dimensional reconstructed images may also be helpful, particularly in patients who have sustained mandibular, zygomatic, or transfacial fractures.

Midfacial Fracture Classification

The following, helpful classification scheme has recently been developed by Gentry.[189] Midfacial fractures are categorized as either *transfacial* fractures, which require fractures of the pterygoid plates, or *limited* fractures, in which the pterygoids are spared (Table 31–21).

Transfacial (LeFort) Fractures

Although other classifications exist, the most widely used system for classifying complex midfacial fractures continues to be the system first described by Rene LeFort in 1901.[190] LeFort identified three inherent areas of weak-

---

TABLE 31–21 Midfacial Fracture Classification

Transfacial Fractures

LeFort I
LeFort II
LeFort III
Complex LeFort

Limited Fractures

Complex Strut Fractures

1. Zygomaticomaxillary complex (tripod) (trimalar)
2. Nasofrontoethmoid
3. Sphenotemporal buttress
4. Nasomaxillary buttress

Solitary Strut Fractures

1. Orbital wall "blowout"
2. Zygomatic arch
3. Nasal arch
4. Isolated orbital rim
5. Localized sinus wall (frontal, maxillary)
6. Orbital rim

ness in the facial skeleton after observing (by dissection) the fractures that resulted in cadavers' heads after he had traumatized them by striking them with wooden clubs and throwing them against the edge of a table.

The LeFort I fracture (first described by Guerin in 1866) is basically a transverse fracture of the maxilla. It results from a blow delivered to the upper lip region, and it extends transversely, at a level above the apices of the teeth, through all three walls of the maxillary sinus and across the nasal septum (Fig. 31–139A). Posteriorly, the fracture extends through the pyramidal process of the palatine bone and the pterygoid process of the sphenoid bone. The resulting "floating palate" is displaced posteriorly, accounting for the malocclusion seen on clinical examination.[191]

The LeFort II fracture (also known as the pyramidal fracture) follows the same course as the LeFort I fracture posteriorly. Anteriorly, however, it curves upward near the zygomaticomaxillary suture and infraorbital foramen; through the inferior orbital rim and onto the orbital floor; up through the medial orbital wall; and across the frontal, nasal bones or nasofrontal suture and nasal septum (Fig. 31–140; see also Fig. 31–139B). The pyramid-shaped fracture segment (the central midface) is posteriorly displaced, resulting clinically in malocclusion and a "dishface" deformity.[192] It usually results from a strong, broad blow over the central facial region.

LeFort III fractures result in complete craniofacial dysjunction. The fracture line extends from the nasofrontal suture through the frontal process of the maxilla, down the medial orbital wall, and across the frontozygomatic suture. The fracture also runs through the zygomatic arch and continues caudally through the pterygoid process of the sphenoid (Fig. 31–141; see also Fig. 31–139C). Thus the distinguishing features between LeFort II and III fractures are the addition of fractures involving the lateral orbital walls and the zygoma in the LeFort III–type injury. LeFort III fractures tend to occur after a blow to the midface in the region of the glabella. These patients have a dishface deformity, cerebrospinal fluid rhinorrhea, damage to the lacrimal apparatus, and malocclusion.[192]

Pure LeFort fractures represent an unusual occurrence clinically, since patients with severe midfacial trauma usually present with multiple fractures and fracture complexes. Thus most patients present with complex LeFort type injury, that is, a hemi–LeFort II (or a LeFort II fracture on one side) and a LeFort III fracture on the contralateral side.[187]

Limited Midfacial Fractures: Complex Strut Fractures

The *tripod* fracture (tetrapod, malar, zygomaticomaxillary-complex, zygomatic-complex fracture) represents one of the most common isolated facial fractures; second only to nasal fractures, it is the most common fracture involving the maxillary sinus.[193] It occurs after a horizontally di-

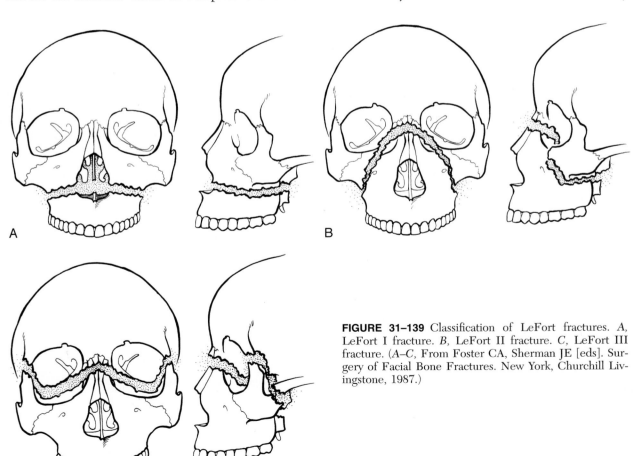

FIGURE 31–139 Classification of LeFort fractures. *A,* LeFort I fracture. *B,* LeFort II fracture. *C,* LeFort III fracture. (*A–C,* From Foster CA, Sherman JE [eds]. Surgery of Facial Bone Fractures. New York, Churchill Livingstone, 1987.)

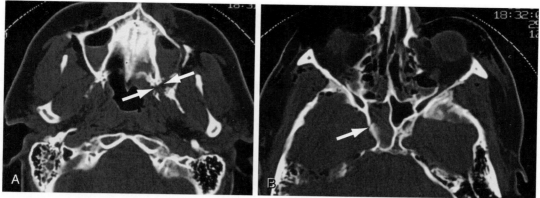

FIGURE 31–140 Axial CT scan. Hemi-LeFort II fracture on the left. *A*, Scan at the level of the hard palate shows air-fluid levels in both maxillary antra. There are comminuted fractures through the anterior and posterolateral walls of the left maxillary sinus. Fractures involving both the medial and the lateral pterygoid plates *(arrows)* on the left are also present, whereas the right hemimaxilla and right pterygoid are intact. *B*, Scan at the level of the orbits, where there are minimally displaced fractures through the nasal bones and a fracture of the bony nasal septum (not shown). Incidentally, note an associated fracture through the lateral wall of the right sphenoid sinus with blood filling the sinus cavity *(arrow)*.

rected blow to the zygoma or zygomatic arch, resulting in disruption of its three major attachments (i.e., the zygomaticomaxillary, zygomaticotemporal, and zygomaticofrontal articulations). The fracture lines extend along the lateral orbital wall (zygomaticofrontal and zygomaticosphenoid sutures) from the inferior orbital fissure to the midorbital floor near the infraorbital canal, then down the anterior maxilla near the zygomaticomaxillary suture and up the posterior maxillary wall back to the inferior orbital fissure (Figs. 31–142 through 31–144). Because of the location of the fracture lines, 94.2% of patients suffer from impairment of the infraorbital nerve.[192]

Nasofrontalethmoid-complex fractures include a wide range of different fracture complexes depending on differences in the initial point of impact as well as the direction and magnitude of the force. As in LeFort III fractures these injuries usually occur as a result of a blow to the midface in the region of the glabella.[194] The nasoethmoid region of the midface is particularly susceptible to trauma because of its fragile nature, with a large number of air spaces separated by thin-walled septa. These fractures can have significant intracranial extension and result in complications such as damage to the nasolacrimal ducts, dural tears, cerebrospinal fluid rhinorrhea, and injury to the anterior ethmoid artery.[194, 195] Fractures in this category include fractures of the lamina papyracea; fractures of the inferior, medial, and supraorbital rims; fractures of the frontal sinuses; fractures of the orbital roofs; nasal fractures; and fractures of the frontal process of the maxilla.

Solitary Strut Fractures

Orbital fractures that solely involve the floor are termed *blowout* fractures and represent the third most common isolated midfacial fracture.[193] The orbital floor is composed of the orbital plate of the maxilla and the orbital processes of the zygomatic and palatine bones (Fig. 31–145). Most people attribute the cause of blowout fractures to the conversion of kinetic energy (from the object) into hydraulic energy by the fluid-filled globe after it has been

struck by an object of greater transverse diameter than itself (Fig. 31–146).[195–197] The energy is then transmitted to the orbital walls in a uniform fashion. The orbital floor is the most common site of fracture, although accompanying fractures involving the medial wall (20% to 50% of cases) and less commonly the orbital roof also occur (Figs. 31–147 through 31–149).[193, 198, 199] Blowout fractures of the orbital floor occur most commonly in the posterior area of the floor, medial to the infraorbital suture and anteromedial to the inferior orbital fissure, the thinnest portion of the orbital floor.

Clinical findings in blowout fractures are variable but include enophthalmos and diplopia. Diplopia occurs in up to 72% of patients with blowout fractures and can be secondary to a number of causes.[200] Transient diplopia may result from edema, hemorrhage, or damage to the nerve supply to the extraocular muscles.[198] Permanent diplopia may result from herniation of periorbital fat or, rarely, the inferior rectus muscle through the fracture defect (see Fig. 31–147).[198] CT is indicated in all patients with either diplopia or plain-film findings suggesting a blowout fracture.[201] The axial images alone may arouse suspicion of an orbital floor fracture (see Fig. 31–149). Direct coronal views provide the best demonstration of the orbital injury (floor, medial wall, and roof fractures, herniation of fat or rectus muscle, and so forth), whereas axial sections usually only demonstrate an osseous fragment or soft tissue mass, or both, in the maxillary antrum.

The medial orbital wall is composed of the frontal process of the maxilla, the lacrimal bone, and the ethmoid bone (lamina papyracea). Isolated medial wall fractures are rare and occur secondary to the same hydraulic mechanisms described for orbital floor fractures. Although isolated fractures are uncommon, medial wall fractures are found in association with 20% to 50% of orbital floor blowout fractures.[198–200] Entrapment of the medial rectus muscle can occur and results in diplopia.[201]

Isolated blowout fractures involving the orbital roof are infrequent but may occur through a hydraulic mechanism similar to that involved in blowout fractures of the medial

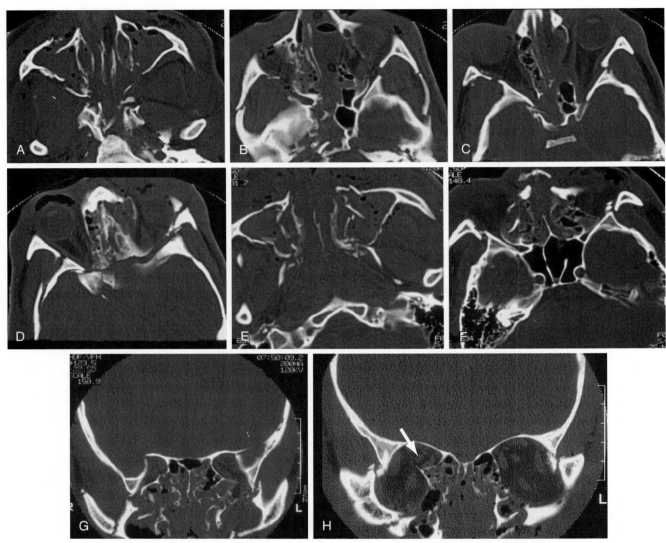

FIGURE 31–141 Bilateral LeFort III fractures. Four axial CT scans (bone windows). *A,* Scan at the level of the maxillary sinuses shows comminuted fractures through all four walls of both maxillary sinuses with associated fractures through the pterygoid plates bilaterally. *B,* Scan at the level of the zygomatic arches demonstrates two minimally displaced fractures through the left zygomatic arch and one through the right zygomatic arch. Comminuted fractures involving the nasoethmoid complex are also present with blood filling the nasal passages. *C,* Scan at the level of the orbits shows fractures through both lateral and orbital walls as well as fractures of the nasal bones and bony nasal septum. *D,* Scan at a level more cephalad than *C* further demonstrates a comminuted fracture of the lateral orbital walls and nasoethmoid complex. This patient also sustained fractures of the temporal sphenoid bones (including the lateral wall of the right sphenoid bones). Axial (*E* and *F*) and coronal (*G* and *H*) CT scans. Bilateral LeFort III fractures in a different patient. Two axial CT scans (bone windows) demonstrate comminuted fractures involving all of the walls of both maxillary sinuses and fractures through the pterygoid plates bilaterally (*E*) as well as comminuted fractures through the lateral orbital walls and nasoethmoid complex (*F*). Two direct coronal scans (bone images) from the same patient also show the maxillary and lateral orbital wall fractures and better delineate the complex, comminuted injury to the nasoethmoid complex. Note the fracture of the lamina papyracea on the right (*H*) with bony spicules that elevate the right medial rectus muscle and come in contact with the inferior aspect of the right optic nerve (*arrow*).

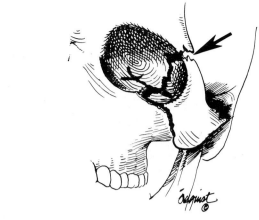

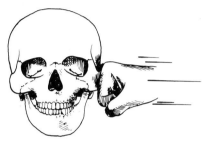

FIGURE 31–142 Schematic drawing of a zygomatic-complex fracture *(arrow)* and the mechanism of injury. (From Langland OE, Langlais RP, McDavid WD, DelBalso AM. Panoramic Radiology, 2nd ed. Philadelphia, Lea & Febiger, 1989.)

FIGURE 31–143 Zygomaticomaxillary-complex fracture. Axial CT scan (bone window) at the level of the zygomatic arches demonstrates a comminuted zygomaticomaxillary-complex fracture on the right. Note the associated sagittally oriented fracture of the right temporal bone that extends through the mandibular fossa *(arrow)*.

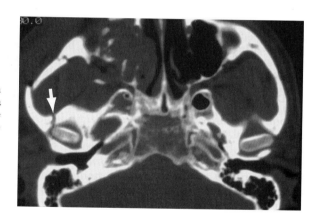

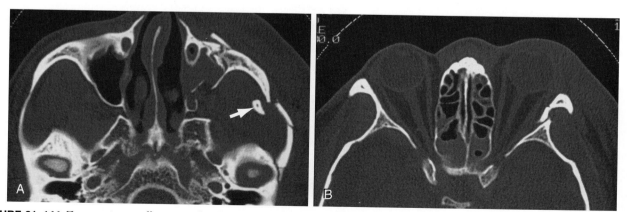

FIGURE 31–144 Zygomaticomaxillary-complex fracture with coronoid impingement. *A*, Axial CT scan (bone window) at the level of the maxillary antra and zygomatic arches. There is a zygomaticomaxillary-complex fracture on the left with fractures through the anterior and posterolateral walls of the maxillary sinus (the pterygoid plates are intact) and a depressed fracture of the left zygomatic arch. The zygomatic fracture fragment is rotated slightly (in a clockwise direction) and is impinging on the coronoid process of the left hemimandible *(arrow)*, demonstrating a potential complication of tetrapod-type fractures. The patient suffered from trismus. *B*, Fracture of the lateral orbital wall.

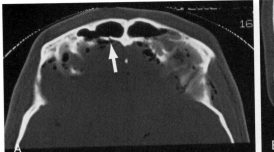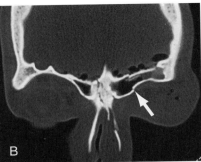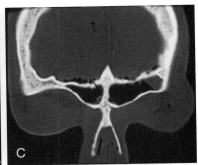

FIGURE 31–150 Frontal sinus fractures with pneumocephalus. Axial (*A*) and coronal (*B* and *C*) CT scans. Several small bubbles of intracranial air are identified bilaterally. On the bone window image (*A*), a minimally displaced fracture (*arrow*) through the posterior wall of the right frontal sinus is shown. The direct coronal (*B* and *C*) bone window images show minimally displaced fractures of both frontal sinuses including the posterior wall of the right frontal sinus and the posterior wall and floor (*arrow*) of the left frontal sinus.

fractures[207]) may be nondepressed, linear, or depressed. Fractures isolated to the posterior wall are relatively rare (representing approximately 5% of fractures[207]) and can be either horizontal or vertical. Fractures that only involve the floor are uncommon and occur as a result of a blowout fracture involving a section of the orbital roof. Fractures that involve both the anterior and posterior walls of the sinus (approximately 28%[207]) are usually the result of massive and penetrating trauma to the area (see Fig. 31–150). Any fracture involving the posterior wall creates communication with the dural spaces, and hence complications such as cerebrospinal fluid leakage, intracranial infection, or pneumocele can develop. Fractures isolated to the anterior wall tend to result in only cosmetic deformities (if untreated), whereas complications of isolated floor fractures are essentially those of orbital injuries.

Sphenoid sinus fractures occur in combination with skull base injuries and radiographically present as an air-fluid level in the sinus or as an opacified sinus. They are best evaluated with CT. Although relatively rare (compared with fractures involving the frontal sinus or cribriform plate, and so forth) the most common complication of sphenoid sinus fractures is the development of a cerebrospinal fluid leak. Rarely the fracture may traumatize the adjacent internal carotid arteries or cavernous sinuses, resulting in a potentially life-threatening injury.

The zygomatic arch is composed of the zygomatic process of the temporal bone and the temporal process of the zygoma. Fractures of the arch usually occur in combination with other injuries (i.e., LeFort III and zygomaticomaxillary complex fractures) and isolated fractures of the arch represent between 10% and 16% of zygomatic fractures.[208] They usually occur as a result of a horizontally directed blow striking the temporal process of the zygoma, posterior to the body of the zygoma. Serious complications of zygomatic arch fractures are rare; however, fractures involving the proximal portion of the zygomatic process of the temporal bone can extend posteriorly to involve the glenoid fossa of the temporal mandibular joint (see Fig. 31–143). Also if sufficient medial displacement of the fracture fragment(s) occurs, impingement on the coronoid process of the mandible (see Fig. 31–144) may result, limiting mandibular motion.

Complications—Cerebrospinal Fluid Rhinorrhea

Apart from potential postoperative complications (i.e., nonunion, malunion, and osteomyelitis), the most common complication of midfacial trauma for which imaging will be requested is likely a cerebrospinal fluid leak. Approximately 80% of all cerebrospinal fluid fistulas are posttraumatic in origin, resulting from fractures involving the skull base or facial bones.[209] The most common site is anteriorly through the region of the cribriform plate or ethmoid roof (fovea ethmoidalis) (Fig. 31–151). As a result, cerebrospinal fluid rhinorrhea is reported in a fairly high percentage (25% to 35%) of LeFort II and LeFort III fractures.[210] The temporal bone represents the second most common site, and if there is associated disruption of the tympanic membrane, cerebrospinal fluid can leak out into the external auditory canal, resulting in otorrhea. However, if the tympanic membrane remains intact, the fluid may pass through the eustachian tube and into the nasal cavity (hence causing rhinorrhea) resulting in a false clinical suspicion of fracture involving the anterior skull base or paranasal sinuses.[188] Fractures of the sphenoid bone that communicate with the sphenoid sinus are the third most common site of cerebrospinal fluid leaks; such leaks are uncommon but do occur.

Various imaging techniques have been advocated for the evaluation of suspected cerebrospinal fluid leaks. Axial and coronal high-resolution (bone algorithm) CT is helpful to identify the fractures but lacks specificity with respect to cerebrospinal fluid fistulas. CT cisternography (high-resolution CT after injection of nonionic contrast material into the subarachnoid space) may actually demonstrate the site of extravasation and at the same time provides excellent anatomic detail (see Fig. 31–151). However, the main disadvantage of CT cisternography is that in order to demonstrate the site of extravasation *cerebrospinal fluid must be actively leaking* at the time of the study. For this reason some authors have advocated the use of radionuclide cisternography ([111In]diethylenetriaminepenta-acetic acid) with imaging at intervals for up to 24 hours. However, this lacks the resolution of CT cisternography and requires nasal packing, which can be uncomfortable.

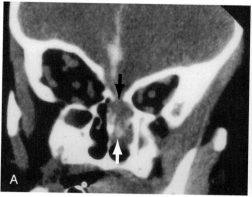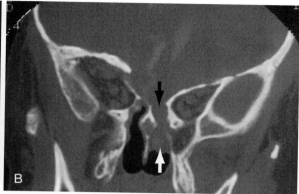

FIGURE 31–151 Posttraumatic cerebrospinal fluid fistula and encephalocele. Two coronal CT images (soft tissue *[A]* and bone window *[B]*) from a CT cisternogram were performed with flowing instillation of 4.5 ml of iohexol (Omnipaque) 180 contrast medium into the lumbar subarachnoid space. This study was performed on a 2-year-old female with cerebrospinal fluid rhinorrhea (left nostril) several months after severe facial trauma. Multiple facial fractures were visualized, including bilateral superior orbital rim fractures and a depressed fracture of the left cribriform plate. Contrast medium *(white arrow)* was identified leaking through the cribriform plate fracture *(black arrow)* and into the nasal passages on the left, confirming the presence of at least one cerebrospinal fluid fistula. A soft tissue mass that was isodense to brain tissue was also identified extending through the cribriform plate defect *(white arrow)*. A posttraumatic left frontal encephalocele was confirmed at the time of surgery for bilateral cerebrospinal fluid fistula repair.

Recently case reports have appeared in various journals illustrating success in identifying cerebrospinal fluid fistulas using a relatively new MRI technique termed MR cisternography.[211] MR cisternography requires the use of heavily T2-weighted (TR of 10,000) fast spin echo techniques with fat suppression, and video reversal of images. In one article, the abilities of both MR cisternography and CT cisternography in identifying fistulas in four patients with cerebrospinal fluid leaks were compared and MR cisternography was found to be superior.

Obviously there continues to be some controversy as to the investigation of choice in evaluating suspected cerebrospinal fluid leaks, and often a combination of imaging modalities (i.e., CT cisternography and radionuclide cisternography) is required to both confirm the presence of a leak and provide precise anatomic identification of the site. Regardless, it is somewhat comforting to realize that most cerebrospinal fluid leaks close spontaneously in a few days, and 95% close within 3 weeks. However, one must remember that persistent leaks may result in meningitis, and cerebrospinal fluid leaks persisting greater than 3 weeks must be identified and treated surgically, usually requiring a dural patch.

MISCELLANEOUS CONDITIONS

Pneumosinus Dilatans and Pneumocele

Pneumosinus dilatans is expansion of an air-filled paranasal sinus. This rare disorder most frequently affects the frontal sinus and may be idiopathic but has been associated with reaction to a planum sphenoidale meningioma, cerebral atrophy, chronic sinus inflammation, atrophy, arachnoid cyst, acromegaly, and spontaneous drainage of a mucocele (Fig. 31–152).[212, 213, 215]

A pneumocele occurs when air within the sinus extends outside the sinus, through a defect in the sinus wall. The epithelium remains intact.[212]

Decompressive Sinus Surgery for Thyroid Ophthalmopathy

The sequelae of thyroid eye disease that remain unresponsive to medical therapy may require surgical decompression. Indications for surgery include compressive optic neuropathy, corneal decompensation from exposure due to severe proptosis, and disfigurement from extreme exophthalmos.[215] The goal of surgery is to enlarge the

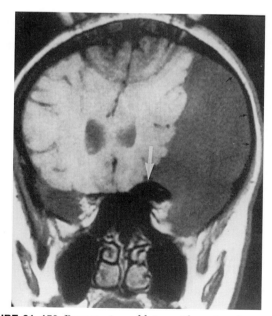

FIGURE 31–152 Pneumosinus dilatans. There is a large arachnoid cyst with "ballooning" of the sphenoid sinus and the pneumatized anterior clinoid *(arrow)*. (From PE Dross, JF Lally, B Bonier. Pneumosinus dilatans and arachnoid cyst: A unique association. AJNR 13[6]:209–211, 1992, © by American Society of Neuroradiology.)

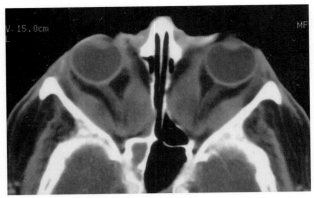

FIGURE 31–153 Decompressive ethmoidectomy for thyroid ophthalmopathy. Axial CT scan shows marked enlargement of the bellies of the extraocular muscles. The medial walls of the orbits have been removed.

bony orbit, usually by removal of the medial or inferior wall (Fig. 31–153).

References

1. Donald PJ. Anatomy and histology, Chapter 3. In Donald PJ, Gluckman JL, Rice DH (eds). The Sinuses, pp. 25–48. Philadelphia, Lippincott-Raven, 1995.
2. Earwacker J. Anatomic variants in sinonasal CT. Radiographics 1993;13:381–415.
3. Som PM, Brandwein M. Sinonasal cavities: Anatomy, physiology, and plain film normal anatomy. In Som PM, Curtin HD (eds). Head and Neck Imaging, pp. 61–96. St. Louis, Mosby–Year Book, 1996.
4. Mafee MF, Carter BL. Nasal cavity and paranasal sinuses. In Valvassori GE, Mafee MF, Carter BL (eds). Imaging of the Head and Neck, pp. 248–328. New York, Thieme Medical, 1995.
5. Castillo M. Congenital abnormalities of the nose: CT and MR findings. AJR 1994;162:1211–1217.
6. Harnsberger HR. Sinonasal imaging: Imaging issues in sinusitis. In Harnsberger HR (ed). Handbook of Head and Neck Imaging, 2nd ed., pp. 339–395. St. Louis, Mosby–Year Book, 1995.
7. Aoki S, Dillon WP, Barkovich AJ, Norman D. Marrow conversion before pneumatization of the sphenoid sinus: Assessment with MR imaging. Radiology 1989;172:373–375.
8. Scuderi AJ, Harnsberger HR, Boyer RS. Pneumatization of the paranasal sinuses: Normal features of importance to the accurate interpretation of CT and MR images. AJR 1993;160:1101–1104.
9. Weed DT, Cole RR. Maxillary sinus hypoplasia and vertical dystopia of the orbit. Laryngoscope 1994;104:758–762.
10. Grossman RI, Yousem DM. Neuroradiology. The Requisites. St. Louis, Mosby–Year Book, 1994.
11. Roithmann R, Shankar L, Hawke M, et al. CT imaging in the diagnosis and treatment of paranasal sinus disease; a partnership between the radiologist and the otolaryngologist. J Otolaryngol 1993;22:253–260.
12. Mafee MF. Preoperative imaging anatomy of nasal-ethmoid complex for functional endoscopic sinus surgery. Radiol Clin North Am 1993;31:1–20.
13. Ritter FN. The Paranasal Sinuses. Anatomy and Surgical Technique, 2nd ed. St. Louis, CV Mosby, 1978.
14. Rice DH, Schaefer SD. Endoscopic Paranasal Sinus Surgery, 2nd ed. Philadelphia, Lippincott-Raven, 1993.
15. Ritter FN, Fritsch MH. Atlas of Paranasal Sinus Surgery. New York, Igaku-Shoin, 1991.
16. Moulin G, Dessi P, Chagnaud C, et al. Dehiscence of the lamina papyracea of the ethmoid bone: CT findings. AJNR 1994;15:151–153.
17. Laine FJ, Smoker WRK. The ostiomeatal unit and endoscopic surgery: Anatomy, variations, and imaging findings in inflammatory disease. AJR 1992;159:849–857.
18. Banberg SF, Harner SG, Forbes G. Relationship of the optic nerve to the paranasal sinuses as shown by computed tomography. Otolaryngol Head Neck Surg 1987;96:331–335.
19. Lang J. Clinical Anatomy of the Nose, Nasal Cavity and Paranasal Sinuses. New York, Thieme Medical, 1989.
20. Babbel RW, Harnsberger HR. A contemporary look at the imaging issues of sinusitis: Sinonasal anatomy, physiology, and computed tomography techniques. Semin Ultrasound CT MR 1991;12:526–540.
21. Silverman FN, Byrd SE, Fitz CR. Face and individual cranial structures. In Silverman FN, Kuhn JP (eds). Caffey's Pediatric X-Ray Diagnosis: An Integrated Imaging Approach, pp. 75–89. St. Louis, Mosby–Year Book, 1993.
22. Mafee MF, Chow JM, Meyers R. Functional endoscopic sinus surgery: Anatomy, CT screening, indications and complications. AJR 1993;160:735–744.
23. Carpenter BLM, Merten DF. Radiographic manifestation of congenital anomalies affecting the airway. Radiol Clin North Am 1991;29:219–240.
24. Sperber GH. Early orofacial development. In Craniofacial Embryology, Dental Practitioner Handbook, 4th ed., pp. 31–57. London, Butterworth Scientific, 1989.
25. Brown OE, Pownell P, Manning SC. Choanal atresia; a new anatomic classification and clinical management applications. Laryngoscope 1996;106:97–101.
26. Brown OE, Burns DK, Smith TH, et al. Bilateral choanal atresia: A morphologic and histologic study, and computed tomographic correlation. Int J Pediatr Otorhinolaryngol 1987;13:125–142.
27. Prescott CA. Nasal obstruction in infancy. Arch Dis Child 1995;72:287–289.
28. Meyer JR, Quint DJ, Holmes JM, et al. Infected congenital mucocele of the nasolacrimal duct. AJNR 1993;14:1008–1010.
29. Peloquin L, Arcand P, Abela A. Endonasal dacryocystocele of the newborn. J Otolaryngol 1995;24:84–86.
30. Berkowitz RG, Grundfest KM, Fitz C. Nasal obstruction of the newborn revisited: Clinical and subclinical manifestations of congenital nasolacrimal duct obstruction presenting as a nasal mass. Otolaryngol Head Neck Surg 1990;103:468–471.
31. Friedman DP, Rao VM, Flanders AE. Lesions causing a mass in the medial canthus of the orbit: CT and MR features. AJR 1993;160:1095–1099.
32. Leopold DA, Hornung DE, Schwob JE. Congenital lack of olfactory ability. Ann Otol Rhinol Laryngol 1992;101:229–236.
33. Truwit CL, Barkovich AJ, Grumbach MM, et al. MR imaging of Kallman syndrome, a genetic disorder of neuronal migration affecting the olfactory and genital systems. AJNR 1993;14:827–838.
34. Barkovich AJ. Congenital malformations of the brain and skull. In Pediatric Neuroimaging, 2nd ed., pp. 177–275. Philadelphia, Lippincott-Raven, 1995.
35. Barkovich AJ, Vandermarck P, Edwards MB, et al. Congenital nasal masses: CT and MR features in 16 cases. AJNR 1991;12:105–116.
36. Naidich TP, Zimmerman RA, Bilaniuk LT. Midface: Embryology and congenital lesions. In Som PM, Curtin HD (eds). Head and Neck Imaging, pp. 3–60. St. Louis, Mosby–Year Book, 1996.
37. David DJ. Cephaloceles: Classification, pathology, and management—A review. J Craniofacial Surg 1993;4:192–202.
38. Zinrich SJ, Borders JC, Eisle DW, et al. The utility of magnetic resonance imaging in the diagnosis of intranasal meningoencephaloceles. Otolaryngol Head Neck Surg 1992;118:1253–1256.
39. Albernaz MS, Horton WD, Adkins WY, et al. Intrasphenoidal encephalocele. Otolaryngol Head Neck Surg 1991;104:279–281.
40. Zinreich SJ. Paranasal sinus imaging. Otolaryngol Head Neck Surg 1990;103:863–869.
41. Hasso AN, Lambert D. Magnetic resonance imaging of the paranasal sinuses and nasal cavities. Top Magn Reson Imaging 1994;6:209–223.
42. Rice DH. Endoscopic sinus surgery. Otolaryngol Head Neck Surg 1994;111:100–110.
43. Som PM, Curtin HD. Chronic inflammatory sinonasal diseases including fungal infections. The role of imaging. Radiol Clin North Am 1993;31:44.
44. Som PM, Curtin HD. Inflammatory lesions and tumors of the nasal cavities and paranasal sinuses with skull base involvement. Neuroimaging Clin N Am 1994;4:499–513.
45. Som PM, Brandwein M. Sinonasal cavities: Inflammatory diseases, tumors, fractures, and postoperative findings. In Som PM, Curtin

HD (eds). Head and Neck Imaging, pp. 126–315. St. Louis, Mosby–Year Book, 1996.

46. Garcia DP, Corbett ML, Eberly SM, et al. Radiographic imaging studies in pediatric chronic sinusitis. J Allergy Clin Immunol 1994;94:523–530.

47. Babbel RW, Harnsberger HR, Sonkens J, et al. Recurring patterns of sinonasal inflammatory disease demonstrated on screening sinus CT. AJNR 1992;13:903–912.

48. Melhem ER, Oliverio PJ, Benson ML et al. Optimal CT evaluation for functional endoscopic sinus surgery. AJNR 1996;17:181–188.

49. Hudgkins PA. Sinonasal imaging. Neuroimaging Clin N Am 1996;6:319–331.

50. Fireman P. Diagnosis of sinusitis in children: Emphasis on the history and physical examination. J Allergy Clin Immunol 1992;90:433–436.

51. Castillo M, Mukherji SK. Paranasal sinuses. In Castillo M, Mukherji SK (eds). Imaging of the Pediatric Head, Neck and Spine, pp. 481–515. Philadelphia, Lippincott-Raven, 1996.

52. Yousem, DM. Imaging of sinonasal inflammatory disease. Radiology 1993;188:302–314.

53. Grant A, von Schoenberg M, Grant HR, et al. Paranasal sinus disease in HIV antibody positive patients. Genitourin Med 1993;69:208–212.

54. Holliday RA. Manifestations of AIDS in the oromaxillofacial region: The role of imaging. Radiol Clin North Am 1993;31:45–60.

55. Gwaltney JM, Phillips CD, Miller RD, et al. Computed tomographic study of the common cold. N Engl J Med 1994;330:25–30.

56. Wald ER, Milmore GJ, Bowen A, et al. Acute maxillary sinusitis in children. N Engl J Med 1981;304:749–754.

57. Rak KM, Newell JD, Yakes WF, et al. Paranasal sinuses on MR images of the brain: Significance of mucosal thickening. AJR 1991;11:381–384.

58. Zinreich SJ, Kennedy DW, Kumar AJ, et al. MR imaging of normal nasal cycle; comparison with sinus pathology. J Comput Assist Tomogr 1988;12:1014–1019.

59. Diament MJ, Senac MO, Gilsanz V, et al. Prevalence of incidental paranasal sinuses opacification in pediatric patients: A CT study. J Comput Assist Tomogr 1987;11:426–431.

60. Diament MJ. The diagnosis of sinusitis in infants and children: X-ray, computed tomography, and magnetic resonance imaging. J Allergy Clin Immunol 1992;90:442–444.

61. Kuhn JP. Imaging of the paranasal sinuses: Current status. J Allergy Clin Immunol 1986;77:6–8.

62. Kovatch AL, Wald ER, Ledesma-Medina J, et al. Maxillary sinus radiographs in children with nonrespiratory complaints. Pediatrics 1984;73:306–308.

63. Lansford BK, Bower CM, Seibert RW. Invasive fungal sinusitis in the immunocompromised pediatric patient. Ear Nose Throat J 1995;74:566–573.

64. Bent JP, Kuhn FA. Diagnosis of allergic fungal sinusitis. Otolaryngol Head Neck Surg 1994;111:580–588.

65. deShazo RD, Swain RE. Diagnostic criteria for allergic fungal sinusitis. J Allergy Clin Immunol 1995;96:24–35.

66. Phillips CD, Platts-Mills TAE. Chronic sinusitis: Relationship between CT findings and clinical history of asthma, allergy, eosinophilia, and infection. AJR 1995;164:185–187.

67. Corey JP, Delsupehe KG, Ferguson BJ: Allergic fungal sinusitis: Allergic, infectious, or both? Otolaryngol Head Neck Surg 1995;113:110.

68. Hartwick RW, Batsakis JG: Sinus aspergillosis and allergic fungal sinusitis. Ann Otol Rhinol Laryngol 1991;100:427.

69. Donald PJ. Fungal infections of the sinuses. In Donald PJ, Gluckman JL, Rice DH (eds). The Sinuses, pp. 271–285. Philadelphia, Lippincott-Raven, 1995.

70. Ashdown BC, Tien RD, Felsberg GJ. Aspergillosis of the brain and paranasal sinuses in immunocompromised patients: CT and MR findings. AJR 1994;162:155–159.

71. Schuknecht B, Simmen D, Panow C, et al. Chronic fungal paranasal sinus inflammation: Radiological diagnostic concept and classification. In American Society of Head and Neck Radiology, 30th Annual Scientific Conference and Postgraduate Course, Los Angeles. Syllabus, p. 73. 1996.

72. Bolger WE, Butzin CA, Parsons DS. Paranasal sinus bony anatomic variations and mucosal abnormalities: CT analysis for endoscopic sinus surgery. Laryngoscope 1991;101:56–64.

73. Vogt-Hohenlinde CH. Topographical anatomy for sinus surgery. Acta Otolaryngol Suppl 1991;484:1–16.

74. Zinrich SJ, Kennedy DW, Rosenbaum AE, et al. Paranasal sinuses: CT imaging requirements for endoscopic surgery. Radiology 1987;163:769–775.

75. Hudgins PA, Browning DG, Gallups J, et al. Endoscopic paranasal sinus surgery; radiographic evaluation of severe complications. AJNR 1992;13:1161–1167.

76. Zinreich SJ, Benson ML, Oliverio PJ. Sinonasal cavities: CT normal anatomy, imaging of the osteomeatal complex, and functional endoscopic surgery. In Som PM, Curtin HD (eds). Head and Neck Imaging, pp. 97–125. St. Louis, Mosby–Year Book, 1996.

77. Calhoun KH, Waggenspack GA, Simpson B, et al. CT evaluation of the paranasal sinuses in symptomatic and asymptomatic populations. Otolaryngol Head Neck Surg 1991;104:480–483.

78. Hudgins PA. Complications of endoscopic sinus surgery. The role of the radiologist in prevention. Radiologic Clin North Am 1993;31:21–32.

79. Neuhaus RW. Orbital complications secondary to endoscopic sinus surgery. Ophthalmology 1990;97:1512–1518.

80. Clayman GL, Adams GL, Paugh DR, et al. Intracranial complications of paranasal sinusitis: A combined institutional review. Laryngoscope 1991;101:234–239.

81. Donald PJ. Orbital complications of sinusitis. In Donald PJ, Gluckman JL, Rice DH (eds). The Sinuses, pp. 173–189. Philadelphia, Lippincott-Raven, 1995.

82. Kendall KA, Senders CW. Orbital and intracranial complications of sinusitis in children and adults. In Gershwin ME, Incaudo GA (eds): Diseases of the Sinuses, pp. 247–271. Totowa, NJ, Humana, 1996.

83. Arjmand EM, Lusk RP, Muntz HR. Pediatric sinusitis and subperiosteal orbital abscess formation: Diagnosis and treatment. Otolaryngology Head Neck Surg 1993;109:886–894.

84. Lew D, Southwick FS, Montgomery WW, et al. Sphenoid sinusitis. N Engl J Med 1983;309:1149–1154.

85. Nemzek W, Postma G, Poirier V, et al. MR features of pachymeningitis presenting with sixth-nerve palsy secondary to sphenoid sinusitis. AJNR 1995;16:960–963.

86. Yuh WTC, Simonsen TM, Wang AM, et al. Venous sinus occlusive disease: MR findings. AJNR 1994;15:309–316.

87. Weissman JL, Tabor EK, Curtin HD. Sphenochoanal polyps: Evaluation with CT and MR imaging. Radiology 1991;178:145–148.

88. Batsakis JG, Sneige N. Choanal and angiomatous polyps of the sinonasal tract. Ann Otol Rhinol Laryngol 1992;101:623.

89. Kerrebijn JDF, Poublon RML, Overbeek SE. Nasal and paranasal disease in adult cystic fibrosis patients. Eur Res J 1992;5:1239–1242.

90. Murphy MJ. Allergy in the Clinical Office. In Donald PJ, Gluckman JL, Rice DH (eds). The Sinuses, pp. 111–122. Philadelphia, Lippincott-Raven, 1995.

91. Drutman J, Babbel RW, Harnsberger HR, et al. Sinonasal polyposis. Semin Ultrasound CT MR 1991;12:561–574.

92. Drutman J, Harnsberger HR, Babbel RW, et al. Sinonasal polyposis: Investigation by direct coronal CT. Neuroradiology 1994;36:469–472.

93. Asmus R, Koltze H, Muhle C, et al. MRI of the head in Wegener's granulomatosis. In Gross WL (ed). Associated Vasculitides, pp. 319–321. New York, Plenum, 1993.

94. Cleary KR, Batsakis JG. Sinonasal lymphomas. Ann Otol Rhinol Laryngol 1994;103:911–914.

95. Allbery SM, Chaljub G, Cho NL, et al. MR imaging of nasal masses. Radiographics 1995;15:1311–1327.

96. Andraca R, Edson RS, Kern EB. Rhinoscleroma: A growing concern in the United States? Mayo Clinic Experience. Mayo Clin Proc 1993;68:1151–1157.

97. Abou-Seif SG, Baky FA, el-Ebrashy F, et al. Scleroma of the upper respiratory passages. J Laryngol Otol 1991;105:198–202.

98. Maldjian JA, Norton KI, Groisman GM, et al. Inflammatory pseudotumor of the maxillary sinus in a 15-year old boy. AJNR 1994;15:784–786.

99. Brihaye P, Clement PAR, Dab I, et al. Pathological changes of the lateral nasal wall in patients with cystic fibrosis (mucoviscidosis). Int J Pediatr Otorhinolaryngol 1994;28:141–147.

100. Schidlow DV. Primary ciliary dyskinesia (the immotile cilia syndrome). Ann Allergy 1994;73:457–468.

101. Elster AD, Theros EG, Key LL, et al. Cranial imaging in autosomal recessive osteopetrosis. Part I. Facial bones and calvarium. Radiology 1992;183:129–135. Part II. Skull base and brain. Radiology 1992;183:137–144.

102. Applegate LJ, Applegate GR, Kemp SS. MR of multiple cranial neuropathies in a patient with Camurati-Engelmann disease: Case report. AJNR 1991;12:557–559.

103. Gandour-Edwards R. Pathology. In Donald PJ, Gluckman JL, Rice DH (eds). The Sinuses, pp. 65–82. Philadelphia, Lippincott-Raven, 1995.

104. Mafee MF. Nonepithelial tumors of the paranasal sinuses and nasal cavity. Role of CT and MR imaging. Radiol Clin North Am 1993;31:75–90.

105. Brown JH, Deluca SA. Imaging of sinonasal tumors. Am Fam Physician 1992;45:1653–1656.

106. Chow JM, Leonetti JP, Mafee M. Epithelial tumors of the paranasal sinuses and nasal cavity. Radiol Clin North Am 1993;31:61–73.

107. Gluckman JL. Tumors of the nose and paranasal sinuses. In Donald PJ, Gluckman JL, Rice DH (eds). The Sinuses, pp. 423–444. Philadelphia, Lippincott-Raven, 1995.

108. Yousem DM, Fellows DW, Kennedy DW, et al. Inverted papilloma: Evaluation with MR imaging. Radiology 1992;185:501–505.

109. Som PM, Shapiro MD, Biller HF, et al. Sinonasal tumors and inflammatory tissues: Differentiation with MR imaging. Radiology 1988;167:803–808.

110. Som PM, Dillon WP, Sze G, et al. Benign and malignant sinonasal lesions with intracranial extension: Differentiation with MR imaging. Radiology 1992;184:25–26.

111. Sigel R, Monnet O, de Baere T, et al. Adenoid cystic carcinoma of the head and neck; evaluation with MR imaging and clinical-pathologic correlation in 27 patients. Radiology 1992;184:95–101.

112. Curtin HD, Williams R. Computed tomographic anatomy of the pterygopalatine fossa. Radiographics 1985;5:429–440.

113. Hutchins LG, Harnsberger HR, Hardin CW, et al. The radiologic assessment of trigeminal neuropathy. AJNR 1989;153:1031–1038.

114. Netter FH. Atlas of Human Anatomy, Plate 39. Summit, NJ, Ciba-Geigy, 1989.

115. Nemzek, WR. The trigeminal nerve. Top Magn Reson Imaging 1996;8:132–154.

116. Diagnosis Pathologic Quiz Case 2. Pathologic diagnosis: Oncocytic schneiderian papilloma. Kaiser Foundation Research Institute, Oakland, Calif. Arch Otolaryngol Head Neck Surg 1994;120:106.

117. Gullane PJ, Davidson J, O'Dwyer T, et al. Juvenile angiofibroma: A review of the literature and a case series report. Laryngoscope 1992;102:928–933.

118. Dillon WP, Som PM, Rosenau W. Hemangioma of the nasal vault: MR and CT features. Radiology 1991;180:761–765.

119. Kapadia SB, Heffner DK. Pitfalls in the histopathologic diagnosis of pyogenic granuloma. Eur Arch Otorhinolaryngol 1992;249:195–200.

120. Kim HJ, Kim JH, Hwang EG. Bone erosion caused by sinonasal cavernous hemangioma: CT findings in two patients. AJNR 1995;16:1176–1178.

121. Enion DS, Jenkins A, Miles JB, Diengdoh JV. Intracranial extension of a naso-ethmoid schwannoma. J Laryngol Otol 1991;105:578–581.

122. Marvel JB, Parke RB. Malignant schwannoma of the nasal cavity. Otolaryngol Head Neck Surg 1990;102:410–412.

123. Buetow MP, Buetow PC, Smirniotopoulos JG. Typical, atypical, and misleading features in meningioma. Radiographics 1991;11:1087–1106.

124. Ductaman BS, Scheithauer BW, Peipgas DG, et al. Malignant peripheral nerve sheath tumor. A clinicopathologic study of 120 cases. Cancer 1986;57:2006–2021.

125. Poirier J, Gray F, Escourolle R. Manual of Basic Neuropathology, 3rd ed., pp. 32–36. Philadelphia, WB Saunders, 1990.

126. Dix JE, Marx WF, Cail WS. Neuroradiology case of the day. Meningioma. AJR 1996;167:260, 264.

127. Som PM, Sachdev VP, Sacher MM, et al. Infrafrontal sinus primary meningioma. Neuroradiology 1991;33:251–252.

128. Osborn AG. Meningiomas and other nonglial neoplasms. In Patterson AS (ed). Diagnostic Neuroradiology, pp. 579–625. St. Louis, Mosby–Year Book, 1994.

129. Iwai Y, Hakuba A, Khosla VK, et al. Giant basal cell prolactinoma extending into the nasal cavity. Surg Neurol 1992;37:280–283.

130. Langford L, Batsakis JG. Pituitary gland involvement of the sinonasal tract. Ann Otol Rhinol Laryngol 1995;104:167–169.

131. Earwaker J. Paranasal sinus osteomas: A review of 46 cases. Skeletal Radiol 1993;22:417–423.

132. Weber AL, Scrivani SJ. Mandible: Anatomy, cysts, tumors, and nontumorous lesions. In Som PM, Curtin HD (eds). Head and Neck Imaging, pp. 319–349. St. Louis, Mosby–Year Book, 1996.

133. Ueno H, Ariji E, Tanaka T, et al. Imaging features of maxillary osteoblastoma and its malignant transformation. Skeletal Radiol 1994;23:509–512.

134. Mafee MF. Fibrooseous lesions of the paranasal sinuses. In American Society of Head and Neck Radiology 30th Annual Course Syllabus, pp. 95–99, 1996.

135. Crim JR, Mirra JM, Eckardt JJ, et al. Widespread inflammatory response to osteoblastoma: The flare phenomenon. Radiology 1990;177:835–836.

136. Camilleri AE. Craniofacial fibrous dysplasia. J Laryngol Otol 1991;105:662.

137. Ruggieri P, Sim FH, Bond JR, Unni KK. Malignancies in fibrous dysplasia. Cancer 1994;73:1411.

138. Barnes L, Verbin RS, Gnepp DR. Diseases of the nose, paranasal sinuses, and nasopharynx. In Barnes L (ed). Surgical Pathology of the Head and Neck, Vol. 1, pp. 883–1044. New York, Marcel Dekker, 1985.

139. Marvel JB, Marsh MA, Catlin FI. Ossifying fibroma of the midface and paranasal sinuses: Diagnostic and therapeutic considerations. Otolaryngol Head Neck Surg 1991;104:803–808.

140. Han MH, Chang KE, Lee CH, et al. Cystic expansile masses of the maxilla: Differential diagnosis with CT and MR. AJNR 1995;16:333–338.

141. Weber AL. Imaging of cysts and odontogenic tumors of the jaw. Radiol Clin North Am 1993;31:101–120.

142. Jones RO, Pillsbury HC. Histiocytosis X of the head and neck. Laryngoscope 1984;94:1031–1035.

143. Appling D, Jenkins HA, Patton GA. Eosinophilic granuloma in the temporal bone and skull. Otolaryngol Head Neck Surg 1983;91:358–365.

144. Lo WM, Solti-Bohman LG. Tumors of the temporal bone and the cerebellopontine angle. In Som PM, Curtin HD (eds). Head and Neck Imaging, pp. 1449–1534. St. Louis, Mosby–Year Book, 1996.

145. Beahrs OH, Henson DE, Hutter RPV, Kennedy BJ (eds). American Joint Committee on Cancer, Manual for Staging of Cancer, 4th ed. pp. 45–48. Philadelphia, JB Lippincott, 1992.

146. Frierson HF, Mills SE, Fechner RE, et al. Sinonasal undifferentiated carcinoma. An aggressive neoplasm derived from schneiderian epithelium and distinct from olfactory neuroblastoma. Am J Surg Pathol 1986;10:771.

147. Deutsch BD, Levine PA, Stewart FM, et al. Sinonasal undifferentiated carcinoma: A ray of hope. Otolaryngol Head Neck Surg 1993;108:697.

148. Conley J, Casler JD. Adenoid Cystic Carcinoma of the Head and Neck. New York, Thieme Medical, 1991.

149. Curtin HD, Williams R, Johnson J. CT of perineural tumor extension: Pterygopalatine fossa. AJNR 1984;5:731–737.

150. Laine FJ, Braun IF, Jensen ME, et al. Perineural tumor extension through the foramen ovale: Evaluation with MR imaging. Radiology 1990;174:65–71.

151. Parker GD, Harnsberger RH. Clinical-radiologic issues in perineural tumor spread of malignant diseases of the extracranial head and neck. Radiographics 1991;11:383–399.

152. Osborn DA. Morphology and the natural history of cribriform adenocarcinoma (adenoid cystic carcinoma). J Clin Pathol 1977;30:195.

153. Kim KH, Sung MW, Chung PS, et al. Adenoid cystic carcinoma of the head and neck. Arch Otolaryngol Head Neck Surg 1994;120:721–726.

154. Perzin KH, Gullane P, Clairmont AC. Adenoid cystic carcinoma arising in salivary glands: A correlation of histologic features and clinical course. Cancer 1978;42:265.

155. Spiro RH, Huvos AG, Strong EW. Adenoid cystic carcinoma of salivary gland origin. Am J Surg 1974;128:512.

156. Suei Y, Tanimoto K, Taguchi A, et al. Radiographic evaluation of bone invasion of adenoid cystic carcinoma in the oral and maxillofacial region. J Oral Maxillofac Surg 1994;52:821–826.

157. Gnepp DR, Heffner DK. Mucosal origin of sinonasal tract adenomatous neoplasms. Mod Pathol 1989;2:365.

158. Barnes L. Intestinal type adenocarcinoma of the nasal cavity and paranasal sinuses. Am J Surg Pathol 1986;10:192.

159. Hyams VJ, Batsakis JG, Michaels L. Tumors of the upper respiratory tract and ear. In Atlas of Tumor Pathology, 2nd Ser., Fasc. 25, pp. 248–251. Washington, DC, AFIP, 1988.

160. Stern SJ, Guillamondegui OM. Mucosal melanoma of the head and neck. Head Neck 1991;13:22.

161. Lee SP, Shimizu KT, Tran LM, et al. Mucosal melanoma of the head and neck: The impact of local control on survival. Laryngoscope 1994;104:121.

162. Crowley JJ, Lupetin AR, Wang SE. Primary nasal amelanotic melanoma: MR appearance. J Magn Reson Imaging 1991;1:601–604.

163. Isiklar I, Leeds NE, Fuller GN, et al. Intracranial metastatic melanoma. Correlation between MR imaging characteristics and melanin content. AJR 1995;165:1503–1512.

164. Derdeyn CP, Moran CJ, Wippold FJ, et al. MRI of esthesioneuroblastoma. J Comput Assist Tomogr 1994;18:16–21.

165. Li C, Yousem DM, Hayden RE, et al. Olfactory neuroblastoma: MR evaluation. AJNR 1993;14:1167–1171.

166. Lloyd GAS, Phelps PD, Michaels L. The imaging characteristics of naso-sinus chondrosarcoma. Clin Radiol 1992;46:189–192.

167. Garrington GE, Scofield HH, Cornyn J, Hooker SP. Osteosarcoma of the jaws. Cancer 1967;20:377.

168. Caron AS, Hajdu SI, Strong EW. Osteogenic sarcoma of the facial and cranial bones. Am J Surg 1971;122:719.

169. Mark RJ, Bailet JW, Tran LM, et al. Dermatofibrosarcoma protuberans of the head and neck. A report of 16 cases. Arch Otolaryngol Head Neck Surg 1993;119:891–896.

170. Laskin WB. Dermatofibrosarcoma protuberans. CA Cancer J Clin 1992;42:116–125.

171. Wenig BM. Neoplasms of the nasal cavity and paranasal sinuses. In Atlas of Head and Neck Pathology, pp. 29–95. Philadelphia, WB Saunders, 1993.

172. Compagno J, Hyams VJ. Hemangiopericytoma-like intranasal tumors. Am J Clin Pathol 1976;66:672.

173. Compagno J. Hemangiopericytoma-like tumors of the nasal cavity: A comparison with hemangiopericytoma of soft tissues. J Laryngol 1978;88:460.

174. Millman B, Brett D, Vrabec DP. Sinonasal hemangiopericytoma. Ear Nose Throat J 1994;73:680–687.

175. Eichorn JH, Dickersin GR, Bhan AK, Goodman ML. Sinonasal hemangiopericytoma: A reassessment with electron microscopy, immunohistochemistry, and long-term follow-up. Am J Surg Pathol 1990;14:856.

176. Han MH, Chang KH, Kim IO, et al. Non-Hodgkin lymphoma of the central skull base: MR manifestations. J Comput Assist Tomogr 1993;17:567–571.

177. Ferry JA, Sklar J, Zukerberg LR, Harris NL. Nasal lymphoma. A clinicopathologic study with immunophenotypic and genotypic analysis. Am J Surg Pathol 1991;15:268.

178. Campo E, Cardesa A, Alos L, et al. Non-Hodgkin's lymphomas of nasal cavity and paranasal sinuses. An immunohistochemical study. Am J Clin Pathol 1991;96:184.

179. Kanavaros P, Lescs MC, Briere J, et al. T-cell lymphoma: A clinicopathologic entity associated with peculiar phenotype and with Epstein-Barr virus. Blood 1993;81:2688.

180. Liang R, Todd D, Chan TK, et al. Nasal lymphoma. A retrospective analysis of 60 cases. Cancer 1990;66:2205.

181. Ho FC, Choy D, Loke SL, et al. Polymorphic reticulosis and conventional lymphomas of the nose and upper aerodigestive tract: A clinicopathologic study of 70 cases, and immunophenotypic studies of 16 cases. Hum Pathol 1990;21:1041.

182. Kikuchi K, Kowanda M, Sasaki J, et al. Large pituitary adenoma of the sphenoid sinus and the nasopharynx: Report of a case with ultrastructural evaluations. Surg Neurol 1994;42:330–334.

183. Wax MK, Yun KJ, Omar RA. Extramedullary plasmacytomas of the head and neck. Otolaryngol Head Neck Surg 1993;109:877–885.

184. Kapadia SB, Desai U, Cheng VS. Extramedullary plasmacytoma of the head and neck. A clinicopathologic study of 20 cases. Medicine 1982;61:317.

185. Norris CM. Case records of the Massachusetts General Hospital. Weekly clinicopathological exercises. Case 21-1992. A 65 year old man with a mass that involved the base of the skull. New Engl J Med 1992;326:1417–1424.

186. Vogl TJ, Steger W, Grevers G, et al. MR characteristics of primary extramedullary plasmacytoma in the head and neck. AJNR 1996;17:1349–1354.

187. Delbalso AM, Hall RE, Margarone JE. Radiographic evaluation of maxillofacial trauma. In Delbalso AM (ed). Maxillofacial Imaging, pp. 35–126. Philadelphia, WB Saunders, 1990.

188. Som PM, Curtin HD. Head and Neck Imaging, 3rd ed., pp. 263–286, 1294–1296. St. Louis, Mosby–Year Book, 1996.

189. Gentry LR. Diagnostic evaluation of facial trauma: Current perspectives. In Harnsberger HR, Curtin HD (eds). 26th Annual Conference and Postgraduate Course, Vancouver, BC. Syllabus, pp. 149–155. American Society of Neuroradiology, 1993.

190. LeFort R. Étude sur les fractures de la machoire superieur. Rev Chir 1901;23:208–227, 360–379, 479–507.

191. Schwenzer N, Kruger E. Midface fracture. In Kruger E, Schilli W, Worthington P (eds). Oral and Maxillofacial Traumatology, Vol 2, pp. 107–136. Chicago, Quintessence, 1986.

192. Rowe NL, Williams JL (eds). Maxillofacial Injuries, Vol. 1, pp. 363–558. Edinburgh, Churchill Livingstone, 1985.

193. Noyek A, Kassel EE, Wortzman G, et al. Contemporary radiologic evaluation in maxillofacial trauma. Otolaryngol Clin North Am 1983;16:473–508.

194. Duval AJ, Banovetz JD. Nasoethmoid fractures. Otolaryngol Clin North Am 1976;9:507–515.

195. Mallen RW. Fractures of the nasofrontal complex. Otolaryngol Clin North Am 1969;2:335–361.

196. Gozum G. Blow-out fractures of the orbit. Otolaryngol Clin North Am 1976;9:477–487.

197. Smith B, Regan WF. Blow-out fractures of the orbit: Mechanism and correction of internal orbital fracture. Am J Ophthalmol 1957;55:733–739.

198. Ball JB. Direct oblique sagittal CT of orbital wall fractures. AJR 1987;148:601–607.

199. Dolan KD, Jacoby CG. Facial fractures. Semin Roentgenol 1978;13:37–51.

200. Johnson DH. CT of maxillofacial trauma. Radiol Clin North Am 1984;22:131–143.

201. Zilkha A. Computed tomography of the blow-out fracture of the medial orbital wall. AJR 1981;137:963–965.

202. Brown OL, Longacre JI, DeStefano GA, et al. Roentgen manifestations of blow-out fractures of the orbit. Radiology 1965;85:908–913.

203. Curtin HD, Wolfe P, Schramm W. Orbital roof blow-out fractures. AJR 1982;139:969–972.

204. McLachlan DL, Flanagan JC, Shannon GM. Complication of orbital roof fractures. Ophthalmology 1982;89:1274–1278.

205. Vinik M, Gargano FP. Orbital fractures. Radiology 1966;97:607–613.

206. Schultz RC. Supraorbital and glabellar fractures. Plast Reconstr Surg 1970;45:227–233.

207. Schockley WW, Stucker FJ Jr, Gage-White L, et al. Frontal sinus fractures: Some problems and some solutions. Laryngoscope 1988;98:18–22.

208. Yanagisawa E. Symposium on maxillofacial trauma. III. Pitfalls in the management of zygomatic fractures. Laryngoscope 1973;83:527–546.

209. Creamer MJ, Blendonophy P, Katz R, Russell E. Coronal computerized tomography and cerebrospinal fluid rhinorrhea. Arch Phys Med Rehab 1992;73:599–602.

210. Morgan BDG, Madan DK, Bergerot JPC. Fractures of the middle third of the face: A review of 300 cases. Br J Plast Surg 1972;25:147.

211. Gammal TE, Brooks BS. MR cisternography: Initial experience in 41 cases. AJNR 1994;15:1647–1656.

212. Bell AF, Ivan DJ, Munson RA. Barosinus pneumocele: Transient visual loss due to sphenoid sinus pneumocele in a U.S. Air Force pilot. Aviat Space Environ Med 1995;66:276–279.

213. Benedikt RA, Brown DC, Roth MK, et al. Spontaneous drainage of an ethmoidal mucocele: A possible cause of pneumosinus dilatans. AJNR 1991;12:729–731.

214. Dross PE, Lally JF, Bonier B. Pneumosinus dilatans and arachnoid cyst: A unique association. AJNR 1992;13:209–211.

215. Kulwin DR, Kersten RC. Orbital decompression for dysthyroid optic neuropathy. In Donald PJ, Gluckman JL, Rice DH. The Sinuses, pp. 563–561. Philadelphia, Lippincott-Raven, 1995.

C H A P T E R

32

Pharynx and Oral Cavity

S U R E S H   K .   M U K H E R J I ,   M.D.

J A N E   W E I S S M A N ,   M.D.

NORMAL ANATOMY

The pharynx consists of a muscular conduit that extends from the skull base to the esophageal verge and is typically subdivided into three distinct regions: nasopharynx, oropharynx, and hypopharynx.[1, 2] The nasopharynx extends from the skull base to the soft palate and is continuous with the oropharynx, which is located between the soft palate and the base of the vallecula. The hypopharynx extends from the base of the vallecula to the undersurface of the cricoid cartilage. On imaging studies, the hyoid bone serves as a good marker for the transition between the oropharynx and hypopharynx. The pharynx is formed by a variety of overlapping musculatures. The nasopharynx and oropharynx are formed by the superior constrictor muscle, which attaches to the caudal aspect of the medial pterygoid muscle; pterygomandibular raphe; posterior portion of the mylohyoid line of the mandible; and lateral aspect of the tongue base. The middle constrictor muscle, which forms the majority of the hypopharynx, is fan-shaped and originates from the cornua of the hyoid bone and inferior portion of the stylohyoid ligament. The inferior constrictor muscle arises from the lateral surfaces of the thyroid and cricoid cartilages. The fibers extend from the cricoid cartilage to the pharynx and form the cricopharyngeus muscle. The fibers also demarcate an area known as the *esophageal verge* that separates the hypopharynx from the cervical esophagus.

Nasopharynx

The nasopharynx constitutes the superior portion of the pharynx. Its primary function is respiratory. The roof of the nasopharynx is formed by the basisphenoid, basiocciput, and first two cervical vertebrae.[1, 3] The floor is formed by the soft palate and the ridge of pharyngeal musculature that the soft palate opposes when it is tensed (Passavant's ridge). The lateral walls are formed by the lateral continuation of the superior constrictor muscle.[1, 3] The posterior border of the nasopharynx is complex and consists of various structures that constitute the characteristic surface anatomy present on cross-sectional imaging (Fig. 32–1). Posteriorly, the nasopharynx is in direct communication with the middle ear cavity via the eustachian tubes, which

are located along the posterolateral wall of the nasopharynx.[3, 4] Just posterior to the orifice of the eustachian tube is the cartilaginous protuberance of the torus tubarius. Posterior and superior to the torus tubarius is a mucosal reflection that overlies the lateral aspect of the longus coli and longus capitis muscles known as the *lateral pharyngeal recess* (fossa of Rosenmüller).

The nasopharynx is surrounded by the buccopharyngeal fascia (visceral fascia) that maintains patency of the airway. This fascia denotes the components of the visceral space (pharyngeal mucosal space) and separates visceral space from the deep fascial spaces. The visceral fascia is also felt to be a barrier to the deep spread of early malignancies.[3, 5, 6] Several small muscles take a portion of their origin from the eustachian tube and are important

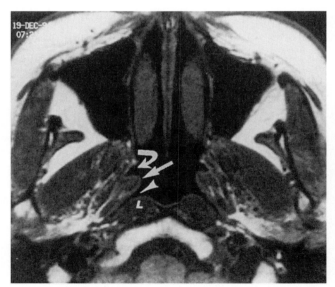

FIGURE 32–1 Axial T1-weighted magnetic resonance imaging (MRI) study shows the normal superficial landmarks of the nasopharynx. *Curved arrow,* Eustachian tube opening; *straight arrow,* torus tubarius; *arrowhead,* fossa of Rosenmüller (lateral pharyngeal recess); L, longus coli muscle. (From Mukherji SK, Weissman JL, Holliday RA. Pharynx. In Som PM, Curtin HD [eds]. Head and Neck Imaging, 3rd ed., p. 441. St. Louis, Mosby–Year Book, 1995.)

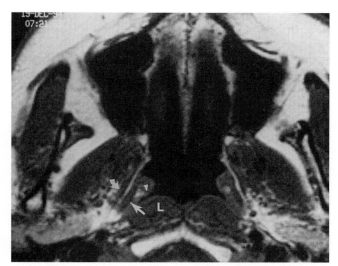

FIGURE 32–2 Axial T1-weighted MRI study illustrates the normal appearance of the deep muscles of the nasopharynx. *Curved arrow,* tensor veli palatini; *straight arrow,* levator veli palatini; *arrowhead,* salpingopharyngeus; L, longus coli. (From Mukherji SK, Weissman JL, Holliday RA. Pharynx. In Som PM, Curtin HD [eds]. Head and Neck Imaging, 3rd ed., p. 441. St. Louis, Mosby–Year Book, 1995.)

potential pathways of tumor spread for malignancies arising within the nasopharynx (Fig. 32–2).[3, 5, 6] The levator veli palatini is a cylindrical muscle supplied by the pharyngeal plexus from fibers of the ninth cranial nerve. This muscle arises from the cartilaginous portion of the eustachian tube and petrous portion of the temporal bone and inserts into the aponeurosis of the soft palate; it elevates the soft palate. The tensor veli palatini is located just lateral to the levator palatini muscle and is innervated by the third division of the trigeminal nerve. Its origin is from the lateral aspect of the eustachian tube, spine of the sphenoid bone, and base of the medial pterygoid process. This muscle hooks around the hamulus of the medial pterygoid muscle and attaches to the lateral aspect of the palatine aponeurosis. It acts to tense the soft palate.[1] A third muscle, the salpingopharyngeus, is thin and arises from the distal aspect of the cartilaginous portion of the eustachian tube and descends into the lateral wall of the pharynx.[1] Because of its size, this muscle is difficult to visualize with magnetic resonance imaging (MRI). All three muscles act to open the eustachian tube during swallowing in order to equilibrate pressure between the pharynx and middle ear cavities. Because of the location of the eustachian tube opening, nasopharyngeal cancer may result in eustachian tube dysfunction with resultant serous otitis media.[3, 4, 6]

An extensive lymphatic plexus drains the nasopharynx and explains the high incidence of cervical nodal metastases associated with nasopharygeal carcinoma.[3, 6] The primary eschelon drainage is to the retropharyngeal nodes and jugulodigastric nodes (group II). However, inconstant lymphatic vessels that pass directly to the spinal accessory and midjugular nodes explain the occasional isolated involvement of these nodal groups.[3, 7]

Oropharynx

The oropharynx consists of the oropharynx proper (pharyngeal constrictor muscles, surrounding mucosa, and lymphoid tissue at the base of the tongue) and the palatine arch complex (oral surface of the soft palate and anterior tonsillar pillars) (Figs. 32–3 through 32–5). The anterior margin is made up of a plane formed by the posterior border of the soft palate, anterior tonsillar pillar, and the circumvallate papilla. The posterior border of the oropharynx is formed by the posterior pharyngeal wall. The lateral margins consist of the tonsils. The tonsils are divided into the anterior tonsillar pillar (palatoglossus muscle), posterior tonsillar pillar (palatopharyngeus muscle), and the lymphoid tissue containing fossa between these two pillars, the palatine (faucial) tonsil. The tonsils and faucial pillars have a similar computed tomography (CT) density,[8, 9] appearing as bilateral symmetric soft tissue densities on either side of the airway. These lymphoid structures are prominent features on MRI studies. They are slightly more intense than muscle on T1-weighted images and increase in signal intensity on T2-weighted images.[10] Tonsils are more prominent in children and young adults; they diminish in size with age and after radiation therapy. Occasionally, dystrophic calcification from previous infections is present on CT scans within the tonsillar beds.

Hypopharynx

The hypopharynx (laryngopharynx) is the portion of the upper aerodigestive tract that extends from the hyoid bone superiorly and to the inferior aspect of the cricoid cartilage inferiorly.[11, 12] Above the hyoid bone is the oro-

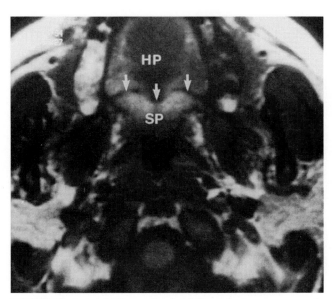

FIGURE 32–3 Axial T1-weighted MRI study demonstrates the normal MRI appearance of the soft palate (SP), the mucosa on the oral surface of the hard palate (HP), and the bony margin at the dorsal aspect of the hard palate *(arrows).* (From Mukherji SK, Weissman JL, Holliday RA. Pharynx. In Som PM, Curtin HD [eds]. Head and Neck Imaging, 3rd ed., p. 442. St. Louis, Mosby–Year Book, 1995.)

pharynx. Below the cricoid cartilage, the hypopharynx becomes the cervical esophagus. Most authors divide the hypopharynx into three regions: the posterior pharyngeal wall (Fig. 32–6), the piriform sinuses (Fig. 32–7), and the postcricoid region (Fig. 32–8).[11–13] Some authors also refer to a fourth or "marginal" area that consists of the lateral pharyngeal wall.

The posterior wall of the hypopharynx starts at the level of the valleculae.[13] Above this, the posterior wall is continuous with the posterior wall of the oropharynx and extends inferiorly to the level of the postcricoid region.

The piriform (pear-shaped) sinus is a lateral recess created by the aryepiglottic fold. There are two piriform sinuses, each with an anterior wall, a medial wall, and a lateral wall.[11] The lowest part of each piriform sinus, called the *apex*, lies at the level of the true vocal cords (see Fig. 32–7). The paired aryepiglottic folds make up the medial walls of the piriform sinuses. The two piriform sinuses merge posteriorly at the level of the cricoid cartilage to form the postcricoid region.

The postcricoid region, also called the *pharyngoesophageal junction,* is the portion of the hypopharynx situated posterior to the cricoid cartilage (see Fig. 32–8).[11–13] This portion of the pharynx allows passage of food from the piriform sinus into the cervical esophagus. The postcricoid hypopharynx abuts the posterior ring of the cricoid cartilage and the arytenoid cartilages.[11] The anterior wall of the postcricoid region is also the posterior

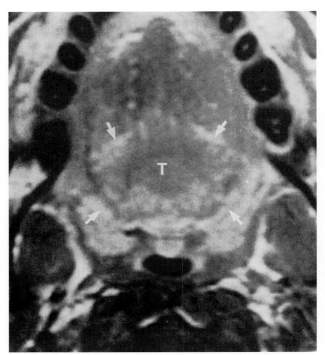

FIGURE 32–5 Axial T1-weighted MRI study shows the normal appearance of the tongue base (T). Note the fat planes surrounding the tongue base *(arrows)*, which are well visualized with MRI. (From Mukherji SK, Weissman JL, Holliday RA. Pharynx. In Som PM, Curtin HD [eds]. Head and Neck Imaging, 3rd ed., p. 443. St. Louis, Mosby–Year Book, 1995.)

wall of the lower larynx. This common wall is sometimes referred to as the *party wall*. The transition from the postcricoid region can be separated from the cervical esophagus by noticing the transition from the relatively flat postcricoid region to the rounded appearance of the cervical esophagus. At this junction, the inferior constrictor muscle is incomplete posteriorly and represents the common location for the origin of a Zenker diverticulum.

The nervous supply of the hypopharynx is from the pharyngeal plexus of nerves that receive contributions from the glossopharyngeal (cranial nerve IX) and vagus (cranial nerve X) nerves. The vagus nerve supplies motor innervation to the constrictors.[14] Sensory information from the hypopharynx travels along the glossopharyngeal nerve[14] and the internal laryngeal branch of the superior laryngeal nerve, which arises from the vagus nerve.[11]

Lymphatic drainage of the hypopharynx is extensive. The piriform sinuses are drained by a network of lymphatics,[13] most of which drain primarily to the upper jugular and midjugular nodes, posterior cervical nodes, and retropharyngeal lymph nodes.[11] Lymphatics of the posterior wall of the hypopharynx drain to the jugular nodes as well as retropharyngeal nodes.[13] Postcricoid lymphatics drain to the midjugular and lower jugular nodes,[14] as well as to paratracheal nodes.[14]

Oral Cavity

The oral cavity is separated from the oropharynx by a plane that is formed by the soft palate, anterior tonsillar

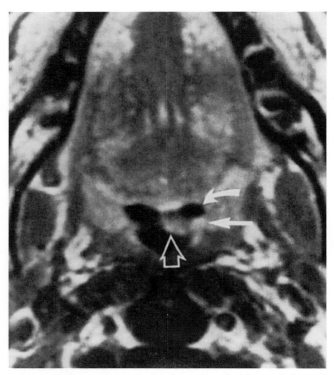

FIGURE 32–4 Axial T1-weighted MRI study obtained through the oropharynx demonstrates the region of the anterior tonsillar pillar *(curved arrow)* and posterior tonsillar pillar *(solid arrow)*. The tip of the uvula is indicated by the *open arrow*. (From Mukherji SK, Weissman JL, Holliday RA. Pharynx. In Som PM, Curtin HD [eds]. Head and Neck Imaging, 3rd ed., p. 443. St. Louis, Mosby–Year Book, 1995.)

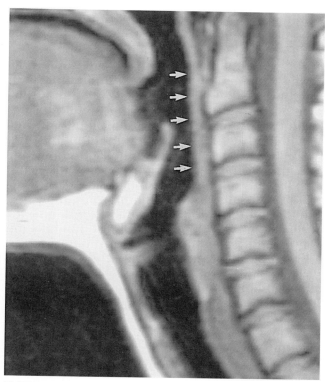

FIGURE 32–6 Sagittal T1-weighted image illustrates the normal appearance of the posterior pharyngeal wall *(arrows)*.

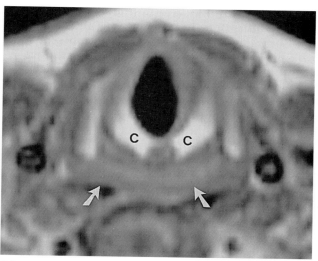

FIGURE 32–8 Axial T1-weighted image obtained at the level of the cricoid cartilage (C) shows the normal appearance of the postcricoid region *(arrows)*.

pillars, and circumvallate papilla. The contents of the oral cavity include the oral tongue, floor of the mouth, gingiva, gingivobuccal and buccomaseteric regions, hard palate, and mandible.[15, 16] The oral tongue is separated from the tongue base by the circumvallate papilla..

The oral tongue (Fig. 32–9) is a mobile muscular structure that consists of mobile symmetric halves separated by a midline septum. The oral tongue is composed of muscular fibers that are arranged in various orienta-

tions and can be separated into intrinsic and extrinsic muscles. The intrinsic muscles are iterdigitating muscles that are difficult to identify individually on imaging studies. These muscles include the superior and inferior longitudinal, the transverse, and the vertical or oblique muscle groups. The extrinsic muscle group forms the foundation of the tongue and anchors the oral tongue to adjacent structures. Their names are derived from their areas of insertion and origin (genioglossus, geniohyoid, hyoglossus, and styloglossus muscles).[16, 17]

The floor of mouth is a U-shaped area, bordered inferiorly by the mylohyoid muscle, laterally by the gingiva overlying the lingual surface of the mandible, superiorly

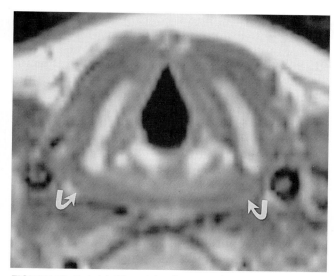

FIGURE 32–7 Axial T1-weighted image shows the normal appearance of the apex of the piriform sinuses *(arrows)*.

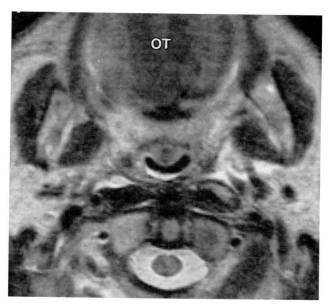

FIGURE 32–9 Axial T1-weighted image obtained through the oral cavity demonstrates the normal appearance of the oral tongue (OT).

by the oral tongue, and posteriorly at the insertion of the anterior tonsillar pillar into the tongue.[15] The submandibular and sublingual spaces are two important landmarks located in the region of the floor of the mouth.[18] These two spaces are separated by the mylohyoid muscle. The submandibular spaces are situated lateral and inferior to the mylohyoid muscle and contain the submandibular glands, lymph nodes, and areolar tissues. The floor of the mouth proper is contained within the sling formed by the mylohyoid muscle. The paired genioglossus and geniohyoid muscles form the midline musculature of the floor of the mouth. The lingual septum of the oral tongue extends inferiorly into the floor of the mouth and separates the two paired genioglossus and geniohyoid muscles. Because these muscles directly overlay each other, they are often difficult to separate on axial CT images and are often referred to as the *geniohyoid-genioglossus complex*.[16]

The sublingual space is bounded laterally by the mylohyoid muscle and medially by the geniohyoid–genioglossus muscle complex. The contents of the sublingual space include the sublingual salivary gland, submandibular duct (Wharton's duct), hyoglossus muscle, fat, lymph nodes, lingual and hypoglossal nerve, and lingual artery. The sublingual glands and surrounding fat are of low attenuation on CT and easily separated from the adjacent muscular structures that are of soft tissue attenuation. The hyoglossus muscle is a small strip of muscle located within the posterior aspect of the sublingual space and has a configuration similar to that of the mylohyoid muscle on axial CT images. The neurovascular supply for the oral tongue and the floor of the mouth is provided by the lingual and hypoglossal nerves and the lingual artery, all of which normally course through the floor of the mouth (Fig. 32–10).[15]

On contrast-enhanced CT, the lingual artery and its proximal branches are normally visualized between the mylohyoid and geniohyoid–genioglossus muscle complex. On CT, this artery is normally surrounded by the low-attenuation tissue present within the sublingual space formed by the sublingual glands and adjacent fat. The lingual and hypoglossal nerves are not visible on CT; however, their positions can be predicted based on an understanding of their anatomic relationships to adjacent structures.[15, 19] The lingual artery and hypoglossal nerve lie medial to the hyoglossus muscle, whereas the lingual nerve lies lateral to this muscle. Anterior to the free margin of the hyoglossus muscle, these three neurovascular structures are closely situated to one another as they course through the sublingual space supplying the oral tongue and the floor of the mouth (Fig. 32–10).[19]

IMAGING TECHNIQUE

Computed Tomography

With CT, the pharynx and oral cavity are best examined with the patient supine and the sections made parallel to the infraorbital-meatal line. The head should be carefully positioned. A localizing lateral scout image should be obtained to avoid artifacts from dental hardware. Imaging should be performed from the skull base to the thoracic inlet (field of view 16 to 18 cm) in order to evaluate for

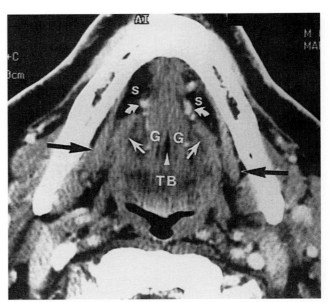

FIGURE 32–10 Axial contrast-enhanced computed tomography (CT) scan illustrates the normal anatomy of the floor of the mouth. *Black arrows*, mylohyoid muscle; *straight white arrows*, hyoglossus muscle; *curved arrows*, lingual vasculature; *arrowhead*, lingual septum; S, low-attenuation area in the sublingual space that may represent fat or the sublingual gland; TB, tongue base; G, paired muscles that compose the genioglossus-geniohyoid complex. (From Mukherji SK, Weeks S, Castillo M, Krishnan LA. Squamous cell carcinomas that arise in the oral cavity and tongue base: Can CT help predict perineural or vascular invasion? Radiology 1996;198:157–162.)

cervical nodal metastases. If the pathologic lesion extends beyond the nasopharynx or if cervical adenopathy is to be assessed, the scan is continued to encompass the full extent of disease. Direct coronal and axial scans should be performed in any patient suspected of having a nasopharyngeal, palatine, or skull base mass.

The pharynx should be studied during suspended respiration. Proper gantry angulation is essential in the oropharynx to avoid dental-related artifacts. Sections that are parallel to the ramus of the mandible should be obtained from the top of the mandibular alveolar ridge to the hyoid bone. This plane or section is usually suitable for surveying the neck. If the larynx and hypopharynx are to be studied in detail, sections must be parallel to the true vocal cords in that portion of the study.

Scans should be contiguous, with a slice thickness of 3 mm or less, and the field of view should be kept as small as possible while still including all essential anatomic areas of interest. Algorithms optimizing bone detail are essential to evaluate pathologic bone conditions. Three-millimeter-thick contiguous sections should be performed through the area of interest. Three-millimeter-thick sections obtained at 5-mm increments should be performed for nodal evaluation. Bone algorithms are required for lesions that abut the skull base or involve the palate or retromolar trigone.

All studies should be performed with intravenous contrast material. Vascular opacification is necessary in order to separate vessels from adjacent lymph nodes. Contrast material should be administered using a power injector. When it is properly administered, adequate vascular opacification should be obtained with 100 to 150 ml of contrast material. We recommend a loading contrast bolus of 50 ml administered at 2 ml/sec. The remainder of the contrast material may be given with intermittent power-injected boluses of 15 to 20 ml.[20]

Magnetic Resonance Imaging

MRI studies of the nasopharynx and oropharynx are obtained with the routine head coil. The floor of the mouth also can often be imaged with this coil, depending on the habitus of the patient. Studies of the neck should use a dedicated neck coil.

A detailed patient history is extremely beneficial for acquiring high-quality imaging studies. Knowledge of the proper location of the lesion allows focusing of the study to the proper area, thereby eliminating unnecessary imaging and reducing overall imaging time. The shorter imaging time also reduces the likelihood of studies being degraded by motion artifact.

The use of intravenous paramagnetic contrast material is essential for evaluating patients with malignancies of the oropharynx and nasopharynx. When the use of an MRI contrast agent is contemplated, it is helpful to acquire a noncontrast T1-weighted sequence in the same plane as the contrast sequence so as not to confuse either high-signal-intensity fat or proteinaceous fluid with an area of enhancement.

MRI studies of the oropharynx, hypopharynx, and oral cavity are performed primarily in the axial plane. Noncontrast T1-weighted coronal images should be performed in patients with nasopharyngeal carcinoma to evaluate for evidence of skull base invasion. Contrast-enhanced T1-weighted images should also be obtained to evaluate for perineural spread of tumor along the mandibular division of the trigeminal nerve and the potential for extension into the cavernous sinus.[20]

CONGENITAL AND DEVELOPMENTAL LESIONS

Dermoid Cyst

The term *dermoid cyst* (DC) is inclusive and used to identify a variety of lesions arising in the extracranial head and neck. The various lesions encompassed by calling a lesion a DC include epidermoid, dermoid, and teratoid cysts. About 7% of DCs occur in the head and neck region. The majority of these lesions (65%) occur in orbital and nasal regions, whereas 24% arise in the oral cavity. DCs are felt to be present from infancy; however, the epidermoid variety usually present at birth, whereas the true dermoid lesion is usually not identified until the second or third decade of life. There is no reported sex predominance for DC.[21]

Histologically, the various lesions denoted under the term *dermoid cyst* are distinct. The epidermoid cyst, which is the most common of these lesions, is encapsulated by a fibrous wall lined by simple squamous epithelium. There are no adnexal structures present within the

wall. The true dermoid cyst is an epithelial-lined cavity that contains a variety of mesodermally derived structures including hair, sebaceous glands, and fat. A teratoid cyst is the least common of these lesions. The lining of these lesions varies from simple stratified squamous epithelium to respiratory-like ciliated epithelium. All these lesions typically contain within the cystic cavity a cheesy keratinaceous material, which may have a high protein content.[21, 22]

Two main theories are used to explain the embryogenesis of DCs. One is that DCs arise from epithelium that has been trapped in an unusual location due to traumatic implantation or some form of anomalous development. Some investigators suggest there is trapping of ectodermal elements during the formation of the tongue and floor of the mouth during fusion of the lateral processes of the mandible and tuberculum impar. A second theory suggests that DCs represent heterotopias or choristomatic cysts.[21, 22]

Oral cavity DCs typically arise in the region of the floor of the mouth and are usually midline lesions; however, it is not uncommon for large lesions to lateralize to one side. Occasionally, DCs may be located on the dorsum of the tongue and hard or soft palate. The clinical presentation usually depends on the location with respect to the mylohyoid muscle. Sublingual DCs centered above the mylohyoid muscle present as a submucosal lesion in the floor of mouth. Because these lesions may elevate the tongue and interfere with glutination, they may be confused clinically with a ranula. Submental DCs are centered below the mylohyoid muscle and typically present as an external swelling situated just above the hyoid bone. Occasionally, these lesions may extend as low as the thoracic inlet.[23]

On physical examination, these lesions tend to have a doughy texture and may demonstrate pitting after palpation. Because these lesions are not fixed to the tongue or hyoid bone, they (unlike thyroglossal duct cysts) do not move when the tongue is protruded.[21]

The treatment of DC is surgical excision with the specific approach based, in part, on the position of the lesion with respect to the mylohyoid muscle. Lesions situated above the mylohyoid may be best resected by an intraoral approach, whereas those located inferior to the mylohyoid would best benefit from a direct cervical approach.[21]

Both CT and MRI may be used to evaluate patients with DC tumors. These lesions typically present as cystic midline lesions located within the floor of the mouth. On CT, the presence of fat within the lesion is pathognomonic of a true dermoid cyst. These lesions are usually sharply demarcated and may contain a thin enhancing rim (Fig. 32–11). Bone erosion or remodeling is a very unusual finding in DC.[21, 24]

On MRI, DCs usually have signal characteristics that are consistent with the cystic nature of these lesions. Occasionally, cysts that contain highly proteinaceous fluid or fat may demonstrate increased T1 and T2 signal shortening. The multiplanar capabilities of MRI are helpful in identifying the exact location of these lesions with respect to mylohyoid muscles. T1-weighted sagittal and coronal

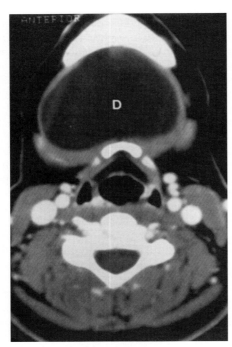

FIGURE 32–11 Axial postcontrast CT scan shows cystic-appearing dermoid (D) in the floor of the mouth. (From Mukherji SK. The neck. In Castillo M, Mukherji SK [eds]. Imaging of the Pediatric Head, Neck, and Spine, p. 582. Philadelphia, Lippincott-Raven, 1996.)

images provide information valuable for planning surgical resection as previously discussed.[21, 24]

Teratoma

Teratomas are tumors of germ cell origin that consist of elements derived from all three germ cell layers. From 7% to 9% of teratomas occur in the extracranial head and neck region. The incidence of teratomas is 1 in 4000 births. Teratomas may occur in numerous locations in the extracranial head and neck including the neck, paranasal sinuses, nasopharynx, orbit, and pharynx. Teratomas that arise in the neck are present at birth and may be seen in full-term, premature, and stillborn infants. The vast majority of teratomas are benign lesions; however, malignant teratomas do occasionally occur. In patients who have undergone prior resection, the risk of malignancy is significantly increased and has been reported to be as high as 20%. Teratomas arising in the nasopharynx have a strong female predilection (6 to 1). There is no reported gender predilection for teratomas situated in the neck. There is no reported increased association with other coexisting congenital anomalies; however, about 20% of cervical teratomas occur in association with maternal hydramnios.[21]

On histologic examination, a variety of tissues arising from all three germ layers are found to be present. Certain lesions may contain as many as 15 separate elements. There is often an abundance of central nervous system tissue with cervical teratomas; however, this is not a distinguishing component of these lesions. These lesions typically have a well-defined capsule.[21]

The vast majority of cervical teratomas present as a large mass arising in the neck. The mass is bulky, with large masses often crossing the midline and involving the contralateral side. The size of lesions tends to vary; however, the majority of lesions vary between 5 and 12 cm in their largest diameter. Because of their large size, they may be associated with considerable morbidity and may be life threatening. Affected infants have symptoms of respiratory obstruction (stridor, cyanosis, and apnea) due to deviation and compression of the trachea. Compression of the esophagus may result in dysphagia. The high incidence of maternal polyhydramnios may in part be due to the inability of the infant to swallow amniotic fluid.[25]

These lesions tend to occur in the region of the thyroid gland, suggesting that they may be of thyroid origin. However, it is currently debatable whether involvement of the thyroid gland is due to invasion by an adjacent lesion or whether the lesion actually arises from the thyroid gland.[21]

The treatment of cervical teratomas is surgical excision. Early resection is essential for proper management of these patients. Delay in resection may result in progression of respiratory symptoms and may lead to atelectasis and pneumonia. Respiratory obstruction is the leading cause of mortality in patients with large cervical teratomas. After treatment, careful follow-up is required of all patients who have undergone previous treatment due to increased risk of malignancy regardless of the location of the lesion and the histologic findings. The cause of the malignant degeneration is thought to be dedifferentiation of the remaining teratomatous elements.[25]

The relationship to adjacent masses is well visualized with both CT and MRI (Fig. 32–12). CT is preferred due to shorter imaging time, which takes on added importance in infants who have underlying respiratory obstruction

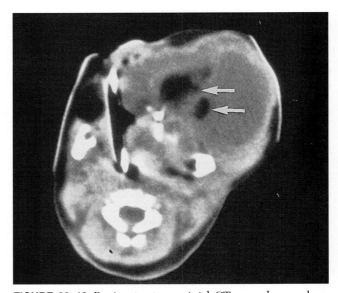

FIGURE 32–12 Benign teratoma. Axial CT scan shows a large heterogeneous exophytic mass involving the left oral cavity. The foci of fat situated within the mass suggest the diagnosis of teratoma (arrows). (Modified from Mukherji SK. The neck. In Castillo M, Mukherji SK [eds]. Imaging of the Pediatric Head, Neck, and Spine, p. 614. Philadelphia, Lippincott-Raven, 1996.)

due to the mass. CT is also beneficial for detecting calcifications and fat within the lesion (Fig. 32–13). The muliplanar capabilities of MRI may be helpful in certain large tumors.[24]

The radiographic appearance is a large, bulky, heterogeneous mass consisting of both solid and cystic components. The tumors are typically located adjacent to the thyroid and are often surrounded by an enhancing rim. These lesions are unilateral but may extend into the contralateral side of the neck and into the thoracic inlet. The presence of fat and calcification within the lesions is a characteristic finding of teratomas. The attenuation of the fluid component is variable depending on the amount of protein and fat within the lesion. The MRI findings are a heterogeneous mass, with the signal intensity dependent on the amount of fat and protein present within the lesion.[24, 26]

Lymphatic Malformations

Lymphatic malformations (LMs), previously termed *lymphangiomas*,[27] are congenital lesions that result from a defect in the embryogenesis of the lymphatic system. LMs occur in equal frequency in males and females. The lesions are most commonly present in newborns, with 65% noted at birth, 80% by 1 year, and 90% by 2 years of age. Ten percent of lesions may present in older children and adults. The extracranial head and neck is the most common site of occurrence for LM (75%). LM has been associated with a number of syndromes, the most common being Turner's syndrome. Other syndromes include Noonan's syndrome, fetal alcohol syndrome, familial pterygium syndrome, distichiasis-lymphedema syndrome, and various chromosomal aneuploidies.[28]

LMs have been classified into three main forms based of the size of the anomalous lymphatic spaces.[29]

Cystic hygroma is the most common form and consists of very large dilated lymphatic spaces lined by a single

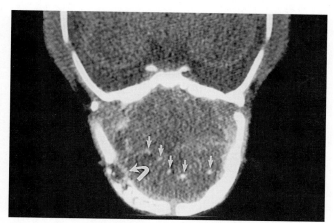

FIGURE 32–13 Malignant teratoma. Coronal CT scan shows an aggressive mass arising within the oral cavity and eroding the adjacent bone (*curved arrow*). Note the scattered foci of calcifications scattered throughout the mass (*straight arrows*). (Modified from Mukherji SK. The neck. In Castillo M, Mukherji SK [eds]. Imaging of the Pediatric Head, Neck, and Spine, p. 614. Philadelphia, Lippincott-Raven, 1996.)

layer of flat endothelium. These lesions are often solitary and occur in the presence of an otherwise normal lymphatic system. Seventy-five percent of these lesions occur in the neck and have a predilection for the posterior triangle.

A *cavernous lymphangioma* is composed of mild to moderately dilated lymphatic spaces, the size of which is between that of the cystic spaces seen in cystic hygromas and that of capillary hemangiomas. These lesions tend to be situated in the oral cavity or salivary glands. Cavernous LMs tend to be subcutaneous lesions and infiltrate adjacent muscular and neurovascular structures without destroying them. The peripheral location and subcutaneous spread are suggestive of a defect in embryogenesis during a later phase of lymphatic development (9 to 10 weeks) when compared with a cystic hygroma.

Capillary hemangioma (simple, lymphangioma simplex) is the least common form of lymphangioma. These lesions are composed of a network of small lymph thin-walled channels the size of capillaries, located predominantly within the epidermis, and may occur anywhere throughout the body. Because of their superficial location, capillary hemangiomas are felt to develop the latest.

A knowledge of the development of the lymphatic system is helpful in order to gain a full understanding of LM. There are two main theories explaining the embryogenesis of the lymphatic system. The *centripetal* theory states that the lymphatic channels develop from rests of primitive mesenchyme; the rests eventually communicate with the venous system. The *centrifugal* theory is the most widely accepted theory and forms the basis of the following explanation of the pathogenesis of LM. This hypothesis states that the lymphatic primordia develop as direct outpouchings from the large central veins located in different regions of the body. These primordia then develop into lymphatic vessels that grow into the surrounding mesenchyme and form the complicated network of the lymphatic system.

The lymphatic primordium begins to develop between the sixth and seventh weeks of gestation and is characterized by the development of six paired primary lymph sacs that arise from the venous system. These sacs consist of two jugular sacs, which arise near the junction of the anterior cardinal vein (future internal jugular vein), two iliac sacs, one retroperitoneal sac, and one cisterna chyli. Some of these sacs temporarily lose their connection with the adjacent vein and become blind sacs. Under normal circumstances, these blind pouches later regain their venous connection. At around 7.5 weeks of gestation, the jugular sacs connect with recently formed paired axillary sacs and form the juguloaxillary complex. At between 8 and 9 weeks of gestation, there is rapid peripheral growth of the juguloaxillary complex resulting in formation of a complex network of lymphatic vessels that extends in a cranial and dorsolateral direction. The main juguloaxillary trunk continues to communicate with the venous system via a communication entering the confluence of the internal and external jugular veins. At about 9 weeks of gestation, the primordium that will eventually form the thoracic duct is present. Eventually, this primordium will anastomose with the left juguloaxillary sac while being continuous inferiorly with the cisterna chyli, thereby forming the thoracic duct. By 10 weeks of gestation, one continuous lymphatic network has formed with the branching of the lymphatic system paralleling that of the vascular system. The juguloaxillary sac has formed a complex plexus predominantly supplying the neck and face, whereas the axillary portion supplies the region of the thoracic inlet and axilla.[28]

LMs are felt to occur from a defect in the normal drainage of the lymphatic channels into the venous system. The result is a progressive enlargement of the isolated lymphatic spaces due to the continued secretion of lymph. There are several proposed explanations of this malformation. The isolated lymphatic network may be due to a portion of the lymphatic network that fails to reestablish a communication with the venous system isolated tissue that is sequestered early in embryogenesis. Early malformations involving the more primitive jugular, subclavian, and axillary sac are felt to result in the formation of cystic hygromas. These lesions occur in soft areolar tissues in areas with wide fascial planes, with the result being sharply demarcated round or oval lesions. The smaller channel lesions occur more peripherally and are felt to occur later in embryogenesis. These malformations have time to grow distally along narrower fascial planes and insinuate themselves along vessels and nerve trunks. Thus, LMs occurring in restrictive areas rich in neurovascular structures, such as the cheeks and lips, tend to contain more of an angiomatous component and cannot enlarge to cystic sizes present in cystic hygromas.[24, 28, 29]

The degree of obstruction and resulting distention of the draining channels is important prognostically. Severe forms result in diffuse lymphangiectasia that may be seen on ultrasonography and are incompatible with life. Reestablishment of a communication between the lymphatic and venous system results in the reduction of edema with redundant skin. This sequence of events is thought to account for the typical phenotype seen in patients with Down's syndrome.[28]

LMs typically present as painless neck masses, which may be found throughout the extracranial head and neck. Cystic hygromas present as soft, doughy, compressible masses situated in the posterior triangle of the neck. Facial lesions are more likely to be cavernous or capillary hemangiomas. LMs tend to enlarge commensurate with the growth of the child. The resultant growth is felt by most to represent excessive secretion from the endothelial lining, although some authors feel that LMs can grow by postnatal endothelial proliferation. Potential complications include disfigurement, respiratory compromise, and recurrent infections. Surgical resection is the treatment of choice for LM. Well-defined cystic hygromas are easily resected. However, distal lesions that extend over several anatomic areas are difficult to completely resect and are prone to recurrence. Such patients need close follow-up and may require multiple surgical procedures.[28]

Both CT and MRI may be used to image patients with LM. CT is the preferred modality to image patients with lesions confined to the neck. However, for extensive lesions involving the face and oral cavity, the full extent of the lesion is best demonstrated with MRI. Contrast-enhanced CT should be performed in order to determine the relationship with the carotid artery and jugular vein

before surgical resection. MRI should be performed before and after contrast administration as the enhancing angiomatous component may be inseparable from the adjacent normal tissue, and this can result in underestimation of the full extent of the lesion. The prenatal diagnosis of LM may also be made with ultrasonography.[24]

It is possible to differentiate cystic hygroma from a capillary or cavernous LM by cross-sectional imaging techniques. The radiographic appearance of a cystic hygroma is a sharply demarcated cyst that does not contain a visible wall. These lesions have a tendency to occur in the posterior compartment of the neck. Large lesions may be multilobular and have considerable mass effect, displacing structures of the carotid sheath and adjacent sternocleidomastoid muscle. Atrophy or invasion of the sternocleidomastoid muscle is an associated finding in patients with cystic hygroma. Lesions that have been partially resected or repeatedly infected may demonstrate an enhancing wall or contain internal septations.[24, 28]

Capillary or cavernous LMs may be found throughout the head and neck but tend to be situated in the face and oral cavity. Radiographically, these lesions are heterogeneous and tend to insinuate themselves around the involved structures (Fig. 32–14). Because of the angiomatous components, these cystic portions of the lesions may enhance with contrast material. The spread pattern of these forms of LM often conforms to the facial planes, with the result being an extensive lesion that involves multiple compartments of the suprahyoid neck. Sagittal and coronal MRI may be very useful for defining the extent of lesions involving the floor of the mouth within the sublingual space.[24]

Ranula

A ranula is a cystic lesion arising in the floor of the mouth that is felt to result from obstruction of a sublingual gland

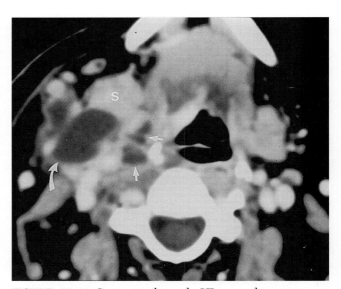

FIGURE 32–14 Contrast-enhanced CT scan demonstrates a multicystic mass (*curved arrow*) involving the right submandibular space that extends deeply and abuts the right lateral wall of the oropharynx (*straight arrows*). Note the anterior displacement of the submandibular gland (S).

or another minor salivary gland. The obstruction is felt to be congenital. The cysts develop from continued secretion from mucous glands into an obstructed duct. Ranulas have also been referred to as *mucoceles* or *pseudocysts* arising in the floor of the mouth. Although ranulas have been reported in every age group, they are most common in children and young adults. There is no reported gender predilection for these developmental lesions.[30, 31]

There are two types of ranulas. A *simple* ranula is the most common form and consists of the lesion contained within the floor of the mouth. These lesions are paramedial and are located in the sublingual space. The *diving ranula* (plunging, complex) is felt by some to arise from rupture of a simple ranula. These lesions extend inferiorly below the level of the mylohyoid muscle either by extending over the free margin of the mylohyoid muscle or directly through it.[32]

These lesions present as mucosa-covered masses arising within the floor of the mouth and have been described by some as having a frog belly appearance. These masses are typically cystic and exhibit a characteristic translucent bluish hue. Ranulas may occasionally rupture, causing expulsion of viscid fluid into the oral cavity. Diving ranulas present as a painless, fluctuant soft tissue neck mass. The majority of diving ranulas are above the hyoid bone; however, large lesions may extend into the thoracic inlet or mediastinum.[32]

Neither simple nor diving ranulas contain an epithelial lining. Secreted mucus is extravasated into the floor of the mouth, which may dissect along the underlying fascial planes. Histologically, recently formed ranulas consist of mucin and histiocytes (mucocytes) surrounded by vascularized connective tissue. Long-standing ranulas are cysts with walls composed of vascularized connective tissue.[32]

The treatment of ranulas depends on the specific type present. Simple ranulas, which are confined to the floor of the mouth, may be treated by marsupialization. Removal of the ipsilateral sublingual gland at the time of surgery is associated with a lower rate of recurrence. Diving ranulas require a more aggressive approach and may require widespread dissection of the floor of the mouth and into the neck depending on the extent of disease.[32]

Both CT and MRI may be used to evaluate patients with ranulas. Multiplanar capabilities may be helpful in evaluating the position of the ranula with respect to the mylohyoid muscle. MRI may also be helpful in localizing the most inferior extent of a diving ranula. Both CT and MRI should be performed with intravenous contrast material.[33, 24]

Simple ranulas are well-defined, low-attenuation, unilocular lesions confined to the floor of the mouth. Simple ranulas conform to the fascial boundaries of the sublingual spaces and are bordered laterally by the mylohyoid muscle and medially by the genioglossus and geniohyoid muscles. Large lesions are often associated with a mass effect, causing medial displacement of these latter muscles. The walls of the ranulas are very thin and often imperceptible and do not enhance with contrast material. Complex ranulas extend into the submandibular or parapharyngeal space by the routes previously described. Ranulas that have been repeatedly infected or have had prior surgery may contain septations or have an enhancing wall.[24, 33]

The MRI appearance of ranulas is a cystic lesion with low to intermediate signal intensity on T1-weighted and increased signal intensity on T2-weighted sequences (Fig. 32–15). The T1-weighted signal may at times vary depending on the protein content of the lesion. The differential diagnosis includes other fluid-containing lesions involving the floor of the mouth, which include dermoid, epidermoid, lyphangioma, hemangioma, or lateral thyroglossal duct cyst. The diagnosis of a ranula is suggested if a cystic lesion with an imperceptible wall is confined to the sublingual space.[24, 33]

Hemangioma

Hemangiomas are the most common tumor in the cervical region in children. They may involve the oropharynx or face, usually as a sessile reddish submucosal mass near the base of the tongue. The cavernous type is most common. CT scans demonstrate a mass of muscle intensity that may or may not enhance. Phleboliths (venous calculi) are diagnostic, if present (Fig. 32–16). MRI studies demonstrate an infiltrative mass of low signal intensity on T1-weighted images and high signal intensity on T2-weighted images.[34] This reflects the pathologic processes of these lesions, which largely consist of stagnant nonclotted blood.[24]

Lingual Thyroid

Lingual thyroid results from incomplete descent of the thyroid gland from the foramen cecum to the lower neck. Lingual thyroid is more common in females (7 to 1) and has been reported in 10% of the population in autopsy studies.[21] By CT, these lesions usually have high attenuation and homogeneously enhance with contrast material (Fig. 32–17). Ninety percent of cases are situated within the tongue base and may extend inferiorly to involve the intrinsic tongue muscles. On MRI, these lesions are

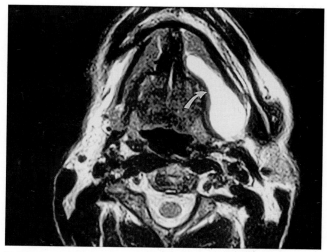

FIGURE 32–15 Axial T2-weighted image through the floor of the mouth shows the characteristic appearance of a ranula (*arrow*).

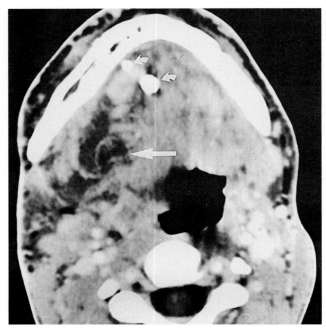

FIGURE 32–16 Axial contrast-enhanced CT scan demonstrates a hemangioma *(straight arrow)* containing focal calcifications *(curved arrows)* involving the floor of the mouth.

typically isointense to hyperintense to tongue musculature on T1- and T2-weighted sequences.[16]

Pharyngoceles

Zenker's diverticulum is an outpouching of the hypopharynx, lined by mucosa. Dyssynergy of the cricopharyngeus muscle seems to play a role in the formation of this pulsion diverticulum.[35] The muscle fails to relax as a bolus passes, generating high pressure "upstream." The diverticulum protrudes through Killian's dehiscence, an area of relative weakness between oblique fibers of the

inferior constrictor muscle and the horizontal cricopharyngeus fibers.[35] A Zenker diverticulum extends posteriorly and often laterally, usually to the left.[35]

A pharyngocele is a benign outpouching of the lumen of the upper piriform sinus. The pharyngocele is lined by normal mucosa. The frontal view of a barium swallow best shows the pharyngocele, which fills with barium. An air-filled pharyngocele may occasionally be seen on CT or MRI (Fig. 32–18) and, when asymptomatic, is often of no clinical significance.[20]

INFECTIONS AND INFLAMMATORY PROCESSES

Retropharyngeal Space Infections

Retropharyngeal space infections (RPIs) are potentially life-threatening processes whose incidence has decreased in the postantibiotic era. Historically, RPIs have been felt to occur almost exclusively in children younger than 6 years. However, RPIs have become more frequently seen in adults. RPIs are more common in males than in females (2 to 1). The cause of diseases of the retropharynx is an infection involving an area whose primary lymphatic drainage is to the retropharyngeal lymph nodes. Potential sites include the sinonasal tract, throat, tonsil, middle ear, or odontogenic disease. RPIs may also occur from direct inoculation from trauma.[36]

The retropharyngeal space (RPS) is found posterior to the pharynx and is a potential space situated between the middle and deep layers of the deep cervical fascia. The anterior boundary of the RPS is formed by the middle layer of the deep cervical fascia (visceral fascia), and the posterior boundary of the RPS is formed by the alar layer of the deep cervical fascia. Laterally, the RPS is limited by the carotid sheath. The RPS extends from the skull base to the level at which the alar fascia fuses with the visceral fascia (C7–T2). A second potential space is found posterior to the RPS and is sometimes referred to as the "danger space." The danger space is bounded anteriorly

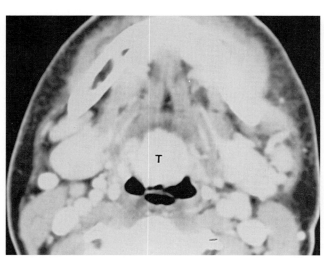

FIGURE 32–17 Contrast-enhanced CT scan shows a densely enhancing lingual thyroid (T) located in the tongue base. (Courtesy of Jeffrey Lang, M.D., and Roy Holliday, M.D.)

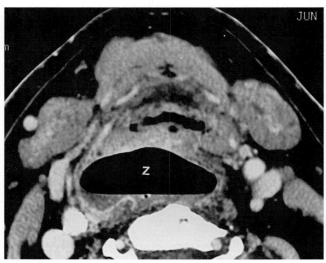

FIGURE 32–18 Axial CT scan shows a large fluid- and air-containing Zenker diverticulum (Z).

by the alar fascia and posteriorly by the prevertebral fascia. Superiorly, it extends to the skull base and is continuous inferiorly with the posterior mediastinum. Because of this communication, infections involving the danger space may extend inferiorly to involve the posterior mediastinum. Infections involving the RPS may enter the danger space because of their close proximity. Radiographically, it is difficult to ascertain if an infection is located within the RPS or the danger space. Therefore, the inferior extent of all infections involving the retropharynx must be determined and mediastinal extension must be excluded in all cases.[36]

The contents of the RPS include fat and lymph nodes. The retropharyngeal lymph nodes are subdivided into lateral and medial groups. The lateral group consists of one to three nodes situated just medial to the carotid sheath. The lateral group lies on the longus coli and longus capitis muscles behind the posterior pharyngeal wall. These lymph nodes usually extend from the skull base to C3. The medial group is an inconstant group located near the midline. When present, these nodes are usually found at the level of the second cervical vertebra, although they may extend inferiorly to C6. The afferent drainage of the retropharyngeal lymph nodes is from the nasopharynx, oropharynx, palate, nasal cavity, paranasal sinuses, middle ear, and eustachian tube and explains the potential sites of infection that can result in RPI. The efferent drainage is to high internal jugular nodes (group 2).[36]

Patients with RPI present with signs and symptoms of an underlying infection involving the upper aerodigestive tract, which at times may be indistinguishable from meningitis. Symptoms include fever, chills, odynophagia, sore throat, dysphagia, nausea, vomiting, respiratory distress, and neck pain and stiffness. On physical examination, patients may be found to be drooling and diaphoretic. Bulging of the posterior oropharyngeal wall is characteristic of infections involving the retropharynx.[37]

Historically, retropharyngeal space abscess was felt to result from efferent spread of infection to involve the retropharyngeal lymph nodes. These nodes were felt to enlarge and then undergo suppuration and develop liquified centers. Retropharyngeal abscesses were felt to be due to the eventual rupture of purulent material contained within the nodes into the RPS.[38] With the development of antibiotics, it appears that the evolution of disease is often slowed so that the disease is diagnosed and treated at an earlier stage before the development of a frank retropharyngeal abscess.[36]

With the development of broad-spectrum antibiotics, a true retropharyngeal abscess appears more likely to result from penetrating trauma of the oropharynx or nasopharynx; direct spread from an osteomyelitis or diskitis involving the vertebral column; or previous surgery. The treatment of this disease process is surgical drainage either by an intraoral or open procedure depending on the size of the lesion and the clinical stability of the patient.[36]

The initial diagnostic evaluation of patients suspected of having RPIs usually consists of a lateral plain film of the neck. An inspiratory film is necessary for adequate evaluation of the prevertebral soft tissues. Fluoroscopy may be helpful in those patients in whom true inspiratory films cannot be obtained. The presence of prevertebral swelling, loss of the normal cervical lordosis, and air in the prevertebral soft tissues are suggestive of an underlying infection. However, the exact location and the extent of the process cannot be determined by plain radiography alone.[24]

CT and MRI permit accurate localization of infections involving the deep neck and help separate infections limited to retropharyngeal lymph nodes from those involving the RPS, thereby permitting differentiation of true retropharyngeal abcesses from suppurative retropharyngeal adenitis with associated RPS edema. CT is preferred to MRI because of its consistently better quality, shorter scan time, lower costs, and better evaluation of associated neck disease. The reduction in scan time with CT is especially advantageous in the pediatric population and may reduce the amount of sedation necessary in infants and young children before imaging when compared with MRI.[24]

Retropharyngeal abscesses consist of midline low-attenuation masses with *enhancing* peripheral capsules located in the RPS (Fig. 32–19). These lesions are often associated with a significant mass effect and displacement of the posterior pharyngeal wall. RPS abscesses resulting from an adjacent diskitis are continuous with the adjacent disk space and associated with erosion of the neighboring vertebral body endplates.[24]

Suppurative retropharyngeal adenitis is characterized by an enlarged retropharyngeal lymph node that contains a low-attenuation center (Fig. 32–20). The presence of a low-attenuation center within a lymph node does not necessarily indicate the presence of pus. Low-attenuation centers may be present in lymph nodes containing early

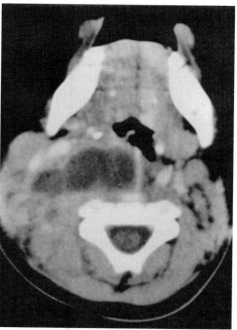

FIGURE 32–19 Postcontrast CT scan shows a large low-attenuation mass in the retropharyngeal space with peripheral enhancement. (From Castillo M. Neuroradiology Companion. Philadelphia, JB Lippincott, 1995.)

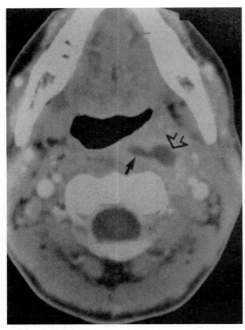

FIGURE 32–20 Axial postcontrast CT scan shows low attenuation in the retropharyngeal lymph node *(open arrow)*, which has ruptured medially, producing a small abscess *(solid arrow)* in the retropharyngeal space. There is wall enhancement. (From Castillo M. Neuroradiology Companion. Philadelphia, JB Lippincott, 1995.)

liquefaction (presuppurative phase) and in those that have undergone complete liquefaction necrosis (suppurative phase). Suppurative retropharyngeal adenitis is often associated with edema within the retropharyngeal space. This edema is characterized by smooth expansion of the retropharyngeal space without evidence of an enhancing rim. The average amount of edema is about 7 to 8 mm in anteroposterior diameter.[39]

Cross-sectional imaging modalities (CT or MRI) permit localization of areas of liquefaction and allow accurate differentiation of suppurative adenitis from retropharyngeal adenitis. Proper identification of low-attenuation material isolated within a single retropharyngeal lymph node in a patient without a life-threatening condition such as respiratory obstruction may be successfully managed with aggressive medical therapy. Close monitoring is required in all these patients. Successfully treated patients should show clinical improvement within 24 to 48 hours.[39] However, the radiologist must be thoroughly familiar with the differences between suppurative retropharyngeal adenitis, retropharyngeal abscess, and retropharyngeal edema before making such recommendations.[24, 38]

Peritonsillar Abscess

Acute tonsillitis is usually a self-limited febrile disease of adolescents or young adults. The most common offending bacterial organisms include beta-hemolytic streptococci, *Staphylococcus, Streptococcus pneumoniae,* and *Haemophilus.* Suppurative uncontrolled infection of the tonsils may result in a peritonsillar abscess (quinsy) or rarely in a tonsillar abscess. A peritonsillar abscess is an accumulation of pus around the palatine tonsils. If the peritonsillar abscess extends outside the tonsillar fossa, it may involve the lateral retropharyngeal or parapharyngeal spaces. Severe sore throat and pharyngeal edema that progress despite antibiotic therapy are the usual clinical presentations. Trismus develops if the medial pterygoid muscle is involved.[40]

On CT scans, the appearance of acute or chronic tonsillitis is nonspecific; focal homogeneous swelling of the palatine tonsil may simulate tumor. The inflammatory process may extend laterally into the parapharyngeal space, medial pterygoid muscle, and soft palate. If mature, the peritonsillar or tonsillar abscess has a low-density center surrounded by an enhanced margin (Fig. 32–21). The abscess may extend from the tonsillar bed superiorly into the retropharyngeal space or inferiorly into the submandibular space.[20, 38]

Ludwig's Angina

Ludwig's angina is a diffuse inflammatory process resulting in a severe cellulitis that involves the sublingual and submandibular spaces and is characteristically caused by oral flora. The majority of cases are due to bacterial infections arising from the mandibular alveolar ridge. Advanced cases lead to airway compromise, deep neck abscess, or, in severe cases, inferior extension along the fascial planes resulting in mediastinitis (Fig. 32–22).[16, 41]

Acquired Immunodeficiency Syndrome and Associated Disorders

Acquired immunodeficiency syndrome (AIDS) is caused by human T-cell lymphotropic virus type III and is a potentially devastating disease of children and adults. The disease may be transmitted by either homosexual or heterosexual contact in adults. In children, 78% of affected

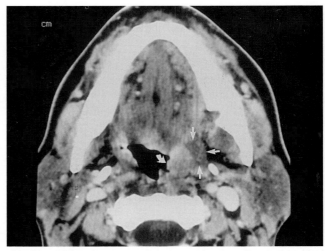

FIGURE 32–21 Contrast-enhanced CT scan performed at the level of the tonsil shows diffuse thickening and abnormal enhancement of the left palatine tonsil *(curved arrow).* Just deep to the tonsil is a low-attenuation mass consistent with a peritonsillar abscess *(straight arrows).*

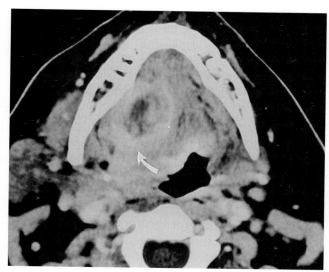

FIGURE 32–22 Contrast-enhanced CT scan shows a large floor-of-mouth abscess situated within the right sublingual space (*arrow*). Note the extensive mass effect associated with this inflammatory process.

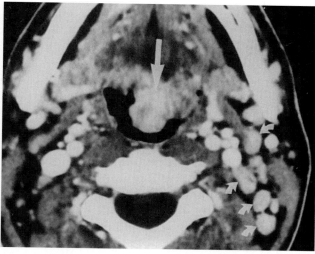

FIGURE 32–24 Axial contrast-enhanced CT scan shows an enhancing mass (*straight arrow*) in the tongue base and multiple enhancing cervical lymph nodes (*curved arrows*). Biopsy showed Kaposi's syndrome. (From Mukherji SK, Weissman JL, Holliday RA. Pharynx. In Som PM, Curtin HD [eds]. Head and Neck Imaging, 3rd ed., p. 469. St. Louis, Mosby–Year Book, 1995.)

individuals are born to parents who are positive for human immunodeficiency virus or who have AIDS, with 55% of infected children succumbing to the disease.[20]

Symptoms include localized or generalized lympadenopathy, thrush, parotid swelling, interstitial pneumonitis, hepatosplenomegaly, and diarrhea. Affected patients also have an increased risk of bacterial superinfection including meningitis and sepsis. The development of certain associated systemic processes are indicative of an underlying immunodeficiency. Infections with *Pneumocystis carinii*, toxoplasmosis, a rare fungal disease, or the development of rare neoplasms such as Kaposi's sarcoma or non-Hodgkin's lymphoma are suggestive of an infected host.[42]

A variety of infectious processes involving the pharynx and oral cavity have been described in AIDS patients. A broad spectrum of viral infections has also been observed in these patients. Unlike herpes simplex virus infections, which are typically self-limited in the intact host, this disease is much more aggressive, producing deep painful ulcerations and requiring treatment with oral acyclovir or

intravenous foscarnet in AIDS patients (Fig. 32–23).[43] Hairy cell leukoplakia is a manifestation of Epstein-Barr virus and presents as a white plaque most often seen on the lateral margin of the tongue. Bacterial infections are characteristically more aggressive in the immunocompromised host. These infections may result in rapid destruction of the mucosa and bone of the maxillary and mandibular ridges and may mimic necrotizing ulcerative gingivitis (trench mouth). Fungal diseases include oral candidiasis, cryptococcosis, and histoplasmosis.[44]

A variety of neoplasms have been reported to have a predilection to occur in AIDS patients. Because of their rarity in the general population, these neoplasms are considered AIDS-defining malignancies in the proper clinical setting and include Kaposi's sarcoma (Fig. 32–24), small noncleaved B-cell (Burkitt's, non-Burkitt's) and large B-cell (immunoblastic) non-Hodgkin's lymphoma. (Fig. 32–25).[42] Involvement of the oropharynx has been

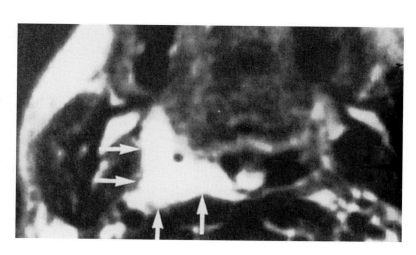

FIGURE 32–23 Axial T2-weighted MRI study shows thickening and increased signal intensity of the posterior and lateral oropharyngeal walls (*arrows*) consistent with a clinical diagnosis of herpes pharyngitis. (From Mukherji SK, Weissman JL, Holliday RA. Pharynx. In Som PM, Curtin HD [eds]. Head and Neck Imaging, 3rd ed., p. 469. St. Louis, Mosby–Year Book, 1995.)

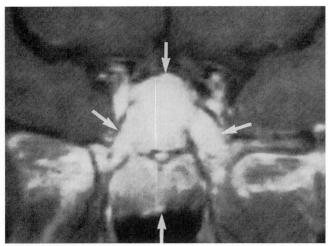

FIGURE 32–25 Coronal-enhanced T1-weighted MRI study performed with a fat saturation shows a large nasopharyngeal mass *(arrows)* that has invaded the sphenoid sinus in this patient who was positive for human immunodeficiency virus. Biopsy showed immunoblastic lymphoma. (From Mukherji SK, Weissman JL, Holliday RA. Pharynx. In Som PM, Curtin HD [eds]. Head and Neck Imaging, 3rd ed., p. 469. St. Louis, Mosby–Year Book, 1995.)

reported in up to 20% of patients with cutaneous Kaposi's sarcoma.[44, 45] Lymphoma most often arises in the lymphoid tissue lining the nasopharynx and tonsil. Early nasopharyngeal lesions may mimic the diffuse adenoid hypertrophy typically seen in immunocompromised hosts and radiographically appear as enhancing soft tissue lying superficial to an intact pharyngobasilar fascia. The contents of the mucosal space of the nasopharynx consist of an epithelial mucosal lining and adenoid tissue. The adenoids are residual lymphatic tissue that occupy the posterior aspect of the mucosal surface of the nasopharynx. Prominent adenoid pads are typically present in children. Gradual involution occurs around puberty, with the majority of individuals having only a thin rim of adenoid tissue by 30 years of age.[15] Prominent adenoid tissue may occasionally be seen in adults and does not necessarily indicate underlying abnormality, especially if the underlying fat planes are intact. However, markedly enlarged adenoid tissue in adults is often present in patients with AIDS.[46] The triad of increased lymphoid tissue

---

TABLE 32–1 AJCC Staging for Nasopharyngeal Cancer

Tis	Carcinoma in situ
T1	Tumor confined to the nasopharynx
T2	Tumor extends to soft tissues of oropharynx and/or nasal fossa
	T2a without parapharyngeal extension
	T2b with parapharyngeal extension
T3	Tumor invades bony structures and/or paranasal sinuses
T4	Tumor with intracranial extension and/or involvement of cranial infratemporal fossa, hypopharynx, or orbit

Abbreviation: AJCC, American Joint Committee on Cancer.

---

in the nasopharynx, parotid masses, and enlarged cervical lymph nodes is suggestive of an infected patient.[42, 46]

Recent studies have suggested that the likelihood of squamous cell carcinoma (SCCA) is increased in patients younger than 40 years who test positive for human immunodeficiency virus. Also, when present in immunocompromised individuals, these malignancies appear to be more aggressive and are extensive at the initial presentation (Roy Holliday, M.D., personal communication). This has been attributed to a deficiency in the host's natural immune defense mechanism.[47]

NEOPLASMS

Squamous Cell Carcinoma

Pharynx

Nasopharynx

SCCA (Table 32–1) is the most common malignancy of the upper aerodigestive tract and accounts for 70% of malignancies arising in the nasopharynx.[3, 4] Lymphomas account for approximately 20%, with the remaining 10% due to a variety of lesions that include adenocarcinoma, rhabdomyosarcoma, adenoid cystic carcinoma, melanoma, plasma cell myeloma, fibrosarcoma, and carcinosarcoma.[4] In North America, nasopharyngeal carcinoma is a relatively rare cancer and constitutes only 0.25% of all malignancies. However, the tumor has a striking prevalence in Asia, where it accounts for 18% of all cancers in China and is the most common cancer in males and third most common cancer in females.[48] In the United States, SCCA is more common in males and is most often diagnosed during the sixth decade of life.[4]

Several factors have been linked with an increased likelihood of developing SCCA of the nasopharynx. IgA antibodies against Epstein-Barr virus have been associated with the undifferentiated form of this tumor. Human leukocyte antigen (HLA)–A2 and HLA-B-Sin histocompatibility loci have been identified as possible markers for genetic susceptibility to SCCA among the Chinese population.[49] The incidence appears to decrease among Chinese born in North America, although the rate is still seven times higher than that of Native Americans.[50] Other risk factors include nitrosamines (present in dry-salted fish), polycyclic hydrocarbons, poor living conditions, and chronic sinonasal infections.[4]

The most commonly used classification for nasopharyngeal carcinoma has been established by the World Health Organization, which divides it into three types based on histopathologic findings. These types are squamous cell carcinoma (type 1), nonkeratinizing carcinoma (type 2), and undifferentiated carcinoma (type 3). Type 1 tumors are keratinized lesions and are similar to other SCCAs found in the remainder of the upper aerodigestive tract. Type 2 lesions have little or no keratin production, and, because of their resemblance to urinary tract tumors, are sometimes referred to as *transitional cell carcinomas.* Type 3 carcinomas often resemble large cell lymphomas and constitute a diverse group of malignancies, which include lymphoepitheliomas, anaplastic lesions, and spindle cell and clear cell varieties of SCCA.[51]

The clinical presentation is based on the size and location of the lesion at the time of initial diagnosis, with most early lesions asymptomatic. The most common presenting complaint is enlarged internal jugular or spinal accessory lymph nodes. Isolated serous otitis media is unusual in adults and, when present, should raise the possibility of eustachian tube dysfunction due to an underlying nasopharyngeal carcinoma. Other symptoms include headaches, nasal obstruction, epistaxis, sore throat, trismus, and proptosis.[3, 4]

Imaging studies alone are usually unable to differentiate SCCA from other malignancies that arise in the nasopharynx. The most reliable finding of a malignancy is an aggressive-appearing enhancing mass that infiltrates the deep fascial planes and spaces of the nasopharynx.[6, 20] The presence of homogeneously enhancing tissue in the nasopharynx localized to the mucosal surface that infiltrates the deep planes can be due to lymphoid tissue or early malignancy. The fossa of Rosenmüller is felt to be the most common site of origin of nasopharyngeal cancer, which, when the lesions are small, is often clinically occult.[3, 4] The presence of asymmetric unilateral effacement of the fossa of Rosenmüller on cross-sectional imaging should be transmitted to the referring otolaryngologist, especially if an adult patient presents with unilateral serous otitis or is suspected of having an occult malignancy of the upper aerodigestive tract (Fig. 32–26).[6, 20]

CT and MRI play complementary roles for imaging patients with nasopharyngeal carcinoma. MRI provides excellent visualization of the soft tissue planes of the nasopharynx and is superior to CT for detecting perineural spread of tumor (see Fig. 32–13). Although both MRI and CT may be used to detect bone erosion, CT is superior to MRI for detecting bone erosion (see Fig. 32–14). This finding is especially important, as up to 25% of cases demonstrate bone erosion that is clinically occult. Advanced lesions may spread to the adjacent cranial nerves and present with neurologic symptoms. Extension

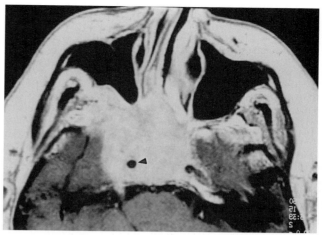

FIGURE 32–27 Contrast-enhanced T1-weighted MRI study shows an advanced nasopharyngeal carcinoma that has invaded the clivus and cavernous sinus. Note the encasement of the right carotid artery (*arrowhead*).

into the cavernous sinus may result in palsies of cranial nerves III to VI (Fig. 32–27). Extension into the parapharyngeal space and skull base may involve cranial nerves IX to XII and the sympathetic chain, which may result in the patient's presenting with otalgia or unilateral Horner's syndrome.

Radiographic evaluation of the entire cervical lymph nodes is essential as 85% to 90% of patients have nodal spread at the time of initial diagnosis.[3, 52, 53] The incidence of bilateral metastases is 50%.[3] The retropharyngeal nodes are usually the first nodes to become involved; however, group II nodes may be involved without radiographic evidence of enlarged retropharyngeal nodes. Submental and occipital nodes typically become affected only when there is an obstruction to the primary lymphatic drainage, such as after radiation therapy.[3]

Oropharynx

The majority of tumors involving the oropharynx (Table 32–2) are SCCA followed by other less common lesions such as lymphoma, minor salivary gland tumors, and other rare mesenchymal lesions. The incidence of SCCA of the oropharynx is increased in patients with a history of tobacco or alcohol abuse or both. Tumors may arise from a variety of locations within the oropharynx including the soft palate, anterior and posterior tonsillar pillars, tonsillar

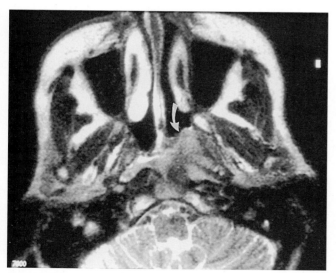

FIGURE 32–26 Nasopharyngeal carcinoma. Axial T2-weighted image shows the appearance of an early nasopharyngeal carcinoma (*arrow*).

TABLE 32–2 AJCC Staging for Oropharyngeal Cancer

Tis	Carcinoma in situ
T1	Tumor is 2 cm or less in greatest dimension
T2	Tumor is more than 2 cm but not more than 4 cm in greatest dimension
T3	Tumor is more than 4 cm in greatest dimension
T4	Tumor invades adjacent structures (e.g., pterygoid muscle[s], mandible, hard palate, deep muscle of tongue, larynx)

Abbreviation: American Joint Committee on Cancer.

fossa, and tongue base. The specific spread patterns and lymphatic drainage vary with the anatomic origin of the lesion.[54]

The majority of malignancies of the soft palate are squamous cell carcinomas (see Fig. 32–19); however, carcinomas of the minor salivary glands have their highest frequency in the posterior soft palate. Carcinomas of the palate tend to be well differentiated and typically affect the oral aspect of the palate (Fig. 32–28). Extension of palatal carcinoma occurs in all directions, but the tonsillar pillars and hard palate are usually affected first.[54] Palatal carcinomas drain first to the high internal jugular and subdigastric nodes with subsequent involvement of the lower internal jugular chain or retropharyngeal nodes. Lymphatic spread is present in 60% of all patients at the time of the diagnosis. Extension up the greater and lessor palatine nerve canals can occur, allowing spread of tumors into the pterygopalatine fossa and cavernous sinus.[54] The CT scan findings of carcinomas of the soft palate depend on the size and extent of the lesions. Subtle lesions along the oral surface of the soft palate may just increase the fullness of the soft palate on axial CT scans. Large lesions may result in unilateral fullness in the region of the tonsil and soft palate and may invade the parapharyngeal space.[55] Direct coronal CT scans must be used to evaluate the soft and hard palate as these structures lie in the axial plane and therefore are poorly examined by axial CT scans. MRI is ideally suited to evaluate the palate in both the sagittal and the coronal planes.[56]

Tumors arising from the anterior tonsillar pillar tend to spread along the muscle and fascial attachments of the palatoglossus muscle. The tumor may spread superiorly to involve the soft palate. From there, malignancies may extend anteriorly to involve the posterior aspect of the hard palate or extend further superiorly along the tensor and levator palatini muscles and pterygoid musculature.[54, 57] Advanced tumor with this spread pattern may eventually reach and potentially invade the skull base. Large tumors invading the skull base may at times be difficult to differentiate from nasopharyngeal carcinomas that have spread inferiorly. Anterior tonsillar pillar lesions may also spread anteromedially along the superior constrictor muscle to involve the pterygomandibular raphe

and, if uncontrolled, the buccinator muscle. Tongue base invasion may result from inferior spread of tumor along the palatoglossus muscle.[54, 57] The lymphatic drainage of anterior tonsillar pillar tumors is primarily to the submandibular and internal jugular nodes. The overall likelihood of positive nodes with anterior tonsillar pillar carcinomas at presentation is 45%.[54-57]

Primary posterior tonsillar pillar lesions are rare. The tumor may extend superiorly along the palatopharyngeus muscle to its origin in the soft palate. Inferior growth may result in extension to structures into which this muscle inserts including the posterior aspect of the thyroid cartilage, middle pharyngeal constrictor, and pharyngoepiglottic fold.[54] The lymphatic drainage is primarily to the internal jugular chain group.

Malignancies of the tonsillar fossa (see Fig. 32–18) are felt to originate from the mucosa of the membrane lining the recess between the anterior and posterior tonsillar pillars or from remnants of the palatine tonsil.[54] This area is also a common site for lesions, which are clinically occult and present with cervical nodal metastases. Given the location, these lesions may spread anteriorly or posteriorly to involve the adjacent tonsillar pillars or deeply and invade the superior constrictor muscle (Fig. 32–29).[54-57] The primary lymphatic drainage for the tonsillar fossa is the ipsilateral internal jugular chain nodes, although the spinal accessory chain and posterior submandibular nodes are also at risk. Tonsillar fossa tumors are associated with a 76% overall chance of having nodes that are clinically positive for containing metastases.

The tongue base is defined as the area posterior to the circumvallate papilla that extends inferiorly to the vallecula. The posterior portion of the tongue base and vallecula contains varied amounts of lymphoid tissue. Because of the varied degree of lingual tonsillar tissue that may normally be present, early tumors may be difficult to detect. Superficial lesions detected by direct visualization may not be seen on imaging studies. Clinically, tongue base carcinomas are often silent and are a common location of occult malignancies arising in the upper aerodigestive tract. Tumors originating in the base of the tongue may spread to the glossotonsillar sulcus and anterior tonsillar pillar.[54] This is different from tonsillar carci-

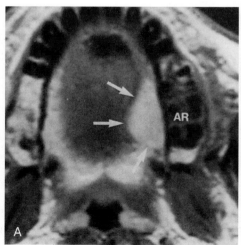
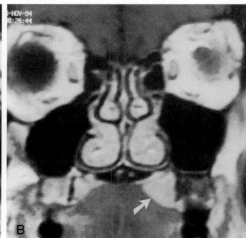

FIGURE 32–28 *A,* Axial contrast-enhanced T1-weighted MRI study shows a well-demarcated enhancing adenocarcinoma *(arrows)* situated along the lateral aspect of the hard palate, which abuts the lingual surface of the maxillary alveolar ridge (AR). *B,* Coronal T1-weighted MRI study demonstrates the lesion situated on the lateral aspect of the hard palate *(arrow).* (*A* and *B,* From Mukherji SK, Weissman JL, Holliday RA. Pharynx. In Som PM, Curtin HD [eds]. Head and Neck Imaging, 3rd ed., p. 453. St. Louis, Mosby–Year Book, 1995.)

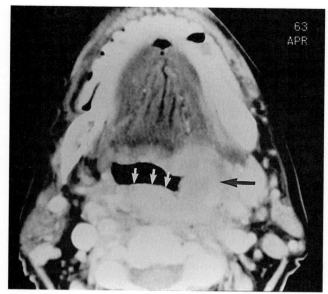

FIGURE 32–29 Contrast-enhanced CT scan shows a large squamous cell carcinoma (SCCA) that has arisen from the tonsillar carcinoma *(black arrow)*, which has extended posteriorly to involve the posterior pharyngeal wall *(white arrows)*.

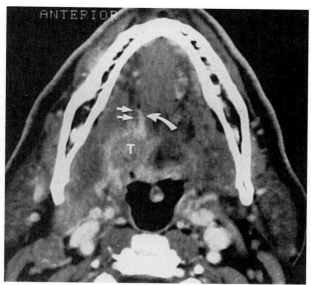

FIGURE 32–30 Axial contrast-enhanced CT scan demonstrates a large (>2 cm in mean diameter) tongue base carcinoma (T) with aggressive margins that invade the sublingual space *(curved arrow)*. Fat planes between the tumor and the vessels that normally course within the sublingual space are obliterated *(straight arrows)*. These findings are suggestive of invasion of the lingual neurovascular bundle. Histopathologic findings indicated perineural invasion. (From Mukherji SK, Weeks S, Castillo M, Krishnan L. Squamous cell carcinomas that arise in the oral cavity and tongue base: Can CT help predict perineural or vascular invasion? Radiology 1996;198:157–162.)

nomas, which have a tendency to invade the tongue base. Because the mucosa of the tongue base is continuous with the vallecula, these tumors have a tendency to spread submucosally.[54] Tumor may spread anteriorly into the sublingual space and encase the lingual neurovasculature (Fig. 32–30). The tongue base has a rich lymphatic network with a significant amount of cross-drainage. This explains the fact that a high percentage of patients (30%) have bilateral metastatic nodes at the time of initial presentation.[54, 58] The primary drainage sites are the internal jugular nodes. Spread to the floor of the mouth places the submandibular nodes at risk for metastases. The spinal accessory chain is also at risk, although the risk is not as great as for the internal jugular group.

Hypopharynx

The hypopharynx is lined by stratified squamous epithelium. More than 95% of all hypopharyngeal tumors are squamous cell cancers.[11, 59] Risk factors include alcohol abuse, smoking, and previous radiation therapy.[61] Hypopharyngeal tumors can remain relatively "quiet" or asymptomatic for a long time.[60] Occasionally, patients with hypopharyngeal carcinomas may present with referred pain. This referred pain travels up from the piriform sinus along the internal laryngeal nerve, then back down the auricular nerve, another branch of the vagus. The auricular nerve (Arnold's nerve) supplies sensory innervation to the external auditory canal and pinna.[11] Tumor originating from the hypopharynx besides those arising from the tongue base, tonsil, and nasopharynx must be included in the differential diagnosis of patients who present with otalgia.[11] At the time of diagnosis, up to 75% of patients with hypopharyngeal tumors have metastases to cervical lymph nodes.[60] From 4% to 15% of patients with SCCA of the hypopharynx have a synchronous or metachronous

second primary tumor.[61, 62] Of these, 25% are diagnosed at the time of the hypopharyngeal tumor, and 40% are diagnosed 6 months or more after diagnosis of the initial primary tumor. Staging of hypopharyngeal carcinoma is based on the American Joint Committee on Cancer Staging TNM system (Table 32–3).

Tumors may arise from any of the anatomic subsites that constitute the hypopharynx. The radiologist should be familiar with these locations as this is the nomenclature routinely used by otolaryngologists and radiation oncologists. SCCA arising from the piriform sinus may be confined to one wall or be more extensive. A piriform

TABLE 32–3 AJCC Staging for Hypopharyngeal Cancer

Tis	Carcinoma in situ
T1	Tumor limited to one subsite of hypopharynx and 2 cm or less in greatest dimension
T2	Tumor involves more than one subsite of hypophyarnx or an adjacent site, or measures more than 2 cm but not more than 4 cm in greatest dimension without fixation of hemilarynx
T3	Tumor measures more than 4 cm in greatest dimension or with fixation of hemilarynx
T4	Tumor invades adjacent structures (e.g., thyroid/cricoid cartilage, carotid artery, soft tissues of neck, prevertebral facial muscles, thyroid, and/or esophagus)

Abbreviation: American Joint Committee on Cancer.

sinus tumor may spread submucosally into the posterior wall of the hypopharynx, the postcricoid region, or the aryepiglottic fold.[60] Large tumors also extend up into the paraglottic fat, the pre-epiglottic fat, and the base of the tongue.[11, 59] Tumors arising from the lateral wall or apex of the piriform sinus often have already invaded the thyroid cartilage at the time of diagnosis.[11, 59, 61] Lesions of the medial wall of the piriform sinus (aryepiglottic fold, or marginal area) may spread along the aryepiglottic fold into the false vocal cord and arytenoid cartilage.[11, 59] Medial wall lesions can, on occasion, invade paraglottic and pre-epiglottic fat. They may also grow posteriorly into the postcricoid region, then cross midline to involve the contralateral piriform sinus. Superficial mucosal lesions in the piriform sinus are best evaluated with barium studies and through direct inspection by the clinician. These lesions are best evaluated by endoscopic evaluation. On CT and MRI studies, a collapsed piriform sinus can mimic a tumor; conversely, it is not always possible to exclude tumor when the piriform sinus is collapsed.[20] Submucosal spread may not be apparent on direct inspection (laryngoscopy) but may be readily detected on CT studies[63, 64] or MRI. CT and MRI are useful for assessing extension of bulk disease into the apex of the piriform sinus, which is located on cross-sectional images at the level of the true vocal cords (Fig. 32–31).

Tumors confined to the postcricoid region are rare (Fig. 32–32).[11, 59] Often, posterior wall tumors invade the posterior larynx (arytenoid and posterior cricoid cartilage), causing vocal cord paralysis and hoarseness. Large tumors concentrically infiltrate and narrow the lumen of the hypopharynx[11, 59] (see Fig. 32–9) and may extend to the inlet of the cervical esophagus (esophageal verge). The junction of the postcricoid region with the esophageal verge should be evaluated for tumor involvement. Inferior extension of tumor to involve the esophageal verge and cervical esophagus may alter the surgical treatment of these tumors and, if undetected preoperatively, may result in a positive surgical margin. A well-known risk factor for cancer of the postcricoid hypopharynx is the Plummer-

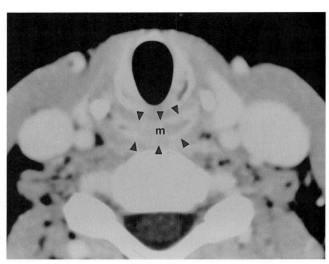

FIGURE 32–32 Contrast-enhanced CT scan demonstrates an SCCA involving the postcricoid region of the hypopharynx (m) separating the enhancing pharyngeal mucosa *(arrowheads)* overlying the anterior and posterior walls of the hypopharynx.

Vinson syndrome, named for two American investigators (also called Paterson-Brown syndrome for the European who described a similar syndrome).[61] The syndrome is more common in women than in men.[61] The four components of Plummer-Vinson syndrome are dysphagia, iron-deficiency anemia, weight loss, and webs in the hypopharynx and cervical esophagus.[61] The carcinomas are usually postcricoid, perhaps related to stasis above the webs.[61]

Carcinomas of the posterior wall of the hypopharynx spread up and down the posterior wall (Fig. 32–33) and may infiltrate deeply. Submucosal tumor may become quite bulky.[11, 59] Tumor may extend up into the posterior wall of the oropharynx and even infiltrate the posterior aspect of the tonsillar pillars.[11, 59] Posterior wall tumor may extend to involve the postcricoid and esophageal

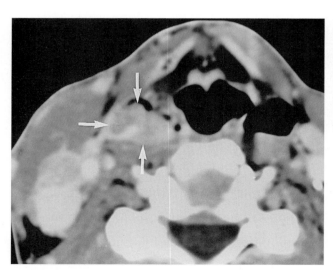

FIGURE 32–31 Contrast-enhanced CT scan shows an SCCA arising in the right piriform sinus *(arrows).*

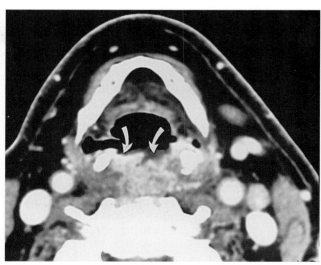

FIGURE 32–33 Contrast-enhanced CT scan illustrates the characteristic appearance of an aggressive SCCA arising from the posterior pharyngeal wall *(arrows).*

verge. Rarely, aggressive and invasive posterior wall tumors extend through the mucosa into the prevertebral muscles and may even invade vertebrae. Obliteration of the prevertebral fat planes by tumor on CT and MRI is suspicious for tumor fixation to the longus coli muscles.[20]

Oral Cavity

SCCA accounts for 90% of all malignant tumors involving the oral cavity (Table 32–4). Other malignancies that may arise in this area include lymphoma, sarcomas, and minor salivary gland tumors. SCCA is more common in males than in females.[16, 17] Ninety-five percent of lesions are diagnosed after 45 years of age with the average age at the time of presentation 60 years. The lips are the most common site of SCCA (44.9%) followed by the oral tongue (16.5%), floor of the mouth (12.1%), lower gingiva (12.1%), palate and upper gingiva (4.7%), and buccal mucosa (9.7%).[16, 65] Risk factors for developing SCCA include abuse of tobacco and alcohol.[17] The fact that the majority of lesions arise along dependent positions of the oral cavity suggests that SCCA may be due to the irritating effects of exogenous carcinogens from long-term smoking and alcohol abuse. The lymphatic drainage of the oral cavity is the submandibular and internal jugular nodal groups.

SCCAs of the floor of the mouth most commonly arise within 2 cm of the anterior midline.[17] Early spread usually occurs medially, along the midline geniohyoid–genioglossus muscle complex; laterally, to involve mylohyoid muscle, gingiva and periosteum of the mandible; and submucosally, to involve the floor of the mouth structures including the sublingual gland and submandibular duct. The periosteum is felt to be a protective barrier against mandibular invasion, and such invasion is typically only present in advanced lesions.[17] Extension into the submandibular duct results in an ipsilaterally obstructed submandibular gland. The role of imaging for floor-of-mouth lesions is not for initial diagnosis, but rather to determine the extent of tumor and evaluate nodal involvement. Both CT and MRI may be used for evaluating such lesions. However, CT is likely more useful than MRI for detecting early cortical mandibular invasion.[16] CT examinations should have a maximal slice thickness of 3 mm acquired contiguously through the area of interest. A high-resolution bone algorithm should be obtained of the mandible in all cases to evaluate for mandibular invasion. MRI may provide better evaluation of the complete extent of tumor. Obliteration of the fat planes surrounding the lingual vessels is suggestive of perineural and perivascular spread and, when present, can correctly identify perineural and perivascular spread in over 90% of cases (Fig. 32–34).[66]

SCCA of the oral tongue most commonly involves the middle and posterior third, with the majority of cases arising from the lateral and undersurfaces of the oral tongue (Fig. 32–35).[17] Early tumors tend to invade the intrinsic tongue muscles and remain localized to the oral tongue.[17] Advanced lesions often extend outside the intrinsic muscle group and invade the extrinsic tongue musculature. Advanced lesions that arise from the anterior and middle third of the oral tongue tend to invade the floor of the mouth. Large tumors involving the posterior third of the tongue may extend into the floor of the mouth, tongue base, anterior tonsillar pillar, glossotonsillar sulcus, and mandible.[17] Imaging studies should specifically determine if the tumor has crossed the midline lingual septum, identify if the tumor extends outside the confines of the intrinsic tongue musculature, and evaluate for the presence of mandibular invasion.[16, 17]

The buccal mucosa is the mucosal lining of the inner surface of the lips and cheeks. The majority of SCCAs that arise from this region are low-grade lesions often occurring on a background of leukoplakia.[17] The majority of lesions arise on the lateral walls of the buccal mucosa. Larger lesions may extend to the gingivobuccal sulcus (Fig. 32–36). Very advanced tumors may invade the adjacent alveolar ridge or extend into the infratemporal fossa. Early lesions are difficult to detect by CT or MRI. Advanced lesions are usually detected by cross-sectional im-

TABLE 32–4 AJCC Staging for Oral Cavity Cancer

TX	Primary tumor cannot be assessed
T0	No evidence of primary tumor
Tis	Carcinoma in situ
T1	Tumor 2 cm or less in greatest dimension
T2	Tumor more than 2 cm but not more than 4 cm in greatest dimension
T3	Tumor more than 4 cm in greatest dimension
T4 (lip)	Tumor invades adjacent structures (e.g., through cortical bone, skin of face, inferior alveolar nerve, floor of mouth)
T4 (oral cavity)	Tumor invades adjacent structures (e.g., through cortical bone, into deep [extrinsic] muscle of tongue, maxillary sinus, skin; superficial erosion alone of bone/tooth socket by gingival primary is not sufficient to classify as T4)

Abbreviation: American Joint Committee on Cancer.

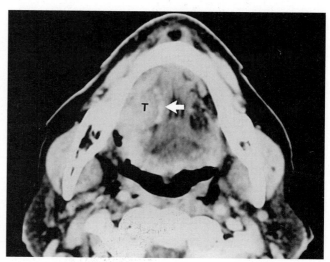

FIGURE 32–34 Contrast-enhanced CT scan demonstrates an aggressive tumor arising from the right side of the floor of the mouth (T). The medial displacement of the lingual vasculature with obliteration of the surrounding low attenuation of the sublingual space *(arrow)* is strongly suggestive of perineural or vasculature invasion.

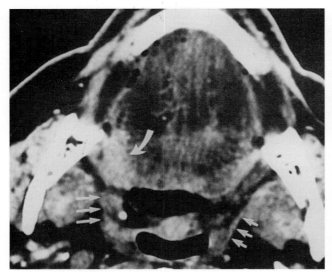

FIGURE 32–35 Axial contrast-enhanced CT scan obtained through the oropharynx demonstrates carcinoma of the tongue base *(curved arrow)* extending posteriorly along the superior constrictor muscle *(large straight arrows)*. Compare the involved superior constrictor muscle with its normal appearance seen on the uninvolved left side *(small straight arrows)*. (From Mukherji SK, Weissman JL, Holliday RA. Pharynx. In Som PM, Curtin HD [eds]. Head and Neck Imaging, 3rd ed., p. 450. St. Louis, Mosby–Year Book, 1995.)

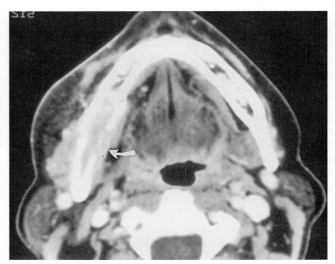

FIGURE 32–37 Axial CT scan shows an aggressive tumor invading the right side of the mandible *(arrow)*.

aging modalities. Specifically, these studies should be evaluated for the presence of bone erosion, extraoral extension, and perineural invasion.[17]

The lips consist of the orbicularis muscle and its various superficial coverings. The orbicularis muscle is covered along its external surface by a thin layer of squamous epithelium, which permits visualization of the underlying vasculature, thereby giving the lips their reddish color.[17] The mucous membrane lining the inside of the lip is the buccal mucosa. The dry lip is the transition from skin to mucous membrane. SCCA of the lip most commonly arises from the vermilion between the commissures and extends deeply to invade the underlying musculature. Advanced lesions often spread to the adjacent commissures, buccal mucosa, and mandible. Perineural invasion of the inferior alveolar nerve has been reported in 2% of cases and results from progressive mandibular invasion.[16, 17]

The gingiva is the mucosal covering of the mandible and maxilla. The spread of SCCA differs depending on whether the lesion arises from the upper or the lower gingiva. The majority of upper gingival lesions extend to invade the hard and soft palate, buccal mucosa, maxillary

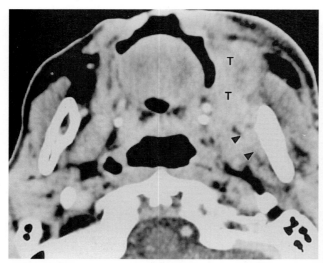

FIGURE 32–36 Contrast-enhanced CT scan shows an aggressive SCCA arising from the left buccal space. The tumor (T) has extended posteriorly along the buccinator muscle to involve the retromolar trigone. The obliteration of fat *(arrowheads)* between the medial pterygoid muscle and the ramus of the mandible is indicative of posterior spread of tumor. (Compare with the contralateral uninvolved side.)

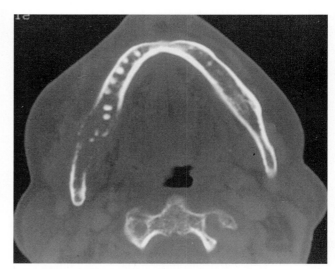

FIGURE 32–38 Bone algorithm of the case shown in Figure 31–37 demonstrates extensive intramedullary and cortical bone erosion associated with this advanced tumor.

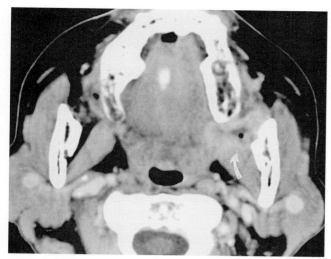

FIGURE 32–39 Contrast-enhanced study demonstrating an SCCA situated within the retromolar trigone (*arrow*).

alveolar ridge, and maxillary antrum. Tumors that originate along the lower gingiva may spread to involve the buccal mucosa, mandible, retromolar trigone, and floor of the mouth (Figs. 32–37 and 32–38). Coronal imaging should be performed for tumors that involve the hard palate. Because of the proximity of tumors to the hard palate, special attention should be given to evaluation of perineural spread along the greater and lesser palatine foramen for tumors involving the hard palate.[16, 17]

The retromolar trigone is a small triangular surface situated between the third molar and the ascending ramus of the mandible.[17] This region is continuous superiorly with the maxillary tuberosity. Tumors that arise in this region have unique spread patterns because of their unusual location (Fig. 32–39). Invasion of the periosteum of the mandible is commonly present because of its close proximity to the retromolar trigone. Tumor may extend posteriorly to involve the pterygomandibular space and medial pterygoid muscle and result in trismus. Tumors may also extend posterolaterally to invade the buccinator muscle and the adjacent buccal fat pad. Superior growth may involve the pterygomandibular raphe. Once this has occurred, tumors may then extend superiorly to invade the maxillary tuberosity and pterygoid plates. From this location, tumors have easy access to the posterior wall of the maxillary sinus; retroantral fat; and rich neurovascular plexus contained within the pterygopalatine fossa. From here, tumors have direct access to the masticator space, skull base, and cavernous sinus. All these regions of potential spread, in addition to nodal evaluation, should be investigated in patients with SCCA of the retromandibular trigone.[17]

Lymphoma

Lymphoma is the most common lymphoproliferative disorder occurring in the extracranial head and neck.[67] Hodgkin's disease (HD) is a malignancy of the hematopoietic system predominantly affecting adolescents and young adults. Males are more frequently affected than

females (2 to 1). The diagnosis of HD is strongly suggested by the presence of Reed-Sternberg cells from a nodal biopsy. While extranodal primary sites are unusual, systemic involvement may result from progression of the disease. Commonly affected organs include liver, spleen, lung, bone, and bone marrow, with the most commonly extranodal site being the spleen. The region of Waldeyer's ring is often uninvolved in patients with HD.

Non-Hodgkin's lymphoma (NHL) is a lymphoproliferative disorder that, unlike HD, is most commonly seen in an older age group, with males more commonly affected than females. Predisposing conditions that increase the likelihood of developing NHL include various congenital and acquired immunodeficiency states. There are a variety of classification schemes that attempt to reflect the heterogeneous group of disorders encompassed under the category of NHL. The most commonly employed systems are the Rappaport and Lukes-Collins classification systems. The former system was based on the resemblance of the various types of malignant cells to their benign counterparts, whereas the latter is based on immunologic markers that separate the cells into B-cell, T-cell, and histiocytic types. Unfortunately, the majority of patients with NHL have advanced disease at the time of presentation. Whereas 98% of HD cases present as nodal masses, 60% of NHL cases present in extranodal sites, with 60% of all extranodal presentations occurring in the head and neck.[68] Areas predisposed for developing lymphoma are those that normally have a high concentration of lymphoid tissue and include cervical nodes, Waldeyer's ring, the palatine tonsil, and the tongue base. Other primary sites in the extracranial head and neck include the parotid gland (15% of patients having a prior history of Sjögren's syndrome), palate, gingiva, lacrimal gland, eyelid, conjunctiva, and paranasal sinuses.[67]

The presenting findings depend on the primary site of

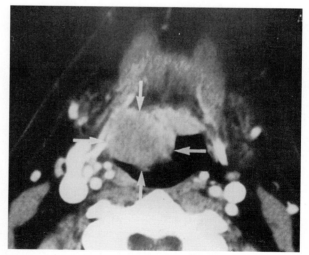

FIGURE 32–40 Axial contrast-enhanced CT scan obtained through the base of the tongue shows an exophytic soft tissue mass (*arrows*) bulging into the right vallecula. Histologic examination showed non-Hodgkin's lymphoma. (From Mukherji SK, Weissman JL, Holliday RA. Pharynx. In Som PM, Curtin HD. [eds]. Head and Neck Imaging, 3rd ed., p. 451. St. Louis, Mosby–Year Book, 1995.)

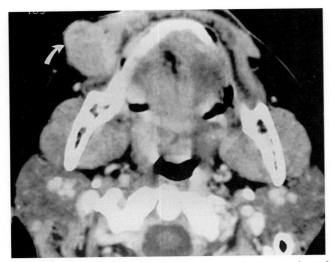

FIGURE 32–41 Contrast-enhanced CT scan shows an adenoid cystic carcinoma arising from the right buccal space (*arrow*). The radiographic findings of adenoid cystic carcinoma are nonspecific and indistinguishable from those of SCCA.

origin. HD typically presents as an asymptomatic mass. Patients may also complain of systemic symptoms, which include night sweats, fever, and weight loss. The clinical symptoms of patients with extranodal presentation of NHL often mimic those of SCCA arising in the same site. Patients with lymphomas arising in the nasopharynx may present with nasal obstruction or unilateral serous otitis media, whereas patients with tonsillar or tongue base lymphoma complain of unilateral sore throat, dysphagia, or other obstructive symptoms. Nodal involve-

ment is present in 80% of patients with NHL who present with extranodal primary lesions.[67]

The imaging findings of extranodal primary lymphoma or other forms of lymphoproliferative disorder arising in the extracranial head and neck are often indistinguishable from those of the more common SCCAs.[24] The diagnosis may be suggested if the lesion is associated with large homogeneously enhancing lymph nodes that do not contain a well-defined area of decreased attenuation. The high concentration of lymphoid tissue in the tongue base and tonsil predisposes these areas for developing lymphoma (Fig. 32–40). Thus, the diagnosis may be suggested by the presence of an endophytic mass arising in an area rich in lymphoid tissue. Large lesions may infiltrate the deep spaces and radiographically mimic advanced SCCAs. Primary nasopharyngeal lesions may invade the skull base (see Fig. 32–25) and spread along nerves in a manner similar to that of SCCA arising in the same location.[24, 67]

Minor Salivary Gland Tumors

Minor salivary gland tumors (MSGTs) are unusual lesions that constitute 2% to 3% of all malignant lesions of the extracranial head and neck.[69] These lesions may occur throughout the oropharynx, as minor salivary glands are normally present within the mucosa of an adult's upper aerodigestive tract (Fig. 32–41). There is no reported sex predilection for these tumors. Neoplasms considered to be MSGTs include adenoid cystic carcinoma, mucoepidermoid carcinoma, adenocarcinoma, malignant mixed carcinoma, acinic cell, oncocytic carcinoma, pleomorphic adenoma, and Warthin's tumor, with adenoid cystic carcinoma the most common histologic malignant variety. The

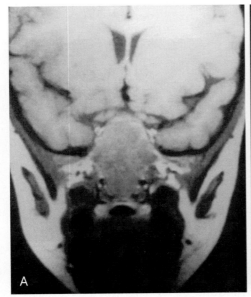

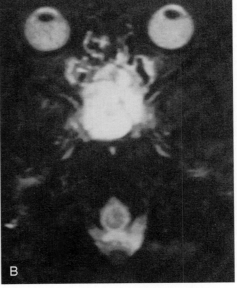

FIGURE 32–42 A 6-year-old girl with rhabdomyosarcoma of the nasopharynx invading the skull base and sphenoid sinus. *A,* Coronal T1-weighted MRI study demonstrates a mass extending into the sphenoid sinus and posterior ethmoid air cells. The mass extends upward to involve the planum sphenoidale. *B,* Axial T2-weighted MRI sequence demonstrates diffuse homogeneous increased signal intensity. The intensity is nonspecific. Rhabdomyosarcoma must be included in the differential diagnosis along with nasopharyngeal lymphoma and SCCA in a young patient with a nasopharyngeal mass. (*A* and *B,* From Mukherji SK, Weissman JL, Holliday RA. Pharynx. In Som PM, Curtin HD [eds]. Head and Neck Imaging, 3rd ed., p. 456. St. Louis, Mosby–Year Book, 1995.)

soft palate is the most common site of origin for MSGT, with the incidence almost equal to that of SCCAs. The majority of lesions arise in the posterolateral portion of the soft palate[70] and occasionally directly extend anteriorly to invade the hard palate. Other extracranial sites of occurrence, besides the soft palate, include the lips, gingiva, buccal mucosa, tongue base, floor of the mouth, paranasal sinuses, nasal cavity, nasopharynx, trachea, and larynx.

CT and MRI play complementary roles for evaluating patients with MSGT of the soft palate. The imaging findings are nonspecific, and the diagnosis is based on endoscopy and biopsy. The full extent of tumors and potential pathways of extension, especially along nerves, is best evaluated with MRI. The presence of bone invasion is best evaluated with CT. Imaging with CT should be performed in both axial and coronal planes (3-mm contiguous sections) after intravenous contrast administration through the palate and reformatted in both soft tissue and bone algorithms. Intraoral films are also recommended for evaluating early bone erosion if the lesion is adjacent to the lingual surface of the maxillary alveolar ridge. Malignant MSGTs have a strong predilection to spread along perineural pathways, with such spread being diagnosed histologically in approximately 50% of cases of adenoid cystic carcinomas. Continued growth may eventually extend into the skull base and cavernous sinus, and, if unrecognized, be a potential cause of treatment failure, both surgically and with radiation therapy. To complicate matters even more, perineural spread may be characterized by skip areas, with uninvolved segments of nerve potentially causing an underestimation of the extent of disease during surgical resection. Because of these factors, close attention must be paid to areas rich in neurovasculature, which are adjacent to sites of malignant MSGT. This is especially true of lesions that arise in the soft palate because of its proximity to the pterygopalatine fossa. Obliteration of the fat in the pterygopalatine fossa and erosion or asymmetric enlargement of the foramina of the greater and lesser palatine nerves are strong indicators of perineural spread. MRI is superior to CT for detecting perineural involvement and spread.

The risk of nodal involvement is related to the size, grade, and location of the primary lesion. The likelihood of metastases increases in sites that are rich in lymphatic drainage. This is reflected in the fact that the incidence of cervical nodal metastases is increased eightfold for lesions located in the nasopharynx and oropharynx, which contain an abundant lymphatic network compared with the paranasal sinuses (59% versus 7%).[69]

Rhabdomyosarcoma

Rhabdomyosarcomas are rare mesenchymal malignant tumors.[70, 71] Approximately 30% of rhabdomyosarcomas involve the head and neck. The orbit and nasopharynx are the most frequent sites of involvement, followed by the paranasal sinuses and middle ear. The tumor occurs primarily in children younger than 6 years but may occur in adolescents.[72] The tumor is thought to arise from rhabdomyoblasts within one of the muscles of the nasopharynx. The initial symptoms may be abrupt or insidious in onset depending on the location of the tumor. Nasopharyngeal rhabdomyosarcomas usually produce rhinorrhea, sore throat, and serous otitis media. Invasion of the skull base is often present. Advanced lesions may extend into the cavernous sinus, resulting in a cavernous sinus syndrome. The long-term prognosis is poor, with 5-year survival rates reported at less than 5%.

By CT scans, nasopharyngeal rhabdomyosarcoma appears as an infiltrating soft tissue mass that often erodes the skull base and posterior wall of the maxillary sinus.[73] The MRI features of rhabdomyosarcoma are nonspecific and similar to those of SCCA (Fig. 32–42). Prolonged T1 and T2 relaxation times are often noted along with frequent involvement of the skull base. Tumors may show a variable amount of enhancement after contrast administration.

Granular Cell Tumors

Granular cell tumors (GCTs) are unusual, benign neoplasms that can be found throughout the body[74] and typically present in the fourth decade of life. The tumors are more common in females and African Americans. Multiple lesions have been reported to occur in approximately 4% to 10% of patients. Fifty percent of GCTs occur within the tongue, and approximately 30% arise in the skin. Other reported primary sites include the larynx and temporal bone. Most of the GCTs found in the upper

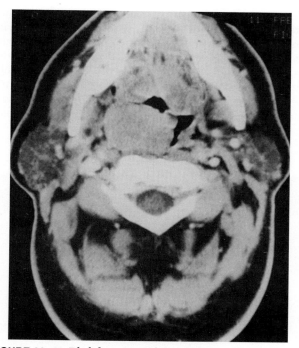

FIGURE 32–43 Rhabdomyoma of the posterior pharyngeal wall. A contrast-enhanced axial CT scan demonstrates a well-circumscribed mass of muscular intensity involving the posterior right lateral wall of the pharynx. Note the sharp interface with the surrounding parapharyngeal space, tongue, and prevertebral muscles. Biopsy proved this to be benign rhabdomyoma. (From Mukherji SK, Weissman JL, Holliday RA. Pharynx. In Som PM, Curtin HD [eds]. Head and Neck Imaging, 3rd ed., p. 458. St. Louis, Mosby–Year Book, 1995.)

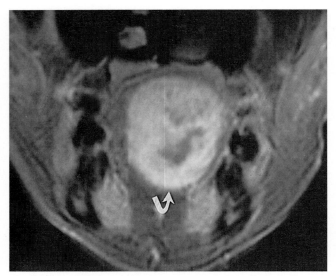

FIGURE 32–44 Coronal fat saturation postgadolinium T1-weighted image shows a large enhancing schwannoma thought to be arising from the lingual nerve *(arrow)*. (Courtesy of David Panush, M.D., and Roy Holliday, M.D.)

aerodigestive tract are intraluminal and solitary. When present, synchronous lesions tend to behave more aggressively.[75]

Imaging shows a soft tissue mass usually arising from the anterior aspect of the cricoid cartilage and extending into the soft tissues of the neck. GCTs are slightly hypointense on T1-weighted MRI studies and show homogeneous contrast enhancement. On T2-weighted MRI studies, GCTs may have either increased or decreased signal. On CT scans, they are solid and relatively homogeneously enhancing lesions. Radiographically, GCTs may mimic a primary SCCA arising within the subglottis or oropharynx.[76]

Other Tumors

Rhabdomyomas are rare benign skeletal tumors that have a predilection to arise in the extracranial head and neck. Whereas cardiac rhabdomyomas affect patients with tuberous sclerosis, extracardiac rhabdomyomas have no relationship to this syndrome. Affected regions include the oropharynx, nasopharynx, larynx, and submandibular triangle. On CT and MRI studies, the tumors are well circumscribed with a density or intensity similar to that of muscle (Fig. 32–43).[21, 24]

Fibrous lesions of the head and neck vary in their biologic activity and histologic appearance. Even though their histologic appearance is benign, some lesions are so locally aggressive that they are considered to be low-grade fibrosarcomas. The term *desmoid* has also been applied to a subgroup of these lesions, which present as well-differentiated but locally infiltrating fibrous masses near the musculoaponeurotic junctions. Twelve percent of desmoids involve the region of the head and neck, most commonly the soft tissues of the supraclavicular region and face.[77] Involvement of the oral cavity or nasopharynx is rare in adults. The CT scan findings of fibromatoses are nonspecific. Desmoids involving the head and neck usually encase and infiltrate the musculature of the supraclavicular region. They may infiltrate fat planes and cannot be differentiated from malignant lesions on the basis of their CT scan findings.

Twenty-five percent of schwannomas are located in the region of the head and neck. Most of these tumors involve cranial nerves in the jugular foramen or lateral neck. The tongue, palate, and floor of the mouth are the most frequent sites in the oral cavity (Fig. 32–44). Most are diagnosed in the second and third decades of life as asymptomatic enlarging masses. They appear on CT scans as focal, well-encapsulated masses.[78] Small lesions are usually homogeneous on CT scans, whereas focal areas of central low density are often present in larger masses. On contrast-enhanced CT scans, these tumors are relatively

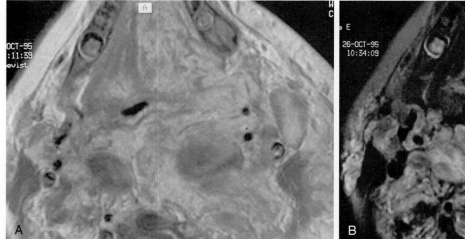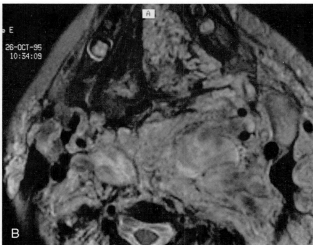

FIGURE 32–45 Plexiform neurofibromas. Axial postgadolinium T1-weighted *(A)* and T2-weighted *(B)* images demonstrate extensive plexiform neurofibromas diffusely involving the pharynx and left side of the floor of the mouth in a patient with neurofibromatosis type 1.

hypovascular compared with the highly vascular paragangliomas.[79] On MRI studies, schwannomas have a low signal intensity on T1-weighted images and high signal intensity on T2-weighted images (Fig. 32–45). Contrast enhancement is typical. Neurofibromas of the oral cavity are rare lesions, usually associated with von Recklinghausen's syndrome.[79] The tongue is the most frequent oral region affected.

References

1. Moore KL. The neck. In Clinically Oriented Anatomy, 2nd ed., pp. 1033–1050. Baltimore, Williams & Wilkins, 1985.
2. Wenig BM, Kornblut AD. Pharyngitis. In Bailey BJ (ed). Head and Neck Surgery—Otolaryngology, pp. 551–553. Philadelphia, JB Lippincott, 1993.
3. Mendenhall WM, Million RR, Mancuso AA, Stringer SP. Nasopharynx. In Million RR, Cassisi NJ (eds). Management of Head and Neck Cancer: A Multidisciplinary Approach, pp. 599–626. Philadelphia, JB Lippincott, 1994.
4. Neel HB, Slavitt DH. Nasopharyngeal cancer. In Bailey BJ (ed). Head and Neck Surgery—Otolaryngology, pp. 1257–1260. Philadelphia, JB Lippincott, 1993.
5. Lederman M. Cancer of the Nasopharynx: Its Natural History and Treatment, pp. 1–50. Springfield, IL, Charles C Thomas, 1961.
6. Mancuso AA, Hanafee WN. Nasopharynx and parapharyngeal space. In Computed Tomography and Magnetic Resonance Imaging of the Head and Neck, 2nd ed., pp. 428–498. Baltimore, Williams & Wilkins, 1985.
7. Rouvierre H (Tobias MJ [trans.]). Anatomy of the Human Lymphatic System, pp. 10–12. Ann Arbor, MI, Edwards Brothers, 1938.
8. Byrd SE, Schoen PJ, Gill G, Richardson M. Computed tomography of palatine tonsillar carcinoma. J Comput Assist Tomogr 1983;7:976–982.
9. Muraki AS, Mancuso AA, Harnsberger HR. CT of the oropharynx, tongue base and floor of the mouth: Normal anatomy and range of variations and applications in staging carcinoma. Radiology 1983;148:725–731.
10. Dillon WP, Mills CM, Kjos B, et al. Magnetic resonance imaging of the nasopharynx. Radiology 1984;152:731–735.
11. Million RR, Cassisi NJ, Mancuso AA. Hypopharynx: Pharyngeal walls, pyriform sinus, postcricoid pharynx. In Million RR, Cassisi NJ (eds). Management of Head and Neck Cancer: A Multidisciplinary Approach, pp. 505–532. Philadelphia, J.B. Lippincott, 1994.
12. American Joint Committee on Cancer. In Fleming ID, Cooper JS, Henson DE, et al. (eds). Manual for Staging of Cancer, 5th ed., pp. 31–41. Philadelphia, Lippincott-Raven, 1997.
13. Barnes L, Gnepp DR. Diseases of the larynx, hypopharynx, and esophagus. In Barnes L (ed). Surgical Pathology of the Head and Neck, pp. 141–226. New York, Marcel Dekker, 1985.
14. Hollinshead WH. Textbook of Anatomy, pp. 928–948. Hagerstown, MD, Harper & Row, 1974.
15. Dillon WP. The pharynx and oral cavity. In Som PM, Bergeron RT (eds). Head and Neck Imaging, pp. 407–465. St Louis, Mosby–Year Book, 1991.
16. Smoker WRK. Oral cavity. In Som PM, Curtin HD (eds). Head and Neck Imaging, 3rd ed., pp. 488–544. St. Louis, Mosby–Year Book, 1995.
17. Million RA, Cassisi NJ, Mancuso AA. Oral cavity. In Million RR, Cassisi NJ (eds). Management of Head and Neck Cancer: A Multidisciplinary Approach, pp. 599–626. Philadelphia, JB Lippincott, 1994.
18. Lederman M. Cancer of the Nasopharynx: Its Natural History and Treatment, pp. 1–50. Springfield, IL, Charles C Thomas, 1961.
19. Mukherji SK, Weeks S, Castillo M, Krishnan LA. Squamous cell carcinomas that arise in the oral cavity and tongue base: Can CT help predict perineural or vascular invasion? Radiology 1996;198:157–162.
20. Mukherji SK, Weissman JL, Holliday RA. Pharynx. In Som PM, Curtin HD (eds). Head and Neck Imaging, 3rd ed., pp. 457–487. St. Louis, Mosby–Year Book, 1995.
21. Batsakis JG. Teratomas of the head and neck. In Tumors of the Head and Neck. 2nd ed., pp. 226–229. Baltimore, Williams & Wilkins, 1979.
22. Reede DL, Holliday RA, Som PM, Bergeron RT. Nonnodal pathologic conditions of the neck. In Som PM, Bergeron RT (eds). Head and Neck Imaging, 2nd ed., p. 544. St. Louis, Mosby–Year Book, 1991.
23. Vogl TJ, Steger W, Ihrler S, et al. Cystic masses in the floor of the mouth: Value of MR imaging in planning surgery. AJR 1993;161:183–186.
24. Mukherji SK. The neck. In Castillo M, Mukherji SK (eds). Imaging of the Pediatric Head, Neck, and Spine, pp. 517–617. Philadelphia, Lippincott-Raven, 1995.
25. Myers EN, Cunningham MJ. Tumors of the neck. In Bluestone CD, Stool SE, Scheetz MD (eds). Pediatric Otolaryngology, Vol. 2, p. 1359. Philadelphia, WB Saunders, 1990.
26. Som PM, Sacher M, Lanzieri CF, et al. Parenchymal cysts of the lower neck. Radiology 1985;157:399–406.
27. Mulliken JB. Vascular malformations of the head and neck. In Mulliken JB, Young AE (eds). Vascular Birthmarks: Hemangiomas and Malformations, pp. 301–307. Philadelphia, WB Saunders, 1988.
28. Zadvinskis DP, Benson MT, Kerr HH, et al. Congenital malformations of the cervicothoracic lymphatic system: Embryology and pathogenesis. Radiographics 1992;12:1175–1189.
29. Batsakis JG. Vasoformative tumors. In Tumors of the Head and Neck, 2nd ed., pp. 301–305. Baltimore, Williams & Wilkins, 1979.
30. Gonzalez C. Tumors of the mouth and pharynx. In Bluestone CD, Stool SE, Scheetz MD (eds). Pediatric Otolaryngology, Vol. 2, p. 964. Philadelphia, WB Saunders, 1990.
31. Som PM. Salivary glands. In Som PM, Bergeron RT (eds). Head and Neck Imaging, 2nd ed., pp. 318–319. St. Louis, Mosby–Year Book, 1991.
32. Batsakis JG, McClatchey KD. Cervical ranulas. Ann Otol Rhinol Laryngol 1988;97:561–562.
33. Coit WE, Harnsberger HR, Osborn AG, et al. Ranulas and their mimics: CT evaluation. Radiology 1987;163:211–216.
34. Itoh K, Nishimura K, Togashi K, et al. MR imaging of cavernous hemangioma of the face and neck. J Comput Assist Tomogr 1986;10:831–835.
35. Graney DO, Marsh B. Trachea/Bronchus/Esophagus: Anatomy. In Cummings CW, Fredrickson JM, Harker LA, et al. (eds). Otolaryngology—Head and Neck Surgery, pp. 2207–2216. St. Louis, Mosby–Year Book, 1993.
36. Gianoli GJ, Espinola TE, Guarisco JL, Miller RH. Retropharyngeal space infection: Changing trends. Otolaryngol Head Neck Surg 1991;105:92–100.
37. Grodinsky M. Retropharyngeal and lateral pharyngeal space abscesses: An anatomical and clinical study with review of the literature. Am J Surg 1979;110:179–199.
38. Batsakis JG, Sneige N. Parapharyngeal and retropharyngeal space disease. Ann Otol Rhinol Laryngol 1989;98:320–321.
39. Mukherji SK, Mancuso AA, Shook J. Retropharyngeal suppurative lymphadenitis: Differentiation from retropharyngeal abscess and treatment implications. [Abstract] Meeting of the Radiological Society of North America, Chicago, 1994.
40. Kornbutt AD. Infections of the pharyngeal spaces. In Paparilla M, Shumrick M (eds). Otolaryngology, Vol. 3, Philadelphia, WB Saunders, 1980.
41. Grodinsky MD. Ludwig's angina: An anatomical and clinical study with review of the literature. Surgery 1939;5:678–696.
42. Holliday RA. Manifestations of AIDS in the oromaxillofacial region: The role of imaging. Radiol Clin North Am 1993;31:45–60.
43. MacPhail LA, Greenspan D, Schiodt M, et al. Acyclovir-resistant, foscarnet-sensitive oral herpes simplex type 2 lesion in a patient with AIDS. Oral Surg Oral Med Oral Pathol 1989;67:427–432.
44. Grepp DR, Chandler W, Hyams V. Primary Kaposi's sarcoma of the head and neck. Ann Intern Med 1984;100:107–114.
45. Abeymayor E, Calcterra T. Kaposi's sarcoma and community acquired immunodeficiency syndrome: An update with emphasis on its head and neck manifestations. Arch Otolaryngol 1983;109:536–542.
46. Stern JC, Lin PT, Lucente FE. Benign nasopharyngeal masses and HIV infection. Arch Otolaryngol Head Neck Surg 1990;116:206–208.
47. Roland JT, Rothstein SG, Khushbakhat RM, Persky MS. Squamous cell carcinoma in HIV-positive patients under age 45. Laryngoscope 1993;103:509–511.
48. Hsu MM, Huang SC, Lynn TC, et al. The survival of patients

with nasopharyngeal carcinoma. Otolaryngol Head Neck Surg 1982;90:289–290.

49. Simons MJ, Wee GB, Day NE, et al. Immunogenetic aspects of nasopharyngeal carcinoma. I. Differences in HLA antigen profiles between patients and control groups. Int J Cancer 1974;13:122–124.

50. Dickson RI. Nasopharyngeal carcinomas: An evaluation of 209 patients. Laryngoscope 1981;91:333–334.

51. Shanmugaratnam K, Sobin LH. Histologic typing of upper respiratory tract tumors. In International Histologic Classification of Tumors, No. 19. Geneva, World Health Organization, 1978.

52. Mesic JB, Fletcher GH, Goepfert H. Megavoltage irradiation of epithelial tumors of the nasopharynx. Int J Radiat Oncol Biol Phys 1981;7:447–453.

53. Fletcher GH, Million RR. Malignant tumors of the nasopharynx. Am J Roentgenol Radium Ther Nucl Med 1965;93:44–45.

54. Million RA, Cassisi NJ, Mancuso AA. Oropharynx. In Million RR, Cassisi NJ (eds). Management of Head and Neck Cancer: A Multidisciplinary Approach, pp. 401–431. Philadelphia, JB Lippincott, 1994.

55. Byrd SE, Schoen PJ, Gill G, Richardson M. Computed tomography of palatine tonsillar carcinoma. J Comput Assist Tomogr 1983;7:976–982.

56. Schaefer SD, Maravilla KR, Close LR, et al. Magnetic resonance imaging versus computed tomography: Comparison in imaging oral cavity and pharyngeal carcinomas. Arch Otolaryngol Head Neck Surg 1985;111:730–734.

57. Mancuso AA, Hanafee WN. Oral cavity and oropharynx including tongue base, floor of mouth and mandible. In Computed Tomography and Magnetic Resonance Imaging of the Head and Neck, 2nd ed., pp. 358–427. Baltimore, Williams & Wilkins, 1985.

58. Lindberg RD. Distribution of cervical lymph node metastases from squamous cell carcinoma of the upper respiratory and digestive tracts. Cancer 1972;29:1448–1449.

59. Mendenhall WM, Parsons JT, Cassisi NJ, Million RR. Squamous cell carcinoma of the pyriform sinus treated with radiation therapy. Radiother Oncol 1987;9:201–208.

60. Barnes L, Gnepp DR. Diseases of the larynx, hypopharynx, and esophagus. In Barnes L (ed). Surgical Pathology of the Head and Neck, pp. 141–226. New York, Marcel Dekker, 1985.

61. Adams GL. Malignant neoplasms of the hypopharynx. In Cummings CW, Fredrickson JM, Harker LA, et al. (eds). Otolaryngology—Head and Neck Surgery, pp. 1955–1973. St. Louis, Mosby–Year Book, 1993.

62. Barnes L. Tumors and tumorlike lesions of the soft tissues. In Barnes L (ed). Surgical Pathology of the Head and Neck, pp. 725–880. New York, Marcel Dekker, 1985.

63. Aspestrand F, Kolbenstvedt A, Boysen M. Carcinoma of the hypopharynx: CT staging. J Comput Assist Tomogr 1990;14:72–76.

64. Mukherji SK, Lee R, Tart RP, Mancuso AA. Can pretreatment computed tomography findings predict local control in T1 and T2 squamous cell carcinoma of the pyriform sinus treated with radiotherapy alone? Preliminary results. Meeting of the Radiological Society of North America, Chicago, 1993.

65. MacComb WS, Fletcher GH, Healey JE. Intra-oral cavity. In Macomb WS, Fletcher GH (eds). Cancer of the Head and Neck, pp. 89–151. Baltimore, Williams & Wilkins, 1967.

66. Mukherji SK, Weeks S, Castillo M, Krishnan LA. Squamous cell carcinomas that arise in the oral cavity and tongue base: Can CT help predict perineural or vascular invasion? Radiology 1996;198:157–162.

67. Mendenhall NP. Lymphomas and related diseases presenting in the head and neck. In Million RR, Cassisi NJ (eds). Management of Head and Neck Cancer: A Multidisciplinary Approach, pp. 857–878. Philadelphia, JB Lippincott, 1994.

68. Wong DS, Fuller LM, Butler JJ, Shullemger CC. Extranodal non-Hodgkin's lymphomas of the head and neck. AJR 1975;123:471–481.

69. Million RR, Cassisi NJ. Minor salivary gland tumors. In Million RR, Cassisi NJ (eds). Management of Head and Neck Cancer: A Multidisciplinary Approach, pp. 737–750. Philadelphia, JB Lippincott, 1994.

70. Lee FA: Rhabdomyosarcoma. In Parker BR, Castellano RA (eds). Pediatric Oncologic Radiology, pp. 33–35. St Louis, CV Mosby, 1977.

71. Canalis RF, Jenkens HA, Hemenway WG, Lincoln C. Nasopharyngeal rhabdomyosarcoma: A clinical perspective. Arch Otolaryngol 1978;104:122–126.

72. Dito WR, Batsakis JG. Intra-oral, pharyngeal and nasopharyngeal rhabdomyosarcoma. Arch Otolaryngol Head Neck Surg 1963;77:123–129.

73. Scotti G, Harwood-Nash DC. Computed tomography of rhabdomyosarcomas of the skull base in children. J Comput Assist Tomogr 1982;6:33–39.

74. Robb PJ, Girling A. Granular cell myoblastoma of the supraglottis. J Laryngol Otol 1989;103:328–330.

75. Cree IA, Bingham BJG, Ramesar KCRB. View from beneath: Pathology in focus granular cell tumour of the larynx. J Laryngol Otol 1990;104:159–161.

76. Mukherji SK, Castillo M, Rao V, Weissler M. Granular cell tumors of the subglottic region of the larynx: CT and MR findings. AJR 1995;164:1492–1494.

77. Masson JK, Soule EH. Desmoid tumor of the head and neck. Am J Surg 1966;112:615–622.

78. Som PM, Lanzieri CF, Sacher M, et al. Extracranial tumor vascularity: Determination by dynamic CT scanning. Parts I and II. Radiology 1985;154:401–412.

79. Das Gupta TK: Tumors of the peripheral nerves. In Das Gupta TK (ed). Tumors of the Soft Tissues, pp. 89–95. East Norwalk, CT, Appleton-Century-Crofts, 1983.

33

Imaging of the Parapharyngeal and Masticator Spaces

JONATHAN S. LEWIN, M.D.
JUNG K. PARK, M.D.

Evaluation of pathologic lesions of the parapharyngeal and masticator spaces represents an important application of modern imaging techniques. The suprahyoid region, extending from the skull base to the hyoid bone, is surrounded for the most part by bone, thereby limiting external clinical examination. In addition, although the superficial extent of mucosal lesions is readily identified by the examining physician, lesions confined to these deeper spaces and also the deep extent of more superficial lesions may be extremely difficult or impossible to evaluate during palpation or endoscopy. Thus, cross-sectional imaging techniques have attained an increasingly important role in the evaluation of pathologic lesions of these spaces.

When a lesion of the parapharyngeal, masticator, or adjacent spaces is encountered, several steps are essential for its characterization and classification, based on a working understanding of the complex anatomy of this area. First, the center or presumed site of origin of the lesion must be determined. Localization of the lesion into one or more of the deep spaces of the suprahyoid neck as defined by fascial anatomy strongly guides the differential diagnosis, as discussed later. Second, imaging characteristics such as the presence or absence of necrosis, cystic components, calcifications, and an estimate of vascularity also enable further limiting of the differential diagnosis. Lesion size; multiplicity; involvement of adjacent bone, cartilage, or neurovascular structures; and the presence of perineural spread must also be carefully evaluated to allow optimal surgical- or radiation-therapy planning and to permit an accurate prognosis. Finally, both an estimate of vascularity and assessment for involvement of the internal carotid and vertebral arteries help to determine whether preoperative angiography, embolization, or balloon test occlusion might be necessary.

Before the modern imaging era, the evaluation of suspected suprahyoid neck abnormality was limited to angiography for detection of vessel encasement or displacement and determination of tumor vascularity, and to sialography for detection of lesions arising within the salivary gland or displacing the duct system. With the advent of computed tomography (CT), the radiologic evaluation of deep space lesions has advanced markedly, providing an improved understanding of the anatomy of the suprahyoid neck and allowing improved differential diagnosis based on characteristic displacement of fascial planes.[1, 2] Further CT refinements include injection of Stensen's duct with contrast material before scanning to aid in the differentiation of deep lobe parotid from parapharyngeal space masses[3, 4] and the dynamic acquisition of CT images during bolus intravenous administration of iodinated contrast material in order to differentiate schwannomas from hypervascular paragangliomas.[5, 6] With the advent of magnetic resonance imaging (MRI), the delineation of tumor margins, evaluation of perineural and intracranial extension, and involvement of adjacent neurovascular structures were further improved as a result of multiplanar-imaging capabilities and improved soft tissue contrast resolution.[7–12] The addition of paramagnetic contrast agents to MRI techniques has further improved the imaging diagnosis of suprahyoid processes and presently yields the best anatomic localization and lesion conspicuity in many cases.[13, 14] The addition of needle-biopsy techniques to cross-sectional imaging has added the capability for minimally invasive histologic diagnosis of head and neck lesions in the radiology department, as well.[15] Presently, both CT and MRI are used in the evaluation of suspected suprahyoid masses at most institutions. Preference for MRI versus CT depends in part on the area of interest in the suprahyoid neck, as discussed later.

ANATOMY

Spaces of the Suprahyoid Neck and Their Fascial Boundaries

Historically, the surgical approach to the neck divided its anatomy into a number of triangles, defined by the sternocleidomastoid, anterior belly of the digastric, and omohyoid muscles. Although localization by triangle and superficial landmarks is helpful to the surgeon for defining the location of a palpable mass, this method of division of the neck is not very helpful to the radiologist attempting to accurately localize a lesion based on cross-sectional images. A preferable method for dividing the suprahyoid neck is based on a division of the anatomy into multiple spaces, defined by layers of cervical fascia. This approach to anatomic compartmentalization of the neck was initially proposed when it was noted that infection tended to spread into well-defined, fascial-bound spaces.[16] Subsequently, it was observed that the division of the suprahyoid neck into a number of distinct spaces based on fascial boundaries considerably simplifies the differential diagnosis of a suprahyoid mass, as each anatomic space tends to produce a relatively unique set of pathologic processes based on its contents.[9, 17, 18]

The fascia of the head and neck are divided into two major components, a fatty, relatively loose superficial cervical fascia and multiple dense complex fascial sheets constituting the layers of the deep cervical fascia. The deep cervical fascia is generally subdivided into three layers, a superficial, or investing, layer; a middle, or visceral, layer; and a deep, or prevertebral, layer.[16] The superficial and middle layers of the deep cervical fascia converge on the hyoid bone, dividing the neck into suprahyoid and infrahyoid portions.[18]

The superficial layer of the deep cervical fascia is a continuous sheet of fibrous tissue that encircles the neck and splits to enclose the trapezius and sternocleidomastoid muscles. Anterior to the sternocleidomastoid muscles, the superficial layer of the deep cervical fascia splits on each side to form the capsule of the parotid gland before reuniting at the posterior margin of the mandible. As the fascia further extends anteriorly and superiorly, it splits again to enclose the mandible, muscles of mastication, and zygomatic arch. Posteriorly, the superficial layer of the deep cervical fascia attaches to the mastoid process of the skull and to the external occipital protuberance.[16]

The deep layer of the deep cervical fascia encircles the vertebral column, paraspinal muscles, and prevertebral muscles, with a firm insertion on the spinous and transverse processes of the vertebral column.[16]

Although there is general agreement on the location and extent of the superficial and deep layers of the deep cervical fascia, there has been considerable confusion in the literature concerning the layers between the two.[16] In the suprahyoid neck, a basic knowledge of three of the fascial components between the superficial and deep layers of the deep cervical fascia is essential to understand the spatial anatomy. The deepest of these layers, usually considered to be the middle layer of the deep cervical fascia, is termed the *buccopharyngeal* or *visceral* fascia. This layer is adherent to the outer surface of the pharyngobasilar fascia superiorly and to the pharyngeal constrictor muscles more inferiorly. The buccopharyngeal fascia thus separates the pharyngeal mucosa, lymphoid tissue, and constrictor muscles, considered to be within the pharyngeal mucosal compartment, from the parapharyngeal space laterally and the retropharyngeal space posteriorly.[16] Anteriorly, the buccopharyngeal fascia attaches

to the pterygoid plate and the pterygomandibular raphe and then continues over the buccinator muscle.

The second important fascial layer between the superficial and deep layers of the deep cervical fascia is a relatively thick fascial sheet that envelops the styloid process and its musculature, extends anteromedially to merge with the fascia associated with the tensor veli palatini muscle, and then continues further anteriorly to fuse with the pterygomandibular raphe and buccopharyngeal fascia.[1, 16, 17] This fascial layer divides the parapharyngeal space into anterolateral (prestyloid) and posteromedial (retrostyloid) compartments.[1, 17]

The third important fascial layer between the deep and superficial layers of the deep cervical fascia is a small fascial slip that extends from the buccopharyngeal fascia anteriorly to the prevertebral fascia posteriorly, near its attachment to the transverse process of the cervical vertebrae. This sagittally oriented fascia has been referred to as the *cloison sagittale* and divides the medially positioned retropharyngeal space from the laterally positioned retrostyloid compartment of the parapharyngeal space.[16] This slip of fascia has also been termed the "alar" fascia; unfortunately, the use of this name can be confusing, as *alar fascia* is more commonly used to describe a slip of the deep layer of the deep cervical fascia that is immediately anterior to the prevertebral fascia, with similar coronal plane of orientation. Thus, to avoid confusion, the term *cloison sagittale* is preferred.[16]

With an understanding of the complex anatomy of the deep layers of fascia, the compartmentalization of the suprahyoid neck becomes relatively simple. The following sections outline the parapharyngeal and masticator spaces and describe their contents.

Parapharyngeal Space

There is controversy in the literature not only with respect to the fascial layers of the suprahyoid neck but also in regard to the nomenclature of the suprahyoid spaces. Many authors divide the parapharyngeal space into a prestyloid compartment, anterior and lateral to the fascia of the tensor veli palatini, and a retrostyloid compartment, posteromedial to the fascia of the tensor veli palatini (Fig. 33–1A–C). Others have suggested that the retrostyloid compartment be considered a separate "carotid space," a suprahyoid analogue to the well-defined carotid space of the infrahyoid neck.[18] With this nomenclature, the term *parapharyngeal space* refers only to the prestyloid compartment. For the purpose of this text, the definition supported by most authors is used and the suprahyoid portion of the carotid sheath and its contents are considered within a larger parapharyngeal space.[16] Recognition of these different nomenclatures is important in order to understand the literature.

The parapharyngeal space is an anatomic recess that is shaped like an inverted pyramid, with its base at the base of the skull and its apex at the greater cornu of the hyoid bone. It occupies the space between the muscles of mastication and the deglutitional muscles.[1, 18, 19] It is bounded laterally by the fascia covering the medial aspect of the medial pterygoid muscle; interpterygoid fascia; deep lobe of the parotid gland; and posterior belly of the digastric muscle.[1, 16] The medial boundary is formed by the buccopharyngeal fascia, or middle layer of the deep cervical fascia, as it covers the pharyngobasilar fascia and the superior pharyngeal constrictor muscle.[1, 20] The anterior boundary of the parapharyngeal space is at the level of the pterygomandibular raphe, where the buccopharyngeal fascia fuses with the interpterygoid fascia and fascia covering the medial aspect of the medial pterygoid muscle.[16] Its posterior margin is the prevertebral fascia covering the vertebral column and prevertebral muscles.[1, 20] Although the caudal extent of the parapharyngeal space is generally described as extending down to the hyoid bone, the sheath of the posterior belly of the digastric and styloid muscles; fascia on the lingual aspect of the mandible; buccopharyngeal fascia; and fascia surrounding the submandibular gland all fuse near the level of the angle of the mandible, thereby limiting the caudal extent of the space.[16] Thus the styloglossus muscle can be considered the functional inferior boundary of the parapharyngeal space.[16] At the level of the mylohyoid muscle, the parapharyngeal space is often continuous with the sublingual and submandibular spaces, allowing lesions to pass from one space to another without crossing a fascial boundary.[21] In addition, although the deep lobe of the parotid gland technically resides within the parotid space, the fascial layer between the deep lobe and the prestyloid parapharyngeal space is often indistinct or absent and presents no barrier to the spread of disease. Thus in many ways the deep lobe of the parotid gland can be considered to reside functionally within the prestyloid compartment of the parapharyngeal space.

As discussed, the parapharyngeal space is divided into an anterolateral prestyloid and posteromedial retrostyloid compartment by the fascia associated with the tensor veli palatini muscle, styloid process, and styloid musculature. The prestyloid compartment contains only fat, the pterygoid venous plexus, and a small branch of the fifth cranial nerve crossing the extreme upper space to reach the tensor veli palatini muscle.[17] Other small neural elements and vessels are also present. The retrostyloid compartment of the parapharyngeal space is much more complex and contains the internal carotid artery, internal jugular vein, cranial nerves IX through XII, sympathetic chain, and styloid musculature.[19] Cranial nerves IX, X, and XII descend between the internal carotid artery and the internal jugular vein; XI resides between and then lateral to the vessels; and the sympathetic chain is posterior and medial to the vascular bundle.[19, 22]

Masticator Space

The masticator space is formed as the superficial layer of the deep cervical fascia splits at the inferior margin of the mandible into medial and lateral layers. This space can be divided into a suprazygomatic compartment, which contains only the bulk of the temporalis muscle, and an infrazygomatic compartment, which includes the remainder of the muscles of mastication; the ramus and posterior body of the mandible; and lingual and inferior alveolar branches of the mandibular division of the trigeminal nerve.[17, 18] The lateral fascial boundary covers the temporalis muscle, attaches to the zygomatic arch, extends infe-

riorly to cover the masseter muscle, and attaches to the posterior and inferior margins of the mandible.[23] The medial fascial boundary of the masticator space is formed by a continuous layer covering the medial aspect of the medial pterygoid muscle, extending anteriorly to the anterior aspect of the mandibular ramus, superiorly to the skull base medial to the medial pterygoid plate and foramen ovale, and posteriorly to the posterior margin of the mandibular ramus.[17, 23] In its course, this fascial layer incorporates the sphenomandibular ligament, which extends from the spine of the sphenoid bone to the lingula of the mandible at the entrance to the mandibular canal.[17, 23] This medial layer separates the prestyloid compartment of the parapharyngeal space from the masticator space. The presence of most of the branches of the mandibular division of the trigeminal nerve within the masticator space, as well as direct contiguity with the foramen ovale, explains the tendency for perineural extension of masticator space malignancy along the mandibular division of the trigeminal nerve, through the foramen ovale, and into the middle cranial fossa (see Fig. 33–1D).[12, 17, 18]

Localization of Pathologic Lesions

As previously noted, the fascial space from which a suprahyoid lesion originates markedly affects the differential diagnosis. Thus it is essential to determine whether the lesion arose within the masticator or parapharyngeal space or simply involved them secondarily. This task can be simplified by assessing the relationship of the lesion to the fat within the prestyloid compartment of the parapharyngeal space, which should be visible in all patients on both CT and MRI examinations. This method is very helpful in assigning lesions to the masticator space or retrostyloid compartment of the parapharyngeal space.[18]

The most difficult distinction in this region is between a lesion of the parotid space arising within the deep portion of the parotid gland medial to the stylomandibular tunnel from that arising primarily within the prestyloid compartment of the parapharyngeal space. In order to define a lesion as primary to the prestyloid compartment of the parapharyngeal space, one must identify fat surrounding the entire circumference of the lesion with an intact fat plane at all levels between the lesion and the deep portion of the parotid gland.[9, 18] The lack of an intervening fat plane at all levels suggests a parotid space mass rather than a prestyloid parapharyngeal tumor. Extension of the mass through the stylomandibular tunnel, which is often widened with posteromedial displacement of the styloid process (see Fig. 33–1E), involvement of the more superficial portions of the parotid gland, or extension of the mass along the facial nerve to the stylomastoid foramen also suggests a parotid space origin.[18]

Factors suggesting the origin of a mass within the retrostyloid compartment of the parapharyngeal space include anterolateral displacement of the prestyloid parapharyngeal fat, extension posterior to the styloid process rather than anteriorly through the stylomandibular tunnel, obliteration of fat planes surrounding the great vessels, anterior or medial displacement of the internal

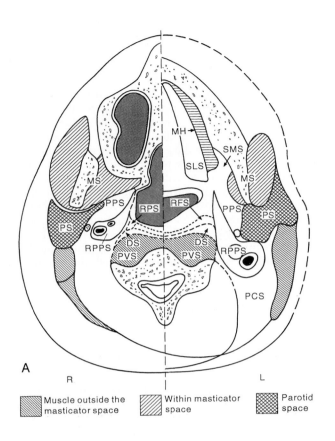

A

R   L

| Muscle outside the masticator space | Within masticator space | Parotid space |

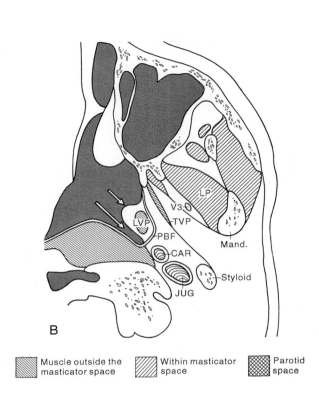

B

| Muscle outside the masticator space | Within masticator space | Parotid space |

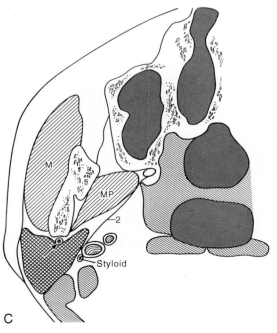

C

FIGURE 33–1 *A,* Diagrammatic representation of suprahyoid spaces at level of nasopharynx (L) and oropharynx (R). *B* and *C,* Diagrammatic representation of fascial layers separating the prestyloid and retrostyloid compartments of the parapharyngeal space and the masticator space.

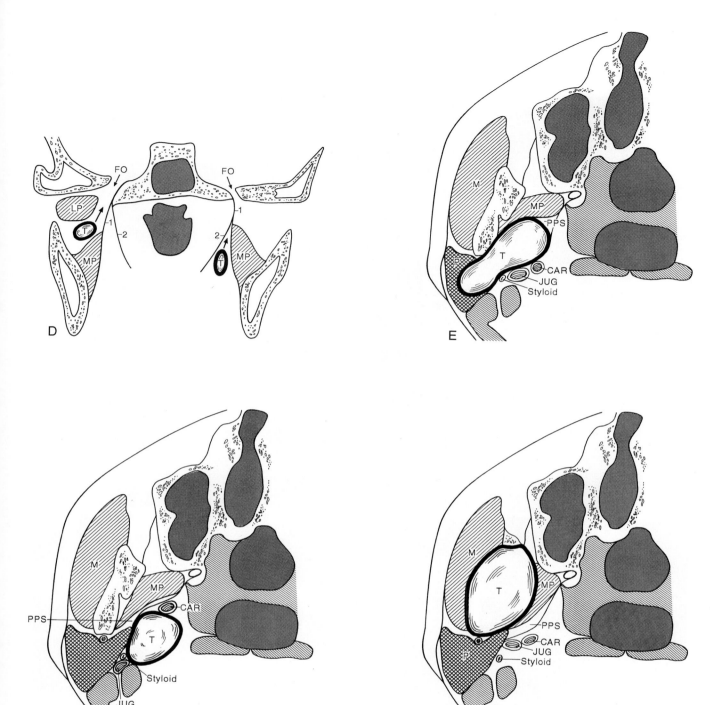

FIGURE 33–1 *Continued. D*, Coronal masticator space. *E*, Deep lobe parotid mass. Extension of the mass through a widened stylomandibular tunnel is noted and is common with deep lobe parotid tumors. When extension through the stylomandibular tunnel is not present, careful search for an intervening fat plane between the mass and the parotid gland at every level is necessary before a mass can be considered prestyloid parapharyngeal in origin. *F*, Retrostyloid compartment parapharyngeal mass. Characteristic anterolateral displacement of the prestyloid parapharyngeal fat, anterior displacement of the internal carotid artery, and extension posterior to the styloid process are typical findings of a retrostyloid parapharyngeal mass. *G*, Masticator space mass. Posteromedial displacement of the prestyloid parapharyngeal fat and obliteration of the normal fat planes within the masticator space are characteristic for a masticator space mass. *Key for diagrams A–G:* 1, fascia attached to the medial pterygoid muscle; 2, fascia of the tensor veli palatini; B, buccinator muscle; CAR, internal carotid artery; DS, danger space; FO, foramen ovale; JUG, internal jugular vein; LP, lateral pterygoid muscle; LVP, levator veli palatini; M, masseter muscle; Mand, mandibular condyle; MH, mylohyoid muscle; MP, medial pterygoid muscle; MS, masticator space; P, parotid gland; PBF, pharyngobasilar fascia; PCS, posterior cervical space; PPS, prestyloid compartment of parapharyngeal space; PS, parotid space; PVS, prevertebral space; RPPS, retrostyloid compartment of parapharyngeal space; RPS, retropharyngeal space; SLS, sublingual space; SMS, submandibular space; Styloid, styloid process; T, tumor; TVP, tensor veli palatini; V3, mandibular division of the trigeminal nerve in the masticator space; *short arrow*, torus tubarius; *long arrow* in *B*, Rosenmüller's fossa; *long arrow* in *C*, external carotid artery. (*A–G*, From Lewin JL. Imaging of the suprahyoid neck. In Valvassori GE, Mafee MF, Carter BL [eds]. Imaging of the Head and Neck, pp. 390–423. Stuttgart, Georg Thieme, 1995.)

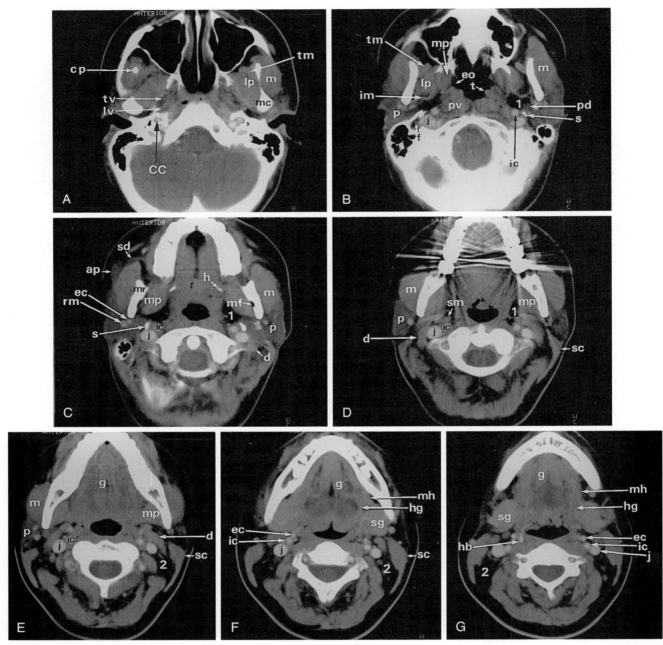

FIGURE 33–2 *A–G*, Normal anatomy: axial 5-mm contrast-enhanced computed tomography (CT) images. *Key for diagrams*: ap, accessory parotid tissue; c, common carotid artery; cc, internal carotid artery in vertical portion of petrous canal; cp, coronoid process of mandible surrounded by superficial (lateral) and deep (medial) heads of temporalis muscle; d, posterior belly of the digastric muscle; e, epiglottis; ec, external carotid artery; eo, eustachian tube orifice; f, fascial nerve surrounded by fat in stylomastoid foramen; fo, foramen ovale; g, genioglossus/geniohyoid muscle; h, hamulus of the medial pterygoid; hb, superior cornu of hyoid bone; hc, hypoglossal canal; hg, hyoglossus muscle; ic, internal carotid artery; im, internal maxillary artery and vein; j, internal jugular vein; lc, longus capitis muscle; lp, lateral pterygoid muscle; lv, levator veli palatini muscle; m, masseter muscle; mc, mandibular condyle; mf, mandibular foramen; mh, mylohyoid muscle; mp, medial pterygoid muscle; mr, ramus of mandible; p, parotid gland; pc, parapharyngeal constrictor muscle; pd, deep lobe of parotid gland extending through stylomandibular tunnel; pv, prevertebral muscle; rm, retromandibular vein; sc, sternocleidomastoid muscle; sd, Stensen's duct; sg, submandibular gland; sm, styloid musculature; t, torus tubarius overlying levator veli palatini muscle; tm, deep head of temporalis muscle; tv, tensor veli palatini muscle; z, zygomatic arch; 1, fat in prestyloid compartment of parapharyngeal space; 2, fat in posterior cervical space. (*A–G*, From Lewin JL. Imaging of the suprahyoid neck. In Valvassori GE, Mafee MF, Carter BL [eds]. Imaging of the Head and Neck, pp. 390–423. Stuttgart, Georg Thieme, 1995.)

carotid artery, and anterolateral displacement of the styloid process (see Fig. 33–1F).[9, 17, 18]

A masticator space mass results in posteromedial displacement of the prestyloid parapharyngeal fat along with obliteration of fat planes within the masticator space, limitation of tumor by the boundaries of the masticator space, and a tendency to spread through the foramen ovale (see Fig. 33–1G).[17] Masticator space lesions may push the medial pterygoid muscle into the prestyloid parapharyngeal fat but are not seen medial to and separate from the muscle.[17]

Normal Imaging Anatomy and Imaging Technique

Anatomy of the parapharyngeal and masticator spaces is well defined on both CT (Fig. 33–2) and MRI (Fig. 33–3). CT examination is best performed with a 3- to 5-mm slice thickness and bolus intravenous contrast enhancement in the axial plane. A high-resolution bone-reconstruction algorithm should be used in addition when perineural spread through the skull base foramina or direct mandibular or skull base invasion is suspected. Direct coronal images are also helpful when a lesion approaches the skull base or when the submandibular and sublingual spaces are involved.

MRI for anatomic localization of an abnormality is best performed with T1-weighted images with their high signal-to-noise ratio and excellent fat/muscle and fat/tumor distinction. Conversely, abnormality is often better detected on T2-weighted images. Recently, fast spin echo T2-weighted images with fat suppression have demonstrated very high lesion conspicuity.[24] T1-weighted studies following gadolinium contrast enhancement are also helpful for the detection of pathologic lesions and provide excellent evaluation of lesion extension and perineural spread. The evaluation of skull base or other bone involvement is often best performed with contrast-enhanced T1-weighted images using fat-saturation techniques.

The axial plane is often most helpful, and both T1- and T2-weighted axial imaging should be performed in all cases. Coronal T1-weighted images improve the evaluation of lesions adjacent to the skull base. Sagittal T1-weighted images are also very helpful when midline lesions are evaluated. The imaging slices should be no more than 3 or 4 mm thick for T1-weighted images and 5 mm thick for T2-weighted images, with an interslice gap of 1 mm or less. For T1-weighted images, the echo time should be kept as short as possible to reduce magnetic-susceptibility artifact. Motion-compensation gradients and spatial-presaturation pulses may be helpful to reduce flow and other motion artifacts. The optimal field of view, matrix size, and number of signal averages depend upon the particular imaging system and field strength but should reflect a compromise between an adequate signal-to-noise ratio, spatial resolution, and total examination length.

Recent advances in computer technology have introduced the use of computer-generated three-dimensional reconstruction of the suprahyoid neck. This can be performed with both CT and MRI (Fig. 33–4). This may help in following tumor volumes, diagnostic imaging, surgical planning, patient education, and medical research.[25]

Additionally, parapharyngeal space and masticator space lesions can be further evaluated using MRI- or CT-guided aspiration (Figs. 33–5 and 33–6). This procedure is minimally invasive and has a high rate of accuracy (90% to 95%), high yield, and low cost.[26] Although the potential for tumor seeding along the needle track exists, it is virtually nonexistent with the use of needles smaller than 20 gauge.[26] As aspiration of head and neck masses before surgery becomes the standard of care, the negligible risk of tumor seeding is outweighed by the information obtained with regard to the surgical approach.[26]

PATHOLOGY

Parapharyngeal Space

A wide variety of pathologic processes can affect the parapharyngeal space; these include congenital lesions, infection, and neoplasm (Tables 33–1 and 33–2). Tumors may arise primarily within the parapharyngeal space, invade from surrounding fascial spaces, or occur as metastatic disease.[27] Benign parapharyngeal masses typically grow slowly and are often asymptomatic, making clinical detection difficult; commonly, they are incidentally discovered on physical examination.[28, 29] When the lesion has grown to 2.5 to 3 cm in diameter, the classic triad of intraoral medial displacement of the lateral pharyngeal wall, tonsil, and palate; retromandibular fullness; and trismus may be present.[6, 28] These findings are seen because growth of a parapharyngeal mass is primarily limited to medial expansion, as the parapharyngeal space is limited by bony structures superiorly and laterally.[27] Although this characteristic displacement of the oropharynx and palate

---

TABLE 33–1 Parapharyngeal Space—Prestyloid Compartment

Congenital Lesions
Second branchial cleft cyst

Inflammatory Disease
Cellulitis
Abscess

Benign Tumors
Benign salivary gland tumors
Uncommon benign tumors
    Lipomas
    Rhabdomyomas
    Teratomas
    Dermoid tumors
    Hibernoma

Malignant Tumors
Malignancies of salivary gland origin
    Mucoepidermoid carcinoma
    Adenoid cystic carcinoma
    Acinic cell carcinoma
Nasopharyngeal carcinoma—direct extension
Uncommon malignant tumors
    Rhabdomyosarcoma
    Leiomyosarcoma
    Synovial cell sarcoma
    Malignant fibrous histiosarcoma
    Chordoma
    Ectomesenchymoma
    Lymphoma—direct extension from parotid gland

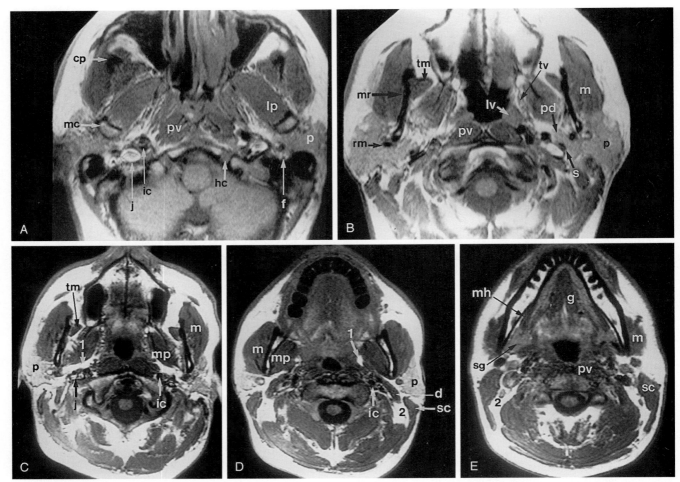

FIGURE 33–3 Normal anatomy: T1-weighted (TR = 700/TE = 14) magnetic resonance imaging (MRI): *A–E,* axial; *F–H,* coronal; *I–K,* sagittal. *Key for diagrams:* ap, accessory parotid tissue; c, common carotid artery; cc, internal carotid artery in vertical portion of petrous canal; cp, coronoid process of mandible surrounded by superficial (lateral) and deep (medial) heads of temporalis muscle; d, posterior belly of the digastric muscle; e, epiglottis; ec, external carotid artery; eo, eustachian tube orifice; f, fascial nerve surrounded by fat in stylomastoid foramen; fo, foramen ovale; g, genioglossus/geniohyoid muscle; h, hamulus of the medial pterygoid; hb, superior cornu of hyoid bone; hc, hypoglossal canal; hg, hyoglossus muscle; ic, internal carotid artery; im, internal maxillary artery and vein; j, internal jugular vein; lc, longus capitis muscle; lp, lateral pterygoid muscle; lv, levator veli palatini muscle; m, masseter muscle; mc, mandibular condyle; mf, mandibular foramen; mh, mylohyoid muscle; mp, medial pterygoid muscle; mr, ramus of mandible; p, parotid gland; pc, pharyngeal constrictor muscle; pd, deep lobe of parotid gland extending through stylomandibular tunnel; pv, prevertebral muscle; rm, retromandibular vein; s, styloid process; sc, sternocleidomastoid muscle; sd, Stensen's duct; sg, submandibular gland; sm, styloid musculature; t, torus tubarius overlying levator veli palatini muscle; tm, deep head of temporalis muscle; tv, tensor veli palatini muscle; z, zygomatic arch; 1, fat in prestyloid compartment of parapharyngeal space; 2, fat in posterior cervical space. (*A–K,* From Lewin JL. Imaging of the suprahyoid neck. In Valvassori GE, Mafee MF, Carter BL [eds]. Imaging of the Head and Neck, pp. 390–423. Stuttgart, Georg Thieme, 1995.)

may suggest a parapharyngeal mass, clinical differentiation between a mass originating within the parapharyngeal space, deep lobe of the parotid, or medial masticator space may be difficult or impossible.[6] As a parapharyngeal mass enlarges, throat discomfort, dysphagia, and hearing loss from encroachment on the pharynx, eustachian tube, and retrostyloid compartment neurovascular structures may occur.[28] When the retrostyloid compartment is affected, cranial nerve involvement may result in the syndrome of Vernet with paralysis of the ninth, tenth, and eleventh cranial nerves.[20] Although problems with speech or swallowing may result from cranial nerve damage, such symptoms are usually due simply to displacement of the

palate by an expansile lesion.[20] A lesion in the parapharyngeal space may also cause severe vasodepressor syncope because of abnormal stimulation of the glossopharyngeal nerve causing complex cardiovascular syncope, including carotid sinus syndrome, glossopharyngeal neuralgia-asystole syndrome, and newly described parapharyngeal space lesion syncope syndrome.[30] A Horner syndrome may occasionally result from involvement of the sympathetic chain by a lesion of this space but is more common with malignant than benign processes.[20] Malignant tumors are also typically associated with pain and cranial nerve palsy much earlier in their course.[28]

In the parapharyngeal space as a whole, major and

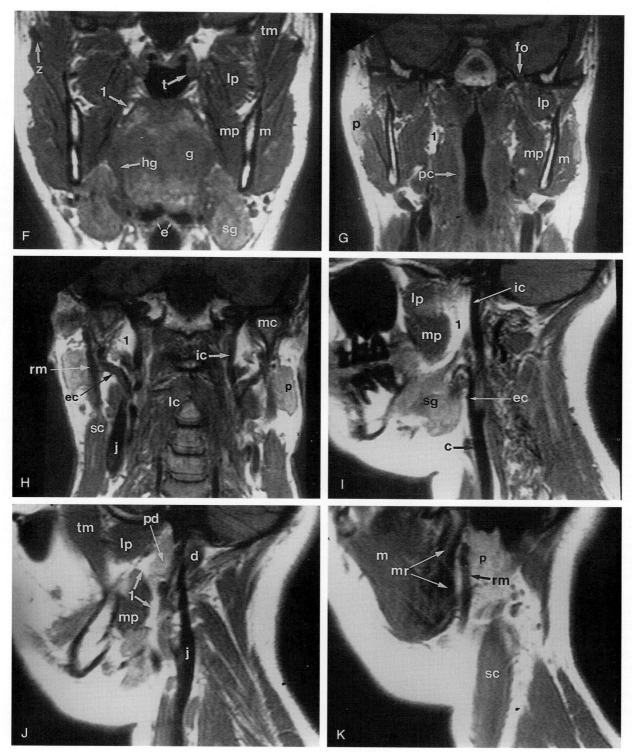

FIGURE 33–3 *Continued*

minor salivary gland tumors constitute 30% to 50% of all masses, including deep lobe parotid tumors extending into the prestyloid compartment of the parapharyngeal space.[9, 29] Neurogenic tumors account for 17% to 30% of parapharyngeal space masses, and glomus tumors constitute 10% to 15%.[9, 29] The remaining parapharyngeal space

lesions include metastases, branchial cleft cysts, lipomas, and rare tumors.[9, 19, 29] Approximately 80% of parapharyngeal space tumors are benign.[9, 19, 29, 31]

This differential diagnosis can be shortened considerably when the mass is identified as being located in either the prestyloid or the retrostyloid compartment of the

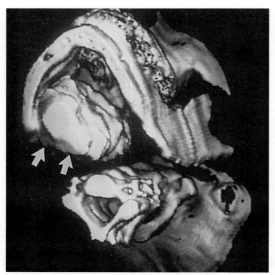

FIGURE 33–4 Reconstructed three-dimensional CT image of mass in the masticator space *(arrows)*. The reconstruction of the segmented mass and surrounding bone is viewed from below.

parapharyngeal space; it can be further limited through evaluation of imaging characteristics.[6, 9, 18] It is particularly important to be able to predict which lesions are likely to be of salivary gland origin, as a potential for recurrence is encountered when a biopsy is performed before removal of a pleomorphic adenoma, the most common salivary gland tumor.[17, 26] In addition, differentiation of a parapharyngeal primary lesion from a tumor of deep lobe parotid origin with extension into the parapharyngeal space ultimately alters the surgical approach.

The following sections discuss the more commonly encountered parapharyngeal space abnormalities.

Prestyloid Compartment of the Parapharyngeal Space

Congenital Abnormalities

Congenital lesions of the prestyloid parapharyngeal space are rare. Although the lesions are unusual, most large series of parapharyngeal space masses include cases of second branchial cleft cysts, which may be the most common low-attenuation lesion in the prestyloid compartment.[6, 8, 20, 32] The second branchial apparatus is the most common source of branchial cleft abnormalities, with cysts more common than sinuses or fistulas.[33] During embryogenesis the second branchial arch overgrows the second, third, and fourth clefts, forming an ectoderm-lined cavity called the *cervical sinus of His*.[33] Incomplete obliteration of the cervical sinus can result in a second branchial apparatus abnormality anywhere along a line from the oropharyngeal tonsillar fossa to the supraclavicular region of the neck.[33–35] Although second branchial cleft cysts most commonly present in a more lateral location, they can atypically present in the parapharyngeal space, arising from the parapharyngeal portion of the embryonic tract.[33, 34] These lesions are low in attenuation on CT, with a thin, smooth wall; however, when infected, the wall may become thickened and irregular, and the surrounding

fat planes may become obscured.[33, 34] Identification of associated sinuses or fistulas and complete excision is important in preventing recurrence of these second branchial cleft anomalies.[35] Other lesions presenting with similar imaging appearances, including cystic or necrotic neural tumors, cystic hygromas, necrotic metastases, or dermoid and epidermoid tumors,[34] are not typically found within the prestyloid compartment of the parapharyngeal space.

Inflammatory Disease

Infection of the prestyloid compartment of the parapharyngeal space most commonly arises from spread of peritonsillar abscesses; retrotonsillar vein thrombophlebitis; third molar extractions with violation of the pterygomandibular raphe; penetrating injury to the lateral pharyngeal wall; or extension of deep lobe parotid abscesses, or as a complication of local anesthesia for tonsillectomy or dental surgery.[36–38] Inflammation may also spread from the submandibular glands, branchial cleft or thyroglossal duct cysts, otitis, mastoiditis, or temporal bone infections through petrous apex air cells.[36, 39]

Patterns of spread of inflammatory changes within the parapharyngeal and adjacent spaces depend upon individual differences in fascial anatomy that may arise from

TABLE 33–2 Parapharyngeal Space— Retrostyloid Compartment

Congenital Lesions
Third branchial cyst—rare
Vascular Lesions
Aneurysm
Pseudoaneurysm
Thrombosis of internal jugular vein or carotid artery
Inflammatory Disease
Septic thrombophlebitis of internal jugular vein
Cellulitis
Abscess
Benign Tumors
Paragangliomas
    Glomus vagale
    Glomus tumor of carotid body
    Glomus jugulare
Nerve sheath origin
    Schwannoma
    Neurofibroma
Uncommon benign tumors
    Meningiomas—extracranial extension
Malignant Tumors
Metastatic disease
    Direct extension
        Nasopharyngeal carcinoma
        Uncommon—intracranial meningioma and clival chordoma
    Nodal extension
        Nasopharyngeal carcinoma
        Hypervascular metastases—kidneys and thyroid gland
Uncommon malignant tumors
    Malignant paraganglioma
    Malignant schwannoma

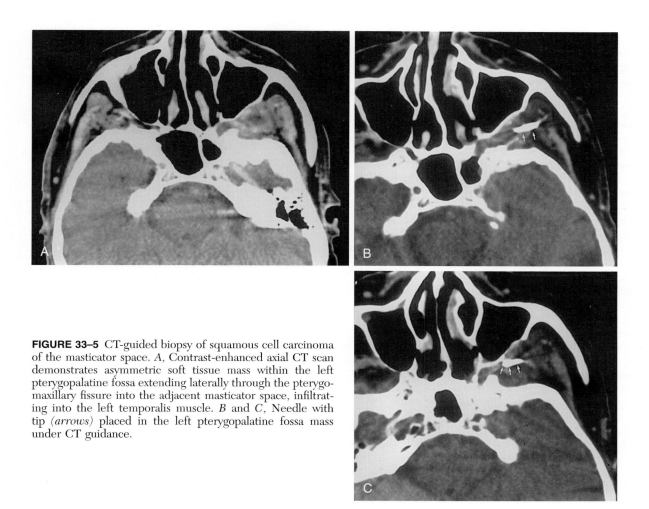

FIGURE 33–5 CT-guided biopsy of squamous cell carcinoma of the masticator space. *A*, Contrast-enhanced axial CT scan demonstrates asymmetric soft tissue mass within the left pterygopalatine fossa extending laterally through the pterygomaxillary fissure into the adjacent masticator space, infiltrating into the left temporalis muscle. *B* and *C*, Needle with tip *(arrows)* placed in the left pterygopalatine fossa mass under CT guidance.

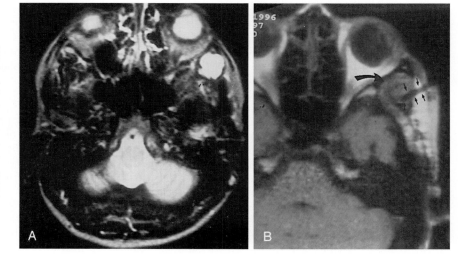

FIGURE 33–6 MRI-guided biopsy of masticator space mass (recurrent odontogenic keratocyst). *A*, T2-weighted axial image (2500/90) demonstrates a mass with homogeneous increased signal involving the left temporal fossa. *B*, Gradient-echo T1-weighted axial image (18/7) demonstrates the mass *(curved arrow)* involving the temporalis muscle. MRI-guided biopsy of this lesion is performed using an MRI-compatible needle *(small arrows)* and a rapid-acquisition gradient-echo "MRI-fluoroscopic" technique.

normal variation, previous trauma, surgery, infection, or radiation therapy.[40] The virulence and antibiotic sensitivity of the invading organism as well as the general health and immunologic status of the host may also affect the spread of infection.[40] Once inside the prestyloid parapharyngeal space, infection can readily extend into the parotid, masticator, submandibular, or retrostyloid compartment of the parapharyngeal space.[36] Common pathogens include *Staphylococcus aureus*, *Streptococcus pyogenes*, anaerobic bacteria, and *Klebsiella pneumoniae*.[38]

The clinical presentation of infection of the parapharyngeal and adjacent spaces includes the sudden onset of fever and chills. Dysfunction of cranial nerves IX through XII or the sympathetic plexus may occur with extension into the retrostyloid compartment, and trismus may occur with masticator space involvement. Painful swelling of the gingival tissues of the maxilla and of the cheek at the level of the mandible on the involved side is the most commonly noted finding in patients with a parapharyngeal abscess.[37, 38] On clinical examination, a medial bulge of the lateral pharyngeal wall is commonly seen.[36, 37]

Complications of parapharyngeal space infection include erosion of the adjacent carotid artery with fatal hemorrhage or pseudoaneurysm formation, as well as extension to the retropharyngeal space with possible asphyxia or dysphagia from the resulting mass effect and inflammation.[37] Paranasal sinus and orbital involvement, intracranial extension with cavernous sinus thrombophlebitis, jugular vein thrombophlebitis, mediastinitis, pericarditis, and osteomyelitis may also result.[38, 39, 41]

Imaging of the parapharyngeal and adjacent spaces may be of great assistance in detecting complications of deep neck infections and determining the optimal timing and approach for surgical drainage.[36] Imaging is most useful when infection is complex, widespread, or difficult to assess clinically.[41] On CT, cellulitis may present as a soft tissue mass with obliteration of adjacent fat planes, often ill-defined, enhancing and extending along fascial planes and into subcutaneous tissues (Fig. 33–7).[37, 41] Involved muscles may enhance and appear enlarged, and overlying subcutaneous tissues often demonstrate linear or mottled increased attenuation beneath thickened skin.[37]

Abscesses of the deep neck spaces, reported to represent up to 9% of masses within the parapharyngeal space, often appear as uni- or multiloculated cystic lesions with air- or fluid-attenuation centers, may have somewhat irregular enhancing walls or surrounding tissue edema, and may conform to the surrounding fascial boundaries.[6, 20, 36, 37] Occasionally, pus formation may be incomplete or may be delayed by antibiotic therapy, and an area of low attenuation on CT suggesting an abscess cavity may not yield pus on aspiration or exploration (see Fig. 33–7). In fact, a false-positive rate of 10% to 15% and a similar false-negative rate have been reported for CT in the prediction of the presence or absence of abscess-cavity formation when compared with intraoperative findings.[37, 39]

Although axial and coronal CT may determine the extent of disease and presence of complications, MRI often provides better localization with its multiplanar capabilities and better soft tissue contrast resolution. Inflammatory exudate is of low to intermediate signal inten-

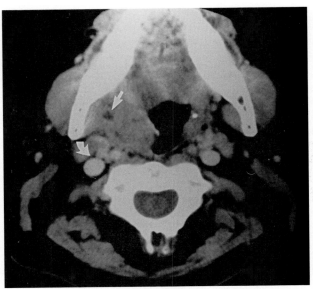

FIGURE 33–7 Prestyloid compartment parapharyngeal space infection from spread of tonsillitis. Axial contrast-enhanced CT scan at the level of the oropharynx demonstrates enlargement of the right faucial tonsil with obliteration of the prestyloid parapharyngeal fat on the right. One small area of decreased attenuation is noted within the inflammatory process, which may represent a small abscess cavity *(straight arrow)*. Fat planes surrounding the contents of the retrostyloid compartment of the parapharyngeal space remain intact *(curved arrow)*. (From Lewin JL. Imaging of the suprahyoid neck. In Valvassori GE, Mafee MF, Carter BL [eds]. Imaging of the Head and Neck, pp. 390–423. Stuttgart, Georg Thieme, 1995.)

sity on T1-weighted images and is often isointense with adjacent muscle.[37] Both cellulitis and abscess cavities exhibit increased signal intensity on T2-weighted images.[37] Gadolinium contrast agents may be helpful to differentiate abscess from cellulitis through demonstration of an enhancing abscess wall.[37] The findings on both MRI and CT are typically unable to differentiate a bacterial versus a granulomatous origin of inflammation.[37]

Antibiotics are an integral part of the management of parapharyngeal space infections. However, early open surgical drainage of abscesses is recommended to avoid life-threatening complications and may allow more rapid recovery.[38] CT-guided or MRI-guided aspiration may also provide a minimally invasive nonsurgical treatment option.[38, 39, 42]

Benign Tumors

The majority of prestyloid parapharyngeal space tumors are benign, and of these, most are of salivary gland origin, with pleomorphic adenoma representing the most common histologic type.[28] Salivary gland tumors in this space most commonly arise from the parotid gland deep to the facial nerve and lateral to the mandible. These commonly extend into the parapharyngeal space through the stylomandibular tunnel, giving a dumbbell configuration.[28, 30]

However, salivary gland tumors can also arise primarily within the prestyloid compartment from congenital rests of salivary gland tissue.[8, 9, 28] The site of origin of prestyloid compartment salivary neoplasms is of importance in the surgical management of these patients, as a lesion arising within the deep lobe of the parotid gland is usually treated with operative control of the facial nerve to prevent nerve damage, whereas a lesion totally confined to the prestyloid parapharyngeal space without connection to the parotid gland may be treated with little concern for facial nerve injury.[6, 43] At some institutions, a submandibular approach without control of the facial nerve also may be used for deep lobe parotid masses when the tumor does not approach the stylomandibular tunnel. The patient typically presents with a painless mass, as benign salivary gland tumors seldom result in other symptoms.[44]

The CT appearance of a benign salivary gland tumor is most often as an ovoid soft tissue mass. The tumors are typically homogeneous when small but when larger may show variable areas of low attenuation representing sites of cystic degeneration or seromucinous collections.[9] In addition, focal areas of high attenuation representing calcification may be present.[9]

The MRI appearance of a benign salivary gland tumor is that of a well-defined mass with low to intermediate signal intensity on T1-weighted and intermediate-weighted (long TR, short TE) images, and intermediate increased signal on T2-weighted images (Fig. 33–8). Smaller lesions are typically homogeneous in appearance, whereas lesions greater than 2.5 cm in diameter are often heterogeneous on all pulse sequences and may have internal foci of low signal or signal void corresponding to areas of calcification or fibrosis (Fig. 33–8C).[8, 9] Areas of high signal intensity on T1- and intermediate-weighted images may also occur in larger tumors and correspond to areas of local hemorrhage.[9] With the prevalence of such findings, mass heterogeneity is not a useful predictor of benign versus malignant neoplasm.[9] The best pre-

dictors of a benign pleomorphic adenoma are the presence of dystrophic calcifications, best detected with CT, or a well-defined highly lobulated tumor contour, best seen on MRI.[9]

To diagnose an extraparotid origin of a prestyloid parapharyngeal tumor, an intact fat plane between the posterolateral margin of the tumor and the deep portion of the parotid gland must be clearly demonstrated.[9] Careful attention is necessary, as this connection may be a very thin isthmus of tissue that is best detected on high-resolution, thin-section axial T1-weighted MRI.[9] When lesions are greater than 4 cm in diameter, the intervening fat plane may be obliterated by mass effect alone, and distinction between intraparotid and extraparotid origin may be impossible (see Fig. 33–8A).[9] In such cases, the surgical approach for a tumor of parotid origin is often used in order to minimize the risk of facial nerve damage.[6, 9]

Benign lesions of the prestyloid compartment of the parapharyngeal space other than those of salivary gland origin are rare, although several series report lipomas of this space.[6, 9, 20, 32] These uncommon lesions are readily identified by their characteristic low attenuation on CT and characteristic signal intensity on all MRI pulse sequences paralleling that of fat. Other rare benign lesions of this space include hibernoma, rhabdomyomas, teratomas, and dermoid tumors.[29, 45]

Malignant Tumors

Malignant tumors of the prestyloid compartment of the parapharyngeal space are much less common than benign lesions and include malignancies of salivary gland origin, such as mucoepidermoid, adenoid cystic, and acinic cell carcinomas, along with direct invasion of malignancies of

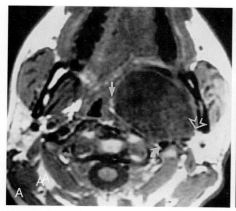 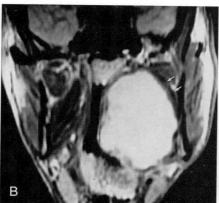 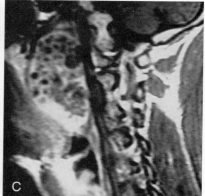

FIGURE 33–8 Pleomorphic adenoma of the prestyloid compartment of the parapharyngeal space. *A*, T1-weighted axial image (500/12) demonstrates a well-defined mass of lower signal intensity than adjacent muscle replacing the prestyloid parapharyngeal fat with minimal residual fat displaced medially *(straight arrow)* and the internal carotid artery displaced posteriorly *(curved arrow)*. No intact fat plane can be demonstrated between the lesion and the deep lobe over the parotid gland *(open arrow)*. *B*, Intermediate-weighted (2500/30) coronal image demonstrates the mass to be relatively homogeneous, of increased signal intensity relative to adjacent muscles and lymphoid tissue, and well defined, with displacement of the oropharyngeal mucosa medially. The left medial pterygoid muscle is compressed and displaced superiorly and laterally *(arrows)*. *C*, Contrast-enhanced T1-weighted (500/15) sagittal image demonstrates marked heterogeneity of the mass, with multiple low-signal-intensity regions, which may represent areas of calcification or fibrosis. Both sagittal and coronal images are useful to demonstrate the craniocaudad extent of the lesion, which fills the majority of the prestyloid parapharyngeal space. The mass is inseparable from the deep lobe of the parotid gland and must be considered arising from the deep lobe for surgical planning. However, the deep lobe of the parotid gland was compressed and displaced laterally with no visible connection to the mass at surgery. (*A–C*, From Lewin JL. Imaging of the suprahyoid neck. In Valvassori GE, Mafee MF, Carter BL [eds]. Imaging of the Head and Neck, pp. 390–423. Stuttgart, Georg Thieme, 1995.)

the adjacent spaces.[9, 19] Differentiation from benign tumors may be difficult, as approximately two-thirds of salivary gland malignancies may have smooth, well-defined margins.[9] However, the presence of an irregular, ill-defined margin or infiltration of surrounding tissues may suggest a more aggressive lesion. Unfortunately, an inflammatory reaction surrounding a benign tumor may occasionally result in a similar appearance.[8] As there is often an incomplete fascial layer between prestyloid parapharyngeal space and the deep lobe of the parotid gland, malignancies of the parotid gland such as lymphoma may easily extend into the prestyloid parapharyngeal space (Fig. 33–9). Other rare malignant tumors in this space include rhabdomyosarcoma, leiomyosarcoma, synovial sarcoma, malignant fibrous histiosarcoma, chordoma, and ectomesenchymoma.[29, 45, 46]

Retrostyloid Compartment of the Parapharyngeal Space

The diagnosis of a mass within the retrostyloid compartment of the parapharyngeal space is based on recognition of the relationship of the mass to the styloid process and internal carotid artery, and observation of the typical displacement of the prestyloid parapharyngeal fat, as discussed previously (see Fig. 33–1F). Masses within the retrostyloid compartment of the parapharyngeal space are most commonly paragangliomas or tumors of nerve sheath origin. However, a variety of masses may arise from the vascular, neural, or lymphoreticular contents of this space (see Table 33–2).

Congenital Abnormalities

Congenital lesions in the retrostyloid compartment of the parapharyngeal space are extremely rare. A third branchial cleft cyst may arise in this space. The internal

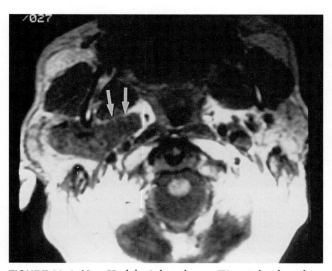

FIGURE 33–9 Non-Hodgkin's lymphoma. T1-weighted axial image (500/15) demonstrates a well-defined mass of heterogeneous signal similar to that of muscle involving the deep and superficial lobes of the parotid gland and extending into the prestyloid parapharyngeal space (*arrows*). There is significant widening of the stylomandibular tunnel with minimal displacement of the fat within the prestyloid compartment of the parapharyngeal space.

carotid artery is a third branchial arch artery, and congenital cysts from this arch may occur anywhere along a tract that passes posterior to the internal carotid artery and inferior to the glossopharyngeal nerve, ultimately entering the pharynx at the piriform sinus.[35, 47] The appearance on CT is similar to that of other cystic lesions, but the unusual location should suggest the correct diagnosis.[47]

Vascular Abnormalities

The internal carotid artery and internal jugular vein can give rise to a variety of lesions within the retrostyloid compartment of the parapharyngeal space. Aneurysm or pseudoaneurysm formation of the internal carotid artery within the space is of particular importance because palpation of a pulsatile mass may clinically mimic a paraganglioma. Preoperative diagnosis of this abnormality is essential for surgical planning to prevent potentially catastrophic hemorrhagic complications. This abnormality should be suggested when a markedly enhancing mass on CT is inseparable from the internal carotid artery in this region, or when flow void or signal intensity suggesting thrombus is noted on MRI.[48] If the diagnosis is in question, angiography can be performed for confirmation. Several nonsurgical vascular pseudotumors may also occur and include a redundant, ectatic, or tortuous internal carotid artery, which may also present clinically as a pulsatile parapharyngeal space mass.[6] On CT, thrombosis of the internal carotid artery or internal jugular vein may mimic a necrotic mass in this region.[48] This potential pitfall may be avoided by noting the tubular configuration of the abnormality, MRI signal intensity characteristics suggesting thrombus, or the absence of a normal internal carotid artery or internal jugular vein. Attention should also be focused to the carotid arteries in patients with history of radiation therapy for nasopharyngeal carcinoma. Incidence of accelerated carotid artery atherosclerosis may be increased in these patients and can be seen on T1-weighted axial MRI.[49]

Inflammatory Disease

Infection of the retrostyloid compartment of the parapharyngeal space often results from extension of cellulitis or abscess from adjacent spaces; it may also result from suppuration and breakdown of internal jugular chain lymph nodes draining areas of submandibular, tonsillar, or pharyngeal infection.[37, 40] Infection of this space may result in a septic thrombophlebitis of the internal jugular vein, which was relatively common in the preantibiotic era, or it may result in internal carotid artery erosion, thrombosis, pseudoaneurysm formation, life-threatening airway obstruction, mediastinitis, pericarditis, or epidural abscess.[39, 40] Findings of cellulitis and abscess are discussed in the previous section on the prestyloid compartment of the parapharyngeal space. MRI is very useful in the assessment of retrostyloid compartment inflammation, as loss of the normal flow void within the internal carotid artery and internal jugular vein assist in the diagnosis of vascular thrombosis.[37] As with the prestyloid compartment, extension to the adjacent deep spaces in common. Extension into the infrahyoid carotid space is relatively uncommon, as there is little room for distention of the fascial space surrounding the vessels. However, inferior extension may occur in the presence of septic thrombosis.

Benign Tumors

Benign tumors represent the most common cause of masses within the retrostyloid compartment of the parapharyngeal space. The most common benign tumors are paragangliomas and schwannomas. Paragangliomas of the head and neck, also known as *chemodectomas* or *glomus cell tumors*, are slowly growing hypervascular tumors composed of nests of cells separated by numerous vascular channels within a fibrous matrix.[10, 50] They most commonly arise at the carotid artery bifurcation, followed by lesions within the jugular foramen or middle ear, and from the ganglion nodosum of the vagus nerve.[50] However, paragangliomas may also arise anywhere along the cervical course of the vagus nerve and its branches to the larynx and trachea, as well as within the mediastinum at the level of the aortic arch and pulmonary artery bifurcation.[50–52] Rarely, they arise along the facial nerve or within the orbit or nasal cavity.[50] The cell of origin acts as a homeostatic chemoreceptor, with tissue hyperplasia at the level of the carotid body and ganglion nodosum of the vagus nerve under hypoxic conditions. This hyperplasia is associated with a markedly increased incidence of paragangliomas in high-altitude regions such as Peru, Colorado, and Mexico City.[44, 50]

Paragangliomas of the retrostyloid compartment of the parapharyngeal space arise most commonly at or just below the ganglion nodosum of the vagus nerve and are termed *glomus vagale* tumors; they may also be secondary to inferior extension of a paraganglioma arising within the jugular foramen (glomus jugulare), or to superior extension of a carotid body tumor (Fig. 33–10).[6, 28, 32, 50–52] Occasionally, paragangliomas also arise from other chemoreceptor tissue located within the parapharyngeal space.[44]

Glomus vagale tumors may present as an asymptomatic mass but more commonly present with symptoms of vagal nerve dysfunction, such as vocal cord paralysis, or with symptoms from involvement of the hypoglossal or glossopharyngeal nerves.[44, 50, 52] Rarely, glomus vagale tumors may secrete catecholamines and cause symptoms of labile hypertension, tremulousness, headache, pallor, palpitations, and sweating.[29] This presentation is in contrast to carotid body paragangliomas, which seldom result in symptoms.[44] The age of patients presenting with paragangliomas varies widely, with the majority younger than 40 years.[32] These lesions are multicentric in approximately 3% to 20% of all patients, and in 25% to 38% of patients with a family history of paragangliomas.[10, 29, 52] Although malignant features with local or distant metastasis are seen in approximately 6% of carotid body tumors, the incidence of malignancy may rise to as high as 19% for glomus vagale tumors.[50, 52]

On CT examination, a glomus vagale tumor presents as a well-marginated mass within the retrostyloid compartment of the parapharyngeal space, almost always displacing the internal carotid artery anteriorly. Enhancement is intense after contrast administration and is homogeneous in the majority of cases.[6, 9] Occasionally, focal nonenhancing areas that are thought to represent areas of hemorrhage or necrosis are noted internally.[6, 9] With dynamic CT scanning during bolus administration of contrast material, rapid initial accumulation of contrast material consistent with a hypervascular mass is strongly suggestive of this diagnosis.[6, 9, 10] Without this dynamic information, CT cannot reliably differentiate a paraganglioma from other tumors that may enhance intensely, including approximately one-third of schwannomas.[5, 6, 10] When paragangliomas arise within the jugular foramen and extend inferiorly into the parapharyngeal space, a CT scan with high-resolution bone algorithm reconstruction best demonstrates the subtle osseous changes and rela-

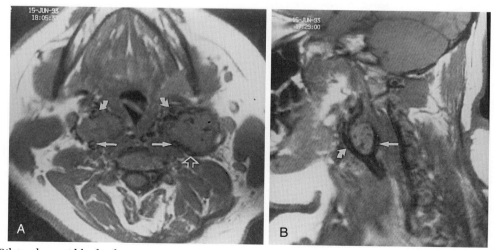

FIGURE 33–10 Bilateral carotid body glomus tumor. *A,* T1-weighted axial image (500/14) demonstrates well-defined bilateral masses isointense to muscle, which displace the external carotid arteries *(curved arrows)* anteriorly and the internal carotid arteries *(straight arrows)* posteriorly. The left internal jugular vein *(open arrow)* is compressed and displaced posteriorly by the mass. *B,* T1-weighted sagittal image (500/14) demonstrates the left-sided carotid body tumor extending superiorly from the carotid bifurcation and displacing the external carotid artery *(curved arrow)* anteriorly and internal carotid artery *(straight arrow)* posteriorly. Multiple areas of flow voids are seen within the mass.

tionship of the tumor to the middle ear and typically reveals a permeative pattern of bone involvement.[10] In addition, the remainder of the neck must be carefully evaluated to exclude multicentric involvement whenever a paraganglioma is suspected.

On MRI evaluation, paragangliomas are clearly outlined and distinguished from adjacent soft tissues and are typically ovoid with slight lobulation of the largest lesions (Fig. 33–11).[9] Again, the internal carotid artery is usually anteriorly or medially displaced. In signal intensity the tumors are approximately equal to or slightly higher than adjacent muscle on T1- and intermediate-weighted images.[8, 10] On T2-weighted images the lesions are moderately high in signal intensity that is greater than that of adjacent muscle.[8, 10] The most characteristic finding of paraganglioma on MRI is the presence of serpentine or punctate very low signal intensity regions, or *signal voids*, which are thought to be secondary to high-velocity flow

and resultant signal loss.[8, 10, 53, 54] These vary in number and distribution within the tumor and may not be present on every slice.[8] However, some areas of signal void should be seen in any lesion greater than 1.5 to 2.0 cm in maximal diameter.[8, 10, 55] Areas of high signal thought to be secondary to slow flow may also be seen interspersed with the areas of signal void.[8, 10] The adjacent high- and low-intensity regions have been described by several authors as having a "salt-and-pepper" appearance.[8, 10] This appearance is highly suggestive of a hypervascular tumor, with the glomus vagale tumor by far the most common lesion giving rise to this appearance in this location.[8] In general, the use of gadopentetate dimeglumine enhancement is not necessary for detection of paragangliomas. However, contrast enhancement is helpful when searching for small postoperative residual tumor.[55] The characteristic pattern of signal intensity, excellent tissue contrast, and anatomic detail, as well as good delineation of adja-

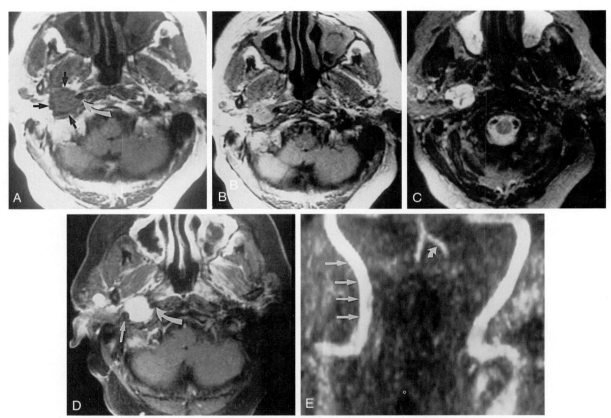

FIGURE 33–11 Glomus vagale tumor. *A*, T1-weighted (570/15) axial MRI demonstrates a lesion (*black arrows*) approximately equal to adjacent muscle in signal intensity, which is displacing the prestyloid parapharyngeal fat and internal carotid artery (*white arrow*) anteromedially. *B*, Intermediate-weighted (2500/15) image demonstrates signal intensity higher than that of adjacent muscle with several punctate areas of decreased signal intensity consistent with flow voids. *C*, T2-weighted (2500/90) image better demonstrates multiple curvilinear signal voids, which likely represent flow within vessels. The lesion has well-defined margins and is much higher in signal intensity than the surrounding tissues. *D*, Contrast-enhanced T1-weighted (600/15) image with fat suppression demonstrates marked enhancement of the lesion. Flow void within the anteromedially displaced internal carotid artery is again noted (*curved arrow*), and the styloid process is visualized (*straight arrow*). *E*, Three-dimensional time-of-flight magnetic resonance angiography (MRA) of the upper cervical internal carotid arteries demonstrates medial displacement of the right internal carotid artery at the level of the tumor (*straight arrows*). There is no evidence of narrowing to suggest encasement. Increased tumor vascularity is only infrequently observed with MRA techniques and is not visualized in this patient. The left internal carotid artery is tortuous, and the basilar and distal vertebral arteries are only partially included on this projection (*curved arrow*). (*A–E*, From Lewin JL. Imaging of the suprahyoid neck. In Valvassori GE, Mafee MF, Carter BL [eds]. Imaging of the Head and Neck, pp. 390–423. Stuttgart, Georg Thieme, 1995.)

cent vascular structures makes MRI the imaging modality of choice in the evaluation of suspected paragangliomas of the suprahyoid neck.[9, 10]

Before dynamic contrast-enhanced CT and MRI, the diagnosis of paraganglioma was established by its characteristic angiographic appearance.[50] The angiographic diagnosis of a glomus tumor was suggested by its profuse vascularity, with tortuous, well-defined nutrient vessels of relatively uniform caliber in the arterial phase and a dense tumor blush in the capillary phase.[50, 56] Characteristically, glomus vagale tumors demonstrate anterior and medial displacement of both the external and internal carotid arteries without involvement of the bifurcation and without direct involvement of the adjacent vessels (Fig. 33–11D).[50, 56] The tumor blush may be less homogeneous than that typical for a carotid body tumor or jugulotympanic paraganglioma; this may be due to the greater degree of sclerosis noted histologically in some glomus vagale tumors.[50] Although no longer necessary for diagnosis, angiography continues to have a role in the treatment of paragangliomas, permitting palliative or preoperative embolization and outlining the vascular supply before surgical resection.[10, 29, 50] Additionally, if carotid artery sacrifice is contemplated, a test balloon occlusion of the internal carotid artery using a radionuclide cerebral perfusion agent (technetium-99m–hexamethylpropyleneamineoxime) may help predict the effect of loss of the involved artery.[29]

Other preoperative tests before resection of paragangliomas include evaluation for catecholamine secretion products such as urine vanillylmandelic acid, metanephrines, dopamine, epinephrine, and norepinephrine. Serum catecholamine levels may also be obtained. This can prevent potential complications from unexpected catecholamine release during surgery.[29] Preoperative barium swallow examination provides baseline functional status since a potential postoperative complication of paraganglioma resection includes injury to cranial nerves IX, X, and XI.[52]

The preferred treatment of a glomus vagale tumor is complete surgical resection; adjunctive radiation therapy may also be useful if complete resection is impossible due to involvement of critical neurovascular structures at the skull base.[50] The postradiation changes of paragangliomas on MRI include a decrease in flow voids, heterogeneously decreased enhancement, and variable signal changes in T2-weighted images. Typically, the size of tumor does not change significantly after radiation therapy.[57]

The second major category of benign retrostyloid parapharyngeal space tumors consists of tumors of nerve sheath origin. Of these, the schwannoma is the most common tumor, followed by the neurofibroma.[28] Schwannomas arise from the Schwann cells of the nerve sheath and typically have both a solid fibrous component (Antoni's type A) and a gelatinous component (Antoni's type B), with both patterns typically present in the same tumor.[44] The schwannoma most commonly arises from the vagus nerve but may arise from the sympathetic trunk or, less commonly, from other adjacent nerves.[27–29, 44] Although this tumor may present as an asymptomatic mass, the nerve of origin is commonly paralyzed, with an ipsilateral vocal cord paralysis representing the most common

symptom of a vagus nerve schwannoma.[44] Pain and rapid growth are unusual in a schwannoma and suggest malignant change and a poor prognosis.[44] When below the angle of the mandible, these tumors are usually mobile from side to side but not in the superior-inferior direction on clinical examination.[56] As with paraganglioma, there is a wide age range at the time of detection, with the majority of patients in their fourth or fifth decade of life.[32] The treatment of choice for schwannomas is enucleation or tumor removal with sparing of the involved nerve. If this is not possible, as in many instances, tumor resection with nerve grafting may be necessary.[29]

Schwannomas are usually ovoid or fusiform masses within the retrostyloid parapharyngeal space and typically displace the internal carotid artery anteriorly when arising from the vagus nerve (Fig. 33–12).[9] This tumor typically has well-delineated margins. It is most commonly higher in attenuation than adjacent muscle on a contrast-enhanced CT scan but may be isodense or, less commonly, of lower attenuation than adjacent muscle.[9] Approximately one-third of schwannomas enhance significantly on CT (Fig. 33–12).[58] However, neurogenic lesions typically demonstrate a hypovascular enhancement time course on dynamic bolus-enhanced CT, differentiating them from hypervascular paragangliomas.[9] When the tumor extends to the level of the jugular foramen, CT typically demonstrates smooth scalloping of the bony margins, as opposed to the permeative changes noted with paraganglioma.[48]

MRI evaluation typically demonstrates a mass of intermediate signal intensity on T1- and intermediate-weighted images and increased signal intensity on T2-weighted images, again with smooth well-delineated contours and a homogeneous overall appearance (Fig. 33–13).[8] Although areas of signal void may occasionally be detected, these lesions do not have the salt-and-pepper appearance noted with paragangliomas.[8] Occasionally, schwannomas may appear cystic on CT and MRI; histologically, these lesions may demonstrate a coalescence of interstitial fluid-forming cystic spaces with prominent Antoni's B tissue, or an abundance of lipid-rich Schwann cells.[59]

Neurofibromas also occur within the retrostyloid compartment of the parapharyngeal space and, although often multiple in patients with neurofibromatosis, may present as a solitary lesion without a history of von Recklinghausen's disease.[28] Medium to large neurofibromas can have significant fatty infiltration and necrosis and can appear on CT as a single mass or as multiple low-attenuation masses that may have either no apparent rim or very thin rim of enhancement.[6] Histologically, the low attenuation appears to be due to the presence of adipocytes (transformed fibroblasts), entrapment of perineural adipose tissue by plexiform neurofibromas, or cystic degeneration secondary to infarction or necrosis.[59]

On MRI, neurofibromas typically have an intermediate signal intensity on T1- and intermediate-weighted images, similar to that of adjacent muscle, and may be somewhat heterogeneous on T2-weighted images.[8] Scattered focal areas of low signal intensity may be seen in larger lesions and may be due to dystrophic calcification, fibrosis, or flow.[8] A salt-and-pepper appearance has been reported in one lesion, but this is atypical for a neurofibroma.[8] On CT,

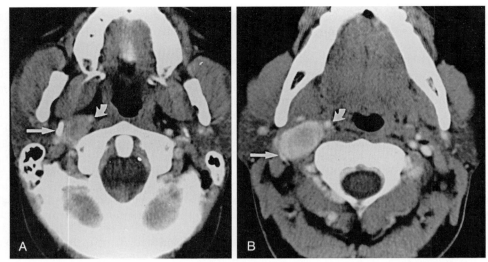

FIGURE 33–12 Vagus schwannoma. *A*, Axial CT scan at the onset of bolus contrast administration demonstrates an ovoid mass displacing the prestyloid parapharyngeal fat and internal carotid artery *(curved arrow)* anteromedially and the styloid process *(straight arrow)* slightly anterolaterally. The mass has relatively well delineated margins and is slightly higher in attenuation than adjacent muscle on this early contrast-enhanced scan. *B*, A slightly lower image again demonstrates displacement of the internal carotid artery medially *(curved arrow)* and internal jugular vein laterally *(straight arrow)*. The mass enhances densely on this image that was acquired later in the course of bolus contrast enhancement. (*A* and *B*, From Lewin JL. Imaging of the suprahyoid neck. In Valvassori GE, Mafee MF, Carter BL [eds]. Imaging of the Head and Neck, pp. 390–423. Stuttgart, Georg Thieme, 1995.)

the presence of multiple low-attenuation, well-defined masses is highly suggestive of this abnormality.

On angiography, neurogenic tumors may present as either vascular or hypervascular lesions.[56] Typically, the vascular stain of a neurogenic tumor is less dense than that of a paraganglioma and is generally more patchy with interspersed hypovascular and hypervascular areas.[56] In addition, the vascular stain of a neurogenic tumor is generally noted later in the angiographic run than is the early arterial stain of a paraganglioma.[56] As with paragangliomas, the preferred method of treatment is surgical resection.[60] Since neurofibromas are intimately associated with the affected nerve, nerve-sparing surgery is generally not possible.[29]

Other benign tumors of the retrostyloid compartment of the parapharyngeal space are uncommon. Extracranial extension of meningiomas, although rare, may spread into this space and typically demonstrate a dumbbell configuration with a small intracranial and larger extracranial component (Fig. 33–14).[6] On CT, the presence of scattered flecks or larger dense areas of calcification is typical, as is significant enhancement after contrast administration.[6] Smooth, scalloped enlargement of the jugular foramen or hyperostosis of the adjacent bone may also occasionally be identified. Rarely, benign tumors of the skull base such as a clival chordoma may extend into the retrostyloid parapharyngeal space (Fig. 33–15).

Malignant Tumors

The most common malignant processes involving the parapharyngeal space are metastatic disease and direct extension from nasopharyngeal or tonsillar carcinoma.[27, 28, 60] In particular, nasopharyngeal carcinoma typically extends superiorly through the sinus of Morgagni, the only lateral opening within the tough pharyngobasilar fascia,

and along the course of the eustachian tube into the parapharyngeal space (Figs. 33–16 through 33–18).[12]

Metastasis to the internal jugular lymph node chain is also common, with demonstration of pathologically enlarged lymph nodes anterolateral to the internal carotid artery and internal jugular vein at or below the level of the posterior belly of the digastric muscle. Although these are generally considered to be below the retropharyngeal compartment of the parapharyngeal space, extranodal spread of malignancy from the uppermost lymph nodes may extend superiorly and present as a mass in this region. Lymph nodes in the upper internal jugular chain are considered abnormal when greater than 1.5 cm in diameter or when there is evidence of central hypodensity suggesting necrosis, frequently encountered with metastatic squamous cell carcinoma.[6] Other primary carcinomas may metastasize to this region as well. In particular, hypervascular metastases from primary lesions of the thyroid gland or kidney may have similar signal intensity characteristics as paragangliomas, with intermediate signal intensity on T1- and intermediate-weighted images and relatively high signal intensity on T2-weighted images.[8] Multiple areas of flow void with a salt-and-pepper appearance may also be noted on T2-weighted images.[8] However, the poorly defined, infiltrative margins and loss of definition of adjacent fat and muscle planes helps distinguish hypervascular metastasis from paraganglioma.[8] Angiographic findings may also suggest a hypervascular mass with these metastases; an irregular arterial caliber suggestive of tumor encasement may be observed and can help differentiate between vascular metastasis and paraganglioma.[56] Occasionally, a malignant paraganglioma or malignant schwannoma may be encountered, as well.

This upper internal jugular lymph node chain may also be involved by lymphoma, which typically demonstrates

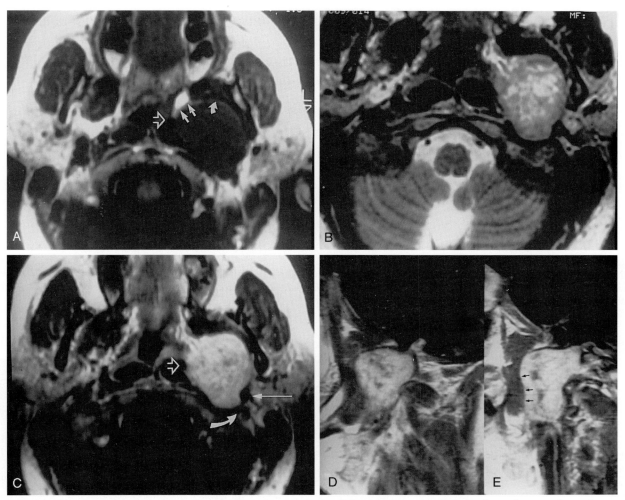

FIGURE 33–13 Vagus schwannoma. *A*, T1-weighted axial image (500/13) demonstrates a well-defined ovoid mass of muscle intensity displacing the fat within the prestyloid parapharyngeal space (*straight arrows*) anteromedially, medial pterygoid muscle (*curved arrow*) anterolaterally, and internal carotid artery (*open arrow*) anteromedially. *B*, T2-weighted axial image (3600/91) demonstrates mixed signal intensity approximately equal to that of cerebrospinal fluid and gray matter. *C*, Contrast-enhanced T1-weighted image (500/13) demonstrates relative homogeneous enhancement of the mass. Internal carotid artery is displaced anteromedially (*open arrow*), and the internal jugular vein (*curved arrow*) is displaced posterolaterally. *Straight arrow* indicates the styloid process. *D*, Contrast-enhanced T1-weighted sagittal (500/13) image of vagus schwannoma. *E*, Contrast-enhanced T1-weighted sagittal image (500/13) demonstrates anterior displacement of the medial and lateral pterygoid muscles (*arrows*) by the mass.

abnormal lymph nodes anterolateral to the vessels within the high internal jugular lymph node chain. The lymph nodes are typically homogeneous on CT and may enhance.[6] On MRI, lymphoma has an intermediate signal intensity on T1- and intermediate-weighted images that is similar to that of muscle; it is moderately higher in signal intensity than muscle on T2-weighted images.[8] The lymph nodes typically are smooth and have homogeneous internal signal intensity.[8] The signal intensity of lymphomatous nodes is usually identical to that of normal lymphoid tissue within the adenoids and faucial tonsils.[8] Most commonly, the diagnosis is suggested by the presence of other involved lymph node chains.

Masticator Space

The masticator space, formed as the superficial layer of deep cervical fascia splits to enclose the mandible and muscles of mastication, may be affected by various lesions of congenital, inflammatory, or neoplastic origin (Table 33–3).

Congenital Abnormalities

Congenital lesions of the masticator space include vascular and lymphatic lesions. The terminology for these lesions has changed over the years, leading to some confusion when interpreting the literature. A simple classification system based on cellular turnover, histologic type, natural history, and physical findings has recently gained increased acceptance; this system divides these malformations into two groups, differentiating *cellular* from *vascular* malformations.[61–64] The cellular malformations, hemangiomas, are also known as *strawberry, capillary, juvenile,* or *cellular* hemangiomas. These present in early infancy and demonstrate rapid growth with endothelial

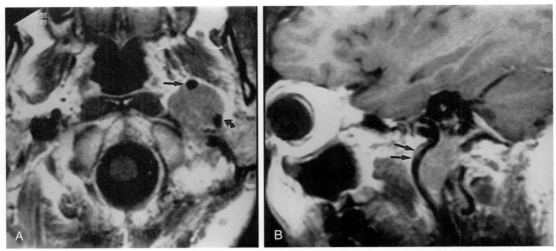

FIGURE 33–14 Intracranial meningioma extending into the retrostyloid parapharyngeal space. *A*, Contrast-enhanced T1-weighted axial image (544/14) demonstrates a well-defined mass with homogeneous enhancement displacing the artery *(straight arrow)* anteriorly and internal jugular vein *(curved arrow)* posteriorly. *B*, Contrast-enhanced T1-weighted sagittal image (672/14) demonstrates anterior displacement of the internal carotid artery *(arrows)* by the mass.

FIGURE 33–15 Clival chordoma extending into the retrostyloid parapharyngeal space. *A*, Contrast-enhanced T1-weighted axial image (800/14) demonstrates an ovoid mass displacing the internal carotid artery *(straight arrow)* anteriorly and the internal jugular vein *(curved arrow)* posterolaterally. *B*, T2-weighted axial image (2500/90) demonstrates homogeneous increased signal similar to that of cerebrospinal fluid. *C* and *D*, T1-weighted sagittal and coronal images (672/14) demonstrate the brightly enhancing mass extending from the clivus to the retrostyloid parapharyngeal space, displacing the internal carotid artery anteriorly *(small arrows)*. The mass also extends intracranially to the cerebellopontine angle *(open arrows)*.

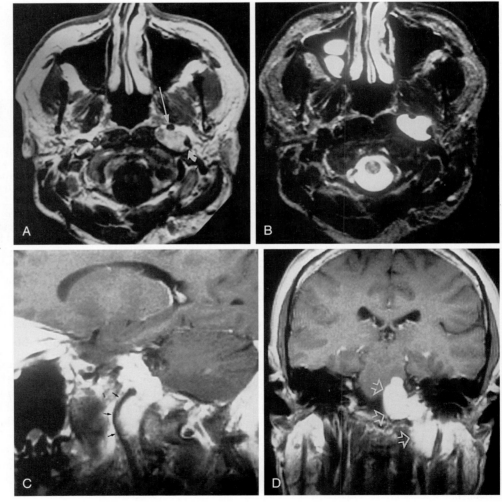

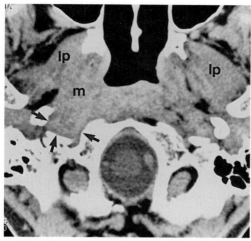

FIGURE 33–16 Squamous cell carcinoma of the nasopharynx. Axial contrast-enhanced CT scan demonstrates parapharyngeal extension of a nasopharyngeal mass with loss of the normal prestyloid parapharyngeal fat medial to the lateral pterygoid muscle. Further extension posteriorly into the retrostyloid compartment of the parapharyngeal space is noted as loss of fat planes separating the neurovascular structures (arrows). In addition, there has been loss of the normal prevertebral fat plane on the right, which suggests extension into the retropharyngeal and prevertebral spaces. lp, lateral pterygoid muscle; m, mass. (From Lewin JL. Imaging of the suprahyoid neck. In Valvassori GE, Mafee MF, Carter BL [eds]. Imaging of the Head and Neck, pp. 390–423. Stuttgart, Georg Thieme, 1995.)

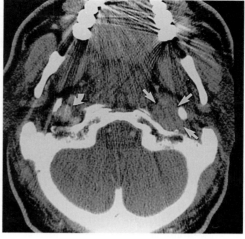

FIGURE 33–18 Metastatic carcinoma to the retrostyloid compartment of the parapharyngeal space. This patient presented with glossopharyngeal neuralgia and syncope several years following treatment for a squamous cell carcinoma of the hypopharynx. Axial contrast-enhanced CT scan demonstrates a soft tissue mass within the retrostyloid compartment of the parapharyngeal space on the left (straight arrows), obliterating the normal fat planes and enhancing vessels. The normal neurovascular structures and surrounding fat planes can be seen on the right (curved arrow). (From Lewin JL. Imaging of the suprahyoid neck. In Valvassori GE, Mafee MF, Carter BL [eds]. Imaging of the Head and Neck, pp. 390–423. Stuttgart, Georg Thieme, 1995.)

cell proliferation. They typically undergo fatty replacement and involution by adolescence.[61, 63, 65]

Vascular malformations can be further divided based on their vascular components: arterial, venous, lymphatic, or combination thereof, such as arteriovenous malformations. As opposed to hemangiomas, vascular malforma-

tions demonstrate no evidence of endothelial cell proliferation, grow at a similar rate as the patient, do not involute or regress, and may not present until late infancy or childhood.[61–64]

Hemangiomas may be well defined on imaging studies or may infiltrate along fascial planes; satellite lesions may

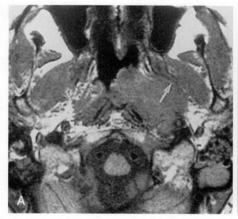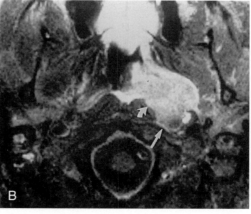

FIGURE 33–17 Squamous cell carcinoma of the nasopharynx with retrostyloid parapharyngeal and prevertebral extension. A, T1-weighted (600/14) axial MRI at the level of the nasopharynx demonstrates a nasopharyngeal mass centered on the left fossa of Rosenmüller with posterolateral extension resulting in loss of the adjacent parapharyngeal fat planes and anterolateral displacement of the lateral pterygoid muscle (arrow). B, Contrast-enhanced T1-weighted (600/15) axial image with fat suppression better demonstrates extension of the enhancing mass posteriorly with obliteration of the normal planes surrounding the neurovascular structures of the retrostyloid compartment of the parapharyngeal space (straight arrow). Loss of definition of the adjacent margin of the left longus capitis muscle suggests prevertebral extension (curved arrow). (A and B, From Lewin JL. Imaging of the suprahyoid neck. In Valvassori GE, Mafee MF, Carter BL [eds]. Imaging of the Head and Neck, pp. 390–423. Stuttgart, Georg Thieme, 1995.)

TABLE 33–3 Masticator Space

Congenital Lesions

Hemangiomas
Vascular malformations
    Arterial
    Venous
    Lymphatic
    Arteriovenous
    Combination of above

Inflammatory Disease

Cellulitis
Abscess
Osteomyelitis

Benign Tumors

Nerve sheath origin
    Schwannomas
    Neurofibroma
Uncommon benign tumors
    Eosinophilic granuloma
    Meningioma
    Osteoblastoma
    Giant cell tumor

Malignant Tumors

Chondrosarcoma
Osteosarcoma
Malignant schwannomas
Rhabdomyosarcoma
Metastatic lesions
    Nasopharyngeal carcinoma
    Salivary gland carcinoma
    Distant primary—lung, breast, kidney
Non-Hodgkin's lymphoma
Uncommon malignant tumors
    Soft tissue Ewing's sarcoma
    Ameloblastoma
    Fibrosarcoma

Pseudotumors

Benign masseteric hypertrophy
Denervation atrophy
Asymmetric accessory parotid gland

---

also be noted.[63] On CT, hemangiomas are relatively dense and typically demonstrate intense enhancement, whereas vascular malformations may not enhance at all.[66, 67] The CT appearance may be characteristic for a vascular malformation when phleboliths are identified within a neck mass. MRI is usually better than CT in defining hemangiomas and vascular malformations due to superior contrast between the lesion and normal surrounding tissues.[41, 63, 64, 68] MRI characteristics for hemangiomas include intermediate signal intensity on T1- and intermediate-weighted images with heterogeneous increased signal intensity on T2-weighted images.[41, 63] Enhancement after gadolinium contrast administration is usually intense.[63, 66] Areas of signal void from associated vascular structures may be identified in hemangiomas during the proliferative phase but are much more common with high-flow vascular lesions such as arteriovenous malformations.[63–65, 69] These may even occasionally give rise to a salt-and-pepper appearance as described with other hypervascular tumors.[8, 41] Slow-flow vascular malformations such as venous

malformation can often be separated from high-flow arteriovenous malformation by MRI. Venous malformations demonstrate homogeneous intermediate signal on T1-weighted images and homogeneous increased signal on T2-weighted images. There is usually an absence of flow voids in the slow-flow venous malformations.[64, 70] Both these lesions have associated muscle atrophy and may demonstrate multifocal involvement.[70]

As the natural course of hemangiomas is regression of the tumor, these usually do not require therapy. Treatment of the vascular malformation varies according to the size, location, and effect of each malformation. Options for therapy include systemic steroids, sclerosing agents, arterial embolization, radiation therapy, and complete surgical excision.[71]

Lymphangiomas are malformations composed of anomalous lymphatic channels and cysts that often extend along the fascial planes of the head and neck and typically infiltrate around rather than compress adjacent structures.[63, 72] They are classified histologically as simple lymphangioma, cavernous lymphangioma, and cystic lymphangioma or hygroma.[73] On CT and MRI examination, they may be unilocular and well circumscribed when small, but typically are multiloculated and less well circumscribed when larger.[72] These lesions exhibit fluid attenuation and signal intensity and have imperceptible, nonenhancing rims (Figs. 33–19 and 33–20).[72] Hemorrhage may occur into a lymphangioma and manifest clinically as rapid enlargement of the lesion; this may be identified by high attenuation on CT and characteristic signal intensity of thrombus on MRI (Fig. 33–20*B*).[63, 72] Lymphangiomas, like hemangiomas and other vascular malformations, frequently do not respect fascial boundaries and commonly involve more than one deep fascial space.

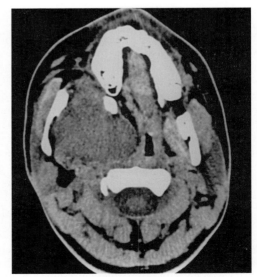

FIGURE 33–19 Lymphangioma of the right masticator space. Contrast-enhanced axial CT scan demonstrates a hypodense mass centered within the masticator space with near complete obliteration of the right medial pterygoid muscle. There is posteromedial displacement of the prestyloid parapharyngeal space.

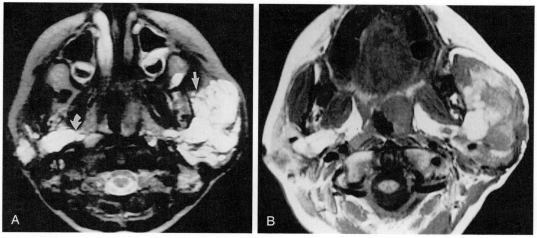

FIGURE 33-20 Lymphangiomas of bilateral parotid spaces and left masticator space. *A*, T2-weighted (5400/90) fast spin echo axial image demonstrates a multiloculated mass involving the superficial and deep portions of the left parotid space extending anteriorly to replace the bulk of the left masseter muscle *(straight arrow)*. A similar multiloculated mass is noted within the right parotid space extending through the stylomandibular tunnel into the prestyloid parapharyngeal space *(curved arrow)*. Both lesions are similar to cerebrospinal fluid in signal intensity and extend through adjacent fascial spaces with an infiltrative appearance. *B*, T1-weighted (750/15) axial MRI at the same level demonstrates varied signal intensity within the loculations of the masses, with many demonstrating increased signal intensity suggesting methemoglobin or highly proteinaceous fluid from prior hemorrhage. The combination of multiloculated fluid-filled masses with areas of internal hemorrhage is highly characteristic of lymphangioma. (*A* and *B*, From Lewin JL. Imaging of the suprahyoid neck. In Valvassori GE, Mafee MF, Carter BL [eds]. Imaging of the Head and Neck, pp. 390-423. Stuttgart, Georg Thieme, 1995.)

Inflammatory Disease

Infection of the masticator space typically follows dental extraction of a lower second or third molar tooth or curettage of a dental socket or infected root.[37] Osteomyelitis of the mandible, zygomatic, or temporal bones after trauma, or due to systemic disease, can also secondarily involve the masticator space.[68, 74] Typically, odontogenic infection results in a subperiosteal abscess, cellulitis, or localized osteomyelitis of the mandible. The infection may then extend to involve the masseter, temporalis, and pterygoid muscles, as well as the fat within the masticator space.[37] Although infection may be confined initially, it tends to spread along fascial and muscle planes, vessels, nerves, salivary gland ducts, and fat pads and can rapidly involve multiple contiguous spaces, following the path of least resistance.[68] Infection typically spreads toward the skull base and suprazygomatic portion of the masticator space most easily.[40, 75] Infection may also spread downward into the floor of the mouth and adjacent spaces.[23, 75]

Clinically, pain, fever, marked trismus, and induration over the angle and ramus of the mandible are often present.[37] Radiologic examination begins with a Panorex view to search for periapical abscesses or granulomas and to evaluate for evidence of osteomyelitis.[37, 74] CT examination may demonstrate a loss of fat planes, with cellulitis or fluid collections suggesting drainable abscesses (Fig. 33-21).[23] In addition to demonstrating involvement of spaces other than those clinically suspected, coronal and axial CT with bone algorithm reconstruction is helpful to detect osteomyelitis of the mandible or skull base.[23, 37, 74] Osteomyelitis is characterized by a loss of definition of the bone cortex associated with increased attenuation within the medullary sequestra. Sclerosis may be seen if the infection is long-standing.[37] On MRI, dis-

ruption of fat planes, multispace involvement, and fluid collections suggesting abscess may be identified. In addition, osteomyelitis may be detected as loss of the normal signal void of cortical bone with obliteration of the normal signal from medullary fat on T1-weighted images.[37] T2-weighted images may demonstrate subperiosteal abscess or increased signal intensity within the medullary cavity of the mandible.[37]

When an abscess is confined to the masticator space, intraoral drainage may provide adequate treatment.[36] However, when infection has spread to contiguous areas, such as the floor of the mouth, parotid, or parapharyngeal spaces, external drainage may be necessary.[68]

Benign Tumors

Benign tumors within the masticator space are most commonly of nerve sheath origin, as the mandibular division of the trigeminal nerve and its major branches pass through the masticator space (Fig. 33-22). The mandibular division of the trigeminal nerve enters through the foramen ovale immediately lateral to the fascial layer separating the prestyloid compartment of the parapharyngeal space from the masticator space.[17] Imaging characteristics of nerve sheath tumors within the masticator space are identical to those arising within the retrostyloid compartment of the parapharyngeal space, as discussed previously. Other benign tumors including meningioma, eosinophilic granuloma, osteoblastoma, and giant cell tumor may occasionally be encountered (Figs. 33-23 and 33-24).[76] Some of these benign tumors may demonstrate perineural spread of tumor, as observed with their malignant counterparts.[76]

Malignant Tumors

Malignant tumors of the masticator space may arise directly from the contents of the space, extend from adja-

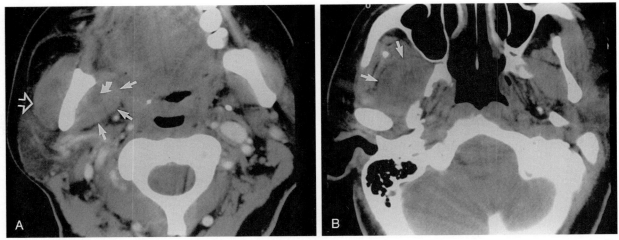

FIGURE 33–21 Masticator space infection following wisdom tooth extraction. *A*, Axial contrast-enhanced CT image at the level of the mandibular ramus demonstrates marked enlargement of the right medial pterygoid muscle *(straight arrows)* with a central region of decreased attenuation suggestive of abscess formation *(curved arrow)*. The posterior aspect of the masseter is also decreased in attenuation and swollen *(open arrow)*. *B*, Axial contrast-enhanced CT image through the level of the mandibular condyle demonstrates involvement of the right lateral pterygoid muscle, which is markedly enlarged and decreased in attenuation *(arrows)*. (*A* and *B*, From Lewin JL. Imaging of the suprahyoid neck. In Valvassori GE, Mafee MF, Carter BL [eds]. Imaging of the Head and Neck, pp. 390–423. Stuttgart, Georg Thieme, 1995.)

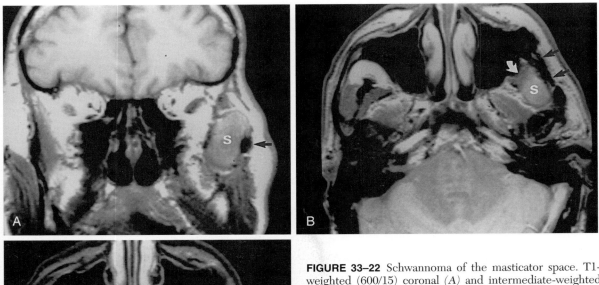

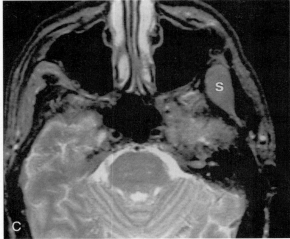

FIGURE 33–22 Schwannoma of the masticator space. T1-weighted (600/15) coronal *(A)* and intermediate-weighted (2500/22) axial *(B)* images demonstrate a lesion of intermediate signal intensity slightly higher than that of adjacent muscle, which is well defined and involves the junction of the suprazygomatic and infrazygomatic compartments of the left masticator space, medial to the zygomatic arch *(black arrows)*. The mass (s) is well delineated and displaces the adjacent temporalis muscle *(white arrow)*. *C*, T2-weighted (2500/90) axial image reveals the lesion (s) to be of intermediate signal intensity, approximately equal in intensity to white matter and adjacent muscle. (From Lewin JL. Imaging of the suprahyoid neck. In Valvassori GE, Mafee MF, Carter BL [eds]. Imaging of the Head and Neck, pp. 390–423. Stuttgart, Georg Thieme, 1995.)

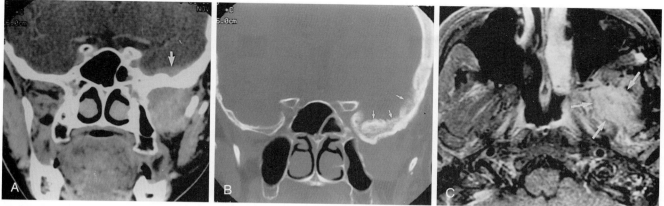

FIGURE 33–23 Meningioma of the masticator space. *A*, Coronal CT scan demonstrates enhancing mass of the masticator space, which obliterates the upper and lower heads of the lateral pterygoid muscle and their surrounding fat planes. Thickening of the greater wing of the sphenoid is noted, with abnormal enhancing soft tissue extending slightly above the sphenoid bone into the middle cranial fossa *(arrow)*. *B*, Coronal CT scan with bone reconstruction demonstrates thickening of the greater wing of the sphenoid bone, consistent with meningioma *(arrows)*. *C*, Gadolinium-enhanced T1-weighted (450/20) axial image with fat suppression demonstrates an enhancing mass that is replacing the lateral pterygoid muscle *(arrows)*. (*A–C*, From Lewin JL. Imaging of the suprahyoid neck. In Valvassori GE, Mafee MF, Carter BL [eds]. Imaging of the Head and Neck, pp. 390–423. Stuttgart, Georg Thieme, 1995.)

cent spaces, or represent metastatic carcinoma. The most common primary malignancies of the masticator space are sarcomas.[23]

Sarcomas within the masticator space include chondrosarcomas, which arise from the mandible near the temporomandibular joint; osteosarcomas, which may originate anywhere along the mandible; malignant schwannomas, which develop in the mandibular division of the trigeminal nerve and its branches; or less commonly, soft tissue and Ewing's sarcomas.[23, 77, 78] Rhabdomyosarcoma may also

involve the masticator space and is more commonly seen in younger patients (Fig. 33–25).[8]

Sarcomas of the masticator space present as intermediate-attenuation lesions on CT, often demonstrating destruction of the adjacent mandible. The different cell types are generally indistinguishable on imaging studies, although the presence of high-attenuation nonossified osteoid or tumor bone formation within osteosarcoma can aid in the diagnosis of this lesion.[72] Identification of chondroid calcification on CT may suggest the diagnosis of

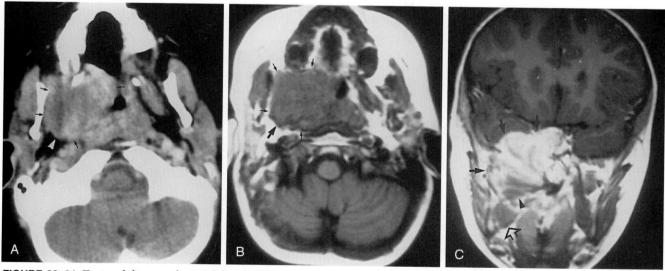

FIGURE 33–24 Eosinophilic granuloma of the skull base extending into the right masticator space. *A*, Contrast-enhanced axial CT image demonstrates an ill-defined mass *(arrows)* of muscle density displacing the prestyloid parapharyngeal space *(arrowhead)* posteriorly. The medial pterygoid muscle is not definable. *B*, T1-weighted (672/14) axial image demonstrates the infiltrating mass *(small arrows)* with signal similar to that of muscle. The medial pterygoid muscle is again not well defined. There is posterior displacement of the prestyloid parapharyngeal space *(large arrow)* and medial displacement of the oropharynx. *C*, Contrast-enhanced T1-weighted (672/14) coronal image demonstrates near homogeneous enhancement of the skull base mass infiltrating into the right masticator space *(straight arrow)*. Inferiorly displaced lateral pterygoid muscle *(arrowhead)* and medial pterygoid muscle *(open arrow)* can be separated from the mass with contrast enhancement.

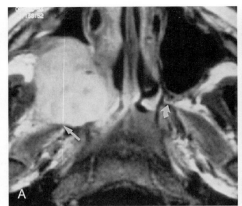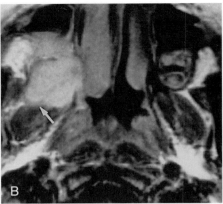

FIGURE 33–25 Ten-year-old child with rhabdomyosarcoma of the inferior orbital fissure with masticator space extension. *A* and *B*, T1-weighted (540/15) contrast-enhanced axial images at the level of the nasopharynx demonstrate an enhancing, slightly heterogeneous mass invading the anterior aspect of the lateral pterygoid muscle (*straight arrows*) and extending anteriorly into the maxillary sinus. The mass obliterates the right pterygopalatine fossa, which is normally seen as a fat-filled cleft at this level, as noted on the left (*curved arrow*). Extension into the orbital apex through the inferior orbital fissure was noted on higher-contrast images. (*A* and *B*, From Lewin JL. Imaging of the suprahyoid neck. In Valvassori GE, Mafee MF, Carter BL [eds]. Imaging of the Head and Neck, pp. 390–423. Stuttgart, Georg Thieme, 1995.)

chondrosarcoma as well.[77] Bone fragments within tumors may be seen within any sarcoma in the presence of significant mandibular invasion. The MRI appearances of the different sarcomas are also often indistinguishable, with intermediate signal intensity on T1- and intermediate-weighted images and moderately increased signal intensity relative to muscle on T2-weighted images.[8]

Malignant schwannoma of the masticator space appears similar to that in the retrostyloid compartment of the parapharyngeal space, often presenting as a tubular mass following the mandibular division of the trigeminal nerve and its primary branches. Extension through the foramen ovale to involve the gasserian ganglion is not uncommon with this lesion, and evaluation of the entire trigeminal nerve to the level of the root entry zone of the pons should be performed to avoid inadequate surgical resection or radiation therapy.[77]

Other primary lesions of the mandible, such as ameloblastoma or fibrosarcoma, are occasionally seen and may extend into the masticator space. The mandibular origin of these lesions is usually evident.

Carcinoma involving the masticator space may be metastatic from a distant primary, such as the lung, breast, or kidney, or may represent spread by squamous cell carcinoma of the oral cavity or salivary gland carcinoma.[23] Hypervascular metastases, such as renal cell and thyroid carcinoma, are usually indistinguishable from other malignancies of this region but may demonstrate a salt-and-pepper appearance on MRI, similar to that noted with paragangliomas.[8] The presence of malignant features such as infiltration of adjacent fat planes and muscles and bone destruction differentiates the hypervascular metastasis from a paraganglioma.

Non-Hodgkin's lymphoma may also occur in this site and may present with better-defined, smooth margins compared with the other malignancies of this space.[8] However, preoperative diagnosis is difficult unless other sites of extranodal or nodal involvement are present to suggest lymphoma.[77]

When the masticator space is involved by malignant tumor, particularly with adenoid cystic carcinoma or recurrent squamous cell carcinoma of the oral cavity or oropharynx, perineural spread of tumor is relatively common and the course of the mandibular division of the trigeminal nerve and its branches should be carefully examined (Figs. 33–26 and 33–27).[11, 18, 23, 76, 78, 79] Perineural extension through the foramen ovale into the middle cranial fossa can be demonstrated on CT examination, although MRI may better demonstrate this entity.[11, 23] Smooth thickening of the trigeminal nerve, concentric expansion of the foramen ovale, obliteration of Meckel's cave, bulging of the lateral dura of the cavernous sinus,

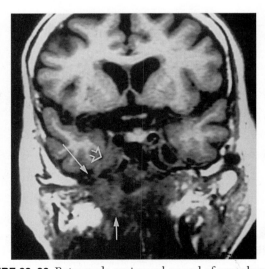

FIGURE 33–26 Retrograde perineural spread of nasopharyngeal carcinoma. Contrast-enhanced T1-weighted (450/12) coronal image demonstrates an infiltrating mass (*short arrow*) isointense to gray matter extending along the mandibular division of the trigeminal nerve from the right masticator space through the foramen ovale (*long arrow*) into Meckel's cave (*open arrow*).

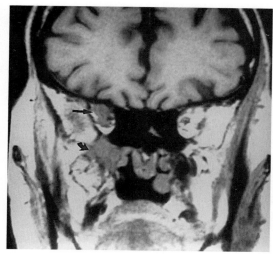

FIGURE 33–27 Antegrade perineural spread of malignant schwannoma along the trigeminal nerve. Contrast-enhanced T1-weighted (600/15) coronal image demonstrates masses isointense to muscle extending into the orbit *(straight arrow)* and pterygopalatine fossa *(curved arrow)* along the ophthalmic and maxillary divisions of the trigeminal nerve, respectively.

antegrade extension of tumor with expansion of foramen rotundum, or atrophy of the muscles of mastication may be observed and suggest perineural tumor extension.[11, 76, 78] Furthermore, abnormal enhancement of the nerve after gadolinium contrast administration is highly suggestive of this diagnosis in the appropriate clinical setting.[13, 80] Perineural spread may also occur into the masticator space and through the foramen ovale from parotid malignancies along the auriculotemporal branch of the trigeminal nerve and result in similar imaging findings. The spread of tumor is in a contiguous manner, following the path of least resistance along the neural planes. The skip lesions seen with perineural spread of tumor are presumably due to macroscopic reappearance of perineural tumor with microscopic continuity through a bony canal or foramen.[78] In addition to detecting perineural spread, imaging allows preoperative evaluation of tumor extent, thereby providing better presurgical prediction of resectability and assisting in surgical and radiation-therapy planning.[23]

Pseudotumors

Several other processes mimicking masses may be found within the masticator space. Benign masseteric hypertrophy is an unusual entity causing a diffuse, homogeneous enlargement of the masseter that is unilateral in half of patients and bilateral in the rest.[68, 81, 82] This may be familial or acquired through habitual grinding of the teeth during sleep; malocclusion may also be contributory.[81, 82] In addition to hypertrophy of the masseter, a rough bony projection of cortical bone may be observed along the anterior surface of the mandible at the site of the masseter insertion.[81, 82] Smooth margins; attenuation and signal intensity identical to those of normal muscle; and lack of abnormal enhancement differentiate this entity from a soft tissue tumor of the masseter.[81] These imaging characteristics and clinical history are important in diagnosing

benign masseteric hypertrophy. Malignant hyperpyrexia has been reported with benign masseteric hypertrophy, making biopsy a potentially hazardous procedure.[82]

Denervation atrophy of the muscles of mastication may result from lesions affecting the brain stem nuclei, trigeminal nerve, or ganglion, or peripheral divisions and branches of the trigeminal nerve; it may also occur in association with underlying systemic diseases, such as myasthenia gravis, polymyositis, progressive systemic sclerosis, or rheumatoid arthritis.[83] Although long-standing denervation results in loss of muscle volume and fatty replacement (Fig. 33–28), during the active phase of muscle resorption, acute denervation can result in muscle edema, which can be observed on CT or MR images (Fig. 33–29).[83] Care must be taken to avoid confusion of this entity with tumor arising within the masticatory muscles. In addition, reflex sympathetic dystrophy can be seen involving the muscles of mastication after skull fracture or craniotomy.[83] Localized edema and inflammation can also be seen associated with contusion, laceration, or temporomandibular joint inflammation.[83]

Asymmetric accessory parotid tissue may also mimic a mass on clinical examination. Accessory parotid tissue is present along the course of Stenson's duct in approximately 21% of the general population.[77] On palpation, this may suggest a mass within the masseter muscle; however, imaging studies clearly define tissue overlying the masseter outside the masticator space that is identical to the parotid gland on CT and MRI examination (see Fig. 33–2C[77]).

SUMMARY

The role of the radiologist in the diagnosis of lesions of the masticator and parapharyngeal spaces has increased

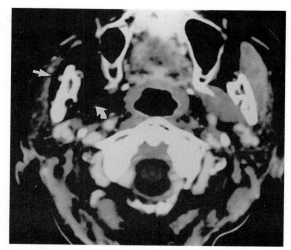

FIGURE 33–28 Chronic atrophy of the muscles of mastication following trigeminal ganglion ablation for treatment of neuralgia. Axial CT scan through the level of the oropharynx demonstrates complete fatty replacement of the right masseter *(straight arrow)* and pterygoid *(curved arrow)* muscles, compared with the normal left side. When atrophy is incomplete, the contralateral normal musculature may be thought to be pathologically enlarged. (From Lewin JL. Imaging of the suprahyoid neck. In Valvassori GE, Mafee MF, Carter BL [eds]. Imaging of the Head and Neck, pp. 390–423. Stuttgart, Georg Thieme, 1995.)

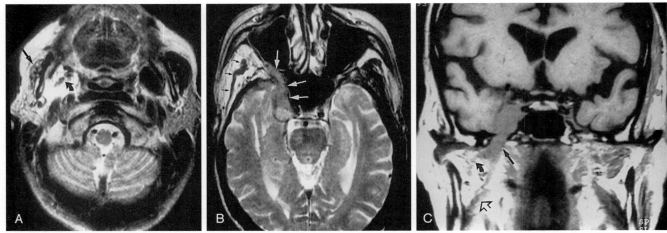

FIGURE 33–29 Denervation atrophy associated with a malignant schwannoma of the trigeminal nerve. *A* and *B*, Axial T2-weighted (3230/90) fast spin echo images demonstrate intermediate signal and volume loss of the right masseter *(straight arrow)*, medial pterygoid *(curved arrow)*, and temporalis muscles. The temporalis tendon and residual muscle tissue are seen outlined by increased signal intensity *(small black arrows)*. The malignant schwannoma of intermediate signal intensity is noted enlarging the right cavernous sinus and extending through the foramen rotundum and into the inferior orbital fissure *(white arrows)*. *C*, T1-weighted (600/15) coronal image demonstrates the mass within the cavernous sinus extending inferiorly through a widened foramen ovale *(straight arrow)* along the mandibular division of the trigeminal nerve. Fatty replacement of the lateral pterygoid *(curved arrow)* and medial pterygoid *(open arrow)* muscles is also noted. (*A–C*, From Lewin JL. Imaging of the suprahyoid neck. In Valvassori GE, Mafee MF, Carter BL [eds]. Imaging of the Head and Neck, pp. 390–423. Stuttgart, Georg Thieme, 1995.)

with the development of more sophisticated imaging techniques. Through distinctive patterns of involvement and displacement to localize the site of origin of a lesion, and intrinsic signal or attenuation to further characterize the abnormality, the construction of a brief and clinically useful list of diagnostic considerations is possible in almost all cases.[84] The anatomic detail provided by modern imaging techniques can also greatly enhance therapeutic planning and prognostication, and endovascular intervention is increasingly useful for preoperative or definitive embolization and balloon test occlusion.

References

1. Som PM, Biller HF, Lawson W. Tumors of the parapharyngeal space: Preoperative evaluation, diagnosis and surgical approaches. Ann Otol Rhinol Laryngol 1981;90(Suppl 80, part 4):3–15.
2. Mancuso AA, Bohman L, Hanafee W, Maxwell D. Computed tomography of the nasopharynx: Normal and variants of normal. Radiology 1980;137:113–121.
3. Som PM, Biller HF. The combined computerized tomography-sialogram: A technique to differentiate deep lobe parotid tumors from extraparotid pharyngomaxillary space tumors. Ann Otolaryngol 1979;88:590–595.
4. Som PM, Biller HF. The combined CT-sialogram. Radiology 1980;135:387–390.
5. Shugar MA, Mafee MF. Diagnosis of carotid body tumors by dynamic computerized tomography. Head Neck Surg 1982;4:518–521.
6. Som PM, Biller HF, Lawson W, et al. Parapharyngeal space masses: An updated protocol based upon 104 cases. Radiology 1984;153:149–156.
7. Lloyd GAS, Phelps PD. The demonstration of tumours of the parapharyngeal space by magnetic resonance imaging. Br J Radiol 1986;59:675–683.
8. Som PM, Braun IF, Shapiro MD, et al. Tumors of the parapharyngeal space and upper neck: MR imaging characteristics. Radiology 1987;164:823–829.
9. Som PM, Sacher M, Stollman AR, et al. Common tumors of the parapharyngeal space: Refined imaging diagnosis. Radiology 1988;169:81–85.
10. Olsen WL, Dillon WP, Kelly WM, et al. MR imaging of paragangliomas. AJNR 1986;7:1039–1042.
11. Laine FJ, Braun IF, Jensen ME, et al. Perineural tumor extension through the foramen ovale: Evaluation with MR imaging. Radiology 1990;174:65–71.
12. Teresi LM, Lufkin RB, Vinuela F, et al. MR imaging of the nasopharynx and floor of the middle cranial fossa. Part II. Malignant tumors. Radiology 1987;164:817–821.
13. Robinson JD, Crawford SC, Teresi LM, et al. Extracranial lesions of the head and neck: Preliminary experience with Gd-DTPA–enhanced MR imaging. Radiology 1989;172:165–170.
14. Hudgins PA, Gussack GS. MR imaging in the management of extracranial malignant tumors of the head and neck. AJR 1992;159:161–169.
15. Duckwiler G, Lufkin RB, Teresi L, et al. Head and neck lesions: MR-guided aspiration biopsy. Radiology 1989;170:519–522.
16. Som PM, Curtin HD. The fasciae and spaces of the head and neck: An analysis of the confusion in the literature with new anatomic correlation, in press.
17. Curtin HD. Separation of the masticator space from the parapharyngeal space. Radiology 1987;163:195–204.
18. Harnsberger HR, Osborn AG. Differential diagnosis of head and neck lesions based on their space of origin. 1. The suprahyoid part of the neck. AJR 1991;157:147–154.
19. Silver AJ, Mawad ME, Hilal SK, et al. Computed tomography of the carotid space and related cervical spaces. Part I. Anatomy. Radiology 1984;150:723–728.
20. Maran AGD, Mackenzie IJ, Murray JAM. The parapharyngeal space. J Laryngol Otol 1984;98:371–380.
21. Coit WE, Harnsberger HR, Osborn AG, et al. Ranulas and their mimics: CT evaluation. Radiology 1987;163:211–216.
22. Thompson HO, Smoker WRK. Hypoglossal nerve palsy: A segmental approach. Radiographics 1994;14:939–958.
23. Hardin CW, Harnsberger HR, Osborn AG, et al. Infection and tumor of the masticator space: CT evaluation. Radiology 1985;157:413–417.
24. Lewin JS, Curtin HD, Ross JS, et al. Fast spin-echo imaging of head and neck neoplasm: Comparison with conventional spin-echo, utility of fat saturation, and evaluation of tissue contrast characteristics. AJNR 1994;15:1351–1357.
25. Lofchy M, Stevens JK, Brown DH. Three-dimensional imaging of the parapharyngeal space. Arch Otolaryngol Head Neck Surg 1994;120:333–336.

26. Yousem DM, Sack MJ, Scanlan KA. Biopsy of parapharyngeal space lesions. Radiology 1994;193:619–622.

27. Work WP. Tumors of the parapharyngeal space. XXXIV Wherry Memorial Lecture. Trans Am Acad Ophthalmol Otol 1969;73:389–394.

28. Lawson VG, LeLiever WC, Makerewich LA, et al. Unusual parapharyngeal lesions. J Otolaryngol 1979;8:241–249.

29. Olsen KD. Tumors and surgery of the parapharyngeal space. Laryngoscope 1994;104:1–28.

30. Cicogna R, Bonomi FG, Curnis A, et al. Parapharyngeal space lesions syncope-syndrome: A newly proposed reflexogenic cardiovascular syndrome. Eur Heart J 1993;14:1476–1483.

31. Work WP, Hybels RL. A study of tumors of the parapharyngeal space. Laryngoscope 1974;84:1748–1755.

32. McIlrath DC, ReMine WH, Devine KD, Dockerty MB. Tumors of the parapharyngeal region. Surg Gynecol Obstet 1963;116:88–94.

33. Harnsberger HR, Mancuso AA, Muraki AS, et al. Branchial cleft anomalies and their mimics: Computed tomographic evaluation. Radiology 1984;152:739–748.

34. Miller MB, Rao VM, Tom BM. Cystic masses of the head and neck: Pitfalls in CT and MR interpretation. AJR 1992;159:601–607.

35. Thaler ER, Tom LWC, Handler SD. Second branchial cleft anomalies presenting as pharyngeal masses. Otolaryngol Head Neck Surg 1993;2109:941–944.

36. Stiernberg CM. Deep-neck space infections. Arch Otolaryngol Head Neck Surg 1986;112:1274–1279.

37. Weber AL, Baker AS, Montgomery WW. Inflammatory lesions of the neck, including fascial spaces—Evaluation by computed tomography and magnetic resonance imaging. Isr J Med Sci 1992;28:241–249.

38. Sethi DS, Stanley RE. Parapharyngeal abscesses. J Laryngol Otol 1991;105:1025–1030.

39. Lazor JB, Cunningham MJ, Eavey RD, Weber AL. Comparison of computed tomography and surgical findings in deep neck infections. Otolaryngol Head Neck Surg 1994;111:746–750.

40. Paonessa DF, Goldstein JC. Anatomy and physiology of head and neck infections (with emphasis on the fascia of the face and neck). Otolaryngol Clin North Am 1976;9:561–580.

41. Faeber EN, Swartz JD. Imaging of neck masses in infants and children. Crit Rev Diagn Imaging 1991;31:283–314.

42. Cole DR, Bankoff M, Carter BL. Percutaneous catheter drainage of deep neck infections guided by CT. Radiology 1984;152:224.

43. Baker DC, Conley J. Surgical approach to retromandibular parotid tumors. Ann Plast Surg 1979;3:304–314.

44. Heeneman H, Maran AGD. Parapharyngeal space tumours. [Review] Clin Otolaryngol 1979;4:57–66.

45. Freije JE, Gluckman JL, Biddinger PW, Wiot G. Muscle tumor in the parapharyngeal space. Head Neck 1992;14:49–54.

46. Bukachevsky RP, Pincus RL, Shectman FG, et al. Synovial sarcoma of the head and neck. Head Neck 1992;14:44–48.

47. Ostfeld EJ, Wiesel JM, Rabinson S, Auslander L. Parapharyngeal (retrostyloid) third branchial cleft cyst. J Laryngol Otol 1991;105:790–792.

48. Harnsberger HR. Handbooks in Radiology: Head and Neck Imaging, pp. 75–88. Chicago, Year Book Medical, 1990.

49. Chung TS, Yousem DM, Lexa F, Markiewicz DA. MRI of carotid angiopathy after therapeutic radiation. J Comput Assist Tomogr 1994;18:533–538.

50. Duncan AW, Lack EE, Deck MF. Radiological evaluation of paragangliomas of the head and neck. Radiology 1979;132:99–105.

51. Cook PL. Bilateral chemodectoma in the neck. J Laryngol Otol 1977;91:611–618.

52. Eriksen C, Girdhar-Gopal H, Lowry LD. Vagal paragangliomas: A report of nine cases. Am J Otolaryngol 1991;12:278–287.

53. Axel L. Blood flow effects in magnetic resonance imaging. AJR 1984;143:1157–1166.

54. Bradley WG, Waluch V. Blood flow magnetic resonance imaging. Radiology 1985;154:443–450.

55. van Gils APG, van den Berg R, Falke THM, et al. MR diagnosis of paraganglioma of the head and neck: Value of contrast enhancement. AJR 1994;162:147–153.

56. Tsai FY, Goldstein JC, Parhad IM. Angiographic features of lateral cervical masses. Trans Am Acad Ophthalmol Otol 1977;84:840–850.

57. Mukherji SK, Kasper ME, Tart RP, Mancuso AA. Irradiated paragangliomas of the head and neck: CT and MR appearance. AJNR 1994;15:357–363.

58. Som PM. Parapharyngeal space. In Som PM, Curtin HD (eds). Head and Neck Imaging, p. 932. St. Louis, Mosby–Year Book, 1996.

59. Kumar AJ, Kuhajda FP, Martinez CR, et al. Computed tomography of extracranial nerve sheath tumors with pathological correlation. J Comput Assist Tomogr 1983;7:857–865.

60. Shoss SM, Donovan DT, Alford BR. Tumors of the parapharyngeal space. Arch Otolaryngol 1985;111:753–757.

61. Mulliken JB, Glowacki J. Hemangiomas and vascular malformations in infants and children: A classification based on endothelial characteristics. Plast Reconstr Surg 1982;69:412–420.

62. Burrows PE, Mulliken JB, Fellows KE, Strand RD. Childhood hemangiomas and vascular malformations: Angiographic differentiation. AJR 1983;141:483–488.

63. Baker LL, Dillon WP, Hieshima GB, et al. Hemangiomas and vascular malformations of the head and neck: MR characterization. AJNR 1993;14:307–314.

64. Gelbert F, Riche MC, Reizine D, et al. MR imaging of head and neck vascular malformations. J Magn Reson Imaging 1991;1:579–584.

65. Barnes PD, Burrows PE, Hoffer FA, Mulliken JB. Hemangiomas and vascular malformations of the head and neck: MR characterization. AJNR 1994;15:193–194.

66. Rossiter JL, Hendrix RA, Tom LWC, Potsic WP. Intramuscular hemangioma of the head and neck. Otolaryngol Head Neck Surg 1993;108:18–26.

67. Aspestrand F, Kolbenstvedt A. Vascular mass lesions and hypervascular tumors in the head and neck. Acta Radiol 1995;36:136–141.

68. Braun IF, Hoffman JC Jr, Reede D, Grist W. Computed tomography of the buccomasseteric region: 2. Pathology. AJNR 1984;5:611–616.

69. Meyer JS, Hoffer FA, Barnes PD, Mulliken JB. Biological classification of soft-tissue vascular anomalies: MR correlation. AJR 1991;157:559–564.

70. Rak KM, Yakes WF, Ray RL, et al. MR imaging of symptomatic peripheral vascular malformations. AJR 1992;159:107–112.

71. Rossiter JL, Hendrix RA, Tom LWC, Potsic WP. Intramuscular hemangioma of the head and neck. Otolaryngol Head Neck Surg 1993;108:18–26.

72. Reede DL, Holliday RA, Som PM, Bergeron RT. Nonnodal pathologic conditions of the neck. In Som PM, Bergeron RT (eds). Head and Neck Imaging, pp. 537–543. St. Louis, Mosby–Year Book, 1991.

73. Caro PA, Soroosh M, Faerber EN. Computed tomography in the diagnosis of lymphangiomas in infants and children. Clin Imaging 1991;15:41–46.

74. Yoshiura K, Hijiva T, Ariji E, et al. Radiographic patterns of osteomyelitis in the mandible. Oral Surg Oral Med Oral Pathol 1994;78:116–124.

75. Ariji E, Moriguchi S, Kuroki T, Kanda S. Computed tomography of maxillofacial infection. Dento-Maxillo-Facial Radiol 1991;20:147–151.

76. Aspestrand F, Boysen M. CT and MR imaging of primary tumors of the masticator space. Acta Radiol 1992;33:518–522.

77. Harnsberger HR. Handbooks in Radiology: Head and Neck Imaging, pp. 46–60. Chicago, Year Book Medical, 1990.

78. Parker GD, Harnsberger HR. Clinical-radiologic issues in perineural tumor spread of malignant diseases of the extracranial head and neck. Radiographics 1991;11:383–399.

79. Curtin HD, Williams R, Johnson J. CT of perineural tumor extension: Pterygopalatine fossa. AJNR 1984;5:731–737.

80. Hudgins PA. Contrast enhancement in head and neck imaging. Neuroimaging Clin North Am 1994;4:101–115.

81. Braun IF, Torres WE, Landman JA, et al. Computed tomography of benign masseteric hypertrophy. J Comput Assist Tomogr 1985;9:167–170.

82. Set PAK, Somers JM, Britton PD, Freer CEL. Pictorial review: Benign and malignant enlargement of the pterygo-masseteric muscle complex. Clin Radiol 1991; 48:57–60.

83. Schellhas KP. MR imaging of muscles of mastication. AJNR 1989;10:829–837.

84. Lewin JL. Imaging of the suprahyoid neck. In Valvassori GE, Mafee MF, Carter BL (eds). Imaging of the Head and Neck, pp. 390–423. Stuttgart, Georg Thieme, 1995.

34

Thyroid and Parathyroid

A L I C E M. S C H E F F, M.D.

R O N A L D L. K O R N, M.D., PH.D.

V I R G I N I A A. L I V O L S I, M.D.

F R A N Ç O I S B E N A R D, M.D.

The thyroid and parathyroid glands regulate critical physiologic processes. Their endocrine hormones modulate diverse metabolic functions and exert exquisite control over serum calcium levels. Only in pathologic states does one truly appreciate their enormous homeostatic significance. Knowledgeably imaging these organs requires an understanding of anatomic features and pathophysiologic changes that encompass a wide spectrum of disease.

In this chapter, the thyroid and parathyroid glands are discussed with reference to pertinent embryology, anatomy, and physiology. Congenital, inflammatory, metabolic, and neoplastic disorders are presented as clinical and pathologic entities with illustrative images. Typical imaging parameters, as well as diagnostic utility, are included to optimize the roles of nuclear medicine scintigraphy, ultrasonography (US), computed tomography (CT), and magnetic resonance imaging (MRI) in clinical practice.

THYROID GLAND

Embryology and Anatomy

The thyroid gland develops early in embryologic life. In humans, the mature gland is believed to derive from two distinct regions of the endodermal pharynx. The median anlage arises in the midline of the anterior pharyngeal floor at approximately the third to fourth week of fetal development. The lateral aspects are thought to develop from the ultimobranchial body (derived from the fourth to fifth pharyngeal complex) at the 5-week stage and fuse bilaterally with the medial thyroid gland by 8 to 9 weeks, producing the definitive bilobed form.[1, 2]

Closely associated with the developing heart, the thyroid begins to descend from its site of origin, the foramen cecum at the base of the tongue, to its final location anterior to the trachea. During this caudal descent, the thyroid gland is attached to the tongue base by a stalk called the *thyroglossal duct*, which rapidly elongates, then fragments and usually degenerates.

In the adult, the thyroid gland weighs approximately 20 gm, and the right and left lobes each measure 4 × 2 × 2 cm. Characteristically, the thyroid isthmus is situated just caudal to the cricoid cartilage. There may be a pyramidal lobe projecting cephalad from the isthmus. The follicular thyroid tissue derives from the median anlage and will secrete thyroid hormones. The ultimobranchial bodies give rise to the parafollicular C cells that are thought to derive from neural crest cells,[2, 3] reside within the basement membrane of follicles, and secrete thyrocalcitonin, which regulates serum calcium levels. Interspersed within the gland are colloid deposits and fibrous septa. In fetal life, the thyroid gland begins to synthesize and release thyroid hormone by the 12th week of gestation.[3]

The thyroid gland has a rich vascular supply. Paired superior thyroidal arteries derive from the external carotid artery, and paired inferior thyroidal arteries branch from the thyrocervical trunks of the subclavian arteries. There is an inconstant thyroidea ima that arises directly from the aorta and supplies a small inferior portion of the gland.[4] The thyroid gland drains into paired superior, middle, and inferior thyroidal veins. The superior and middle veins drain into the internal jugular vein, and the inferior veins drain into the brachiocephalic veins.[4] Innervation is supplied by the vagus nerve and sympathetic plexus.

Abnormalities of thyroid development during fetal life can lead to a variety of conditions. Most developmental abnormalities result from morphogenic errors that lead to displacement of cells derived from the median anlage. Ectopic thyroid tissue can be found in the lingual, high cervical, or mediastinal regions as well as within myocardium or ovaries (struma ovarii).[2] In addition, the thyroglossal duct may not degenerate and instead may persist as a fistulous tract.

If the thyroid gland fails to descend, the median thyroid may give rise to a mass of tissue at the base of the tongue termed a *lingual thyroid*. Such individuals may have no functioning thyroid tissue in the neck and become acutely hypothyroid if the mass is removed surgically. Thyroid scintigraphy is extremely important in demonstrating function in a lingual thyroid. Other individuals may have a thyroglossal duct cyst if the thyroid duct does not completely degenerate. These cysts may become infected but usually just present with a mass that is excised. As many as 60% of thyroglossal duct cysts contain normal thyroid follicles in their walls.[1]

Additional developmental anomalies include hemiagenesis of one lobe, more commonly the left lobe, with persistence of the right lobe and isthmus. This has been referred to as a "hockey stick" sign.[5] It has been stated that 30% to 75% of people[4, 5] may have a pyramidal lobe, which usually arises from the isthmus and ascends superiorly toward the midline. A pyramidal lobe can also project from the medial aspect of the body of the right or left lobe. The pyramidal lobe is more frequently visualized during scintigraphy in the presence of a hyperthyroid state such as Graves' disease. Malformations of branchial pouch differentiation may result in intrathyroidal sites for the thymus or parathyroid gland.

Hormonogenesis

The primary function of the thyroid gland is the synthesis and thyroid-stimulating hormone (TSH)–mediated release of two hormones, triiodothyronine (T_3) and thyroxine (T_4), which control metabolic function throughout the body. Pituitary secretion of TSH is in turn regulated by the hypothalamic release of thyroid-releasing hormone (TRH).

Thyroid hormone synthesis is a six-step process. The first step involves iodide trapping. Iodide is actively extracted from the plasma and concentrated in follicular cells. In humans, the thyroid to serum iodide ratio is approximately 50 to 1.[6] The second step involves iodide oxidation. Iodide is oxidized by thyroid peroxidase in the presence of hydrogen peroxide to a chemically reactive form. Steps 3 and 4 are termed *organification of iodide into thyroid hormone*. In step 3, tyrosine residues on thyroglobulin molecules stored within the follicles are iodinated to form monoiodotyrosine and diiodotyrosine. In step 4, T_3 is formed by coupling monoiodotyrosine and diiodotyrosine and T_4 is formed by coupling two molecules of diiodotyrosine. Step 5 involves release of thyroid hormones under the control of TSH. Release of T_3 and T_4 from thyroglobulin involves endocytosis and proteolysis of thyroglobulin within the follicular cell. Microvilli extend from the apical surface of follicular cells and enclose small fragments of colloid-forming membrane-bound vesicles. After these vesicles fuse with lysosomes they become phagolysosomes, which migrate to the basal surface of the follicular cell. During this passage, lysosomal proteases and peptidases split out T_3 and T_4, which are discharged into capillaries.[6] Simultaneously, deiodination of free monoiodotyrosine and diiodotyrosine occurs for iodide salvage and recycling within the thyroid (step 6).

Pathologically organification defects can occur. Usually they involve enzymatic defects interfering with oxidation of iodide or iodination of tyrosine. A rare congenital defect causes absence of iodide uptake.[5]

In the circulation, thyroid hormones are transported by several carrier proteins: thyroxine-binding globulin carries approximately 70% of T_3 and T_4, thyroxine-binding pre-

globulin carries 20% to 30% of T_4 and 5% of T_3, and albumin carries most of the remaining hormones. The active form of each hormone is the free form, with free T_4 and free T_3 representing 0.03% and 0.3%, respectively. T_3 is three to five times more active physiologically than T_4. T_4 is entirely synthesized in the thyroid and disappears from peripheral blood with a half-time of 7 to 8 days. In contrast, T_3 is 80% to 95% synthesized by peripheral conversion from T_4 and has a blood half-time of 1 day. Blood clearance rates have important implications for patients undergoing thyroid hormone withdrawal before radionuclide scanning. Likewise, medications that interfere with organification of iodide, such as propylthiouracil and methimazole (Tapazole), alter radioactive iodine uptake measurements in hyperthyroid patients and must be withdrawn before scanning. High concentrations of dietary iodine (seaweed, shellfish), a recent contrast-enhanced CT scan, or topical application of povidone-iodine (Betadine) solution usually diminishes radioiodine uptake and prevents acceptable thyroid scintigraphy.

Clinical Syndromes Associated with Thyroid Disease: Thyrotoxicosis and Hypothyroidism

Thyrotoxicosis

Thyrotoxicosis is a common thyroid disturbance with multiple causes. Thyrotoxicosis is the clinical syndrome that develops when circulating levels of T_4 or T_3 are increased. Hyperthyroidism is sustained thyroid hyperfunction with increased thyroid hormone biosynthesis and release.[7] Although many people presenting clinically with thyrotoxicosis have hyperthyroidism, thyroid inflammation or exogenous hormone administration can produce similar symptoms. Thyrotoxicosis is manifested by a wide range of symptoms that vary in relative severity (Table 34–1).

On physical examination there are multiple findings. The skin is warm, smooth, moist, and flushed, reflecting peripheral vasodilatation and increased heat loss due to the hyperdynamic circulatory state. Patients are often hyperactive and demonstrate hyperreflexia. Cardiac manifestations are common and may present early in the disease. Tachycardia, palpitations, cardiomegaly, or arrhythmias may be observed. Patients may have a wide-eyed stare with upper eyelid retraction and lid lag on slow downward gaze. In Graves' disease, the globe may protrude, termed *proptosis*, secondary to immunoinflammatory changes in the retro-orbital tissues.

Thyrotoxicosis associated with hyperthyroidism is most

TABLE 34–1 Clinical Manifestations of Thyrotoxicosis

Nervousness, hyperactivity, emotional lability
Palpitations, tachycardia, atrial fibrillation
Fatigue, muscular weakness
Weight loss with good appetite
Diarrhea, menstrual changes
Heat intolerance, warm skin, excessive perspiration
Fine tremor (outstretched hand), hyperreflexia
Eye changes

often caused by Graves' disease (diffuse toxic hyperplasia), toxic multinodular goiter, or toxic adenoma. Occasionally, it is due to a TSH-secreting pituitary adenoma, hyperfunctioning thyroid carcinoma, or thyroid-stimulating trophoblastic tumor (choriocarcinoma or hydatidiform mole). Thyrotoxicosis not associated with hyperthyroidism (low radioactive iodine uptake) may reflect release of preformed thyroid hormones during inflammatory thyroid disease (subacute or silent thyroiditis), exogenous hormone use, or ectopic thyroid tissue (dermoid tumor–struma ovarii).[6, 7]

Manifestations of thyrotoxicosis are determined more by the patient's age[8] and the presence of coexisting disease than by biochemical severity.[9] Younger patients often present with anxiety and hyperactivity, whereas older patients develop cardiovascular dysfunction. Elderly patients may present with cardiac symptoms but have only mild or subclinical hyperthyroidism (normal serum total and free T_4 and free T_3 levels with subnormal serum TSH levels).[10] With the introduction of modern, sensitive TSH assays using a sandwich monoclonal antibody technique plus chemiluminescent tracers,[11, 12] subnormal serum TSH levels less than 0.1 μU/ml can be measured. Normal TSH values range from 0.5 to 5.0 μU/ml in a euthyroid person younger than 60 years.[13]

Documentation of subclinical hyperthyroidism by laboratory measurement of a suppressed TSH level is extremely important. A woman older than 60 years with a TSH value below 0.1 μU/ml is three times more likely to develop atrial fibrillation than a peer whose TSH value is normal.[14] Also, women with autonomous thyroid nodules or multinodular goiter who have normal T_3 and T_4 levels but low TSH values tend to have a lower average bone mineral density and increased osteoporosis risk.[15] Accordingly, clinical management of patients with subclinical hyperthyroidism, documented by subnormal TSH levels, may require radioactive iodine-131 administration to decrease thyroid function and lower the risk of cardiac dysfunction.

Thyroid crisis or storm may occur as a clinical emergency in patients with unrecognized or inadequately treated thyrotoxicosis. Severe hypermetabolism erupts, characterized by fever, tachycardia, hypertension, extreme anxiety, and eventually hypotension, coma, and death. Thyroid storm is thought to result from an acute adrenergic outburst in a person oversensitized to the effects of adrenergic amines by thyroid hormone.[16] Sympatholytic treatments have been effective, but thyroid storm may be fatal in 20% to 25% of patients.[6]

Hypothyroidism

Hypothyroidism is the most common disorder of thyroid function. *Primary* or *thyroidal hypothyroidism* is decreased thyroid hormone production. This may be due to the absence of a thyroid gland or may reflect a structural or functional derangement. *Central hypothyroidism* is decreased thyroid stimulation by TSH secondary to pituitary disease (secondary hypothyroidism) or hypothalamic TRH deficiency (tertiary hypothyroidism).

If hypothyroidism occurs prenatally or in infancy, cretinism with its associated physical and mental retardation follow unless treatment is initiated within weeks. Hypo-

TABLE 34–2 Clinical Manifestations of Hypothyroidism

Fatigue, slow movement, hyporeflexia
Bradycardia
Mental impairment, slow speech, depression
Cold intolerance, dry skin, hoarseness
Decreased appetite, weight gain, constipation
Menstrual disturbances
Nonpitting edema (myxedema), lethargy

thyroidism appearing in older children or adults is termed *myxedema*. Clinical expression can range from subtle fatigue to coma (Table 34–2), and the course may be indolent or rapid.[17] Even prolonged hypothyroidism is reversible in children and adults. Primary hypothyroidism usually results from diseases that destroy thyroid tissue such as chronic autoimmune (Hashimoto's) thyroiditis or iodine-131–induced hypothyroidism.

Thyroid Imaging

Thyroid Scintigraphy (Nuclear Medicine)

Most routine thyroid scintigrams are performed with iodine-123 or technetium-99m–pertechnetate. Iodine-131 is useful in the evaluation of substernal goiter (1 mCi orally) and metastatic thyroid cancer (3 to 5 mCi orally).

Routine thyroid scintigraphy is usually performed with a gamma scintillation camera, fitted with a 3- to 5-mm pinhole collimator, 20 minutes after the intravenous injection of 5 to 10 mCi (185 to 370 MBq) of technetium-99m–pertechnetate or 4 to 24 hours after the oral ingestion of 200 to 400 μCi (7.4 to 14.8 MBq) of iodine-123. Images are obtained in multiple views (200,000 to 250,000 counts per image) and correlated with palpatory findings during scanning (Table 34–3).[18]

Radioactive iodine uptake is measured with a dedicated probe. The percentage of thyroid uptake is determined relative to the dose given to the patient, corrected for radioactive decay.

The normal thyroid gland is faintly palpable. On scintigraphy, the gland shows homogeneous tracer distribution. Normal uptake ranges from 10% to 30% at 24 hours.

Ultrasonography

High-resolution linear array transducers ranging from 7.5 to 10 MHz are used for thyroid US. With the patient's neck hyperextended, the thyroid gland is entirely imaged in transverse and longitudinal planes. The normal gland is uniformly hyperechoic. On transverse scans, the two major lobes lie on each side of the trachea, bridged by the isthmus. The carotid arteries and the more lateral jugular veins flank the thyroid gland. The gland is anterior to the longus colli and posterior to the strap muscles (Fig. 34–1).[19]

Computed Tomography

In CT, the patient is scanned supine with the neck hyperextended. Contiguous 5-mm-thick axial slices are usually obtained from the hyoid bone to the aortic arch. Thinner (1.5 to 2 mm) sections may be required to delineate small

TABLE 34-3 Radiopharmaceuticals Used for Thyroid Imaging

Tracer	Physical Half-Life	Photon Energy (keV)	Administered Dose and Route	Dose to Thyroid Gland
^{123}I	13 hr	159	200–400 μCi, PO	0.38 Gy/200 μCi (15% uptake)
^{131}I	8 days	364	20–100 μCi, PO	0.78 Gy/100 μCi (15% uptake)
^{99m}Tc	6 hr	140	1–10 mCi, IV	0.0013 Gy/mCi
^{201}Tl	73 hr	80	2–5 mCi, IV	0.013 Gy/2 mCi
^{99m}Tc-sestamibi	6 hr	140	10–25 mCi, IV	0.0023 Gy/10 mCi
^{111}In-pentetreotide	67 hr	173 247	3–6 mCi, IV	0.0074 Gy/3 mCi

lesions. The thyroid gland is usually visible 6 to 8 mm below the vocal cords and terminates proximal to the thoracic inlet. However, substernal extension can occur, requiring scanning into the thorax in order to evaluate the caudal extent of the gland. Contrast injection followed by scanning may provide additional information. The normal thyroid gland has a density of approximately 80 to 130 Hounsfield units (HU), approximately 1.5- to 2-fold greater than that of muscle. Contrast enhancement usually increases the density by 30 to 40 Hounsfield units in normal tissue, and uptake often correlates with function.[20]

When scintigraphy and contrast-enhanced CT scans are required, the nuclear medicine procedure must be performed first as iodinated contrast material blocks the uptake of radioiodine (iodine-123, iodine-131) and technetium-99m–pertechnetate.

Magnetic Resonance Imaging

When MRI is used to scan the thyroid, a dedicated surface coil centered over the gland provides the highest-quality images. If the field to be imaged is larger, the head or body coil may be employed. The patient is

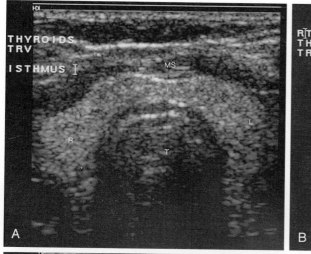
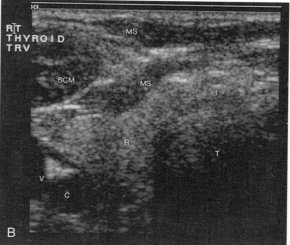
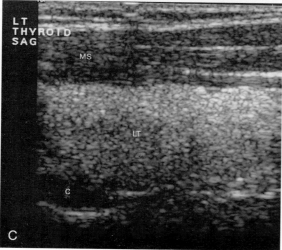

FIGURE 34–1 Normal anatomy of the thyroid gland on ultrasonography. *A*, Transverse ultrasound image at the level of the isthmus reveals homogeneous echotexture of the right (R) and left (L) lobes of the gland and isthmus (I). The trachea is in the midline (T) and casts a posterior acoustic shadow. The strap muscles (MS) are anterior to the gland. The great vessels are posterior and lateral and are best seen in *B*. *B*, Close-up evaluation of the right (R) lobe of the thyroid gland. The internal jugular vein (V), which is just in the field of view, and carotid artery (C) are labeled. SCM, sternocleidomastoid muscle. *C*, Sagittal view of the left lobe (LT) of the thyroid gland demonstrates its homogeneous echotexture as it lies just posterior to the longitudinally oriented strap muscles and anterior to the carotid artery.

scanned supine with quiet breathing, and with swallowing suspended, if possible. Scanning sequences depend on the clinical question but can be obtained in multiple planes with T1, T2, proton-density weighting, fat saturation, and contrast enhancement. Techniques that reduce motion and pulsation artifact, employ respiratory or cardiac gating or both, shorten imaging time, and optimize the field of view improve lesion conspicuity.

On T1-weighted images, the normal thyroid gland shows a nearly homogeneous signal with an intensity usually brighter than that of adjacent neck muscles. On T2-weighted images, the thyroid gland is hyperintense relative to adjacent muscle (Fig. 34–2). Normal parathyroid glands are not seen on routine thyroid images.[20]

Graves' Disease

Graves' disease is one of several autoimmune thyroid disorders. Hashimoto's thyroiditis (chronic lymphocytic thyroiditis) and silent or postpartem thyroiditis (subacute lymphocytic thyroiditis) are also autoimmune disorders but are totally different from Graves' disease in pathophysiology and clinical presentation.

In Graves' disease the TSH or thyrotropin receptor on follicular cells is the target for thyroid-stimulating antibodies. The TSH receptor is an adenylate cyclase–linked cell surface receptor. The autoantibodies bind to follicular cells via the receptor, stimulating them as though the receptor were being triggered by TSH. This induces constant function and autonomy—thyrotoxicosis with hyperthyroidism. The thyroid gland enlarges and is referred to as a *diffuse toxic goiter*.

Graves' disease is relatively common, occurring in 0.4% of the U.S. population.[6] Although it may occur at any age, the peak incidence is in the third and fourth decades, with a female to male ratio of 5 to 1. There is familial predisposition, and there is an association between Graves' disease and Hashimoto's thyroiditis. Hyperthyroidism supervening on preexisting Hashimoto's thyroiditis is sometimes called *Hashi-toxicosis*.

Pathologically in Graves' disease, there is diffuse hyperplasia of the gland. The tissue is usually uniform. Although the thyroid gland typically triples or quadruples its weight (60 to 80 gm), occasionally the gland may enlarge and weigh as much as 200 gm.[1] When present, exophthalmos is related to an increase in the volume of extraocular muscles and orbital tissues, secondary to edema, increased deposits of hydrophilic mucopolysaccharides, fibrosis, and lymphocytic infiltrates. Later in the disease, contractures of the extraocular muscles can develop and may lead to incoordination of eye movement.

Clinically, Graves' disease presents principally in young women as thyrotoxicosis with increased output of T_3 and T_4 and suppression of TSH release by the pituitary. Serologic tests for autoantibodies such as the TSH receptor autoantibody (previously known as the thyroid-stimulation immunoglobulin) may show elevated levels, confirming the autoimmune phenomena. In addition to Graves' disease, the differential diagnosis of thyrotoxicosis includes toxic adenoma; toxic multinodular goiter; transient elevation of serum T_3 and T_4 levels secondary to thyroid inflammation and injury in thyroiditis; exogenous hormone; and rarely, ectopic thyroid tissue.

Radionuclide scintigraphy may be very useful in evaluating the patient with suspected Graves' disease and differentiating that process from thyroiditis. In Graves' disease, the gland is homogeneously enlarged and shows intense tracer uptake well above the normal range of 30%, often reaching 60% to 85% uptake at 24 hours (Figs. 34–3 and 34–4). In thyroiditis, tracer uptake is usually less than 10% (normal range 10% to 30%) but may be normal. On scintigraphy, tracer uptake in inflammatory thyroiditis is often inhomogeneously reduced in a patchy pattern.

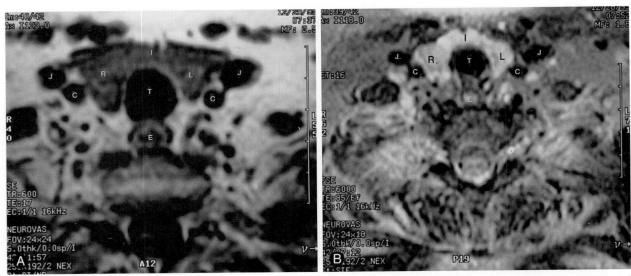

FIGURE 34–2 Normal anatomy of the thyroid gland on magnetic resonance imaging (MRI). *A* and *B*, Axial T1- and T2-weighted images of the thyroid gland. On T1-weighted sequences the thyroid gland is of low to medium signal intensity. The gland becomes high in signal intensity on T2-weighted sequences. R, right lobe of thyroid gland; L, left lobe of thyroid gland; I, thyroid isthmus; J, internal jugular vein; C, carotid artery; T, trachea; E, esophagus.

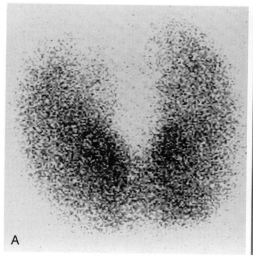

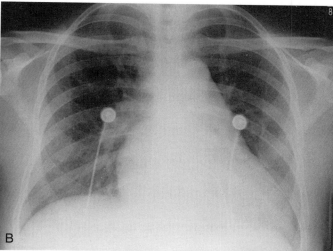

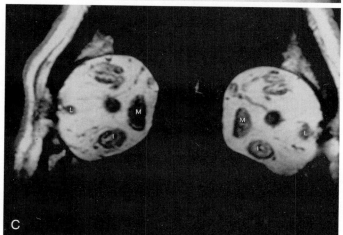

FIGURE 34–3 Graves' disease. *A*, Two-hour ^{123}I scintigraphy reveals diffusely increased uptake in both lobes of an enlarged thyroid gland. The 24-hour uptake is 75% (normal 10% to 30%). This particular patient presented with severe thyroid ophthalmopathy and thyroid storm. *B*, Chest radiograph from the same patient demonstrates cardiomegaly. Cardiac manifestations of thyrotoxicosis are common in the elderly. Thyroid storm is uncommon but can be life threatening and is a medical emergency. *C*, Coronal T1-weighted sequences through the orbits demonstrate bilateral enlargement of the inferior (I) and medial (M) rectus muscles and proliferation of the orbital fat in a different patient with thyroid ophthalmopathy. The lateral (L) rectus muscles are normal. In Graves' ophthalmopathy the inferior and medial rectus muscles are the most frequently affected, and the lateral rectus muscles are the least commonly involved. Thyroid ophthalmopathy can occur in euthyroid and hyperthyroid states of Graves' disease. (*C*, Courtesy of Frank Lexa, M.D., University of Pennsylvania Medical Center, Philadelphia, PA.)

Differentiating Graves' disease from subacute thyroiditis is vital for proper patient management. Patients with Graves' disease require medical treatment with β blockers and antithyroid medication. They may undergo radioiodine ablation of the thyroid gland or even surgery to control this autoimmune disorder and prevent cardiac complications or thyroid storm.

On US, the findings are relatively nonspecific. The gland is usually enlarged and diffusely hypoechoic. Visualization of a thyroid isthmus thickened by a few millimeters helps to suggest a diffusely enlarged gland. There may be overall contour lobulation, but there usually are no palpable nodules.[21] A characteristic increase in thyroid vasculature is observed on color Doppler in both systole and diastole; this has been termed the *thyroid inferno*.[22]

On CT and MRI, patients with Graves' disease usually show diffuse glandular enlargement with avid enhancement. The CT density, measured in Hounsfield units, is actually decreased, reflecting a decrease in iodine concentration even though there is an overall increase in iodine content in the gland.[20] Even with treatment, the density may not return to normal levels.[23] Carcinoma of the

thyroid gland is relatively rare in patients with Graves' disease.

Thyroiditis

Thyroiditis is infiltration of the thyroid gland by inflammatory cells caused by a diverse group of infectious and inflammatory disorders. The inflammatory process may be acute and self-limiting or chronic and progressive. It may be organ-specific (limited to the thyroid gland) or part of a multisystem process.

The term *thyroiditis* refers to several clinical syndromes of differing causes. Classification is somewhat confusing as many of these syndromes have two or three names—an eponym, a pathologic signature, and a clinical descriptor. Characteristics of the major types of thyroiditis are presented in Table 34–4. Hashimoto's thyroiditis and silent thyroiditis, which is termed *postpartum thyroiditis* if it occurs in the postpartum period, are autoimmune thyroid diseases.

De Quervain's thyroiditis is thought to have a viral cause. Acute suppurative thyroiditis usually has a bacterial

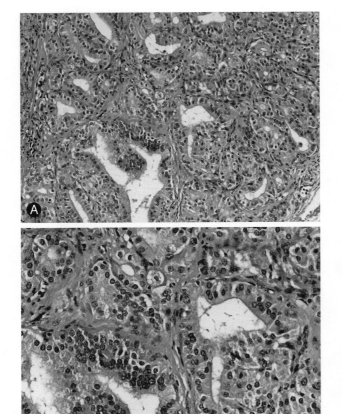

FIGURE 34–4 Graves' disease. *A,* Photomicrograph shows follicular, papillary, and solid patterns of growth. Note rare lymphocytes in stroma *(left).* (H&E 400×.) *B,* On higher power, note round, dark nuclei. (H&E 400×.)

or, less commonly, a fungal cause. Riedel's thyroiditis (struma) is characterized by extensive fibrosis. The last two categories are very rare.

Hashimoto's Thyroiditis (Chronic Lymphocytic)

Hashimoto's thyroiditis, also known as *chronic lymphocytic thyroiditis,* is the prototype of autoimmune thyroiditis. In 1912, Hashimoto[24] described several goitrous patients whose firm, rubbery thyroid glands demonstrated lymphocytic infiltration, fibrosis, and follicular cell atrophy. Additionally, some follicular cells showed eosinophilic change (Hürthle's or Askanazy's cells). The goitrous form of autoimmune thyroiditis is the most prevalent and retains the name *Hashimoto's thyroiditis.* Variant conditions include a chronic fibrous form and lymphocytic thyroiditis of childhood and adolescence.[25]

In Hashimoto's thyroiditis, both cellular and humoral immune mechanisms are involved in pathogenesis. Autoantibodies have been identified against thyroglobulin (which is stored in the follicles and is the matrix on which T_3 and T_4 are formed), thyroperoxidase (which is the heme-containing peroxidase involved in T_3 and T_4 biosynthesis that has been defined as the antigen target on thyroid microsomes),[26] and the TSH receptor. TSH-re-

ceptor blocking antibodies also have a role in Hashimoto's thyroiditis. In reported cases, when TSH-receptor blocking antibodies disappeared, normal thyroid function returned.[27]

Hashimoto's thyroiditis is predominantly a disease of women, with a female to male ratio of 10 to 1. Most cases occur in persons between 30 and 50 years of age. Some are noted in children. Hashimoto's thyroiditis is associated with other autoimmune diseases, such as systemic lupus erythematosus, pernicious anemia, and Graves' disease. Patients with Hashimoto's disease present with typical features of primary hypothyroidism. The serum TSH level is high, and T_3 and T_4 values are low.

Antibody titers are markedly elevated during the acute phases of the disease. The inflammatory process may involve the thyroid gland inhomogeneously over weeks, months, or years. During phases of gland destruction with hormone release, clinical symptoms of thyrotoxicosis may be superimposed on hypothyroidism. Ultimately, hypothyroidism prevails after substantial gland destruction has occurred. Despite the observed autoimmune phenomenon, the precise mechanisms of follicular cell destruction are uncertain.

On scintigraphy, there is no characteristic scan pattern in Hashimoto's thyroiditis. Uptake of iodine-123 or technetium-99m–pertechnetate may be mildly to severely reduced and is often heterogeneous.[28] On US, the thyroid gland is diffusely abnormal, demonstrating decreased and

TABLE 34–4 Thyroiditis

Clinical Syndrome	Clinical Presentation and Course
Hashimoto's thyroiditis (chronic lymphocytic—autoimmune)	Goiter and hypothyroidism Progressive thyroid replacement Fibrous variant with atrophy Increased risk of non-Hodgkin's lymphoma Associated with other autoimmune diseases
Silent (painless) thyroiditis (subacute lymphocytic thyroiditis—autoimmune)	± Goiter Transient hyperthyroid symptoms with resolution
Postpartum thyroiditis (subacute lymphocytic thyroiditis—autoimmune)	Goiter Transient hyperthyroid symptoms Usually resolves, but may progress to chronic thyroiditis
De Quervain's thyroiditis (subacute granulomatous—viral)	Neck pain, usually follows viral upper respiratory infection Transient hyperthyroid symptoms with resolution
Acute suppurative thyroiditis (infectious—bacterial, fungal—very rare)	Extreme swelling and tenderness of thyroid Skin erythema, sepsis, thyrotoxicosis
Riedel's (struma) thyroiditis (extensive fibrosis, very rare)	Extreme fibrosis of thyroid gland and surrounding neck structures

inhomogeneous echogenicity. The gland may be normal or enlarged. There may be multiple, ill-defined hypoechoic areas separated by thickened fibrous strands,[21] giving a coarse texture to the gland. Small hyperechoic foci associated with acoustic shadowing represent punctate calcifications.[20] Small discrete nodules are common. Large nodules raise the possibility of neoplasia. Color Doppler usually demonstrates increased vascularity.[21] At the end stage the gland may be small, heterogeneous in echotexture, and fibrotic.

On CT scans, the enlarged thyroid gland has an irregular surface and an inhomogeneous distribution of iodine. T2-weighted MRI images show increased signal intensity, sometimes with linear low-intensity bands thought to represent fibrosis.[29]

US may be used to follow Hashimoto's thyroiditis patients for unsuspected malignancy. Although there is an increased incidence of non-Hodgkin's lymphoma,[30, 31] thyroid carcinoma is rarely observed clinically[25] but has been reported.[32] Thyroid lymphoma can produce focal hypoechoic lesions or diffuse disease[34–35] that may be difficult to differentiate from the hypoechoic pattern of Hashimoto's thyroiditis. The presence of associated lymphadenopathy raises the suspicion of superimposed lymphoma (Fig. 34–5). Lymphadenopathy can be detected more accurately by CT or MRI than by US because of superior definition of extrathyroidal structures.

Silent (Painless) Thyroiditis, or Postpartum Thyroiditis (Subacute Lymphocytic)

Silent (painless) thyroiditis and postpartum thyroiditis are two clinical manifestations of subacute lymphocytic thyroiditis. When this disease occurs unrelated to pregnancy, it is referred to as *silent* or *painless* thyroiditis. Subacute lymphocytic thyroiditis is usually self-limited. Low-titer antithyroid antibodies are present, and the disorder is considered to be autoimmune.[25]

The patient typically presents with thyrotoxicosis that progresses to transient hypothyroidism before returning to the euthyroid state. Some individuals with painless thyroiditis do not experience glandular enlargement, whereas others develop goiter. During the initial period of follicular disruption, the patient has hyperthyroid symptoms as preformed hormone is released into the circulation (T_3 and T_4 levels are elevated and TSH levels are suppressed). Antithyroid antibodies can be identified, and there is infrequent association with a prior viral infection. In contrast to Graves' disease, the radioactive iodine uptake is low and the pattern on scintigraphy varies from no tracer uptake to diffuse or heterogeneous reduction. Scan patterns normalize when the process resolves.

Subacute lymphocytic thyroiditis typically occurs in the postpartum period 4 to 6 weeks after delivery. As in silent thyroiditis, women with postpartum thyroiditis present with goiter, thyrotoxicosis, and antithyroid antibodies. The process usually resolves after transient hypothyroidism. However, some patients progress to chronic lymphocytic thyroiditis. Postpartum thyroiditis develops in 5% of postpartum women and can recur with subsequent pregnancies.[36]

De Quervain's Thyroiditis (Subacute Granulomatous Thyroiditis)

Subacute granulomatous thyroiditis is a self-limited inflammation of the thyroid gland that usually follows a viral upper respiratory infection. The peak incidence is in the teens to the 40s, with a female to male ratio of 3 to 1. The patient presents with pain in the thyroid and neck, painful, tender enlargement of the thyroid gland, pain radiating to the jaw or ears, thyrotoxicosis, fatigue, and variably fever. Viruses involved have included mumps virus, coxsackievirus, influenza virus, adenovirus, and echoviruses.[1, 6] Early in the inflammatory phase, scattered follicles may be replaced by neutrophils forming microabscesses. Later, macrophages and multinucleate giant cells form around damaged follicles. Their resemblance to

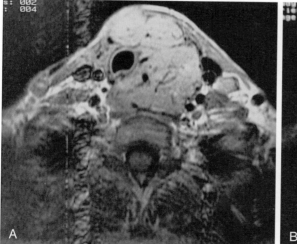
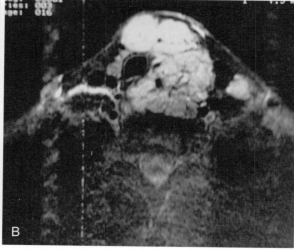

FIGURE 34–5 Hashimoto's thyroiditis. Axial T1- (*A*) and T2- (*B*) weighted sequences show a complex thyroid mass with mixed signal inhomogeneity. This proved to be Hashimoto's thyroiditis. The ^{123}I scintigraph showed areas of hot and cold nodules (not shown), which can be seen in approximately 30% of Hashimoto's patients. Hashimoto's thyroiditis is the great mimicker on imaging studies and should be considered in the differential diagnosis of most thyroid diseases. There is also an increased risk of non-Hodgkin's lymphoma, which was suspected clinically in this patient.

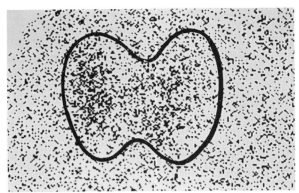

FIGURE 34–6 De Quervain's thyroiditis. Anterior pinhole image from ^{123}I scintigraphy demonstrates heterogeneous and reduced uptake in both lobes of the thyroid gland. This is a nonspecific pattern and can be seen in Hashimoto's (approximately 50% of the time) as well as in other causes of thyroiditis. This patient had a viral prodrome 3 weeks before the study: sore throat and tender gland. The clinical symptoms and the ^{123}I scan shown here are typical of subacute granulomatous thyroiditis. Although the 24-hour uptake was abnormally low (2% to 3%) in this patient, hyperthyroid, euthyroid, or hypothyroid states can be seen depending on the stage of the disease. Full thyroid function usually returns within 6 to 12 months.

granulomas has fostered the term *granulomatous thyroiditis*.[6]

Clinically, the patient presents with symptoms of thyrotoxicosis, elevated T_3 and T_4 levels, and low radioactive iodine uptake. Scintigraphy demonstrates variable patterns that usually resolve within 6 to 12 months as the patient returns to the euthyroid state (Fig. 34–6).

Acute Suppurative Thyroiditis

Acute suppurative (infectious) thyroiditis is relatively rare. Microbial seeding of the thyroid by bacteria and less

frequently by *Mycobacterium, Aspergillus, Candida,* and *Cryptococcus* species[1] tends to occur in debilitated or immunocompromised individuals. The thyroid gland may show suppurative inflammation and occasionally abscess formation. On imaging, the affected lobe(s) shows enlargement and inhomogeneity (Fig. 34–7). With disease progression, loculated abscesses and adjacent soft tissue edema and cellulitis may be present.

Riedel's Thyroiditis (Struma)

Riedel's struma is a very rare form of chronic thyroiditis, characterized by an extensive fibrosing reaction that destroys most of the thyroid gland while simultaneously extending into the surrounding neck structures. The thyroid gland has a woody hardness. The female to male ratio is 3 to 1. The incidence is greatest in the 30s to 60s. Patients may have manifestations of an obstructive, invasive process that can be confused with a thyroid malignancy, or they may just have a painless lump in the neck.[37] Stridor, dysphagia, recurrent laryngeal nerve paralysis, dyspnea, and even suffocation can occur.[6] The cause is unknown, and the process does not appear to be autoimmune. This entity is associated with other fibrosing processes such as retroperitoneal fibrosis, mediastinal fibrosis, sclerosing cholangitis, and orbital pseudotumor. From 30% to 40% of patients may show progression to hypothyroidism.

The typical features of Riedel's thyroiditis on imaging studies include an infiltrative process that causes obliteration of tissue planes and matting of adjacent structures. On noncontrast CT, fibrosis can appear hypodense, whereas other benign and malignant processes tend to be more heterogeneous.[37] On MRI, the features of the fibrotic process usually demonstrate low signal intensity on T1- and T2-weighted images. There have been reports of a more focal masslike process.[38] In this example, the

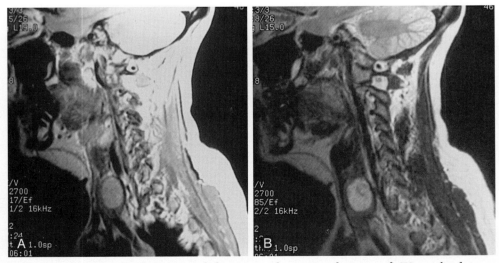

FIGURE 34–7 Tuberculous abscess. *A* and *B*, Sagittal fast spin echo proton-density and T2-weighted images reveal a well-circumscribed mass in the left lobe of the thyroid gland. This mass was detected incidentally during a routine examination of the cervical spine for disk disease. Fine-needle biopsy was positive for acid-fast bacilli. Most cases of acute suppurative thyroiditis are associated with systemic manifestations and are most frequently due to *Staphylococcus aureus, Staphylococcus haemolyticus,* or pneumococci. Patients are usually euthyroid; ^{123}I uptake is normal, and the scintigram reveals regions of decreased uptake at the site of tenderness. (*A* and *B*, Courtesy of Evan Siegelman, M.D., and Jeff Goldmann, M.D., University of Pennsylvania Medical Center, Philadelphia, PA.)

T2-weighted images demonstrated low signal intensity, reflecting the fibrosing reaction characteristic of Riedel's thyroiditis. The low T2-weighted signal property is in contradistinction to the heterogeneous hyperintense signal of thyroid malignancy[39] and homogeneously bright signal of thyroid lymphoma.[40]

Goiter: Diffuse Nontoxic, Multinodular (Adenomatous), and Toxic Multinodular Goiter

The term *goiter* refers to any enlargement of the thyroid gland. The enlargements may be diffuse or nodular. To compensate for inadequate thyroid hormone output, follicular epithelium undergoes compensatory hypertrophy and hyperplasia and the thyroid gland enlarges to achieve a euthyroid state. In some instances hypo- or hyperthyroidism may develop. Initially the goitrous enlargement is diffuse, but with time it usually becomes nodular. If the impediment to thyroid hormone output abates, the thyroid gland may even revert to normal during the diffuse state.

Diffuse Nontoxic (Simple) Goiter

A simple nontoxic goiter is a thyroid gland that is enlarged diffusely and does not demonstrate nodularity or hyper- or hypofunction. Enlarged follicles are filled with colloid, hence the term *colloid goiter.* Diffuse goiter is endemic if it affects more than 10% of the population in a particular geographic location, or it may be sporadic. Endemic goiter is prevalent in iodine-deficient areas. Accordingly, the incidence has been markedly reduced with the use of iodized salt. In simple sporadic goiter, there is a female preponderance, with a ratio of 8 to 1, and a peak incidence at puberty.[6] Sporadic goiter is less common than endemic goiter, with the latter affecting approximately 200 million individuals worldwide.

There are two stages in the evolution of diffuse nontoxic goiter—hyperplasia and colloid involution.[6] During hyperplasia, the gland enlarges modestly with diffuse, symmetric involvement and marked hyperemia. The newly generated follicles, lined by columnar epithelium, are small and contain scant colloid. The duration of the hyperplastic stage is variable. However, when a euthyroid state is maintained, follicular cell growth ceases and is followed by colloid involution. As follicles fill with colloid and enlarge, the epithelium flattens. Follicular enlargement is not uniform. Some follicles become overdistended whereas others remain small.[1] During colloid involution the thyroid gland may show marked enlargement and ultimately weigh more than 500 gm.

Multinodular (Adenomatous) Goiter

With time, most simple goiters become transformed into multinodular goiters. The multinodular goiter may remain nontoxic or may induce thyrotoxicosis. The hypermetabolism is usually less severe than in Graves' disease, and there is no associated ophthalmopathy. Multinodular goiters are rarely associated with hypothyroidism. Differentiating a large multinodular goiter from a neoplastic process can be challenging.

The multinodular, or adenomatous, goiter is markedly heterogeneous. Characteristic features include nodularity caused by colloid-filled or hyperplastic follicles, irregular scarring, focal hemorrhage with hemosiderin deposition, focal calcifications, and microcysts (Fig. 34–8). Glandular enlargement may be asymmetric, involving one lobe more than the other, with compression of adjacent structures such as the trachea and esophagus. The goitrous enlargement may even extend substantially into the anterior mediastinum and less commonly into the posterior mediastinum.

Clinically, multinodular goiters may present with cosmetic disfigurement, dysphagia, inspiratory stridor, or even venous obstruction. Hemorrhage into the goiter may induce sudden painful enlargement. The patient with thyrotoxicosis may have cardiovascular dysfunction, particularly atrial fibrillation, tachycardia, and occasionally heart failure. Serum TSH levels are markedly suppressed (<0.1 μU/ml), even though serum levels of T_3 and T_4 are only slightly elevated. Differentiation of multinodular goiter from a neoplasm may be difficult if the enlargement of a single focus exceeds the overall rate of enlargement of the gland.

On imaging, one may observe a variety of patterns. With nuclear medicine scintigraphy (Fig. 34–9) radioiodine or technetium-99m–pertechnetate may accumulate in patchy foci throughout the gland or, less commonly, in one or a few nodules. Some of these nodules may even demonstrate autonomous function. If the patient has symptoms of thyrotoxicosis, therapeutic doses of radioiodine (iodine-131) may be required to reduce overall thyroid function. Although it was previously thought that a solitary cold nodule in a multinodular goiter was less likely to be malignant than a solitary nodule in a normal gland, some studies have demonstrated similar rates of malignancy.[41] In a review of more than 5000 patients with nodular goiter, the rate of malignancy for patients with a solitary cold nodule was 4.7%, and the rate for patients with multiple nodules was 4.1%. This observation supports older surgical series that reported the prevalence of cancer in a dominant cold nodule in a multinodular goiter to be almost as high as in a solitary nodule in a normal gland.[42, 43]

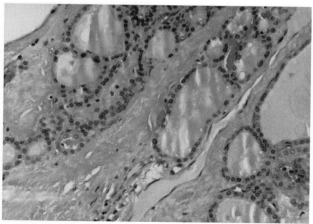

FIGURE 34–8 Nodular goiter. The photomicrograph shows variable-sized follicles and fibrosis. (H&E 150×.)

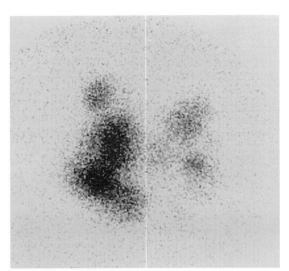

FIGURE 34–9 Multinodular goiter on ¹²³I scintigraphy. Anterior pinhole images obtained 2 hours after the administration of ¹²³I demonstrate multiple hot and cold nodules. This is a typical example of a multinodular goiter.

On US (Fig. 34–10), a simple goiter demonstrates diffuse enlargement with uniform or irregular echotexture that may be increased or decreased in intensity. A multinodular goiter is often irregular and demonstrates either diffuse inhomogeneity or relatively normal thyroid tissue with nodules. Approximately 60% of glands have punctate calcifications that manifest as hyperechoic foci with distal acoustic shadowing.

On CT scanning, a multinodular goiter again shows an enlarged symmetric or asymmetric gland with multiple low-density areas of varying discreteness and varied CT density. The gland may enhance uniformly with contrast material (simple goiter) but often contains poorly enhancing areas that reflect hemorrhage, necrosis, or cyst formation. Focal calcifications are common. CT examination can identify compression of the trachea, esophagus, or adjacent vessels and may demonstrate extension of the

thyroid gland into the thorax, which occurs in approximately 20% of patients (Fig. 34–11A and B). In contrast to scintigraphy, which may fail to show continuity between the cervical thyroid and mediastinal goiter, CT scanning demonstrates the thyroidal origin of the mediastinal mass. In addition, prolonged contrast enhancement (>2 minutes), focal calcifications, and a CT density greater than that of muscle help to differentiate the mediastinal goiter from an aneurysm or lymphoma.[44]

On MRI (Fig. 34–11C–G), the multinodular (adenomatous) goiter may show minimal to moderate heterogeneity on T1-weighted images with multiple high-intensity foci representing cystic areas containing colloid (proteinaceous) or hemorrhage (methemoglobin). The extent of the goiter, including the intrathoracic component and its relation to adjacent structures, is clearly delineated. On T2-weighted images heterogeneity is more evident. Nodules as small as 3 to 5 mm may be visualized owing to high-intensity signal contrast. Calcifications are visualized as scattered low-intensity foci on T1- and T2-weighted sequences. After gadolinium administration, glandular enhancement is inhomogeneous.

Toxic Multinodular Goiter (Plummer's Disease)

In 1913, Plummer[45] reported hyperthyroidism resulting from nodular goiter. This was different from the diffuse toxic goiter known as Graves' disease. He did not differentiate between what is now recognized as two types of toxic nodular goiter—the toxic multinodular goiter and the toxic autonomously functioning thyroid nodule (see Benign Neoplasms). In clinical practice, this differentiation is useful.

Toxic multinodular goiter frequently develops in people older than 50 years. The thyroid gland may contain one or several large, hyperfunctioning nodules. Clinically, the patient has symptoms of thyrotoxicosis, often including tachycardia or atrial fibrillation. The patient may stare and demonstrate lid lag on downward gaze but does not develop infiltrative ophthalmopathy or proptosis. If the goiter is large, there may be symptoms of pressure or

FIGURE 34–10 Multinodular goiter on ultrasonography and ¹²³I scintigraphy. A, Transverse ultrasound image shows bilateral nodular masses. The lesions seen on this single image are hypoechoic (L and R), but the mass on the left (L) has a more complex character. B, Anterior pinhole images obtained 4 hours after the administration of ¹²³I demonstrate bilateral hot and cold nodules with intense uptake in the more complex nodule.

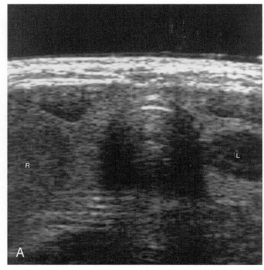
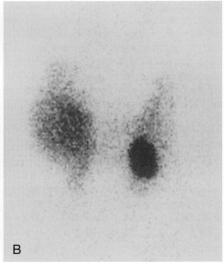

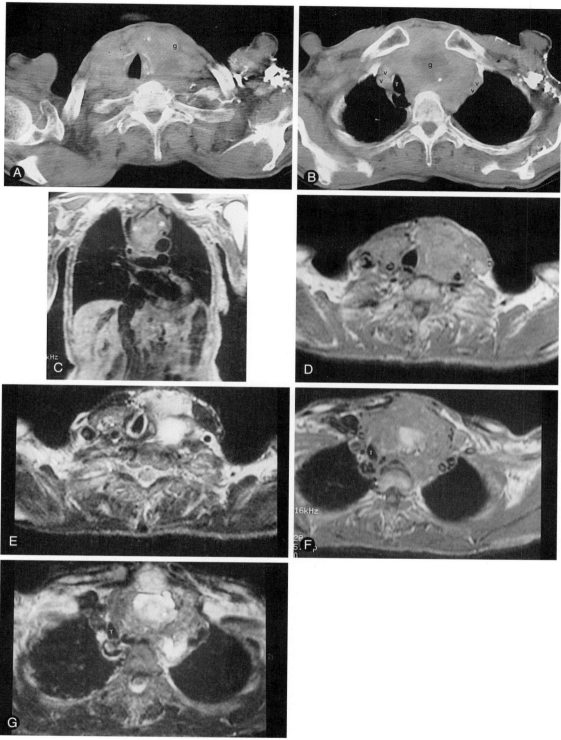

FIGURE 34–11 Large substernal goiter on computed tomography (CT) and MRI. *A* and *B*, Contrast-enhanced axial CT images demonstrate a large complex mass (g) extending from the thyroid bed into the superior mediastinum. The mass is displacing the trachea (T) and great vessels (v). Notice areas of hypodensity and calcification within the mass (the calcifications were also seen on precontrast images). Coronal *(C)* and axial *(D–G)* T1- and T2-weighted images reveal the complex nature of the mass. There are mixed areas of hyperintensity and hypointensity on both T1- and T2-weighted sequences. These signal characteristics are not specific enough to make a definitive diagnosis, and any one of these findings may be present in malignant disease. However, tissue sampling would be necessary to exclude malignancy in the absence of adenopathy and infiltration of adjacent structures. The axial MRI images correspond in location to the axial CT images. The small punctate foci of calcification seen on the CT scan are not well appreciated on the MRI images.

obstruction of the aerodigestive tract. Radioiodine therapy may diminish hyperfunction in toxic multinodular goiter and reduce the risk of a significant cardiac event.

Nodular Thyroid Disease

The thyroid gland has a tendency to develop nodules that are often discovered by a patient or palpated as an incidental finding on physical examination. In the United States, the prevalence of such palpable nodules in the adult population is estimated to be 4% to 7%. Most of the nodules are follicular (colloid) nodules that develop in an adenomatous goiter after cycles of hyperplasia and colloid involution. Some are benign adenomas. To put this in perspective, in a recent review,[13] it was estimated that approximately 75 to 120 million people in the United States have thyroid nodules, 10 to 18 million of which are palpable.

Fortunately, thyroid cancer is relatively rare, and differentiated forms such as papillary and follicular tend to have a favorable prognosis. The annual incidence of newly diagnosed thyroid cancer in the United States is approximately 12,000 cases, and the annual death rate is roughly 1000 people.[46] The incidence is greater in women than men and increases with advancing age. Another curious feature about thyroid cancer is the prevalence of incidental (occult) carcinomas identified at autopsy (prevalence, 3.9%)[47] or surgery (prevalence, 10.5%; size, 2 to 10 mm).[48] Therefore, since any thyroid nodule, including the tiny (<1 cm) nodules identified by high-resolution US, could potentially be malignant, the challenge lies in identifying the malignant lesions that require surgical exploration and appropriate cancer therapy without performing unnecessary interventions on benign nodules.

The incidence of thyroid cancer has been increasing in both men and women from approximately 1935 through 1975, corresponding to years in which low-level radiation treatments were applied to the head and neck, particularly in children, for such benign processes as acne, enlarged thymus, recurrent otitis media, adenoidal hypertrophy, and tinea capitis. Duffy and Fitzgerald in 1950[49] first recognized the relationship between radiation and thyroid cancer. In their report of 28 cases, they found an unusually large fraction of children with thyroid cancer after therapeutic irradiation. Although initially doubted, evidence that low-level radiation causes thyroid cancer has since been confirmed by a wide variety of studies that are summarized in an excellent review by Schneider.[50] A linear dose-response relationship exists between 1 and 20 Gy.[5, 51, 52] It has not been possible to determine whether there is a dose below which no increased risk of developing thyroid cancer exists.

Approximately 15% to 30% of patients who received radiation in this dose range will develop a thyroid nodule, and 6% to 8% of these people will develop thyroid cancer, usually with a well-differentiated papillary or follicular histologic appearance. Early detection is essential because carcinoma in this population is more biologically aggressive and may require more extensive surgical procedures to achieve a cure rate equal to that in nonirradiated patients.[53] Long-term follow-up is mandatory, as the latent period for the development of carcinoma may be as long

as 30 years. After high-dose irradiation (>20 Gy) thyroid carcinoma is rare, most likely because radiation in this dose range is actually killing the thyroid tissue.[5]

Attempts to determine that a thyroid nodule is likely to be a carcinoma based on the patient's history and physical findings have yielded poor results and subjected patients to unnecessary surgery. The differential diagnosis of a thyroid mass encompasses benign adenomas, cysts (hemorrhagic, colloid), hemorrhage into an adenoma, parathyroid cysts, carcinoma and lymphoma of the thyroid, metastasis, localized thyroiditis, abscess, and extrathyroidal disease. Factors that make the nodule more likely a carcinoma include age (<20 or >60 years); male sex (cancer frequency is three to four times greater in women, but they have a much greater incidence of nodules than men); an ipsilateral enlarged lymph node; a history of long-standing goiter; residence in an iodine-deficient region; hoarseness (secondary to vocal cord paralysis on the same side as the thyroid nodule); low-dose radiation during childhood for benign conditions; a family history of thyroid carcinoma or of multiple endocrine neoplasia (risk of medullary carcinoma of the thyroid); and chronic lymphocytic thyroiditis (increased risk of non-Hodgkin's lymphoma).[53]

However, as most thyroid nodules occur sporadically and are not associated with these findings, it is important to have an efficient diagnostic approach to identify malignancy. Historically, radionuclide scintigraphy was performed to determine whether a nodule demonstrated radioactive iodine uptake. A palpable nodule that did not demonstrate radioactive iodine uptake relative to the normal gland was termed a *cold* nodule with malignant potential. As such, it required biopsy or surgical removal. A lesion that demonstrated relatively increased uptake was called a *hot*, or functioning, nodule. If adjacent normal thyroid tissue was suppressed, and if in turn the nodule could not be suppressed with exogenous thyroid hormone, it was considered to have autonomous function. In either case, as the incidence of carcinoma is very low, the lesion was followed or treated (radioiodine or surgery) to reduce the autonomous function.

With the advent of high-resolution US techniques, the architecture of a nodule has been exquisitely delineated, but no findings have conclusively differentiated a benign nodule from a carcinoma. A sonolucent halo around the nodule favored, but did not guarantee, benignity.[54]

Fine-needle–aspiration biopsy, initially introduced in 1930[55] but fraught with conflicting results regarding accuracy during the past 50 years or more, has gained acceptance as the pre-eminent diagnostic method for evaluating thyroid nodules worldwide.[56] With technical refinement using a 22- to 25-gauge, 1.5-inch needle, an aspiration technique or a slight in-and-out excursion of the needle through the nodule without aspiration, it is usually possible to obtain a satisfactory specimen with minimal contamination by blood. Frequently the procedure is performed four to six times to obtain an adequate specimen (at least six clusters of cells on two slides). Specimens may be stained and examined while the patient waits. Interpretation requires a skilled cytopathologist.[56]

In addition to providing a safe, accurate, minimally invasive diagnostic procedure for the management of patients with thyroid nodules, the fine-needle–aspiration biopsy is extremely cost-effective. Gharib and Goellner's[57] review of the 1982 to 1991 literature on the utility of fine-needle–aspiration biopsy in nodular thyroid disease revealed high diagnostic accuracy and significant cost savings. The percentage of patients undergoing thyroidectomy decreased by 25%, and the yield of carcinoma in patients who underwent surgery increased from 15% to at least 30%. These authors stated that fine-needle–aspiration biopsy decreased the cost of care by 25%.

In these series, four cytologic diagnostic categories were used: benign, suspicious for malignancy, malignancy, and nondiagnostic. These authors demonstrated that an algorithm that included fine-needle–aspiration biopsy, T_4 levels, and TSH levels but omitted radionuclide and high-resolution US scans reduced the cost of nodule evaluation without sacrificing diagnostic accuracy. In cases in which the initial fine-needle–aspiration biopsy was nondiagnostic, rebiopsy was performed. If this was nondiagnostic, a radionuclide scan could be performed to determine whether the nodule was functioning. If the nodule was nonfunctioning, the patient went to surgery. If the nodule was functioning, the patient was observed.

When the biopsy was satisfactory, benign nodules were observed and malignant or suspicious nodules were further evaluated with surgery. The authors felt that because a suspicious aspirate had a 30% chance of malignancy, surgical exploration was preferable to performing a scintigraph to determine whether the nodule was functioning and unlikely to be malignant. Thus, fine-needle–aspiration biopsy is the procedure of choice to evaluate a palpable thyroid nodule in a patient who does not demonstrate symptoms of thyrotoxicosis or suppression of serum TSH levels.

Benign Neoplasms: Adenomas

Adenomas of the thyroid gland are benign, encapsulated neoplasms that are usually solitary and nonfunctioning and are detected in young and middle-aged adults. Thyroid adenomas are usually small (<4 cm) and discrete, surrounded by a complete fibrous capsule, and distinctly separated from the adjacent thyroid tissue. These solitary nodules are true neoplasms, developing from monoclonal proliferation,[1] and differ histologically from the adenomatous nodules that develop in a multinodular goiter. However, both follicular adenomas and follicular (colloid) nodules can undergo hemorrhage, fibrosis, and cyst formation.

Histologically, there are several patterns ranging from microfollicular adenomas, composed of tiny follicles, to macrofollicular or colloid adenomas, composed of dilated, colloid-filled follicles. Follicular adenomas are differentiated from encapsulated follicular carcinomas by failing to demonstrate capsular or vascular invasion (Fig. 34–12).

A less common variant has been described with branching papillary excrescences protruding into microcystic spaces. This lesion had been referred to as a *papillary cystadenoma* but now apparently is considered a carcinoma.[6] There is also a rare lesion called the *Hürthle cell adenoma*, histologically composed of large granular cells, with pink-staining cytoplasm, arranged in a trabecu-

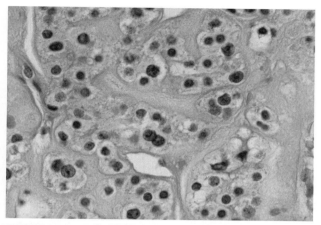

FIGURE 34–12 Follicular adenoma. A photomicrograph shows focal groups and nests of cells with clear cytoplasm. One cannot determine a benign from a malignant lesion by examining only the center of the lesion. The presence of capsular and vascular invasion must be demonstrated to establish malignancy. (H&E 400×.)

lar pattern. Additional rare lesions include dermoid cysts, lymphomas, hemangiomas, and teratomas, the latter found primarily in infants.

Follicular adenomas slowly increase in size and plateau between 3 and 4 cm as expansile pressure restricts their blood supply.[6] If a follicular adenoma suddenly enlarges and becomes painful, the acute change usually reflects intralesional hemorrhage.

Although most adenomas are nonfunctioning (Fig. 34–13), autonomously functioning thyroid adenomas can occur at any age and are usually nontoxic, that is, the patient does not have symptoms of hyperthyroidism. These nodules usually remain relatively small and seldom become toxic if they are less than 3 cm.[58] The transition to toxicity is usually very gradual and occurs more frequently with advancing age (>60 years). TSH suppression, measured by a high-sensitivity technique, may be the first indication of evolving toxicity. Spontaneous degeneration can occur with significant reduction in nodule size. The presence of carcinoma is rare.[59]

On scintigraphy, the hyperfunctioning nodule appears more intense than the surrounding gland. If the nodule is truly autonomous (independent of TSH), it may suppress the surrounding normal thyroid tissue (Fig. 34–14) and in turn may not be suppressed by exogenous levothyroxine (Synthroid; T_4) or triiodothyronine (Cytomel; T_3). Typically, when a T_3 thyroid-suppression test is performed after a baseline iodine-123 scan and uptake, the patient takes 75 mg of triiodothyronine daily for 7 to 10 days and the study is repeated. The normal response demonstrates a reduction of radioiodine uptake by 50% and a drop in the serum T_4 level. If the uptake in the hot nodule is not accordingly reduced, the test indicates that the nodule has autonomous function.

In addition to demonstrating the presence of a hyperfunctioning nodule, radioiodine has a role in the ablation of an autonomously functioning thyroid adenoma. For therapeutic procedures iodine-131 is utilized, as the short-acting β radiation will deposit in the nodule and

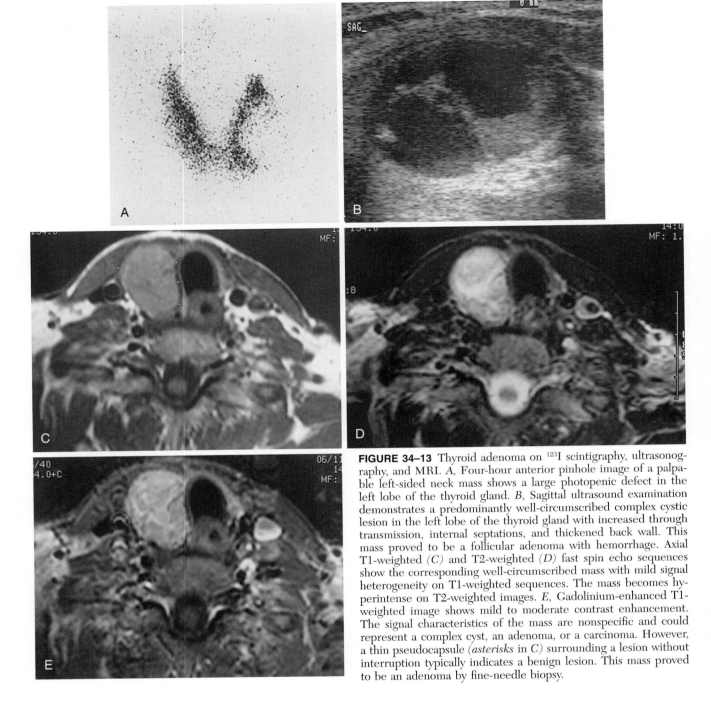

FIGURE 34–13 Thyroid adenoma on ^{123}I scintigraphy, ultrasonography, and MRI. *A,* Four-hour anterior pinhole image of a palpable left-sided neck mass shows a large photopenic defect in the left lobe of the thyroid gland. *B,* Sagittal ultrasound examination demonstrates a predominantly well-circumscribed complex cystic lesion in the left lobe of the thyroid gland with increased through transmission, internal septations, and thickened back wall. This mass proved to be a follicular adenoma with hemorrhage. Axial T1-weighted *(C)* and T2-weighted *(D)* fast spin echo sequences show the corresponding well-circumscribed mass with mild signal heterogeneity on T1-weighted sequences. The mass becomes hyperintense on T2-weighted images. *E,* Gadolinium-enhanced T1-weighted image shows mild to moderate contrast enhancement. The signal characteristics of the mass are nonspecific and could represent a complex cyst, an adenoma, or a carcinoma. However, a thin pseudocapsule *(asterisks* in *C)* surrounding a lesion without interruption typically indicates a benign lesion. This mass proved to be an adenoma by fine-needle biopsy.

ablate this tissue. Since radioiodine uptake in the nodule may be relatively low, iodine-131 doses in the range of 25 to 29 mCi or higher may be needed. Alternatively, the autonomous nodule may be removed surgically. In either case, the risk of postprocedure hypothyroidism is low. The previously suppressed normal thyroid tissue is relatively protected from injury by iodine-131 and resumes normal function when the nodule has been ablated.

There have been reports from Italy describing the successful treatment of autonomously functioning thyroid adenomas (toxic and nontoxic) and parathyroid adenomas with 95% ethanol injection. In most protocols, 2 to 4 ml of 95% ethanol is injected into the nodule, 1 to 2 times a week for a total of 3 to 10 injections, depending on the size of the nodule. The results vary but generally show resolution of the hyperthyroid state without development of hypothyroidism.[60–65] One potential complication is the inadvertent injection of ethanol into the recurrent laryngeal nerve, producing either transient or permanent vocal cord paralysis.[66] Transient pyrexia has been reported.[61] As

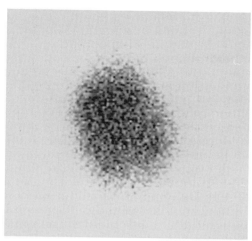

FIGURE 34–14 Autonomously functioning nodule on ^{123}I scintigraphy. A 24-hour anterior pinhole image demonstrates a large, solitary, hyperfunctioning nodule in the right lobe of the thyroid with suppression of radionuclide uptake in the remainder of the gland. Note that the 24-hour uptake is abnormally elevated at 42% (normal range 10% to 30%). This is a typical example of an autonomously functioning nodule leading to a toxic goiter.

with iodine-131 therapy, stored thyroid hormone is released into the circulation and can exacerbate thyrotoxicosis.

Malignant Neoplasms

Although primary carcinoma of the thyroid is a relatively rare disease, with approximately 12,000 new cases identified in the United States annually, it continues to stimulate considerable academic and clinical interest. Differentiated thyroid carcinoma arises from both follicular and parafollicular C cells. The malignant potential ranges from low grade (papillary carcinoma) to extraordinarily malignant (anaplastic carcinoma). Metastatic lesions in the thyroid usually derive from melanoma or from breast, kidney, or lung cancer.

Classification is based on histologic examination. For prognosis, the biologic behavior, tumor size, extent of disease, and tendency toward hematogenous or lymphatic metastases are important considerations. As previously discussed, low-level radiation to the neck region is associated with an increased incidence of thyroid cancer (see Nodular Thyroid Disease).

There is increasing evidence supporting a genetic basis for several thyroid carcinomas. The *ret* oncogene on the long arm of chromosome 10 has been implicated in papillary carcinoma (which originates from thyroid follicular cells) and in familial forms of medullary carcinoma (which originates from calcitonin-secreting parafollicular C cells).[13] The *ret* oncogene has tyrosine kinase activity. Familial cases of medullary thyroid carcinoma have been identified in type II multiple endocrine neoplasia syndromes (MEN-IIa and MEN-IIb). MEN-IIa includes medullary thyroid carcinoma, pheochromocytoma, and parathyroid hyperplasia, and MEN-IIb includes medul-

lary thyroid carcinoma, mucosal neuromas, and a marfanoid habitus.

The major categories of thyroid cancer include papillary, follicular, medullary, and anaplastic carcinoma. Traditionally, it was stated that papillary carcinoma accounted for approximately 60% to 70% of thyroid cancers and follicular carcinoma accounted for 20% to 25%. With subclassification of papillary carcinoma to include the follicular variant, and stricter definition of capsular and vascular invasion to differentiate follicular carcinoma from other lesions, the relative distribution may more accurately be 80% papillary carcinoma and 5% follicular carcinoma.[1]

It is generally thought that medullary carcinoma accounts for 5% to 10% of thyroid cancer and undifferentiated anaplastic carcinoma accounts for 5% to 15%. Again, relative distribution varies depending on the author.[1, 6]

Thyroid carcinoma demonstrates a wide range of behavior, as indicated by the mortality rates: papillary carcinoma, 8% to 11%; follicular carcinoma, 24% to 33%; medullary carcinoma, 50%; anaplastic carcinoma, 75% to 90%.[53] Lymphoma associated with Hashimoto's thyroiditis may represent malignant transformation of B-cell lymphocytes.[30, 31]

Papillary Carcinoma

The most common type of thyroid cancer is papillary carcinoma. It is a low-grade malignancy that occurs in children and adults and has a female to male ratio of 3 to 1.[67] The presentation peaks at approximately 30 years of age. Papillary carcinoma encompasses lesions that demonstrate a pure papillary pattern, a mixed papillary and follicular pattern, and a totally follicular pattern, providing that histologic and cytologic characteristics suggest papillary carcinoma.[1] Papillary carcinomas may be very small (<1 cm), appropriately termed *microcarcinomas*, or occult lesions. Intrathyroidal tumors may be encapsulated or diffusely infiltrating. Papillary carcinomas may also be extrathyroidal.

On histologic examination, one sees papillae consisting of epithelial cells arranged around a fibrovascular core. Almost all papillary carcinomas contain some follicular elements. The follicular areas may be scant or may predominate. However, the key to the diagnosis of papillary carcinoma is the presence of optically clear, ground-glass nuclei with nuclear grooves.[1, 67] Approximately 40% of papillary carcinomas contain psammoma bodies, which are the laminated calcified "ghosts" of papillae.[1]

The follicular variant of papillary carcinoma (Fig. 34–15) demonstrates a predominantly follicular pattern that has features and biologic behavior characteristic of papillary carcinoma. Although the tumors were at one time classified under follicular carcinoma, the follicular variant was redescribed in a study by Chen and Rosai.[68] The tumor may have clear nuclei, psammoma bodies, and an infiltrating growth pattern. It usually has a favorable prognosis and a propensity for lymph node metastasis rather than hematogenous dissemination.

Several histologic subtypes of papillary carcinoma have been described that seem to have more aggressive biologic behavior. In this group are the tall cell variant

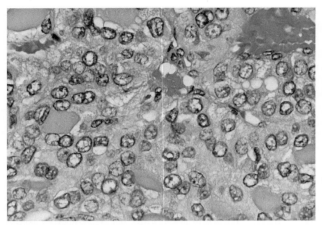

FIGURE 34–15 Follicular variant of papillary carcinoma. Despite the follicular pattern, the nuclei are those of papillary cancer: enlarged, cleaned out, nuclear grooves. (H&E 400×.)

(Fig. 34–16), the columnar cell type, and the diffuse sclerosis variant.[1]

Papillary cancers have been termed *multifocal*, as it is common to identify multiple tumor foci within a thyroid gland. Clonality studies have demonstrated that these sites represent intraglandular lymphatic spread rather than multiple clones of tumor.[1]

Papillary carcinoma is a slow-growing neoplasm with 20-year survival rates greater than 90%.[1] Metastatic spread to the regional lymph nodes occurs via lymphatics, and distant metastases are relatively rare. Papillary carcinoma presents with cervical lymph node metastases 40% of the time. Children younger than 18 years have an even-higher incidence of regional node metastases at presentation.[69] Nevertheless, their outcome is usually excellent.[70]

It is intriguing to note that the prevalence of papillary carcinoma has increased in populations where iodine supplements have been added to the diet, whereas the prevalence of goiter and the incidence of follicular and anaplastic carcinomas have declined.[71] Recurrence rates are highest in individuals younger than 20 years or older than 60 years. Mortality, however, increases markedly with advancing age (>60 years).

Follicular Carcinoma

Follicular carcinoma is a well-differentiated, relatively low grade malignancy. Peak presentation occurs at approximately 45 years of age. In most series, it is thought to represent 10% to 25% of thyroid carcinoma. However, when strict criteria are applied to the pathologic interpretation of capsular and vascular invasion, this neoplasm may actually represent only 5% of thyroid carcinomas.[1] These two criteria must be unequivocal. Ideally, the capsule will be transversed and the involved vessels will be the size of small veins. Tumor thrombus should be visualized within their lumina.

Follicular carcinomas are solitary lesions that may be encapsulated or may show gross invasion. The tumor does not appear to be induced by radiation and spreads hematogenously. Metastases are most commonly identi-

fied in the lungs or skeleton. If the tumor is grossly encapsulated, the 5-year survival rate is high, approaching 85% to 90%. However, late recurrences and metastases can occur even after an interval of 10 to 15 years. Obviously, invasive tumors have a more guarded prognosis.

In general, follicular carcinomas tend to behave more aggressively than papillary carcinomas and have a lower survival rate. Both carcinomas concentrate radioiodine and can be scanned with tracer doses of iodine-131. Likewise, metastatic and recurrent lesions can be eradicated with therapeutic doses of radioiodine.

Hürthle's Cell Tumors

Hürthle's cell tumors are surrounded by controversy regarding nomenclature and treatment. They occur in persons from their late teens into advanced age, with a mean age of 40 to 50 years and a female predominance of 2 to 1.[67] Histologically, Hürthle's cell tumors have abundant, granular, pink cytoplasm that contains numerous mitochondria. Nuclei are enlarged and frequently pleomorphic with prominent nucleoli.

In contrast to follicular and papillary carcinomas, Hürthle's cell tumors do not concentrate radioiodine well. However, they can be imaged with technetium-99m–sestamibi,[72] a myocardial perfusion tracer that has a high avidity for mitochondria-rich cells and has demonstrated clinical utility in imaging a variety of benign and malignant tumors.[73] Technetium-99m–sestamibi uptake in Hürthle's cell adenomas and carcinomas is intense and persistent, which differentiates them from other carcinomas and benign lesions that show relatively rapid tracer washout.

Although Hürthle's cell adenomas and carcinomas are considerably less common than follicular cell carcinomas, their behavior is more aggressive. They tend to involve cervical lymph nodes and may present with distant metastases. There has been considerable controversy about the ability to differentiate benign Hürthle's cell tumors from malignant tumors. This discussion has fostered the con-

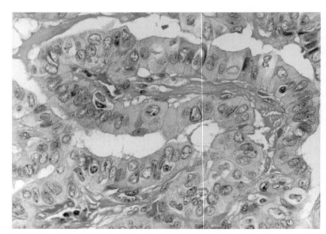

FIGURE 34–16 Tall cell variant of papillary carcinoma. The photomicrograph shows papillae with a fibrovascular core (*center*). Lining cells are tall (twice as tall as they are wide) and show characteristic clear, grooved nuclei of papillary cancer. (H&E 400×.)

cept that all of these tumors should be treated as potentially malignant.

However, there seems to be a growing opinion that one can differentiate benign from malignant Hürthle's cell tumors by applying the guidelines for malignancy used in differentiating other lesions, that is, capsular and vascular invasion.[67] Adenomas are encapsulated tumors without capsular or vascular invasion, and carcinomas demonstrate capsular, vascular, or thyroid parenchymal invasion. This distinction is more than academic, as benign Hürthle's cell tumors can be removed by lobectomy with an excellent prognosis.

Medullary Thyroid Carcinoma

Medullary carcinoma is derived from the parafollicular C cells and accordingly secretes a unique tumor marker, the hormone calcitonin. This is an aid in diagnosis and prognostication after surgery. Medullary carcinoma is relatively rare and associated with a higher mortality than the more differentiated papillary and follicular carcinomas. The majority of cases of medullary carcinoma occur sporadically, presenting at a mean age of 45 years, and consist of a solitary, unilateral mass. Histologically, the cells may be spindle-shaped. The stroma typically contains amyloid, and the architectural growth patterns are varied.[67] The tumor may invade locally, metastasize to regional or distant lymph nodes, or disseminate distantly to lungs, bone, and liver.

Medullary carcinoma may be familial (approximately 10% to 20% of cases) and inherited as an autosomal dominant component of MEN-II. Patients with MEN-IIa have a better prognosis than patients with sporadic medullary carcinoma or MEN-IIb. The presence of a palpable mass is associated with increased mortality, whereas the presence of cervical lymph nodes reduces the cure rate to less than 50%.[53]

Medullary carcinoma of the thyroid does not concentrate radioiodine but can be imaged with radiotracers that identify neuroendocrine tissue such as iodine-131–metaiodobenzylguanidine (^{131}I-MIBG) or the somatostatin analogue indium-111–pentetreotide (OctreoScan 111).[74, 75] Primary medullary carcinoma of the thyroid and metastatic lesions have been identified with somatostatin receptor scintigraphy.

Anaplastic Carcinoma

In contrast to the well-differentiated papillary and follicular carcinomas, anaplastic carcinoma of the thyroid is an extremely aggressive lesion that usually manifests in elderly patients, predominantly women, who have a long-standing history of goiter. The tumor enlarges rapidly, frequently obstructing the airway or the digestive tract, and is almost always fatal. The poorly differentiated, or anaplastic, tumors account for approximately 10% to 15% of thyroid cancer. Histologically, they may be difficult to differentiate from lymphomas (Fig. 34–17). Metastatic disease is widespread, involving regional lymph nodes, lungs, bones, and other distal sites. Anaplastic carcinomas do not concentrate radioiodine.

Lymphoma

Primary lymphoma of the thyroid is relatively uncommon. Like anaplastic carcinoma, it has a female predominance

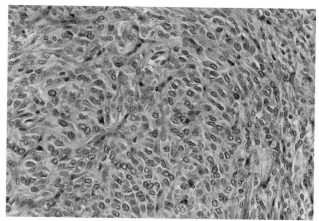

FIGURE 34–17 Poorly differentiated carcinoma. The photomicrograph reveals spindled cell type with prominent vascularity. Papillary cancer was seen in other areas. In the absence of necrosis and giant cells, this is not diagnosable as anaplastic carcinoma. (H&E 200×.)

and tends to occur in older individuals with a history of goiter.[53] Most of the lymphomas are of the non-Hodgkin type. Lymphoma may develop in patients with Hashimoto's thyroiditis, perhaps secondary to long-standing antigen stimulation of B-cell lymphocytes.[30, 31] Many of these lymphomas can be evaluated using gallium-67 scans.

Clinical Considerations

In evaluating the patient with a thyroid nodule or mass, certain clinical findings might favor malignancy. Among these are a hard, fixed, or rapidly enlarging nodule, associated hoarseness (perhaps due to vocal cord paralysis), development of a nodule in a person younger than 20 or older than 60 years, a history of low-dose ionizing radiation, male sex, and ipsilateral lymphadenopathy. As discussed previously, most patients require a diagnostic procedure (fine-needle–aspiration biopsy) to determine the presence of malignancy.

In patients with a history of low-dose ionizing radiation (<20 Gy) and a new dominant nodule, a subtotal thyroidectomy should be a therapeutic consideration. These people have a 40% chance of having cancer somewhere in the thyroid gland and approximately a 60% likelihood that it is in the presenting nodule.[50] Their overall incidence of cancer is 7%, versus the rest of the population, in whom the risk of developing a nodule is 5% to 7%. Children in this population are particularly worrisome, as the incidence of malignancy may be as high as 50% if the child is younger than 14 years.[76]

In terms of prognosis, the size and extent of involvement are usually more important than morphology in the patient with differentiated thyroid cancer. If the primary papillary carcinoma is small (<1.5 cm), the prognosis is excellent. Recurrence rates after initial therapy are low, and the disease is seldom fatal.[77] When the tumor is moderate to large (>1.5 cm), the risk of recurrence or death increases progressively with tumor size.[71] Mortality rates can be as high as 50% with tumors that are initially 7 cm, versus 6% if the lesion ranges from 2 to 3.9 cm.[78] In another series,[79] the cancer mortality rate from

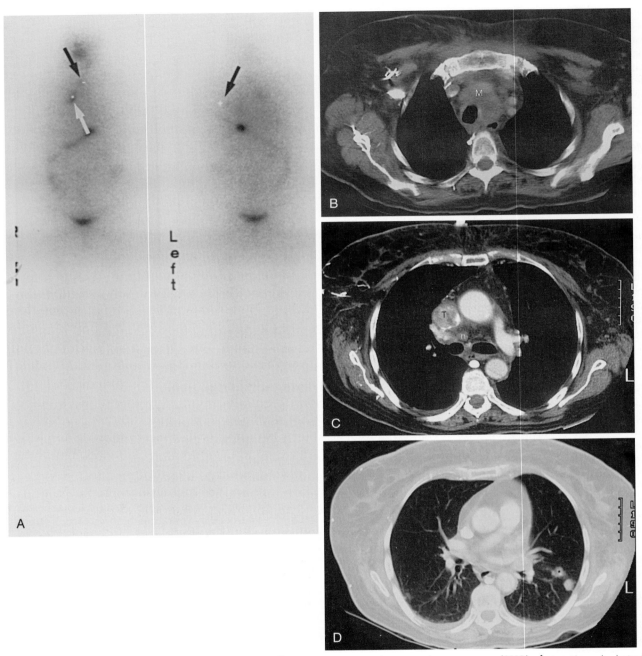

FIGURE 34–18 Metastatic pulmonary disease from papillary carcinoma causing superior vena cava (SVC) obstruction. *A,* Anterior and posterior images from a whole body scan in a patient with new onset of facial and upper extremity edema and a history of papillary carcinoma reveal metastatic disease in the neck on the right side *(black arrow on left),* and mediastinum *(white arrow).* Posterior image also shows a subtle focus of increased activity in the left lung thought to represent pulmonary metastasis *(black arrow on right).* Occlusion of the SVC was suspected on the clinical grounds. Normal distribution of ^{131}I includes the choroid plexus, nasopharynx, salivary glands, lactating breasts, stomach, bowel, kidneys, bladder, and occasionally the liver. *B–D,* Contrast-enhanced axial CT images at the level of the sternoclavicular joint *(B),* carina *(C),* and hila *(D)* confirm the presence of extensive metastatic disease (M in *B*), including adenopathy (n in *C*) in the mediastinum, displacing the trachea toward the right lung. Notice the thrombus (T in *C*) in the SVC, which confirmed SVC obstruction. One of the pulmonary nodules has peripheral, clumplike calcification *(asterisk in D).*

have been correlated with a poor outcome for patients with medullary carcinoma. Although children with papillary carcinoma may present with extensive cervical lymph node metastases, their outcome is better than that of adults with comparable disease.[53]

Distant metastases occur more frequently with advancing age and involve, in order of decreasing frequency, the lung, skeleton, and central nervous system (Figs. 34–18 through 34–20). At least 50% of the adults with distant metastases die within 5 years, regardless of whether they

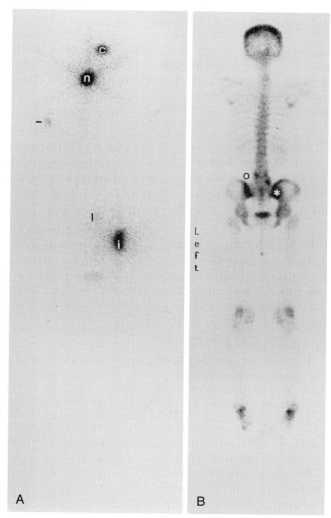

FIGURE 34–19 Metastatic thyroid disease to the bones. *A,* Posterior whole body image from ^{131}I scintigraphy reveals abnormal uptake in the region of the cervical spine (c), neck (n), left chest *(minus sign),* lumbar spine (l), and right iliac bone (i). *B,* Subtle changes of increased activity and asymmetry are noted in the corresponding iliac bone *(asterisk)* and lumbar spine (o) region on a posterior view from bone scintigraphy. Bone, lungs, lymph nodes, and sometimes liver are sites for metastatic thyroid carcinoma. This example illustrates that ^{131}I scanning is a more sensitive study for osseous lesions than is bone scintigraphy in patients with differentiated thyroid carcinomas but that it does not have the resolution of the latter. This is because many metastatic lesions are osteolytic and appear on the bone scan only after fracture or therapy (healing).

differentiated thyroid carcinoma was 5% when the lesion was less than 5 cm and 39% if the lesion was larger. Distant metastases also occurred more frequently when the primary tumor was larger than 5 cm. In other reports,[80, 81] the recurrence rate increased from 5% to 10.8% in lesions greater than 2.5 cm in diameter.

Primary tumor encapsulation is a prognostically favorable sign. If the primary tumor has extended through the thyroid capsule, the recurrence rate can be in the range of 40% and the death rate may vary from 5% to 35%.[82, 83]

Regional lymph node metastases may actually improve the prognosis for patients with papillary carcinoma but

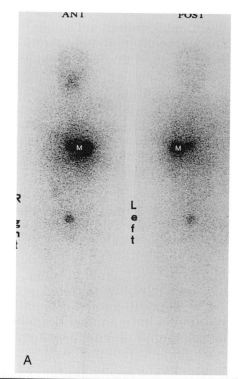

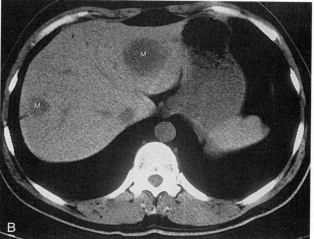

FIGURE 34–20 Liver metastasis from thyroid carcinoma detected on ^{131}I whole body images. *A,* Anterior and posterior images of a whole body scan 48 hours after ^{131}I ingestion (5 mCi, orally) demonstrate increased uptake in the left upper quadrant, which is due to hepatic metastasis (M). *B,* Hepatic metastatic (M) disease is confirmed on the axial CT examination. It is unusual for thyroid carcinoma to metastasize to the liver before bone or the lungs.

have papillary or follicular carcinomas.[71] Pulmonary metastases from papillary carcinoma may be compatible with longer survival. Bone and central nervous system metastases have a more serious prognosis.

Considerable controversy exists in the literature and among experienced thyroid surgeons regarding the type of operation to perform in patients with differentiated thyroid cancer. Surgical injury to the recurrent laryngeal nerve with resultant vocal cord paralysis and inadvertent removal of all of the parathyroid glands are the major risks of total thyroidectomy.

There is debate prognostically whether a total thyroidectomy or a more limited procedure is optimal. Thyroid cancers exhibit a wide spectrum of biologic behavior, and many patients have done well with minimal surgery. However, the contralateral lobe can contain microscopic cancer foci, and clinically, recurrence after lobectomy may be as high as 25%.[76] Mazzaferri and coworkers[80] documented that total thyroidectomy reduced the recurrence of thyroid cancer compared with lesser procedures. In their 10-year study of 576 patients with papillary carcinoma, the recurrence rate for patients with a presenting tumor greater than 1.5 cm was lowest in the group that underwent total thyroidectomy, radioiodine ablation of residual thyroid tissue, and thyroid hormone replacement. For smaller papillary lesions, the recurrence rate was not statistically different if less extensive surgery was performed.

Postoperatively, the patient who has undergone a total or subtotal thyroidectomy is easier to monitor for recurrence. The serum thyroglobulin determination is a more sensitive indicator of recurrent disease in the absence of native tissue. Radioiodine (iodine-131) has a greater likelihood of detecting and treating recurrence when normal thyroid tissue has been removed since the native tissue has approximately a 100-fold greater affinity for iodine than does metastatic disease (Fig. 34–21). Tumors that incorporate iodine-131 poorly or not at all may be imaged with thallium-201 (Fig. 34–22) or technetium-99m–sestamibi.[73]

Therefore, most thyroid experts recommend a total or subtotal thyroidectomy as the preferred operation for patients with papillary carcinoma greater than 1.5 cm in diameter or follicular carcinoma. If a patient has a smaller papillary carcinoma (<1.5 cm), ipsilateral total lobectomy and isthmusectomy can be performed.[76]

Imaging

There is extensive literature pertaining to imaging strategies in thyroid cancer. Historically, as previously discussed, nuclear scintigraphy was performed to determine whether a palpable neck mass or nodule was intrathyroidal, and if so, whether it took up less radioiodine than adjacent normal thyroid tissue (cold nodule) or exhibited increased function (hot nodule). Cold nodules required further evaluation as 10% to 25% could harbor a malignancy. This risk was greater in children, men of all ages, and people older than 60 years. Hot nodules, which were often autonomously functioning thyroid adenomas, rarely harbored malignancy[59] and could be followed (see Benign Neoplasms).

With the advent of high-resolution US, CT, and MRI,

many investigators tried to define a cancer signature. However, there are no imaging features that always differentiate benign from malignant thyroid lesions. The presence of ipsilateral lymphadenopathy, extrathyroidal invasion, or the rare distant metastasis favors the diagnosis of carcinoma. Unless the patient has a true simple cyst, which probably accounts for less than 1% of thyroid nodules, or a stable autonomously functioning adenoma, tissue diagnosis should be made by fine-needle–aspiration biopsy (see Nodular Thyroid Disease).

Benign Cyst or Nodule

US examination of the thyroid is routinely performed to evaluate a thyroid nodule.[19, 21] A pure cyst is usually round and demonstrates a smooth, discrete wall. These simple cysts have an epithelial lining and are usually filled with fluid that is anechoic (does not reflect echoes). The tissues behind the cyst have increased echogenicity, termed *acoustic enhancement.*

In contrast, complex cysts (without an epithelial lining) demonstrate cystic and solid components, some of which may be septated (see Fig. 34–13*B*). These "complex cysts" may actually be degenerating colloid cysts (follicular nodules), hemorrhagic cysts (degenerating follicular adenomas), or carcinomas.

Calcifications may be present that, if sufficiently large, demonstrate increased echogenicity with acoustic shadowing (loss of echogenicity behind the calcification). Thyroid US may be useful in assisting fine-needle–aspiration biopsy, especially when the solid component is a small or mural nodule, or when the initial biopsy failed to reveal carcinoma and there is uncertainty about the region that was actually sampled.

Thyroid US is particularly useful in children in whom the cause of a neck mass could easily be nonthyroidal.[84] It may be the preferred study to evaluate a pregnant woman for whom radioiodine scanning would be undesirable, since the fetal thyroid gland concentrates iodine by the 12th week of gestation.

Likewise, CT scanning demonstrates a simple cyst as a discrete, smooth-walled, homogeneous, hypodense lesion surrounded by normal thyroid tissue. Simple cysts do not enhance with contrast material. CT scanning of complex cysts demonstrates solid components, tissue fronds, and frequently calcification and hemorrhage. Although a thick-walled cyst with an irregular inner margin could represent a carcinoma, it could just as easily indicate hemorrhage into a follicular adenoma.[20]

On MRI, simple cysts are usually low intensity on T1-weighted images and high intensity on T2-weighted images. Cysts with a high protein content, such as a thyroglossal duct cyst, show heterogeneously increased intensity on both T1- and T2-weighted images.[29] Complex cysts, such as hemorrhagic and colloid cysts (Fig. 34–23), have homogeneous high-intensity signal on T1-weighted images and very high intensity on T2-weighted images. The increased signal intensity in hemorrhagic cysts is due to the presence of methemoglobin, whereas the increased signal intensity in colloid cysts reflects the highly proteinaceous fluid content.[29]

As discussed previously, benign nodules are usually either follicular adenomas or follicular (colloid or adeno-

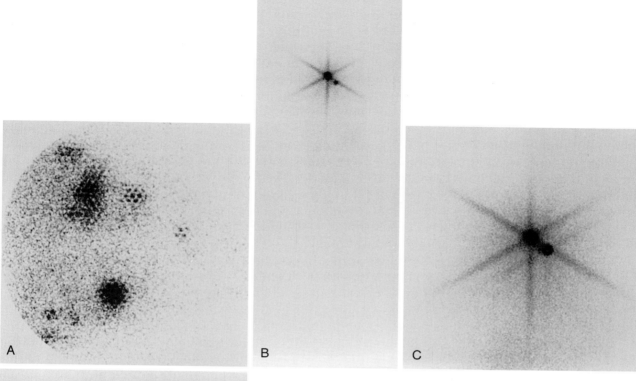

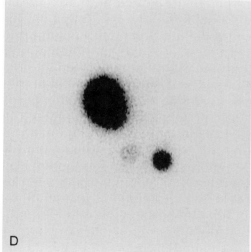

FIGURE 34–21 Artifacts revealed using ^{131}I and the value of pinhole imaging. *A,* Multiple foci of increased ^{131}I uptake are identified in the lungs bilaterally owing to metastatic pulmonary nodules present on a chest radiograph. The mosaic pattern of activity in areas of increased uptake represents attenuation of the high-energy ^{131}I photon (364 keV) by the hexagonal-shaped lead septa of a medium-energy collimator. A high-energy collimator is preferable with high-energy photons. *B,* In another patient with a subtotal thyroidectomy for thyroid carcinoma, a whole body image obtained 48 hours after ^{131}I administration reveals at least two foci of increased uptake in the neck. Note that this starburst artifact from septal penetration could potentially obscure accurate evaluation of residual tissue in the thyroid bed, adenopathy, or both. *C* and *D,* The starburst artifacts seen in *B* and *C* can be eliminated by the use of pinhole collimation, which resolved three lesions in *D.*

matous) nodules. Follicular adenomas are monoclonal, benign, well-encapsulated neoplasms with a variable degree of colloid (macrofollicular adenomas) and cellularity (cellular adenomas). Follicular nodules are usually incompletely encapsulated and may be poorly demarcated from adjacent thyroid tissue. They can contain abundant colloid or be hemorrhagic.

On US, follicular adenomas are discrete nodules of variable size and echogenicity. Small, solid adenomas with uniformly low echogenicity may be mistaken for cysts. However, they lack acoustic enhancement. Often a sonolucent rim (halo) surrounds a follicular adenoma (Fig. 34–24), demarcating the adenoma from adjacent thyroid tissue. Although this halo often denotes a benign nodule, it can be observed in the presence of carcinoma.[54] Follicular adenomas may demonstrate a complex cystic pattern as they undergo hemorrhage, necrosis, and calcification. Likewise, follicular nodules may be homogeneous or complex.

On CT scans, follicular adenomas may demonstrate areas of hemorrhage, necrosis, or cyst formation and cannot be differentiated from carcinoma.[20] Adenomas are usually single, whereas follicular nodules are frequently multiple. On MRI (see Fig. 34–13C–E), follicular adenomas are usually round or oval lesions with heterogeneous signal on T1-weighted images and increased signal on T2-

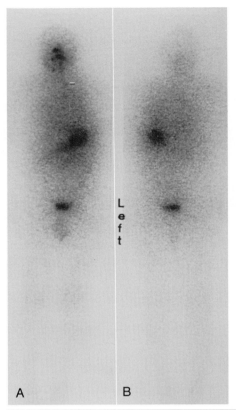

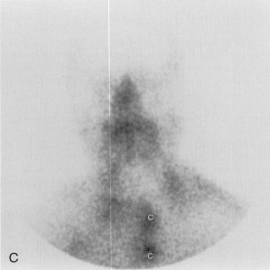

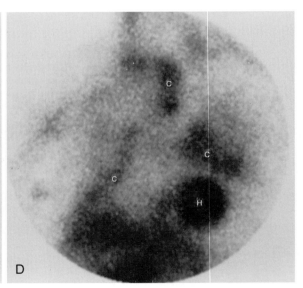

FIGURE 34–22 Use of thallium-201 for detection of metastatic thyroid carcinoma. *A* and *B,* Whole body image 48 hours after the administration of ^{131}I in a patient with papillary carcinoma fails to reveal any appreciable area of increased uptake, except for a very faint area in the right neck (*minus sign;* the subtle but real lesion is just to the left of the marker) on the anterior projection *(A)* but not the posterior view *(B). C* and *D,* This patient was rescanned 2 weeks later using thallium-201. *C* illustrates the anterior view over the neck. *D* shows the anterior view over the chest. Note in *D* the areas of abnormal uptake in the neck on the left and lungs bilaterally from metastatic disease (C). It is not uncommon to see metastatic disease take up thallium-201 or ^{99m}Tc-sestamibi but not [131]I. The sensitivity of thallium-201 for detection of thyroid metastasis has been reported to be 60% to 90%. H, heart.

weighted images.[29] If present, subacute hemorrhage is of higher signal intensity (methemoglobin) than the adenoma. Chronic hemorrhage is dark (hemosiderin).

Carcinoma

Given that there are no pathognomonic features of thyroid carcinoma on US, CT, or MRI, what imaging parameters might favor carcinoma (Table 34–5)? On US, thyroid cancer is usually hypoechoic relative to normal thyroid.[19, 21] However, lesions that are isoechoic and occasionally even hyperechoic (Fig. 34–25) have been reported. In a large series (401 patients with solitary cold

nodules on scintigraphy), solid hypoechoic lesions predominated.[54] The breakdown was as follows: papillary carcinoma, solid hypoechoic 77%, solid isoechoic 14%, solid hyperechoic 4%; follicular carcinoma, solid hypoechoic 44%, solid isoechoic 52%; medullary carcinoma, solid hypoechoic 67%, solid isoechoic 33%; anaplastic carcinoma, solid hypoechoic 85%, solid isoechoic 15%; lymphoma, solid hypoechoic 100%. In this series, if a perinodular sonolucent halo was incomplete, the lesion was more likely to be malignant. If it was complete, the nodule was more apt to be benign.

Occasionally, a thyroid cancer can present as a small

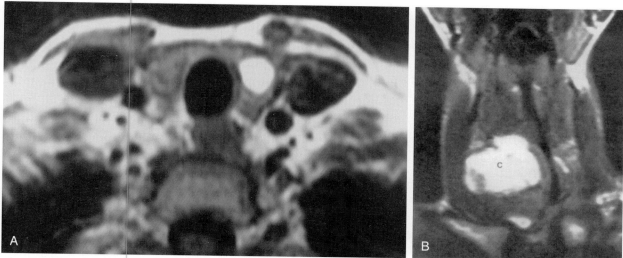

FIGURE 34–23 Colloid cyst. *A,* Axial T1-weighted sequence reveals a well-circumscribed hyperintense mass in the left lobe of the thyroid gland. This proved to be a colloid cyst. *B,* Coronal image from another patient demonstrates a similar hyperintense colloid cyst (C) on the T1-weighted MRI scan. Hemorrhage, fat, colloid, hyperproteinaceous secretions, melanin, and sometimes calcium are hyperintense on T1-weighted sequences. (*B,* From Yousem DM, Scheff AM. Thyroid and parathyroid gland pathology: Role of imaging. Otolaryngol Clin North Am 1995;28:621–649.)

nodule or frond protruding into a large cyst. The nodule may be calcified. The authors termed this image the *sonographic sign of cystic papillary carcinoma.*[85]

Patients with medullary carcinoma may demonstrate bright echogenic foci within the primary intrathyroidal tumor as well as within metastatic cervical lymph nodes.

Pathologically, calcium deposits surrounded by amyloid in medullary carcinoma produce this characteristic echogenicity.[86]

Thyroid lymphomas are usually hypoechoic and may spread into both lobes and to regional lymph nodes.[20] Both benign and malignant thyroid lymphomas may have irregular borders, be single or multiple, and present as a solid or complex mass. In patients with Hashimoto's thyroiditis, prominent or discrete hypoechoic lesions that may demonstrate rapid enlargement should raise the possibility of lymphoma.

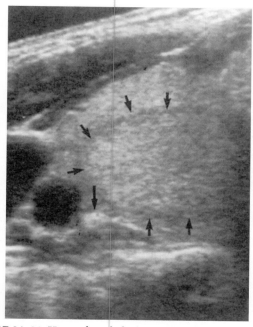

FIGURE 34–24 Hypoechoic halo *(arrows)* surrounding a thyroid mass on ultrasonography. A hypoechoic halo entirely surrounds a large thyroid mass on a longitudinal scan. Any thyroid mass that is surrounded by an intact hypoechoic halo is at least 10 times more likely to be benign than malignant. (From Yousem DM, Scheff AM. Thyroid and parathyroid gland pathology: Role of imaging. Otolaryngol Clin North Am 1995;28:621–649.)

TABLE 34–5 Radiographic Features Suggestive of Primary Thyroid Malignancy

Modality	Findings
Ultrasonography	Adenopathy
	Invasion or infiltration into surrounding structures
	Metastasis
	Calcifications in patients at risk for medullary carcinoma
Computed tomography	Adenopathy
	Hyperdense nodes
	Calcified nodes
	Invasion or infiltration into surrounding structures
	Metastasis
	Calcifications in patients at risk for medullary carcinoma
Magnetic resonance imaging	Adenopathy
	Central enhancement after gadolinium administration
	Invasion or infiltration into surrounding structures
	Metastasis
Scintigraphy	Cold nodule

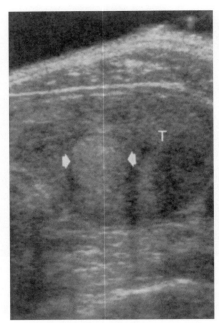

FIGURE 34–25 Thyroid carcinoma on ultrasonography. A well-circumscribed hyperechoic lesion is identified in the right lobe of the thyroid gland on the longitudinal view *(arrows)* adjacent to the trachea (T). Biopsy results proved it to be papillary carcinoma. The chance of malignancy in a solid echogenic lesion is less than 5%. (From Yousem DM, Scheff AM. Thyroid and parathyroid gland pathology: Role of imaging. Otolaryngol Clin North Am 1995;28:621–649.)

On CT scans (Figs. 34–26 and 34–27), carcinomas are usually low-density masses relative to normal thyroid tissue and may contain calcification, cysts, or hemorrhage. The presence of lymphadenopathy or infiltration of adjacent tissues suggests malignancy.

Metastatic lymph nodes in papillary carcinoma can have multiple discrete calcifications. They may appear as benign cysts or as hyperplastic or hypervascular nodes or have areas of high attenuation secondary to intranodal hemorrhage or high concentrations of thyroglobulin or colloid, or both.[87] If cervical lymph nodes with these findings are identified in a woman between the ages of 20 and 40 years, the diagnosis of papillary thyroid carcinoma should be suggested even in the absence of a thyroid mass. Calcifications are also prominent in medullary carcinoma and regional metastatic nodes.

Thyroid lymphomas are usually low to intermediate in density and show poor contrast enhancement.[33] Differentiating thyroid lymphoma that develops in a gland already altered by Hashimoto's thyroiditis may be difficult as both processes reduce the CT density. Compression, invasion, or displacement of adjacent structures and lymphadenopathy suggest lymphoma.

Anaplastic carcinoma is usually a large, irregular low-attenuation mass that may have areas of calcification and necrosis. Invasion of adjacent tissues is common. Differentiating a very large multinodular goiter from anaplastic carcinoma may be difficult. However, the presence of normal thyroid tissue favors the goiter,[20] whereas a more invasive appearance favors carcinoma.

CT scanning has utility in detecting pulmonary metastases. Minute lung nodules can be detected on high-resolution CT scans, even in patients with negative chest radiographs. The extent of tumor mass on CT correlates with serum thyroglobulin levels.[88]

MRI can reveal exquisite detail. Anatomic resolution of small structures within the thyroid gland has improved significantly with the application of a high-field-strength surface coil and a small field of view to improve the signal-to-noise ratio.[29] Even though lesions as small as 4 to 5 mm can be identified, benign and malignant lesions may have similar imaging characteristics. All tumor types are typically isointense to slightly hyperintense on T1-weighted and hyperintense on T2-weighted images. Metastatic lymph nodes have similar imaging characteristics.[20] As with CT scanning, MRI is most useful in demonstrating the extrathyroidal extent of disease and associated lymphadenopathy. The ability to obtain coronal images may enhance the preoperative evaluation of anatomic changes produced by tumor compression or invasion of adjacent structures.[20] Gadolinium does not aid in distinguishing benign from malignant lymph nodes in thyroid disease.

Congenital Lesions

As discussed under Embryology and Anatomy, the two most common congenital abnormalities of the thyroid gland are the thyroglossal duct cyst and the lingual thyroid. A thyroglossal duct cyst can form when there is persistence of part of the tract of migration of the thyroid gland from the foramen cecum (at the base of the tongue) to the lower neck (anterior to the thyroid cartilage; Fig. 34–28). As this is an epithelium-lined tract, a cyst with retained secretions may develop and can become infected. Occasionally, a carcinoma may develop in a thyro-

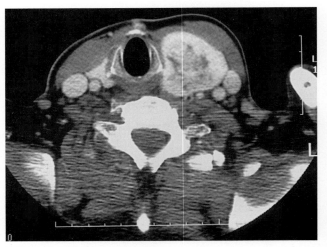

FIGURE 34–26 Thyroid carcinoma on CT scan. An axial contrast-enhanced image reveals a well-defined hyperdense mass with a low-density center involving the left lobe of the thyroid gland. This was shown to be a follicular carcinoma with central necrosis. There are no characteristic features for malignancy on CT except for lymphadenopathy or infiltration of adjacent tissues, or both.

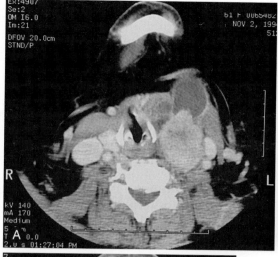

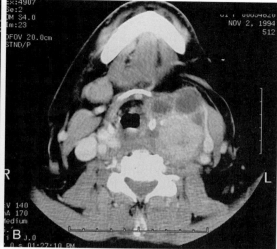

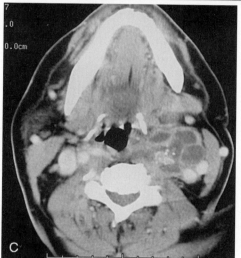

FIGURE 34–27 Various characteristics of thyroid carcinoma. This complex lesion originating from the left lobe of the thyroid gland is papillary carcinoma. It extends into the paralaryngeal and hypopharyngeal structures on the contrast-enhanced CT image. *A,* Note the predominately solid hyperdense mass with central necrosis and cystic components at the level of the thyroid cartilage. *B* and *C,* Axial images obtained more cephalad demonstrate regions of punctate and rimlike calcifications. The presence of calcifications, hyper- or hypodense masses, cystic areas, hemorrhage, or necrosis on CT is not specific for malignancy or a particular histologic type of thyroid carcinoma. However, the invasion and destruction of the hyoid bone seen in this example are highly suggestive of malignancy.

glossal duct cyst. The incidence is less than 1%, and the histologic type is usually papillary (Fig. 34–28*F*).[89, 90]

A thyroglossal duct cyst can be identified as a midline cystic mass situated at the infrahyoid level in 65% of cases and at the hyoid and suprahyoid levels in 15% and 20%, respectively.[91] Classically, infrahyoidal thyroglossal duct cysts are identified embedded in the strap muscles (Fig. 34–28*E*) at the base of the tongue in the midline, and within the hyoid bone above the insertion of the strap muscles.

On US, the thyroglossal duct cyst may be predominantly anechoic with scattered internal echoes reflecting the proteinaceous fluid. On CT (Fig. 34–28*D*), the density may be low if the cyst has a low protein content or mildly increased if the fluid is proteinaceous or contains hemorrhage. MRI images may demonstrate either low or high signal intensity on T1-weighted images (reflecting protein content and hemorrhage) but usually show high signal intensity on T2-weighted images. Contrast enhancement usually indicates the presence of trauma or infection that generally involves only the peripheral rim. After surgical removal of the thyroglossal duct cyst (which includes removal of the entire duct including the midpor-

tion of the hyoid bone and the region at the base of the tongue that includes the foramen cecum—Sistrunk's procedure), the recurrence rate is approximately 4%.[92]

The lingual thyroid gland is usually identified as a midline mass that represents failure of the thyroid gland to migrate from its origin at the base of the tongue. If thyroid migration was not completely arrested, functioning thyroidal tissue may be present in the lower neck. Diagnostic imaging studies are performed to determine whether the midline mass is a lingual thyroid and to localize any functioning thyroid tissue along the normal path of migration. On technetium-99m–pertechnetate or iodine-123 scintigraphy (Fig. 34–29), a lingual thyroid demonstrates focal tracer uptake in the midline mass. On CT scanning, thyroidal tissue within the tongue is identified by high density, reflecting iodine content, or by intense contrast enhancement. On MRI, lingual thyroid tissue is isointense to the thyroid gland and also demonstrates intense enhancement.[20]

In the evaluation of congenital hypothyroidism, thyroid ectopia, which includes lingual thyroid, as well as thyroid aplasia, hemiaplasia, and dyshormonogenesis, should be considered. There are proponents for neonatal assessment

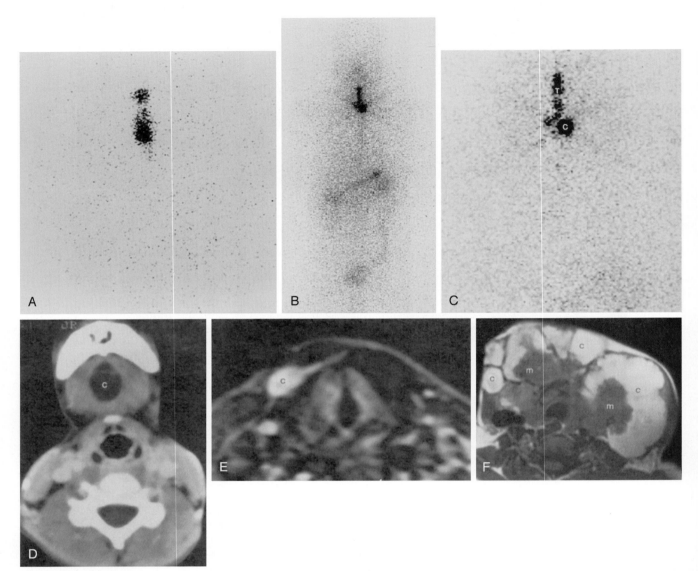

FIGURE 34–28 Thyroglossal duct pathology. *A,* Pinhole images from ^{123}I scintigraphy demonstrate a tubular-shaped region of activity in the midline of the neck, which represents ectopic thyroid tissue in a persistent thyroglossal duct. *B* and *C,* A structure that appears similar is identified in another patient with a history of Graves' disease on a whole body image from an ^{131}I scan during a metastatic workup for thyroid carcinoma. *C* is a magnification view. T, thyroid tissue in thyroglossal duct; C, carcinoma. *D,* Thyroglossal duct cyst (C) is seen in the midline in the floor of the mouth on an axial CT image. Most thyroglossal duct cysts are midline and infrahyoid (65%), but they can be found anywhere from the foramen cecum of the tongue to the anterior mediastinum, as well as in a paramedian location. Approximately 25% of them contain functioning thyroid tissue. *E,* Axial T2-weighted MRI scan shows a cystic lesion (C) in the strap muscle just anterior to the larynx. The appearance and location of this lesion are virtually pathognomonic for a thyroglossal duct cyst. *F,* Carcinoma in a thyroglossal duct cyst is seen on this axial T1-weighted MRI scan, which reveals solid elements in hyperintense cysts (C). This proved to be papillary carcinoma in a thyroglossal duct cyst. The incidence of carcinoma within a thyroglossal duct cyst that contains thyroid tissue is less than 1%. (*D–F,* From Yousem DM, Scheff AM. Thyroid and parathyroid gland pathology: Role of imaging. Otolaryngol Clin North Am 1995;28:621–649.)

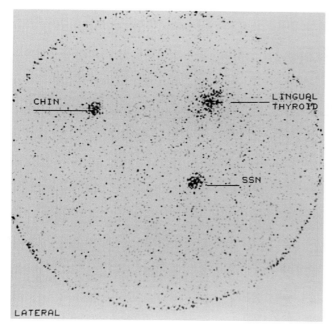

FIGURE 34–29 Lingual thyroid. A lateral image from ^{123}I scintigraphy demonstrates increased uptake in the posterior portion of the tongue, which is due to a lingual thyroid. Note that there is no thyroid tissue in the expected location in the neck near the suprasternal notch (SSN) marker. Approximately 70% of cases with lingual thyroid tissue are associated with absence of thyroid tissue in the neck. The primary roles of imaging are to determine whether there is functioning thyroid tissue in the lingual mass and to determine whether there is thyroid tissue in the neck.

by US,[93, 94] but only thyroid scintigraphy can demonstrate that the presumed thyroid tissue is functioning. This information is essential to differentiate thyroid ectopia from thyroid agenesis. Clinically, this distinction is important, as the neurointellectual prognosis in thyroid ectopia may be higher than in thyroid agenesis.[95] Prompt initiation of thyroid hormone replacement after birth is mandatory.

PARATHYROID GLANDS

Hyperparathyroidism

Primary hyperparathyroidism is a relatively frequent disorder, occurring in approximately 1 in 700 adults older than 45 years.[96] This disease is characterized by hypersecretion of parathormone (PTH), with resulting hypercalcemia. The classic clinical features include stones (renal calculi), groans (abdominal pain), bones (demineralization or arthritis), and moans (psychiatric disturbances).[97] In addition, several radiographic and scintigraphic abnormalities are seen in patients with parathyroid disorders and oftentimes can be dramatic (Fig. 34–30).

The causes of primary hyperparathyroidism include parathyroid hyperplasia (10% to 15%), isolated parathyroid adenoma (80% to 85%; Fig. 34–31), multiple adenomas (2% to 3%), and parathyroid carcinoma (<1%).[98] Hyperplasia typically involves multiple parathyroid glands. Solitary adenomas usually weigh between 0.5 and 5 gm

but can vary from 100 mg to over 40 gm.[99] Their size can vary from 1 to over 3 cm.[1] Parathyroid carcinoma is a rare cause of hyperparathyroidism. As these tumors tend to be highly malignant, the possibility of such an occurrence should not be overlooked.

There are secondary and tertiary forms of hyperparathyroidism. In the former, parathyroid gland enlargement is secondary to renal insufficiency. In tertiary hyperparathyroidism, hypercalcemia occurs as a progression of secondary hyperparathyroidism owing to the autonomous secretion of PTH from chronically overstimulated parathyroid glands.

The treatment of primary hyperparathyroidism is surgical excision of the diseased parathyroid gland(s). Surgery has a 95% success rate when an experienced head and neck surgeon performs the operation.[100, 101] Although the need for an imaging procedure before primary exploration has been questioned,[102] some authors report fewer complications and shorter operating times when abnormal glands are localized before surgery.[103–105] However, most surgeons advocate thorough bilateral cervical exploration, since small lesions or hyperplasia may easily be missed by current imaging techniques. In selected high-risk patients, imaging may permit the surgeon to excise the abnormal gland with unilateral exploration and then abort the procedure if complications occur. When hyperparathyroidism recurs after successful surgery, imaging is indicated, as ectopic glands are prevalent in this group of patients.

Embryology, Anatomy, and Physiology

The parathyroid glands develop from the third and fourth branchial pouches. The thymus and inferior parathyroid glands are derived from the third branchial pouch and migrate caudally. The superior glands are derived from the fourth branchial pouch. Since they are closely related to the thyroid, they tend to be more constant in location than the inferior glands, which can migrate into the mediastinum.

Although most individuals have four parathyroid glands, the incidence of a supernumerary gland ranges from 2% to 6%.[106] Only 1% of the superior parathyroid glands reside in an ectopic location. The inferior glands have a more variable location. Most can be found below the lower thyroid pole or in the thyrothymic tract. Some normal glands are located significantly below the sternal notch (2%) or at another unpredictable location in the mediastinum (2%). Intrathyroidal parathyroid glands are observed in only 2% to 5% of patients.

The normal parathyroid gland weighs less than 70 mg and measures $5 \times 4 \times 2$ mm.[106] The parathyroid glands are composed of chief cells, oxyphil cells, fibrous stroma, and a variable amount of fat. Oxyphil cells are rarely found in childhood. They tend to appear around puberty and increase with age. These cells are rich in mitochondria, but their exact function is unknown.

Chief cells secrete PTH to regulate calcium ion concentration in interstitial fluids by a classic feedback loop with serum calcium levels. PTH is not stored for subse-

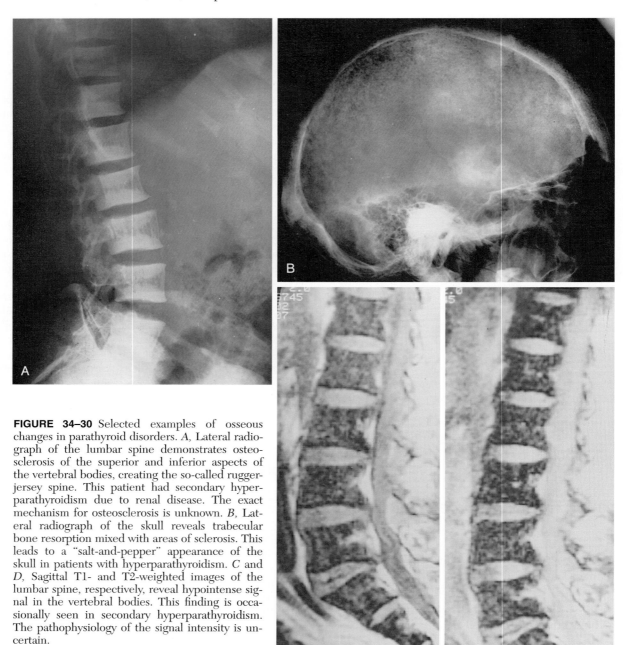

FIGURE 34–30 Selected examples of osseous changes in parathyroid disorders. *A,* Lateral radiograph of the lumbar spine demonstrates osteosclerosis of the superior and inferior aspects of the vertebral bodies, creating the so-called rugger-jersey spine. This patient had secondary hyperparathyroidism due to renal disease. The exact mechanism for osteosclerosis is unknown. *B,* Lateral radiograph of the skull reveals trabecular bone resorption mixed with areas of sclerosis. This leads to a "salt-and-pepper" appearance of the skull in patients with hyperparathyroidism. *C* and *D,* Sagittal T1- and T2-weighted images of the lumbar spine, respectively, reveal hypointense signal in the vertebral bodies. This finding is occasionally seen in secondary hyperparathyroidism. The pathophysiology of the signal intensity is uncertain.

quent release like thyroid hormones but is synthesized after direct stimulation. PTH acts predominantly on the skeleton, kidneys, and gastrointestinal tract to mobilize skeletal calcium, reduce renal calcium excretion, and increase gastrointestinal calcium absorption.[107]

PTH is cleaved in the circulation into a physiologically active, rapidly cleared, amino-terminal fragment and an inactive, slowly cleared, carboxy-terminal fragment. Most radioimmunoassays measure the inactive fragment. If a normal PTH level is measured in a patient with hypercalcemia, this suggests hyperparathyroidism. PTH should be suppressed and undetectable in the presence of an elevated serum calcium concentration.

Parathyroid Imaging

Adenoma

Noninvasive imaging modalities that may be used to detect parathyroid adenomas include US, radionuclide scintigraphy, CT, and MRI. More invasive methods, such as arteriography, digital subtraction angiography, and selective parathyroid venography with PTH measurements, are very reliable techniques but have the disadvantage of associated risks and higher costs.[108]

The use of US to evaluate the parathyroid gland requires a linear-array, high-resolution transducer (7.5 to 10 MHz) and an experienced sonographer. The patient is

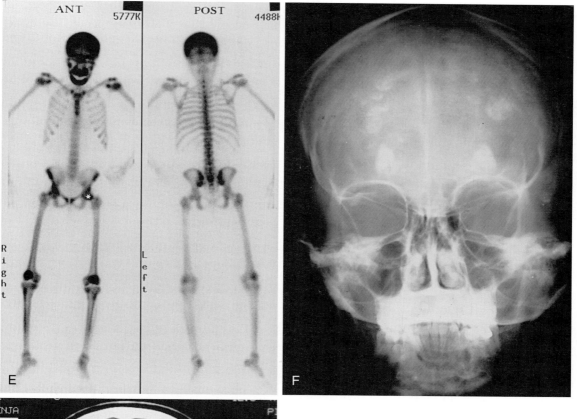

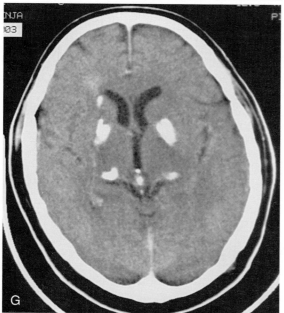

FIGURE 34–30 *Continued E,* Whole body bone scintigraphy using ^{99m}Tc–methylene diphosphonate (MDP) reveals diffusely increased uptake in the axial and appendicular skeleton with little or no observed soft tissue or renal activity. This is an example of a superscan (or beautiful scan) and can be seen in patients with hyperparathyroidism. This patient had secondary hyperparathyroidism due to chronic renal insufficiency. Note the mildly increased uptake in the left hip due to avascular necrosis *(asterisk). F* and *G,* Frontal skull radiograph demonstrates paramedian clumplike calcifications. The corresponding non–contrast-enhanced axial CT image demonstrates extensive basal ganglia calcifications bilaterally. Basal ganglia calcifications can be seen in a variety of infectious, toxic, and metabolic conditions including hypoparathyroidism, hyperparathyroidism, pseudohypoparathyroidism, and pseudopseudohypoparathyroidism. (*A–C, E,* and *F,* Courtesy of Larry Neustadter, D.O., Veterans Administration Hospital, Philadelphia, PA.)

supine with the neck hyperextended. Examination must include the evaluation of the thyroid and the region of the carotid sheath extending from the thyroid cartilage cranially to the sternal notch caudally.

The typical appearance of a parathyroid adenoma is a homogeneous mass of low echogenicity (Fig. 34–32).[109, 110] Adenomas are usually solid, oval, or oblong but occasionally present with cystic components. US is an excellent

modality for imaging a perithyroidal adenoma. Differential considerations include a hyperplastic lymph node and esophagus and an eccentric thyroid adenoma. Color Doppler can occasionally aid in the distinction between thyroid and parathyroid lesions. Thyroid lesions tend to have some vascularity on color Doppler, whereas small parathyroid lesions are more likely to lack Doppler signal. However, larger parathyroid lesions can be vascular.[111] US

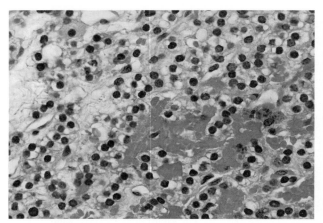

FIGURE 34–31 Parathyroid adenoma. The photomicrograph shows nests of chief cells with fresh stromal hemorrhage (*upper left*). No fat is visible in this totally cellular gland. (H&E 400×.)

is less accurate than other techniques in localizing ectopic adenomas that reside in the neck or anterior mediastinum beyond the acoustic imaging window.

With the introduction of the thallium-201–technetium-99m–pertechnetate subtraction scintigraphic technique in the early 1980s,[112] radionuclide scintigraphy offered a unique diagnostic study for parathyroid adenoma detection. Thallium-201 is taken up by both the thyroid and the parathyroid glands. As the sole imaging agent, it cannot easily differentiate a parathyroid adenoma from the adjacent or overlapping thyroid gland. Technetium-99m is trapped in thyroid tissue but not in parathyroid lesions. When the thallium-201 (thyroid + parathyroid) and technetium-99m–pertechnetate (thyroid) images are coregistered and normalized, computer-based subtraction

techniques can remove the thyroid component, permitting identification of abnormal parathyroid tissue.

There are a variety of imaging protocols. Typically 2 to 5 mCi of each tracer is administered intravenously, and either sequential or dual isotope imaging is performed. The mediastinum must be included in the field of view to assess the possibility of ectopic parathyroid adenomas. Motion artifacts can degrade the images, make subtraction unreliable, and confuse interpretation. After thyroid subtraction, the abnormal perithyroidal parathyroid adenoma appears as a moderate-to-intense focus of thallium uptake (Fig. 34–33).

The reported sensitivity of thallium-201–technetium-99m subtraction scintigraphy varies but is approximately 80%, with an overall diagnostic accuracy of 78% and a positive predictive value of 94% as reported in a comprehensive review of 14 studies.[113] False-positive results include some inflammatory conditions, lymphoma, and thyroid nodules, although as seen on Figure 34–34, adenomas can still be identified despite the presence of a thyroid nodule. Size is an important factor in determining the sensitivity of thallium-201–technetium-99m–pertechnetate imaging, and lesions smaller than 0.3 to 0.5 gm are rarely visualized. The histologic content of parathyroid adenomas also influences the sensitivity, with greater accuracy in lesions having a high concentration of mitochondria.[114]

Technetium-99m–sestamibi parathyroid scintigraphy was introduced in 1989[115] and provides images that are superior to those obtained with thallium-201–technetium-99m–pertechnetate subtraction scintigraphy. Technetium-99m–sestamibi is a positively charged, lipid-soluble myocardial-perfusion tracer. The intracellular distribution is determined by the negative transmembrane charge po-

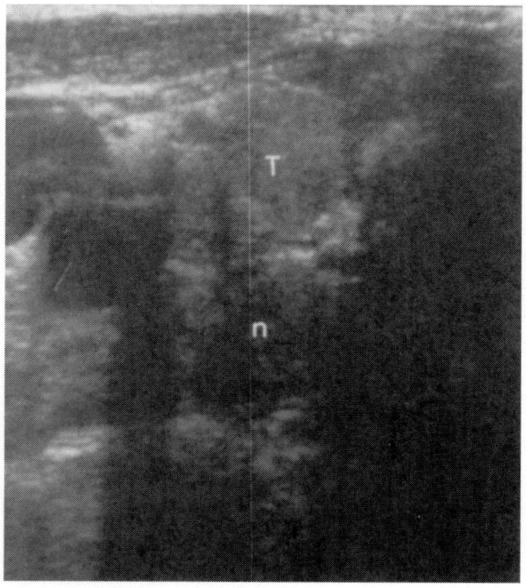

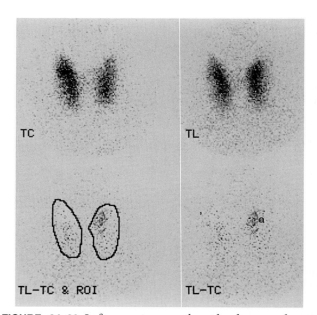

FIGURE 34–32 Ultrasonographic appearance of parathyroid adenoma. A transverse sonogram reveals a hypoechoic mass (n) posterior to the right lobe of the thyroid gland (T) that is due to a parathyroid adenoma. (From Yousem DM, Scheff AM. Thyroid and parathyroid gland pathology: Role of imaging. Otolaryngol Clin North Am 1995;28:621–649.)

FIGURE 34–33 Left superior parathyroid adenoma demonstrated on ²⁰¹Tl-⁹⁹ᵐTc–pertechnetate subtraction scintigraphy. Note that the adenoma, poorly resolved on the thallium study, becomes clearly delineated (a) on the subtraction image (*lower right scintigraph*). (Courtesy of N. Laurin, M.D., Hospital St-Joseph, Trois-Rivières, Quebec, Canada.)

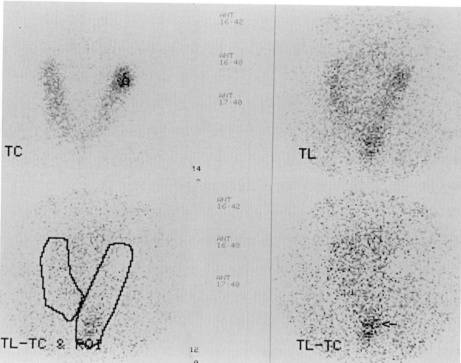

FIGURE 34–34 Parathyroid adenoma. Left inferior parathyroid adenoma (*arrow* in *lower right panel*) demonstrated on ^{201}Tl-^{99m}Tc–pertechnetate subtraction scintigraphy in a patient with a "hot" thyroid nodule on the superior portion of the left lobe (O). This case illustrates that although nodules can produce false-positive results on subtraction scintigraphy, most do not take up thallium avidly. (Courtesy of N. Laurin, M.D., Hospital St-Joseph, Trois-Rivières, Quebec, Canada.)

tential of the cellular and mitochondrial membranes. Thus, cells with a high mitochondrial content retain the positively charged tracer.

Technetium-99m–sestamibi can be used in single-tracer studies, taking advantage of rapid washout of the tracer from the thyroid, whereas there is avid retention in parathyroid lesions. Initial images are obtained immediately after tracer injection and encompassing the neck and chest. Delayed images of the same sites are obtained 2 to 3 hours later.[116] Perithyroidal parathyroid lesions are identified as areas of radiotracer retention (Fig. 34–35). Technetium-99m–sestamibi parathyroid scintigraphy can also image ectopic lesions as shown in Figures 34–36 and 34–37. Some authors use a subtraction technique with technetium-99m–sestamibi, substituting iodine-123 to identify the thyroid.[117]

The reported sensitivities of technetium-99m–sestamibi vary between 80% and 100%, with consistently high specificity[99, 118, 119] and accuracy. Sestamibi parathyroid scintigraphy appears more accurate than US, CT, and thallium-201–technetium-99m–pertechnetate subtraction scintigraphy, but few studies have compared it directly with MRI. In a study on 23 patients with persistent or recurrent hyperparathyroidism, the sensitivities, positive predictive values, and accuracies of MRI and sestamibi techniques were comparable and superior to those of US.[120] Potential pitfalls in technetium-99m–sestamibi scintigraphy include the occasional adenoma with rapid washout (Fig. 34–38), attributed to a low content of oxyphil (mitochondria-rich) cells,[121] poor conspicuity of lesions close to the heart, and the occasional thyroid nodule or Hürthle's cell tumor[72] that can behave like a parathyroid adenoma and retain technetium-99m–sestamibi.

The use of CT in evaluating the neck and mediastinum

for parathyroid adenomas can be helpful when US or radioscintigraphy, or both, are inconclusive. The advantage of CT over US is in its superior evaluation of the mediastinum. Because of the small size and vascularity of parathyroid adenomas, an optimal CT protocol is essential in the evaluation of the parathyroid glands; for example, it should include thin sections (3 to 5 mm) through the neck and the use of bolus contrast injection, as up to 25% of all parathyroid adenomas exhibit contrast enhancement.[110] The ability to detect parathyroid abnormalities with CT is diminished, however, by streak artifacts, swallowing artifacts, and distortion of normal anatomy in patients who have had prior surgery. In addition, cervical lymph nodes, tortuous vessels, thymus, and esophagus can be confused with parathyroid adenomas on contrast-enhanced studies. The sensitivity of CT has been reported from 41% to 86%,[122] which is generally comparable to that of US.

MRI has a role similar to that of CT in evaluating the mediastinum. This method offers superior tissue discrimination and is more sensitive than CT for identifying parathyroid adenomas. MRI should be obtained on a high-field-strength system using a surface coil. Electrocardiographic gating can be used to improve accuracy and reduce artifacts due to heart motion. In addition, gadolinium administration can help to increase lesion conspicuity. With an appropriate coil, MRI is able to image the entire neck and anterior mediastinum.

Parathyroid adenomas can have a variable appearance on MRI.[104] Typically, adenomas are of intermediate signal intensity compared with thyroid and muscle but low signal intensity compared with fat on T1-weighted sequences and hyperintense on T2-weighted sequences (Fig. 34–39). They usually enhance after gadolinium ad-

Text continued on page 1240

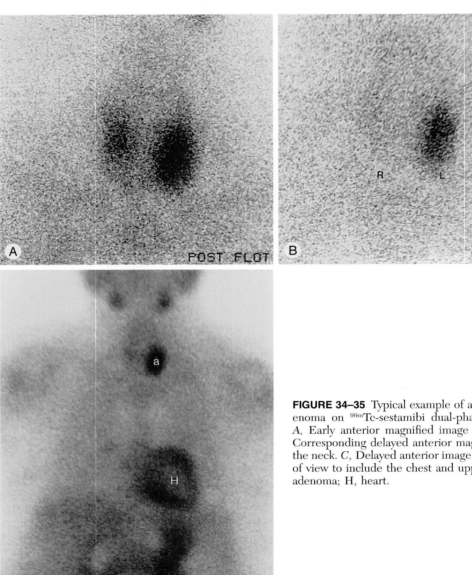

FIGURE 34–35 Typical example of a parathyroid adenoma on ^{99m}Tc-sestamibi dual-phase scintigraphy. *A,* Early anterior magnified image of the neck. *B,* Corresponding delayed anterior magnified image of the neck. *C,* Delayed anterior image with larger field of view to include the chest and upper abdomen. a, adenoma; H, heart.

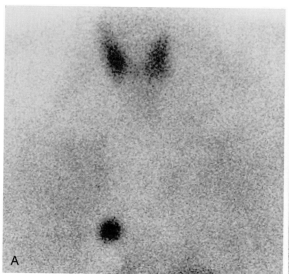
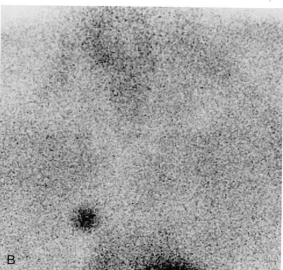
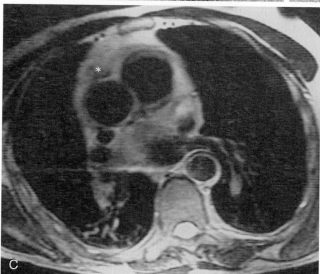

FIGURE 34–36 Ectopic parathyroid adenoma demonstrated on dual-phase ^{99m}Tc-sestamibi scintigraphy and T2-weighted MRI. *A* and *B*, Intense focus of activity is seen in the region of the right mediastinum just superior to the heart on both early *(A)* and late *(B)* images. *C,* T2-weighted axial image reveals the corresponding lesion embedded in the mediastinal fat *(asterisk)* anterior to the aorta and superior vena cava. Despite cardiac gating, the lesion is better detected on the scintigraphic images than on MRI. Contrast enhancement, fat saturation techniques, or both may have made this lesion more conspicuous. Cross-sectional imaging is still necessary to identify the precise anatomic location of the ectopic tissue for surgical excision. (*A* and *B,* Courtesy of Libby Cone, M.D., Graduate Hospital, Philadelphia, PA.)

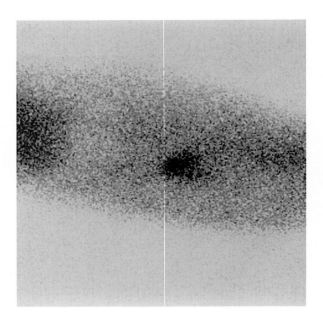

FIGURE 34–37 Demonstration of recurrence of hyperparathyroidism due to a transplanted parathyroid adenoma in the forearm. The presence of a parathyroid adenoma at this site was confirmed at surgery.

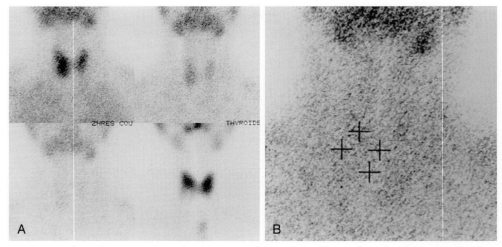

FIGURE 34–38 *A* and *B*, Right inferior parathyroid adenoma with an unusually rapid washout on sequential imaging. *Upper left panel*, immediately after injection; *upper right panel*, 1 hour after injection; *lower left panel*, 3 hours after injection; *lower right panel*, 99mTc-sestamibi demonstrates a cold defect in the inferior right portion of the thyroid that corresponded to a palpable lesion indicated by the cross-hair marks in *B*. No oxyphil cells were found on histologic examination of the parathyroid adenoma.

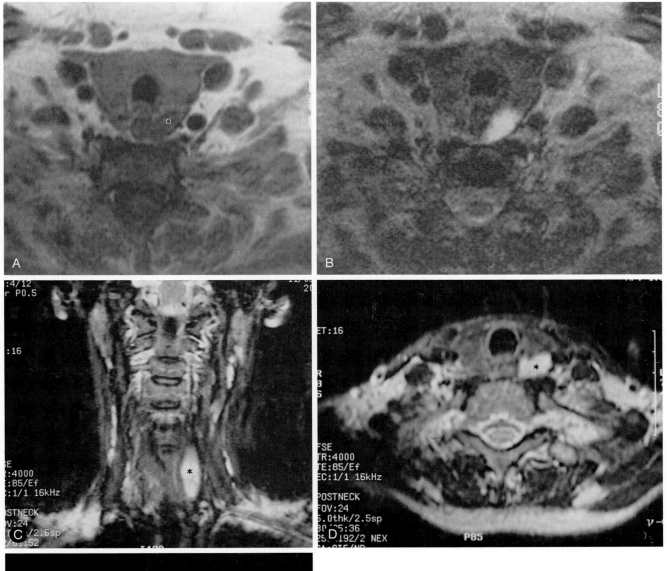

FIGURE 34–39 Examples of parathyroid adenomas on MRI from two different patients. *A* and *B,* There is a 1-cm parathyroid adenoma (o) posterior to the left lobe of the thyroid gland that is hypointense to muscle on T1-weighted sequences *(A)* and hyperintense on T2-weighted sequences *(B).* Coronal *(C)* and axial *(D)* fat-saturated fast spin echo T2-weighted and dynamic gadolinium-enhanced fat-saturated T1-weighted images (fast multiplanar spoiled gradient shown in *E*) demonstrate a 1.5-cm parathyroid adenoma. The T1-weighted image (not shown) revealed a hypointense lesion similar in appearance to the abnormality in *A,* just posterior to the left lobe of the thyroid gland. This lesion is hyperintense on T2-weighted sequences *(asterisks)* and enhances after gadolinium administration. Parathyroid adenomas can be hypo-, iso-, or hyperintense on T1- and T2-weighted sequences depending on the degree of cellularity, hemorrhage, or fibrosis present in the lesion. (*A–E,* Courtesy of Evan Siegelman, M.D., and Jeff Goldman, M.D., University of Pennsylvania Medical Center, Philadelphia, PA.)

ministration. Occasionally, however, these lesions may be iso- or hyperintense on T1-weighted sequences and hypointense on T2-weighted sequences depending on the degree of fibrosis, hemorrhage, and hemosiderin deposition present in the adenoma. Pitfalls in the detection of parathyroid adenomas include confusion with cervical lymph nodes, large cervical ganglia, and multiplicity of ectopic sites.[104] Distinction between abnormal gland and vessel is less of a problem with MRI owing to the numerous pulse sequences available that can confirm the identity of vascular structures. In patients with hyperparathyroidism using state-of-the-art technology, MRI has a sensitivity and accuracy for parathyroid adenoma of about 90%.[120]

Parathyroid Hyperplasia

Parathyroid hyperplasia is very difficult to image successfully with any modality owing to the small size of the hyperplastic gland. In addition, when there is a discrepancy in the size of the gland, the diagnostician may conclude that a single parathyroid adenoma is responsible for the biochemical abnormalities. The sensitivity for the detection of parathyroid hyperplasia is low for all imaging modalities. For example, nuclear medicine techniques may have a sensitivity ranging from 40% to 60%, compared with 30% to 57% for US, 45% for CT, and up to 80% for MRI.[5, 119, 120] Although these studies suffer from small sample size, MRI appears to be superior to other modalities. Additional studies, however, will be required for confirmation.

Conclusions

Multiple modalities that can complement each other in a unique way are available for parathyroid imaging. Because of its high sensitivity and high accuracy, scintigraphic imaging with sestamibi is an excellent choice as the first-line imaging study. MRI has comparable accuracy in identifying adenomas and is unsurpassed in providing anatomic information that is invaluable to the surgeon. US is less expensive and moderately sensitive in the cervical region but is not well suited to assess abnormal ectopic parathyroid glands. In difficult cases an integrated approach may be essential to localize recurrent and ectopic parathyroid adenomas.

References

1. LiVolsi VA. The thyroid and parathyroid. In Sternberg SS (ed). Diagnostic Surgical Pathology, 2nd ed., pp. 523–560. New York, Raven, 1994.
2. Pintar JE, Toran-Allerand CD. Normal development of the hypothalamic-pituitary-thyroid axis. In Braverman LE, Utiger RD (eds). Werner and Ingbar's The Thyroid, 6th ed., pp. 7–21. Philadelphia, JB Lippincott, 1991.
3. Moore KL. The branchial apparatus. In The Developing Human, 2nd ed., pp. 156–187. Philadelphia, WB Saunders, 1977.
4. Lyerly HK. The thyroid gland. I. Historical aspects and anatomy. In Sabiston DD Jr (ed). Textbook of Surgery, 14th ed., pp. 556–597. Philadelphia, WB Saunders, 1991.
5. Price DC. Radioisotopic evaluation of the thyroid and parathyroids. Radiol Clin North Am 1993;31:991–1015.
6. De Lellis RA. The endocrine system. In Cotram R, Kumar V, Robbins SL (eds). Robbins Pathologic Basis of Disease, 4th ed., pp. 1214–1242. Philadelphia, WB Saunders, 1989.
7. Braverman LE, Utiger RD. Introduction to thyrotoxicosis. In Braverman LE, Utiger RD (eds). Werner and Ingbar's The Thyroid, 6th ed., pp. 645–647. Philadelphia, JB Lippincott, 1991.
8. Nordyke RA, Gilbert FI Jr, Harada ASM. Graves' disease: Influence of age on clinical findings. Arch Intern Med 1988;148:626–631.
9. Trzepacz PT, Klien I, Robert M, et al. Graves' disease: An analysis of thyroid hormone levels and hyperthyroid signs and symptoms. Am J Med 1989;87:558–561.
10. Ross DS. Subclinical hyperthyroidism. In Braverman LE, Utiger RD (eds). Werner and Ingbar's The Thyroid, 6th ed., pp. 1249–1253. Philadelphia, JB Lippincott, 1991.
11. Spencer CA, LoPresti JS, Patel A, et al. Application of a new chemiluminometric thyrotropin assay to subnormal measurement. J Clin Endocrinol Metab 1990;70:453–460.
12. Spencer CA, Schwartzbein D, Guttler RB, et al. Thyrotropin (TSH)-releasing hormone stimulation test responses employing third and fourth generation TSH assays. J Clin Endocrinol Metab 1993;76:494–498.
13. Dworkin HJ, Meier DA, Kaplan M. Advances in the management of patients with thyroid disease. Semin Nucl Med 1995;25:205–220.
14. Sawin CT, Geller A, Wolf PA, et al. Low serum thyrotropin concentration as a risk factor for atrial fibrillation in older persons. N Engl J Med 1994;331:1249–1252.
15. Ross DS. Hyperthyroidism, thyroid hormone therapy, and bone. Thyroid 1994;4:319–326.
16. Lyerly HK. Hyperthyroidism. The thyroid gland. III. Hyperthyroidism. In Sabiston DD Jr (ed). Textbook of Surgery, 14th ed., pp. 568–576. Philadelphia, WB Saunders, 1991.
17. Braverman LE, Utiger RD. Introduction to hypothyroidism. In Braverman LE, Utiger RD (eds). Werner and Ingbar's The Thyroid, 6th ed., pp. 919–920. Philadelphia, JB Lippincott, 1991.
18. Thrall JH, Ziessman HA. Endocrine system. In Nuclear Medicine: The Requisites, pp. 321–343. St. Louis, Mosby–Year Book, 1995.
19. Gooding GAW. Sonography of the thyroid and parathyroid. Radiol Clin North Am 1993;31:967–989.
20. Jennings AS. Non-isotopic techniques of thyroid imaging. In Braverman LE, Utiger RD (eds). Werner and Ingbar's The Thyroid, 6th ed., pp. 525–543. Philadelphia, JB Lippincott, 1991.
21. Hopkins CR, Reading CC. Thyroid and parathyroid imaging. Semin Ultrasound CT MR 1995;16:279–295.
22. Ralls PW, Mayekawa DS, Lee KP, et al. Color flow Doppler sonography in Graves' disease: Thyroid inferno. AJR 1988;150:780–784.
23. Kaneko T, Matsumoto N, Fukui K, et al. Clinical evaluation of thyroid: CT values in various thyroid conditions. J Comput Tomogr 1979;3:1–4.
24. Hashimoto H. Zur Kenntnis der lymphomatosen Veränderungen der Schilddruese (struma lymphomatosa). Arch Klin Chir 1912;97:219–248.
25. Volpé R. Autoimmune thyroiditis. In Braverman LE, Utiger RD (eds). Werner and Ingbar's The Thyroid, 6th ed., pp. 921–932. Philadelphia, JB Lippincott, 1991.
26. Kaufman KV, Rapoport B, Seto P, et al. Generation of recombinant enzymatically active human thyroid peroxidase and its recognition by antibodies in sera of patients with Hashimoto's thyroiditis. J Clin Invest 1989;84:394–403.
27. Takasu N, Yamada T, Takasu M, et al. Disappearance of thyrotropin-blocking antibodies and spontaneous recovery from hypothyroidism in autoimmune thyroiditis. N Engl J Med 1992;326:513–518.
28. Intenzo CM, Park H, Kim SM, et al. Clinical, laboratory, and scintigraphic manifestations of subacute and chronic thyroiditis. Clin Nucl Med 1993;18:302–306.
29. Gefter WB, Spritzer CE, Eisenberg B, et al. Thyroid imaging with high-field-strength surface-coil MR. Radiology 1987;164:483–490.
30. Clark OH, Greenspan FS, Dunphy JE. Hashimoto's thyroiditis and thyroid cancer: Indications for operations. Am J Surg 1980;140:65–71.
31. Ott RA, Calandra DB, McCall A, et al. The incidence of thyroid carcinoma in patients with Hashimoto's thyroiditis and solitary cold nodules. Surgery 1985;98:1202–1206.
32. Nordmeyer JP, Shafeh TA, Heckmann C. Thyroid sonography in autoimmune thyroiditis. A prospective study on 123 patients. Acta Endocrinol 1990;122:391–395.
33. Takashima S, Ikezoe J, Morimoto S, et al. Primary thyroid lymphoma. Evaluation with CT. Radiology 1988;168:765–768.

34. Takashima S, Morimoto S, Ikezoe J, et al. Primary thyroid lymphoma: Comparison of CT and US assessment. Radiology 1989;171:439–443.

35. Kasagi K, Hatabu H, Tokuda Y, et al. Lymphoproliferative disorders of the thyroid gland: Radiological appearances. Br J Radiol 1991;64:569–575.

36. Hamburger JI. The various presentations of thyroiditis: Diagnostic considerations. Ann Intern Med 1986;104:219–224.

37. Takashima S, Morimoto S, Ikezoe J, et al. CT evaluation of anaplastic thyroid carcinoma. AJR 1990;154:1079–1085.

38. Perez Fontan FJ, Carballido FC, Felipe FP, et al. Riedel thyroiditis: US, CT, and MR evaluation. J Comput Assist Tomogr 1993;17:324–325.

39. Higgins CB, Auffermann W. MR imaging of thyroid and parathyroid glands: A review of current status. AJR 1988;151:1095–1106.

40. Takashima S, Ikezoe J, Morimoto S, et al. Case report: MR imaging of primary thyroid lymphoma. J Comput Assist Tomogr 1989;13:517–518.

41. Belfiore A, LaRose GL, LaPorta GA, et al. Cancer risks in patients with cold thyroid nodules: Relevance of iodine intake, sex, age, and multinodularity. Am J Med 1992;93:363–369.

42. Cerise EJ, Spears R, Ochsner A. Carcinoma of the thyroid and nontoxic nodular goiter. Surgery 1952;31:552–561.

43. McCall A, Jarosz H, Lawrence AM, et al. The incidence of thyroid carcinoma in solitary cold nodules and in multinodular goiters. Surgery 1986;100:1128–1132.

44. Glazer GM, Axel L, Moss AA. CT diagnosis of mediastinal thyroid. AJR 1982;138:495–498.

45. Plummer HS. The clinical and pathological relationship of simple and exophthalmic goiter. Am J Med Sci 1913;146:790–803.

46. Mazzaferri EL. Management of a solitary thyroid nodule. N Engl J Med 1993;328:553–559.

47. Mazzaferri EL, de los Santos ET, Rofagha-Keyhani S. Solitary thyroid nodules: Diagnosis and management. Med Clin North Am 1988;72:1177–1211.

48. Pelizzo MR, Piotto A, Rubello D, et al. High prevalence of occult papillary thyroid carcinoma in a surgical series for benign thyroid disease. Tumori 1990;76:255–257.

49. Duffy BJ Jr, Fitzgerald PJ. Cancer of the thyroid in children: A report of 28 cases. J Clin Endocrinol Metab 1950;10:1296–1311.

50. Schneider AB. Carcinoma of follicular epithelium. Pathogenesis. In Braverman LE, Utiger RD (eds). Werner and Ingbar's The Thyroid, 6th ed., pp. 1121–1137. Philadelphia, JB Lippincott, 1991.

51. Favus MJ, Schneider AB, Stachura ME, et al. Thyroid cancer occurring as a late consequence of head-and-neck-irradiation. Evaluation of 1,056 patients. N Engl J Med 1976;294:1019–1025.

52. Maxon HR, Thomas SR, Saenger EL, et al. Ionizing irradiation and the induction of clinically significant disease in the human thyroid gland. Am J Med 1977;63:967–978.

53. Harvey HK. Diagnosis and management of the thyroid nodule: An overview. Otolaryngol Clin North Am 1990;23:303–337.

54. Solbiati L, Volterrani L, Rizzatto G, et al. The thyroid gland with low uptake lesions: Evaluation by ultrasound. Radiology 1985;155:187–191.

55. Martin HE, Ellis EB. Biopsy by needle puncture and aspiration. Ann Surg 1930;92:169–181.

56. Hamberger JI, Kaplan MM, Husain M. Diagnosis of thyroid nodules by needle biopsy. In Braverman LE, Utiger RD (eds). Werner and Ingbar's The Thyroid, 6th ed., pp. 544–559. Philadelphia, JB Lippincott, 1991.

57. Gharib H, Goellner JR. Fine needle aspiration of the thyroid: An appraisal. Ann Intern Med 1993;11:282–289.

58. Hamberger JI. Evolution of toxicity in solitary nontoxic autonomously functioning thyroid nodules. Clin Endocrinol Metab 1980;50:1089–1093.

59. Ross DS. Evaluation of the thyroid nodule. J Nucl Med 1991;32:2181–2192.

60. Livraghi T, Paracchi A, Ferrari C, et al. Treatment of autonomous thyroid nodules with percutaneous ethanol injection: Preliminary results. Radiology 1990;175:827–829.

61. Monzani F, Goletti O, Caraccio N, et al. Percutaneous ethanol injection treatment of autonomous thyroid adenoma: Hormonal and clinical evaluation. Clin Endocrinol 1992;36:491–497.

62. Mazzeo S, Toni MG, DeGaudio C, et al. Percutaneous injection of ethanol to treat autonomous thyroid nodules. AJR 1993;161:871–876.

63. Papini E, Panunzi C, Pacella CM, et al. Percutaneous ultrasound-guided ethanol injection: A new treatment of toxic autonomously functioning thyroid nodules. J Clin Endocrinol Metab 1993;76:411–416.

64. Livraghi T, Paracchi A, Ferrari C, et al. Treatment of autonomous thyroid nodules with percutaneous ethanol injection: 4-year experience. Radiology 1994;190:529–533.

65. Ozdemir H, Ilgit ET, Yucel C, et al. Treatment of autonomous thyroid nodules: Safety and efficacy of sonographically guided percutaneous injection of ethanol. AJR 1994;163:929–932.

66. Solbiati L, Pra LD, Ierace T, et al. High-resolution sonography of the recurrent laryngeal nerve: Anatomic and pathologic considerations. AJR 1985;145:989–993.

67. Schwartz MR. Pathology of the thyroid and parathyroid gland. Otolaryngol Clin North Am 1990;23:175–215.

68. Chen KTK, Rosai J. Follicular variant of thyroid papillary carcinoma. A clinicopathologic study of 6 cases. Am J Surg Pathol 1977;1:123–130.

69. DeKeyser LFM, VanHerle AJ. Differentiated thyroid cancer in children. Head Neck Surg 1985;8:100–109.

70. Buckwalter JA, Gurll NJ, Thomas CG Jr. Cancer of the thyroid in youth. World J Surg 1981;5:15–25.

71. Mazzaferri EL. Radioiodine and other treatment outcomes. In Braverman LE, Utiger RD (eds). Werner and Ingbar's The Thyroid, 6th ed., pp. 1138–1165. Philadelphia, JB Lippincott, 1991.

72. Vattimo A, Bertelli P, Cintorino N, et al. Identification of Hürthle cell tumor by single-injection, double-phase scintigraphy with technetium-99m-sestamibi. J Nucl Med 1995;36:778–782.

73. Abdel-Dayem HM, Scott AM, Macapinlac HA, et al. Role of Tl-201 chloride and 99m-Tc sestamibi in tumor imaging. In Freeman LM (ed). Nuclear Medicine Annual, pp. 181–234. Philadelphia, Lippincott-Raven, 1994.

74. Krenning EP, Kwekkeboom DJ, Bakker WH, et al. Somatostatin receptor scintigraphy with [111-In-DTPA-D-Phe¹]- and [I123-Tyr³]-octeotide: The Rotterdam experience with more than 1,000 patients. Eur J Nucl Med 1993;20:716–731.

75. Dörr U, Sautter-Bihl M-L, Heiner B. The contribution of somatostatin receptor scintigraphy to the diagnosis of recurrent medullary carcinoma of the thyroid. Semin Oncol 1994;21:42–45.

76. Siperstein AE, Clark OH. Carcinoma of follicular epithelium. Surgical therapy. In Braverman LE, Utiger RD (eds). Werner and Ingbar's The Thyroid, 6th ed., pp. 1129–1137. Philadelphia, JB Lippincott, 1991.

77. Hubert JP, Kiernan PD, Beahrs OH, et al. Occult papillary carcinoma of the thyroid. Arch Surg 1980;115:394–398.

78. Hay ID. Papillary thyroid carcinoma. Endocrinol Metab Clin North Am 1990;19:545–576.

79. Cady B, Rossi R. An expanded view of risk-group definition in differentiated thyroid carcinoma. Surgery 1988;104:947–953.

80. Mazzaferri EL, Young RL, Ortell JE, et al. Papillary thyroid carcinoma: The impact of therapy on 576 patients. Medicine 1977;56:171–196.

81. Mazzaferri EL. Papillary thyroid carcinoma: Factors influencing prognosis and current therapy. Semin Oncol 1987;14:315–332.

82. Carcangiu ML, Zampi G, Pupi A, et al. Papillary carcinoma of the thyroid: A clinical pathologic study of 241 cases treated at the University of Florence, Italy. Cancer 1985;55:805–828.

83. Cody HS III, Shah JP. Locally invasive well-differentiated thyroid cancer: 22 years' experience at Memorial Sloan-Kettering Cancer Center. Am J Surg 1981;142:480–483.

84. Sherman NH, Rosenberg HK, Heyman S, et al. Ultrasound evaluation of neck masses in children. J Ultrasound Med 1985;21:127–134.

85. Hatabu H, Kasagi K, Yamamoto K, et al. Cystic papillary carcinoma of the thyroid gland: A new sonographic sign. Clin Radiol 1991;43:121–124.

86. Gorman B, Charboneau JW, James EM, et al. Medullary thyroid carcinoma: Role of high-resolution US. Radiology 1987;162:147–150.

87. Som PM, Brandwein M, Lidov M, et al. The varied presentations of papillary thyroid carcinoma cervical nodal disease: CT and MR findings. AJR 1994;15:1123–1128.

88. Piekarski J-D, Schlumber M, Leclere J, et al. Chest computed tomography (CT) in patients with micronodular lung metastases of differentiated thyroid carcinoma. Int J Radiat Oncol Biol Phys 1985;11:1023–1031.

89. Hays LL, Marlow SF Jr. Papillary carcinoma arising in a thyroglossal duct cyst. Laryngoscope 1968;78:2189–2193.

90. Silverman PM, Degesys GE, Ferguson BJ, et al. Papillary carcinoma in a thyroglossal duct cyst: CT findings. J Comput Assist Tomogr 1985;9:806–808.

91. Batsakis JG. Tumors of the Head and Neck: Clinical and Pathological Considerations. Baltimore, Williams & Wilkins, 1979.

92. Hawkins DB, Jacobsen BE, Klatt EC. Cysts of the thyroglossal duct. Laryngoscope 1982;92:1254–1258.

93. Takashima S, Nomura N, Tanaka H, et al. Congenital hypothyroidism: Assessment with ultrasound. AJNR 1995;16:1117–1123.

94. Verelst J, Chanoine J-P, Delange F. Radionuclide imaging in primary permanent congenital hypothyroidism. Clin Nucl Med 1991;16:652–655.

95. Rovet J, Ehrlich R, Sorbara D. Intellectual outcome in children with fetal hypothyroidism. J Pediatr 1987;110:700–704.

96. Clark OH, Duh QY. Primary hyperparathyroidism, a surgical perspective. Endocrinol Metab Clin North Am 1989;268:943–953.

97. Castleman B, Kibbee BU (eds). Case records of the Massachusetts General Hospital: Case 29. N Engl J Med 1990;322:1106–1112.

98. Yousem DM, Scheff AM. Thyroid and parathyroid gland pathology: Role of imaging. Otolaryngol Clin North Am 1995;28:621–649.

99. Taillefer R. Tc-99m sestamibi parathyroid scintigraphy. In Freeman LM (ed). Nuclear Medicine Annual 1995, p. 54. Philadelphia, Lippincott-Raven, 1995.

100. Edis AJ, Sheedy PF, Bearhs OH, et al. Results of reoperation for hyperparathyroidism, with evaluation of preoperative localization studies. Surgery 1978;84:384–391.

101. Satava RM, Beahrs OH, Scholz DA. Success rate of cervical exploration for hyperparathyroidism. Arch Surg 1975;110:625–627.

102. Thompson CT. Localization studies in patients with hyperparathyroidism. Br J Surg 1988;75:97–98.

103. Lundgren EC, Gillott AR, Wiseman JS, Beck J. The role of preoperative localization in primary hyperparathyroidism. Am Surg 1995;61:393–396.

104. Higgins CB. Role of magnetic resonance imaging in hyperparathyroidism. Radiol Clin North Am 1993;31:1017–1028.

105. Russell CF, Laird JD, Ferguson WR. Scan-directed unilateral cervical exploration for parathyroid adenoma: A legitimate approach? World J Surg 1990;14:406–409.

106. Zwas ST, Czerniak A. The parathyroids. In Wagner HN Jr, Szabo Z, Buchanan JW (eds). Principles of Nuclear Medicine, 2nd ed., p. 642. Philadelphia, WB Saunders, 1995.

107. Rosenblatt M, Kronenberg HM, Pots JT. Parathyroid hormone. Physiology, chemistry, biosynthesis, secretion, metabolism and mode of action. In DeGroot LJ (ed). Endocrinology, Vol. 2, pp. 848–891. Philadelphia, WB Saunders, 1989.

108. Miller DL, Doppman JL, Krudy AG, et al. Localization of parathyroid adenomas in patients who have undergone surgery. Part II. Invasive imaging methods. Radiology 1987;162:138–141.

109. Reading CC, Charboneau JW, James EM, et al. High resolution parathyroid ultrasonography. AJR 1982;139:539–546.

110. Stark DD, Gooding GAW, Moss AA. Parathyroid imaging: Comparison of high-resolution CT and high-resolution sonography. AJR 1983;141:633–638.

111. Gooding GAW, Clark OH. Use of color Doppler imaging in the distinction between thyroid and parathyroid lesions. Am J Surg 1992;164:51–56.

112. Winzelberg GG, Hydovitz JD. Radionuclide imaging of parathyroid tumors: Historical perspectives and newer techniques. Semin Nucl Med 1985;15:161–170.

113. Hauty M, Swartz K, McKlung M, et al. Technetium-thallium scintiscanning for localization of parathyroid adenomas and hyperplasia, a reappraisal. Am J Surg 1987;153:479–486.

114. Sandrock D, Merino MJ, Norton JA, et al. Ultrastructural histology correlates with results of thallium-201/technetium-99m parathyroid subtraction scintigraphy. J Nucl Med 1993;34:24–29.

115. Coakley AJ, Kettle AG, Wells CP, et al. Technetium-99m-sestamibi—A new agent for parathyroid imaging. Nucl Med Commun 1989;10:791–794.

116. Taillefer R, Boucher Y, Potvin C, et al. Detection and localization of parathyroid adenomas in patients with hyperparathyroidism using a single radionuclide imaging procedure with technetium-99m-sestamibi (double-phase study). J Nucl Med 1992;33:1801–1807.

117. O'Doherty MJ, Kettle AG, Wells P, et al. Parathyroid imaging with technetium-99m-sestamibi: Pre-operative localization and tissue uptake studies. J Nucl Med 1992;33:313–318.

118. McBiles M, Lambert AT, Cote MG, Kim SY. Sestamibi parathyroid scintigraphy. Semin Nucl Med 1995;25:221–234.

119. Lee VS, Wilkinson RH Jr, Leight GS Jr, et al. Hyperparathyroidism in high-risk surgical patients: Evaluation with double-phase technetium-99m sestamibi imaging. Radiology 1995;197:627–633.

120. Numerow LM, Morita ET, Clark OH, et al. Persistent/recurrent hyperparathyroidism: A comparison of sestamibi scintigraphy, MRI, and ultrasonography. J Magn Reson Imaging 1995;5:702–708.

121. Bénard F, Lefebvre B, Beuvon F, et al. Rapid washout of technetium-99m-MIBI from a large parathyroid adenoma. J Nucl Med 1995;36:241–243.

122. Miller DL. Preoperative localization and interventional treatment of parathyroid tumors: When and how? World J Surg 1991;15:706–715.

CHAPTER

35

Salivary Glands and Lymph Nodes

BRIAN C. BOWEN, Ph.D., M.D.
MICHELLE L. WHITEMAN, M.D.

SALIVARY GLANDS

Embryology and Anatomy

All the salivary glands develop from an ingrowth of local proliferations of surface epithelium, and they have a similar overall structure. The parotid anlagen are the first to develop, between the fourth and sixth weeks of embryonic life, and are of ectodermal origin. The submandibular gland anlagen appear in the sixth week and are probably of endodermal origin. The sublingual glands arise in the seventh to eighth week, and the minor salivary glands develop later, in the twelfth week of embryonic life.[1-5] The epithelial buds of each gland enlarge, elongate, and branch. The distal ends of the buds have bulbous terminals that develop into acini. The acinar cells do not assume their secretory function during fetal development.[6]

The ductal organization within the salivary glands has a treelike branching pattern. The main duct gives rise to the excretory ducts, which branch into the striated ducts, which in turn divide into the intercalated ducts. The pattern of arborization progresses from proximal to distal, with an increase in the number of side branches and a decrease in the size of the ducts. The intercalated ducts terminate in the acinar cells, which produce saliva.

The parotid anlagen become encapsulated after the submandibular and sublingual glands have become encapsulated. The lymphatic system emerges after this encapsulation of the submandibular and sublingual glands but before that of the parotid glands. Thus there are lymphatic channels and lymph nodes within the capsule of the fully developed parotid gland and not within the submandibular or sublingual glands.[5] The paired parotid, submandibular, and sublingual glands are considered the major salivary glands.

Parotid Gland

The parotid gland is the largest of the salivary glands and overlies the ramus and angle of the mandible. The gland is surrounded by the superficial layer of deep cervical fascia, which also extends into the gland, dividing it into lobules. A small portion of the gland extends deep, lying within the stylomandibular tunnel, and forms part of the lateral margin of the parapharyngeal space. The gland is not anatomically divided into deep and superficial lobes, but by convention, the course of the facial nerve is used as a reference, with that portion of the gland deep to the facial nerve termed the *deep lobe* and the portion of the gland overlying the facial nerve referred to as the *superficial lobe*.[7] The parotid gland lies below and anterior to the external auditory canal and mastoid tip, inferior to the zygomatic arch, and extends down to the level of the angle of the mandible.[1, 2] In the adult, the parotid gland is purely a serous gland. In the neonate, some mucous cells are also present.[1, 2, 5]

The main trunk of the facial nerve exits the mastoid at the stylomastoid foramen and gives off three small branches, the posterior auricular, the posterior digastric, and the stylohyoid nerves. The facial nerve then runs laterally around the styloid process and courses along the lateral surface of the posterior belly of the digastric muscle. The facial nerve then pierces the posterior capsule of the parotid gland and runs lateral to the retromandibular vein. The retromandibular vein lies just lateral to the external carotid artery within the parotid gland. The nerve subsequently divides into the temporal, zygomatic, buccal, mandibular, and cervical branches.[5, 8]

The main parotid duct, Stensen's duct, emerges from the anterior aspect of the gland, courses over the masseter muscle and buccal fat pad, and then turns medially to pierce the buccinator muscle and buccal mucosa (Fig. 35–1). This duct opens intraorally opposite the second upper molar tooth.[5] In about 20% of the population, accessory parotid tissue is present and lies along the course of Stensen's duct, anterior to the main parotid gland and usually on or above the duct. The intraparotid lymph nodes and immediately adjacent nodes drain into the superior deep cervical lymph node chain (see later).[5]

Submandibular Gland

The submandibular gland, the second largest salivary gland, wraps around the posterior edge of the mylohyoid muscle. The lingual nerve lies above it and the hypoglos-

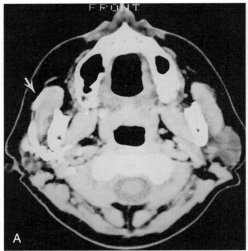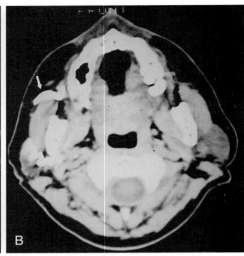

FIGURE 35–1 Computed tomography (CT) sialogram. *A* and *B*, The course of Stensen's duct is shown as it loops over the masseter muscle and pierces the buccinator muscle (*arrows*).

sal nerve below it. The main duct is Wharton's duct, which exits the gland anteriorly and runs forward and upward, lying medial to the mylohyoid muscle and sublingual gland and lateral to the genioglossus muscle. The duct opens into the anterior floor of the mouth just lateral to the frenulum, behind the lower incisor teeth. The submandibular gland is a mixed serous and mucous gland, and its lymph drains into the submandibular nodes.

Sublingual Gland

The sublingual gland is the smallest of the major salivary glands and lies just under the sublingual mucosa of the floor of the mouth, situated between the mylohyoid muscle (which is inferolateral to the gland) and the genioglossus-geniohyoid muscle complex (which is medial to the gland). The gland is oval and usually about 2.5 cm in length. The sublingual gland is a mixed serous and mucous gland. Approximately 20 individual minor ducts (ducts of Rivinus) open onto the floor of the mouth along the sublingual papilla and fold. Some of these minor ducts may fuse to form Bartholin's duct, which opens into Wharton's duct.[2] The lymphatic drainage of the sublingual gland is to the submental and submandibular lymph nodes.

Minor Salivary Glands

Hundreds of minor salivary glands lie beneath the mucosa of the oral cavity, palate, pharynx, larynx, trachea, and paranasal sinuses. These are predominantly mucous glands.[5] The greatest numbers are in the soft and hard palate.

The total daily production of saliva is between 1000 and 1500 ml. The parotid glands contribute approximately 45%, the submandibular glands about 45%, the sublingual glands 5%, and the minor salivary glands 5%.[9] The fluid is formed in the acini and modified within the ductal system. The normal pH range of saliva is 5.6 to 7.0, and a variety of substances contained within saliva provide it with antibacterial properties.[2] Since the parotid is composed of serous cells, its secretion is watery, high in enzymes, and low in mucin. In contrast, the sublingual gland is predominantly composed of mucous cells, and its

secretions are therefore high in mucin and quite viscous. Saliva performs a number of crucial functions. Lubrication of the oral and pharyngeal surfaces protects them from chemical, thermal, and mechanical trauma. The presence of amylase aids in the digestion of carbohydrates. Saliva aids in the prevention of dental caries by cleaning the teeth and gums of foreign material. Saliva not only has antibacterial properties but also promotes dental calcification.

Aberrant salivary gland tissue refers to salivary tissue in an ectopic location. This heterotopic tissue (choristoma) has been reported in a number of locations in the head and neck, including the middle ear (Fig. 35–2), neck, and mandible (Stafne's cyst).[2, 10]

Imaging

A variety of imaging modalities are available for the evaluation of salivary gland disease, including plain films, ultrasonography, sialography, computed tomography (CT), and magnetic resonance imaging (MRI). The clinical presentation usually dictates which approach is chosen. Acute, painful, and diffuse swelling of a gland likely indicates an inflammatory process, as does a history of recurrent subacute episodes of painful glandular swelling. A focal mass is more suggestive of a neoplasm, either benign or malignant.

Plain Films

Plain films are used primarily for the detection of radiopaque sialolithiasis (Fig. 35–3), mandibular erosion, and dystrophic calcifications. Noncontrast CT detects some calcifications that are not apparent on plain films. A survey examination for the parotid gland includes an open-mouth lateral film, posteroanterior views, and oblique views. To detect submandibular gland calculi, an open-mouth lateral view is taken with the patient's finger depressing the tongue, as well as oblique views and an intraoral occlusal film.[5]

Sialography

Sialography requires the injection of a radiopaque contrast material into the parotid or submandibular gland via

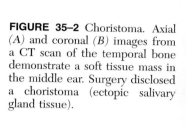
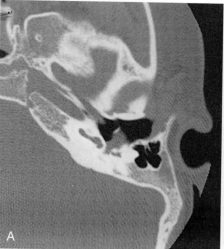
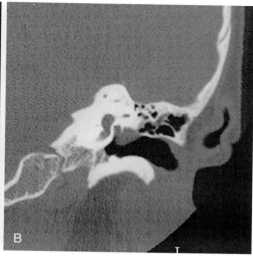

FIGURE 35–2 Choristoma. Axial *(A)* and coronal *(B)* images from a CT scan of the temporal bone demonstrate a soft tissue mass in the middle ear. Surgery disclosed a choristoma (ectopic salivary gland tissue).

the intraoral opening of Stensen's or Wharton's duct. The sublingual and minor salivary glands have openings that are too numerous and small for routine cannulation. Sialography is the only modality that reveals the detailed anatomy of the salivary ductal system. Thus, sialography is the study of choice for those diseases affecting primarily the ductal system, such as sialadenitis, sialosis, and autoimmune-related diseases. A sialogram may also be obtained to detect a small sialolith; to evaluate for fistula, stricture, diverticulum, or trauma; and rarely, as a dilating procedure for ductal stenosis.[5, 11]

The main duct is cannulated with a sialographic cannula. For the parotid gland, 0.5 to 1.5 ml of diatrizoate meglumine and iodipamide meglumine (Sinografin), a water-soluble contrast agent, is injected with hand pressure. For the submandibular gland, only 0.2 to 0.5 ml is needed. If there is active infection, the procedure is contraindicated since it may propagate infection back into the gland. A secretogogue, such as lemon juice, is often helpful in identifying the intraoral location of Stensen's or Wharton's duct, as a drop of saliva may be seen at the opening of the duct. A diffuse pattern of arborization should be seen, without a focal filling defect (Fig. 35–4). The injection should be monitored with fluoroscopy. In some cases, CT is added to better define intraparotid masses, although these lesions are usually better imaged with MRI or contrast (intravenous) CT (Fig. 35–5).

Computed Tomography

CT and MRI are the studies of choice for the evaluation of mass lesions. The characterization of a mass lesion includes the location of the lesion within the gland (and position relative to the facial nerve, for parotid masses), the margins of the lesion, whether the mass has extended outside the gland capsule and involves other structures, and if the mass appears homogeneous versus heterogeneous, with necrotic, cystic, or solid components. The pattern of enhancement should be evaluated on contrast studies. Multiplicity or bilaterality should also be noted and is often helpful in narrowing the differential diagnosis. Gross involvement of the mandible or skull base is well seen with CT or MRI, but subtle bone erosion is unquestionably better imaged with CT.

The normal parotid gland has a fatty interstitial structure and produces serous secretions. The CT attenuation of the gland (-25 to 15 Hounsfield units [HU]) is therefore much lower than that of muscle, and slightly higher than that of fat. In children, however, the gland may appear homogeneously increased in density. With age, the gland becomes increasingly fatty in appearance. Stensen's duct can be seen on CT in up to 94% of normal patients, using 3-mm-thick sections.[12] The external carotid artery and retromandibular vein are usually seen posterior to the mandibular ramus. Within the parotid gland, the facial nerve courses lateral to the retromandibular vein and external carotid artery but is not usually seen on routine CT studies. CT is quite sensitive for calcification, and if a calculus cannot be identified on plain film it may be detected on CT. The submandibular glands are more

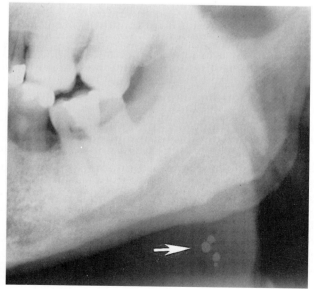

FIGURE 35–3 Submandibular calculi. Lateral radiograph of the submandibular region discloses several radiopaque calculi *(arrow)*.

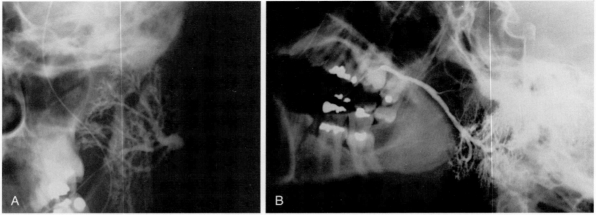

FIGURE 35–4 Normal parotid sialogram. Anteroposterior *(A)* and lateral *(B)* views of a normal parotid sialogram demonstrate the normal branching pattern of the ductal system. The main parotid duct is smooth in contour and not enlarged.

cellular than the parotid glands and thus appear higher in density on CT and lower in signal intensity on T1-weighted MRI images, compared with the parotid glands.

High-grade malignancies within the salivary glands often have irregular, infiltrative margins, whereas most benign lesions are smooth in contour and sharply delineated from adjacent glandular tissue on both CT and MRI. However, some malignancies may also have a benign appearance, and thus morphology is not consistently reliable in differentiating benign from malignant lesions. The CT or MRI appearance correctly differentiates benign from malignant lesions in approximately 87% of cases.[13] This is similar to the predictive ability of clinical examination combined with history.[13] In comparison, positron emission tomography with fluorine-18–labeled fluoro-

deoxyglucose (FDG PET) reliably differentiates benign from malignant salivary gland lesions in 69% of cases.[14]

The goal of CT and MRI is not to identify the specific histologic type (although this is possible in some cases) but to define the extent of the lesion for the surgeon, evaluate for adenopathy (which may not be palpable), and, if possible, distinguish a malignant process from a benign lesion.

Magnetic Resonance Imaging

The usual sequences employed for imaging of the salivary glands include T1-weighted axial and coronal images along with dual-echo axial sections. In some cases, gadolinium-enhanced fat suppression studies may provide additional information, especially regarding perineural or intracranial spread. On MRI, the parotid gland is intermediate to bright on T1-weighted images due to its fatty content, and intermediate in signal on T2-weighted images. Stensen's duct can be identified in up to 90% of normal subjects using meticulous technique.[12] Unless it is enlarged, the facial nerve is not consistently identified on routine MRI scans.[15]

Because of greater soft tissue contrast resolution, MRI may better define the margins of a salivary gland lesion compared with CT, and the multiplanar capability of MRI is often helpful. In addition, image degradation from dental amalgam is limited compared with the extensive streak artifact seen on CT. However, CT is often better at detecting associated adenopathy and is usually less expensive than MRI. CT is also more reliable for the detection of calcium. Not only is the presence of calcification important in the evaluation of inflammatory disease, but a tumor containing calcification is likely to be a pleomorphic adenoma. In addition, the longer acquisition time of conventional spin-echo MRI renders the images more sensitive to motion artifact than CT. Thus, each modality offers some benefit over the other, and they often provide complementary information.

MRI has shown a definite advantage over CT in differentiating intraparotid masses from parapharyngeal space masses. Because the deep lobe extends to the lateral aspect of the prestyloid parapharyngeal space, it is some-

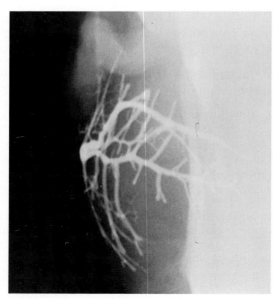

FIGURE 35–5 Abnormal parotid sialogram. This sialogram was performed to evaluate a mass lesion of the parotid gland. Note stretching and displacement of the ducts, which are draped around a soft tissue mass. Surgical resection revealed an acinic cell tumor.

times difficult to define the true origin of a mass in this region. This distinction, however, is crucial since the surgical approach depends on the space of origin. A deep lobe parotid lesion necessitates a transparotid approach with control of the facial nerve. Parapharyngeal masses may be approached via a submandibular or transoral resection, without localization of the facial nerve. A mass can be localized to the parotid gland on MRI or CT if the epicenter of the lesion is clearly lateral to the parapharyngeal space, if the fat of the parapharyngeal space is displaced medially, or if the stylomandibular tunnel appears widened (Fig. 35–6). If a clear fat plane between the parotid gland and the mass cannot be delineated, the mass is either of parotid origin or of extraparotid origin but so large that the fat planes are completely effaced. A third possibility, although less likely, is that the lesion is extraparotid in origin but infiltrates the adjacent parotid gland. If the mass cannot be clearly separated from the parotid gland, a parotid approach is indicated so that the facial nerve is identified.

Many cellular tumors tend to have intermediate to low signal intensity on all sequences, whereas benign lesions and some low-grade malignancies tend to have increased signal intensity on T2-weighted images.[5, 16, 17] However, signal intensity on T2-weighted images is not predictive of the specific histologic type.[18, 19] Malignant lesions demonstrate a variety of signal patterns ranging from hypo- to iso- to hyperintense.[18-20] Benign lesions, such as Warthin's tumors, are often intermediate or mixed in signal intensity.[18, 21] Thus, benign lesions cannot be reliably differentiated from malignant lesions solely on the basis of MRI signal characteristics. Because the parotid gland is fatty, most benign and malignant lesions are relatively hypointense on T1-weighted images. Thus, radiographic findings need to be correlated with the clinical presentation. Benign tumors are usually slow growing, painless, mobile masses and do not cause facial paralysis. Malignant tumors may enlarge over several weeks, may be painful, are "rock hard" to palpation, and may be fixed. Facial nerve paralysis in association with a mass lesion of the parotid gland is highly suspicious for a malignant process and the lesion should be presumed malignant unless proved otherwise.

Ultrasonography

Ultrasonography is helpful in differentiating solid from cystic masses. It can also be used to identify calculi. However, the greater resolution of CT and MRI for visualization of deeper structures and the skull base has established CT and MRI as the primary imaging modalities, especially for imaging of neoplastic disease of the salivary glands.

Nuclear Medicine

Technetium-99m pertechnetate studies normally reveal symmetric uptake in the salivary glands with a "washout" after administration of a secretogogue that promotes excretion of isotope into the oral cavity. Diffuse glandular dysfunction, as seen in Sjögren's syndrome, radiation sialadenitis, diabetes mellitus, malnutrition, and cirrhosis, results in diffusely decreased activity of the salivary glands. Focally increased activity is seen in Warthin's tumor and in oncocytoma, which occurs less frequently. Warthin's tumors are the most common tumors to be present bilaterally, so that focally increased activity, if seen bilaterally, is strongly suggestive of Warthin's tumors.

Nonneoplastic Conditions

Acute Inflammatory Diseases

Viral and bacterial inflammatory disorders are the most common abnormalities of the salivary glands. Most bacte-

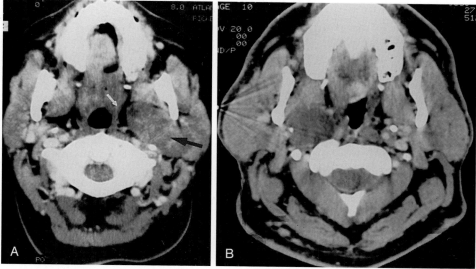

FIGURE 35–6 Intraparotid versus extraparotid mass. *A*, A large, inhomogeneous mass is seen in the deep lobe of the left parotid gland. Note the medial displacement of the parapharyngeal fat *(white arrow)*. Also note the marked widening of the left stylomandibular tunnel *(black arrow)* compared with the right. Surgical resection disclosed a pleomorphic adenoma. *B*, Axial postcontrast CT scan reveals a hypodense, well-circumscribed mass in the right poststyloid parapharyngeal space (carotid space). The lesion appears to be completely separate from the parotid gland. The parapharyngeal fat of the prestyloid parapharyngeal space is displaced anteromedially. The carotid artery is also displaced anteromedially. This patient was known to have neurofibromatosis. Atrophy of the right tongue was noted on other images (not shown), suggesting a 12th nerve neuroma.

rial infections ascend from the oral cavity and are often related to a diminished salivary flow. The maintenance of a normal salivary flow is the best deterrent to such infections. A number of disorders may reduce the production of saliva including radiation, dehydration, trauma, surgery, prior infections, and some medications.[22] These infections are more common in the parotid gland than in the submandibular gland and are termed *acute suppurative sialadenitis*. They occur most often in debilitated, dehydrated patients with poor oral hygiene.[23] Many of the cases are seen in the postoperative period, after surgery unrelated to the oral cavity.

In *parotid sialadenitis*, the gland is acutely swollen and tender with overlying erythema and a purulent discharge from the affected duct. The most common organisms are *Staphylococcus aureus*, *Streptococcus viridans*, and *Streptococcus pneumoniae*. Treatment is with hydration, warm compresses, and antibiotics. Submandibular sialadenitis is usually secondary to sialolithiasis. Clinically, there is painful swelling of the gland and adjacent nodes, and a calculus is present. When acute sialadenitis goes undiagnosed or is inadequately treated, an abscess or multiple abscesses may develop and may extend outside the gland. Surgical drainage with antibiotic therapy is the usual treatment.

Suppurative sialadenitis involving the parotid gland is also seen in neonates, primarily affecting premature infants with dehydration.[24] The onset is usually 1 to 2 weeks after delivery, and erythema of the skin overlying the parotid may be seen.[24] Again, hydration and antibiotics are the appropriate treatment.

CT imaging of acute suppurative sialadenitis reveals an enlarged gland with increased attenuation as a result of inflammation. Postcontrast studies often show enhancement. Sialography is contraindicated, since the procedure can propagate the acute infection further into the gland. Sialolithiasis is clearly evident if the calculus is radiopaque.

The most common cause of viral parotitis is *mumps*, a frequent viral infection seen in children 4 to 10 years of age. There is acute, painful swelling of the gland that is unilateral in ⅓ of cases and bilateral in ⅔, associated with malaise and trismus. Although the parotid glands are primarily affected, the submandibular glands may also be involved. The incubation period is 2 to 3 weeks, and the duration of the infection is 7 to 10 days. The clinical diagnosis can be confirmed with serum antibody titers. The condition is usually self-limited. Rarely, other organ systems may become infected, resulting in orchitis, pancreatitis, nephritis, encephalitis, cochleitis, or meningitis. Once infected, there is immunity to future bouts of infection. Other viral agents can rarely precipitate parotid infection as well.

Sialodochitis is inflammation of the main salivary duct. The duct is often dilated secondary to a distal obstruction. On CT, the walls of the duct are thickened and enhancing and the duct itself is enlarged. A diameter of 3 mm or greater suggests possible obstruction.

Sialolithiasis

Approximately 80% to 90% of salivary gland stones are seen in the submandibular gland, 10% to 20% occur in the parotid glands, and only 1% to 7% in the sublingual glands.[22] About 25% of patients with sialolithiasis have multiple stones, and 2.2% have bilateral salivary stones (Fig. 35–7).[22, 25] Eighty percent of submandibular and 60% of parotid stones are radiopaque on plain films.[4]

The increased incidence of calculi in the submandibular gland compared with the parotid gland is related to the thicker nature of submandibular secretions, the more alkaline pH, a higher concentration of hydroxylapatite and phosphatase, and the anatomy of Wharton's duct.[1, 4, 22] Approximately 85% of submandibular gland calculi occur in Wharton's duct. Symptomatic parotid stones are usually located in Stensen's duct, although asymptomatic small calculi may also be found throughout the parotid gland. Most calculi can be seen on plain films, although CT has far greater sensitivity for small calcifications. Noncalcified stones are best demonstrated by sialography.

Chronic Inflammatory Diseases

Chronic Recurrent Sialadenitis

Chronic recurrent sialadenitis is recurrent painful swelling of the salivary gland that is usually associated with an incomplete ductal obstruction.[23] A stricture may be present in the main duct, and if that is treated, the gland may return to normal function. In more severe cases, saliva production is reduced and sialography demonstrates focal narrowing of the main duct, central ductal dilatation (sialectasia), and lack of visualization of the peripheral ducts and acini, which are inflamed or destroyed (Fig. 35–8). Scattered, focal collections of contrast material may be seen, representing microabscess formation (Fig. 35–9). When multiple, these collections vary in size and are distributed irregularly within the gland.[5]

Autoimmune Diseases

The autoimmune diseases share a common underlying disease process. A lymphoid infiltrate surrounds the intra-

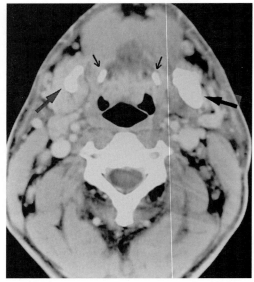

FIGURE 35–7 Sialolithiasis. Axial postcontrast CT scan reveals chunky calcification of both submandibular glands (*large arrows*) and within Wharton's duct, bilaterally (*small arrows*).

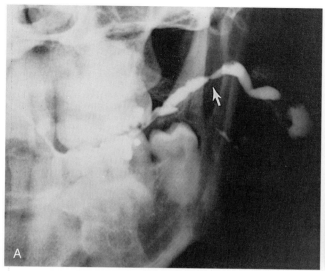
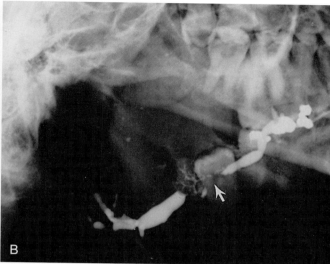

FIGURE 35–8 Sialectasia. Anteroposterior *(A)* and lateral *(B)* views from a patient with chronic sialadenitis who underwent sialography. There is irregular ductal dilatation centrally, and the peripheral ducts are not visualized. Stricture formation is noted *(arrows)*. Findings are compatible with chronic sialadenitis, sialectasia, and stricture.

lobular ducts, eventually replacing the acinar tissue and resulting in glandular atrophy. There is an associated proliferation of ductal epithelium that results in obliteration of the ductal lumen and the production of myoepithelial islands.[5, 22, 26]

Salivary or lacrimal gland enlargement, or both, on an inflammatory basis has been termed *Mikulicz's disease.* The *sicca syndrome (primary Sjögren's syndrome)* is an autoimmune disorder that is characterized by keratoconjunctivitis sicca, xerostomia (dry mouth), altered taste, dry tongue, and intermittent unilateral or bilateral salivary gland enlargement. *Secondary Sjögren's syndrome* refers to patients who have a systemic connective tissue disorder (rheumatoid arthritis, scleroderma, lupus) associated with the sicca syndrome. Over 90% of adults with Sjögren's syndrome are female[22] and are usually over 40 years of age. These patients are at increased risk for the development of non-Hodgkin's lymphoma.[2, 26]

Clinically, these patients may have recurrent acute episodes or may have glandular enlargement without pain. There may also be chronic glandular enlargement with superimposed acute exacerbation of disease.[27] Enlargement of the submandibular glands is far less common than parotid enlargement.

Sialography of patients with autoimmune disease initially reveals a normal central collecting system and numerous punctate (1 mm or less) collections of contrast material uniformly distributed throughout the gland (Fig. 35–10). These are the earliest diagnostic sialographic findings of Sjögren's syndrome.[5] These punctate collections can progress to larger, more globular collections. Superimposed infection may result, and abscess formation can occur.[5] At the end of the sialogram, a secretogogue is given to promote contrast drainage from the main ducts. However, in these patients contrast material remains within the small collections. This picture is fairly specific

FIGURE 35–9 Chronic sialadenitis. Anteroposterior *(A)* and lateral *(B)* views of a parotid sialogram reveal scattered, focal collections of contrast material with an irregular distribution within the gland.

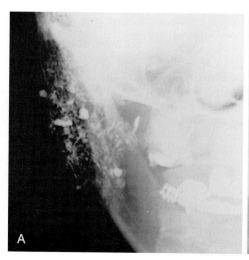
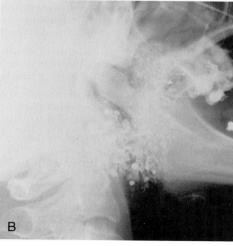

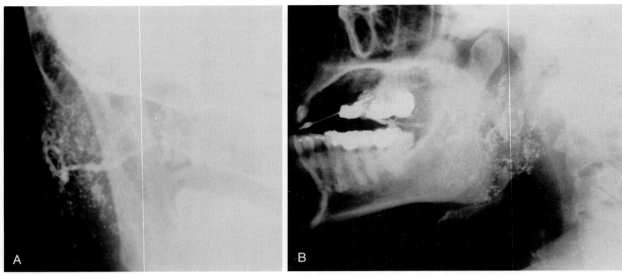

FIGURE 35–10 Sjögren's syndrome. Anteroposterior (A) and lateral (B) views from a sialogram of a patient with autoimmune disease. Note the "speckled" appearance with multiple, uniform, punctate collections of contrast material, with a homogeneous distribution throughout the gland.

for the diagnosis of autoimmune disease and distinguishes these patients from those with sialosis or chronic sialadenitis.[5]

CT imaging reveals a gland that is often enlarged and of increased attenuation, similar in appearance to that of chronic sialadenitis. The sialographic findings are, therefore, far more specific. MRI reveals an enlarged gland with a heterogeneous, speckled (honeycomb-like) appearance, seen best on T2-weighted images.[28] Others have termed this MRI pattern *salt and pepper* because of the mixed appearance of focal hypo- and hyperintensities. The hypointensities represent aggregates of lymphocytes and collagenous fibrous tissue, whereas the hyperintensities reflect dilated intraglandular ducts.[29]

Sialosis (Sialadenosis)

Sialosis denotes a nonneoplastic, noninflammatory, nontender chronic or recurrent enlargement of the parotid glands.[2, 5] The other salivary glands are only rarely involved.[22] The glandular swelling is usually bilateral and symmetric but can be unilateral or asymmetric. In some cases, diminished salivary flow is seen.[5] Sialosis is associated with a variety of endocrinopathies, metabolic disturbances, and a number of medications. Predisposing conditions include diabetes mellitus, alcoholism, chronic malnutrition, hypertension, obesity, hyperlipidemia, pregnancy, and celiac disease.[5] Pathologically, acinar hypertrophy is seen early followed by fibrosis and fatty replacement, without inflammation. Sialography reveals parotid enlargement with a fairly normal ductal system, differentiating sialosis from chronic sialadenitis and the autoimmune disorders.[5]

Radiation Sialadenitis

Postirradiation sialadenitis may occur acutely or on a more chronic basis. The chronic form is far more common and may be seen after radiation therapy for a head or neck cancer. The gland becomes atrophic, with xero-

stomia. Sialography reveals focal ductal pruning and patchy areas where there is a lack of acinar filling.[5] The acute form of radiation sialadenitis, which is associated with a single dose of 10 gy or more, is rarely seen. Within 24 hours, there is a painful swelling of the gland that subsides in 3 to 4 days. A transient xerostomia may occur.[5]

Granulomatous Diseases

A variety of granulomatous diseases may involve the salivary glands, usually arising from adjacent lymph nodes or intraparotid nodes. These include sarcoidosis, tuberculosis, syphilis, cat-scratch fever, toxoplasmosis, and actinomycosis.[22] There is usually nontender, chronic glandular enlargement that is often multinodular. The parotid glands are abnormal in 10% to 30% of patients with sarcoid. This is usually bilateral with parotid swelling and decreased salivary flow. CT or MRI may reveal multiple small lesions that represent parotid granulomas. Tuberculous infection of the salivary glands may be primary or as a result of systemic infection. Sialographic findings are similar to those of bacterial sialadenitis, and abscess formation may occur.

Salivary Gland Cysts

True cysts of the salivary glands may be congenital or acquired. The congenital cysts include branchial cleft cysts, lymphoepithelial cysts, and, rarely, dermoid cysts.[5] Although present at birth, these cysts are usually asymptomatic until much later. Clinical presentation is usually a painless mass. If infected, the cyst may become painful. The most common congenital cyst of the parotid gland is the first branchial cleft cyst. CT or MRI reveals a cystic mass that can be superficial to the parotid gland, within it, or deep to the gland (Fig. 35–11). If the cyst connects to the external auditory canal, the patient may complain of otorrhea. In the region of the submandibular gland, second branchial cleft cysts are more common. These may be detected in children when a mass is found at the

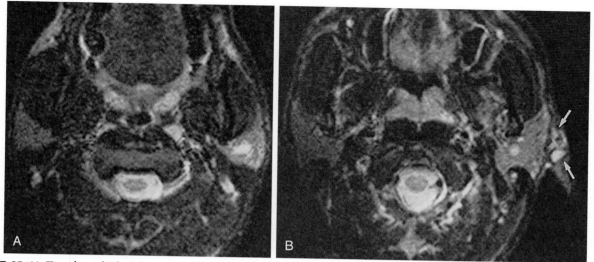

FIGURE 35–11 First branchial cleft cyst. *A*, T2-weighted axial image (2873/80) reveals a small fluid collection in the left parotid gland. *B*, A multiloculated extension *(arrows)* is seen in the overlying soft tissues, just deep and anterior to the left auricle. Surgical resection disclosed a first branchial cleft cyst.

angle of the mandible. If there is an associated sinus tract or fistula, the tract extends downward with an opening in the anterior neck, just above the clavicle, that is visible at birth. These lesions may also present in young adults. The second branchial cleft cysts are more commonly seen without associated tract or fistula. Ninety-five percent of all branchial cleft anomalies arise from a remnant of the second branchial apparatus. Normally, the second branchial cleft apparatus completely involutes by the ninth week of gestation. When involution is incomplete, the remnant tissue creates a potential for the growth of a branchial cleft anomaly.

On CT, the true cysts are sharply marginated, smooth-walled masses with a density slightly higher than that of water. The wall is thin and uniform. If the contents are very proteinaceous, the cyst has higher attenuation (Fig.

35–12). If the cyst becomes infected, the cyst wall may appear thickened and less distinct and demonstrate enhancement, simulating an abscess.[5] On MRI, typical cysts are hypointense on T1-weighted images (approaching the signal of water) and hyperintense on T2-weighted studies. Proteinaceous fluid can appear hyperintense to cerebrospinal fluid on all sequences. The second branchial cleft cyst can be seen just posterior to the submandibular gland, which is usually displaced anteromedially. The cyst is often located anterior to the sternocleidomastoid muscle and displaces the carotid artery and jugular vein posteromedially. A diagnostic clue is a "beak," which can be seen along the medial aspect of the cyst, extending between the internal and external branches of the carotid artery.

Acquired cysts usually develop as a result of incom-

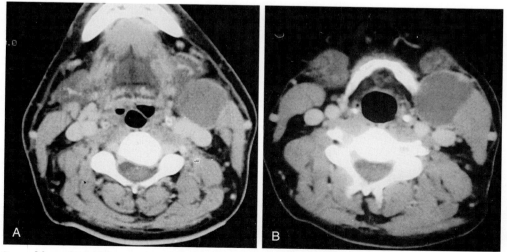

FIGURE 35–12 Second branchial cleft cyst. *A* and *B*, Axial postcontrast CT images reveal a fluid-density mass lesion adjacent to the left submandibular gland, with slight ventral displacement of the submandibular gland. This location is quite characteristic of a second branchial cleft cyst, along the anterior margin of the sternocleidomastoid muscle, anterolateral to the vascular structures. There is a slight thickening of the wall of the cyst. The cyst fluid is of greater density than water because this cyst was infected.

plete or intermittent ductal obstruction. The underlying cause may be a postinflammatory stricture, a calculus, trauma, surgery, or a mass, either benign or malignant. Acquired cysts have a layer of cuboidal, columnar, or squamous epithelium. These may also be called *mucous retention cysts* or *salivary mucoceles*.

If a duct ruptures, there is escape of mucus into the adjacent tissues and a salivary mucocele is formed. In these cases there is no epithelial lining and the mucocele is actually a pseudocyst. Usually, this is a consequence of trauma.[5] A sialocele is a focal accumulation of saliva as a result of complete or incomplete traumatic disruption of the ductal system. The sialocele may or may not communicate with the ductal system, and this communication can be demonstrated by sialography. If there is no communication, the sialocele appears as a smooth mass lesion that displaces adjacent ducts.

Lymphoepithelial cysts in patients with human immunodeficiency virus (HIV) are multiple cysts within the parotid gland and may be seen unilaterally or bilaterally. These cysts are lymphoepithelial in origin and probably arise from incomplete ductal obstruction as a result of adjacent lymphocytic infiltration or arise from cysts within parotid lymph nodes (Fig. 35–13). There is often associated lymphadenopathy. These parotid cysts may be the

first sign that the patient is HIV-seropositive and may be seen before a diagnosis of an acquired immunodeficiency disease. Although these cysts are almost always benign, a solid parotid mass in an HIV-seropositive patient should be viewed with suspicion, as there is a 40% chance of malignancy, most likely a lymphoma or Kaposi's sarcoma.[30]

Ranulas

A ranula is a mucous retention cyst occurring in the sublingual gland. A *simple ranula* remains in the floor of the mouth, above the level of the mylohyoid muscle, and has an epithelial lining. A *plunging or diving ranula* results from rupture of a simple ranula through the posterior aspect of the sublingual space into the submandibular space. This diving ranula does not have an epithelial lining and is, in reality, a pseudocyst.

A simple ranula presents as a mass in the floor of the mouth, in the region of the sublingual glands. The overlying mucosa often has a bluish coloration. On CT, it is unilocular and cystic in appearance measuring 10 to 20 HU. The cyst wall is thin and may be imperceptible. The simple ranula is lateral to the genioglossus muscle and medial to the mylohyoid muscle. On MRI, the ranula is low in signal intensity on T1-weighted images, intermediate on proton-density scans, and hyperintense on T2-

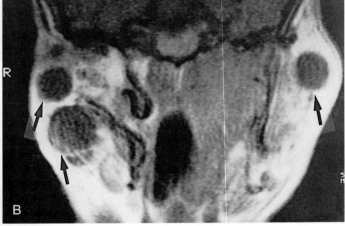

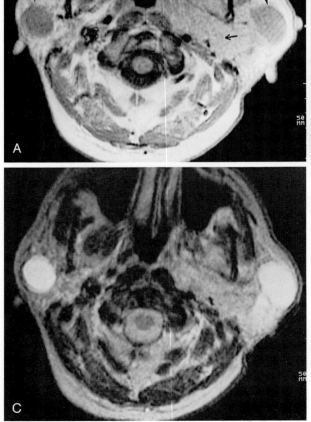

FIGURE 35–13 Lymphoepithelial cysts. This 53-year-old man was referred for imaging because of parotid enlargement. Axial *(A)* and coronal *(B)* T1-weighted (400/16) magnetic resonance imaging (MRI) studies reveal cystic lesions of both parotid glands that are hyperintense to cerebrospinal fluid *(large arrows)*. Results of biopsies performed on these were consistent with a lymphoepithelial origin. Human immunodeficiency virus infection was suspected and eventually confirmed. Also incidentally noted was a large soft tissue mass infiltrating the left parapharyngeal space and extending into the deep lobe of the parotid, with widening of the stylomandibular tunnel *(small arrow)*. Biopsy of this lesion revealed lymphoma. *C*, T2-weighted (2000/85) axial image demonstrates the hyperintense lymphoepithelial cysts. The lymphoma is of intermediate signal intensity.

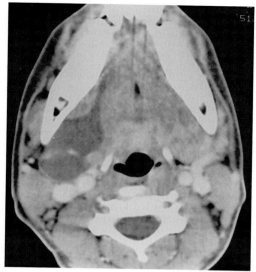

FIGURE 35–14 Diving (plunging) ranula. Axial postcontrast CT scan reveals a flask-shaped fluid-density mass on the right. The lesion involves the sublingual space anteriorly and projects posteriorly into the submandibular space, with a septation. This configuration is characteristic of a diving (or plunging) ranula.

A *pneumocele of the salivary gland* is caused by retention of air in the gland parenchyma. This is seen in patients with elevated intrabuccal pressures, such as trumpet players or glassblowers. There is retrograde insufflation of the gland via Wharton's or Stensen's duct.[31]

Tumors and Tumorlike Lesions

Most causes of salivary gland enlargement are nonneoplastic in nature. Salivary gland tumors are relatively uncommon and constitute less than 3% of all head and neck tumors.[32] Parotid tumors are by far the most common of the salivary gland neoplasms. From 75% to 80% of parotid gland tumors are benign. However, the tumors that arise in the smaller salivary glands tend to be more aggressive, and thus 40% to 50% of submandibular tumors are benign, 20% to 40% of the minor salivary gland tumors are benign, and only 15% of sublingual gland tumors are benign.[33, 34] In children, 30% to 35% of salivary tumors are malignant, which is a slightly higher percentage than that seen in adults.[1, 33] Overall, however, salivary gland tumors are uncommon in the pediatric population, with hemangioma the one most commonly encountered.

A variety of epithelial and nonepithelial tumors, as well as metastatic lesions, may arise within the salivary glands (Table 35–1). Epithelial tumors are staged using the TNM system (Table 35–2). In many cases, imaging studies are helpful in differentiating benign from malignant lesions, as well as in defining the extent of disease and any associated adenopathy. However, many low-grade malignancies cannot be reliably differentiated from benign tumors, and determination of the specific histologic type is not possible on the basis of imaging characteristics alone (with a few exceptions). Thus, fine-needle aspiration is usually performed preoperatively to establish a histologic diagnosis and to allow more complete preoperative planning. These aspirations are performed using a 22- to 25-gauge needle without significant morbidity. The larger-core needle biopsies provide a larger sample of tissue;

weighted studies. The differential diagnosis includes lymphangioma, epidermoid, and a lateral thyroglossal duct cyst. Dermoid and lipoma can be differentiated from a ranula on the basis of signal characteristics, since both dermoid and lipoma appear increased in signal intensity on T1-weighted images due to their fatty content.

A plunging ranula appears clinically as a painless mass in the submandibular triangle, with or without evidence of a mass in the floor of the mouth. The plunging ranula has a very characteristic appearance on imaging studies (Fig. 35–14). A linear collection is seen within the sublingual space, which extends posteriorly into a more rounded pseudocyst (Fig. 35–15).

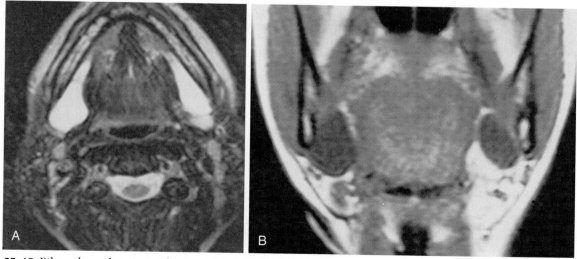

FIGURE 35–15 Bilateral ranulas. *A*, Axial T2-weighted (2500/102) MRI study reveals bilateral masses in the floor of the mouth, arising from the sublingual space with posterior extension to the submandibular space. *B*, T1-weighted (333/10) coronal view reveals the lesions to be isointense to water.

TABLE 35–1 Salivary Gland Tumors

Epithelial Tumors	Nonepithelial Tumors	Metastatic Disease
Pleomorphic adenoma Benign mixed tumor Carcinoma ex pleomorphic adenoma Monomorphic adenoma Warthin's tumor Oncocytoma Basal cell adenoma Clear cell adenoma Sebaceous lymphadenoma Adenoid cystic carcinoma Mucoepidermoid carcinoma Acinic cell carcinoma Adenocarcinoma Squamous cell carcinoma Adenosquamous carcinoma Undifferentiated carcinoma	Hemangioma Lymphangioma° Lymphoma Lipoma Neurogenic tumors Schwannoma Neurofibroma Dermoid and epidermoid	Metastases to salivary glands Metastases to intraparotid lymph nodes

°Lymphangioma is considered a vascular malformation in the classification of vascular lesions by Mulliken and Glowacki.[44]

however, they carry a small but definite risk of tumor seeding.

Epithelial Tumors

Pleomorphic Adenoma

Pleomorphic adenoma (benign mixed tumor) is the most common tumor of the salivary glands, accounting for 70% to 80% of all benign tumors occurring in the major salivary glands. Over 80% of pleomorphic adenomas arise in the parotid gland, 8% in the submandibular gland, 6.5% in the minor salivary glands, and 0.5% in the sublingual glands. Of those in the parotid gland, 90% arise lateral to the course of the facial nerve.[10, 33] The clinical presentation is that of a slow-growing, painless mass that may be several millimeters or several centimeters when detected. Women older than 40 years are more often affected. As the name implies, pleomorphic adenomas have an extremely diverse histologic pattern.

On CT, these benign mixed tumors are smoothly marginated and usually solitary, although the lesion may appear multilobulated. The larger lesions may reveal necrosis, cystic change, hemorrhage, or focal calcification.[35] This dystrophic calcification is not always present, but when it is, it is highly suggestive of pleomorphic adenoma.[5] Areas of increased attenuation within the mass are likely to represent intratumoral hemorrhage and may be associated with a sudden enlargement of the mass or localized pain, or both.

On MRI, pleomorphic adenoma is intermediate in signal on T1- and proton-density-weighted images, and intermediate to bright on T2-weighted images (Fig. 35–16). The lesion is usually heterogeneous in appearance. Focal areas of increased signal within the tumor on T2-weighted images probably represent myxoid tissue and are very typical of pleomorphic adenoma.[36] Recurrence of this tumor after surgical resection is reported to be between 1% and 50% and relates directly to the extent of the initial surgical procedure.

Three types of malignant tumors may be associated with pleomorphic adenomas: carcinoma ex pleomorphic adenoma, malignant mixed tumor, and metastasizing benign mixed tumor.[1] The malignant mixed tumor is quite rare, containing both epithelial and stromal neoplastic elements. This lesion has a poor prognosis.[5] The carci-

TABLE 35–2 Summary of TNM Staging of Salivary Gland Tumors and Cervical Lymph Nodes

Tumors (T)°

T0 = no evidence of primary tumor
T1 = tumor ≤2.0 cm in dimension
T2 = tumor >2.0 cm but ≤4.0 cm in dimension
T3 = tumor >4.0 cm but ≤6.0 cm in dimension
T4 = tumor >6.0 cm in dimension

Regional Lymph Nodes (N)

N0 = no regional lymph node metastasis
N1 = single ipsilateral metastatic lymph node ≤3 cm in dimension
N2a = single ipsilateral metastatic lymph node >3 cm in dimension but ≤6 cm in dimension
N2b = multiple ipsilateral metastatic lymph nodes, each ≤6 cm in dimension
N2c = bilateral or contralateral metastatic lymph nodes, each ≤6 cm in dimension
N3 = metastatic lymph node >6 cm in dimension

Stage Groupings

Stage I = T1a or T2a N0M0
Stage II = T1b or T2b or T3a N0M0
Stage III = T1 or T2 N1M0
    T3b or T4a N0M0
Stage IV = T4b, any N, M0
    Any T, N2 or N3, M0
    Any T, any N, M1

From the tumor, node, metastasis (TNM) staging guidelines for head and neck tumors. Used with the permission of the American Joint Committee on Cancer, Chicago, Illinois. The original source for this material is the AJCC Manual for Staging of Cancer, 4th edition (1992), published by J. B. Lippincott Company, Philadelphia.

°Additionally, the lesion is defined as (a) or (b): (a) = no local extension; (b) = local extension to skin, soft tissues, bone, or lingual or facial nerves.

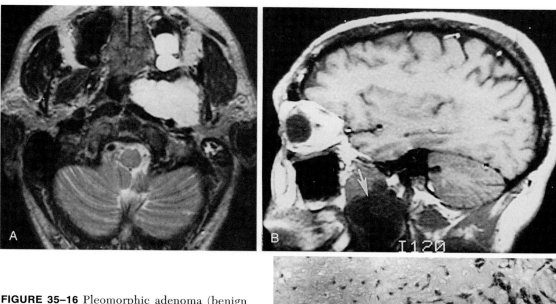

FIGURE 35–16 Pleomorphic adenoma (benign mixed tumor). *A,* A large, hyperintense mass lesion is identified in the left parapharyngeal space with extension to the deep lobe of the parotid on this T2-weighted (3600/102) axial image. Note that there is no widening of the stylomandibular tunnel. *B,* The lesion *(arrow)* is hypointense on T1-weighted images (500/11). At surgery, the lesion was found to be separate from the parotid gland, probably of minor salivary gland origin within the parapharyngeal space. The pathologic diagnosis was pleomorphic adenoma. As the name implies, pleomorphic adenomas demonstrate a diverse histologic appearance. *C,* Both stromal (upper left) and glandular (lower right) elements are apparent on this section. (H&E, ×200.)

noma ex pleomorphic adenoma arises within a benign mixed tumor. This is usually an adenocarcinoma but can be another epithelial subtype. Patients are often in their sixties and have a chronic history of a benign mixed tumor that suddenly demonstrates rapid growth. Pain and facial nerve paralysis may be present. The carcinoma ex pleomorphic adenoma is an aggressive lesion with a high rate of recurrence and a high rate of metastasis.[35] Regional lymph nodes, lung, bone, and brain are the most common sites of metastases.[34] The malignant transformation from benign mixed tumor to carcinoma is likely related to the length of time the lesion is present. It has been estimated that if all pleomorphic adenomas were left untreated, nearly 25% would undergo malignant degeneration.[35] The imaging appearance of the carcinoma ex pleomorphic adenoma is variable. The lesion may be indistinguishable from a benign mixed tumor or may resemble a benign mixed tumor with a focus that has a more aggressive appearance. Alternatively, the entire lesion may have an aggressive appearance with a necrotic center, thick, irregular walls, and infiltrating margins.[5] The metastasizing benign mixed tumor is a very rare lesion that has been described in association with pleomorphic adenoma. Although this lesion metastasizes, both the primary site and the metastases reveal no histologic evidence of malignancy.[10, 35]

Monomorphic Adenomas

Monomorphic adenomas are a group of benign neoplasms that probably arise from ductal epithelium. The presence of a uniform epithelial pattern and the absence of a chondromyxoid stroma distinguish these lesions from the more common pleomorphic adenoma.[5] The predominant tumors in this group are Warthin's tumor and oncocytoma. Also included are basal cell adenoma, clear cell adenoma, and sebaceous lymphadenoma, which are rare lesions.[10]

After benign mixed tumor, Warthin's tumor is the second most common benign neoplasm of the parotid gland, representing 5% to 10% of all parotid tumors. Unlike most salivary gland tumors, there is a male predominance of 3:1 to 5:1, and patients are older than 50 years. Facial nerve paralysis is distinctly unusual with a Warthin's tumor. Within the parotid gland, the most common site for this tumor is in the tail of the superficial lobe. It is most often a solitary lesion but can be multiple and bilateral. Multiplicity is seen in approximately 30% of cases, and

10% are bilateral.[5] Warthin's tumor is the most common parotid tumor to demonstrate multiplicity, and the most common to occur bilaterally.

On CT, Warthin's tumors are small, ovoid lesions with smooth margins in the tail of the superficial lobe of the parotid gland. These tumors often undergo cystic change. If multiple masses are seen in one parotid gland or are present bilaterally, Warthin's tumor is the most likely diagnosis. The differential diagnosis also includes lymphoma, granulomatous disease, and intraparotid adenopathy. If the multiple lesions are cystic in appearance, HIV-related lymphoepithelial cysts may also be considered in the differential diagnosis. On MRI, Warthin's tumors are low to intermediate in signal intensity on T1-weighted images (Fig. 35–17) and intermediate or mixed on T2-weighted images.[21] Cyst formation is common, and proteinaceous cysts containing cholesterol crystals may be seen as foci of increased signal intensity on the T1-weighted images. Hemorrhage may be seen as well. On T2-weighted images, Warthin's tumors may be homogeneously intermediate in signal or of mixed signal, with high-intensity foci intermixed with areas of intermediate signal intensity.[21]

Warthin's tumors are known to accumulate ^{99m}Tc pertechnetate on salivary radionuclide scans. Warthin's tumors contain oncocytes, and it is those cells that probably accumulate the radioisotope. The only other salivary gland tumor with uptake on ^{99m}Tc study is the oncocytoma.[37]

Oncocytoma consists entirely of oncocytes and most commonly occurs in the parotid gland. Oncocytes are large cells with a granular eosinophilic cytoplasm that may be seen scattered throughout normal major and minor salivary glands. These cells are rarely present in patients younger than 50 years but are commonly seen in older patients.[1, 10] The oncocytoma represents less than 1% of all salivary gland tumors. Most patients are between 55 and 70 years of age. These are slow-growing tumors that are rarely multiple. In the major salivary glands they are well encapsulated, but in the minor salivary glands there may be local invasion, despite a benign histologic appearance. Very rarely, these lesions may become malignant and even metastasize. On imaging studies, these tumors have a nonspecific appearance similar to that of a Warthin's tumor or pleomorphic adenoma. The treatment is surgical, as these lesions are radioresistant.[1, 10]

Basal cell adenomas are benign, slow-growing lesions that account for 2% of all salivary gland tumors. Most arise within the superficial lobe of the parotid gland. The mean age of these patients is 60 years. The lesions in the major salivary glands are well encapsulated, whereas those in the minor salivary glands are less commonly encapsulated.

Clear cell adenomas are rare lesions, most often found in the parotid gland. These tumors arise from the intercalated ducts of the salivary glands. Although benign, these tumors have been reported to demonstrate infiltrative growth as well as metastases, and some investigators regard these lesions as low-grade carcinomas.

Mucoepidermoid Carcinoma

Approximately 0.3% of all malignant tumors arise in salivary gland tissue. These are equally common in men and women. Of the malignant lesions arising in the minor salivary glands, those occurring in the cheek and lips have the best prognosis, whereas those occurring in the paranasal region have the worst prognosis.

Mucoepidermoid carcinoma is the most common malignancy of the parotid gland and the second most common malignancy of the submandibular gland (after adenoid cystic carcinoma). Mucoepidermoid carcinoma accounts for less than 10% of all salivary gland tumors but constitutes 30% of malignant salivary tumors. Approximately 60% of mucoepidermoid tumors arise in the parotid gland, and 30% arise from the minor salivary glands, primarily those in the palate and buccal mucosa.[10] This lesion is also the most common malignant salivary gland tumor found in children.[10, 33] Most patients are in the third to fifth decade, however.

These tumors are classified histologically as low-, intermediate-, or high-grade tumors.[38] The low-grade tumors have an excellent prognosis, with the 5-year survival rate nearly 90%. These lesions are well circumscribed although not completely encapsulated. Hemorrhage and necrosis may be seen, and these tumors often contain cystic areas. Recurrence after surgery is about 6%.[10] The recurrence rate for intermediate-grade lesions is 20%.[39]

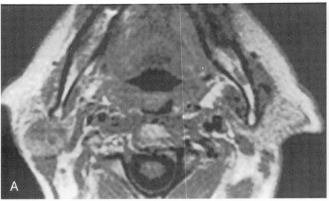 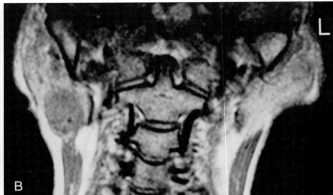

FIGURE 35–17 Warthin's tumor. Axial *(A)* and coronal *(B)* T1-weighted (550/25) MRI studies reveal a well-circumscribed mass lesion in the tail of the right parotid gland. Pathologic findings were consistent with those of Warthin's tumor.

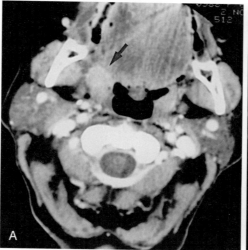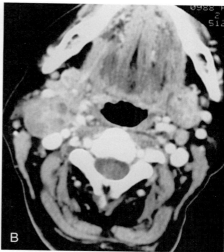

FIGURE 35-18 Mucoepidermoid carcinoma. *A,* Postcontrast axial CT scan reveals focal enhancement in the right tonsillar region *(arrow).* *B,* At a slightly more caudal level, adenopathy is identified in the right jugular chain. Surgical removal with neck dissection revealed a high-grade mucoepidermoid carcinoma arising from minor salivary glands in the tonsil. Metastatic disease to the lymph nodes was confirmed.

High-grade mucoepidermoid carcinomas have irregular, infiltrative margins. These are aggressive lesions with a 5-year survival rate of only 41.6%.[32] Metastases may be seen to lymph nodes, bone, and lung (Fig. 35–18). Surgery is the primary treatment, with radical neck dissection.[1, 10]

The imaging appearance of mucoepidermoid carcinoma varies with the histologic grade. Low-grade lesions are benign in appearance with smooth margins and cystic areas. The appearance may simulate that of a benign mixed tumor. On MRI, the lower-grade lesions tend to have areas of increased signal intensity on T2-weighted images, whereas the high-grade tumors are more cellular and less cystic, with intermediate signal intensity on both T1- and T2-weighted images (Fig. 35–19).[5]

Adenoid Cystic Carcinoma

Adenoid cystic carcinoma (cylindroma) accounts for 4% to 8% of all salivary gland tumors and is the most common malignant tumor of the submandibular and minor salivary glands. Adenoid cystic carcinoma accounts for 3% of parotid tumors, 15% of submandibular tumors, and 30% of minor salivary gland tumors. Most patients are in the fifth or sixth decade. This tumor has a high rate of recurrence but may have a slow growth rate so that prolonged survival has been reported even after metastatic disease has been documented. The 5-year survival rate is 69%, and the 15-year survival rate is 38%. The prognosis for adenoid cystic carcinoma is far worse when the site of origin is in the minor salivary glands.[10, 40]

Cyst formation and hemorrhage are rarely seen in association with these tumors. Nodal metastases are not common, but hematogenous metastases to lungs and bones may occur in 20% to 50% of cases.[10, 33]

The pathologic hallmark of adenoid cystic carcinoma is perineural invasion, which is a primary factor in the high recurrence rate of this malignancy. There may be "skip" areas, where the proximal nerve appears intact while a more distal segment of the nerve is involved. This results in great difficulty in obtaining clear surgical margins. The surgical margins may appear to be free of disease, whereas occult disease may be present along distal portions of the nerve. Perineural disease also ac-

counts for the frequent complaint of pain at clinical presentation. Prognosis relates directly to the predominant histologic pattern (tubular, cribriform, or solid).[41, 42] The degree of cellularity increases from the tubular to the solid form. With increasing cellularity, the prognosis worsens.[41] Most tumors demonstrate a mixed pattern.[20]

On imaging studies, the lesions in the parotid gland have a more benign appearance, whereas those in the minor salivary glands are more infiltrative. Extension to the skull base via the facial or mandibular nerve is not uncommon, and this region should be carefully inspected when evaluating for recurrent disease (Fig. 35–20). MRI reveals the more cellular tumors (with worse prognosis) to be low to intermediate in signal intensity on T2-weighted images, whereas less cellular tumors have increased signal intensity.[20] Approximately 20% to 25% of adenoid cystic carcinomas appear bright on T2-weighted images, whereas the remainder are low to intermediate in signal intensity.[20]

Acinic Cell Carcinoma

Acinic cell carcinoma represents only 2% to 4% of all major salivary gland tumors and occurs chiefly in the parotid gland (Fig. 35–21). This lesion is seen primarily in patients in the fifth or sixth decade but can be seen in children and is the second most common childhood parotid malignancy (after mucoepidermoid carcinoma).[43] In 3% of cases, bilateral parotid tumors may be seen.[10] This is usually a painless, slow-growing tumor and may be solid or cystic. Nodal metastases occur in 10% of patients, and distant metastases (to lung and bone) may be seen in 15%.[38]

Prognosis depends on the extent of surgical resection. Local excision of a parotid acinic cell carcinoma results in a 67% recurrence rate and a 22% mortality rate. However, total parotidectomy results in a 10% recurrence rate with survival of nearly 100%.[10]

Adenocarcinoma

Adenocarcinoma may be low or high grade and can arise in major or minor salivary glands. These tumors constitute 2% to 4% of all parotid neoplasms and 20% of minor

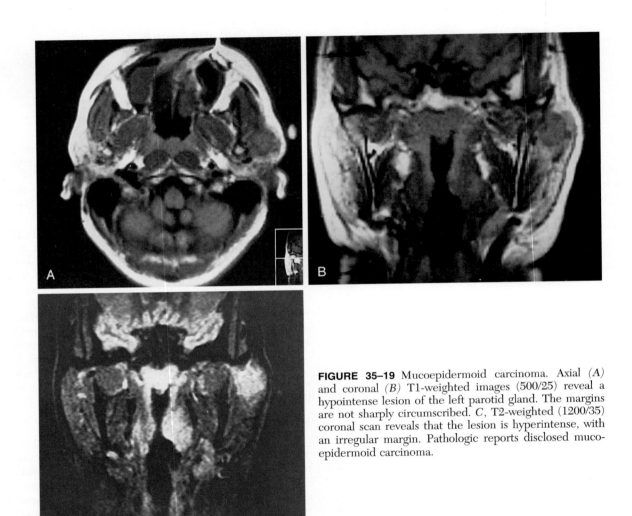

FIGURE 35–19 Mucoepidermoid carcinoma. Axial *(A)* and coronal *(B)* T1-weighted images (500/25) reveal a hypointense lesion of the left parotid gland. The margins are not sharply circumscribed. *C*, T2-weighted (1200/35) coronal scan reveals that the lesion is hyperintense, with an irregular margin. Pathologic reports disclosed mucoepidermoid carcinoma.

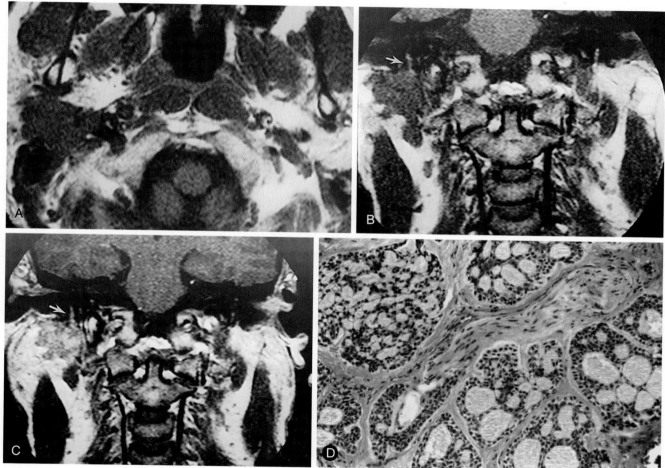

FIGURE 35–20 Adenoid cystic carcinoma. *A*, T1-weighted (700/20) axial MRI section reveals a hypointense mass lesion of the right parotid gland, involving portions of both the superficial and the deep lobes of the parotid. Posteriorly, there is extension toward the skull base in the region of the stylomastoid canal. *B*, T1-weighted coronal (700/20) image again reveals a poorly circumscribed hypointense lesion with ill-defined margins. There is evidence of perineural spread along the facial nerve within the stylomastoid canal (*arrow*). *C*, Postcontrast T1-weighted coronal image (700/20) reveals enhancement of the parotid lesion and of the perineural extension (*arrow*). *D*, High-power view from a different patient with perineural growth of adenoid cystic carcinoma demonstrates the nerve coursing obliquely across the field. Surrounding the nerve is the glandular formation of adenoid cystic carcinoma with perineural infiltration. (H&E, ×200.)

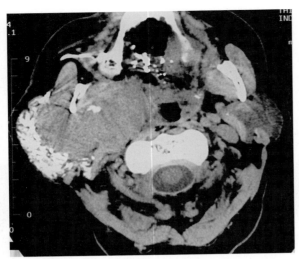

FIGURE 35–21 Acinic cell tumor. Postsialography CT scan reveals lateral displacement of the normal glandular tissue due to a large mass arising from the deep lobe of the parotid. The mass effaces the parapharyngeal fat. Note widening of the stylomandibular tunnel. The course of Stensen's duct is also well demonstrated.

salivary gland tumors. The prognosis is poor for the high-grade lesions, with a 5-year survival rate of 46%, but only 15% are disease-free at 5 years.[1]

Squamous Cell Carcinoma

Although squamous epithelium is not ordinarily a component of the salivary glands, chronic inflammation can result in squamous metaplasia. Primary squamous cell carcinoma arises from this squamous metaplasia and accounts for less than 0.5% of all parotid tumors and 3% of submandibular gland neoplasms.[5] Patients are usually in the sixth or seventh decade and most often male. Facial paralysis is common. These tumors show rapid growth and local infiltration. Metastases to regional nodes, lung, and liver may be seen, and nodal metastases are present in 47% of cases. The 5-year cure rate is 30%.[10] The imaging appearance is that of an infiltrative tumor that is hypointense on T1-weighted images and hypo-, iso-, or hyperintense on T2-weighted images.[18]

Adenosquamous Carcinoma

Adenosquamous carcinoma is a rare lesion, occurring almost exclusively in the minor salivary glands. It is a highly aggressive tumor, with 80% of patients developing regional nodal or distant metastases or both. The 5-year survival rate is 25%.

Nonepithelial Tumors and Vascular Lesions

Nonepithelial salivary gland tumors account for less than 5% of all salivary gland neoplasms and include lipoma, lymphoma, and the neurogenic tumors. Hemangioma and lymphangioma are also included in this group by some authors; however, others classify these vascular lesions differently.[44]

Vascular Lesions

A currently accepted classification scheme for vascular lesions is that of Mulliken and Glowacki.[44] It separates vascular malformations (capillary, venous, arterial, lymphatic, or combined) from vascular tumors, specifically the hemangioma of infancy. *Vascular malformations* are present at birth, grow proportionately with the patient, do not involute, and may involve bone. They may not be clinically evident until late infancy or childhood. *Capillary, venous,* and *lymphatic malformations* of the head and neck are considered "low-flow" lesions. *Venous malformations* (often termed "cavernous hemangiomas") are predominantly solid soft tissue masses that may be superficial and well defined or may infiltrate deeply across fascial planes. They have features in common with lymphaticohemangiomas and lymphangiomas.[45] Venous malformations have intermediate signal intensity on T1-weighted images, heterogeneous high signal intensity on T2-weighted images, and homogeneous or mildly heterogeneous, prominent enhancement on postgadolinium T1-weighted images. More specific features that may be present on T2-weighted images are discrete areas of homogeneous increased signal representing venous lakes and punctate low signal representing phleboliths.[46] "Flow voids" on conventional spin-echo images and flow-related enhancement on motion-compensated gradient-echo images are generally absent.

In contrast to vascular malformations, the *hemangioma of infancy* usually appears in the first 3 months of life. It rapidly enlarges (proliferative stage) and then begins to involute at approximately 12 months of age. Involution can be expected to occur in over 95% of patients and is usually completed by 7 years of age. It is composed of masses of endothelial cells whose histologic appearance varies as the tumor grows and then regresses. Angiographically, there is an organized pattern of arterial supply with venous drainage via dilated superficial veins that empty into normal veins; however, arteriovenous shunt formation can occur. During the proliferative phase, the hemangioma is a mass with "high-flow" arterial and venous components manifested as flow voids on conventional spin-echo images (Fig. 35–22) and flow-related enhancement on motion-compensated gradient-echo images (e.g., time-of-flight MR angiography). Involuted hemangiomas with low-flow characteristics may resemble venous malformations on MRI studies.[45, 46] Both types of vascular lesions demonstrate intense enhancement on postcontrast CT.

Hemangioma of the parotid gland is the most common salivary gland tumor seen in children,[1, 10] accounting for over 50% of all pediatric salivary gland tumors (Fig. 35–23). This lesion is far more common in girls. It is soft and compressible and often multilobulated in appearance. A bluish coloration may be seen in the overlying skin, and there may be an associated cutaneous hemangioma.

Lymphangiomas are considered vascular malformations by Mulliken and Glowacki.[44] Lymphangiomas have traditionally been classified as capillary, cavernous, or cystic. *Cystic lymphangiomas*, called *cystic hygromas*, are composed of cysts ranging in size from a few millimeters to several centimeters. Because all three histologic types may present in one lesion, the dominant type determines classification. Most lymphangiomas occur in early childhood, with 50% to 60% present at birth and 80% to 90% detected by 2 years of age. Lymphangiomas account for

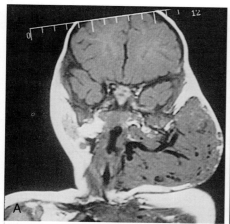
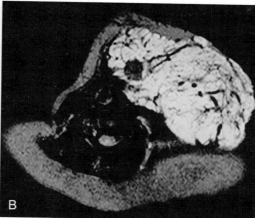
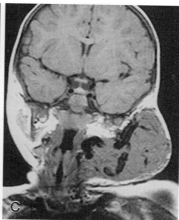

FIGURE 35–22 Hemangioma of infancy. This 7-month-old infant had a left face-neck mass that had been present since birth. *A*, T1-weighted coronal image reveals multiple signal voids within the lesion, consistent with a highly vascular mass. *B*, On T2-weighted (3000/80) images, the lesion is markedly hyperintense, quite extensive, and again reveals numerous signal voids, representing prominent vasculature. *C*, Repeat MRI study 1 year later, after treatment with steroids and interferon, reveals significant regression of the mass.

5% to 6% of all benign tumors of infancy and childhood.[47] The most common location for a lymphangioma in an infant is the posterior triangle of the neck and superior mediastinum. In adults, it is more commonly identified in the submandibular, parotid, and sublingual spaces.

Cystic hygromas are typically asymptomatic, compressible soft tissue masses, but they may encroach on the laryngopharynx, causing dyspnea, or undergo a rapid increase in size owing to infection or hemorrhage. Cystic hygromas tend to insinuate themselves between structures. Large hygromas can traverse fascial planes.

On CT, cystic hygromas appear as multilocular, thin-walled, nonenhancing masses of low (water) density (Fig. 35–24). With infection, there is thickening and enhancement of the walls of the cysts. The signal characteristics of the fluid within cystic hygromas on T1- and T2-weighted MRI images are similar to those of cerebrospinal fluid, unless hemorrhage or infection is present. T2-weighted images may show the relatively low intensity septations within larger hygromas.

Lymphoma

The salivary glands are a very rare site for primary lymphoma. Secondary involvement may occur, but it is also unusual. The salivary glands are secondarily involved by lymphoma in 1% to 8% of all cases of lymphoma. In 80% of cases in which the salivary glands are affected, the parotid gland is the site involved. Both Hodgkin's and non-Hodgkin's lymphomas have been reported.[33]

The most common imaging appearance is due to involvement of intraparotid lymph nodes. One or more benign-appearing, homogeneous masses are seen within the gland. Extraparotid nodal disease may also be seen and can aid in the diagnosis. These nodes tend to be large

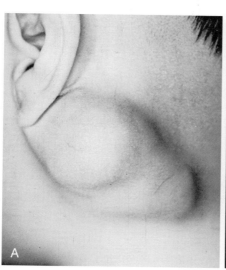
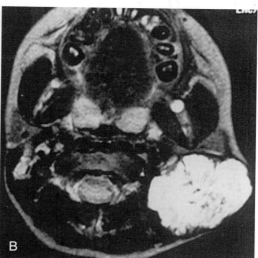

FIGURE 35–23 Hemangioma. *A*, Oblique view of this older child reveals a lobulated mass posterior and inferior to the auricle. Note the small vascular markings on the skin surface. *B*, T2-weighted axial MRI study reveals the lesion to be markedly hyperintense with central flow voids suggestive of a vascular lesion.

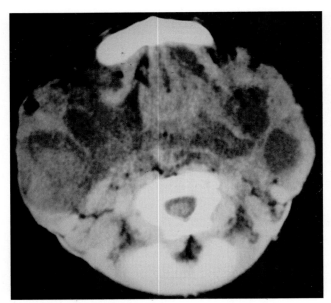

FIGURE 35–24 Lymphangioma (cystic hygroma). Axial CT scan obtained through the floor of the mouth reveals an extensive bilateral multilobulated cystic lesion consistent with cystic hygroma.

and multiple and are very homogeneous in appearance. A less common pattern of lymphomatous involvement is diffuse infiltration of the gland. On MRI, lymphoma tends to be intermediate in signal on all sequences (Fig. 35–25). Disease involvement by Hodgkin's disease may be less homogeneous.[48]

Lipomas

Lipomas account for 1% of parotid gland tumors. These lesions are homogeneous in appearance with very low density (-65 to -125 HU) and are usually well circumscribed. On MRI, there is high signal intensity on T1-weighted images and decreased signal intensity on T2-weighted studies. Hemorrhage and fibrotic changes can occur and may cause a focus of increased attenuation. If

these changes are dominant, the possibility of a liposarcoma should be considered.

Neurogenic Tumors

The neurogenic tumors include neuromas (schwannomas) and neurofibromas. These are usually well-circumscribed masses arising from the facial nerve or its branches. Schwannomas are solitary, whereas neurofibromas may be multiple and may be seen in association with other stigmata of neurofibromatosis. These neurogenic tumors can be cystic in appearance and usually enhance. On CT, the neurofibromas can demonstrate a very low attenuation, simulating a lipoma.

Dermoid or Epidermoid

Dermoid or epidermoid of the salivary glands usually presents as a slow-growing mass beneath the oral tongue. Epidermoids are more often associated with the sublingual gland, whereas dermoids more often involve the submandibular gland. If lined by a simple squamous epithelium, the mass is considered an epidermoid. A dermoid contains, in addition to the epithelial lining, a variable number of skin appendages.

On imaging these are unilocular masses. Epidermoids have fluid density on CT and are close to water signal intensity on MRI. Dermoids may be of mixed density (or intensity) or may have a fatty appearance (very low density on CT, high intensity on T1-weighted MR images, and low intensity on T2-weighted images).

Metastatic Disease

Of the major salivary glands, the parotid is the most frequently affected by metastatic disease (Fig. 35–26). This is due primarily to the presence of lymph nodes within the parotid gland. The nodes drain the scalp, face, and external ear. Consequently, melanoma of the scalp is a common lesion to metastasize to these nodes. Squamous cell carcinoma of the oral cavity, pharynx, ear, and paranasal sinuses may also metastasize to these intraparotid nodes. If a fine-needle aspiration reveals squamous cell carcinoma or melanoma, very careful inspection of the scalp and external auditory canal is warranted. Metastases

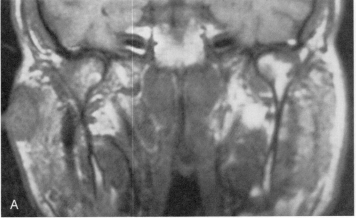
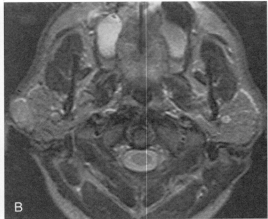

FIGURE 35–25 Lymphoma. *A,* T1-weighted (700/20) coronal MRI study reveals a nodular lesion along the lateral margin of the parotid gland. *B,* The lesion is intermediate in signal intensity on T2-weighted (2200/80) images. Biopsy revealed lymphoma.

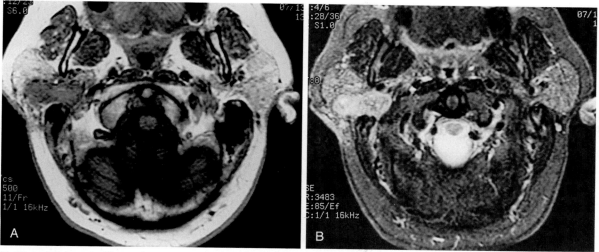

FIGURE 35–26 Malignant fibrous histiocytoma. *A*, T1-weighted (500/11) axial MRI study reveals a dumbbell-shaped lesion of the right parotid, involving superficial and deep lobes. *B*, T2-weighted (3483/85) scan demonstrates the lesion to be hyperintense. Histopathologic studies revealed malignant fibrous histiocytoma.

to the parotid from distant sites have also been reported, including lung, breast, renal cell, and gastrointestinal carcinomas (Fig. 35–27).[10, 32, 49]

Prognosis and Treatment

The single most important prognostic factor is the stage of the salivary gland tumor at presentation. The second most important determinant of prognosis is the grade of the tumor. Facial nerve paralysis is a poor prognostic sign.

Benign tumors limited to the superficial parotid can be removed with a superficial parotidectomy. Subtotal or total parotidectomy is necessary for most malignant lesions as well as for benign lesions involving superficial and deep lobes of the parotid. Facial nerve sacrifice

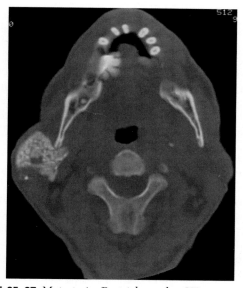

FIGURE 35–27 Metastasis. Postsialography CT scan reveals an irregular filling defect in the posterior aspect of the right parotid gland. Further investigation revealed a metastatic lesion from a neuroendocrine tumor elsewhere in the head-neck region.

becomes necessary if a malignancy involves the nerve. Submandibular gland tumors are treated by resection of the gland, and adjacent structures may also be removed in order to achieve clear margins. Minor salivary gland tumors are primarily treated surgically, and the site of origin and the extent of disease determines the particular type of resection required.

A clear survival advantage for combined surgery and radiation therapy at 5 and 10 years has been determined when removal is incomplete.[50] Postoperative radiotherapy is usually employed for intermediate- and high-grade mucoepidermoid carcinoma, malignant mixed tumors, adenocarcinoma, high-grade acinic cell carcinoma, all squamous cell carcinomas, cases in which clear margins were not achieved, and any malignant tumor stage II or greater.[51, 52]

Conclusion

Although sialography is now performed infrequently, it is indicated in the evaluation of a patient with recurrent parotid swelling. Dilatation of Stensen's duct and the central ducts suggests sialadenitis with or without obstruction. CT may be helpful to visualize calculi. Scattered, irregular collections of contrast material on sialography suggest abscess formation, whereas punctate collections, uniform in size and distribution, suggest autoimmune disease.

A well-circumscribed, homogeneous mass lesion within the salivary gland suggests a benign cause, whereas an irregular mass with infiltrative margins and areas of necrosis is highly suspicious for malignancy. On T2-weighted MRI images, malignant lesions demonstrate a varied appearance, ranging from hypo- to hyperintense. Benign lesions, such as pleomorphic adenomas, are usually hyperintense, but Warthin's tumors are intermediate or mixed in signal intensity. The absolute histologic type is very difficult to predict on the basis of imaging alone, although a reasonable differential diagnosis can be constructed.

The goal of salivary gland imaging is to accurately describe the location and extent of the lesion and the presence or absence of adenopathy, rather than to predict the specific histologic type. In most cases, a preoperative fine-needle aspiration provides a specific histologic diagnosis. Multiple masses suggest Warthin's tumor, acinic cell tumors, lymphoma, metastases, or granulomatous disease. Multiple cystic parotid masses, especially in association with nasopharyngeal lymphoid hyperplasia and cervical adenopathy, suggest that the patient may be HIV-seropositive. Calcification within a mass suggests a pleomorphic adenoma or, less commonly, a mucoepidermoid carcinoma.

CERVICAL LYMPH NODES

There are approximately 300 cervical lymph nodes, and these are divided into 5 to 10 major groups depending on the classification system.[53] Lymph flows to each group from the salivary glands and visceral structures, from somatic areas, or from other nodal groups, and drains into an adjacent group or groups or into neck veins. In filtering the lymph, the nodes may become the depository of pathologic substrates such as metastatic or infected cells. Identification of these abnormal nodes on physical examination or on imaging studies, combined with a knowledge of the drainage patterns, is important for diagnosis and prognosis.[54]

Anatomy: Lymph Node Groups

Cervical nodes are classified into groups based primarily on the work of Rouvière.[55] Modification of this older classification[53, 56] has resulted in a clinicoanatomic-level system (Figs. 35–28 and 35–29; see also later discussion) that has become the standard for reporting of nodal disease. Rouvière proposed 10 major lymph node groups: occipital, mastoid, facial, retropharyngeal, submandibular, sublingual, submental, parotid, anterior cervical, and lateral cervical. Each of the first several groups listed normally has fewer than 5 to 10 nodes for each side of the neck. The facial nodes follow the course of the external maxillary artery and the anterior facial vein in the subcutaneous tissues of the face. The retropharyngeal nodes are divided into medial and lateral subgroups. The lateral retropharyngeal nodes can extend the entire length of the pharynx. They are located anteromedial to the internal carotid artery and are often enlarged in infants and children (Fig. 35–30). There are only one or two medial retropharyngeal nodes. These are located near the midline, usually in the nasopharynx at the level of C2. The submandibular (or submaxillary) nodes are located within the submandibular space[57] and are typically anterior or lateral to the submandibular gland (Fig. 35–31). The sublingual lymph nodes, or nodules,[53] are divided into two groups: one medial to the ipsilateral genioglossus muscle and one lateral to it. The lateral group is situated along the anterior lingual vessels in the sublingual space.[57] The submental nodes are situated between the anterior bellies of the digastric muscles and superficial to the mylohyoid muscle, in the submental triangle (Fig. 35–31).

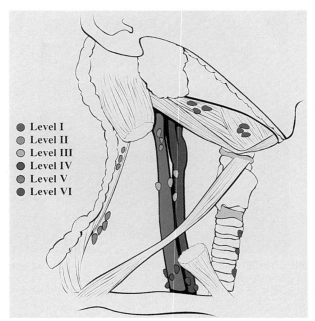

- Level I
- Level II
- Level III
- Level IV
- Level V
- Level VI

FIGURE 35–28 Clinicoanatomic classification of lymph node groups into levels (see text). Level I, submental-submandibular groups. Levels II, III, and IV, upper, middle, and lower internal jugular groups, respectively. Level V, posterior triangle (spinal accessory) group. Level VI, anterior compartment (juxtavisceral) group. (From Wester DJ, Whiteman MLH, Singer S, et al. Imaging of the postoperative neck with emphasis on surgical flaps and their complications. AJR 1995;164:989–993.)

Up to approximately 20 nodes may be located within the parotid gland (intraglandular) or superficial to it.[53]

The anterior and lateral cervical groups in Rouvière's classification may be subdivided into chains of nodes that have classical names based on adjacent structures. Thus, the anterior cervical group, located between the two carotid sheaths in the infrahyoid neck, is composed of the anterior jugular chain (1 to 4 nodes), which follows the course of the anterior jugular vein in the superficial fascia overlying the strap muscles, and the juxtavisceral chain (6 to 16 nodes) in the visceral space (see Fig. 35–29).[58, 59] From superior to inferior, the juxtavisceral chain consists of prelaryngeal, perithyroidal, pre-/paratracheal, and tracheoesophageal nodes (Fig. 35–32). The Delphian node is the prelaryngeal node that is situated on the cricothyroid membrane and receives lymph from the infraglottic larynx.

The lateral cervical group, encompassing both the suprahyoid and infrahyoid neck, is composed of deep and superficial chains.[53] The superficial chain (1 to 4 nodes) is superficial to the sternocleidomastoid muscle and follows the course of the external jugular vein (see Fig. 35–31). There are several deep chains: internal jugular (15 to 40 nodes), spinal accessory (4 to 20 nodes), and transverse cervical (or supraclavicular, 1 to 10 nodes). The internal jugular nodes lie close to the internal jugular vein, from its junction with the posterior belly of the digastric muscle superiorly to the level of the clavicle inferiorly (see Fig. 35–31). Compared with adjacent internal jugular nodes, two nodes are usually larger: the jugu-

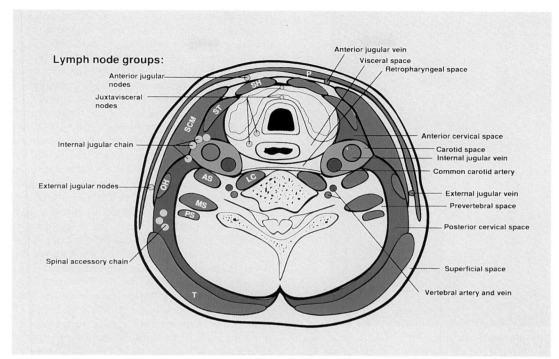

FIGURE 35–29 Schematic axial diagram of the infrahyoid neck at the level of the thyroid gland. The major lymph node groups, indicated on the left, correspond to lymph node levels: IV (infraomohyoid, or infracricoid, internal jugular chain), V (spinal accessory chain), VI (juxtavisceral nodes). The fascial spaces, indicated on the right, are bordered by layers (*darker lines*) of the deep cervical fascia, except for the superficial space, which has an outer margin formed by the superficial cervical fascia. The abbreviations for muscles are platysma (P), sternohyoid (SH), sternothyroid (ST), sternocleidomastoid (SCM), inferior belly of the omohyoid (OH), anterior scalene (AS), middle scalene (MS), posterior scalene (PS), longus colli (LC), and trapezius (T). (Adapted from Bowen BC. Brachial plexus and lower neck masses. In Ramsey RG [syllabus ed]. Core Curriculum Course in Neuroradiology, p. 182. Chicago, American Society of Neuroradiology, 1994. © by American Society of Neuroradiology.)

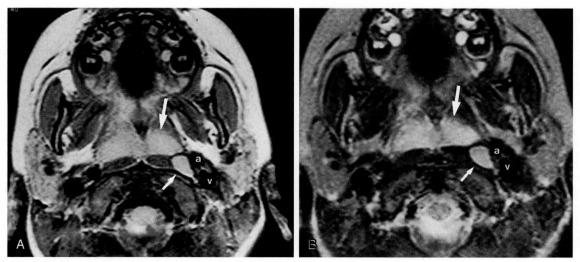

FIGURE 35–30 Retropharyngeal lymph node. Proton density (*A*) and T2-weighted (*B*) axial MRI studies demonstrate a uniformly hyperintense lateral retropharyngeal lymph node (*short arrows*) located anteromedial to the internal carotid artery (a) and internal jugular vein (v). The soft palate (*long arrows*), containing lymphoid tissue, also demonstrates normal hyperintense signal.

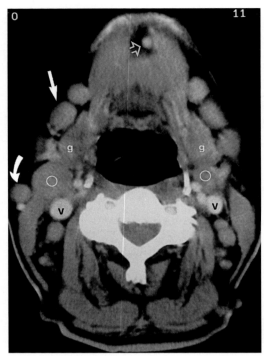

FIGURE 35–31 Submandibular-submental (level I) and upper internal jugular (level II) lymph nodes in a patient with non-Hodgkin's lymphoma. Postcontrast CT scan demonstrates bilateral homogeneous, nonenhancing nodes. The submandibular nodes are located anterior and lateral to the submandibular glands (g), and the internal jugular nodes (*open circles*) are anterior to the internal jugular vein (v). The nodes posterior to the vein at this level are part of the internal jugular or spinal accessory chains, or both. The largest submandibular node (*closed arrow*) measures 1.7 cm in greatest axial diameter. A single left submental node (*open arrow*) is present. An external jugular node (*curved arrow*) is also shown.

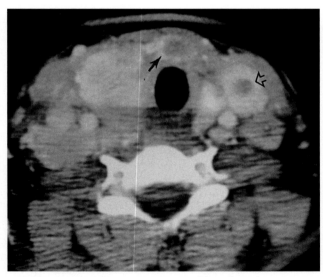

FIGURE 35–32 Metastatic juxtavisceral lymph node. Metastatic nodes with central hypodensity (necrosis) and peripheral enhancement are present at level VI (pretracheal group, *closed arrow*) and level IV (internal jugular group, *open arrow*). The primary tumor was a papillary thyroid carcinoma.

lodigastric node (Fig. 35–33), situated at the junction of the internal jugular vein and the posterior belly of the digastric; and the jugulo-omohyoid node at the junction of the internal jugular vein and omohyoid muscle (approximately the level of the cricoid cartilage). The supraomohyoid internal jugular nodes, that is, those above the jugulo-omohyoid junction, lie predominantly anterolateral to the internal jugular vein. The infraomohyoid nodes are found either anterior, posterior, or lateral to it (see Fig. 35–29).[53] When the highest of the supraomohyoid internal jugular nodes are located posterior to the vein, they are inseparable from the highest nodes of the spinal accessory (or posterior triangle) chain (see Fig. 35–31).

The spinal accessory chain follows the oblique course of the spinal accessory nerve in the posterior triangle, or posterior cervical space.[58, 59] The nerve and accompanying nodes lie on the levator scapulae muscle, and posteroinferiorly they course beneath the trapezius muscle. Thus, they have a more posterolateral location inferiorly in the neck, distinguishing them from the internal jugular nodes located deep to the sternocleidomastoid muscle (Fig. 35–34; see also Fig. 35–29). In the supraclavicular region the spinal accessory nodes blend with the transverse cervical nodes. The transverse cervical chain (Fig. 35–35) follows the transverse cervical vessels, running posterolaterally in front of the anterior scalene muscle and brachial plexus across the base of the posterior triangle to course beneath the trapezius muscle.

Clinicoanatomic Classification

Lymph Node Levels

A simplified classification based on the anatomic location of clinically palpable nodes, which drain most of the primary sites for head and neck cancers, is commonly used today to describe nodal disease (see Figs. 35–28 and 35–29).[60] In this classification, regional lymph nodes are described by levels, which are related to anatomic landmarks identifiable clinically and on imaging studies. There are six[56] or seven[53] levels, designated by Roman numerals:

I = submental and submandibular nodes

II = upper internal jugular chain, from the skull base (jugulodigastric region) to the hyoid bone (clinical and imaging landmark) or carotid bifurcation (surgical landmark)

III = middle internal jugular chain, from the hyoid bone to the cricoid cartilage (clinical and imaging landmark) or omohyoid muscle (surgical landmark)

IV = lower internal jugular chain, from the cricoid cartilage to the clavicle

V = posterior triangle nodes, primarily the lower half of the spinal accessory chain and transverse cervical nodes

VI = nodes within the visceral space (see Fig. 35–29), or anterior compartment,[62] from the hyoid bone to the suprasternal notch, including the precricoid, perithyroidal, and paratracheal nodes, as well as those along the course of the recurrent laryngeal nerve;[56] or alternatively, nodes related to the thyroid gland[53]

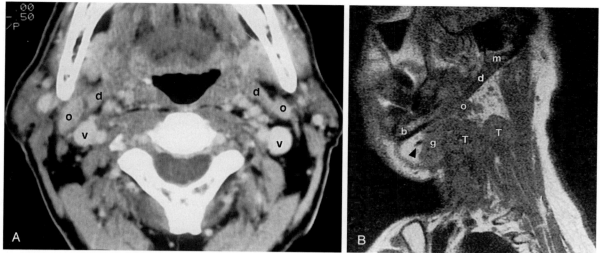

FIGURE 35–33 Jugulodigastric lymph node relative to the posterior belly of the digastric muscle. *A*, Postcontrast CT scan demonstrates bilateral, enhancing jugulodigastric nodes in a 58-year-old man with anaplastic carcinoma of the thyroid metastatic to regional lymphatics. The digastric muscles (d) have already crossed the internal jugular veins (v) and now lie anterior to the veins and anteromedial to the jugulodigastric nodes (o) in axial section. The right jugulodigastric node measures 2 cm in greatest axial diameter. *B*, Left parasagittal, T1-weighted MRI study in a different patient. The posterior belly of the digastric muscle (d) inserts on the medial aspect of the mastoid process (m) and courses anteriorly and inferomedially toward the hyoid bone (low-signal focus indicated by *arrowhead*). The digastric lies primarily superior to the jugulodigastric node (o) in this section. The patient has extensive metastatic tumor (T) from a previously treated papillary carcinoma of the thyroid. Submandibular gland (g). The cortical bone of the body of the mandible (b) has low signal intensity.

VII = nodes in the tracheoesophageal groove and para-esophageal region extending down to the superior mediastinium[53, 61]

This level system has several advantages over previous nonstandardized classification systems. First, since the regional lymphatics at each level constitute a drainage pathway for certain primary tumor sites, the detection of abnormal nodes at a given level on CT or MRI may suggest the most likely primary site in a patient with a clinically inapparent primary cancer.[60] Second, use of the level system has led to a uniform nomenclature for neck

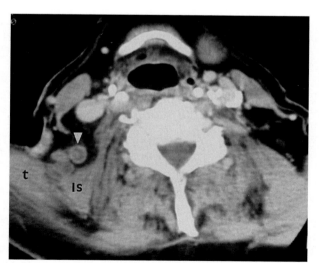

FIGURE 35–34 Posterior triangle (spinal accessory) lymph nodes. A cluster of four nodes is seen with the largest (*arrowhead*) measuring 1.1 cm maximally and demonstrating partial necrosis. These are biopsy-proven metastatic nodes from a primary renal cell carcinoma. The trapezius (t) and levator scapulae (ls) muscles are indicated. Skin enhancement is due to recent open biopsy of nearby nodes.

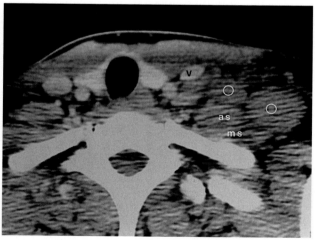

FIGURE 35–35 Transverse cervical lymph nodes. Two homogeneous, nonenhancing nodes (*open circles*) located anterior and lateral to the left anterior scalene (as) and middle scalene (ms) muscles in a 30-year-old woman with Hodgkin's disease. The largest node measures 3 cm in greatest axial diameter at the level of the T1 vertebra. Posterior to the left internal jugular vein (v) is a smaller internal jugular node (level IV).

dissection procedures.[56] Third, this system provides a common language for nodal disease that can be used by both surgeons and radiologists.

Nodal Levels and Primary Malignancy

The patterns of dissemination of epithelial cancers of the upper aerodigestive tract have been summarized by Som[53] and Mancuso,[62] and more recently by Shah and Lydiatt.[60] The most frequent sites of primary tumors that drain into the nodes at each level include

1. Level I, submental nodes — lower lip, floor of mouth, and anterior gingiva
   Level I, submandibular nodes — face, nose, paranasal sinuses, oral cavity, and submandibular gland
2. Level II nodes — oral cavity, oropharynx, nasopharynx, hypopharynx, and supraglottic larynx
3. Level III nodes — thyroid, larynx, hypopharynx, and cervical esophagus
4. Level IV nodes — thyroid, esophagus, breast, lung, and intra-abdominal organs
5. Level V nodes — nasopharynx, thyroid, esophagus, breast, and lung
6. Level VI and VII nodes — thyroid, larynx, and lung

Nasopharyngeal carcinoma is associated with the highest percentage (86% to 90%) of patients presenting initially with metastases, and also the highest percentage (33%) of patients with bilateral metastatic nodes.[53] The retropharyngeal, sublingual, and parotid nodal groups are not included in the level system. The retropharyngeal nodes receive lymphatic drainage from the nasal fossae, paranasal sinuses, oro- or nasopharynx, palate, and middle ear, and drain into the level II and III internal jugular nodes. The sublingual nodes receive drainage from the tongue and floor of the mouth and drain into the level I, II, and III nodes. The parotid nodes receive drainage from the skin of the face and periauricular region as well as the posterior gingiva, buccal space, and parotid gland itself. These nodes drain into upper internal jugular (level II) and external jugular nodes.

Nodal Levels and Neck Dissection

The nomenclature for neck dissection[56] that uses the lymph node level system is as follows:

1. Radical neck dissection — removal of all lymph nodes from levels I through V. The spinal accessory nerve, internal jugular vein, and sternocleidomastoid muscle are also removed. It does not include removal of occipital, buccal, retropharyngeal, paratracheal, and periparotid nodes (except infraparotid nodes located posteriorly in the submandibular triangle).
2. Modified radical neck dissection — removal of all lymph nodes from levels I through V, with preservation of spinal accessory nerve, internal jugular vein, and sternocleidomastoid muscle or some of these.
3. Selective neck dissection
   (a) Supraomohyoid neck dissection — removal of level I through III nodes.
   (b) Posterolateral neck dissection — removal of level II through V nodes, as well as occipital and retro-auricular nodes. This procedure is mostly used

in the treatment of cutaneous melanoma of the posterior scalp and neck.
   (c) Lateral neck dissection — removal of level II through IV nodes.
   (d) Anterior compartment neck dissection — removal of level VI nodes, including the Delphian node. This procedure is frequently indicated for treatment of thyroid cancer.
4. Extended radical neck dissection — removal of one or more lymph node groups or nonlymphatic structure(s) not included in the radical neck dissection or both. The additional lymph node groups include parapharyngeal, superior mediastinal, and paratracheal.

Using the level system, the location of recurrent disease in the postoperative neck may be related to the preserved or resected nodal groups.[63]

Imaging

Patients presenting with a neck mass of uncertain cause usually undergo CT first since it is considered superior to MRI in the evaluation of cervical metastatic disease (see later). For conventional CT of the neck, 3- to 4-mm-thick axial sections are obtained from the skull base (level of external auditory canal) to the thoracic inlet (level of manubrium), and a bolus-drip technique for intravenous contrast infusion is used. If the mass is suprahyoid, the suprahyoid CT sections are contiguous and the infrahyoid sections are separated by a gap of 1 to 2 mm (or are thicker). If the mass is infrahyoid, then the infrahyoid CT sections are contiguous and the suprahyoid sections separated by a gap. Vascularity of a lesion may be assessed with rapid-sequence (dynamic CT) scanning during a bolus infusion of contrast material. The attenuation-time curve for the lesion can help in distinguishing a hypervascular mass (such as paraganglioma, with an arterial pattern of enhancement) from a minimally vascular nodal mass.[64] Preliminary studies suggest that spiral CT is comparable to conventional CT in the evaluation of head and neck lesions.[65] Although spiral scans have more noise (quantum mottle) than conventional scans, motion artifact is minimal and less contrast medium is required.

MRI of the neck in a patient with nodal disease is typically performed using a circumferential, volume radiofrequency coil. Preliminary studies have shown that multiple overlapping surface coils, which use phase-array technology and follow the curvature of the lateral neck, allow detailed (in-plane resolution of 0.3 × 0.3 mm) images of the soft tissues and vessels of the carotid space to be obtained.[66] In studies using conventional spin-echo sequences, T1-weighted and T2-weighted axial images are usually obtained, supplemented with T1-weighted or T2-weighted coronal images or both. Sagittal images are reserved for preliminary localization and midline lesions. The utility of gadolinium enhancement can vary with the degree of vascularity and the location of a nodal lesion. Enhancement may decrease visibility of a lesion if it becomes isointense to surrounding fat on postcontrast T1-weighted images. This shortcoming is avoided if fat-suppression methods are employed. One method is frequency-selective, or chemical shift–selective, suppression that uses a preparatory radiofrequency pulse to saturate the fat resonance. Using this method, Tien and colleagues[67] found that postcontrast fat-suppression T1-weighted images improved detection of head and neck tumors compared with standard T1-weighted and T2-weighted images, whereas fat-suppression T2-weighted images were superior in demonstrating lymphadenopathy. There are, however, disadvantages with this method of fat suppression since magnetic field inhomogeneities may result in areas of incomplete fat suppression or even suppression of water signal, increased magnetic-susceptibility artifact, and lower signal-to-noise ratio.

Dynamic contrast-enhanced MRI of neck lesions using a spin-echo technique produces signal intensity–time curves that are similar to the contrast-enhancement curves obtained with dynamic CT.[68] The curves are useful for confirming a diagnosis of benign hypervascular mass but contribute little to nondynamic MRI in predicting malignancy.

Fast spin-echo (FSE) imaging is an alternative to conventional spin-echo imaging. Zoarski and coworkers[69] reported that FSE T2-weighted images were equal to or better than conventional T2-weighted images when evaluated for lesion conspicuity, motion artifact, number of lesions seen, and image quality. Also, the FSE images were obtained in less than half the scan time of the conventional images. Except for fat, tissue signal characteristics are similar on conventional and FSE images obtained with comparable TEs and effective TEs, respectively.[70] The disadvantage of FSE is that fat remains relatively hyperintense on the T2-weighted images, so that the borders of a hyperintense lesion may be obscured by surrounding fat unless fat suppression is used.[69] Inversion-recovery FSE imaging, in which a 180-degree inversion pulse is added to the beginning of the FSE sequence, provides more uniform fat suppression and has been shown to improve conspicuity of small hyperintense lymph nodes adjacent to fat, and to improve early detection of tumor spread across fascial planes.[70] Nevertheless, inversion-recovery FSE acquisitions are recommended only as a supplement to FSE imaging because both fat and muscle have markedly decreased signal intensity, thus obscuring anatomic detail, and because pathologic tissues (lymphoma, sarcoid, some highly cellular carcinomas, blood products) with shortened T2 relaxation time have decreased visibility on inversion-recovery FSE images.

An alternative to CT and MRI in the detection of lymph node metastases from head and neck squamous cell carcinoma is ultrasonography combined with ultrasound-guided fine-needle aspiration biopsy.[71] The examination and biopsy are performed with a 7.5-MHz probe on the largest node, or on the nodes showing central hypoechogenicity. This technique tends, however, to detect metastases in levels II, III, and IV nodes better than those in level I and V nodes. Although interobserver variability in detection has been of concern in ultrasound evaluations, a recent multicenter study[71] found no statistically significant difference between a group of experienced sonologists and a larger group who performed the examinations much less frequently. Whereas sensitivity (77%) was less than that usually reported for CT (see later), specificity, determined by the ultrasound-guided biopsy, was 100%.

Newer physiologic or biochemical methods for assessing nodal disease in the head and neck, including radioimmunoscintigraphy,[72] FDG PET, and ferrimagnetic MRI contrast agents,[73, 74] remain to be tested in multicenter clinical trials.

Normal and Abnormal Lymph Nodes
Histopathology

Normal lymph nodes are oval or bean-shaped with an indentation, or hilum, on the side where blood vessels enter and leave the node. On histologic examination, fatty tissue is often found at the hilus, which is also the site where efferent lymphatic vessels leave the node. Afferent lymphatics may enter the node anywhere along its fibrous capsule, opening into the marginal sinus that surrounds the cortex of the node.[75] The cortex is partly compartmentalized by radially oriented fibrous septa from the capsule and contains the spherical aggregations of lymphocytes known as *primary nodules* or *follicles* (Fig. 35–36). These contain the germinal, or reaction, centers, which are the most active sites of lymphocyte proliferation in the node. Lymph nodes involved in an inflammatory response, which is characterized by enlargement of the follicles, are thus termed *reactive* nodes. The follicles are continuous centrally with the medullary cords of lymphatic tissue. In the central, medullary portion of the node, the medullary sinuses are located between the medullary cords and the connective tissue septa or trabeculae, resulting in looser arrangement of cells. The medullary sinuses drain into the one or two efferent lymphatic vessels at the hilum. Thus, the node consists of a loosely arranged medulla surrounded by a densely packed cortex except at the hilum (Fig. 35–36). In the patient with head and neck cancer metastatic to the regional lymph nodes, tumor cells can enter the lymph node via the afferent lymphatics and lodge in the marginal sinus. As they proliferate, the malignant cells invade the nodal medulla, blocking the flow of lymph and eventually producing medullary necrosis. They may also penetrate the nodal capsule, resulting in invasion of perinodal tissues (Fig. 35–36). Central necrosis and extracapsular extension are relatively late events in the evolution of tumor in the metastatic node.[76]

Computed Tomography and Magnetic Resonance Imaging

On CT, normal cervical lymph nodes have homogeneous density (10 to 20 HU), an ovoid shape, and typically measure less than or equal to 1 cm in largest cross-sectional diameter.[77] The occipital, mastoid, facial, lingual, and median retropharyngeal nodes are at most a few millimeters in diameter and difficult to detect on CT. Mancuso and associates[77] found that 20% of the level II internal jugular nodes, more than any other group, measured at the upper limit of 1 cm. A lower-attenuation area, representing adipose metaplasia, may be observed within normal nodes, particularly those of the submandibular group.[78] It usually has an eccentric location,[77] near the hilus (Fig. 35–37). Rarely, this fatty replacement occurs centrally and measures more than 3 mm, simulating tumor necrosis.[77] Fatty replacement has been observed in nodes particularly after inflammation or irradiation.

On conventional spin-echo MRI, normal lymph nodes

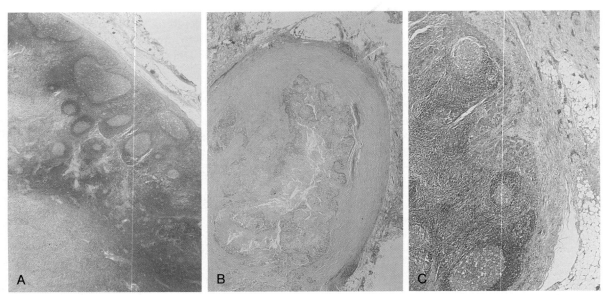

FIGURE 35–36 Histopathology of cervical lymph nodes. *A,* Normal lymph node. There is darker staining of the densely packed cortex *(upper right),* containing follicles with germinal centers, compared with that in the more loosely arranged medulla *(lower left).* The cortex is separated from surrounding fibroadipose tissue by a thin fibrous capsule. (H&E, ×200.) *B,* Central nodal necrosis. Abnormal lymph node with thickened fibrovascular capsule peripherally and tumor plus necrotic debris centrally. On CT or MRI studies, the rim enhancement accompanying central necrosis is likely due to perfusion of the vascularized, thickened capsule. (H&E, ×100.) *C,* Extranodal spread of tumor. Abnormal lymph node with tumor invasion of marginal sinus, capsule, and surrounding adipose tissue. From left to right at the center of the image: normal cortex (bluish stain), tumor within thickened marginal sinus (reddish blue), infiltrated and thickened capsule (pink), and disrupted capsular margin with tumor invading adipose tissue (white). (H&E, ×200.) *(A–C,* Courtesy of Dr. Joyce Young-Ramsaran, Department of Pathology, University of Miami School of Medicine.)

have homogeneous signal intensity. It is less than that of fat and equal to or greater than that of muscle on T1-weighted images. On T2-weighted images, the intensity of normal nodes is equal to or greater than that of fat, which is much greater than that of muscle. Again, eccentric fatty replacement may be observed within a normal node.

Criteria for determining abnormal lymph nodes are well established on contrast-enhanced CT. These are based on size, shape, and grouping of nodes, as well as central nodal necrosis and extranodal tumor spread:

1. *Size:* The size criteria are used to assess homogeneous, well-marginated nodes. In general, one of three approaches is taken. In the first and most common approach, submandibular (level I) and jugulodigastric nodes (low-level II and high-level III) larger than 1.5 cm in greatest diameter in the axial CT plane are considered abnormal, whereas any other cervical nodes larger than 1 cm are judged abnormal (see Figs. 35–31, 35–33, and 35–35). By these criteria, approximately 80% of enlarged nodes will be infiltrated by tumor and 20% will be hyperplastic.[79–81] In the second approach, all cervical nodes larger than 1-cm maximal axial diameter are considered abnormal.[82, 83] This improves sensitivity at the expense of specificity. A variation on the maximal size criteria is to consider any retropharyngeal node greater than 0.8 cm abnormal (Fig. 35–38).[84] In the third approach, nodes with a minimal diameter in the axial plane greater than or equal to 1 cm are considered abnormal, except for subdigastric nodes

(low-level II and high-level III), which are abnormal if greater than or equal to 1.1 cm.[78] Using these criteria, van den Brekel and colleagues[78] reported that sensitivity and specificity in the detection of metastatic nodes were each 82% when abnormal size alone was considered.

2. *Shape:* Metastatic nodes tend to be more rounded (maximal and minimal axial diameters approximately equal) than hyperplastic nodes, which are oblong. When the criterion of rounded shape is combined with that of nodal size, though, the sensitivity of CT in detecting abnormal nodes is improved only slightly[61] or not at all.[78]

3. *Nodal grouping:* A cluster of three or more contiguous nodes, each with borderline normal size (8- to 15-mm maximal diameter or 8- to 10-mm minimal axial diameter) in the drainage pathway of a primary tumor, is at increased risk of harboring metastasis.[78, 84, 85] Van den Brekel and colleagues[78] found that when this criterion was combined with the minimal-axial-diameter criterion, there was an increase of about 5% in sensitivity at high specificity.

4. *Central nodal necrosis:* Use of this criterion improves both sensitivity and specificity in the detection of metastatic nodes.[61, 78, 82] When the combined CT criteria of nodal size and central necrosis are applied, most authors have reported sensitivities ranging from 87% to 97% and specificities ranging from 71% to 100%.[78, 81–83, 85–87] The higher values for sensitivity and specificity have been reported in the more recently published

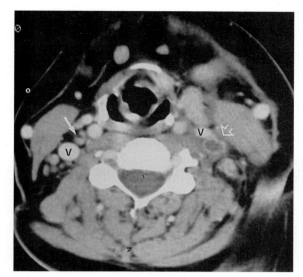

FIGURE 35–37 Normal node with fatty replacement compared with a node with central necrosis and extranodal tumor spread. Level III internal jugular nodes in a 52-year-old woman with metastatic breast carcinoma. The 1-cm right-sided node (closed arrow) has eccentric low density with attenuation similar to that of adjacent fat. The 1.4-cm left-sided node (open arrow) demonstrates central hypodensity with attenuation similar to that of spinal fluid. The enhancing margin of the node is unsharp, and the surrounding fat planes are obscured. The internal jugular veins (v) are labeled.

studies. The central necrosis criterion is particularly useful in identifying metastatic nodes that are normal or borderline in size but have an abnormal central hypodensity (see Figs. 35–34 and 35–37). Although called "necrosis," the central hypodensity can represent aggregates of tumor cells in the nodal medulla or necrotic tissue resulting from tumor infiltration or both. The hypodensity is accentuated by enhancement of the peripheral, cortical portion of the node. Larger metastatic nodes may demonstrate a patchy, inhomogeneous enhancement rather than the more common thick, irregular peripheral rim of enhancement.

5. *Extranodal spread*: Extranodal or extracapsular spread refers to extension of metastatic tumor to tissues outside the lymph node and is a criterion like central necrosis that improves accuracy by facilitating identification of metastatic nodes that are not pathologic by size criteria. On CT, extranodal spread results in poorly defined margins around the enhancing nodal capsule (see Fig. 35–37).[61] Spread becomes more evident when there is obliteration of fat surrounding a node and invasion of nearby muscle, vessels, or fascial boundaries, with irregular contrast enhancement (Fig. 35–39).

Contrast-enhanced CT is preferred to spin-echo MRI in the evaluation of neoplastic lymphadenopathy because of the ability of CT to more accurately detect central nodal necrosis and to better show extranodal spread of tumor.[88] Lymph node size, shape, and grouping are equally well evaluated on MRI and CT images with comparable section thicknesses; however, metastatic nodes

with central necrosis on CT may have low, intermediate, or high signal intensity on T2-weighted MRI images and intermediate to low signal intensity on T1-weighted images (Fig. 35–40). The variability in signal overlaps that of hyperplastic nodes, limiting accurate identification of metastatic nodes (Fig. 39–41).[89] Yousem and associates[88] attribute the variable signal on MRI to the admixture of tumor cell aggregates, which have intermediate signal on T1-weighted and T2-weighted images, and necrotic tissue, which has low T1-weighted and very high T2-weighted signal intensity. They also found that enhancement with gadolinium did not significantly increase the sensitivity or accuracy of MRI compared with CT in detecting central necrosis. Relative to surgical pathologic examination (*n* = 23 nodes), the accuracy of CT was 94%; that of T1-weighted and T2-weighted unenhanced MRI was 87%; and that of postgadolinium, fat-suppressed T1-weighted MRI was 80% (average for two readers).[88] Similarly, MRI was not as accurate in detecting extranodal tumor spread. There has been no conclusive evidence to date that the actual T1 or T2 relaxation times of individual lymph nodes can differentiate neoplastic infiltration from inflammatory enlargement.[90–92]

Pathologic Conditions

The patient's age is an important factor when formulating a differential diagnosis for a neck mass of nodal origin. In children, lymphadenopathy is likely to be secondary to infection; lymphoma is the most common head and neck malignancy. Excluding thyroid lesions, a unilateral neck mass in an adult younger than 40 years is usually malignant, and the most common malignancy is lymphoma. In adults older than 40 years, metastatic disease (squamous cell or thyroid carcinoma) is the most common cause of a nodal mass.[58]

Neoplastic Disease

Greater than 90% of all head and neck cancers are *squamous cell carcinomas*. Most of the remaining cancers are

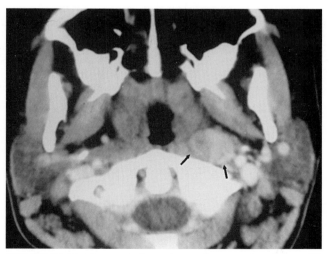

FIGURE 35–38 Metastatic lateral retropharyngeal node in a 15-year-old girl with papillary carcinoma of the thyroid. The node (arrows) is abnormal by size criteria, measuring 2 cm × 1.2 cm.

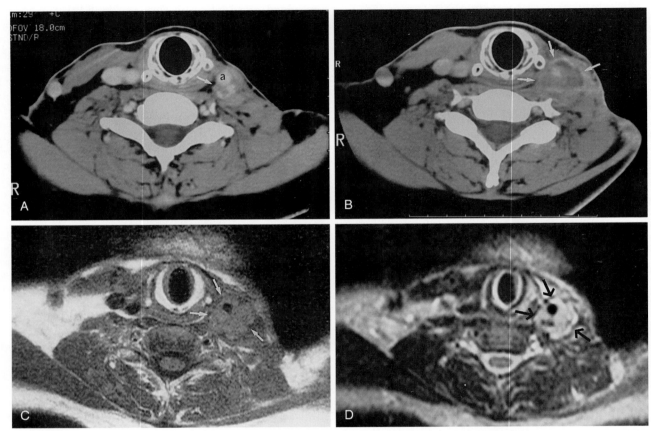

FIGURE 35–39 Extranodal spread of tumor with encasement of the common carotid artery in a 59-year-old man with recurrent papillary carcinoma of the thyroid. *A,* Previous left-sided neck dissection with sacrifice of the internal jugular vein. This postoperative CT scan reveals a clinically occult, irregularly enhancing nodal mass *(arrow)* posterior to the left common carotid artery (a) and anterior to the anterior scalene muscle. *B,* A CT scan obtained 9 months later demonstrates further growth of tumor. The enhancing margins *(arrows)* of the tumor encase the artery and are confluent with the scalene muscles. T1-weighted *(C)* and T2-weighted *(D)* images obtained at the same time as the CT scan in *B* also show the encasement *(arrows)* of the carotid artery by tumor, which is hyperintense to muscle. The low-signal area within the tumor mass posterior to the artery in *D* is isointense to tumor in *C* but is slightly hyperdense or enhancing in *B.* The area most likely represents calcification, old intratumoral hemorrhage, or scar.

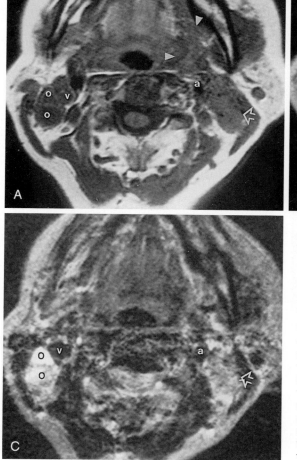

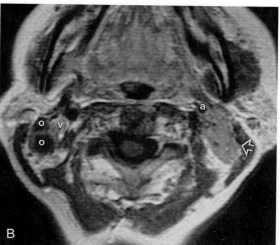

FIGURE 35–40 Variable signal characteristics of metastatic nodes on MRI. A 65-year-old woman presented with bilateral neck masses and a clinically occult head and neck cancer. MRI suggested a left tongue base lesion (*arrowheads* in A), which was later confirmed by biopsy results. Precontrast (*A*) and postcontrast (*B*) T1-weighted images demonstrated bilateral level II nodal masses. The left-sided mass (*open arrow*) is slightly hyperintense to muscle, shows solid enhancement, and has ill-defined margins that are confluent with the overlying sternocleidomastoid muscle and the internal carotid artery (a). The left internal jugular vein is compressed and not demonstrated. The right-sided mass is multilobulated, with areas of central low signal intensity and peripheral enhancement: two areas represent metastatic "necrotic" nodes (o), and the third is the internal jugular vein (v). *C*, The T2-weighted image at the same level demonstrates both high and intermediate signal intensity for the "necrotic" nodes (o), signal void for the right internal jugular vein (v), and intermediate signal intensity for the left-sided, tumor-replaced node(s) (*open arrow*) with extracapsular spread.

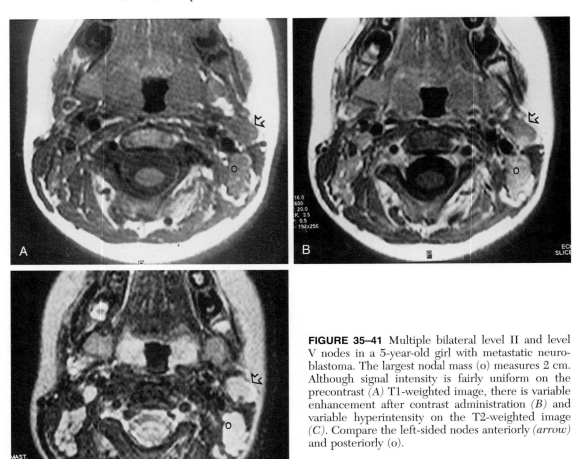

FIGURE 35–41 Multiple bilateral level II and level V nodes in a 5-year-old girl with metastatic neuroblastoma. The largest nodal mass (o) measures 2 cm. Although signal intensity is fairly uniform on the precontrast (A) T1-weighted image, there is variable enhancement after contrast administration (B) and variable hyperintensity on the T2-weighted image (C). Compare the left-sided nodes anteriorly (*arrow*) and posteriorly (o).

adenocarcinomas of salivary origin, melanomas, or *tumors of somatic soft tissues.*[93] The most important prognostic factor in squamous cell carcinoma of the head and neck is the presence of metastatic disease in the regional lymph nodes.[94] The presence of a single metastatic node in either the ipsilateral or contralateral side of the neck relative to the primary tumor reduces the 5-year survival rate by about 50%, and the presence of single bilateral nodes reduces the rate by 75%. If there is extranodal tumor spread, the rate of survival is further reduced by one-half. Thus, detection of one metastatic lymph node in each side of the neck, combined with evidence that tumor has spread beyond the nodal capsule, reduces the survival rate to 12.5% of that of a patient with the same primary tumor but without nodal metastases.[61] Thus, clinical staging of regional lymph nodes is an important part of the TNM system of tumor staging (see Table 35–2), and the accurate detection of metastatic nodes provides optimal staging.

Patients with primary head and neck squamous cell carcinoma who have no evidence of nodal metastases on palpation are staged as N0. Between 15% and 39% of these patients have regional lymph node metastasis, that is, clinically occult disease, by histologic examination or

clinical outcome.[54, 78, 79, 83, 94, 95] Most studies have shown that CT[81, 83, 85–87, 96] and MRI[83, 86, 97] improve the accuracy of detection of metastatic lymph nodes compared with palpation. In two studies, the accuracy of CT was equal to[98] or less than[99] that of the clinical examination. When combined with physical examination, CT results in more accurate lymph node staging in the neck.[83, 84, 87, 96, 100] The improvement may be gauged by the decrease in overall error rate ([false-positive cases + false-negative cases / total cases] × 100) for assessing the presence or absence of nodal metastases. In reviewing the radiologic and otolaryngologic literature, van den Brekel and coworkers[78] reported that the overall error rate decreased from a range of 20% to 28% for palpation to a range of 7.5% to 19% for CT. Van den Brekel and associates[97] also reported that MRI reduced the error rate to 16% compared with 32% for palpation in detecting nodal metastases in each side of the neck (nodal levels I to V). The decreased error rate with the use of CT or MRI imaging is important because it may alter the decision to perform an elective neck dissection. In most institutions, it is currently considered acceptable to perform an elective dissection in a patient with a stage N0 neck if the rate of clinically occult disease is likely to exceed 20% to 30%.[83, 97] If CT (or

MRI) lowers the error rate, and correspondingly the occult disease rate ([false-negative cases / total cases] × 100), the indication for elective dissection is brought into question and a different approach to treatment may be considered. Thus, Friedman and colleagues[83] have suggested that in patients undergoing surgical treatment of a primary tumor, neck dissection (radical or modified) be performed for all CT- or MRI-positive necks, even if no nodes are palpable. For the CT-negative neck, radiation therapy may be adequate, or alternatively no treatment may be an option, depending on the "philosophy of the surgeon." This approach remains controversial.[77]

Papillary carcinoma of the thyroid that metastasizes to regional lymph nodes is capable of producing a spectrum of imaging findings: enlarged homogeneous nodes, necrotic or cystic nodes, enhancing or calcified nodes (Fig. 35–42). The calcifications, better seen on CT than MRI,

are usually small or psammomatous.[61] Nodes with cystic necrosis may mimic a benign cyst, appearing well margined and hypodense on CT; however, increased protein content or hemorrhage in the metastatic nodes can result in a distinct high signal on T1-weighted as well as T2-weighted images. The differential diagnosis for nodal hemorrhage includes metastatic renal cell carcinoma and Kimura's disease (soft tissue eosinophilic granuloma).[101, 102]

Hodgkin's and non-Hodgkin's lymphomas commonly present with enlarged nodes that are homogeneous in density or intensity, mimicking hyperplastic nodes (Fig. 35–43). Typically, level III and IV nodes are involved, but isolated involvement of level II or external or anterior jugular nodes also occurs. Central nodal necrosis is rare, occurring more often with non-Hodgkin's than with Hodgkin's lymphoma. Peripheral nodal enhancement is also an unusual finding. Calcification has been observed in

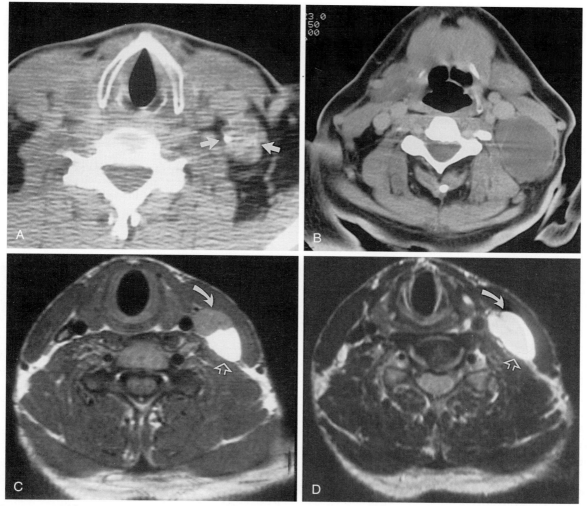

FIGURE 35–42 Variable appearance of papillary adenocarcinoma of the thyroid metastatic to regional lymph nodes. *A* and *B*, CT scan of a 54-year-old man with nodal metastases. *A*, Cluster of necrotic and nonnecrotic level III nodes with calcifications *(arrows)*. *B*, Cystic (12 Hounsfield units), 5 cm maximal level II or V node. *C* and *D*, MRI studies of a 37-year-old man with nodal metastases. *C*, T1-weighted (600/20) image demonstrates level III-IV junction. The anterior component *(curved arrow)* is hypointense to fat and slightly hyperintense to muscle. The posterior component *(open arrow)* is approximately isointense to fat. *D*, T2-weighted (2000/75) image shows that both components are hyperintense to fat. The MRI appearance of the mass is consistent with confluent nodes containing solid tumor anteriorly *(curved arrow)* and hemorrhage or proteinaceous material (thyroid protein) posteriorly *(open arrow)*.

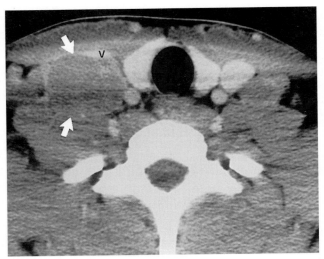

FIGURE 35–43 Homogeneous, nonenhancing level IV lymph node (*arrows*) in a 20-year-old man with Hodgkin's disease. The node measures 4.2 cm in maximal axial diameter. The right internal jugular vein (v) is compressed.

TABLE 35–3 Differential Diagnosis Based on Computed Tomography Findings for Cervical Nodes

Homogeneous Density with Postcontrast Enhancement

Hyperplastic nodes
Granulomatous disease (tuberculosis, sarcoid)
Lymphoma
Castleman's disease
Vascular metastases (thyroid and renal cell carcinomas, melanoma, Kaposi's sarcoma)

Calcification

Granulomatous disease (tuberculosis, histoplasmosis, sarcoidosis)
Lymphoma (especially after radiation or chemotherapy)
Metastasis (thyroid carcinoma, seminoma, mucin-producing carcinomas)
Sinus histiocytosis with massive lymphadenopathy ("eggshell" calcification)

Mixture of Homogeneous, Necrotic, Enhancing, and Calcified Nodes

Thyroid carcinoma
Tuberculosis
Lymphoma

both forms of lymphoma, both before and after radiation treatment or chemotherapy, yet is more commonly observed after treatment and in patients with the nodular sclerosing type of Hodgkin's lymphoma.[103, 104] It is impossible to differentiate nodal disease secondary to Hodgkin's or non-Hodgkin's lymphoma, or metastatic carcinoma based on the CT or MRI appearance. Nevertheless, large (>2 to 3 cm in diameter), nonnecrotic, homogeneous node(s) should suggest diseases other than metastatic squamous cell carcinoma (Fig. 35–43). These include large cell lymphoma, as well as sarcoidosis, Castleman's disease (lymphoproliferative disorder secondary to lymphoid follicle hyperplasia and marked capillary proliferation with endothelial hyperplasia), and sinus histiocytosis with massive lymphadenopathy.[61] Hyperplastic (reactive) nodes are usually less than 2 cm in their greatest diameter.[53] The ultrasound appearance of non-Hodgkin's lymphoma is reportedly more homogeneous and slightly more echogenic than that of Hodgkin's lymphoma or metastatic disease.[105] In adolescents and young adults, CT evidence of a naso- or oropharyngeal mass, in association with lymphadenopathy, should suggest not only lymphoma but also infectious mononucleosis or HIV infection.

Inflammatory and Infectious Disease

Cervical tuberculous adenitis (scrofula) is uncommon in the United States.[106] Most cases are caused by *Mycobacterium tuberculosis* and atypical mycobacteria (e.g., *Mycobacterium avium-intracellulare*, *Mycobacterium scrofulaceum*, *Mycobacterium kansasii*), rather than the classic agent *Mycobacterium bovis*. Adenitis due to atypical mycobacteria is histologically indistinguishable from that caused by *M. tuberculosis*; however, the former more commonly occurs in children without evidence of old or active tuberculosis and demonstrates unilateral involvement of nodes (levels I and II, as well as parotid and preauricular groups) in the direct drainage pathway of

oropharyngeal or orbital (conjunctival) infection. *M. tuberculosis* adenitis is a manifestation of systemic disease. It is more commonly seen in young adults 20 to 30 years old and tends to involve bilateral level III to V nodes (Fig. 35–44). The more inferior the involvement in the neck, the more likely the presence of concomitant pulmonary tuberculosis.[107] Clinically, the lymph nodes are firm and nontender, and local inflammatory changes are absent unless there is a fistula or superimposed pyogenic (bacterial) infection. The purified protein derivative test is

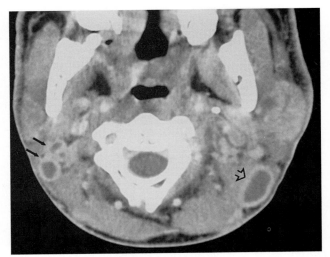

FIGURE 35–44 Tuberculous adenitis in a 27-year-old man with acquired immunodeficiency syndrome. *Closed arrows* show a cluster of right level V necrotic nodes. The left-sided node (*open arrow*), superficial to the trapezius muscle, has no associated inflammatory changes in the overlying subcutaneous fat or skin. The nodal necrosis is indistinguishable from that due to metastatic squamous cell carcinoma.

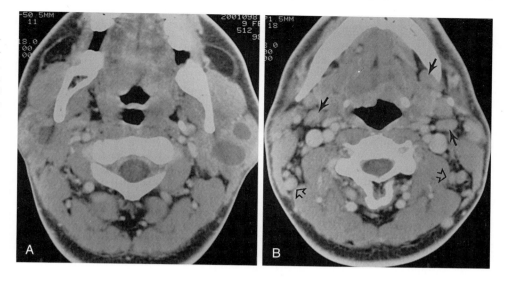

FIGURE 35–45 Multiple hyperplastic cervical nodes and bilateral parotid lymphoepithelial cysts in a 31-year-old man with human immunodeficiency virus infection. *A*, The parotid cysts are hypodense and without rim enhancement (compare with MRI characteristics in Fig. 35–13). *B*, Several submandibular (level I) and internal jugular (level II) nodes *(closed arrows)* are equal to or slightly greater than 1.5 cm. Some spinal accessory (level V) nodes *(open arrows)* measure 1.0 cm or greater. All are homogeneous in density.

strongly positive, except in the anergic patient. Excisional biopsy is recommended for diagnosis since fistula formation and poor wound healing are complications of incisional biopsy in these patients.

On CT, the findings are variable.[108] Involved nodes may be enlarged, homogeneous in density, and enhancing or nonenhancing. Alternatively, they may have central necrosis and a thick rim of enhancement. Either nonnecrotic or necrotic nodes can be partly calcified. When cervical nodes with these varied findings coexist in one patient, the differential diagnosis should include lymphoma and thyroid carcinoma (Table 35–3). Coalescence of several necrotic nodes results in a "cold abscess." Tuberculous adenitis is rarely accompanied by subcutaneous and dermal manifestations of inflammation, such as thickening of adjacent fascial boundaries and muscles or infil-

tration of lymphatics (reticular densities within adipose tissue), unless there is superimposed infection or fistula, as mentioned previously.

Cervical lymph node calcification is uncommon but has been reported for several neoplastic and inflammatory conditions, in addition to tuberculosis (see Table 35–3). The pattern of calcification is typically irregular, and only rarely is there an eggshell configuration.[109]

As described in the section on salivary glands cysts, the combination of diffuse cervical lymphadenopathy and multiple, unilateral, or bilateral parotid (lymphoepithelial) cysts is associated with HIV infection (Fig. 35–45).[110] On CT, the cysts are hypodense with minimal or no peripheral enhancement. They may coexist with intraparotid hyperplastic nodes; however, a solid parotid mass should be viewed with suspicion considering the risk of large cell

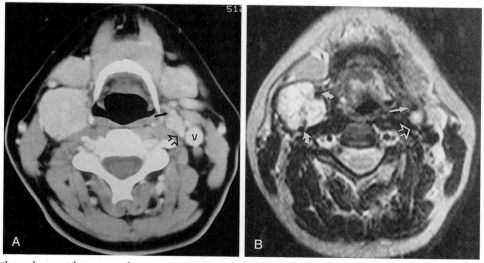

FIGURE 35–46 Bilateral carotid paragangliomas. *A*, Postcontrast CT scan demonstrates bilateral, markedly enhancing masses. Splaying of the carotid bifurcation is difficult to identify on the right. On the left, the mass is located between the left external carotid artery *(closed arrow)* and internal carotid artery *(open arrow)*, which is anteromedial to the left internal jugular vein (v). *B*, T2-weighted MRI study demonstrates the "flow void" within the external and internal carotid arteries on the right *(curved arrows)* and on the left *(closed and open arrows as in A)*. The paragangliomas are predominantly hyperintense, like lymph nodes, although the right-sided tumor has linear hypointensities that suggest vessels.

lymphoma in these patients.[30] In general, the cervical nodes are homogeneous, less than or equal to 2 cm in their greatest diameter, and show no preferential involvement of any level.

Conclusion

Familiarity with the distribution and appearance of cervical lymph nodes is valuable to the radiologist whether the imaging is performed for characterization of a palpable neck mass of unknown cause or for staging of a known primary head and neck cancer. The precise location of the unknown mass may suggest a vascular or neurogenic origin rather than a nodal lesion. For example, a markedly enhancing mass that splays the carotid bifurcation is more likely to be a carotid paraganglioma (Fig. 35–46). An interscalene mass in the prevertebral space is likely to be a schwannoma of the brachial plexus and not a spinal accessory or internal jugular nodal metastasis (see Fig. 35–29).[62]

In staging of primary squamous cell carcinoma of the head and neck, the use of the level method of describing nodal metastases ensures that the findings described by the radiologist are understood by the surgeon. Furthermore, the use of all the accepted criteria —size, grouping, central necrosis, extranodal spread—to identify metastatic nodes on CT should result in improved accuracy of staging, and consequently greater reliance of the surgeon on diagnostic imaging and greater collaboration with the radiologist. Finally, the radiologist can also aid the clinician by recognizing certain CT patterns of nodal disease (see Table 35–3). Although aspiration cytologic examination or excisional biopsy is ultimately necessary for histologic diagnosis,[111] CT or MRI, perhaps accompanied by functional or biochemical studies in the future, will continue to provide the optimal means for assessing the location and extent of cervical adenopathy that may be clinically occult.

References

1. Batsakis JG. Tumors of the Head and Neck: Clinical and Pathological Considerations, 2nd ed., pp. 1–120. Baltimore, Williams & Wilkins, 1979.
2. Mason DK, Chisholm DM. Salivary Glands in Health and Disease, pp. 3–206. London, WB Saunders, 1975.
3. Johns ME. The salivary glands: Anatomy and embryology. Otolaryngol Clin North Am 1977;10:261.
4. Moss-Salentijn L, Moss ML. Development and functional anatomy. In Rankow RM, Polayes IM (eds). Diseases of the Salivary Glands, pp. 17–31. Philadelphia, WB Saunders, 1976.
5. Som PM. Salivary glands. In Som PM, Bergeron RT (eds). Head and Neck Imaging, 2nd ed., pp. 277–348. St. Louis, Mosby–Year Book, 1991.
6. Thackray AC. Salivary gland tumors. Proc R Soc Med 1968; 61:1089.
7. Hollinshead WH. Anatomy for Surgeons: The Head and Neck, Vol. I, 3rd ed., p. 20. Philadelphia, Harper & Row, 1982.
8. Davis RA. Surgical anatomy of the facial nerve and parotid gland based upon a study of 350 cervico-facial halves. Surg Gynecol Obstet 1956;102:385.
9. Wotson S, Mandel ID. The salivary secretions in health and disease. In Rankow RM, Polayes IM (eds). Diseases of the Salivary Glands, pp. 32–53. Philadelphia, WB Saunders, 1976.
10. Peel RZ, Gnepp DR. Diseases of the salivary glands. In Barnes L (ed). Surgical Pathology of the Head and Neck, Vol. I, pp. 533–645. New York, Marcel Dekker, 1985.
11. Osmer JC, Pleasants JE. Distension sialography. Radiology 1966;87:116.
12. Tart RP, Kotzur IM, Mancuso AA, et al. CT and MR imaging of the buccal space and buccal space masses. Radiographics 1995;15:531.
13. McGuirt WF, Keyes JW Jr, Greven KM, et al. Preoperative identification of benign versus malignant parotid masses: A comparative study including positron emission tomography. Laryngoscope 1995;105:579.
14. Keyes JW Jr, Harkness BA, Greven KM, et al. Salivary gland tumors: Pretherapy evaluation with PET. Radiology 1994;192:99.
15. Thibault F, Halimi P, Bely N, et al. Internal architecture of the parotid gland at MR imaging: Facial nerve or ductal system? Radiology 1993;188:701.
16. Casselman JW, Mancuso AA. Major salivary gland masses: Comparison of MR imaging and CT. Radiology 1987;165:183.
17. Mandelblatt SM, Braun IF, Davis PC. Parotid masses: MR imaging. Radiology 1987; 163:411.
18. Schlakman BN, Yousem DM. MR of intraparotid masses. AJNR 1993;14:1173.
19. Freling NJM, Molenaar WM, Vermey A, et al. Malignant parotid tumors: Clinical use of MR imaging and histologic correlation. Radiology 1992;185:691.
20. Sigal R, Monet O, de Baere T, et al. Adenoid cystic carcinoma of the head and neck: Evaluation with MR imaging and clinical-pathologic correlation in 27 patients. Radiology 1992;184:95.
21. Minami M, Tanioka H, Oyama K, et al. Warthin tumor of the parotid gland: MR-pathologic correlation. AJNR 1993;14:209.
22. Rabinov K, Weber AL. Radiology of the Salivary Glands, pp. 1–264. Boston, GK Hall, 1985.
23. Travis LW, Hecht DW. Acute and chronic inflammatory diseases of the salivary glands: Diagnosis and management. Otolaryngol Clin North Am 1977;10:329.
24. Leake D, Leake P. Neonatal suppurative parotitis. Pediatrics 1970;46:203.
25. Levy DM, ReMine WH, Devine KD. Salivary gland calculi. JAMA 1962;181:1115.
26. Som PM, Shugar JM, Train JS, Biller HF. Manifestations of parotid gland enlargement: Radiographic, pathologic, and clinical correlations. Part I. The autoimmune pseudosialectasias. Radiology 1981;141:415.
27. Godwin J. Benign lymphoepithelial lesion of the parotid gland (adenolymphoma, chronic inflammation, lymphoepithelioma, lymphocytic tumor, Mikulicz disease): Report of eleven cases. Cancer 1952;5:1089.
28. Spath M, Kruger K, Dresel S, et al. Magnetic resonance imaging of the parotid gland in patients with Sjögren's syndrome. J Rheumatol 1991;18:1372.
29. Takashima S, Takeuchi N, Morimoto S, et al. MR imaging of Sjögren syndrome: Correlation with sialography and pathology. J Comput Assist Tomogr 1991;15:393.
30. Huang RD, Pearlman S, Friedman WH, et al. Benign cystic vs. solid lesions of the parotid gland in HIV patients. Head Neck 1991;13:522.
31. Som PM. Cystic lesions of the neck. Postgrad Radiol 1987;7:211.
32. Eneroth CM. Salivary gland tumors in the parotid gland, submandibular gland and the palate region. Cancer 197;27:1415.
33. Rabinov K, Weber AL. Radiology of the Salivary Glands, pp. 292–367. Boston, GK Hall, 1985.
34. Rankow RM, Polayes IM. Surgical treatment of salivary gland tumors. In Rankow RM, Polayes IM (eds). Diseases of the Salivary Glands, pp. 239–283. Philadelphia, WB Saunders, 1976.
35. Som PM, Shugar JM, Sacher M, et al. Benign and malignant parotid pleomorphic adenomas: CT and MR studies J Comput Assist Tomogr 1988;12:65.
36. Tsushima Y, Matsumoto M, Endo K, et al. Characteristic bright signal of parotid pleomorphic adenomas on T2-weighted MR images with pathological correlation. Clin Radiol 1994;49:485.
37. Shugar JMA, Som PM, Biller HF. Warthin's tumor, a multifocal disease. Ann Otol Rhinol Laryngol 1982;9:246.
38. Batsakis JG, Chinn E, Regezi JA, Repola DA. The pathology of head and neck tumors: Salivary glands. Part 2. Head Neck Surg 1978;1:167.
39. Healey WV, Perzin KH, Smith L. Mucoepidermoid carcinoma of salivary gland origin. Cancer 1970;26:368.
40. Conley J, Dingman DL. Adenoid cystic carcinoma in the head and neck (cylindroma). Arch Otolaryngol 1974;100:81.

41. Perzin K, Gullane P, Clairmont A. Adenoid cystic carcinomas arising in salivary glands: A correlation of histologic features and clinical courses. Cancer 1978;42:265.

42. Nascimento AG, Amaral ALP, Prado LAF, et al. Adenoid cystic carcinoma of the salivary glands: A study of 61 cases with clinico-pathologic correlation. Cancer 1986;57:312.

43. Batsakis JG, Chinn EK, Weimert TA, et al. Acinic cell carcinoma: A clinicopathologic study of 35 cases. J Laryngol Otol 1979;93:325.

44. Mulliken JB, Glowacki J. Hemangiomas and vascular malformations in infants and children: A classification based on endothelial characteristics. Plast Reconstr Surg 1982;69:412.

45. Meyer JS, Hoffer FA, Barnes PD, et al. Biological classification of soft-tissue vascular anomalies: MR correlation. AJR 1991;157:559.

46. Baker LL, Dillon WP, Hieshima GB et al. Hemangiomas and vascular malformations of the head and neck: MR characterization. AJNR 1993;14:307.

47. Barnes L. Surgical Pathology of the Head and Neck, Vol. 1, pp. 725–880. New York, Marcel Dekker, 1985.

48. Johns ME. The salivary glands: Anatomy and embryology. Otolaryngol Clin North Am 1977;10:261.

49. Johns ME. Parotid cancer: A rational basis for treatment. Head Neck Surg 1980;3:132.

50. Spiro RH, Armstrong J, Harrison L, et al. Carcinoma of the major salivary glands. Recent trends. Arch Otolaryngol 1989;115:316.

51. Elkon D, Colman M, Hendrickson FR. Radiation therapy in the treatment of malignant salivary gland tumors. Cancer 1978;41:502.

52. Reinfuss M, Korzeniowski S. Role of radiotherapy in the treatment of malignant tumors of the salivary glands. Tumor 1980;66:467.

53. Som PM. Lymph nodes of the neck. Radiology 1987;165:593.

54. Shah JP. Patterns of cervical lymph node metastasis from squamous carcinomas of the upper aerodigestive tract. Am J Surg 1990;160:405.

55. Rouvière H. Lymphatic system of the head and neck. In Tobias MJ (trans). Anatomy of the Human Lymphatic System, pp. 5–28. Ann Arbor, MI, Edwards Brothers, 1938.

56. Robbins KT, Medine JE, Wolfe GT, et al. Standardizing neck dissection terminology. Arch Otolaryngol Head Neck Surg 1991;117:601.

57. Dillon WP. The pharynx and oral cavity. In Som PM, Bergeron RT (eds). Head and Neck Imaging, 2nd ed., pp. 407–466. St. Louis, Mosby–Year Book, 1991.

58. Bowen BC. Brachial plexus and lower neck masses. In Ramsey RG (syllabus ed). Core Curriculum Course in Neuroradiology, pp. 181–191. Chicago, American Society of Neuroradiology, 1994.

59. Smoker WRK, Harnsberger HR. Differential diagnosis of head and neck lesions based on their space of origin. 2. The infrahyoid portion of the neck. AJR 1991;157:155.

60. Shah JP, Lydiatt W. Treatment of cancer of the head and neck. CA Cancer J Clin 1995;45:352.

61. Som PM. Detection of metastasis in cervical lymph nodes: CT and MR criteria and differential diagnosis. AJR 1992;158:961.

62. Mancuso AA. Workbook of MRI and CT of the Head and Neck, 2nd ed., pp. 197–220. Baltimore, Williams & Wilkins, 1989.

63. Wester DJ, Whiteman MLH, Singer S, et al. Imaging of the postoperative neck with emphasis on surgical flaps and their complications. AJR 1995;164:989.

64. Michael AS, Mafee MF, Valvassori GE, et al. Dynamic computed tomography of the head and neck: Differential diagnostic value. Radiology 1985;154:413.

65. Suojanen JN, Mukherji SK, Dupuy DE, et al. Spiral CT in evaluation of head and neck lesions: Work in progress. Radiology 1992;183:281.

66. Hayes CE, Mathis CM, Yuan C. Surface coil phased arrays for high-resolution imaging of the carotid arteries. J Magn Reson Imaging 1966;6:109.

67. Tien RD, Hesselink JR, Chu PK, et al. Improved detection and delineation of head and neck lesions with fat suppression spin-echo MR imaging. AJNR 1991;12:19.

68. Takashima S, Noguchi Y, Okumura T, et al. Dynamic MR imaging in the head and neck. Radiology 1993;189:813.

69. Zoarski GH, Mackey JK, Anzai Y, et al. Head and neck: Initial clinical experience with fast spin-echo MR imaging. Radiology 1993;188:323.

70. Panush D, Fulbright R, Sze G, et al. Inversion-recovery fast spin-echo MR imaging: Efficacy in the evaluation of head and neck lesions. Radiology 1993;187:421.

71. Takes RP, Knegt P, Manni JJ, et al. Regional metastasis in head and neck squamous cell carcinoma: Revised value of US with US-guided FNAB. Radiology 1996;198:819.

72. van Dongen GAMS, Leverstein H, Roos JC, et al. Radioimmuno-scintigraphy of head and neck cancer using ^{99m}Tc-labeled monoclonal antibody E48 F(ab')$_2$. Cancer Res 1992;52:2569.

73. Anzai Y, Lufkin R. New imaging techniques for nodal disease in the head and neck. In Syllabus of the Postgraduate Course, pp. 39–41. American Society of Head and Neck Radiology, 26th Annual Conference, Vancouver, BC, 1993.

74. Lee AS, Weissleder R, Brady TJ, et al. Lymph nodes: Microstructural anatomy at MR imaging. Radiology 1991;178:519.

75. Copenhaver WM, Kelly DE, Wood RL. Bailey's Textbook of Histology, 17th ed., pp. 392–397. Baltimore, Williams & Wilkins, 1978.

76. Feinmesser R, Freeman JL, Feinmesser M, et al. Role of modern imaging in decision-making for elective neck dissection. Head Neck 1992;14:173.

77. Mancuso AA, Harnsberger HR, Muraki AS, et al. Computed tomography of cervical and retropharyngeal lymph nodes: Normal anatomy, variants of normal, and applications of staging head and neck cancer. I. Normal anatomy. Radiology 1983;148:709.

78. van den Brekel MWM, Stel HV, Castelijns JA, et al. Cervical lymph node metastasis: Assessment of radiologic criteria. Radiology 1990;177:379.

79. Sako K, Pradier RN, Marchetta FC, et al. Fallibility of palpation in the diagnosis of metastases to cervical nodes. Surg Gynecol Obstet 1964;118:989.

80. Cinberg JZ, Silver CE, Molnar JJ, et al. Cervical cysts: Cancer until proven otherwise. Laryngoscope 1982;92:27.

81. Stevens MH, Harnsberger HR, Mancuso AA, et al. Computed tomography of cervical lymph nodes: Staging and management of head and neck cancer. Arch Otolaryngol Head Neck Surg 1985;111:735.

82. Friedman M, Roberts N, Kirshenbaum GL, et al. Nodal size of metastatic squamous cell carcinoma of the neck. Laryngoscope 1993;103:854.

83. Friedman M, Mafee MF, Pacella BL, et al. Rationale for elective neck dissection in 1990. Laryngoscope 1990;100:54.

84. Mancuso AA, Harnsberger HR, Muraki AS, et al. Computed tomography of cervical and retropharyngeal lymph nodes: Normal anatomy, variants of normal, and applications of staging head and neck cancer. II. Pathology. Radiology 1983;148:715.

85. Close LG, Merkel M, Vuitch MF, et al. Computed tomography evaluation of regional lymph node involvement in cancer of the oral cavity and oropharynx. Head Neck 1989;11:309.

86. Hillsamer PJ, Schuller DE, McGhee RB, et al. Improving diagnostic accuracy of cervical metastases with computed tomography and magnetic resonance imaging. Arch Otolaryngol Head Neck Surg 1990;116:1297.

87. Friedman M, Shelton V, Mafee M, et al. Metastatic neck diseases: Evaluation by CT. Arch Otolaryngol 1984;110:443.

88. Yousem DM, Som PM, Hackney DB, et al. Central nodal necrosis and extracapsular neoplastic spread in cervical lymph nodes: MR imaging versus CT. Radiology 1992;182:753.

89. Mancuso AA, Dillon WP. The neck. Radiol Clin North Am 1989;27:407.

90. Dooms GC, Hricak H, Moseley ME, et al. Characterization of lymphadenopathy by magnetic resonance relaxation times: Preliminary results. Radiology 1985;155:691.

91. Glazer GM, Orringer MB, Chenevert TL, et al. Mediastinal lymph nodes: Relaxation time/pathologic correlation and implications in staging of lung cancer with MR imaging. Radiology 1988;168:429.

92. Wiener JL, Chako AC, Merten CW, et al. Breast and axillary tissue MR imaging: Correlation of signal intensities and relaxation times with pathologic findings. Radiology 1986;160:299.

93. Cotran RS, Kumar V, Robbins SL. Diseases of the head and neck. In Robbins SL (ed): Pathologic Basis of Disease, 4th ed., pp. 811–826. Philadelphia, WB Saunders, 1989.

94. Johnson JT. A surgeon looks at cervical lymph nodes. Radiology 1990;175:607.

95. Ali S, Tiwari RM, Snow GB. False positive and false negative neck nodes. Head Neck 1985;8:78.

96. Stern WBR, Silver CE, Zeifer BA, et al. Computed tomography of the clinically negative neck. Head Neck 1990;12:109.

97. van den Brekel MWM, Castelijns JA, Croll GA, et al. Magnetic

resonance imaging vs palpation of cervical lymph node metastasis. Arch Otolaryngol Head Neck Surg 1991;117:666.

98. Feinmesser R, Freeman JL, Nojek AM, et al. Metastatic neck disease: A clinical/radiographic/pathologic correlative study. Arch Otolaryngol Head Neck Surg 1987;113:1307.

99. Moreau P, Goffart Y, Collignon J. Computed tomography of metastatic cervical lymph nodes: A clinical, computed tomographic, pathologic correlative study. Arch Otolaryngol Head Neck Surg 1990;116:1190.

100. Mancuso AA, Maceri D, Rice D, et al. CT of cervical lymph node cancer. AJR 1981;136:381.

101. Som PM, Biller HF. Kimura disease involving parotid gland and cervical nodes: CT and MR findings. J Comput Assist Tomogr 1992;16:320.

102. Smith JRG, Hadgis C, Van Hasselt A, et al. CT of Kimura disease. AJNR 1989;10(suppl):34.

103. Brereton ND, Johnson RE. Calcification in mediastinal lymph nodes after radiation therapy of Hodgkin's disease. Radiology 1973;112:705.

104. Bertrand M, Chen JT, Libschitz HI. Lymph node calcification in Hodgkin's disease after chemotherapy. AJR 1977;129:1108.

105. Bruneton JN, Roux P, Caramella E, et al. Ear, nose, and throat cancer: Ultrasound diagnosis of metastasis to cervical lymph nodes. Radiology 1984;152:771.

106. Levin-Epstein AA, Lucente FE. Scrofula—The dangerous masquerader. Laryngoscope 1982;92:938.

107. Wong ML, Jefek BW. Cervical mycobacterial disease. Trans Am Acad Ophthalmol Otolaryngol 1974;78:75.

108. Reede DL, Bergeron RT. Cervical tuberculous adenitis: CT manifestations. Radiology 1985;154:701.

109. Silvers AR, Som PM, Meyer RJ. Egg shell nodal calcification in a patient with sinus histiocytosis with massive lymphadenopathy treated with interferon. AJNR 1996;17:361.

110. Holliday RA, Cohen WA, Schinella RA, et al. Benign lymphoepithelial parotid cysts and hyperplastic cervical adenopathy in AIDS-risk patients: A new CT appearance. Radiology 1988;168:439.

111. Yousem DM. Dashed hopes for MR imaging of the head and neck: The power of the needle. Radiology 1992;184:25.

CHAPTER

36

Essential and Advanced Temporomandibular Joint Imaging: A Study of Cases

EDWIN L. CHRISTIANSEN, D.D.S., Ph.D.
JOSEPH R. THOMPSON, M.D.

Nothing spoils a party so much as pain. One can imagine Visigoths tending to wounds inflicted by an encounter with marauding Norwegian "Berserks,"* the wounded Visigoth warriors unable to feast or boast because of jaw pain and dysfunction resulting from some Viking's massive fist in their faces. Probably then, as now, the average level of facial pain measured on a visual analogue scale (VAS) (zero to 100) was 83 VAS units (Fig. 36–1).

More contemporaneously, possibly less interesting, but certainly citable, Sir Astley Cooper, writing several centuries later in his 1823 opus *A Treatise on Fractures and Dislocations,* tells us that "the mandibular condyle will occasionally quit its cartilage . . . creating a snapping sound within the joint just in front of the ear."[1]

Although not uppermost in the minds of 19th- and early-20th-century physicians, temporomandibular joint (TMJ) disorders (TMDs) received their share of attention in the medical literature of the day, enough so that we know that TMDs are neither a recent nor a passing phenomenon.[2–5]

Medical literature from the 1800s and early 1900s highlights problems of mandibular ankylosis, joint anomalies, mandibular fractures, and so forth, that involve this unique articulation.[6, 7] In 1914, Blair[8] presented a fascinating retrospective summary of 212 TMJ surgical cases, some dating back to 1854. For each case, he systematically collected the following data: the age of the patient; the diagnosis; the causation; the presurgical mandibular movements; the surgical procedure; and the postsurgical mandibular movements. Even by today's standards, it is an impressive piece of work. One surgery, performed in 1875, intended to restore jaw function with an autogenous

interpositional flap of temporalis muscle between the fossa and the condyle as a disk replacement.[8] The procedure reads much like its modern descendant.[9]

Discussions of the cause of TMDs written in the 1800s and early 1900s read differently from the modern menu of causes. The focus was chiefly on the medical (infections) and mechanical (trauma), and virtually nothing was said about stress, the dental occlusion, or myofascial pain trigger points.

The essential contemporary perspective on TMDs is that this unique (ginglymoarthrodial) articulation is subject to the continuum of diseases that affect virtually every other joint.[10–15] The concept of one joint, one painful or annoying (or both) disorder manifesting as clicking or popping (an onomatopoetic point here), or both, is misleading and myopic.

This chapter presents fundamental concepts indicative of, and justifiable for, TMJ imaging. The greater goal is to direct the medical mind beyond the apparent "popularity" and sometime superficialities of clicking and popping jaw joints. We hope to give a broader perspective of, more knowledge of, and greater credibility to the authentic TMD pain patient.

With that as introduction, in the plainest of terms regarding chronically popping, painless joints: Who really cares? Should someone care? Someone should care. We just do not think that every clicking or popping TMJ deserves exotic imaging or treatment. According to Mejersjö and Carlsson,[16, 17] most TMD patients do quite well with conservative therapy. Their symptoms often resolve with minimal intervention and may or may not recur.

Some would dismiss the TMD pain patient as a

---

*According to nonbiased Norwegian history courtesy of Dr. Thor Bakland, the "Berserks" were fierce warriors from the Trondheim region of Norway. The Norwegian word comes from two roots, *bjorn* (bear) and *serk* (ancient word for an outer garment), thus the origins of our modern English word. Clad in bearskins, the *Bjornserk* would attack, banging their shields with their swords, screaming, and yelling. It is said that the French used to pray for protection from the Berserk warriors who were often recruited as mercenaries.

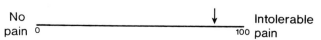

FIGURE 36–1 Average pain level of temporomandibular joint disorder patients expressed in visual analogue scale units (zero to 100) is 83 *(arrow).*

"crank," a "crock," a psychologic case beyond the reach of medical and dental rescue. In defense of these "cranks" and their sometime lack of response to treatment, we find that this is more often due to improper or inappropriate diagnosis as well as ineffective, inadequate treatment rendered too late rather than because of their brittleness as patients.

Since the early 1970s, the trunk of the TMD diagnostic tree has more aggressively pushed a root or two into both conventional and advanced imaging. In our experience, it is unlikely that improper diagnosis and ineffective treatment are the result of a frank imaging or reading error. How then would adequate imaging and accurate interpretation lead to improper or inadequate treatment?

The answer to that question has to do with teeth. Consider this: Just as the energy of an earthquake spreads radially from its origin, there are some dentists who consider the TMJ to be the epicenter of a myriad of symptoms, some too ludicrous to list. Just as some referring dentists may focus on the joint as they do on the teeth, it is the wise physician or radiologist who maintains a wider perspective.

BACKGROUND

In our (defensible) opinion, most of what comes through the clinic door posing as *TMJ* is, either in whole or in part, an expression of myofascial pain. Headache is the chief complaint of the majority of so-called TMJ patients, exceeding 76%.[18] After headache, others on this list—in descending order—include TMJ pain, TMJ noises, and earache.[18] Although this short list may appear contradictory to the opening of this paragraph, it is not. This is because three of these four symptoms—and in many cases all four—can be explained solely on the basis of myofascial pain. And if myofascial pain is the culprit, then why would one exhaust diagnostic resources on advanced imaging and inappropriate treatment of the TMJ?

Over the years, as we learn and begin asking ourselves this question, fewer patients are being referred for advanced imaging and fewer still for surgical intervention. More are referred for physical therapy; more are receiving myofascial trigger point injections; more are receiving specially compounded topical medications absorbed transdermally; and more are treated with extremely low dose antidepressants, for example, 5 to 10 mg of amitriptyline at bedtime.

In defense of this position consider the nearly omnipresent headache. Is there such a thing as a TMJ headache? Probably. How would such a headache manifest? Would the headache be temporal, occipital, frontal, periorbital, retro-orbital, or vertex? Possibly. Which one of these, then, is a TMJ headache? One of these? All of these?

In the typical myofascial (TMJ) pain patient, it is possible clinically to elicit or exacerbate *all of the headaches listed by the palpation of specific muscle trigger points, all of which are anatomically remote from the TMJ.* This strongly suggests that the so-called TMJ headache is most probably overrated, overemphasized, overdiagnosed, and not clearly understood. Because of this it is probable that the real cause(s) of the so-called TMJ headache are often poorly and ineffectively treated.

Many patients are referred solely because of popping joints in coincidence (rather than in concert) with one or more pain complaints. And because the headaches, earaches, or even perceived painful joints are coincident with obvious joint noises, a correlation is assumed and the patient may be referred for diagnostic imaging followed by extensive and expensive therapy. When displacement of the articular disk is confirmed by the radiologist, the "correlation" is cemented in the mind of the referring physician that "The headaches are due to the displaced disk"; we would respond, "Not necessarily."

Because the ear is close to the TMJ, many presume that earache is somehow explained by way of this proximity or Pinto's ligament.[19] To our knowledge, no functional relationship has yet been demonstrated between the TMJ and the middle ear via Pinto's ligament.[20] Earache can usually be attributed to one or more of three muscles: (1) medial pterygoid, (2) masseter (deep fibers), or (3) sternocleidomastoid.[21] Specific treatment of the offending muscle almost always resolves the earache.

When the patient is asked, "Where does it hurt?" and she or he points one finger directly at one or both TMJs, what is there to doubt? To begin with, one should doubt whether the pain is really resident in the TMJ. Those who understand myofascial pain will go beyond the subjective symptom and will palpate the lateral pterygoid muscle because they know that it refers to the TMJ and this referred pain may be perceived as intra-articular pain.[22]

The reader may be thinking that clicking and popping *are* specific for a TMD and that these signs are, without argument, pathognomonic for an intra-articular disorder, an internal derangement if you please. Well, yes and no. Yes, because the clicking or popping can be isolated to the joint per se, and no, because these noises often begin secondary to myofascial pain trigger points that go undiagnosed and untreated.

Repeatedly in our clinic, by the use of trigger point injections into (more so) the lateral pterygoid muscle and (less so) the deep fibers of the masseter muscle, clicking and pain have been halted.

In conclusion, we have explained four out of four of the most frequent symptoms—supposedly attributable to a TMD—almost entirely on the basis of myofascial pain; we hedge a bit with the qualifier *almost* because we recognize that not *all* TMD is due to myofascial pain, just most.

Cases to Consider

CASE ONE: A 72-year-old woman is referred because of chronic migraine headache unresponsive to medical treatment. The referring neurologist believes that the noisy TMJs are the cause of her headaches. Her *daily* medications include (1) a sublingual caffeine tablet on waking and hydrocodone bitartrate–acetaminophen (Vicodin) as needed; (2) 120 mg of propranolol (Inderal LA) three times daily; (3) 350 mg of carisoprodol (Soma) three times daily; (4) 250 mg of amitriptyline (Elavil) at bedtime. A retired nurse, she describes her headaches as suboccipital and frontal. Utilizing this information, the examiner finds that palpation of the trapezius and splenius cervicis muscles reproduces and exacerbates her headache. Not satisfied with this sign, the examiner administers an additional diagnostic test. The patient is placed supine and the weight of her head is supported by the fingertips at the base of the occiput (applying pressure and stretch) on the culprit muscles for 90 seconds. When seated upright again, she reports her headache essentially gone.[18]

Conclusion. The headache is myofascial rather than migrainous, and it is certainly not secondary to a TMJ disorder, clicking aside. The patient is referred for physical therapy in which her headaches are successfully treated and resolved.

CASE TWO: A 63-year-old man is referred with chronic, unresponsive earache, having been treated at least three times with antibiotics for possible ear infection, and all without result. Because of the anatomic proximity of the ear to the TMJ, the referring physician had concluded or diagnosed or surmised that the earache originated in, or was somehow related to, the (coincidentally) popping TMJ. Justifiable reasoning? Perhaps. Some might be inclined to deem such reasoning more forgivable than justifiable.

In the absence of an identifiable problem from some other cause, it is more likely that the earache is referred from one or more of the three specific muscles mentioned earlier that are known to refer as earache: (1) the sternocleidomastoid, (2) the medial pterygoid, and (3) the deep fibers of the masseter. Palpation of the left medial pterygoid reproduces and exacerbates the earache. For diagnostic confirmation and initial treatment, the muscle is injected with local anesthetic (without vasoconstrictor) via an extraoral route,[23] and this provides complete relief of the earache for the first time in more than 8 months. The patient is referred back to his primary care physician with definitive recommendations for treatment.[18]

We find that patients with headache and earache—both of myofascial origin—who undergo advanced TMJ imaging do so because the referring practitioner is, as we have discussed, focused on the TMJ. He or she is unaware of the classic patterns of referred myofascial pain. Quite simply, any TMJ diagnosticians unfamiliar with classic myofascial pain referral routes are seriously limited in their ability to diagnose and therefore are limited in their ability to treat the patient effectively.

The TMJ-TMD clinical form at Loma Linda University* has a section titled *Symptom Review,* which lists 17 typical symptoms.[24] The patient is asked to select the one or ones that best describe the experience. The list includes

1. Headache
2. TMJ pain
3. TMJ noise
4. Earache
5. Upper jaw pain

6. Lower jaw pain
7. Hearing loss
8. Ear fullness
9. Eye pain
10. Neck pain
11. Shoulder pain
12. Ringing in ears
13. Forehead pain
14. Dizziness
15. Nausea
16. Tongue or throat pain
17. Difficulty swallowing

In our experience, symptoms 1 through 17 can be attributed to muscles. Those interested in explanations and illustrations of each of these referral patterns are referred to the classic work of Travell and Simons: *Myofascial Pain and Dysfunction; The Trigger Point Manual,* Vol. I.[21–23]

Given the elusive and often overlapping patterns of joint pain and myofascial pain, how does one determine or diagnose whether the alleged TMJ pain is due to (1) solely a joint disorder, (2) solely myofascial pain, or (3) a combination of joint and myofascial pain?

For the clinician, this is the most difficult part of the management of TMD patients. In our opinion, learning the variations of functional and dysfunctional TMJs is the easier part of the challenge; that is, myofascial pain patterns are the more difficult part. To be effective diagnosticians, it is absolutely essential that clinicians be fully acquainted with the spectrum of myofascial trigger points and their specific pain referral patterns.

CASE THREE: A 14-year-old boy is playing basketball and takes an elbow in the right cheek. There is persistent pain in the right masseter muscle 4 weeks after the incident. Clicking begins in the right TMJ during the fifth week. No treatment has been rendered. The mother is concerned that her son has "TMJ" and arranges a consult. Clinical findings reveal two things: (1) a clicking right joint of 2 days' duration and (2) a prominent, painful trigger point in the right masseter muscle of 5 weeks' duration. The patient is directed to use moist heat and ice (conservative therapy) 20 and 10 minutes respectively twice daily on the painful muscle and to return for consult in 2 days. At the return appointment, it is learned that both the pain and the clicking have disappeared. There are no residuals 2 years after the trauma.[18]

CASE FOUR: A 33-year-old woman comes to the dental clinic for routine dental care by a junior dental student. The patient returns for a second appointment the following week when it is learned that she has had unilateral pain and clicking since the previous appointment.

When asked where she "feels" the pain, she points directly to the left TMJ as the pain site. She (correctly) associates her present pain with the previous extended appointment. The perplexed student seeks a consultation for his perplexed patient.

During the consultation, it is learned that the patient had her mouth opened for more than 3 hours for a dental procedure. Clinical examination reveals a very painful right lateral pterygoid muscle. (The patient is nearly lifted out of

*With thanks to Drs. Bill Solberg and Glenn Clark for their generosity in sharing their clinical forms.

the dental chair on the end of the examiner's index finger.) The student is directed to inject the painful muscle with mepiracaine (Polocaine) plain local anesthetic without vasoconstrictor. Both clicking and pain are diminished as the anesthetic takes effect but persist at a lesser level for 3 more days. The student is directed to repeat the injection. All symptoms subside, with no recurrence after 3 months.[18]

CASE FIVE: A 44-year-old woman is referred for examination of her "TMJ" pain because after 4 years of TMJ treatment and physical therapy she continues to experience essentially disabling pain on a daily basis.

During the interview, the patient begins to grimace with obvious severe pain while holding the left side of her face. She says, "There goes the TMJ now." (Judging by body language and facial expressions, the pain is obviously very intense.) The clinician is keenly observing all this and thinking, regarding the claimed TMJ problem, "I don't think so." The pain lasts for less than 1 minute.

The clinician is not impressed that this is a TMD. It is apparent that her pain is unrelated to her jaw joints, and when told this she finds it difficult to accept because of 4 years of (unsuccessful) treatment for "TMJ." This patient has been programmed to "believe" she has a disordered TMJ, and the treating or referring dentist has also been programmed to "treat" a TMJ disorder, amazingly, for 4 years. Two days of carbamazepine (Tegretol) suspension, 100 mg twice daily, totally relieve her pain and she no longer debates the diagnosis. She is referred to a neurologist in her hometown.[18]

Which of these five cases represents a true TMD? Solely on the basis of painless clicking or popping joints, cases 2, 3, and 4 certainly qualify. Yet in a more specific sense with regard to the *pain and causation,* none of them qualify as such. The remaining two cases were clearly misdiagnosed.

Which of these cases *could* have undergone TMJ imaging? Possibly those with noisy TMJs. Which of these cases should have been imaged? None of them; and none of them were.

To run the risk of iteration, when a practitioner is focused on the clicking or popping joint, treatment too often begins with the obviously displaced disk rather than on the less obvious, but probably culprit, painful muscles. In our opinion, if any of these cases had been treated as a TMJ-TMD problem with conventional conservative therapy, for example, occlusal splints, occlusal adjustment, medications—let us trust that TMJ surgery would never have been a consideration—resolution would most probably have been delayed or missed altogether.

Although a technically correct radiographic or magnetic resonance imaging (MRI) report regarding the osseous joint conditions and the articular disk may have been issued in each of these cases, the fact that the report was accurate regarding the anatomic relationship of the TMJ elements would not have contributed to the appropriate and adequate treatment of the patient. And is not accurate diagnosis the key to accurate and indicated treatment? Of course it is.

Dilemmas such as these are managed when the prac-

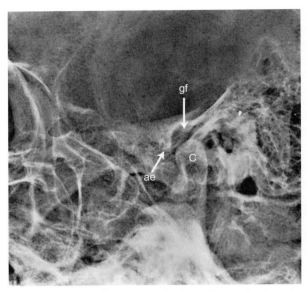

FIGURE 36–2 Lateral transcranial plain film projection shows the condyle (C) within the glenoid fossa (gf) and articular eminence (ae). Transcranial projections display the lateral one-fourth to one-third of the condyle.

titioner is well rounded and reminded in all manner of TMDs. This is the best way to avoid trivial and unproductive referrals. Please remember, *a clicking joint does not mean a painful joint.*

RADIOGRAPHIC METHODOLOGY

Transcranial Plain Film Projections

The earliest reference to, and published illustration of, a TMJ radiograph was in 1913.[25] This was a transcranial

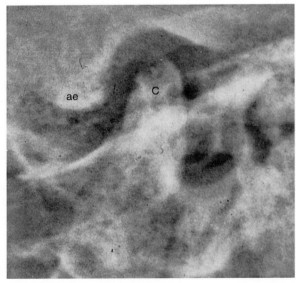

FIGURE 36–3 Although it displays the condyle (C) and the articular eminence (ae), the lateral pharyngeal projection subjects the thyroid to unnecessary radiation; thus, it is not recommended.

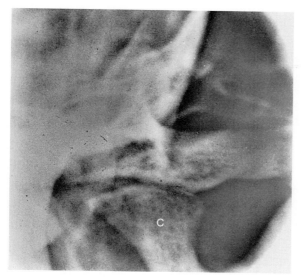

FIGURE 36–4 Transorbital plain film projection reveals coronal condylar (C) morphology. The lens of the eye is unnecessarily exposed to radiation; thus, this projection is not recommended.

projection similar to that shown in Figure 36–2. Over the decades, variations on the theme of transcranial projections have included at least six interpretations of *transcranial* as well as transpharyngeal (Fig. 36–3) and transorbital projections (Fig. 36–4).[26–31]

However adequate or inadequate these early radiographs may have been, most did not escape the scrutiny of contemporary medical radiologists such as Bishop,[32] who opined that "they are conspicuous by their absence or unconvincing by their presence."

As late as 1950, Updegrave,[33] a dentist, presented an allegedly "improved technique" that was essentially the same as that used by medical radiologists more than 30 years earlier.

Transcranial projections continue to be used, particularly in private dental offices where intraoral dental equipment is readily available and adaptable for this purpose. In our opinion, one major problem with the "dental office TMJ radiologist" (lack of training aside) is that some techniques use the typical intraoral x-ray film (43 × 32 mm), an area too small to provide adequate diagnostic information.

Some of the most definitive work published on the transcranial projection was presented by Petersson[34] in his 1976 doctoral dissertation comparing information obtained from different transcranial techniques. In the absence of superior alternatives, transcranial TMJ radiograms have the potential to provide important information regarding the lateral third of the mandibular condyle. Some continue to advocate the transcranial plain film TMJ projection, but with each passing year their number diminishes. The chief limitation of this projection is that two-thirds of the condylar process is not clearly seen. The significance of this limitation is illustrated in the distribution of condylar degenerative joint disease: 50% laterally, 25% centrally, and 25% medially (Fig. 36–5).[35]

The lateral head plain film (Fig. 36–6) is inadequate for the TMJs but is included here to illustrate the open bite in a patient with TMJ rheumatoid arthritis.

CASE SIX: A 47-year-old man is referred for evaluation for TMJ symptoms. His chief complaints are that he cannot now chew as he did previously because his teeth no longer fit together and that his speech is becoming increasingly awkward and difficult. During the initial questions regarding history, the patient is observed to be markedly prognathic. It is obvious to the clinician that a marked malocclusion is present and that maximal intercuspation of the teeth is neither normal nor possible; it appears as though the mandible has outgrown the maxilla.

The clinician's suspicion is aroused. On more specific questioning, the patient denies that his hat, shoe, or hand

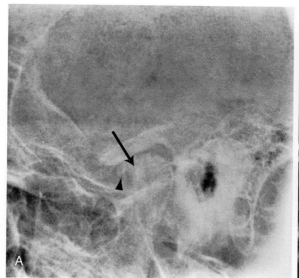
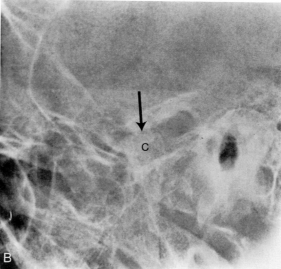

FIGURE 36–5 Lateral plain film projection (A), showing the mouth closed, demonstrates degenerative changes as an absence of superior joint space (*arrow*) and marked osteophytosis (*arrowhead*) on the mandibular condyle (C). With the mouth opened (B) translation is evident, but the joint space remains narrowed (*arrow*).

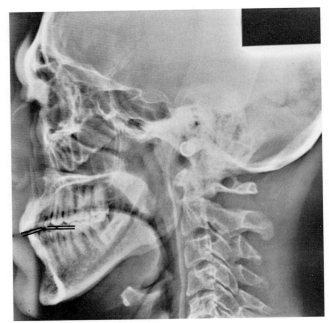

FIGURE 36–6 Lateral skull plain film projection shows a patient with rheumatoid arthritis affecting the temporomandibular joints (not clearly seen), resulting in an anterior open bite (*parallel lines*).

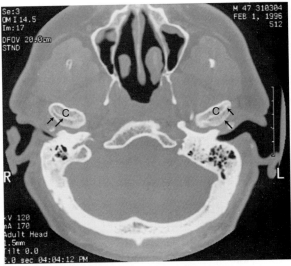

FIGURE 36–8 Axial bone detail, computed tomographic section shows dual cortical margins (*arrows*) on condyles (C) of an acromegaly patient. The bony overgrowth most probably accounts for much of the mandibular advancement.

size has changed. His explanations are that although his cap no longer fits, it had become wet and shrunk; although he can no longer wear his old shoes, it is because so many shoes are imported and one can no longer rely on the stated size; and finally, his wedding ring is too small because of weight gain.

His wife then reminds him of a recent family gathering at which, when measured against his childhood growth pole, it was discovered that he had grown 2 inches taller. TMJ tomograms (Fig. 36–7) and eventually computed tomography (CT) (Fig. 36–8) are ordered. Blood work for growth hormone is ordered, and the results are more than five times normal. The patient is referred to an endocrinologist for more adequate workup and treatment.

MRI reveals an inferior pituitary mass approximately 7 × 7 × 6 mm.

The "TMJ" significance of this case pivots on two points: first, the diagnosis had eluded one or more practitioners, and when action was finally taken it was based on a "TMJ" problem. Second, and truly of TMJ significance, the overgrowth of the mandibular condyles and the resulting malocclusion was such that the patient could not chew easily or efficiently, and this in turn caused pain in the masticatory muscles that led to his appearance at the clinic as a "TMJ" patient.[18]

Tomography: Linear and Pluridirectional

Transcranial TMJ projections were the "gold standard" by virtue of being the only standard from approximately 1913 until 1939 when Petrilli and Gurley[36] (a pediatrician

FIGURE 36–7 Linear tomograms, showing the mouth partially open, depict the glenoid fossa (gf) and articular eminence (ae) of the temporomandibular joints of an acromegaly patient whose condyle (C) is enlarged dorsoventrally (*A*) (*arrow*) and superiorly (*B*) (*arrowheads*).

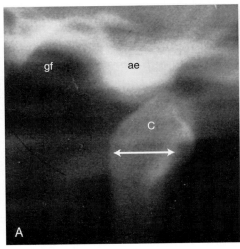
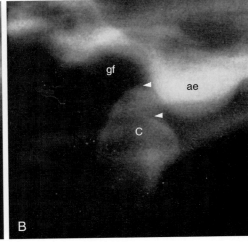

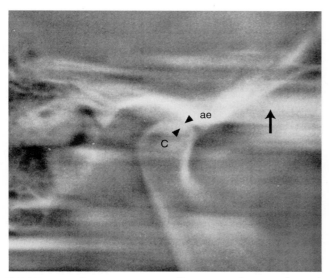

FIGURE 36–9 Linear tomogram illustrates a horizontal streak artifact in the condyle (C) and ventral of the articular eminence (ae) *(arrow)*. The mouth is partly opened, and the joint space is less than normal *(arrowheads)*.

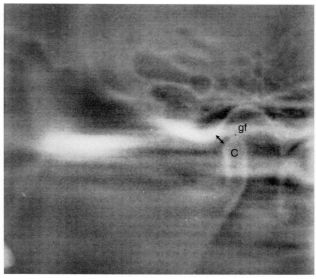

FIGURE 36–11 Linear tomographic projections show the jaw positioned to minimize the influence of linear streak artifact in the glenoid fossa (gf). The joint space *(arrow)* is greater than normal. C, condyle.

and dentist, respectively) published the first paper on TMJ tomography.

There are essentially two categories of tomography—linear (Fig. 36–9) and pluridirectional (Fig. 36–10)—with five motion configurations: (1) linear, (2) circular, (3) elliptic, (4) hypocycloidal, and (5) helical. Hypocycloidal tomography is most often used because it produces the least motion artifact, whereas linear tomography produces significant motion artifact (Fig. 36–11).

Clicking or popping within the joint often results in

focal osteosclerosis (Fig. 36–12) on the dorsal slope of the articular eminence. In linear tomography, the adjacent osseous auditory meatus can create the effect of osseous rarefaction when exposure is made with the mouth closed (Fig. 36–13). To avoid this problem, more than one exposure should be made, at least one of which has the mouth partially or completely open (Fig. 36–14). Some investigators have believed that the steepness of the slope of the articular eminence (Fig. 36–15) in some way predisposes to clicking or popping joints. Both widening (Fig.

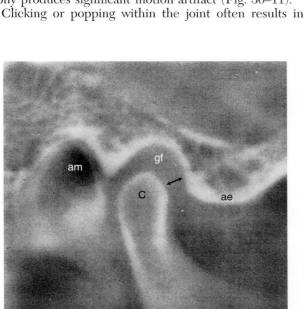

FIGURE 36–10 Pluridirectional tomogram, sagittal projection, illustrates the clarity of the auditory meatus (am), glenoid fossa (gf), articular eminence (ae), and mandibular condyle (C). The anterosuperior joint space *(arrow)* is greater than normal.

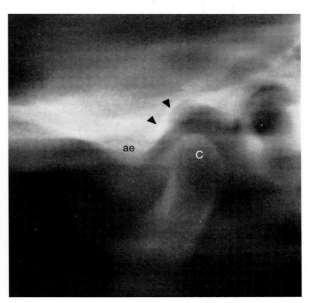

FIGURE 36–12 Linear tomogram, sagittal projection, shows the focus of sclerosis *(arrowheads)* on the articular eminence (ae), most probably resulting from chronic clicking or popping within the joint. C, condyle.

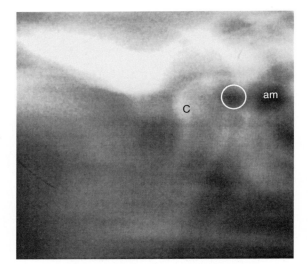

FIGURE 36–13 The proximity of the auditory meatus (am) imposes an apparent osseous rarefaction *(circle)* of the mandibular condyle (C).

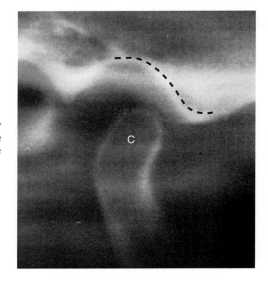

FIGURE 36–14 Linear tomogram, sagittal projection, shows the mouth partly open. Note the uniform thickness of the condylar (C) cortical margin and the more diffuse mild osteosclerosis *(dotted line)* on the articular eminence. The ventral limit of osteosclerosis coincides with the limit of condylar translation.

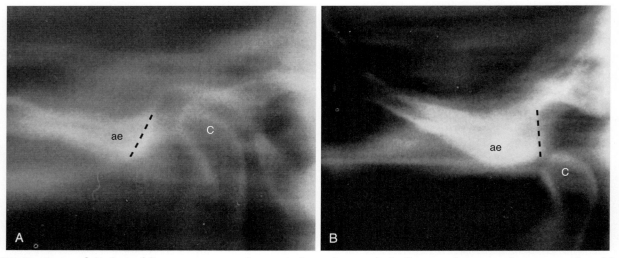

FIGURE 36–15 *A* and *B,* Sagittal linear tomograms show articular eminences (ae) of greater-than-normal steepness *(dotted lines).* Some investigators think that such morphologic variations may contribute to the onset of unprovoked clicking or popping. C, condyle.

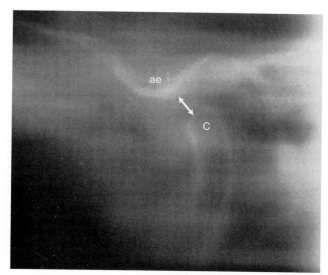

FIGURE 36–16 Linear tomogram shows markedly increased joint space *(arrow)* between the condyle (C) and the articular eminence (ae), suggesting a thickened or displaced disk, or both. The joint space is approximately three times normal.

36–16) and narrowing (Fig. 36–17) of the joint space are significant in terms of indirect signs of diskal position and condition. Degenerative changes within the joint, both primary (Fig. 36–18) and secondary (Fig. 36–19), are seen within the TMJ, secondary changes more so than primary changes.

The most exhaustive investigation into the adequacy of tomography for TMJ imaging was the postdoctoral work undertaken in the early 1970s by Ekerdal.[37, 38]

CASE SEVEN: A 23-year-old woman complains of *painful* popping in her right TMJ secondary to spousal battery.

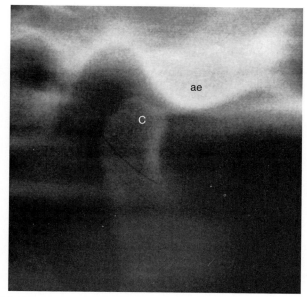

FIGURE 36–17 In contrast to the widened joint space shown in Figure 36–16, there is a mild narrowing of the joint space between the condyle (C) and the articular eminence (ae).

Clinical examination confirms the clicking and suggests an internally deranged joint manifesting as a displaced and reducing articular disk. Linear tomographic examination of the right joint (Fig. 36–20) reveals osteosclerosis on the dorsal slope of the articular eminence and narrowing of the superior joint space. Both of these are common findings in clicking joints.

Although direct and obvious findings may be the most helpful to the radiologist, indirect findings can be equally so with regard to the TMJ. One should evaluate condylar position and joint spacing with the mandible in more than one position. When the joint space is too narrow, the articular disk is either thinned or absent at that point in the tomographic plane. Alternatively, if the joint space is widened, the articular disk is misplaced or misshapen, or both.

The position of the jaw can enhance the visualization of such findings. With the mouth closed and the teeth in maximal contact, one can evaluate the joint spaces posterior and superior to the mandibular condyle. When the mandible is advanced in the protrusive position, one can evaluate the consistency of the anterosuperior joint space, which is probably the most relevant joint space. With the mouth opened maximally, one can again evaluate for consistency of joint space and adequacy of condylar translation. Typically, when patients undergo TMJ radiography, the jaw is routinely placed in three positions for examination: the mouth closed and the teeth in maximal intercuspation; the mandible protruded and the mouth opened maximally; and some position of clinical significance such as the point of pain.

In the case of the 23-year-old woman, the consistency of the history, the symptoms, and the clinical and radiographic signs do not indicate advanced imaging in order that the impression or diagnosis be underscored. Treatment proceeds on the basis of the foundation previously described.

Pantomography

The lowly pantomogram, although inadequate and inappropriate for the routine or detailed examination of the TMJ, is quite adequate in cases of fracture or as a screening modality for chronic pain that is inconsistent with typical TMD or myofascial presentation. The geometric nature of the pantomogram is such that it tends to simulate the following abnormal features: anterior condylar flattening, osteophytes, joint space narrowing, and left or right condylar asymmetry.[39]

Rarely, one encounters a patient already experiencing a disordered TMJ when something additional and certainly more insidious is occurring (Figs. 36–21 and 36–22). The pantomogram is quite adequate as a screening radiograph. We would suggest to the medical radiologist as we do to the dentist to look at the teeth last. We can think of unfortunate cases in which the teeth were evaluated to the exclusion of more significant findings.

CASE EIGHT: A 26-year-old man—brother of a dental student—complains of jaw pain after being beaten by a gang of thugs. His face is bruised, his eye is swollen shut, and he is unable to open his mouth. Pantomography is

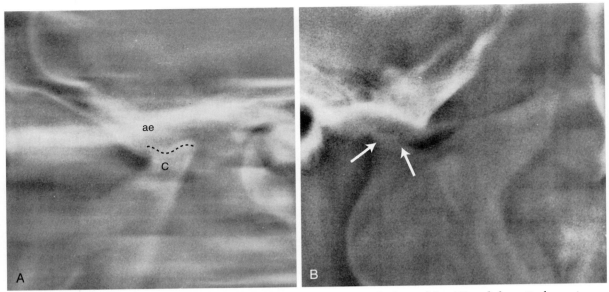

FIGURE 36–18 Marked (A) to severe (B) rheumatoid degenerative changes on both condyles (C) and the articular eminences (ae) are depicted on sagittal linear tomograms. A shows partial condylar loss (dotted line), whereas B shows complete loss of the condyle (arrows).

ordered (Fig. 36–23), and the findings indicate a fractured mandibular condyle. This radiographic modality is completely adequate for screening purposes such as these. The patient is referred to maxillofacial surgery for immediate care.

Arthrography

In the latter part of the 1930s, when the majority of American dental investigators were debating ad nauseam the most "precise" radiographic modality or the most "precise" adaptation of a particular modality, investigators in Denmark[40] and Germany[41] were pursuing the indirect soft tissue imaging technique of TMJ arthrography. In search of an answer to the question of articular disk position, positive contrast arthrography seemed a logical step in the sequence of TMJ radiographic research.

For the ofttimes imaginative and creative Germans, the problem of TMJ arthrography proved too difficult to solve, and it fell to the ingenuity of Flemming Norgaard in Denmark, working amidst bombs and blackouts, to successfully produce the first known definitive TMJ

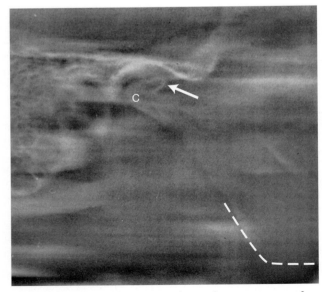

FIGURE 36–19 Secondary osteoarthritic changes in an aged patient are illustrated by the increased obtuse angle of the mandibular ramus (dotted lines) relative to the mandibular body and condylar (C) osteophytic changes (arrow).

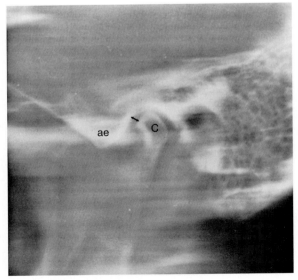

FIGURE 36–20 Sagittal linear tomogram of a battered woman shows generalized osteosclerosis over the articular eminence (ae), loss of condylar (C) superior joint space, and a widened anterosuperior joint space (arrow), which point to disk displacement and correlate with clinical findings.

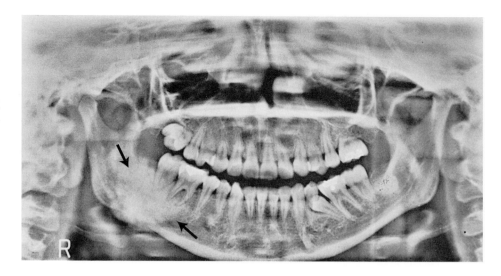

FIGURE 36–21 Pantomogram of a 12-year-old girl who as a very young child had been treated for retinoblastoma. The mandibular lesion (*arrows*) is osteogenic sarcoma, possibly resulting from therapeutic ionizing radiation administered years earlier.

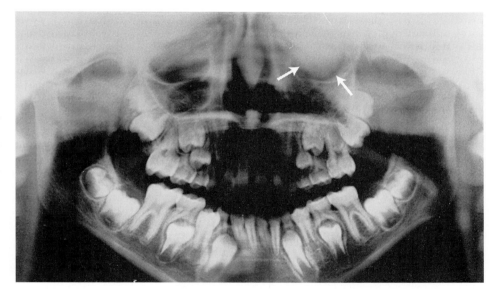

FIGURE 36–22 A 10-year-old boy with definitive symptoms of temporomandibular joint disorder (unable to open his mouth adequately) also had a nasopharyngeal mass (*arrows*).

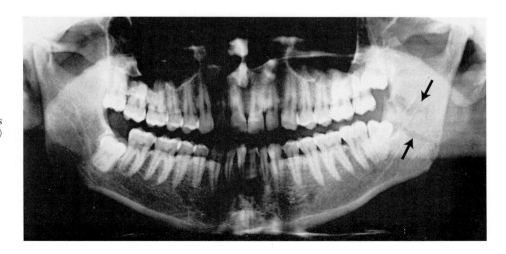

FIGURE 36–23 Pantomogram shows mandibular fracture lines (*arrows*) secondary to battery.

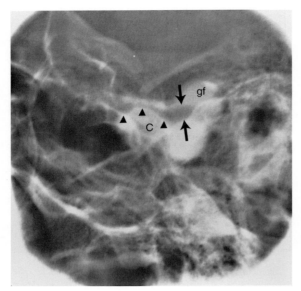

FIGURE 36–24 Transcranial plain film dual joint space arthrography reveals an articular disk *(arrowheads)* and a bilaminar zone dorsal to the disk *(arrows)*. Contrast material fills space in the glenoid fossa (gf). The condyle (C) rests on the ventral slope of the articular eminence in this open-mouth view.

arthrogram. Norgaard's work lay largely unappreciated until TMJ arthrography was "rediscovered" in the late 1970s.[42–44]

The evolution of arthrography was moved from inferior to dual joint space plain film studies (Fig. 36–24), and thence to arthrotomography (Fig. 36–25).

Refinements to arthrotomography included Westesson's[45] double-contrast methodology in which both air and contrast medium were injected into the joint spaces. In our opinion, the most definitive investigations on the mechanism of joint clicking or popping were carried out by Isberg[46] in Sweden.

Early in the dental involvement in TMJ disorders, collective dental wisdom held that clicking and popping were caused by the disk's moving over the *anterior* or ventral border of the disk. It is now known that this is not the case, as the most prominent popping in the mandibular translatory cycle occurs as the condyle negotiates the *posterior* or dorsal diskal margin of the disk when it is (most often) ventromedially displaced. Cases of posterior diskal displacement are rare.[47]

In the early 1980s, among medical and dental radiologists, it was held that if contrast material were retained in the ventral compartment of the inferior joint space when the mouth was maximally opened, this was a sign of a displaced articular disk. Kaplan and others,[48, 49] pondering whether this assumption was valid, designed an investigation and subsequently presented and published the results of their work in which inferior joint space arthrography was performed on asymptomatic (and presumably normal) volunteers. Their most significant finding was that contrast material may be *retained* in the ventral compartment of the inferior joint space in normal TMJs.

Variations on the theme of arthrography included CT-assisted arthrography (Fig. 36–26), which for a while was explored as a means of extracting more information from the arthrographic procedure. This was abandoned, however, because it was felt that the returns did not justify the cost and additional room time.[50]

CASE NINE: A 13-year-old boy presents for evaluation with complaints of an inability to open his mouth. The patient and his parent state that over the past year his

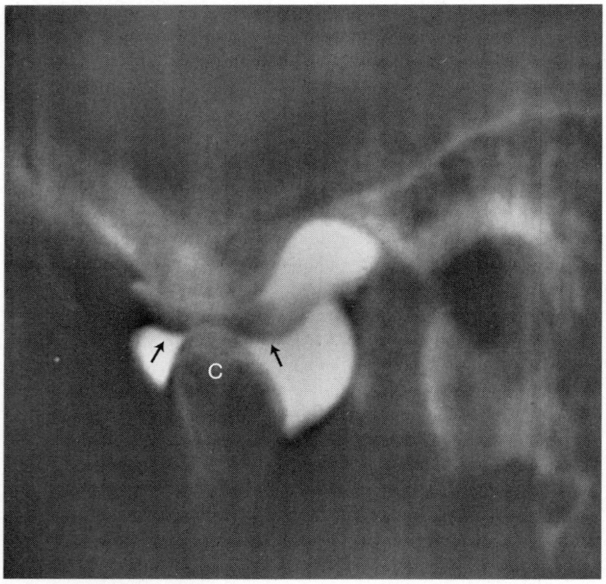

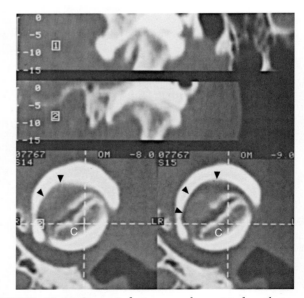

FIGURE 36–25 Arthrotomogram, showing the mouth opened, with contrast material in the upper and lower joint spaces, clearly outlines the normally positioned articular disk *(arrows)* on the mandibular condyle (C).

FIGURE 36–26 Computed tomography–assisted arthrogram, axial section (below) with sagittal (upper) and coronal (middle) vertical reconstructions. The articular disk *(arrowheads)* is best seen in the axial section ventral to the condyle (C).

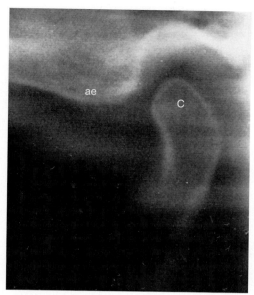

FIGURE 36–27 Linear tomogram of a teenaged boy shows marked restriction of the condylar (C) translation relative to the summit of the articular eminence (ae). The condyle should translate to the summit of the eminence or slightly beyond.

maximal opening has steadily decreased. The patient is tall for his age, 5 feet 10 inches. Clinical evaluation reveals maximal opening of 15 mm. Further testing discloses a very solid feel when the boy tries to open his mouth. Linear tomograms do not clearly disclose the suspected problem (elongated coronoid processes) (Fig. 36–27). Vertically re-formatted computed tomograms clearly show the elongation (Fig. 36–28). Osteosclerotic changes are present in the zygomatic arch where the coronoid processes have been contacting bilaterally. The patient is referred to maxillofacial surgery for evaluation and probable coronoidectomy.

X-Ray CT

The earliest publication of any attempt to utilize x-ray CT (Fig. 36–29) for TMJ disorders is best attributed to Suarez and associates.[51] This work was followed by numerous papers that were, for the greater part, more illustrative than definitive.[52–61] For a period of more than 6 years, we explored many aspects of advanced TMJ imaging with CT,[62–68] and the work culminated in a textbook.[69]

Our conclusions about the efficacy of CT as a modality for TMJ imaging are summarized as follows.

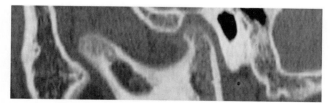

FIGURE 36–28 Vertically re-formatted sagittal osseous computed tomography section shows an elongated coronoid process, which prevented wide opening of the mouth.

CT is

Unsurpassed for osseous imaging
Inadequate for imaging thinned or normal articular disks
Adequate for imaging thickened or misshapen articular disks
Unsurpassed for manipulation of display data
Unsurpassed for reconstruction of three-dimensional images
Adequate for presurgical planning
Inappropriate (overkill) for routine TMJ imaging
Ideal for research of the stomatognathic system
An acceptable risk for patients with regard to radiation dose
Probably superior to MRI based on total returns (disk aside)
Inadequate for real-time dynamic imaging
A modality that produces images that are too noisy in the presence of dental restorations

The first attempts at using CT for imaging the position of the articular disk were very promising, until it was learned that the attenuation value of the articular disk is essentially the same as that of the tendinous attachment of the superior and inferior parts of the lateral pterygoid muscle to the madibular pterygoid fovea.[70]

The reason that CT is inadequate for a thinned or normal disk, whether it may be normally or abnormally positioned, is related to the edge response function. The anatomic transition from bone to soft tissue to bone occurs in too small a distance to permit the computer to display these abrupt changes in attenuation. Therefore, instead of a distinct edge to the attenuation values, there is a slope. It is in the slope of this edge response that the image of the normal or thinned disk is lost. However, when the disk is thickened and the distance across bone-disk-bone is increased, the disk is usually visible.

Three-dimensional reconstructions[71–73] of the TMJ (Fig. 36–30), although they are interesting and dynamic in presentation, are not generally helpful in the routine TMJ CT study. They seem to be most helpful in presurgical planning and in other special cases in which spatial relations must be considered.

In cases of degenerative joint disease or other osseous abnormalities, nothing surpasses CT for image detail, flexibility, and manipulation of the display data (Fig. 36–31).

CASE TEN: A 15-year-old girl is referred to the TMJ clinic from Loma Linda University Medical Center after undergoing intravenous antibiotic therapy for an infection. The CT scans accompanying the patient are the first either of us has seen of a TMJ intra-articular infection (Fig. 36–32). The patient is seriously medically compromised with numerous ailments. It is concluded, in the absence of any obvious joint destruction, the resolution of the infection, and the presence of complicating factors such as dialysis three times weekly, and so forth, that the patient has been adequately cared for and that nothing further would be accomplished by any manner of conservative TMJ therapy. The patient is referred for much-needed dental repair and restorations in a hospital setting.

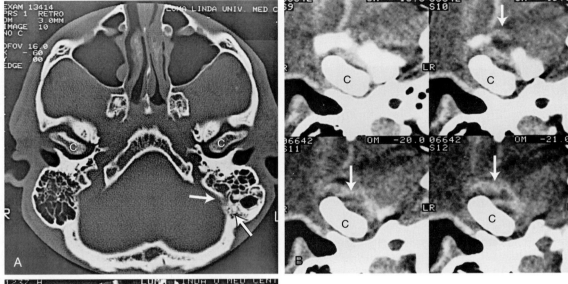

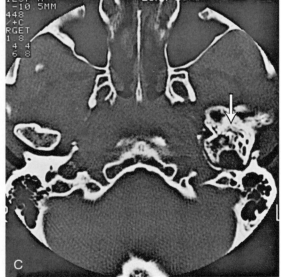

FIGURE 36–29 Axial computed tomography (CT) section of osseous detail *(A)* held promise of greater diagnostic detail when applied to temporomandibular joint (TMJ) studies. Note the metastatic tumor in the left mastoid *(arrows)*. The patient underwent a TMJ study because it was first believed that his pain represented a TMJ disorder. Axial soft tissue sections *(B)* taken each 1.0 mm best show the anterolateral displaced disk in the upper right, lower left, and lower right *(arrows)*. Axial bone detail CT section *(C)* of a large osteochondroma in the left TMJ.

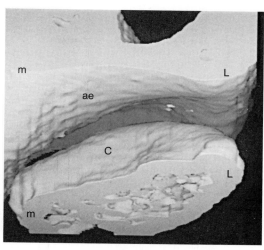

FIGURE 36–30 Three-dimensional image reconstructed from display data matrix. Gradient shading gives an impression of depth. Note the condylar head (C) viewed from the front, articular eminence (ae), and joint space lateral (L) and medial (m) to the condyle. (Photograph courtesy of Dr. David Roberts.)

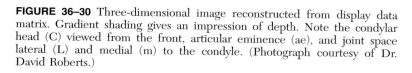

FIGURE 36–31 *A* shows three corrected sagittal vertically reformatted images (upper left [UL], lower left [LL], and lower right [LR]) of a degenerated condyle (C) constructed along dotted cursor lines in the upper right (UR) axial image. Vertically reformatted sagittal and coronal sections, respectively *(B and C),* of degenerated joint with condylar (C) osteophytosis *(arrowheads),* loss of joint space, and erosive changes.

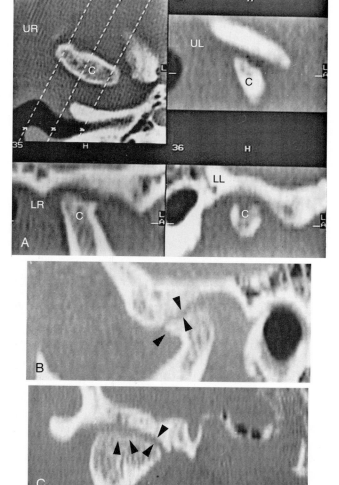

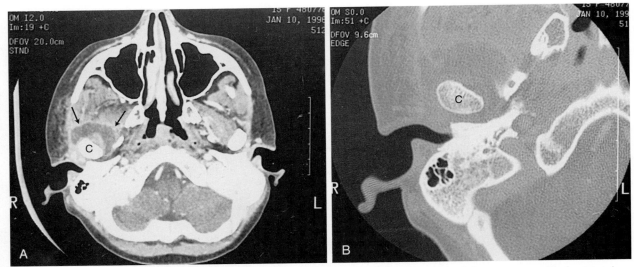

FIGURE 36–32 Axial computed tomography sections show an infectious invasion of the right *(A)* temporomandibular joint *(arrows)* but without resultant damage to the mandibular condyle (C) *(B)*. The patient was treated with intravenous antibiotics.

In any thin-section imaging technique, a description of the size, shape, and position of the articular disk must be assumed accurate *only* for that section location (Fig. 36–33), as each of these disk descriptors can change dramatically in less than the length (average 2 cm) of the mandibular condyle.

Magnetic Resonance Imaging

MRI was welcomed as a breakthrough in TMJ imaging because early studies suggested that not since arthrography had the articular disk been so readily and elegantly displayed (Fig. 36–34). Studies have been carried out

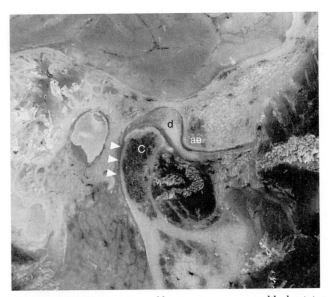

FIGURE 36–33 Cryosection of human temporomandibular joint illustrates a degenerated condyle (C), loss of joint space dorsal to the condyle *(arrowheads)*, the articular eminence (ae), and a displaced articular disk (d). Conditions illustrated in this section may change dramatically over the width of the condyle.

comparing MRI findings with clinical and surgical findings,[74, 75] determining the optimal imaging plane[76–78] and optimal section thickness,[79] optimizing disk contrast,[80] and measuring the influence of temporal artery flow artifact.[81]

More recent studies have looked at the nuances of imaging technique in search of improved images.[82–84] Broader applications of MRI to the stomatognathic system include *evidence* of pain based on joint effusion,[85] spectroscopy of the muscles of mastication,[86, 87] the diagnosis of such entities as myositis ossificans,[88] and rheumatic disease affecting the TMJ.[89] MRI is also being applied to the study of energy metabolism in the masseter muscles,[90] a muscle often associated with myofascial pain and mandibular dysfunction.

The tendinous insertion of the inferior belly of the lateral pterygoid muscle may be mistaken for the articular disk in some cases (Fig. 36–35). In the medial portion of the joint the articular disk, in its ventral aspect, attaches directly to fibers of the superior belly of the lateral pterygoid muscle, whereas as one moves centrally and laterally within the joint the insertion is more tendinous.

Although one may rely more on an MRI for diskal identification, the same principles of indirect findings that apply to other imaging modalities such as joint space and condylar position should be applied to MRI in order to minimize confusion of the articular disk with similarly hydrated tissue such as the lateral pterygoid tendons described previously (Fig. 36–36). Similarly, it is important to image with the patient's mouth both opened and closed, not so much to determine whether disk reduction occurs (because that is most usually readily determined during clinical examination), but rather to determine whether there are significant changes in the shape, condition, and position of the disk during different jaw excursions (Fig. 36–37). Before any contemplated definitive and irreversible procedure, such information would be valuable to the practitioner and the patient with regard to prognosis.

Although in most (60%) patients[69] the disk dislocates

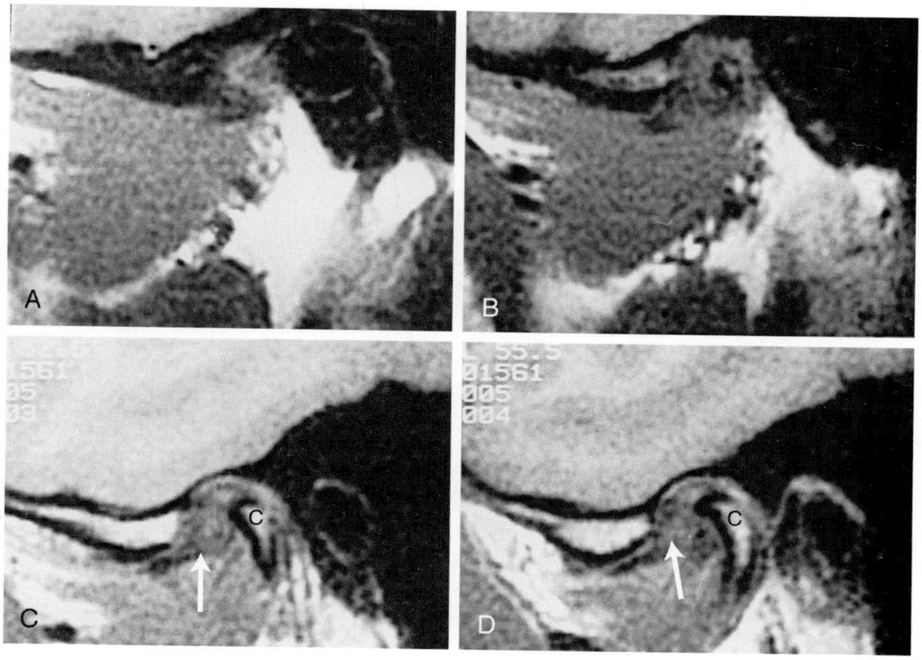

FIGURE 36–34 Sagittal serial magnetic resonance images medial to the joint space *(A and B)* to the medial condylar (C) pole *(C and D)* show a displaced and thickened disk *(arrows).*

anteromedially and diskal visibility improves or is maintained as one moves medially through the joint, in some patients the disk slips laterally (Fig. 36–38).

In MRI, there is no radiation dose to the patient, as with all ionizing radiation studies, and there is no invasiveness or pain. The additional possible postprocedural complications of arthrography have led to MRI being considered its rightful successor.

MRI, like every other modality, has its drawbacks and

its detractors. One of the principal drawbacks to MRI is cost; it is clearly the most expensive modality used in TMJ imaging. Although there is a basis for confidence in TMJ MRI, one should not ignore the strength and validity of the less sophisticated modalities when appropriately applied.

Research has contributed to strengthening the diagnostic reliability of MRI. The diagnostician should

Obtain both direct coronal and sagittal images
Be aware of the effects of flow phenomena from the superficial temporal artery on image interpretation
Be aware that accurate diagnosis of disk position many be no better than 89%
Understand the subjective superiority of high-resolution thin-section (1.5-mm) images compared with routine 3-mm images
Understand that MRI tends to underdiagnose perforation and overdiagnose nonreducibility
Understand the relationship between disk position, joint effusion, and probable pain

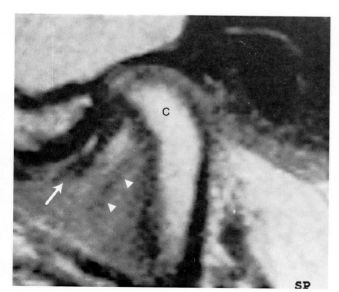

FIGURE 36–35 Sagittal magnetic resonance image shows two areas of decreased signal intensity ventral to the mandibular condyle (c). The inferior area *(arrowheads)* represents a tendinous attachment of the lateral pterygoid muscle to the condylar pterygoid fovea, and the superior area *(arrow)* represents the articular disk.

CASE ELEVEN: A high school cheerleader, aged 16 years, is referred for evaluation after an incident in which during a cheerleading routine, instead of being caught, the girl slipped from the grasp of her partners, landing on her chin from a height of approximately 6 feet. There are no fractures, but since the incident she has been unable to open her mouth more than 15 mm. Conservative therapy does not benefit her, either with increased mandibular mobility or with relief of pain. The decision is made to pursue advanced imaging in the form of MRI in order to assist in the decision of how to proceed with future therapy. On the basis of the position and shape of the articular disk (Fig. 36–39), the decision is made that mandibular manipulation with the patient under general anesthesia will most probably not be successful in

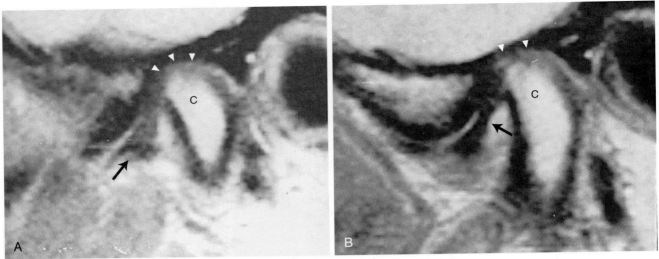

FIGURE 36–36 Note the loss of both the anterosuperior and superior joint spaces *(arrowheads)* in this sagittal magnetic resonance image *(A)* with the disk ventral (anterior) *(arrow)* to the condyle (C). *B* depicts the diminished joint space superior *(arrowheads)* to the condyle (C) with a typically described "bow tie" displaced articular disk *(arrow)*.

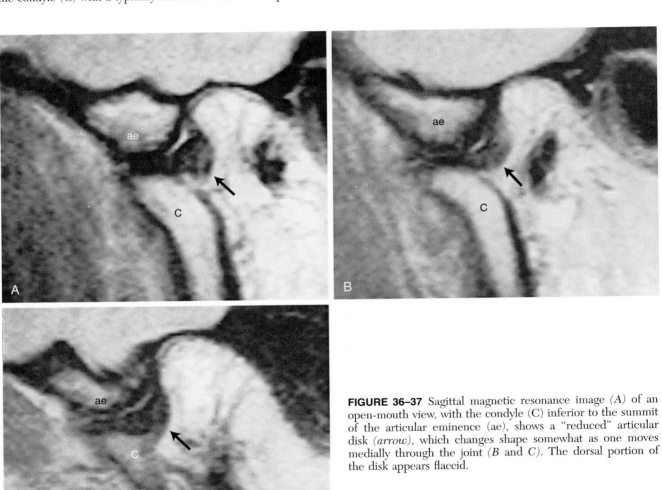

FIGURE 36–37 Sagittal magnetic resonance image *(A)* of an open-mouth view, with the condyle (C) inferior to the summit of the articular eminence (ae), shows a "reduced" articular disk *(arrow)*, which changes shape somewhat as one moves medially through the joint *(B* and *C)*. The dorsal portion of the disk appears flaccid.

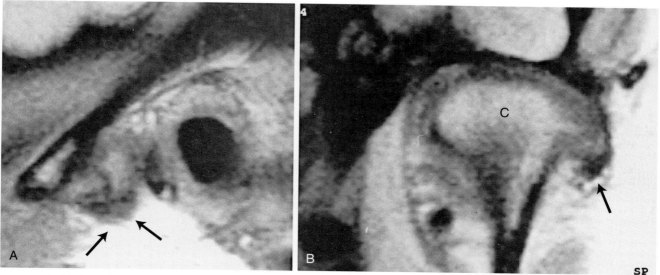

FIGURE 36–38 Sagittal magnetic resonance imaging (MRI) study in the lateral joint shows an area of low signal intensity *(arrows)* consistent with a laterally displaced disk. The condyle is not seen. Corrected coronal MRI section *(B)* shows the condyle (C) with the articular disk slipped laterally *(arrow)*.

remobilizing the mandible. The consulting oral and maxillofacial surgeons decide that the best result will most probably be realized with arthroscopy.

A PHILOSOPHY FOR IMAGING

For us, the working word in selecting the optimal imaging modality is *adequacy.* In matters of TMJ imaging, the foundation of the "adequate" image is based largely on

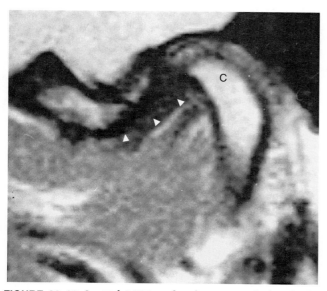

FIGURE 36–39 Sagittal MRI study of a teenaged cheerleader who was dropped on her chin by team members. The result was a traumatically displaced articular disk *(arrowheads)* and dramatically reduced maximal mouth opening of 15 mm. C, condyle.

the questions: What is the clinical question? What is it that the practitioner needs to know in order to provide the most effective treatment?

Is it necessary to confirm disk displacement with imaging? In most cases probably not, as this can be determined with a high degree of clinical confidence without imaging of any kind.

Is it necessary to know the precise position of the articular disk? There are three choices: arthrography, CT-assisted arthrography, and MRI.

Is it necessary to know the condition or shape of the articular disk? This may be the most important single piece of information the clinician or surgeon can have, as there are more ramifications stemming from this than from other data one might collect. Disk shape and condition are best determined with dual-compartment arthrography, which will more clearly reveal areas of thickening, thinning, and perforation.

We have specified one's "need to know" as distinguished from one's "wishing to know" these matters. When speaking of the need to know we are placing this need within the context and process of indicated and definitive treatment alternatives, the choice of which is most likely to be determined by the report of the radiologist.

If one is merely curious concerning the position or condition of the disk and if this knowledge neither influences nor alters therapy, then where is the justification for imaging, advanced or otherwise? In our opinion, it does not exist.

There is another important element to consider, what McNeill refers to as a *paradigm shift.*[91] Over the past several years, TMD therapy has shifted gradually, and wisely, from a philosophy of "fixing" the problem to, in many cases, allowing the disorder to exhaust itself in a known and predictable manner. In a case managed in this manner, is there an urgency to image? Most probably not. It may be wisest to await those conditions in which imaging is appropriate and necessary rather than to succumb to curiosity.

To close somewhat as we opened, pain is one of the great, if not the greatest, motivators on the part of both the patient and the practitioner. But TMD pain can most often be resolved by conservative and inexpensive modalities. Thus, although there is a place for advanced imaging in the diagnosis and treatment of TMD patients, it is not for all patients, nor is it even for most patients. It is for the few who do not respond to conservative therapy, whose pain is such that it prevents them from having a normal life with normal activities and whose practitioner wisely selects the most productive imaging time and modality for each stop on the pain-dysfunction continuum.

References

1. Cooper A.: A Treatise on Fractures and Dislocations. 1st American ed., 2nd London ed. London, 1823.
2. Baer WS. Arthroplasty with the aid of animal membrane. Am J Orthop Surg 1918;16:1–29.
3. Humphry GM. Excision of the condyle of the lower jaw. Br Assoc Med J 1856;60:61.
4. Murphy JB. Cicatrical fixation of mandible following noma release; interposition of mucous flaps. Surg Clin Phila 1916;5:855–859.
5. Annandale T. Displacement of the inter-articular cartilage of the lower jaw, and its treatment by operation. Lancet 1887;1:411.
6. Murphy JB. Temporomandibular arthroplasty. Ann Surg 1914; 60:127–129.
7. Murphy JB. Arthroplasty for intra-articular bony and fibrous ankylosis of temporomandibular articulation. JAMA 1914;62:1784–1794.
8. Blair VP: Operative treatment of ankylosis of the mandible. Trans South Surg Gynecol Assoc 1914;26:436–465.
9. Meyer RA. The autogenous dermal graft in temporomandibular joint disk surgery. J Oral Maxillofac Surg 1988;46:948–954.
10. Davidson C, Wojtulewik JA, Bacon PA, Winstock D. Temporomandibular joint disease in ankylosing spondylitis. Ann Rheum Dis 1975;34:87–91.
11. DelBalso AM, Pyatt RS, Busch RF, et al. Synovial cell sarcoma of the temporomandibular joint: Computed tomographic findings. Arch Otolaryngol 1982;108:520–522.
12. Flurr E, Haverling M, Molin C. Gout in the temporomandibular joint; report of case. Otorhinolaryngology 1974;36:16–20.
13. Harris RJ. Lyme disease involving the temporomandibular joint. J Oral Maxillofac Surg 1985;43:629.
14. Jonsson R, Lindvall A-M, Nyberg G. Temporomandibular joint involvement in systemic lupus erythematosus. Arthritis Rheum 1983;26:474–477.
15. Larheim TA. Comparison between three radiographic techniques for the examination of the temproromandibular joints in juvenile rheumatoid arthritis. Acta Radiol Diagn 1981;22:195–201.
16. Mejersjo C, Carlsson GE. Long-term results of treatment for temporomandibular joint pain-dysfunction. J Prosthet Dent 1983; 49:809–815.
17. Mejersjo C. Long-term development after treatment of mandibular dysfunction and osteoarthritis. Thesis for doctorate in odontology. University of Goteborg, Sweden. Swed Dent J Suppl 1984;22:1–58.
18. Clinical data, Loma Linda, CA, 1980–1995. Temporomandibular Joint Clinic, School of Dentistry, Loma Linda University.
19. Pinto OF. A new structure related to the temporomandibular joint and middle ear. J Prosthet Dent 1962;12:95–103.
20. Komori E, Sugasaki M, Ranabe H, Kato S. Discomalleolar ligament in the human adult. J Craniomand Pract 1986;4:299–305.
21. Travell J, Simons D. Myofascial Pain and Dysfunction: The Trigger Point Manual, p. 167. Baltimore, Williams & Wilkins, 1983.
22. Travell J, Simons D. Myofascial Pain and Dysfunction: The Trigger Point Manual, p. 203. Baltimore, Williams & Wilkins, 1983.
23. Travell J, Simons D. Myofascial Pain and Dysfunction: The Trigger Point Manual, pp. 220, 250, 261. Baltimore, Williams & Wilkins, 1983.
24. University of California, Los Angeles, School of Dentistry, temporomandibular joint clinical form. Appropriated and adapted for use at Loma Linda University School of Dentistry.
25. Murphy JB. Bony ankylosis of jaw, with interposition of flaps from temporal fascia. Clin John B Murphy, MD, 17 April, 1913; pp. 659–664.
26. Kern MJ. Complete roentgenological survey of the head. AJR 1926;16:264–265.
27. Lindblom G. Technique for roentgen-photographic registration of the different condyle positions in the temporomandibular joint. Dent Cosmos 1936;78:1227–1235.
28. Sproull J. Technique for roentgen examination of the temporomandibular articulation. AJR 1933;30:262–264.
29. McQueen WW. Radiography of the temporomandibular articulation. Minneapolis Dist Dent J 1937;21:28–30.
30. Higley LB. Practical application of a new and scientific method for producing temporomandibular roentgenograms. J Am Dent Assoc 1937;24:222.
31. Ivy RH. Interpretation of Dental and Maxillary Roentgenograms. St. Louis, CV Mosby, 1918.
32. Bishop PA. Roentgenographic consideration of the temporomandibular joint. AJR 1929;21:556.
33. Updegrave WJ: Improved roentgenographic technique for the temporomandibular articulation. J Am Dent Assoc 1950;40:391–401.
34. Petersson A. Radiography of the Temporomandibular Joint. A Comparison of Information Obtained from Different Radiographic Techniques. [Doctoral dissertation] Malmo, University of Lund, Lund, Sweden, 1976.
35. Christiansen EL, Thompson JR, Kopp S, et al. Radiographic signs of temporomandibular joint diseases: An investigation utilizing x-ray computed tomography. Dentomaxillofac Radiol 1985;14:83–92.
36. Petrilli A, Gurley JF. Tomography of the temporomandibular joint. J Am Dent Assoc 1939;26:218.
37. Ekerdal O. Tomography of the temporomandibular joint; correlation between tomographic image and histologic sections in a three-dimensional system. Acta Radiol (Stockh) 1973;329(Suppl):1–107.
38. Ekerdal O. Tomography of the temporomandibular joint. Medica Mundi 1971;16:144.
39. Ruf S, Pancherz H. Is orthopantomography reliable for TMJ diagnosis? An experimental study on a dry skull. J Orofacial Pain 1995;9:365–374.
40. Norgaard F. Arthrography of the mandibular joint. Acta Radiol 1944;23:740.
41. Zimmer EA. Die Roentgenologie des Kiefergelenke. SSO Schweiz Monatsschr Zahnheild 1941;51:949.
42. Wilkes CH. Arthrography of the temporomandibular joint in patients with the TMJ pain-dysfunction syndrome. Minn Med 1978;61:645.
43. Farrar WB, McCarty WL Jr. Inferior joint space arthrography and characteristics of condylar paths in internal derangements of the TMJ. J Prosthet Dent 1979;41:548.
44. Katzberg RW, Dolwick MF, Bales DJ, Helms CA. Arthrotomography of the temporomandibular joint: New technique and preliminary observations. A J R 1979;132:949–955.
45. Westesson PL. Double-contrast arthrography and internal derangement of the temporomandibular joint. Swed Dent J Suppl 1982;13:1–57.
46. Isberg A. Temporomandibular Joint Clicking. [Doctoral thesis] Stockholm, Sweden, Karolinska Institutet, School of Dentistry, 1980.
47. Gallagher DM. Posterior dislocation of the temporomandibular joint meniscus. Report of three cases. J Am Dent Assoc 1986;113:411–415.
48. Kaplan P. Inferior joint space arthrography of normal temporomandibular joints: A reassessment of diagnostic criteria. Scientific Paper £592, presented at the 71st Scientific Assembly and Annual Meeting of the Radiological Society of North America, Chicago, November 17–22, 1985.
49. Kaplan P. Inferior joint space arthrography: Reassessment of diagnostic criteria. Radiology 1986;159:585.
50. Katzberg RW Dolwick MF, Keith DA, et al. New observations with routine and CT-assisted arthrography in suspected internal derangements of the temporomandibular joint. Oral Surg 1981;51:569–574.
51. Suarez FR. A preliminary study of computerized tomographs of the temporomandibular joint. Compend Contin Educ Dent 1980;1:217.
52. Blankestun J, Goering G, Thun CJP. Arthrography, arthrotomogra-

phy and computed tomography in the differential diagnosis of temporomandibular joint dysfunction. J Oral Rehabil 10:499;1983.

53. Cohen H, Ross S, Gordon R. Computerized tomography as a guide in the diagnosis of temporomandibular joint disease. J Am Dent Assoc 1985;110:57–60.

54. Helms CA, Katzberg RW, Moorish R, Dolwick MF. Computerized tomography of the temporomandibular joint. J Oral Maxillofac Surg 1983;41:512–517.

55. Helms CA, Richardson ML, Vogler JB III, Hoddick WL. Computed tomography for diagnosing temporomandibular joint disk displacement. J Craniomand Pract 1984–1985;3(1):23–26.

56. Manzione JV, Seltzer SE, Katzberg RW, et al. Internal derangement of the temporomandibular joint: Diagnosis by direct sagittal computed tomography. Radiology 1984;150:111–115.

57. Avrahami E, Horowitz Y, Cohn DF. Computed tomography of the temporomandibular joint. Comput Radiol 1984;8:211–216.

58. Blankestun J, Boering G, Thun CJP. Arthrography, arthrotomography and computed tomography in the differential diagnosis of temporomandibular joint dysfunction. J Oral Rehabil 1983;10:449.

59. Cohen H, Ross S, Gordon R. Computerized tomography as a guide in the diagnosis of temporomandibular joint disease. J Am Dent Assoc 1985;110:57–60.

60. Fjellstrom CA, Olofsson O. Computed tomography of the temporomandibular joint meniscus; a report of preliminary tests. J Maxillofac Surg 1985;13:24–27.

61. Helms CA, Moorish RB, Kircos LT, et al. Computed tomography of the temporomandibular joint meniscus: Preliminary observations. Radiology 1982;145:719–722.

62. Christiansen EL, Thompson JR, Kopp S. Intra- and inter-observer variability and accuracy in the determination of linear and angular measurements in computed tomography: An in-vitro and in-situ study of human mandibles. Acta Odontol Scand 1986;44:221–229.

63. Christiansen EL, Moore RJ, Thompson JR, et al. Radiation dose in radiography, CT, and arthrography of the temporomandibular joint. AJR 1987;148:107–109.

64. Christiansen EL, Thompson JR, Zimmerman G, et al: Computed tomography correlation of condylar and articular disc positions within the temporomandibular joint. Oral Surg 1987;64:757–767.

65. Christiansen EL, Chan TT, Thompson JR, et al: Computed tomography of the normal temporomandibular joint. Scand J Dent Res 1987;95:499–509.

66. Christiansen EL, Thompson JR, Hasso AN, et al. CT number characteristics of malpositioned TMJ menisci: Diagnosis with CT number highlighting (blinkmode). Invest Radiol 1985;22:315–321.

67. Thompson JR, Christiansen EL, Sauser DD, et al. Contrast arthrography versus computed tomography for the diagnosis of dislocation the temporomandibular joint meniscus. AJNR 1984;5:747–750.

68. Christiansen EL. Temporomandibular Joint X-Ray Computed Tomography. [Dissertation] Stockholm, Karolinska Institutet, 1988.

69. Christiansen EL, Thompson JR. Temporomandibular Joint Imaging. St. Louis, Mosby–Year Book, 1990.

70. Christiansen EL, Thompson JR, Hasso AN, Hinshaw DB Jr. Correlative thin section temporomandibular joint anatomy and computed tomography. Radiographics 1986;6:703–723.

71. Pettigrew J, Roberts D, Riddle R, et al. Three-dimensional imaging of the temporomandibular joint meniscus. J Dent Res 1984;63:195.

72. Roberts D, Pettigrew J, Udupa J, Ram C. Three-dimensional imaging and display of the temporomandibular joint. Oral Surg Oral Med Oral Pathol 1984;58:461–474.

73. Udupa J, Roberts D, Christiansen EL. Quantified three-dimensional imaging techniques for biomechanical analysis of skeletal joints. Proceedings of the IEEE Eighth Annual Conference, Fort Worth, November 7–10, 1986.

74. Marguelles-Bonner RE, Farpentier P, Yung P, et al. Clinical diagnosis compared with findings of magnetic resonance imaging in 242 patients with internal derangement of the TMJ. J Orofacial Pain 1995;9:244–253.

75. Raustia AM, Pyhtinen J, Pernu H. Clinical magnetic resonance imaging and surgical findings in patients with temporomandibular joint disorder—A survey of 47 patients. Rofo Fortschr Geb Rontgenstr Neuen Bildgeb Verfahr 1994;160:406–411.

76. Tasaki MM, Westesson PL. Temporomandibular joint: Diagnostic accuracy with sagittal and coronal MR imaging. Radiology 1993;186:723–729.

77. Brooks SL, Westesson PL. Temporomandibular joint; value of coronal images. Radiology 1993;188:317–321.

78. Musgrave MT, Westesson PL, Tallents RH, et al. Improve magnetic resonance imaging of the temporomandibular joint by oblique scanning planes. Oral Surg Oral Med Oral Pathol 1991;71:525–528.

79. Westesson PL, Kwok E, Barsotti JB, et al. Temporomandibular joint: Improved MR image quality with decreased section thickness. Radiology 1992;182:280–282.

80. Chen YJ, Gallo LM, Palla S. Contrast optimization in magnetic resonance imaging of the TMJ disc. [Abstract] J Orofacial Pain 1996;10:186.

81. Crabbe JP, Brooks SL, Lillie JH. Gradient-echo MR imaging of the temporomandibular joint: Diagnostic pitfall caused by the superficial temporal artery. AJR 1995;164:451–454.

82. Rao VM, Vinitski S, Liem M, Rapoport R. Fast spin-echo imaging of the temporomandibular joint. J Magn Reson Imaging 1995;5:293–296.

83. Niitsu M, Hirohata H, Yoshioka S, et al. Magnetization transfer contrast on gradient echo MR imaging of the temporomandibular joint. Acta Radiol 1995;36:295–299.

84. Crabbe JP, Brooks SL, Lillie JH. Gradient-echo MR imaging of the temporomandibular joint. AJR 1995;164:451–454.

85. Westesson PL, Brooks SL. Temporomandibular joint; Relationship between MR evidence of effusion and the presence of pain and disk displacement. AJR 1992;159:559–563.

86. Minowa K, Abe S, Sawamura T, et al. Magnetic resonance spectroscopy of normal human masseter muscles. Poster presentation at the Second International Congress on Orofacial Pain and Temporomandibular Disorders, Paris, May 24–25, 1996.

87. Marcell T, Chew W, McNeill C, et al. Magnetic resonance spectroscopy of the human masseter in nonbruxing and bruxing subjects. J Orofacial Pain 1995;9:116–130.

88. Tong KA, Christiansen EL, Heisler W, et al. Asymptomatic myositis ossificans of the medial pterygoid muscle: A case report. J Orofacial Pain 1994;8:223–226.

89. Larheim TA, Smith HJ, Apestrand F. Rheumatic disease of temporomandibular joint with development of anterior disk displacement as revealed by magnetic resonance imaging; a case report. Oral Surg Oral Med Oral Pathol 1991;71:246–249.

90. Yamaguchi T, Satoh K, Komatsu K, et al. Evaluation of energy metabolism in masseter muscles of TMD patients using (31)P magnetic imaging spectroscopy. [Abstract] J Orofacial Pain 1996;10:185.

91. McNeil C. Paradigm shift. J Orofacial Pain 1996;11:1.

37

Degenerative Diseases of the Spine

ROBERT DOWNEY BOUTIN, M.D.

H. JOSEPH SPAETH, M.D.

DONALD RESNICK, M.D.

Degenerative processes occur in the spines of all people who are fortunate enough to celebrate their 70th birthdays. The severity and site of this "degenerative disease," however, vary immensely. Although it may be asymptomatic, age-related degeneration may become severe enough to contribute to some of the most common causes of impairment in adults: spine stiffness, neck pain, and back pain.[1] The role of imaging symptomatic patients is primarily to diagnose the source of symptoms, direct appropriate therapy, and help in determining the patient's prognosis. In this chapter, we review the imaging of the major types of spinal articulations, the major classes of disease affecting them, and the various complications of these processes.

ANATOMY OF THE VERTEBRAL COLUMN

The individual segments of the vertebral column are interconnected by the intervertebral disks, the uncovertebral joints, the facet joints, and the spinal ligaments. Each *intervertebral disk* is composed of a central nucleus pulposus and a peripheral anulus fibrosus. The nucleus pulposus at birth is composed of a gelatinous matrix, which is gradually replaced by fibrocartilage. The anulus fibrosus contains an inner zone of fibrocartilage and an outer zone of collagenous fibers. These outer fibers are primarily anchored to the cartilaginous endplate and periosteum of the adjacent vertebral bodies. The periosteal fibers, termed *Sharpey's fibers*, are remarkable for their strength.

The intervertebral disks between the cervical vertebrae do not extend to the lateral edges of the vertebral bodies. Articulation in this area occurs at the *uncovertebral joints* or *joints of Luschka,* which are articular clefts found between the superior uncinate process of one vertebra and the inferior articulating surface of the vertebra above. The uncovertebral joints form postnatally by fibrillation in the marginal fibers of the anulus fibrosus or by slow absorption of loose fibrous tissue. Interestingly, these joints are only present from the C3 through C7 vertebrae and may not even be present in all persons.

Apophysis (Greek, an offshoot) refers to a bony process or facet, such as that extending from the junction of the pedicle and lamina in the posterior elements of the spine. The superior articulating process of one vertebra is separated from the inferior articulating process of the vertebra above by a true synovial joint, termed a *facet* (or *apophyseal*) *joint.* Facet joints contain a meniscus-like structure and are surrounded by a loose, thin articular capsule.

The eight principle *spinal ligaments* provide additional support to the articulations that connect the individual segments of the vertebral column (Fig. 37–1). These ligaments are the

Anterior longitudinal ligament, extending along the anterior surface of the vertebral column

Posterior longitudinal ligament, intimate with the posterior aspects of the vertebral bodies and intervertebral disks

Ligamentum flavum, connecting the laminae of adjacent vertebrae

Interspinous ligament, connecting adjacent spinous processes

Supraspinous ligament, attaching to the apices of the spinous processes

Ligamentum nuchae, passing from the occiput to the cervical spinous processes

Intertransverse ligament, connecting transverse processes

Iliolumbar ligament, connecting the lowest lumbar vertebra to the iliac crest

MAJOR TYPES OF DEGENERATIVE DISEASES OF THE SPINE

Degenerative diseases of the spine may be divided into those affecting predominantly the anterior aspect of the spinal column, the posterior aspect of the spinal column,

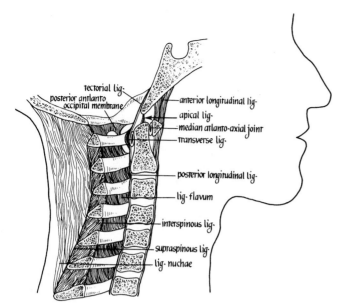

FIGURE 37–1 The spinal ligaments in the sagittal plane. (From Banna M [ed]. Clinical Radiology of the Spine and the Spinal Cord. Rockville, MD, Aspen Systems Corporation, 1985.)

Labels in figure: tectorial lig.; posterior antlanto occipital membrane; anterior longitudinal lig.; apical lig.; median atlanto-axial joint; transverse lig.; posterior longitudinal lig.; lig. flavum; interspinous lig.; supraspinous lig.; lig. nuchae

or both (Table 37–1). The conditions affecting the anterior elements most commonly relate to the intervertebral disk and are generally referred to as *degenerative disk disease* (DDD). DDD is characterized by several alterations in the intervertebral disk and the adjacent vertebral body, including loss in disk fluid or proteoglycan, loss in disk height, disk displacement, and vertebral body hyperostosis. As discussed later, DDD is actually a generic designation for two interrelated but different processes: *intervertebral osteochondrosis* (primarily affecting the nucleus pulposus) and *spondylosis deformans* (primarily affecting the anulus fibrosus). In contrast, *arthrosis* and *osteoarthrosis* are the degenerative processes that primarily affect the uncovertebral and the facet joints, respectively, and are manifest by joint space narrowing, subchondral sclerosis, and bone hypertrophy. *Ligamentous degeneration* can develop in any of the spinal ligaments located anteriorly or posteriorly and is associated with calcification or ossification.

Although each of the various degenerative disorders of the spine has fundamental anatomic and radiologic characteristics that differentiate them, it is important to recognize that some of the processes are related, that they frequently coexist at the same vertebral level, and that the presence of one process may influence the natural history of another. In short, the integrity of one structure depends on the integrity of neighboring structures. Intervertebral osteochondrosis, for example, produces a loss in height of the disk space with consequent posterior displacement of the vertebral body; then, telescopic subluxation of the facet joints can occur and contribute to facet joint osteoarthrosis. Conversely, hypertrophic abnormalities in the facet joints can be associated with anterior displacement of one vertebra on another, predisposing those vertebral levels to intervertebral osteochondrosis and spondylosis deformans. In the discussion that follows,

we summarize the degenerative disorders afflicting each of the various types of spinal connections: intervertebral disks, uncovertebral joints, synovial joints, and spinal ligaments.

Degenerative Disk Disease

DDD may be related, at least in part, to the poor diskal nutrition that tends to occur with advancing age. In infants and young children, a vascular network supplies blood to the intervertebral disk and cartilaginous endplate. (Whether the endplate should be considered part of the vertebral body or part of the intervertebral disk is a matter of debate.)[2] By the age of 12 years, the vascular network atrophies and the metabolism of the disk becomes primarily anaerobic.[3] Nutrients then must reach the metabolically active disk by diffusion, either from the marrow of the vertebrae (across the subchondral bone and cartilaginous endplate) or from nearby blood vessels (across the anulus fibrosus). When morphologic changes occur in the vertebrae and endplates with advancing age, normal diskal nutrition may be compromised and predispose a patient to DDD. Indeed, decreasing nutrition of the central disk may be the single most important mechanism responsible for age-related degeneration of intervertebral disks, as this allows accumulation of cell waste products and causes a fall in pH levels that further compromises cell function and may lead to cell death. Other biochemical explanations for DDD relate to fatigue failure of the matrix proteins, excess accumulation of degraded matrix molecules, and cell senescence.[1]

Water represents the major component of the normal disk. In young persons, water makes up approximately 80% of the anulus fibrosus and 90% of the nucleus pulposus. The remainder of the disk is composed largely of an extracellular matrix of proteoglycan and collagen. The proteoglycans of the intervertebral disk are similar to those of articular cartilage, consisting of a protein core with many different glycosaminoglycan side chains. These glycosaminoglycans attract water molecules and generate a substantial osmotic pressure that helps to expand the disk, especially the nucleus.[4] Collagen fibers also help to resist axial compression but, in addition, confer on the anulus the ability to resist radial tension induced by axial loading.

Intervertebral Osteochondrosis

Intervertebral chondrosis is dehydration and loss of tissue resiliency in the intervertebral disk, particularly in the nucleus pulposus, that occurs with aging. When this process also involves the neighboring bone, it has been termed *intervertebral osteochondrosis*.[5] As the process of intervertebral osteochondrosis progresses, clefts within the nucleus and anulus enlarge and the intervertebral disk diminishes in height. This height loss results in bulging of the outer fibers of the anulus fibrosus. The cause of intervertebral osteochondrosis probably relates to longstanding stress at the diskovertebral junction, although it is unclear whether excessive strain is a fundamental cause or merely an aggravating factor. Evidence exists that genetic factors may play an important role in influencing the development of intervertebral osteochondrosis.[6]

TABLE 37–1 Intervertebral Disk Space Loss and Adjacent Sclerosis

Disease	Mechanism	Radiographic Appearance
Intervertebral (osteo)chondrosis	Degeneration of the nucleus pulposus and cartilaginous endplate Cartilaginous nodes	Disk space narrowing Vacuum phenomena Well-defined sclerotic vertebral margins
Infection	Osteomyelitis and "diskitis"	Disk space narrowing Poorly defined sclerotic vertebral margins Soft tissue mass
Trauma	Diskal injury and degeneration Cartilaginous nodes	Disk space narrowing Well-defined sclerotic vertebral margins Fracture Soft tissue mass
Neuropathic osteoarthropathy	Loss of sensation and proprioception with repetitive trauma	Disk space narrowing Extensive sclerosis of vertebrae Osteophytosis Fragmentation Malalignment
Rheumatoid arthritis°	Apophyseal joint instability with recurrent diskovertebral trauma or Inflammatory tissue extending from neighboring articulations	Disk space narrowing Poorly or well-defined sclerotic vertebral margins Subluxation Apophyseal joint abnormalities
Calcium pyrophosphate dihydrate crystal deposition disease	Crystal deposition in cartilaginous endplate and intervertebral disk with degeneration	Disk space narrowing Calcification Poorly or well-defined sclerotic vertebral margins Fragmentation Subluxation
Alkaptonuria	Crystal deposition in cartilaginous endplate and intervertebral disk with degeneration	Disk space narrowing Vacuum phenomena Well-defined sclerotic vertebral margins Calcification

From Resnick D, Niwayama G. Degenerative disease of the spine. In Resnick D (ed). Diagnosis of Bone and Joint Disorders, Vol. 3, 3rd ed., pp. 1372–1462. Philadelphia, WB Saunders, 1995.
° Usually involves cervical spine.

Radiographically, intervertebral osteochondrosis is manifested by the vacuum disk phenomenon, disk space narrowing, and reactive sclerosis of the vertebral body (Fig. 37–2). The *vacuum disk phenomenon* refers to radiolucent collections of gas that accumulate in clefts that form within the disk as it degenerates. It deserves special emphasis because it is a prevalent, distinctive, and dependable finding. These radiolucent collections within the disk can be demonstrated in approximately 20% of elderly persons.[7] These intervertebral gas collections are most prominent in the nucleus pulposus, although they can occur in the anulus fibrosus. Gas occasionally can be seen in disk material that has extended through an adjacent endplate or longitudinal ligament. Gas overlying the spinal canal, for example, supports the diagnosis of disk protrusion when there is no history of trauma.[8] The accumulation of intervertebral diskal gas, which is 90% nitrogen,[9] is accentuated in spinal extension and may disappear in spinal flexion. In extension, the intervertebral disk is distracted, which results in negative pressure that attracts

gas from the surrounding extracellular spaces. In flexion, the disk space is compressed and gas tends to be resorbed.[10] Knowledge of this process is helpful, for example, when the cause of disk space narrowing and destruction in two adjacent vertebral bodies is unknown. In this setting, the elicitation of a vacuum disk phenomenon during trunk extension strongly suggests degenerative, not infectious, disease.[11] Vacuum phenomena can also occur in the other articulations that undergo degenerative processes, such as the facet joints, as well as in normal peripheral joints under traction.

The radiographic differential diagnosis of intradiskal gas may include other, less common categories of disease: diskal infection, neoplasm, trauma, and osteonecrosis. Very rarely, diskal infection with gas-producing organisms can produce an appearance similar to that of the vacuum phenomenon.[12] Usually, however, diskitis is caused by pyogenic or granulomatous infections that cause increased—not decreased—intradiskal pressure. Neoplastic processes may result in intradiskal gas only in exceptional

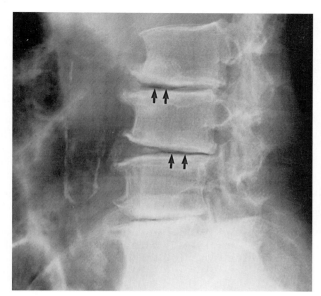

FIGURE 37–2 Vacuum disk phenomenon *(arrows)* on a lateral view of the lumbar spine with the patient positioned in extension. Linear rarefactions, projecting within the intervertebral disk, represent the vacuum phenomenon and often become more prominent on extension views, virtually excluding the possibility of septic diskitis.

cases.[13] Posttraumatic intradiskal gas collections most commonly occur in the cervical spine, presumably related to the defect caused by avulsion of peripheral disk fibers from the adjacent vertebral body.[14, 15] Finally, gas collections in the intervertebral disk must be differentiated from those in the paravertebral soft tissues (which may be infected)[16] or arising within the vertebral body itself (which is highly suggestive of osteonecrosis).[17]

Degenerative disk calcification is another manifestation of disk degeneration, in which calcium is deposited in the intervertebral disk. Degenerative disk calcification usually is localized to one or two disk levels, predominates in the thoracic and lumbar spine, and is seen on approximately 5% of chest and abdominal radiographs in adults.[18, 19] At autopsy, the prevalence of calcification is approximately 7% in the nucleus pulposus and 70% in the anulus fibrosus.[20] These calcific deposits are composed predominantly of hydroxyapatite.[21] Degenerative disk calcification is usually permanent and asymptomatic. However, disk degeneration may be followed by proliferation of blood vessels through fine clefts in the cartilaginous endplate. This hypervascularity has been implicated as a potential route for hematogenous spread of infection or tumor to the intervertebral disks that are otherwise avascular in adults. Disk vascularization also may stimulate ossification in the anulus fibrosus or in the nucleus pulposus, which may eventually lead to intervertebral ankylosis. In addition to vascularization and ossification, disk fibrosis may also occur after disk degeneration or trauma. If present at multiple levels, this fibrosis can lead to decreased mobility in the vertebral column.[5]

The differential diagnosis of degenerative disk calcification includes many systemic disorders,[22] including acromegaly, amyloidosis, alkaptonuria, hemochromatosis, hyperparathyroidism, poliomyelitis, and calcium pyrophosphate dihydrate crystal deposition disease. The precise location, appearance, and chemical characteristics vary among these systemic disorders, but unlike degenerative calcification, all these systemic disorders are associated with disk calcification in multiple intervertebral disks.

Standardized atlases with validated radiographic index descriptions of disk degeneration have been developed to optimize interobserver and intraobserver agreement in interpretation.[23] No such standard exists for magnetic resonance imaging (MRI), despite evidence of disappointing interobserver variability in the interpretation of disk degeneration.[24] With MRI of DDD, however, a characteristic constellation of findings in the intervertebral disk and adjacent portions of the vertebral body may be demonstrated. These findings were elaborated by Modic, Ross, and their coworkers[25–27] and are summarized here. As a general rule, the signal intensity of the normal intervertebral disk is lower than that of the vertebral body on T1-weighted images. On T2-weighted images, the normal disk has a central area of low signal intensity, with the remainder of the disk displaying a higher signal intensity than that of the vertebral body.

Modifications in this normal MRI appearance of the disk and the adjacent vertebral body occur with DDD (Fig. 37–3). The earliest changes involve loss of signal intensity in the intervertebral disk on T2-weighted images. This loss of T2 signal intensity is thought to be secondary to disk dehydration or alterations in proteoglycan composition, or both. This finding often appears first in the anterior third of the disk and progresses to involve the entire disk. Widespread abnormalities of diskal signal intensity may occur when fissures develop between the cartilaginous endplate, the anulus fibrosus, and the nucleus pulposus. Although calcification and intradiskal fissures usually produce a signal void on all pulse sequences, this is not always the case. Fissured areas within the disk characteristically contain gas, but they can fill with fluid and therefore be displayed as hypointense on T1-weighted images and hyperintense on T2-weighted images. Intradiskal calcification may cause a hyperintense appearance on T1-weighted images; the actual appearance of calcific tissue on MRI studies depends on the degree and the particular structure of the calcification.[28–30] Whereas T2-weighted spin-echo sequences are most sensitive to abnormalities in disk hydration and proteoglycan content, signal voids from intradiskal gas are better delineated on gradient-echo sequences. Correlation with conventional radiography or computed tomography (CT) usually makes the differentiation between these types of abnormalities elementary.[29, 30]

In the vertebral body, three types of signal intensity changes commonly accompany DDD. *Type I bone marrow changes* are visualized as low T1 signal intensity and high T2 signal intensity, with contrast enhancement after intravenous administration of gadolinium chelates. This enhancement occurs because fibrovascular tissue has replaced the normal cellular marrow in the vertebral body. Type I changes may regress or may progress to type II changes.

Type II bone marrow changes are manifested by high

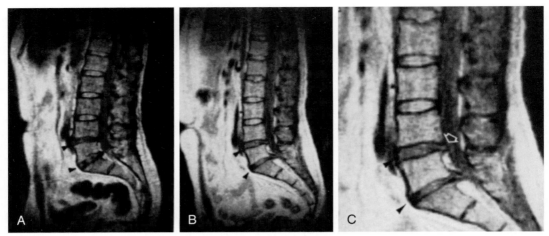

FIGURE 37–3 *A–C,* Intervertebral osteochondrosis or degenerative disk disease. T2-weighted MRI studies reveal decreased signal *(arrowheads)* within the disk relative to the normal high signal intensity in adjacent disks. *(A–C, Courtesy of M. Solomon, M.D., Los Gatos, California.)*

T1 signal intensity and relatively diminished T2 signal intensity. When a sequence is fat saturated, these sites remain isointense with fat elsewhere. No contrast enhancement is observed. Histologically, type II changes in the bone marrow represent sites of fatty marrow. Type II changes typically occur after type I changes. Unlike type I changes, type II changes usually do not regress, and may progress further to type III changes.

Type III changes in the vertebral body demonstrate low signal intensity on both T1-weighted and T2-weighted images. These changes reflect the absence of normal bone marrow that has been replaced with regions of considerable hyperostosis, corresponding to sclerotic changes evident on conventional radiographs. Type III changes are the most common type of bone marrow changes observed in patients undergoing MRI for lumbar

disk disease (80%); type II (15%) and type I (5%) changes are considerably less common.

With regard to differential diagnosis, type I bone marrow changes may resemble the MRI findings of vertebral osteomyelitis. Although both these processes display increased T2 signal intensity in the bone marrow, diskitis routinely accompanies osteomyelitis and would cause the disk to have increased, not decreased, T2 signal intensity. Common ancillary findings with diskitis would include a characteristic history (e.g., intravenous drug abuse), physical examination (e.g., low-grade fever, spinal tenderness), laboratory results (e.g., elevated erythrocyte sedimentation rate), and imaging findings (e.g., epidural abscess).

Differential diagnosis of type I bone marrow changes of intervertebral osteochondrosis also may include *idiopathic segmental sclerosis of the vertebral body.* This term

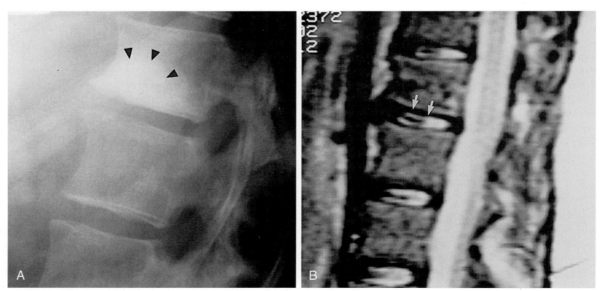

FIGURE 37–4 Idiopathic segmental sclerosis of the vertebral body in a 37-year-old woman. *A,* Lateral radiograph demonstrates a hemispherical region of vertebral body sclerosis abutting the inferior endplate of T12 *(arrowheads). B,* T2-weighted MRI study fails to demonstrate any of the characteristic signal changes associated with disk degeneration *(arrows).*

is applied to the increased radiodensity in the peridiskal bone that occurs when a specific cause cannot be identified (Fig. 37–4). Pathologic findings suggest that the bone eburnation is reactive in type and is perhaps related to trauma.[31, 32] Histologic data do not support an infectious or neoplastic cause. Idiopathic segmental sclerosis of the vertebral body predominates in the mid to lower lumbar spine of young and middle-aged women.[33] Occasionally, a history of trauma or back pain is elicited, but neither is a universal finding.

The importance of idiopathic segmental sclerosis of the vertebral body lies in its differentiation from other patterns of vertebral body sclerosis. The predominant radiographic feature of this entity is a hemispheric band of sclerosis, sometimes accompanied by osteolytic foci and new bone formation.[31, 34] Some investigators speculate that bone lysis is an initial manifestation and reactive bone formation occurs secondarily.[35] The sclerosis typically extends from the anterior or posterior portion of the vertebral body, and the margins of the abnormality commonly are well defined. MRI of idiopathic segmental sclerosis reveals hypointensity on T1-weighted images, with hyperintensity on T2-weighted images predominantly at the periphery of the lesion.[36, 37] The adjacent vertebral body may or may not be affected.

Spondylosis Deformans

Spondylosis deformans (Fig. 37–5) begins with deterioration in the anulus fibrosus and is characterized by spinal osteophytosis that is most profound along the anterior and lateral aspects of the vertebral column. *Spondylosis* is distinguished from *spondylitis* (an inflammatory process of the vertebrae) and from osteoarthrosis (a degenerative process of the synovial joints).

Spondylosis becomes extremely common with increasing age. By the age of 50 years, up to 80% of men demonstrate osseous excrescences in the spine. Besides age, risk factors for spinal osteophytosis are said to include male gender and occupations that require heavy physical labor.

The pathogenesis of spondylosis is thought to begin with breakdown of fibers that anchor the outer portion of the anulus fibrosus to the adjacent vertebra. Resultant laxity allows minor degrees of disk displacement anteriorly and anterolaterally. As this microdisplacement is accentuated by weight bearing and spinal motion, traction occurs at the site of anchorage of the outermost fibers (i.e., Sharpey's fibers) of the intervertebral disk to the vertebral body. Osteophytes develop at these areas that are several millimeters from the diskovertebral junction, first growing in a horizontal direction and then in a vertical direction.

This relationship between the formation of osteophytes and the disruption of the outer, anchoring annular fibers is generally accepted. The cause of degeneration in the peripheral fibers of the anulus fibrosus that attach to the adjacent vertebral body, however, has not been determined. In some cases, trauma appears to be an important factor. Localized osteophytes, for example, can develop 1 to 3 months after a single traumatic episode. In other cases, genetic factors also may be significant by influencing multiple variables, including the shapes of the vertebral bodies.[38] In general, a period of 1 to 3 years is required before osseous excrescences enlarge to such an

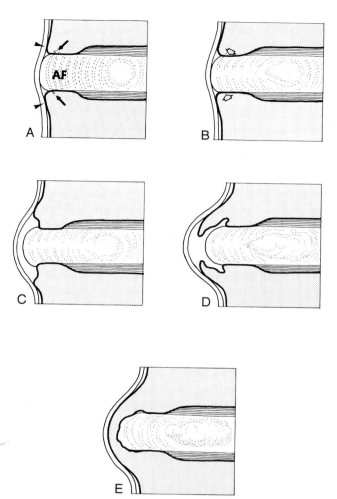

FIGURE 37–5 Spondylosis deformans: Concept of its pathogenesis according to Schmorl. Progressive stages of spondylosis deformans. The normal situation is depicted at the upper left (*A*) with sequential abnormalities demonstrated in the other drawings (*B–E*). Observe the normal attachment of the anulus fibrosus (AF) to the vertebral rim by strong fibers (*solid arrows* in *A*). Also note the attachment of the anterior longitudinal ligament to the anterior edge of the vertebral bodies (*arrowheads* in *A*). With breakdown in the site of attachment of the anulus fibrosus to the vertebral body (*arrows* in *B*), anterior protrusion of intervertebral disk material produces elevation of the anterior longitudinal ligament and enlarging osteophytes at the point at which this ligament attaches to the vertebral body (*B–D*). Eventually, the osteophytes may bridge the intervertebral disk space (*E*). (*A–E*, From Resnick D. Diagnosis of Bone and Joint Disorders, Vol. 3, 3rd ed., p. 1388. Philadelphia, WB Saunders, 1995.)

extent that they are recognizable on radiographic examinations.[39]

The clinical manifestations of spondylosis depend, in part, on the size and location of the osteophytes. Although some patients do not complain of problems, others experience pain, stiffness, restricted motion, and dysphagia. Interestingly, neurologic deficits are relatively uncommon given the nearly universal nature of vertebral osteophytosis in the aged. This fact can be explained by the relative infrequency of prominent osteophyte formation on the posterior aspect of the vertebral bodies. Whereas the major attachments of the anterior longitudinal ligament are to the vertebral bodies, the major attachments of the posterior longitudinal ligament are to the intervertebral disks. Posterior diskal displacement, which certainly may be associated with significant neurologic abnormalities, does not lead to severe stretching and traction of the posterior longitudinal ligament and, thus, is not associated with prominent osteophytosis. Minor fibrous connections between the posterior margin of the vertebral body and the outer layers of the anulus fibrosus, however, may result in small bony excrescences posteriorly.

With regard to differential diagnosis, spinal osteophytes accompanying spondylosis must be differentiated from other bony outgrowths of the vertebral column, including primarily spinal infection, spinal trauma, seronegative spondyloarthropathies, and diffuse idiopathic skeletal hyperostosis (DISH) (see Fig. 37–5). *Spinal infection* or *trauma* can produce outgrowths that are identical to those of spondylosis. In fact, their pathogenesis may be similar if the infectious or traumatic insult disrupted the attachment of the anulus fibrosus to the vertebral body. Differentiation from spondylosis is usually made on the basis of history and localization of the osteophytosis to only one (or two) levels.

Seronegative spondyloarthropathies can lead to osseous excrescences that must be differentiated from spondylosis. Ankylosing spondylitis is characterized by ossifi-cation within the outer portion of the anulus fibrosus, resulting in outgrowths that are termed *syndesmophytes*. In contrast to spinal osteophytes (broad-based, beaklike excrescences that arise from the vertebral body several millimeters from the disk), syndesmophytes typically are thin and vertically oriented as they extend from the edge of one vertebral body to the next. Attention to other sites—such as the sacroiliac, facet, and costovertebral articulations—allows accurate differentiation of the two disorders; these joints are affected commonly and severely in ankylosing spondylitis but are uninvolved in spondylosis. Bony outgrowths in psoriasis and Reiter's syndrome may resemble typical syndesmophytes of ankylosing spondylitis or may appear as distinct paravertebral ossifications. In the latter circumstance, they are separated from the vertebral surface and, initially, possess a poorly defined or irregular contour.

DISH is a common entity characterized by flowing ossification along the anterior and lateral aspects of at least four contiguous vertebral bodies. The diagnosis of DISH can be excluded if there are extensive radiographic changes of intervertebral disk degeneration, facet joint fusion, or sacroiliac joint erosions or ankylosis. Additional causes of bone excrescences of the spine that may resemble or appear identical to those in spondylosis are fluorosis, hypoparathyroidism, sternocostoclavicular hyperostosis, acne conglobata, paralysis, and certain medications such as vitamin A derivatives (Fig. 37–6).

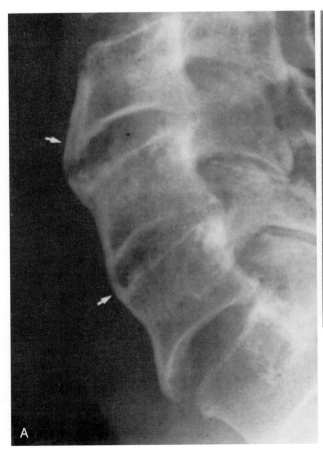

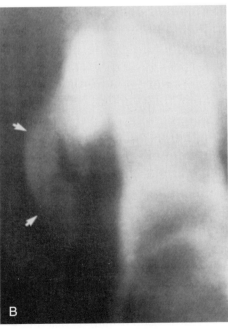

FIGURE 37–6 Isotretinoin hyperostosis. In two different patients, prominent ligamentous ossification is apparent (*arrows*) in the midcervical spine (*A*) and about the anterior arch of the atlas (*B*). (*A*, Courtesy of J. Mink, M.D., Los Angeles, CA. *B*, courtesy of J. Lawson, M.D., New Haven, CT.)

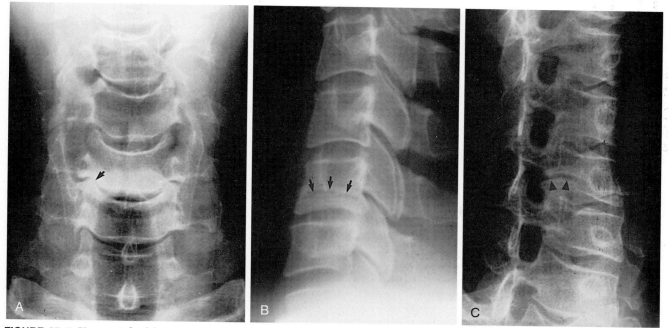

FIGURE 37–7 Uncovertebral hypertrophy. Anteroposterior *(A)*, lateral *(B)*, and oblique *(C)* radiographs reveal hypertrophy of the uncovertebral process *(arrows* and *arrowheads)* with neuroforaminal narrowing. The margin of the uncovertebral joint, made more prominent by the hypertrophied uncovertebral process, can appear on the lateral view as a pseudofracture.

Uncovertebral (Neurocentral) Joint Arthrosis

The five lowest cervical vertebral bodies (C3–C7) contain bony ridges extending from each side, termed *uncinate processes.* The uncovertebral (or neurocentral) joints of Luschka are formed at the articulation between the superior and the inferior uncinate processes of adjacent vertebral bodies. Although the uncovertebral joints are primarily considered cartilaginous, they also possess anatomic features resembling those of synovial articulations.

As the intervertebral disk degenerates, there is progressive loss in height of the disk space, and the uncinate processes approach each other. Eventually, these articular processes may be pressed together, and the intervening uncovertebral joint may degenerate.[40–42] Osteophytes often form, projecting from the posterior edge of the vertebral bodies into the spinal canal, the intervertebral foramina, and the foramina transversarium;[43] this hyperostosis can compromise the spinal cord, nerve roots, and vertebral arteries, respectively. Once the uncinate processes impinge on one another, further loss in intervertebral disk height can occur only anteriorly. This process produces a segmental loss of normal cervical lordosis and usually results in compensatory hyperextension at higher levels.

Radiographically, the diagnosis of arthrosis (Fig. 37–7) is accomplished when there is joint space narrowing, sclerosis, and osteophytosis about the uncovertebral articulations. In some cases, the space between adjacent uncovertebral osteophytes can create a thin radiolucent line that projects over a cervical vertebral body in lateral radiographs and should not be misinterpreted as a fracture.[44]

Synovial Joint Osteoarthrosis

Facet Joint

Degenerative changes in the facet joints (Fig. 37–8) are induced by abnormal stress across the articulation, a situation that can be related to a variety of primary processes including trauma, kyphosis, and scoliosis.[45] Although any level may be affected, these changes predominate in the

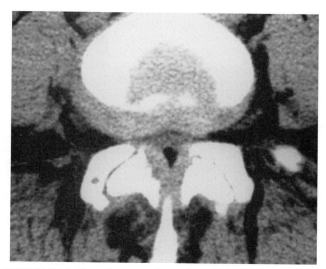

FIGURE 37–8 Facet hypertrophy and spinal stenosis. Transverse computed tomography (CT) scan reveals osteoarthrosis of the apophyseal joints. Facet osteophytes encroach on the spinal canal and contribute to the spinal stenosis. (From Hart BL, Benzel EC, Ford CC [eds]. Fundamentals of Neuroimaging. Philadelphia, WB Saunders, 1997.)

middle and lower cervical spine, upper thoracic and midthoracic spine, and lower lumbar spine.[5, 46–48]

The term *osteoarthritis* refers to inflammation of a synovial joint secondary to degenerative disease, whereas *osteoarthrosis* is a more general term that refers to degenerative changes that may or may not reveal inflammatory cells on histopathologic examination. Interestingly, spinal osteoarthrosis is associated with a generalized increase in bone mineral density, suggesting to some investigators that the decreased bone turnover in patients with spinal osteoarthrosis may exert a protective effect against osteoporosis.[39]

The pathologic and radiologic characteristics of osteoarthrosis of the facet joints are similar to those accompanying degenerative disease of other synovial joints.[5, 49, 50] Fibrillation and erosion of articular cartilage that progress to irregularity and denudation of the cartilaginous surface are responsible for radiographically detectable joint space narrowing. Bony eburnation and osteophytes are frequent and may be accompanied by intra-articular osteocartilaginous bodies. Joint space narrowing and capsular laxity permit anterior subluxation of a superior vertebra on an inferior one, a process known as *degenerative anterior spondylolisthesis*. This osteoarthritic subluxation creates traction between the apposing articulating surfaces, which may be manifest as a vacuum phenomenon. Synovial irritation and hyperplasia can also be encountered. Occasionally, intra-articular bony ankylosis can result and simulate the appearance of ankylosing spondylitis or juvenile chronic arthritis, especially in the cervical spine.

CT or MRI, by virtue of cross-sectional display, readily demonstrates the key findings of facet joint osteoarthrosis: joint space narrowing and osteophytosis. Ancillary findings of osseous fragmentation and vacuum phenomena may also be identified. Most importantly, the potential complications of facet joint osteoarthrosis can be analyzed, including synovial cyst formation and hyperostosis in the spinal canal, lateral recesses, and neural foramina. *Synovial cysts* presumably are related to dissection of synovium or synovial fluid through tears in the capsule of the facet joint, which result in a well-defined cystic structure seen on cross-sectional imaging. Synovial cysts are reported most frequently in the lower lumbar spine and the cervical spine, where they may be responsible for neurologic deficits. Spontaneous collapse of the cyst before or at the time of surgery has been reported.[51]

Prominent clinical symptoms and signs may accompany osteoarthrosis of the facet joints.[52, 53] The synovial membrane, capsules, and ligaments of these articulations are richly supplied by nerves,[54–56] which explains the common, although controversial, occurrence of pain in patients with degenerative joint disease at these sites.[46, 47] The existence of menisci in the facet joints has been emphasized in several publications,[57–59] although the histologic composition of these structures and their contribution to spinal symptoms are debated. Investigators generally agree, however, that facet joint osteoarthrosis—alone or in combination with degeneration of the intervertebral disk—plays a role in the production of various types of spinal stenosis with resultant spinal cord and nerve root compression. Pain, tenderness, and restricted motion are

recognized sequelae of such neurologic compromise. In the lumbar spine, the technique of injecting long-acting anesthetic agents or corticosteroids into the facet joints may document the precise spinal level from which the pain is arising.[60] Contrast material may be added as well, to document the intra-articular location of the injection.[61]

Costovertebral and Costotransverse Joints

The *costovertebral joints* are located between the heads of the ribs and the vertebral bodies, whereas the *costotransverse joints* are between the necks and tubercles of the ribs and the transverse processes of the vertebrae. As synovial joints, they are subject to degenerative joint disease even as early as the third decade of life, although few pathologic descriptions exist regarding this process.[62] Degenerative changes predominate in the articulations of the 11th and 12th ribs.[5] Joint space narrowing, bony eburnation, and osteophytosis are the expected alterations, although radiographic demonstration of these changes may be difficult because of overlying bony structures, namely the ribs and vertebrae.

Osteoarthrosis of the costovertebral joints (Fig. 37–9) may lead to diminished mobility or ankylosis between the ribs and vertebrae. When this occurs, the muscles attaching to the hypomobile or immobile rib exert increased forces. In accordance with Wolff's law (i.e., a bone develops the structure most suited to resist the forces acting on it), stress-related hyperostosis in the affected rib results. If one is not aware of this process, the increased radiodensity in the rib might be mistaken for evidence of Paget's disease or even osteoblastic metastases. Similar hyperostosis of the ribs is observed in a variety of spinal diseases that lead to new bone formation and costovertebral joint ankylosis, such as ankylosing spondylitis, psoriatic spondylitis, and DISH.

Transitional Lumbosacral Joint

Congenital variations at the lumbosacral junction are commonplace.[63, 64] Newly formed articulations may exist between the enlarged transverse process of the transi-

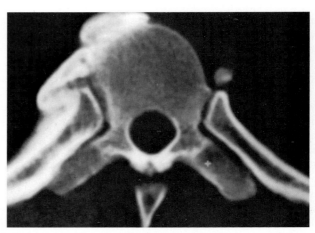

FIGURE 37–9 Costovertebral joint osteoarthrosis resulting in hypertrophic changes of the adjacent rib that can simulate Paget's disease or osteoblastic metastasis. (Courtesy of J. Haller, M.D., Vienna, Austria.)

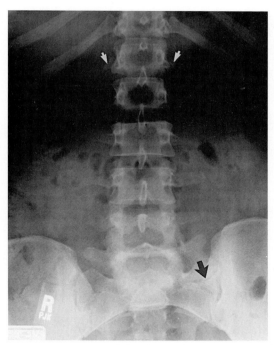

FIGURE 37–10 Transitional lumbosacral segment. Small T12 ribs are present *(white arrows)*. The left transverse process of the L5 segment is broadened and articulates with the sacrum *(black arrow)*. This configuration may be associated with low back pain.

tional vertebra and the wings of the sacrum (or rarely the ilium). These joints may be unilateral or bilateral and may possess synovium.

The relationship of low back pain to transitional vertebrae is a matter of considerable debate. Potential causes of symptoms include osteoarthritis[63, 65, 66] and diskal herniation[67–69] as well as bursitis, periostitis, and neuritis.[5] Transitional vertebrae that articulate with only one side of the sacrum may have a higher association with symptoms and signs.[62] Osteoarthrosis is known to result from abnormal stress and movement, such as the type that may exist between the transitional vertebra and the sacrum. When present, osteoarthrosis may be manifest by articular space narrowing, sclerosis, osteophytosis, and even bony ankylosis.

The relationship between transitional lumbosacral joints and disk herniation may depend on the type of transitional segment (Fig. 37–10). Castellvi and associates[69] defined four different types of transitional segments: type I, dysplastic transverse process; type II, incomplete lumbarization or sacralization; type III, complete lumbarization or sacralization; and type IV, mixed. When compared with a control population, patients with type I transitional lumbosacral segments had the same frequency and distribution of disk herniation. In individuals with type III and IV transitional segments, there were no examples of herniated disks, either at the level of the transition or just proximal to this level. However, with type II transitional vertebrae, there was an increased prevalence of disk herniation at the transitional level and at the level immediately above the transitional

segment. These outcome differences may be related to the presence or absence of a vestigial disk (which is devoid of nuclear material), as well as the expected variations in the biomechanics at the transitional segment. Hemisacralization is also thought to predispose patients to degenerative spondylolisthesis, because diminished mobility at the L5–S1 level shifts mechanical stresses to the adjacent L4–L5 level.[70]

Atlantoaxial Joint

As with synovial joints elsewhere, degenerative changes may occur in the atlantoaxial (or atlanto-odontoid) joint. Atlantoaxial joint osteoarthrosis (Fig. 37–11) may be responsible for complaints such as suboccipital headache and neck stiffness.[71–73]

Radiography can reveal narrowing of the interosseous space between the anterior arch of the atlas and the odontoid process, as well as cortical thickening and osteophytosis.[73] Lateral radiography is most accurate in distinguishing absent to mild disease from severe disease (83% sensitivity; 84% specificity) but tends to overestimate mild degenerative involvement when none is present (52% specificity).[74] CT provides the best radiographic detail necessary for accurate diagnosis. This method can demonstrate a vacuum phenomenon within the joint in approximately 2% of adults.[74] CT also facilitates the observation of several other degenerative findings including small ossicles, transverse ligament calcification, and osteophytosis of the median facet of the atlas.[72]

Ligamentous Degeneration

Many problems in the spine that cause pain are attributed to instability. Although the effect of muscle activity on spine stability is well recognized,[75] several spinal ligaments contribute to the stability of the vertebral column and thereby inhibit abnormal motion. With age, however, ligamentous integrity is commonly affected by the decline in elastic tissue in ligaments, the accumulated effects of repetitive microtrauma, and the concurrent degenerative changes in other supporting spinal structures. As ligaments contain a rich supply of nerves, degenerative processes affecting the ligaments may be associated with pain and tenderness. Degenerative abnormalities may affect essentially any spinal ligament, including the anterior longitudinal ligament, the posterior longitudinal ligament, the ligamenta flava, the interspinous and supraspinous ligaments, the ligamentum nuchae, the intertransverse ligaments, and the iliolumbar ligaments.

Anterior Longitudinal Ligament

The anterior longitudinal ligament most commonly undergoes calcification and ossification in the setting of DISH. As the name implies, the cause of DISH is unknown. DISH is a common disorder of middle-aged and older persons, with a reported prevalence of 28% in one autopsy study (in which the average age at the time of death was approximately 65 years).[76] DISH affects men more than women, by a ratio of approximately 2 to 1.[77] Besides advanced age and male gender, additional risk factors that predict susceptibility to DISH include diabetes mellitus, above-average alcohol intake, and below-

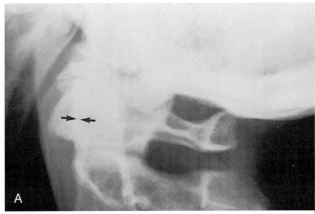

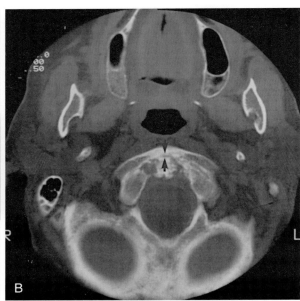

FIGURE 37–11 Atlantoaxial osteoarthrosis. A lateral radiograph (A) and transverse CT scan (B) reveal joint space narrowing (arrows), hypertrophy, and subchondral sclerosis involving the atlanto-odontoid articulation.

average dietary intake of calcium, carotene, and vitamins A, C, and E.[78]

Three strict radiographic criteria are prerequisites for the diagnosis of DISH: (1) flowing calcification or ossification along the anterolateral aspect of at least four contiguous vertebral bodies; (2) a relative absence of intervertebral disk degeneration; and (3) absence of facet joint ankylosis and sacroiliac joint ankylosis or erosion (Fig. 37–12).[79] The first criterion is helpful in separating DISH from typical spondylosis; the second criterion distinguishes DISH from intervertebral osteochondrosis; the third criterion eliminates patients with ankylosing spondylitis (Table 37–2).[51–56]

Although the majority of patients with DISH have symptoms and signs, a direct cause-and-effect relationship

has not been proved.[78, 80] Clinical complaints generally are initially apparent in the thoracolumbar spine and are characterized by intermittent discomfort and stiffness. Within several years of onset, thoracolumbar spinal stiffness and pain can progress, with involvement of lumbar and cervical segments.[80] Additional specific symptoms in patients with DISH relate to prominent cervical osteophytosis causing dysphagia and to extraspinal enthesopathic abnormalities predisposing patients to recurrent tendinitis.[81–83] Although the clinical findings are mild in comparison with the often spectacular radiographic findings, there is frequently a close correlation between the clinical abnormalities and the underlying radiographic and radionuclide findings.

DISH may represent a vulnerable state in which exten-

FIGURE 37–12 Diffuse idiopathic skeletal hyperostosis. Lateral radiographs of the thoracic (A) and cervical (B) spine show the typical exuberant ossification with the anterior longitudinal ligament (arrows). The large anterior excrescences in the latter case indent on the pharynx and can be associated with dysphagia.

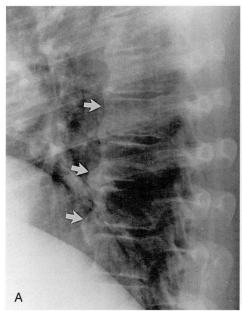

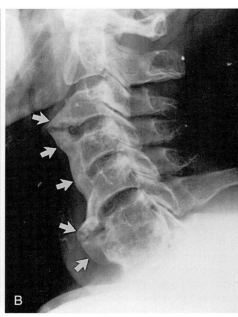

TABLE 37–2 Differential Diagnosis of Radiographic Findings in DISH, Ankylosing Spondylitis, and Intervertebral Osteochondrosis

Site	DISH	Ankylosing Spondylitis	Intervertebral (Osteo)chondrosis
Vertebral bodies	Flowing ossification and hyperostosis; large osteophytes; bony ankylosis frequent radiographically, less frequent pathologically	Thin syndesmophytes; osteitis with "squaring"; extensive bony ankylosis radiographically and pathologically	Sclerosis of superior and inferior surfaces
Intervertebral disk	Normal or mild decrease in height	Normal or convex in shape	Moderate to severe decrease in height; vacuum phenomena
Apophyseal joints	Normal or mild sclerosis; occasional osteophytes	Erosions; sclerosis; bony ankylosis	Normal
Sacroiliac joints	Para-articular osteophytes	Erosions; sclerosis; bony ankylosis	Normal
Peripheral skeleton	"Whiskering"; para-articular osteophytes; ligament calcification and ossification; hyperostosis	"Whiskering"; arthritis	Normal

From Resnick D, Niwayama G. Diffuse idiopathic skeletal hyperostosis (DISH). In Resnick D (ed). Diagnosis of Bone and Joint Disorders, Vol. 3, 3rd ed., pp. 1463–1495. Philadelphia, WB Saunders, 1995.
Abbreviation: DISH, diffuse idiopathic skeletal hyperostosis.

sive ossification results from an exaggerated response to certain stimuli that would normally produce only modest new bone formation. As such, DISH could be considered to represent an ossifying diathesis that causes excessive bone formation at skeletal sites subject to normal or abnormal stresses. Affected sites generally are where tendons and ligaments attach to bone, in both the axial and the extra-axial skeleton. Such bone production predominates in the spine, but similar bone formation occasionally may predominate in extraspinal sites. Further evidence that a bone-forming tendency is present in patients with DISH is the propensity of these persons to develop heterotopic ossification after surgery.[84] DISH is also associated with an increased prevalence of ossification of the posterior longitudinal ligament.

Posterior Longitudinal Ligament

The posterior longitudinal ligament extends from the axis and membrana tectoria above to the sacrum below, within the vertebral canal. Its fibers are attached to the posterior margins of the vertebral bodies and intervertebral disks. The association of chronic cervical myelopathy and extensive ossification of the posterior longitudinal ligament (OPLL) was recorded first in Japan in 1960.[85] Subsequent reports documented a prevalence of approximately 1% to 2% in the Japanese population,[86, 87] and increased awareness of this condition has revealed a more global distribution. OPLL is more frequent in men than in women, occurring in a ratio of approximately 2 to 1. The disease is most frequently diagnosed in patients between 50 and 60 years of age.

The cause of OPLL is unknown, although numerous possibilities have been advanced that include infectious agents, trauma, fluoride intoxication, diabetes mellitus, and an immunologic disorder, perhaps related to a particular type of human leukocyte antigen.[88–91] The observation

that OPLL occurs frequently in patients with DISH suggests a common cause and pathogenesis of these conditions. OPLL is present in approximately 50% of patients with DISH; conversely, DISH has been observed in over 20% of patients with OPLL.[92] Both of these ossifying diatheses are characterized by ligamentous calcification or ossification, osteophytosis, and hyperostosis at multiple skeletal sites.

Although persons with OPLL may be entirely asymptomatic,[93, 94] a variety of symptoms and signs have been associated with this disorder. Indeed, OPLL is said to be responsible for more than 20% of cervical myelopathy cases observed in the United States.[95] Clinical complaints are initiated by trauma in approximately 20% of cases. The principal neurologic symptoms can be divided into three groups: (1) cord signs, manifested by dominant motor and sensory disturbances in the lower extremity (56%); (2) segmental signs, manifested by dominant motor and sensory disturbances in the upper extremity (16%); and (3) cervicobrachialgia, causing no obvious neurologic deficits but associated with pain in the neck, the shoulder, and the arm (28%).[89] Additional symptoms may include neck pain and stiffness, urinary and rectal dysfunction, and loss of libido. Cord signs generally are noted in those cases in which the thickness of the ligament is greater than 30% to 60% of the sagittal diameter of the cervical spinal canal.[89, 94]

The diagnosis of OPLL is established by its characteristic radiographic appearance: a dense band of ossification measuring 1 to 5 mm along the anterior aspect of the spinal canal (Fig. 37–13). The ossification may exhibit a continuous distribution, extending in an uninterrupted fashion along the posterior margin of several vertebral bodies and intervertebral disks; alternatively, the ossification may be segmental, confined to the vertebrae only. Anterior vertebral osteophytes frequently are identifiable,

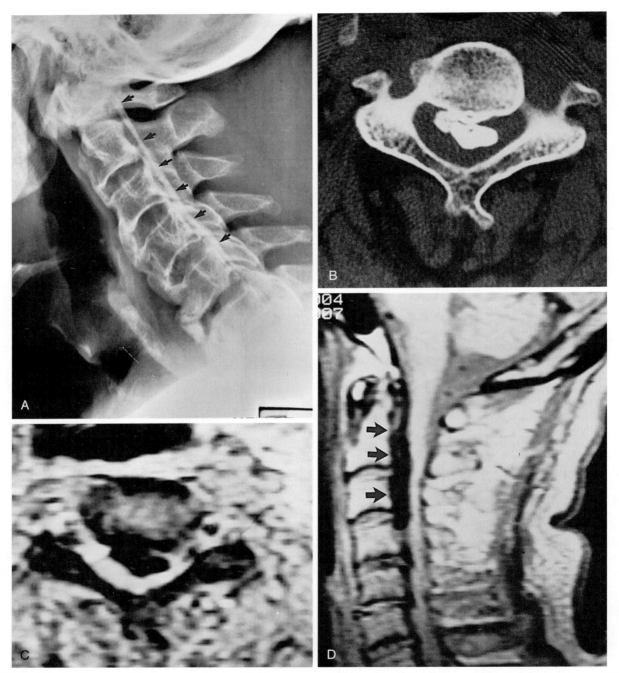

FIGURE 37–13 Ossification of the posterior longitudinal ligament. A lateral radiograph *(A)* in one patient and a transverse CT scan *(B)*, transverse gradient-echo MRI study *(C)*, and sagittal T1-weighted MRI study *(D)* in another patient demonstrate posterior longitudinal ligament ossification *(arrows)*. There is a radiolucent cleft between the ligament ossification and the vertebral body in both cases. CT and MRI reveal significant spinal stenosis.

but the intervertebral disk height generally is preserved. Although any vertebral level may be involved, it is the cervical spine that is classically affected.

MRI is the procedure of choice to demonstrate the encroachment of the ossified ligament on the spinal cord. In a study of 100 patients with OPLL, Yamashita and coworkers[96] emphasized the following MRI features: OPLL was generally seen as a band of low signal intensity on all pulse sequences between the bone marrow of the

vertebral body and the dural sac; signal intensity that corresponded to that of marrow fat was observed within the area of ossification in approximately 55% of cases with the continuous type of OPLL and 10% of the cases of segmental OPLL; the degree of spinal cord compression was more severe in the cases of continuous OPLL; and disk degeneration frequently was an associated feature.

The differential diagnosis of a vertical band of low

signal intensity on both T1- and T2-weighted images in the spinal canal may include OPLL, hypertrophy of the posterior longitudinal ligament, hemosiderin deposition, flowing blood or cerebrospinal fluid, and calcified meningioma. When high signal intensity is also present, diagnostic considerations include OPLL, osteophyte formation, and disk displacement.

Ligamentum Flavum

The ligamenta flava are attached to the laminae and the articular capsule of the facet joints. The ligaments from each side approximate each other at the base of the spinous process, where small clefts exist to allow the passage of veins. The ligamenta flava are thickest in the lumbar spine, somewhat thinner in the thoracic spine, and thinnest in the cervical spine.

Degenerative changes in the ligamenta flava are frequent and generally of no clinical significance. Occasionally, extensive calcification or ossification in hypertrophied

ligamenta flava occur in patients with myelopathy or radiculopathy in the cervical, thoracic, and lumbar spine.[97-106] Enthesophytes are most common and most prominent in the middle cervical and lower thoracic regions. In the cervical spine, calcific collections consist of calcium hydroxyapatite crystals in the majority of cases; calcium pyrophosphate dihydrate crystals are occasionally encountered. In the thoracic spine, ossification (rather than calcification) of the ligamentum flavum predominates. Regardless of the site, intervertebral osteochondrosis and facet joint osteoarthrosis are commonly associated.[5]

Radiographically, degenerative changes are manifested as ossification in the ligamenta flava, often with proliferative changes in adjacent bone, which produce dense areas overlying the spinal canal in the lateral projection (Fig. 37-14). These changes occasionally resemble proliferative abnormalities accompanying ankylosing spondylitis and, rarely, POEMS (polyneuropathy, organomegaly, endocrinopathy, M protein, skin changes) syndrome.[107]

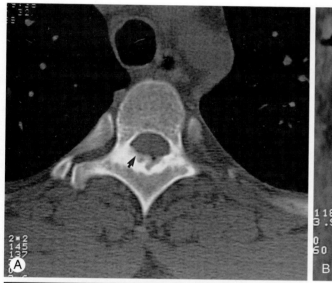
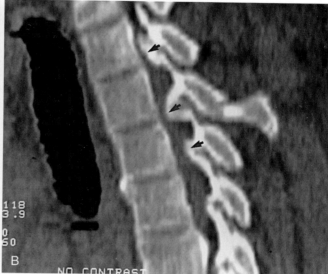
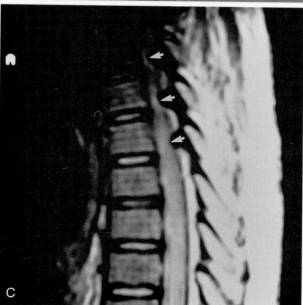

FIGURE 37–14 Ossification of the ligamentum flavum. A transverse CT scan (A) with sagittal reconstruction images (B) and a sagittal MRI (C) study demonstrate ligamentum flavum ossification with indentation on the spinal canal (arrows).

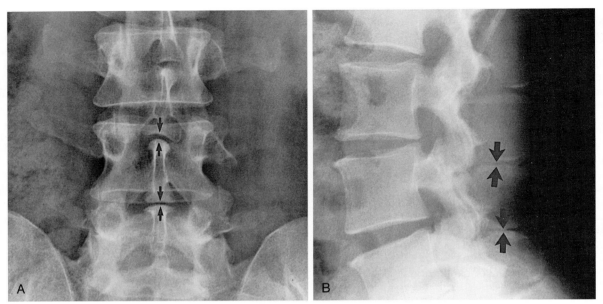

FIGURE 37–15 Baastrup's disease. Radiographs demonstrate hypertrophied "kissing" spinous processes. The anteroposterior view (*A*) shows hypertrophy and the lateral view (*B*) eburnation of the subcortical bone (*arrows*). Bursitis that may develop between the spinous processes can be a cause of back pain.

Interspinous and Supraspinous Ligaments

The interspinous ligaments extend from the root to the apex of each spinous process, connecting adjoining processes. The supraspinous ligaments lie slightly more posteriorly and connect the apices of the spinous processes from the level of the C7 vertebra to the sacrum. Interspinous and supraspinous ligament abnormalities frequently coexist. Excessive lordosis or extensive disk degeneration leads to close approximation of spinous processes and to degeneration of intervening ligaments. *Spinous process impingement syndrome*, also known as *Baastrup's disease*, develops when adjacent spinous processes abut one another (Fig. 37–15).[108, 109] These "kissing spines" may develop reactive eburnation and adventitial

bursae (which may become inflamed) and be associated with considerable pain.[110–112] The diagnosis of spinous process impingement syndrome requires lateral radiographs of the lumbar spine, preferably accomplished during flexion and extension. The characteristic radiologic abnormalities are abnormal contact of adjacent spinous processes, combined with sclerosis at the superior and inferior margins of apposing processes.

Hypertrophy of the tips of the lumbar spinous processes is not infrequent in patients with low back pain and a history of occupational stress related to long periods of back flexion (e.g., agricultural field workers). Chronic repetitive stress presumably leads to fibrosis and periostitis, with a resultant enthesopathy in the supraspinous and

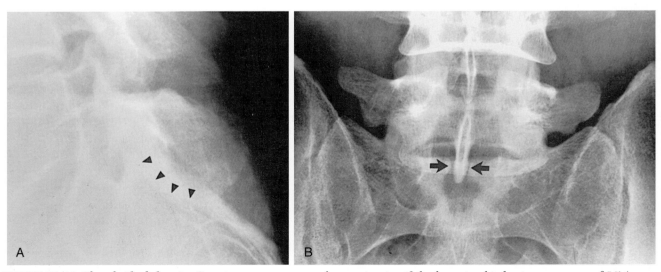

FIGURE 37–16 Clasp-knife deformity. Symptoms may occur on hyperextension if the hypertrophied spinous process of L5 (*arrowheads* in *A*) extends through the small spina bifida defect at S1 (*arrows* in *B*).

interspinous ligaments. Hypertrophic change in the L5 spinous process, combined with spina bifida of the upper sacral segments, is termed a *clasp-knife deformity* (Fig. 37–16).[113] Symptoms may result with hyperextension of the back, as the enlarged spinous process may extend through the defect into the spinal canal.

Ligamentum Nuchae

The triangular ligamentum nuchae is the cephalad extension of the supraspinous ligament, passing from the C7 vertebra to the external occipital protuberance. Fibers of the ligamentum nuchae attach to cervical spinous processes and paracervical muscles. The function of the ligamentum nuchae may be to assist in head position and control.[114] It possesses few elastic fibers, however, and appears to provide only minimal structural support to the spine. Ossicles resembling sesamoid bones are common in the ligamentum nuchae and have no clinical significance (Fig. 37–17).

Intertransverse Ligaments

Intertransverse ligaments connect the transverse processes of adjacent vertebrae. Degenerative changes presumably can accompany altered stress in these ligaments but are uncommon, even in the setting of substantial scoliosis. Trauma may lead to osseous bridging of transverse processes, particularly in the lumbar spine.[115–119] Patients usually are adults who have sustained fractures of the transverse processes and develop heterotopic ossification in the surrounding soft tissues.

Iliolumbar Ligament

The iliolumbar ligament extends from the transverse process of the lowest lumbar vertebra to the iliac crest. Occasionally, this ligament calcifies or ossifies (Fig. 37–18). The pathogenesis of this process is unknown, but it may be related to traumatic factors, congenital factors, or an ossifying diathesis such as DISH. Although the clinical

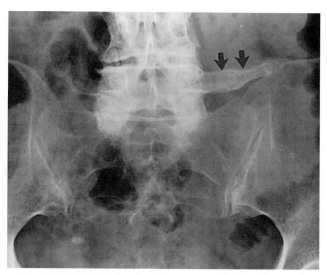

FIGURE 37–18 Iliolumbar ligament ossification *(arrows)*.

consequences are not always clear, local pain produced by deep palpation has been described.[120] Radiographically, this degenerative process is visualized as a horizontal band of calcific density in the distribution of the iliolumbar ligament.

DEGENERATIVE DISEASES OF SPECIFIC SEGMENTS OF THE SPINE

Cervical Spine

Cervical spondylitic myelopathy, a spectrum of degenerative changes occurring in the cervical spine, is the most common cause of spinal cord dysfunction in patients over 50 years of age.[121] Perhaps the most prevalent type of cervical spondylitic myelopathy is DDD, which is commonplace after the age of 40 years and affects more than 70% of patients older than 70 years.[122] Both men and women demonstrate a similar frequency of abnormality, although changes may be more severe in men.[123] The most commonly involved site is the intervertebral disk at the C5–C6 level, followed by the intervertebral disk at the C6–C7 level.[43] The intervertebral disk at the C2–C3 level is affected least often. Degenerative changes in the uncovertebral joints (of Luschka) and the facet joints are common, especially in the middle and lower cervical spine.

Encroachment on the intervertebral neural foramina may occur secondary to hyperostosis adjacent to the intervertebral disks, uncovertebral joints, and facet joints. The foramina most frequently involved are at the C3–C4, C4–C5, and C5–C6 levels. When these foramina are evaluated by conventional radiography, oblique projections are required.[124]

Numerous publications have implicated degenerative changes in the cervical spine with a variety of symptoms and signs; these include pain, stiffness, and radicular symptoms,[125] as well as pathologic reduction in vertebrobasilar blood flow velocities[126] and vestibular system dis-

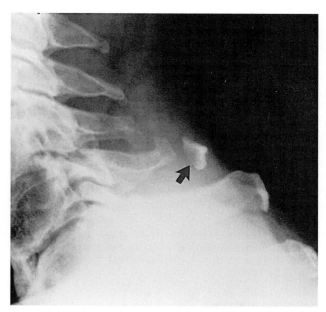

FIGURE 37–17 Ligamentum nuchae ossification *(arrow)*.

turbances.[127] Although many investigators have found a positive correlation between patients' symptoms and degenerative signs demonstrated with radiography,[128] considerable caution must be applied to the interpretation of the clinical significance of observed radiographic abnormalities.[129] In a study of two large groups of patients, one symptomatic and one asymptomatic, no differences were detected in the frequency of abnormalities of the uncovertebral joints, the intervertebral foramina, and the facet joints. In the asymptomatic group, degenerative changes were observed in 25% of patients in their fifth decade of life and in 75% of patients in their seventh decade of life. Even exuberant osteophytosis was not necessarily associated with significant clinical manifestations. In both the symptomatic and the asymptomatic groups, abnormalities were detected most frequently at the C5–C7 levels, although the prevalence of disk space narrowing at these levels was higher in the symptomatic group of patients.[130] In another study comparing symptomatic and asymptomatic patients, there was a fair correlation between radiographic and clinical abnormalities below the age of 40 years, but poor correlation between these abnormalities after the age of 40 years.[131] As MRI is more sensitive than conventional radiography in the detection of soft tissue processes, it is not surprising that many MRI findings of spine deterioration may be observed in asymptomatic people.[132, 133]

Thoracic Spine

Degenerative diseases in the thoracic spine appear to be less frequent and less debilitating than those in the cervical and lumbar spine. Intervertebral osteochondrosis has a predilection for the midthoracic area, whereas spondylosis predominates in the middle and lower thoracic region. Disk protrusions into the spinal canal are far less common in the thoracic spine than in the lumbar spine. A distinctive pattern of disk degeneration that is virtually confined to the thoracic spine and associated with kyphosis in elderly persons is termed *senile thoracic kyphosis* (see later discussion). Costovertebral osteoarthrosis, obviously, is confined solely to the thoracic region.

Lumbar Spine

Degenerative changes in the lumbar spine are ubiquitous in the elderly. By the age of 70 years, approximately 100% of subjects have intervertebral osteochondrosis, spondylosis, or facet joint osteoarthritis on pathologic examination. Although habitual physical activity may correlate with a lower prevalence of osteoarthrosis in the knee joints, the same physical activity may be associated with a greater prevalence of degenerative changes in the lumbar spine.[134]

On radiographic examination, virtually every elderly patient reveals at least minor degenerative changes of the lumbar spine, particularly between the L4 and the S1 segments. Disk space narrowing is very common in these areas, although the radiologist must be careful in regarding such narrowing as abnormal if a transitional type of distal lumbar vertebra is present. As discussed previously, a vestigial disk (devoid of a nucleus pulposus) may be

found at this level, and disk degeneration may be more frequent proximally at the adjacent level.[69]

The clinical significance of radiographic findings of DDD in the lumbar spine is debated. Numerous investigators believe that back symptoms and signs are associated with abnormalities visualized on radiographic examinations.[135–137] In one study comparing radiographs of symptomatic and asymptomatic persons,[138] disk space narrowing was more prevalent in symptomatic patients (56%) than in asymptomatic patients (22%); the difference between the two groups was particularly striking in younger patients. Osteophytosis, however, was almost as common in asymptomatic patients (47%) as in symptomatic patients (57%). These data suggest that intervertebral osteochondrosis is a cause of low back pain and spondylosis is not.

Other investigators have failed to document the usefulness of radiography in the evaluation of low back pain.[139] Two large studies that compared symptomatic and asymptomatic persons observed an inconsistent relationship between low back pain and radiographic signs of spinal degeneration.[140, 141] In another study, there was little correlation between radiographic changes of facet joint osteoarthrosis and low back pain.[123] Although MRI has proved superior to other methods in many respects, the results of several studies document frequent MRI abnormalities of the lumbar spine in asymptomatic persons.[142] As with the cervical spine, imaging findings in the lumbar spine must be correlated with clinical ones before performing any interventional procedure.

MAJOR COMPLICATIONS OF DEGENERATIVE DISEASES OF THE SPINE

Alignment Abnormalities

Segmental Instability

Motion of the vertebral column is complex, influenced by the integrity of the intervertebral disks, facet joints, and surrounding ligaments and muscles. This motion is governed by the anatomic characteristics of these structures, which are not constant from one segment of the spine to another. A brief overview of normal and abnormal spinal mobility, based on the work of others,[143–151] is contained here.

The biomechanics of the lumbar spine have been studied sedulously. Unique anatomic features in this vertebral segment generally allow a great deal of freedom in extension, somewhat less in flexion, a considerable amount of lateral bending, and only small degrees of rotation. The prominent thickness of the intervertebral disks in the lumbar region allows a relatively large degree of spinal mobility. During flexion and extension of the lumbar spine, the nucleus pulposus within each disk serves in a manner analogous to that of a ball bearing, allowing a rolling motion in which the vertebral body appears to glide over the nucleus. The posterior joints guide and steady this movement.[152] In the presence of intervertebral osteochondrosis, this smooth pattern of movement is transformed into one that is uneven, jerky, and either

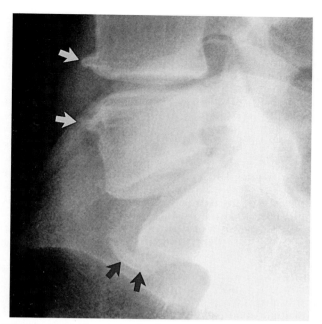

FIGURE 37–19 Traction and "claw" osteophytes. Traction osteophytes *(white arrows)*, whose bases are positioned slightly away from the endplate, extend horizontally. Marginal or claw osteophytes *(black arrows)* have a broader base and a hooked shape.

excessive[145, 152] or restricted.[147] Osteoarthrosis in the posterior articular facets presumably also has a direct effect on the extent and pattern of spinal motion.

Radiologic evaluation of the pattern of motion in the lumbar spine is made difficult by the three-dimensional nature of the movements. Conventional radiography is a useful tool, in that various positions may be employed in the evaluation of spinal instability. In addition to lateral radiographs obtained in the neutral position, lateral radiographs are commonly obtained during spinal flexion and extension. An alternative approach employs lateral radiography after the application of a standard axial load and then again after traction. The difference in displacement between compression and traction radiographs may correlate significantly with back pain, lumbar instability, and the patient's prognosis.[153] For some indications, other investigators also include frontal radiographs in the neutral position and with the patient bent to either side, as well as additional images obtained during spinal rotation.[154–156]

Although accurate appraisal of minor aberrations in movement requires the use of numerous anatomic landmarks,[144, 149, 154] general radiographic observations are indicative of degenerative instability,[151] including traction osteophytes on adjacent vertebral bodies and the presence of gas within the intervertebral disk. Traction osteophytes are osseous excrescences arising from the anterior aspect of the vertebral body, several millimeters from the diskovertebral junction.[152, 157, 158] This type of osteophyte is said to maintain a horizontal shelflike configuration, which allows differentiation from the more common marginal beaklike or "claw" osteophyte that has a broad base and terminal arch (Fig. 37–19). According to Macnab,[152] intervertebral instability results in traction on the outermost (Sharpey's) fibers that attach to the vertebral body

surface, thus inducing the formation of "traction" osteophytes. Unfortunately, differentiation between a claw osteophyte and a traction osteophyte commonly is not possible.[158] Indeed, both types of outgrowths appear to develop at approximately the same location on the vertebral body, consistent with the pathogenesis of spondylosis deformans that has been offered previously.

Lateral radiographs obtained in flexion and in extension should be regarded as positive when they reveal forward or backward displacement of one vertebra on another exceeding 5 mm,[70] an abrupt change in the length of the pedicles, narrowing of the intervertebral foramina, or loss of height of an intervertebral disk. On frontal radiographs obtained with the patient bending laterally in one direction and then in the other, additional abnormalities include asymmetry in the person's ability to bend in both directions, loss of normal vertebral rotation and tilt, an abnormal degree of disk closure or opening, malalignment of spinous processes and pedicles, and lateral translation of one vertebra on another.[151]

Degenerative Anterolisthesis

The term *spondylolysis* (Fig. 37–20) refers to an interruption of the pars interarticularis of the vertebra. Spondylolysis is now thought to be an acquired abnormality in the vast majority of cases, occurring when abnormal stress is applied to the vertebra and mechanical failure results (i.e., stress fracture). *Spondylolisthesis* refers to displacement of one vertebra on another. Formerly, the term *spondylolisthesis* was used only when a spondylolysis existed as well. At present, however, it is known that substantial spondylolisthesis may exist without vertebral arch disruption. Indeed, the most common cause of spondylolisthesis occurs with facet joint osteoarthritis—without spondylolysis—a situation termed *degenerative anterior spondylolisthesis* or simply *degenerative anterolisthesis* (Fig. 37–21).[159–165]

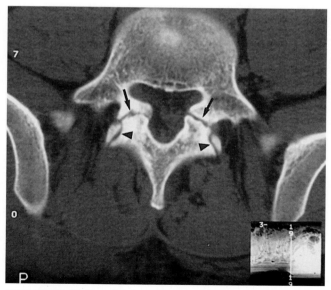

FIGURE 37–20 Spondylolysis. Transverse CT scan reveals bilateral pars interarticularis defects *(arrows)* distinct from the facet joints *(arrowheads)*.

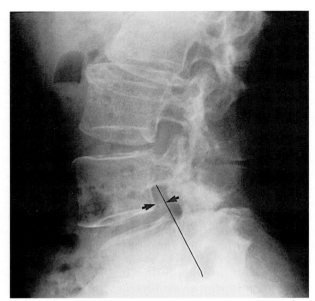

FIGURE 37–21 Degenerative anterior spondylolisthesis. Narrowing of the apophyseal joints from osteoarthrosis along with the resultant capsular laxity allows the mild subluxation of L4 on L5 *(arrows)* seen on this lateral radiograph.

Degenerative anterolisthesis occurs in approximately 4% of elderly patients[166] and predominates at the L4–L5 level.[159, 167–170] Unlike the L5 vertebra—with its broad posterior elements and its firm support provided by the iliac crest and iliolumbar ligaments—the L4 vertebra is at the apex of the lumbar curve and has relatively small transverse processes, less ligamentous support,[159] and more mobility.[171] Furthermore, developmental or acquired alterations in the neural arch[167, 172] at this spinal level may lead to undue stress on the L4 vertebra and consequent osteoarthritis of the adjacent facet joints. The facets at the L4–L5 level are oriented more sagittally than those at the L5–S1 level[173, 174] and therefore are more capable of allowing anterior spondylolisthesis. In most cases, the degree of forward slipping is between 10% and 25% of the anteroposterior diameter of the L5 vertebral body. A greater degree of anterolisthesis can result in cases in which there are bilateral pars interarticularis defects or in which the intervertebral disk is almost completely destroyed.[166]

Although forward displacement of L4 on L5 is by far the most common site of degenerative anterolisthesis, other levels may be affected, including the L5–S1 and L3–L4 segments. In the presence of a transitional lumbosacral vertebra, the predilection for L4–L5 involvement may be even more striking. In the cervical spine, hyperlordosis[175, 176] and stiff lower cervical segments[177] have been associated with degenerative anterolisthesis. Although unstable degenerative spondylolisthesis of the cervical spine is not common, it usually occurs at C3–C4 or C4–C5. Cervical spine subluxations can cause myelopathy, cervicobrachial pain, or neck pain alone.[177]

Clinical abnormalities associated with degenerative anterolisthesis include backache with or without leg pain, sciatica with signs of nerve root compression, and inter-

mittent claudication of the cauda equina.[167, 178, 179] Symptoms and signs related to bulged or herniated intervertebral disks are not uncommon.[164, 180] Many patients with degenerative anterolisthesis are, however, symptom free.[162]

Radiographic findings of degenerative anterolisthesis include anterior displacement of a superior vertebra on an adjacent inferior one, in addition to facet joint osteoarthritis (with joint space narrowing, sclerosis, and osteophytosis). In most cases, the forward displacement is between 10% and 25% of the anteroposterior dimension of the vertebral body. Abnormal motion between adjacent vertebrae is best detected using flexion-extension radiographs in the lateral projection and lateral bending radiographs in the frontal projection.[181] Myelography demonstrates deformity in the column of intrathecal contrast medium due to anterolisthesis or other causes of spinal stenosis such as facet joint osteophytosis.[182]

CT—with or without intrathecal contrast medium—is considered superior to conventional myelography. This method facilitates diagnosis of the presence and severity of multiple abnormalities including spinal stenosis, lateral disk protrusion, lateral recess narrowing, and facet joint osteoarthrosis.[183] The use of spiral CT may improve the length of time for diagnostic evaluation, as well as optimize the capacity for multiplanar analysis. The ability to manipulate re-formations to correct for an individual patient's position and rotation, for example, aids in analysis of vertebral alignment.[184]

MRI can also be applied to the assessment of degenerative anterolisthesis. Advantages of this technique are numerous and include multiplanar capability; delineation of pathologic changes in the intervertebral disks; and direct visualization of the spinal canal, spinal cord, and nerve roots. Specific morphologic alterations occurring in the setting of degenerative anterolisthesis that are well demonstrated with MRI include buckling of the ligamentum flavum, intervertebral disk displacement, compression of nerve roots or ganglia, and hypertrophy of the articular facets. Fluid within osteoarthritic facet joints and, not uncommonly, in nearby synovial cysts appears as high signal intensity on T2-weighted images.

Degenerative Retrolisthesis

Whereas degenerative anterolisthesis is secondary to facet osteoarthrosis, *degenerative retrolisthesis* (Fig. 37–22) is caused by intervertebral osteochondrosis.[185–187] Both types of degenerative spondylolistheses are notable by virtue of their intact neural arches; no spondylolysis need be present.

The pathogenesis of degenerative retrolisthesis relates to the disk space narrowing that occurs with intervertebral disk degeneration. With a decrease in the height of a disk space, the adjacent vertebrae become more closely approximated. Because the superior articular process has an oblique inclination, it moves in an inferoposterior direction and leads to posterior displacement of the superior vertebra relative to the inferior vertebra.

Degenerative retrolisthesis is most frequent in mobile segments of the spine. In particular, the most common sites of degenerative retrolisthesis are in the upper lumbar spine and in the middle to lower cervical spine.

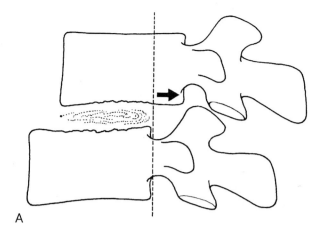

A

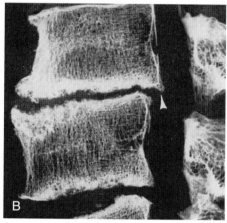

B

FIGURE 37–22 Spondylolisthesis without spondylolysis: Degenerative retrolisthesis. *A,* As the intervertebral disk space narrows owing to intervertebral (osteo)chondrosis, telescoping of the apophyseal joints allows backward displacement of the upper lumbar vertebra on the lower one. *B,* Retrolisthesis of L2 in relationship to L3 *(arrowhead)* is related to severe intervertebral (osteo)chondrosis in the intervening intervertebral disk. (*A,* From Resnick D [ed]): Diagnosis of Bone and Joint Disorders, Vol. 3, 3rd ed., p. 1416. Philadelphia, WB Saunders, 1995. *B,* From Resnick D. Degenerative diseases of the vertebral column. Radiology 1985;156:3–14.)

Clinical findings include pain, rigidity, a restricted range of motion, and neurologic abnormalities related to spinal cord compression.

Radiographic findings include posterior displacement of a superior vertebra on an adjacent inferior one, as well as typical changes of intervertebral osteochondrosis (with disk space loss, vacuum disk phenomena, and marginal vertebral body sclerosis). Neurologic complications related to degenerative retrolisthesis are best investigated with MRI.

Senile Thoracic Kyphosis

An accentuated thoracic kyphosis is common in older persons. This deformity may be due to osteoporotic kyphosis or senile thoracic kyphosis (Fig. 37–23), or both. With *osteoporotic kyphosis,* the weakened vertebral body collapses anteriorly where the greatest stress is borne. In

contradistinction, *senile thoracic kyphosis* results from degeneration in the anulus fibrosus. As the disk degenerates in patients with senile thoracic kyphosis, the resistant anterior edges of the vertebral bodies may concentrate force on the adjacent anterior fibers of the anulus fibrosus. With consequent injury, blood vessel proliferation and hemorrhage in annular tears can become evident on pathologic examination. As part of the reparative process, fibrosis, sclerosis, and even osseous bridging may occur.[5]

Senile thoracic kyphosis classically occurs in men, who are less likely to have significant vertebral osteoporosis. Senile thoracic kyphosis and osteoporotic thoracic kyphosis, however, are similar in many ways: both are observed in older patients; both produce a progressive kyphosis; and both involve mechanical failure in the anterior aspects of the thoracic spine. In senile thoracic kyphosis, the failure occurs in the intervertebral disk; in osteoporotic kyphosis, the failure occurs in the weakened vertebral bodies. Senile thoracic kyphosis can be differentiated from other processes (e.g., intervertebral osteochondrosis) because the disk space narrowing and reactive sclerosis predominantly are located anteriorly.

Degenerative Lumbar Scoliosis

Scoliosis in the spine of elderly persons is a common occurrence.[188-190] The relationship between degenerative

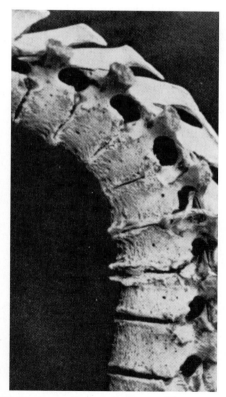

FIGURE 37–23 Senile thoracic kyphosis. The macerated spine of a 63-year-old woman reveals senile kyphosis with ossification of multiple intervertebral disks. Osteophytes are evident in the nonossified segments of the spine. (From Schmorl G, Junghanns H. The Human Spine in Health and Disease, 2nd American ed. New York, Grune & Stratton, 1971. Courtesy of Georg Thieme Verlag.)

lumbar scoliosis (Fig. 37–24) and clinical abnormalities is, however, debated. Some investigators report that these patients have disabling low back and lower extremity pain, weakness, and neurogenic claudication;[191] other researchers indicate that there is a lack of important clinical manifestations.[190] One specific pattern of neurologic compromise in patients with degenerative lumbar scoliosis has been termed the *far-out syndrome*. This syndrome is reportedly caused by impingement of the L5 spinal nerve between the L5 transverse process and the top of the sacrum.[192]

The precise cause of degenerative lumbar scoliosis is not clear. In some cases, senile scoliosis may represent the persistence of its adolescent counterpart. Any condition leading to asymmetric loading of the spine (e.g., anomalies, spondylolysis, leg length discrepancy) also could be an important factor in the genesis or progression of lumbar scoliosis.[111] Although degenerative diseases of the spine typically do not progress to scoliosis, the presence of scoliosis may contribute to the following degenerative diseases of the spine:

Intervertebral osteochondrosis complicating degenerative lumbar scoliosis is manifest by asymmetric disk degeneration, predominantly affecting disk tissue on the concave aspect of the curve. As asymmetric disk space loss occurs and the scoliotic deformity worsens, the abnormal stress at the inner aspect of the curve intensifies, and a vicious circle of events becomes apparent.

Spondylosis deformans in the setting of degenerative lumbar scoliosis leads to characteristic beaklike osteophytes along the concave aspect of the curve. As with other degenerative vertebral osteophytes, they appear to form after the attachment between the vertebral body and the anulus fibrosus is damaged. It is not clear, however, why osteophytosis is not encountered on the convex side where a similar process resulting from distraction might be expected.

Osteoarthritis of the facet joints leads to joint space narrowing, sclerosis, and osteophytosis. These findings are typically most severe along the concave aspect of the curve, near its apex.

Degenerative Lumbar Kyphosis

After the age of 40 years, increasing age is correlated with a loss of distal lumbar lordosis in asymptomatic adults.[193] When extreme, the normal lumbar lordosis actually may become reversed and symptomatic. Although it is a well-recognized occurrence, the initiating event in this degenerative condition is not clear.[194, 195] Affected persons walk with a forward-bending posture and often complain of low back pain. Radiographs typically reveal a marked loss of sacral inclination, marked disk space narrowing, and loss of height at the anterior aspect of the lumbar vertebral bodies. Atrophy and fatty infiltration in the lumbar extensor muscles may be demonstrated with CT or MRI.

Intervertebral Disk Displacement

Normally, the intervertebral disk is a load-bearing structure with hydrostatic properties related to its high water content. The anatomic arrangement of a centrally located nucleus pulposus surrounded by concentric fibers of the anulus fibrosus converts axial loading forces into tensile strains on the annular fibers and cartilaginous endplates.[196] The precise pressure in the disk is influenced by the patient's position and activity even in normal circumstances.[197] When the nucleus is subjected to elevated pressure, it attempts to prolapse from its confined space. The direction of disk displacement may be influenced by the type of stress, as well as the integrity of the nucleus and anulus. For example, axial loading usually leads to bursting of the disk contents in either a superior or an inferior direction.[198] This mechanism can, however, result in posterior protrusion of disk material into the spinal canal when there is weakness in the posterolateral aspect of the anulus or an abnormally (posteriorly) positioned nucleus. Disk displacement may occur in virtually any direction: superiorly or inferiorly (cartilaginous nodes), anteriorly or anterolaterally (spondylosis deformans), or posteriorly or posterolaterally (intraspinal or intraforaminal displacement).

Superior and Inferior Disk Displacement

Cartilaginous nodes, also referred to as *Schmorl's nodes*, occur secondary to intravertebral disk displacement. In the setting of intervertebral osteochondrosis, cartilaginous nodes most commonly involve the lower endplate. Several disease processes can weaken or disrupt the endplate or subchondral bone, however, and the distribution of cartilaginous nodes in these cases depends on the site of the primary process (Table 37–3).

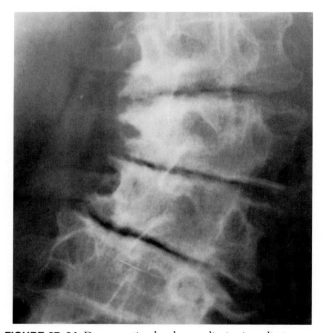

FIGURE 37–24 Degenerative lumbar scoliosis. A scoliotic curve in the lumbar region is associated with intervertebral (osteo)-chondrosis (vacuum phenomena, disk space narrowing, sclerosis) and spondylosis deformans (osteophytes). Both processes are more exaggerated on the concave aspect of the curve. (From Resnick D [ed]. Diagnosis of Bone and Joint Disorders, Vol. 3, 3rd ed., p. 1418. Philadelphia, WB Saunders, 1995.)

TABLE 37–3 Disk Displacement

Direction	Resulting Abnormality
Anterior displacement	Spondylosis deformans
Posterior displacement	Intraspinal herniation
Superior displacement	Cartilaginous (Schmorl's) node
Inferior displacement	Cartilaginous (Schmorl's) node

From Resnick D, Niwayama G. Degenerative disease of the spine. In Resnick D (ed). Diagnosis of Bone and Joint Disorders, Vol. 3, 3rd ed., pp. 1372–1462. Philadelphia, WB Saunders, 1995.

Radiographically, the appearance of cartilaginous nodes is fundamentally similar, regardless of the specific cause.[199-202] A radiolucent lesion within the vertebral body surrounded by helmet-shaped sclerosis that borders on the intervertebral disk corresponds to a site of disk displacement contained by eburnated or thickened bony trabeculae. In the presence of intervertebral osteochondrosis, some specific characteristics are seen. Degenerative clefts and collapse of the nucleus pulposus cause the vacuum disk phenomenon and disk space narrowing. The displaced disk material may not extend deeply into the vertebral body unless considerable osseous fragmentation and erosion have allowed the disk to be ground into the substance of the vertebra.

A distinct type of cartilaginous node formation is the *limbus vertebra*, characterized by intraosseous penetration of disk material at the junction of the cartilaginous endplate and the bony rim.[203, 204] This abnormality originates in childhood, when the developing apophyses may not fuse with the remaining portion of the vertebral body. In these situations, displaced pieces of intervertebral disk may extend along an oblique course toward the outer surface of the vertebral body, isolating a small triangular segment of bone.[205] The most common site is at the anterosuperior corner of a single lumbar vertebral body. Less commonly, the posteroinferior vertebral margin of other spinal segments are affected. CT and MRI can demonstrate the small bone fragments, the adjacent disk material, and the sclerosis of the adjacent cortex of the vertebral body.[206]

Anterior and Anterolateral Disk Displacement

The anterior longitudinal ligament usually prevents complete displacement of disk contents anteriorly. The mechanism whereby microdisplacement of disk material—secondary to breakdown of the outer annular fibers at their attachment site to the vertebral margin—causes spondylosis deformans has been detailed earlier in this chapter. Occasionally, however, tears in the anterior longitudinal ligament permit anterior and anterolateral protrusion of disk material, sometimes with cephalad or caudad migration.[207, 208]

Posterior and Posterolateral Disk Displacement

Displacement of disk material in a posterior or posterolateral direction is of great clinical significance because of the intimate relationship between the intervertebral disk and important neurologic structures. Anatomic features predisposing to such disk displacement include the relatively posterior position of the normal nucleus pulposus, the existence of fewer and weaker annular fibers in this region, and a posterior longitudinal ligament that is not as strong as the anterior longitudinal ligament.[209]

Although the terminology that is used to indicate the extent of disk displacement is not uniform, consistent descriptive designations are important to avoid miscommunication and potential legal misadventures. Four increasing stages of disk displacement (Fig. 37–25) are described in the following paragraphs.

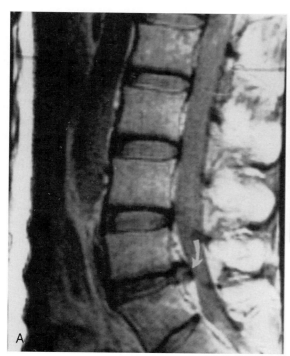

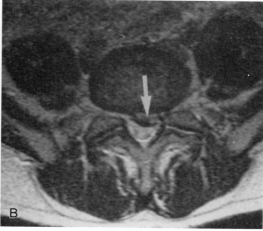

FIGURE 37–25 Disk extrusion. Sagittal *(A)* and axial *(B)* MRI demonstrates extrusion of disk material *(arrows)* through a tear in the anulus fibrosus. The disk material is contained within an elevated posterior longitudinal ligament. (*A,* and *B,* From Hart BL, Benzel EC, Ford CC [eds]. Fundamentals of Neuroimaging, p. 163. Philadelphia, WB Saunders, 1997.)

Disk bulge, in which the annular fibers remain intact but disk material is displaced into the spinal canal in a typically diffuse, nonfocal, broad-based, and circumferential fashion. The disk is thought to bulge outward beyond the vertebral body margins because the nucleus loses its turgor and anulus fibers diminish in elasticity.

Disk protrusion, in which nucleus pulposus extends through a partial tear in the anulus fibers but is still confined by the intact outermost fibers. In contrast to the disk bulge, disk protrusion is generally visualized as a broad-based asymmetric extension of disk material. The dimension of the connection with the parent disk is greater than the dimension of the extending component.

Disk extrusion, which is a focal, asymmetric extension of disk material beyond the interspace such that the largest dimension of the fragment in the anteroposterior plane is greater than the base of connection to the parent disk. With a disk extrusion, the nucleus pulposus penetrates all the fibers of the anulus fibrosus but is connected by a pedicle with the parent disk and may be confined by the posterior longitudinal ligament. Although some authors define *extrusion* as displaced disk material that has passed completely through the posterior longitudinal ligament,[210] other investigators define extrusion as displaced disk material that is *not* contained by the displaced posterior longitudinal ligament.[211] Perhaps the best solution to this discrepancy is to specify whether an extrusion is subligamentous or transligamentous when this determination can be made, recognizing that some data suggest that MRI is not reliable in accessing the integrity of the posterior longitudinal ligament.[212]

Disk sequestration, in which a free fragment of disk material is displaced through a full-thickness tear in the anulus and is no longer contiguous with the parent disk. The sequestered (or free) fragment may migrate from the level of the disk space to lie either anterior or posterior to the posterior longitudinal ligament. The recognition of a sequestered fragment is of paramount importance. Appropriate preoperative diagnosis alerts the surgeon to explore in a more cephalad or caudad direction in order to remove the free fragment. A sequestered fragment is a potential cause of failed back surgery syndrome and is generally a contraindication to chymopapain injection, percutaneous diskectomy, and, for many surgeons, microdiskectomy.[213]

The label *herniation* may be defined as any situation in which the nucleus pulposus extends through some or all of the fibers of the anulus fibrosus. Using this definition, disk prolapse, extrusion, and sequestration are all forms of herniation. Conversely, by this definition, an annular bulge would not represent a true disk herniation. With either a bulge or herniation of the disk, the disk height is commonly diminished. Because of the sagittally oriented midline septum in the anterior epidural space,[214] herniations usually occur at the posterolateral aspect of the anulus. The herniated disk material may contain, in addition to the nucleus pulposus, a portion of the anulus fibrosus and the cartilaginous endplate.[215] Approximately 90% of lumbar disk herniations occur at the L4–L5 and L5–S1 levels, with an additional 7% at the L3–L4 level.

Three distinct types of anular tears have been described.[216] *Concentric tears* are caused by delamination of longitudinal annular fibers and characterized by fluid-filled spaces between annular lamellae. *Transverse tears* involve the insertion of Sharpey's fibers into the ring apophysis. *Radial tears* involve all layers of the anulus from the nucleus to the disk surface. Both concentric and transverse tears are common regardless of whether degenerative changes are present in the nucleus; these types of tears probably represent incidental findings. In contradistinction, radial tears are hypothesized to be the essential lesion in the pathogenesis of disk space loss and an important factor in disk herniation. Both transverse and radial tears are seen as linear areas of increased signal intensity on both enhanced T1-weighted and T2-weighted images.[217–219] Annular tear enhancement can be explained on the basis of ingrowth of vascularized granulation tissue.[27] Although gadolinium-enhanced sequences are probably more sensitive for the detection of annular tears than T2-weighted sequences,[220] the routine application of the former technique is not recommended.[221] Gadolinium enhancement of nerve roots has correlated with radicular symptoms in some reports,[222, 223] but other authors have found that nerve root enhancement correlates poorly with clinical radiculopathy.[224, 225]

The precise relationship between annular tears and diskogenic pain is not clear. Low back pain in the absence of neurologic signs may originate within the musculoskeletal tissues of the spine such as the disk itself, rather than within the nerve root from displacement or compression.[226] Indeed, there is some evidence that pain can occur when the intrinsic architecture of the disk is altered, even though the external shape of the disk remains normal and the nerve roots are not compressed.[227] An injury to the vertebral endplate, for example, might expose antigenic nuclear material to the vertebral body, eliciting an inflammatory response.[228, 229] Findings during CT diskography have supported a relationship between the extent of annular disruption and the reproduction of a patient's pain during the injection of contrast material.[226] Fissures restricted to the inner third of the anulus fibrosus rarely are accompanied by a painful injection during diskography, whereas those extending to the outer surfaces of the anulus regularly are associated with a painful injection of contrast material.[230–232]

The imaging diagnosis of posterior disk displacement is best accomplished with three methods: CT, CT myelography, and MRI. All three methods have demonstrated statistically similar accuracy in the detection of disk herniations.[233, 234] The choice of an imaging method in any given patient is influenced by reported data describing the advantages of one technique over another, the spinal segment to be imaged, the patient's limitations (e.g., cardiac pacemaker, spinal instrumentation), and physician considerations (e.g., the specific expertise of the radiologist, experience of the referring physician).

Conventional myelography and CT myelography, discussed in great detail elsewhere, are invasive procedures requiring intrathecal contrast injection with potential discomfort and complications. Conventional myelographic criteria of a bulging anulus include a rounded and symmetric extradural deformity that does not extend above or below the intervertebral disk space; the nerve roots remain uniform in caliber and normal in size. With disk herniation, an angular extradural deformity may extend from the intervertebral space in a cranial or caudal direction, and the nerve roots may appear thickened.[235] With CT myelography, the morphologic findings of disk displacement are the same as with conventional CT, but contrast resolution is optimized with the former technique.

With CT, bulging of the anulus fibrosus is typically associated with generalized extension of the disk contour beyond the margins of the vertebral body in a symmetric and uniform fashion, whereas a focal extension is more typical of a herniated nucleus pulposus.[237–239] Diagnostic difficulty may arise when there is localized or asymmetric annular bulging, which has a propensity to occur in patients with scoliosis. In such cases, re-formatted images in the sagittal plane may facilitate detection of focal disk displacement at the interspace.[238] A herniated disk in a central or paracentral location produces a smooth, focal radiodense area that deforms or displaces the epidural fat. It has been suggested that the larger the disk herniation, the more likely the presence of sequestration,[240] and that a sequestered fragment tends to travel a greater distance in a superior than in an inferior direction.[241]

Both CT and MRI are superior to conventional myelography in many respects. Besides the noninvasive nature of these cross-sectional techniques, they permit the detection of lateral herniations located either within or lateral to the neural foramina. Lateral herniations are not routinely detected with conventional myelography and yet represent 12% of all herniations.[242, 243] With CT or MRI, pertinent findings include focal protrusion of the disk margin near or in the intervertebral foramen, as well as displacement or deformity of the nerve root, epidural fat, dural sac, and epidural veins. Ancillary CT and MRI findings of disk herniation in any location include swelling and dilatation of nerve roots, calcification or gas within displaced disk material, and a soft tissue mass in the posterior portion of the involved intervertebral disk.[244–247] With the administration of intravenous contrast material, enhancement is commonly observed at the margins of the herniated disk, a phenomenon that may relate to the presence of displaced epidural veins and irritated edematous tissue.[248–251]

Differential diagnosis of disk herniation on myelography and CT may at times include conjoined nerve roots, arachnoid diverticulae (dilated nerve root sleeves), synovial cysts, osteophytosis, postsurgical fibrosis, and various neoplasms and infections. The finding of osseous erosion tends to favor many of these alternative diagnoses, although this finding is occasionally associated with disk herniation.[252–253] With MRI, differential considerations may include anatomic variants (e.g., conjoined nerve root, dilated nerve root sleeve, perineural cyst) and nerve root tumors (e.g., schwannoma, neurofibroma). Sequestered fragments may occasionally produce an appearance similar to that of other epidural abnormalities, such as fibrotic tissue, synovial cyst, abscess, and neoplasm. Intravenous contrast administration can be helpful in distinguishing among these entities, because the central portion of a disk or synovial cyst will not enhance.

Synovial Cyst

Intraspinal synovial cysts arise adjacent to facet joints, with which they commonly communicate. Although the pathogenesis remains unclear, they most commonly occur in the setting of facet joint osteoarthrosis or trauma. Elevated intra-articular pressure likely results in extrusion of fluid and other joint contents into the periarticular soft tissues. It is not clear whether a synovial cyst (with synovial fluid) may evolve into a ganglion cyst (with mucinous fluid) by loss of the communication with the joint capsule, or whether synovial and ganglion cysts are unrelated lesions.[254] Both types of cysts are variable in size and may occasionally appear and enlarge rapidly.[255, 256]

Routine radiography may be normal or show nonspecific findings such as disk degeneration and degenerative spondylolisthesis. Conventional myelography may show a rounded, extradural filling defect in the posterolateral spinal canal.[257]

CT provides far more diagnostic information, typically demonstrating a fluid-density or soft tissue–density mass adjacent to a degenerative facet joint. The cyst may contain gas, which is thought to originate from a vacuum phenomenon in the nearby facet joint. Occasionally, the cyst may contain hemorrhage or possess a partially or completely calcified rim.[258–261] CT may also reveal erosion of the lamina or pedicle adjacent to the synovial cyst.[262] After the injection of contrast material into the adjacent facet joint, free communication with the cyst may be demonstrated. When such a communication exists, the injection of corticosteroid medication into the joint may be an efficacious alternative[263] to the more traditional surgical treatment: laminectomy or hemilaminectomy with cyst excision.[264]

With MRI, intraspinal cysts are typically also seen as mass lesions adjacent to degenerative facet joints. The signal intensity of synovial and ganglion cysts is variable. On T1-weighted images, they may be isointense or hyperintense when compared with cerebrospinal fluid; on T2-weighted images, they may be hyper- or hypointense when compared with CSF. Signal void on all pulse sequences may be related to gas within the cyst or calcification in the rim of the cyst.[254, 258, 265] After the intravenous injection of gadolinium compounds, enhancement may occur in the rim of the cyst.[266]

Spinal Stenosis

Spinal stenosis is constriction of the neural elements in the spinal canal, lateral recesses, and neural foramina. Spinal stenosis may be congenital or acquired or may result from a combination of congenital abnormalities with superimposed degenerative changes. Although congenital disorders such as achondroplasia are classic causes of narrowing of the spinal canal, spinal stenosis is far more frequent in middle-aged and elderly persons. Indeed, the degenerative diseases of the spine detailed previously commonly contribute to compromise of neural contents: spondylosis related to the degenerating disk, facet joint osteoarthrosis, ligamentous degeneration, spondylolisthesis, disk displacement, or a combination of these disorders. As abnormal mobility from degenerative changes at one level predisposes to abnormal stress at another level,[267] spinal stenosis initially confined to one level may subsequently be acquired at multiple levels.

In one retrospective study of 158 patients with surgically proved lumbar spinal stenosis,[268] the cause was most commonly degenerative (70%); less commonly, the cause was congenital (16%) or a combination of degenerative and congenital abnormalities (14%). In this same patient population, patients with spinal stenosis reported low back pain (87%), radicular pain (82%), polyradicular claudication (58%), and neurologic deficits (37%). After surgery, radicular pain and polyradicular claudication were relieved in approximately 90% of the patients, whereas relief from low back pain and neurologic deficits was achieved in only 60% and 50% of the patients, respectively.

Radiographic evaluation of spinal stenosis is notoriously insensitive. In the cervical spinal canal, radiographic measurement of the canal in the sagittal dimension (measured from the posterior surface of the vertebral body to the spinolaminar line) may be used.[269] Although the normal diameter of the spinal canal varies with age and race, cord compression may occur in adults if this diameter is 10 mm or less; it is unlikely to occur if this diameter is 13 mm or more.[270–273] Since this absolute measurement is subject to error introduced by magnification during radiography, comparing the anteroposterior diameter of the spinal canal with that of the adjacent vertebral body may be helpful. Normally, the ratio between these two measurements is about 1, with a value of 0.8 or less indicative of developmental canal stenosis.[274] Of course, this method is flawed in that it does not take into account stenosis that is secondary to ligamentous degeneration, disk displacement, and bony excrescences arising from the vertebral spondylosis, uncovertebral joint osteoarthrosis, and facet joint osteoarthrosis.

In the lumbar spine, analogous factors may be considered. By radiography, the lower limit of normal for the transverse interpediculate diameter is 20 mm and for the midsagittal diameter (between the posterior surface of the vertebral body and the base of the superior portion of the spinous process) is 15 mm.[275] The L4–L5 and L5–S1 segments are most commonly affected.

Because several of the abnormalities causing spinal stenosis are soft tissue rather than osseous, the limitations of conventional radiography must be emphasized. CT and MRI represent far more sensitive techniques in the evaluation of stenosis.[27, 276–282] Although specific measurements have been reported as criteria for the diagnosis of spinal canal stenosis,[276, 283] simply noting whether the thecal sac is compressed (rather than rounded) may be a reliable indicator of spinal stenosis.[213] Extradural defects can be identified as narrowing in the subarachnoid space. With severe stenosis, the subarachnoid space may be completely effaced and the nerve roots may become so edematous and redundant that they may mimic a vascular malformation. With chronic stenosis, severely compressed nerve roots may enhance after contrast administration.[284] Criteria for the normal dimension of the nerve root tunnels are not firmly established.

Spinal stenosis in the lumbar segment can be divided into three groups on the basis of its anatomic location. Any or all of the following locations may be affected.

1. *Central canal stenosis* is characterized by distortion or compression of the thecal sac with obliteration of the adjacent epidural fat.[285] Whereas osseous abnormalities are visualized more easily when CT is used, MRI appears superior to CT in the demonstration of narrowing of the thecal sac. The classic configuration of the stenosed canal is that of a trefoil, although a trefoil shape occasionally may be a normal variant at the L4 or L5 level.[286]

2. *Lateral recess (or subarticular) stenosis* occurs immediately ventral to the superior articular process and pars interarticularis. The lateral recess is bordered laterally by the medial margin of the pedicle and anteriorly by the posterior surface of the vertebral body.[245, 287, 288] The anteroposterior dimension varies from one spinal level to another, although a measurement of 3 mm or less is definitely abnormal, whereas a measurement of 3 to 5 mm is said to be highly suggestive of lateral recess stenosis.[287] The recess should be measured at its superior portion close to the superior articular facet, where bone hypertrophy about the facet joint is a leading cause of neural encroachment. In contrast to patients with central canal stenosis due to disk herniation who present with symptoms that are aggravated by sitting and a variety of Valsalva's maneuvers, patients with lateral recess syndrome have leg pain that is characteristically initiated or aggravated by standing and walking and relieved completely by sitting or squatting.[289]

3. *Neural foraminal stenosis* occurs as the lumbar nerve passes laterally just below the pedicle of the upper vertebrae. Diminution of the lower part of the intervertebral foramen is not as important because no nerve traverses this region.[290] Causes of foraminal narrowing include disk herniation, synovial cyst formation, and osteophytosis arising from the vertebral body or articular process, as well as proximal placement of nerve root ganglia, focal inflammatory disease, tumors, and postoperative fibrosis.[291–293] Neural foramina may also be distorted in the setting of spondylolisthesis, which may be related to bilateral spondylolysis, degenerative anterolisthesis (due to facet joint osteoarthrosis), or degenerative retrolisthesis (due to intervertebral osteochondrosis). CT and MRI are clearly superior to myelography in delineating neural foraminal encroachment,[291] demonstrating distortion of the exiting nerve and surrounding epidural fat and displaying the soft tissue or bony mass responsible for the stenosis.[292, 294] With MRI, signal abnormalities in the spinal cord may be observed at the site of severe stenosis. On T2-weighted images, these abnormalities appear as intramedullary foci of high signal intensity. Histologically, these foci probably represent edema, inflammation,

vascular ischemia, myelomalacia, gliosis, or some combination of these abnormalities. After surgical decompression of spinal stenosis, some of the signal intensity abnormalities may resolve.[295]

As with other degenerative diseases of the spine, asymptomatic patients may have anatomic abnormalities: 4% to 28% of CT or MRI examinations in asymptomatic adults may show changes of lumbar stenosis.[296]

IMAGING GUIDELINES FOR LOW BACK PAIN AND RADICULOPATHY

Low back pain is common, costly, and controversial. This affliction affects up to 80% of people during their lifetimes and sends patients to physicians more often than any other chief complaint except the common cold. The cost of low back pain is substantial as well, estimated at more than $50 billion annually.[297–299] Epidemiologic studies have implicated a number of risk factors, including obesity, smoking, repetitive twisting motions, and whole body vibration.[300, 301] Physical, psychosocial, and workplace factors are clearly potential variables that may contribute to patient symptoms.

Clinically, low back pain is commonly associated with buttock and lower extremity pain. *Lumbar radiculopathy* is characterized by pain in the posterior or lateral part of the lower extremity that may radiate below the knee. *Neurogenic claudication* refers to leg pain with weakness or sensory symptoms worsened by walking and relieved by sitting.

The natural history of a first episode of low back pain or radiculopathy is generally characterized by a short duration of symptoms. Fortunately, conservative (nonsurgical) therapy results in complete resolution of symptoms in 50% of patients within 1 week, and 90% of patients within 12 weeks.[300] Most cases of low back pain are not attributable to herniated disks. When it is present, spontaneous regression of disk herniations may occur and be documented by CT or MRI.[302, 303] Unfortunately, however, recurrent symptoms are common, occurring in approximately 25% of conservatively treated patients and 15% of surgically treated patients within 4 years.[304] In addition to a lower recurrence rate, surgery generally offers a more rapid relief of symptoms. Surgery is usually performed in the setting of definitive radiologic evidence of herniation, a corresponding pain syndrome with associated neurologic deficits, and a failure to respond to 6 weeks of conservative therapy. Only 5% to 10% of patients with long-standing sciatica require surgery.[305]

Guidelines have been advanced to aid clinical physicians in choosing the appropriate time to order an appropriate imaging examination. Conventional radiographs in the anteroposterior and lateral projections are a relatively inexpensive means of screening patients to exclude degenerative, congenital, infectious, and neoplastic causes of pain. Advanced imaging techniques are generally not recommended for patients with low back pain or radiculopathy before 6 weeks of conservative therapy because it is unlikely to alter clinical management in the vast majority of patients and may suggest anatomic signs of trouble when none exists. Exceptions to this general rule

may prevail when the patient has disabling pain, a major neurologic deficit, progressive weakness, or clinical findings worrisome for infection or neoplasm (e.g., a history of cancer, intravenous drug abuse, immunocompromised status, unexplained fever, or an elevated erythrocyte sedimentation rate). In the postoperative setting, MRI with gadolinium is indicated after conventional radiography in those patients with recurrent or worsening radicular symptoms or signs. In other patients—after 6 weeks of conservative therapy—spine imaging may be indicated for evaluation of unremitting low back pain or radiculopathy.

Once the decision has been made to obtain an advanced imaging study, MRI generally is considered the best initial imaging examination to evaluate the spectrum of conditions that might be responsible for symptoms, including infection, neoplasm, and the various degenerative diseases of the spine. Indeed, data from multiple studies suggest that MRI is the single best test to confidently detect and distinguish among these differential diagnostic possibilities. Not only does MRI display diseases of the disk and bone marrow accurately,[306] but also it is more sensitive and specific than CT in detecting various types of neurologic lesions.[307]

Although MRI provides the best global assessment of diseases of the bone marrow, disk, spinal cord, and nerve roots, inaccuracies do exist. In particular, one must recall that when morphologic abnormalities of the intervertebral disks are present, they of course do not always produce symptoms. In one study of 67 persons who had never had low back pain or sciatica, disk herniation was reported in 21% of patients less than 40 years of age and in 28% of those more than 40 years old.[308] In a different study, prospective evaluation of disk herniation and spinal stenosis by MRI was 83% accurate when compared with surgical findings.[27] Other authors report that MRI yields up to 20% false-negative and 15% false-positive studies in the evaluation of disk displacement.[309]

If MRI does not satisfactorily document a source of pain or radicular symptoms, CT or CT myelography may be necessary. Conventional CT scanning is commonly diagnostic for various degenerative diseases of the spine, but many surgeons prefer CT myelography for presurgical planning, considering it the best test for demonstrating the soft tissue and bony changes that result in nerve root and spinal cord compression syndromes.[310]

SUMMARY

Degenerative processes occur in the spine as a normal consequence of the aging process. Radiologic investigation of the spine should be performed only after a thoughtful evaluation of the clinical symptoms and signs. Conventional radiography remains the mainstay screening examination to evaluate those symptoms and signs that may result from degenerative diseases of the spine. Although there are several complementary imaging methods available in our diagnostic armamentarium, MRI has emerged as the single best presurgical decision-making tool and has resulted in an improved understanding of the frequency and spectrum of anatomic findings that can be present as part of the aging process.

References

1. Buckwalter JA. Aging and degeneration of the human intervertebral disc. Spine 1995;20:1307.
2. Higuchi M, Kaneda K, Abe K. Postnatal histogenesis of the cartilage plate of the spinal column. Electron microscopic observations. Spine 1982;7:89.
3. King AG. Functional anatomy of the lumbar spine. Orthopedics 1983;12:1588.
4. Weidenbaum M, Foster RJ, Best BA, et al. Correlating magnetic resonance imaging with the biochemical content of the normal human intervertebral disc. J Orthop Res 1992;10:552.
5. Schmorl G, Junghanns H (Besemann EF, trans). The Human Spine in Health and Disease, 2nd ed., p. 138. New York, Grune & Stratton, 1971.
6. Battie MC, Haynor DR, Fisher LD, et al. Similarities in degenerative findings on magnetic resonance images of the lumbar spines of identical twins. J Bone Joint Surg 1995;77A:1662.
7. Gershon-Cohen J, Schraer H, Sklaroff D, et al. Dissolution of the intervertebral disk in the aged normal. The phantom nucleus pulposus. Radiology 1954;62:383.
8. Khodadadyan C, Hoffmann R, Neumann K, et al. Unrecognized pneumothorax as a cause of intraspinal air. Spine 1995;20:838.
9. Ford LT, Gilula LA, Murphy WA, et al. Analysis of gas in vacuum lumbar disc. AJR 1977;128:1056.
10. Knutsson F. The vacuum phenomenon in the intervertebral discs. Acta Radiol 1942;23:173.
11. Goobar JE, Pate D, Resnick D, et al. Radiography of the hyperextended lumbar spine: An effective technique for demonstration of discal vacuum phenomena. J Can Assoc Radiol 1987;38:271.
12. Kröker P. Sichtbare Rissbildungen in den Bandscheiben der Wirbelsäule. Rofo Fortschr Geb Rontgenstr Neuen Bildgeb Verfahr 1949;72:1.
13. Schabel SI, Moore TE, Rittenberg GM, et al. Vertebral vacuum phenomenon. A radiographic manifestation of metastatic malignancy. Skel Radiol 1979;4:154.
14. Reymond RD, Wheeler PS, Perovic M, et al. The lucent cleft, a new radiographic sign of cervical disc injury or disease. Clin Radiol 1972;23:188.
15. Bohrer SP. The annulus vacuum sign. Skeletal Radiol 1986;15:233.
16. Jeffrey RB, Callen PW, Federle MP. Computed tomography of psoas abscesses. J Comput Assist Tomogr 1980;4:639.
17. Maldague BE, Noel HM, Malghem JJ. The intravertebral vacuum cleft: A sign of ischemic vertebral collapse. Radiology 1978;129:23.
18. Cohen JA, Abraham E. The calcified intervertebral disc. J Med Soc NJ 1973;70:459.
19. Bywaters EGL, Hamilton EBD, Williams R. The spine in idiopathic hemochromatosis. Ann Rheum Dis 1971;30:453.
20. Rathcke L. Cysten in den Zwischenwirbelscheiben. Beitr Pathol Anat 1931;87:737.
21. Taylor TK, Little K. Calcification in the intervertebral disc. Nature 1963;199:612.
22. Weinberger A, Myers AR. Intervertebral disc calcification in adults: A review. Semin Arthritis Rheum 1978;8:69.
23. Lane NE, Kremer LB. Radiographic indices for osteoarthritis. Rheum Dis Clin North Am 1995;21:379.
24. Raininko R, Manninen H, Battie MC, et al. Observer variability in the assessment of disc degeneration on magnetic resonance images of the lumbar and thoracic spine. Spine 1995;20:1029.
25. Modic MT, Masaryk TJ, Ross JS, et al. Imaging of degenerative disk disease. Radiology 1988;168:177.
26. Modic MT, Steinberg PM, Ross JS, et al. Degenerative disk disease: Assessment of changes in vertebral body marrow with MR imaging. Radiology 1988;166:193.
27. Ross JS, Modic MT. Current assessment of spinal degenerative disease with magnetic resonance imaging. Clin Orthop 1992;279:68.
28. Major NM, Helms CA, Genant HK. Calcification demonstrated as high signal intensity on T1-weighted MR images of the disks of the lumbar spine. Radiology 1993;189:494.
29. Bangert BA, Modic MT, Ross JS, et al. Hyperintense discs on T1-weighted MR: Correlation with calcification. Radiology 1995;195:437.
30. Kucharczyk W, Henkelman RM. Visibility of calcium on MR and CT: Can MR show calcium that CT cannot? AJNR 1994;15:1145.
31. Martel W, Seeger JF, Wicks JD, et al. Traumatic lesions of the discovertebral junction in the lumbar spine. AJR 1976;127:457.
32. McCarthy EF, Dorfman HD. Idiopathic segmental sclerosis of vertebral bodies. Skeletal Radiol 1982;9:88.
33. White AA III, McBride ME, Wiltse LL, et al. The management of patients with back pain and idiopathic vertebral sclerosis. Spine 1986;11:607.
34. Dihlmann SW, Eisenschenk A, Mayer, et al. The "mirror image" and "two-thirds" types of hemispherical spondylosclerosis. Eur Spine J 1995;4:110.
35. Dihlmann W. Hemispherical spondylosclerosis—A polyetiologic syndrome. Skeletal Radiol 1981;7:99.
36. Jensen ME, CW, DeBlois GG, et al. Hemispherical spondylosclerosis: MR appearance. J Comput Assist Tomogr 1989;157:416.
37. Sobel DF, Zyroff J, Thorne RP. Diskogenic vertebral sclerosis: MR imaging. J Comput Assist Tomogr 1987;11;855.
38. Palmer PES, Stadalnick R, Arnon S. The genetic factor in cervical spondylosis. Skeletal Radiol 1984;11:178.
39. Peel NF, Barrington NA, Blumsohn A, et al. Bone mineral density and bone turnover in spinal osteoarthrosis. Ann Rheum Dis 1995;54:867.
40. Payne EE, Spillane JD. Cervical spine: Anatomico-pathological study of 70 specimens (using special technique) with particular reference to the problem of cervical spondylosis. Brain 1957;80:571.
41. Bradshaw P. Some aspects of cervical spondylosis. Q J Med 1957;26:177.
42. Macnab I. Cervical spondylosis. Clin Orthop 1975;109:69.
43. Lestini WF, Weisel SW. The pathogenesis of cervical spondylosis. Clin Orthop 1989;239:69.
44. Goldberg RP, Vine HS, Sacks BA, et al. The cervical split: A pseudofracture. Skeletal Radiol 1982;7:267.
45. Taylor JR, Twomey LT. Age changes in lumbar zygapophyseal joints. Observations on structure and function. Spine 1986;11:739.
46. Ghormley RK. Low back pain with special reference to the articular facets, with presentation of an operative procedure. JAMA 1933;101:1773.
47. Epstein JA, Epstein BS, Lavine LS, et al. Lumbar nerve root compression at the intervertebral foramina caused by arthritis of the posterior facets. J Neurosurg 1973;39:362.
48. Kirkaldy-Willis WH, Wedge JH, Yong-Hing K, et al. Pathology and pathogenesis of lumbar spondylosis and stenosis. Spine 1978;3:319.
49. Hadley LA. Anatomico-roentgenographic studies of the posterior spinal articulations. AJR 1961;86:270.
50. Fletcher G, Haughton VM, Ho K-C, et al. Age-related changes in the cervical facet joints: Studies with crymicrotomy, MR, and CT. AJNR 1990;11:27.
51. Hemminghytt S, Daniels DL, Williams AL, et al. Intraspinal synovial cysts: Natural history and diagnosis by CT. Radiology 1982;145:375.
52. Hourigan CL, Bassett JM. Facet syndrome: Clinical signs, symptoms, diagnosis, and treatment. J Manipulative Physiol Ther 1989;12:293.
53. Bogduk N, Marsland A. The cervical zygapophyseal joints as a source of neck pain. Spine 1988;13:610.
54. Auteroche P. Innervation of the zygoapophyseal joints of the lumbar spine. Anat Clin 1983;5:17.
55. Giles LGF, Taylor JR. Innervation of lumbar zygapophyseal synovial folds. Acta Orthop Scand 1987;58:43.
56. Giles LGF, Taylor JR. Human zygapophyseal joint capsule and synovial fold innervation. Br J Rheumatol 1987;26:93.
57. Engel R, Bogduk N. The menisci of the lumbar zygapophysial joints. J Anat 1982;135:795.
58. Giles LGF, Taylor JR. Intra-articular synovial protrusions in the lower lumbar apophyseal joint. Bull Hosp Jt Dis 1982;42:248.
59. Yu S, Sether L, Haughton VM. Facet joint menisci of the cervical spine: Correlative MR imaging and cryomicrotomy study. Radiology 1987;164:79.
60. Mooney V, Robertson J. The facet syndrome. Clin Orthop 1975;115:149.
61. Lynch MC, Taylor JF. Facet joint injection for low back pain. A clinical study. J Bone Joint Surg 1986;68B:138.
62. Hadley LA. Anatomico-roentgenographic Studies of the Spine, 2nd ed., p. 447. Springfield, IL, Charles C Thomas, 1973.
63. Tini PG, Weiser C, Zinn WM. The transitional vertebra of the

lumbosacral spine: Its radiological classification, incidence, prevalence, and clinical significance. Rheumatol Rehabil 1977;16:180.

64. Wigh RE. The thoracolumbar and lumbosacral transitional junctions. Spine 1980;5:215.

65. Tabor ML. Etude statistique des anomalies du rachis lombaire et lombosacre. Constatations radiologiques sur 7500 malades orthopediques. J Radiol 1968;49:713.

66. Nachemson A. Towards a better understanding of low-back pain. Rheumatol Rehabil 1975;14:129.

67. DePalma AF, Rothman RH. Congenital and acquired abnormalities of the lumbar spine. In The Intervertebral Disc, p. 260. Philadelphia, WB Saunders, 1970.

68. Wigh R, Anthony HF. Transitional lumbosacral discs: Probability of herniation. Spine 1980;6:168.

69. Castellvi AE, Goldstein LA, Chan DPK. Lumbosacral transitional vertebrae and their relationship with lumbar extradural defects. Spine 1984;9:493.

70. Frymoyer JW. Degenerative spondylolisthesis: Diagnosis and treatment. J Am Acad Orthop Surg 1994;2:9.

71. Genez BM. Atlantoodontoid osteoarthritis. Crit Rev Diagn Imaging 1991;32:301.

72. Genez BM, Willis JJ, Lowrey CE, et al. CT findings of degenerative arthritis of the atlantoodontoid joint. AJR 1990;154:315.

73. Harata S, Tohno S, Kawagishi T. Osteoarthritis of the atlantoaxial joint. Int Orthop 1981;5:277.

74. Zapletal J, Hekster RE, Wilmink JT, et al. Atlantoodontoid osteoarthritis: Comparison of lateral cervical projection and CT. Eur Spine J 1995;4:238.

75. Gardner-Morse M, Stokes IA, Laible JP. Role of muscles in lumbar spine stability in maximum extension efforts. J Orthop Res 1995;13:802.

76. Boachie-Adjei O, Bullough PG. Incidence of ankylosing hyperostosis of the spine (Forestier's disease) at autopsy. Spine 1987;12:739.

77. Forestier J, Lagier R. Ankylosing hyperostosis of the spine. Clin Orthop 1971;74:65.

78. Lenchik L, Andresen R, Sartoris DJ, et al. Risk factors for diffuse idiopathic skeletal hyperostosis (DISH). [Abstract] AJR 1996;166(Suppl):173.

79. Resnick D, Niwayama G. Radiographic and pathologic features of spinal involvement in diffuse idiopathic skeletal hyperostosis (DISH). Radiology 1976;119:559.

80. Julkunen H, Heinonen OP, Pyörörälä K. Hyperostosis of the spine in an adult population: Its relationship to hyperglycemia and obesity. Ann Rheum Dis 1971;30:605.

81. Resnick D, Shaul SR, Robins JM. Diffuse idiopathic skeletal hyperostosis (DISH): Forestier's disease with extraspinal manifestations. Radiology 1975;115:513.

82. Meeks LW, Renshaw TS. Vertebral osteophytosis and dysphagia. Two case reports of the syndrome recently termed ankylosing hyperostosis. J Bone Joint Surg 1973;55A:197.

83. Utsinger PD, Resnick D, Shapiro RF. Diffuse skeletal abnormalities in Forestier's disease. Arch Intern Med 1976;136:763.

84. Resnick D, Linovitz RJ, Feingold ML. Postoperative heterotopic ossification in patients with ankylosing hyperostosis of the spine (Forestier's disease). J Rheumatol 1976;3:313.

85. Tsukimoto H. An autopsy report of syndrome of compression of spinal cord owing to ossification within spinal canal of cervical spine. Arch Jpn Chir 1960;29:1003.

86. Onji Y, Akiyama H, Shimomura Y, et al. Posterior paravertebral ossification causing cervical myelopathy: Report of eighteen cases. J Bone Joint Surg 1967;49A:1314.

87. Yokoi K. Ectopic calcification in the epidural space. Orthop Surg 1963;14:1262.

88. Bakay L, Cares HL, Smith RJ. Ossification in the region of the posterior longitudinal ligament as a cause of cervical myelopathy. J Neurol Neurosurg Psych 1970;33:263.

89. Ono K, Ota H, Tada K, et al. Ossified posterior longitudinal ligament. Spine 1977:2:126.

90. Okamoto Y, Yasuma T. Ossification of the posterior longitudinal ligament of the cervical spine with or without myelopathy. J Jpn Orthop Assoc 1967;40:1349.

91. Tsuyama N. The ossification of the posterior longitudinal ligament of the spine (OPLL). J Jpn Orthop Assoc 1981;55:425.

92. Tsuyama N. Ossification of the posterior longitudinal ligament of the spine. Clin Orthop 1984;184:71.

93. Nakanishi T, Mannen T, Toyokura Y. Asymptomatic ossification of the posterior longitudinal ligament of the cervical spine. J Neurol Sci 1973;19:375.

94. Nose T, Egashira T, Enomoto T, et al. Ossification of the posterior longitudinal ligament: A clinico-radiological study of 74 cases. J Neurol Neurosurg Psych 1987;50:321.

95. Epstein N; The surgical management of ossification of the posterior longitudinal ligament in 51 patients. J Spinal Disord 1993;6:432.

96. Yamashita Y, Takahashi M, Matsuno Y, et al. Spinal cord compression due to ossification of ligaments: MR imaging. Radiology 1990;175:843.

97. Hukuda S, Mochizuki T, Ogata M, et al. The pattern of spinal and extraspinal hyperostosis in patients with ossification of the posterior longitudinal ligament and the ligamentum flavum causing myelopathy. Skeletal Radiol 1983;10:79.

98. Miyasaka K, Kaneda K, Ito T, et al. Ossification of spinal ligaments causing thoracic radiculopathy. Radiology 1982;143:463.

99. Nakajima K, Miyaoka M, Sumie H, et al. Cervical radiculopathy due to calcification of the ligamenta flava. Surg Neurol 1984;21:479.

100. Iwasaki Y, Akino M, Abe H, et al. Calcification of the ligamentum flavum of the cervical spine. Report of four cases. J Neurosurg 1983;59:531.

101. Kubota M, Baba I, Sumida T. Myelopathy due to ossification of the ligamentum flavum of the cervical spine. A report of two cases. Spine 1981;6:553.

102. Omojola MF, Cardoso ER, Fox AJ, et al. Thoracic myelopathy secondary to ossified ligamentum flavum. Case report. J Neurosurg 1982;56:448.

103. Miyasaka K, Kaneda K, Sato S, et al. Myelopathy due to ossification or calcification of the ligamentum flavum: Radiologic and histologic evaluations. Am J Neuroradiol 1983;4:629.

104. Kubota T, Kawano H, Yamashima T, et al. Ultrastructural study of calcification process in the ligamentum flavum of the cervical spine. Spine 1987;12:317.

105. Okada G, Hosoi S, Kato K, et al. Case report 779. Skeletal Radiol 1993;22:211.

106. Hodge J, Ghelman B, DeCarlo EF, et al. Case report 781. Skeletal Radiol 1993;22:218.

107. Bardwick PA, Zvaifler NJ, Gill GN, et al. Plasma cell dyscrasia with polyneuropathy, organomegaly, endocrinopathy, M protein, and skin changes: The POEMS syndrome. Medicine 1980;59:311.

108. Yamada K, Nichiwaki I, Yasukawa H. Supplemental study upon the pathogenesis of low back pain in Baastrup's disease. Arch Jpn Chir 1954;23:384.

109. Resnick D. Degenerative diseases of the vertebral column. Radiology 1985;156:3.

110. Baastrup CI. On the spinous processes of the lumbar vertebrae and the soft tissue between them and on pathological changes in that region. Acta Radiol Scand 1933;14:52.

111. Jacobson HG, Tausend ME, Shapiro JH, et al. The "swayback" syndrome. AJR 1958;79:677.

112. Goobar JE, Clark GM. Sclerosis of the spinous processes and low back pain ("cock spur" disease). AIR 1962;5:587.

113. Goobar JE, Erickson F, Pate D, et al. Symptomatic clasp-knife deformity of the spinous processes. Spine 1988;13:953.

114. Fielding JW, Burstein AH, Frankel VH. The nuchal ligament. Spine 1976;1:3.

115. Hyman G. A case of pseudarthrosis following fractures of the lumbar transverse processes. Br J Surg 1945;32:503.

116. Sutro CJ. Ossification of the intertransverse tissues of the lumbar vertebrae (an anomaly). Bull Hosp Jt Dis 1961;22:137.

117. Yoslow W, Becker MH. Osseous bridges between the transverse processes of the lumbar spine. Report of three cases and review of the literature. J Bone Joint Surg 1968;50A:513.

118. Jackson DW. Unilateral osseous bridging of the lumbar transverse processes following trauma. Case report. J Bone Joint Surg 1975;57A:125.

119. Billet FPJ, Schmitt WGH, Böhmer E. Knöcherne Sprangen der Lendenwirbelquerfortsätze. Rofo Fortschr Geb Rontgenstr Neuen Bildgeb Verfahr 1991;155:171.

120. Broudeur P, Larroque CH, Passeron R, et al. Le syndrome iliolombaire. [French with English abstract] Rev Rhum Mal Osteoartic 1982;49:693.

121. Ross JS. Myelopathy. Neuroimaging Clin N Am 1995;5:367.
122. DePalma A, Rothman R. The Intervertebral Disc. Philadelphia, WB Saunders, 1970.
123. Lawrence JS, Bremner JM, Bier F. Osteoarthrosis: Prevalence in the population and relationship between symptoms and x-ray changes. Ann Rheum Dis 1966;25:1.
124. Marcelis S, Seragini FC, Taylor JAM, et al. Cervical spine: Comparison of 45° and 55° anteroposterior oblique radiographic projections. Radiology 1993;188:253.
125. Hardin JG, Halla JT. Cervical spine and radicular pain symptoms. Curr Opin Rheumatol 1995;7:136.
126. Machala W, Gaszynski W, Olszewski J, et al. The effect of degenerative cervical spine lesions and blood flow velocity in vertebrobasilar system in Doppler measurement. Neurol Neurochi Pol 1995;29:17.
127. Rzewnicki I. The examination of vestibular system in patients with degenerative changes of the cervical spine. Otolaryngol Pol 1995;49:332.
128. Radanov BP, Sturzenegger M, Di Stefano G. Long-term outcome after whiplash injury. A 2-year follow-up considering features of injury mechanism and somatic, radiologic, and psychosocial findings. Medicine 1995;74:281.
129. Gore DR, Sepic SB, Gardner GM. Roentgenographic findings of the cervical spine in asymptomatic people. Spine 1986;11:521.
130. Friedenberg ZB, Miller WT. Degenerative disc disease of the cervical spine. J Bone Joint Surg 1963;45A:1171.
131. McRae DL. The significance of abnormalities of the cervical spine. AJR 1960;84:3.
132. Boden SD, McCowin PR, David DO, et al. Abnormal magnetic resonance scans of the cervical spine in asymptomatic subjects. A prospective investigation. J Bone Joint Surg 1990;72A:1178.
133. Teresi LM, Lufkin RB, Reicher MA, et al. Asymptomatic degenerative disk disease and spondylosis of the cervical spine: MR imaging. Radiology 1987;164:83.
134. White JA, Wright V, Hudson AM. Relationships between habitual physical activity and osteoarthrosis in ageing women. Public Health 1993;107:459.
135. Hirsch C. Studies of the pathology of low back pain. J Bone Joint Surg 1959;41B:237.
136. Badgley CE. Clinical and roentgenological study of low back pain with sciatic radiation. A clinical aspect. AJR 1937;37:454.
137. Ford LT, Goodman FG. X-ray studies of the lumbosacral spine. South Med J 1966;59:1123.
138. Torgerson WR, Dotter WE. Comparative roentgenographic study of the asymptomatic and symptomatic lumbar spine. J Bone Joint Surg 1976;58A:850.
139. Splithoff CA. Lumbosacral junction. Roentgen comparison of patients with and without backaches. JAMA 1953;152:1610.
140. Frymoyer JW, Newberg A, Pope MH, et al. Spine radiographs in patients with low-back pain. An epidemiological study in men. J Bone Joint Surg 1984;66A:1048.
141. Collee G, Kroon HM, Dijkmans BAC, et al. Radiological findings in relation to clinical features in low back pain. J Orthop Rheumatol 1990;3;147.
142. Boden SD, David DO, Dina TS, et al. Abnormal magnetic resonance scans of the lumbar spine in asymptomatic subjects. A prospective investigation. J Bone Joint Surg 1990;72A:403.
143. Allbrook D. Movements of the lumbar spinal column. J Bone Joint Surg 1957;39:339.
144. Gianturco C. A roentgen analysis of the motion of the lower lumbar vertebrae in normal individuals and in patients with low back pain. AJR 1944;52:261.
145. Knutsson F. The instability associated with disc degeneration in the lumbar spine. Acta Radiol 1944;25:593.
146. Matteri RE, Pope MH, Frymoyer JW. A biplane radiographic method of determining vertebral rotation in postmortem specimens. Clin Orthop 1976;116;95.
147. Mensor MV, Duvall T. Absence of motion at the fourth and fifth lumbar interspaces in patients with and without low back pain. J Bone Joint Surg 1959;41A:1047.
148. Pennal GF, Conn GS, McDonald G, et al. Motion studies of the lumbar spine. J Bone Joint Surg 1972;54B:442.
149. Hanley EN, Matteri RE, Frymoyer JW. Accurate roentgenographic determination of lumbar flexion-extension. Clin Orthop 1976;115:145.
150. Morgan FP, King T. Primary instability of lumbar vertebrae as a common cause of low back pain. J Bone Joint Surg 1957;39B:6.
151. Kirkaldy-Willis WH, Farfan HF. Instability of the lumbar spine. Clin Orthop 1982;165:110.
152. Macnab I. The traction spur. An indicator of segmental instability. J Bone Joint Surg 1971;53A:663.
153. Friberg O. Lumbar instability: A dynamic approach by traction-compression radiography. Spine 1987;12:119.
154. Stokes IAF, Wilder DG, Frymoyer JW, et al. Assessment of patients with low back pain by biplanar radiographic measurement of intervertebral motion. Spine 1981;6:233.
155. Pope MH, Wilder DG, Frymoyer JW. Experimental measurement of vertebral motion under load. Orthop Clin North Am 1977;8:155.
156. Pope MH, Wilder DG, Stokes IAF, et al. Biomechanical testing as an aid to decision making in low back pain patients. Spine 1979;4:135.
157. Malmivaara A. Disc degeneration in the thoracolumbar junctional region. Evaluation by radiography and discography in autopsy. Acta Radiol 1987;28:755.
158. Pate D, Goobar J, Resnick D, et al. Traction osteophytes of the lumbar spine: Radiographic-pathologic correlation. Radiology 1988;166:843.
159. Rosenberg NJ. Degenerative spondylolisthesis. Predisposing factors. J Bone Joint Surg 1975;57A:467.
160. Rosenberg NJ. Degenerative spondylolisthesis. Surgical treatment. Clin Orthop 1976;117:112.
161. Wiltse LL, Newman PH, Macnab I. Classification of spondylolysis and spondylolisthesis. Clin Orthop 1976;117:23.
162. Fitzgerald JAW, Newman PH. Degenerative spondylolisthesis. J Bone Joint Surg 1976;58B:184.
163. Cauchoix J, Benoist M, Chassaing V. Degenerative spondylolisthesis. Clin Orthop 1976;115:122.
164. Epstein JA, Epstein BS, Lavine LS, et al. Degenerative lumbar spondylolisthesis with an intact neural arch (pseudospondylolisthesis). J Neurosurg 1976;44:139.
165. Epstein BS, Epstein JA, Jones MD. Degenerative spondylolisthesis with an intact neural arch. Radiol Clin North Am 1977;15:275.
166. Farfan Hf. The pathological anatomy of degenerative spondylolisthesis. A cadaver study. Spine 1980;5:412.
167. Macnab I. Spondylolisthesis with an intact neural arch—The so-called pseudospondylolisthesis. J Bone Joint Surg 1950;32B:325.
168. Adkins EWO. Spondylolisthesis. J Bone Joint Surg 1955;37B:48.
169. Newman PH, Sone KH. The etiology of spondylolisthesis. J Bone Joint Surg 1963;45B:39.
170. Imada K, Matsui H, Tsuji H. Oophorectomy predisposes to degenerative spondylolisthesis. J Bone Joint Surg 1995;77B:126.
171. Junghanns H. Spondylolisthesen ohne Spalt in Zwischengelenkstuck. Arch Orthop Unfallchir 1930;29:118.
172. Allbrook D. Movements of the lumbar spinal column. J Bone Joint Surg 1957;39B:339.
173. Van Schaik JPJ, Veriest H, Van Schaik FDJ. The orientation of laminae and facet joints in the lower lumbar spine. Spine 1985;10:59.
174. Grobler LJ, Robertson PA, Novotny JE, et al. Etiology of spondylolisthesis. Assessment of the role played by lumbar facet joint morphology. Spine 1993;18:80.
175. Epstein JA, Carras R, Epstein BS. Myelopathy in cervical spondylosis with vertical subluxation and hyperlordosis. J Neurosurg 1970;32:421.
176. Lee C, Woodring JH, Rogers LF, et al. The radiographic distinction of degenerative slippage (spondylolisthesis and retrolisthesis) from traumatic slippage of the cervical spine. Skeletal Radiol 1986;15:439.
177. Deburge A, Mazda K, Guigui P. Unstable degenerative spondylolisthesis of the cervical spine. J Bone Joint Surg 1995;77A:122.
178. Moiel R, Ehni G. Cauda equina compression due to spondylolisthesis with an intact neural arch. Report of two cases. J Neurosurg 1968;28:262.
179. Epstein NE, Epstein JA, Carras R, et al. Degenerative spondylolisthesis with an intact neural arch: A review of 60 cases with an analysis of clinical findings and the development of surgical management. Neurosurgery 1983;13:555.
180. Scoville WB, Corkill G. Lumbar spondylolisthesis with ruptured disc. J Neurosurg 1974;40:529.
181. Dupuis PR, Yong-Hing K, Cassidy JD, et al. Radiologic diagnosis of degenerative lumbar spinal instability. Spine 1985;10:262.

182. Newman PH. Stenosis of the lumbar spine in spondylolisthesis. Clin Orthop 1976;115;116.
183. Rothman SLG, Glenn WV Jr, Kerber CW. Multiplanar CT in the evaluation of degenerative spondylolisthesis. A review of 150 cases. Comput Radiol 1985;9:223.
184. Gorbea ET, Olan WJ, Matsumoto MA, et al. Multiplanar reformation of helical computed tomography for cervical myelography. [Abstract] AJR 1996;166(Suppl):176.
185. Gillespie HW. Vertebral retroposition (reversed spondylolisthesis). Br J Radiol 1951;24:193.
186. Johnson R. Posterior luxations of the lumbosacral joint. J Bone Joint Surg 1934;16:867.
187. Willis TA. Lumbosacral retrodisplacement. AJR 1963;90:1263.
188. Benner B, Ehni G. Degenerative lumbar scoliosis. Spine 1979;4:548.
189. Epstein JA, Epstein BS, Jones MD. Symptomatic lumbar scoliosis with degenerative changes in the elderly. Spine 1979;4:542.
190. Robin GC, Span Y, Steinberg R, et al. Scoliosis in the elderly. A follow-up study. Spine 1982;7:355.
191. Edeiken J, Wallace JD, Curley RF, et al. Thermography and herniated lumbar disks. AJR 1968;102:790.
192. Wiltse LL, Guyer RD, Spencer CW, et al. Alar transverse process impingement of the L5 spinal nerve: The far-out syndrome. Spine 1984;9:31.
193. Gelb DE, Lenke LG, Bridwell KH, et al. An analysis of sagittal spinal alignment in 100 asymptomatic middle and older aged volunteers. Spine 1995;20:1351.
194. Milne JS, Lauder IJ. Age effects in kyphosis and lordosis in adults. Ann Hum Biol 1974;1:327.
195. Takemitsu Y, Harada Y, Iwahara T, et al. Lumbar degenerative kyphosis. Clinical, radiological and epidemiological studies. Spine 1988;13:1317.
196. Lipson SJ, Muir H. Proteoglycans in experimental intervertebral disc degeneration. Spine 1981;6:194.
197. Nachemson AL. Disc pressure measurements. Spine 1981;6:93.
198. Jayson MIV, Herbert CM, Barks JS. Intervertebral discs. Nuclear morphology and bursting pressures. Ann Rheum Dis 1973;32:308.
199. Resnick D, Niwayama G. Subchondral resorption of bone in renal osteodystrophy. Radiology 1976;118:315.
200. Hilton RC, Ball, Benn RT. Vertebral endplate lesions (Schmorl's nodes) in the dorsolumbar spine. Ann Rheum Dis 1976;35:127.
201. Begg AC. Nuclear herniations of the intervertebral disc: Their radiological manifestations and significance. J Bone Joint Surg 1954;36B:180.
202. Martel W. A radiologically distinctive cause of low back pain. Arthritis Rheum 1977;20:1014.
203. Kozlowski K. Anterior intervertebral disc herniations (report of six cases). Rofo Fortschr Geb Rontgenstr Neuen Bildgeb Verfahr 1978;129:47.
204. Kozlowski K. Anterior intervertebral disc herniations in children. Unrecognized chronic trauma to the spine. Aust Radiol 1979;23;67.
205. Niedner F. Zur Kenntnis der normalen und pathologischen Anatomie der Wirbelkörperrandleiste. Rofo Fortschr Geb Rontgenstr Neuen Bildgeb Verfahr 1932;46:628.
206. Yagan R. CT diagnosis of limbus vertebra. J Comput Assist Tomogr 1984;8:149.
207. Kemmler H. Vorderer Bandscheibenprolaps der Halswirbelsäule auf traumatischer Grundlage. Monatsschr Unfallheilkd 1938;45:194.
208. Cloward R. Anterior herniation of a ruptured lumbar intervertebral disk. Comments of the diagnostic value of the discogram. Arch Surg 1952;64:457.
209. Postacchini F, Bellocci M, Massobrio M. Morphologic changes in annulus fibrosus during aging. An ultrastructural study in rats. Spine 1984;9:596.
210. Mink JH. Imaging evaluation of a candidate for percutaneous lumbar discectomy. Clin Orthop 1989;238:83.
211. Onik G, Helms CA. Automated percutaneous lumbar diskectomy. AJR 1991;156:531.
212. Silverman CS, Lenchik L, Shimkin PM, et al. The value of MR in differentiating subligamentous from supraligamentous lumbar disk herniations. AJNR 1995;16:571.
213. Helms CA. CT of the lumbar spine, p. 197. In American Roentgen Ray Society Categorical Course Syllabus, 1994 Annual Meeting, San Francisco, 1994.
214. Schellinger D, Manz HJ, Vidic B, et al. Disk fragment migration. Radiology 1990;175:831.
215. Yasuma T, Makino E, Saito S, et al. Histological development of intervertebral disc herniation. J Bone Joint Surg 1986;68A:1066.
216. Yu S, Haughton VM, Sether LA, et al. Criteria for classifying normal and degenerating disks. Radiology 1989;170:523.
217. Ross JS, Modic MT, Masaryk TJ. Tears of the anulus fibrosus: Assessment with GD-DTPA–enhanced MR imaging. AJR 1990;154:159.
218. Sether LA, Yu S, Haughton VM, et al. Intervertebral disk: Normal age-related changes in MR signal intensity. Radiology 1990;177:385.
219. Schiebler ML, Grenier N, Fallon M, et al. Normal and degenerated intervertebral disk: In vivo and in vitro MR imaging with histopathologic correlation. AJR 1991;157:93.
220. Ross JS, Modic MT, Masaryk TJ. Tears of the annulus fibrosus: Assessment with Gd-DTPA-enhanced MR imaging. AJNR 1989;10:1251.
221. Ross JS, Modic MT, Masaryk TJ, et al. Assessment of extradural degenerative disease with Gd-DTPA-enhanced MR imaging: Correlation with surgical and pathologic findings. AJR 1990;154:151.
222. Crisi G, Carpeggiani P, Trevisan C. Gadolinium-enhanced nerve roots in lumbar disk herniation. AJNR 1993;14:1379.
223. Jinkins JR. MR of enhancing nerve roots in the unoperated lumbosacral spine. AJNR 1993;14:193.
224. Lane JI, Koeller KK, Atkinson JLD. Enhanced lumbar nerve roots in the spine without prior surgery: Radiculitis or radicular veins? AJNR 1994;15:1317.
225. Lane JI, Koeller KK, Atkinson JL. Contrast-enhanced radicular veins on MR of the lumbar spine in an asymptomatic study group. AJNR 1995;16:269.
226. Aprill C, Bogduk N. High-intensity zone: A diagnostic sign of painful lumbar disc on magnetic resonance imaging. Br J Radiol 1992;65:361.
227. Crock HV. Internal disc disruption: A challenge to disc prolapse. Spine 1986;11:650.
228. Bogduk N, Twomey LT. Clinical Anatomy of the Lumbar Spine, pp. 141–142. Melbourne, Churchill Livingstone, 1987.
229. Hsu KY, Zucherman JF, Derby R, et al. Painful lumbar end-plate disruptions: A significant discographic finding. Spine 1988;13:76.
230. Vanharanta H, Guyer RD, Ohnmeiss DD, et al. Disc deterioration in low-back syndrome. A prospective multicenter CT/discography study. Spine 1988;13:1349.
231. Vanharanta H, Sachs BL, Spivey MA, et al. The relationship of pain provocation to lumbar disc deterioration as seen by CT/discography. Spine 1987;12:295.
232. Sachs BL, Vanharanta H, Spivey MA, et al. Dallas discogram description. A new classification of CT/discography in low-back disorders. Spine 1987;12:287.
233. Modic MT, Masaryk TJ. Lumbar herniated disc disease and canal stenosis: Prospective evaluation by surface coil MR, CT, and myelography. AJR 1986;147:757.
234. Thornbury JR, Frybacks DG, Turski PA, et al. Disk-caused nerve compression in patients with acute low back pain: Diagnosis with MR, CT myelography, and plain CT. Radiology 1993;186:731.
235. Kieffer SA, Sherry RG, Wellenstein DE, et al. Bulging lumbar intervertebral disk: Myelographic differentiation from herniated disk with nerve root compression. AJR 1982;138:709.
236. Williams AL, Haughton VW, Meyer GA, et al. Computed tomographic appearance of the bulging annulus. Radiology 1982;142:403.
237. Kieffer SA, Sherry RG, Wellenstein DE, et al. Bulging lumbar intervertebral disk: Myelographic differentiation from herniated disk with nerve root compression. AJR 1982;138:709.
238. Williams JP, Joslym JN, Butler TW. Differentiation of herniated lumbar disc from bulging annulus fibrosis. Use of reformatted images. J Comput Assist Tomogr 1982;6:89.
239. Haughton VM, Syvertsen A, Williams AL. Soft-tissue anatomy within the spinal canal as seen on computed tomography. Radiology 1980;134:649.
240. Dillon WP, Kaseff LG, Knackstedt VE, et al. Computed tomography and differential diagnosis of the extruded lumbar disc. J Comput Assist Tomogr 1983;7:969.
241. Fries JW, Abodeely DA, Vijungco JG, et al. Computed tomography of herniated and extruded nucleus pulposus. J Comput Assist Tomogr 1982;6:874.

242. Abdullah AF, Ditto EW III, Byrd EB, et al. Extreme lateral lumbar disc herniation: Clinical syndrome and special problems of diagnosis. J Neurosurg 1974;41:229.

243. Osborn AG, Hood RS, Sherry RG, et al. CT/MR spectrum of far lateral and anterior lumbosacral disk herniations. AJNR 1988;9:775.

244. Jahnke RW. Low density in the posterior portion of the lumbar disk: A new CT finding in disk herniations. J Comput Assist Tomogr 1983;7:313.

245. Dorwart RH. Computed tomography of the lumbar spine: Techniques, normal anatomy, pitfalls, and clinical applications. Crit Rev Diagn Imaging 1984;22:1.

246. Chafetz N, Genant HK. Computed tomography of the lumbar spine. Orthop Clin North Am 1983;14:147.

247. Dorwart RH, DeGroot J, Sauerland EK, et al. Computed tomography of the lumbosacral spine: Normal anatomy, anatomic variants, and pathologic anatomy. Radiographics 1982;2:459.

248. Russell EJ, D'Angelo CM, Zimmerman RD, et al. Cervical disk herniation: CT demonstration after contrast enhancement. Radiology 1984;152:703.

249. Baleriaux D, Noterman J, Ticket L. Recognition of cervical soft disk herniation by contrast-enhanced CT. AJNR 1983;4:607.

250. Raininko R, Torma T. Contrast enhancement around a prolapsed disk. Neuroradiology 1982;24:49.

251. DeSantis M, Vici FF. Late contrast enhancement in the CT diagnosis of herniated lumbar disk. Neuroradiology 1984;26:303.

252. Flak B, Li DKB, Knickerbocker WJ. Case report 567. Skeletal Radiol 1989;18:481.

253. Norfray JF, Gado M, Becker RL, et al. Extruded nucleus pulposus causing osseous erosion of a lumbar vertebral body. A report of three cases. Spine 1988;13:941.

254. Jackson DE Jr, Atlas SW, Mani JR, et al. Intraspinal synovial cysts: MR imaging. Radiology 1989;170:527.

255. Cameron SE, Hanscom DA. Rapid development of a spinal synovial cyst. A case report. Spine 1992;17:1528.

256. Sampson MA, Warren SJ. Acute extradural compression due to an intraspinal synovial cyst: CT and myelogram appearances. Clin Radiol 1990;41:433.

257. Onofrio BM, Mih AD. Synovial cysts of the spine. Neurosurgery 1988;22:642.

258. Silbergleit R, Gebarski SS, Brunberg JA, et al. Lumbar synovial cysts: Correlation of myelographic, CT, MR, and pathologic findings. AJNR 1990;11:777.

259. Maupin WB, Naul LG, Kanter SL, et al. Synovial cyst presenting as a neural foraminal lesion: MR and CT appearance. AJR 1989;153:1231.

260. Reust P, Wendling D, Lagier R, et al. Degenerative spondylolisthesis, synovial cyst of the zygapophyseal joints, and sciatic syndrome: Report of two cases and review of the literature. Arthritis Rheum 1988;31:288.

261. Fardon DF, Simmons JD. Gas-filled synovial cyst. A case report. Spine 1989;14:127.

262. Marce S, Schaeverbeke T, Vital JM, et al. Facet joint synovial cyst causing sciatica and lamina erosion. Rev Rhum Engl Ed 1993;60:144.

263. Mariette X, Glon Y, Clerc D, et al. Medical treatment of synovial cysts of the zygapophyseal joints: Four cases with long-term followup. Arthritis Rheum 1989;32:660.

264. Yarde WL, Arnold PM, Kepes JJ, et al. Synovial cysts of the lumbar spine: Diagnosis, surgical management, and pathogenesis. Report of eight cases. Surg Neurol 1995;43:459.

265. Liu SS, Williams KD, Drayer BP, et al. Synovial cysts of the lumbosacral spine: Diagnosis by MR imaging. AJR 1990;154:163.

266. Chaing KS, Lee Y-Y, Mawad ME. MR of intraspinal synovial cyst: Rim enhancement with gadopentetate dimeglumine. AJR 1991;157:416.

267. Sullivan JD, Farfan HF, Kahn DS. Pathological changes with intervertebral joint rotational instability in the rabbit. Can J Surg 1971;14:71.

268. Lemaire JJ, Sautreaux JL, Chabannes J, et al. Lumbar canal stenosis. Retrospective study of 158 operated cases. Neurochirurgie 1995;41:89.

269. Hinck VC, Sachdev NS. Developmental stenosis of the cervical spinal canal. Brain 1966;89:27.

270. Wolf BS, Khilnani M, Malis L. The sagittal diameter of the bony cervical canal and its significance in cervical spondylosis. J Mt Sinai Hosp 1956;23:283.

271. Payne EE, Spillane JD. The cervical spine: An anatomico-pathological study of seventy specimens (using a special technique) with particular reference to the problem of cervical spondylosis. Brain 1957;80:571.

272. Murone I. The importance of the sagittal diameters of the cervical spinal canal in relation to spondylosis and myelopathy. J Bone Joint Surg 1974;56B:30.

273. Gupta SK, Roy RC, Srivastava A. Sagittal diameter of the cervical canal in normal Indian adults. Clin Radiol 1982;33:681.

274. Pavlov H, Torg JS, Robie B, et al. Cervical spine stenosis: Determination with vertebral body ratio method. Radiology 1987;164:771.

275. Eisenstein S. The morphometry and pathological anatomy of the lumbar spine in South African Negroes and Caucasoids with specific reference to spinal stenosis. J Bone Joint Surg 1977;59B:173.

276. Ullrich CG, Binet EF, Sanecki MG, et al. Quantitative assessment of the lumbar spinal canal by computed tomography. Radiology 1980;134:137.

277. Postacchini F, Pezzeri G, Montanaro A, et al. Computerized tomography in lumbar stenosis. A preliminary report. J Bone Joint Surg 1980;62B:78.

278. Carrera GF, Haughton VM, Syversen A, et al. Computed tomography of the lumbar facet joints. Radiology 1980;134:145.

279. Yousem DM, Atlas SW, Goldberg HI, et al. Degenerative narrowing of the cervical spine neural foramina: Evaluation with high-resolution 3DFT gradient-echo MR imaging. AJNR 1991;12:229.

280. Brown BM, Schwartz RH, Frank E, et al. Preoperative evaluation of cervical radiculopathy and myelopathy by surface-coil MR imaging. AJR 1988;151:1205.

281. Hedberg MC, Drayer BP, Flom RA, et al. Gradient echo (GRASS) MR imaging in cervical radiculopathy. AJR 1988;150:683.

282. Kent DL, Haynor DR, Larson EB, et al. Diagnosis of lumbar spinal stenosis in adults: A metaanalysis of the accuracy of CT, MR, and myelography. AJR 1992;158:1135.

283. Weisz GM, Lee P. Spinal canal stenosis. Concept of spinal reserve capacity: Radiologic measurement and clinical applications. Clin Orthop 1983;179:134.

284. Jinkins JR. Gd-DTPA enhanced MR of the lumbar spinal canal in patients with claudication. J Comput Assist Tomogr 1993;17:555.

285. Bolender N-F, Schonstrom NSR, Spengler DM, et al. Role of computed tomography and myelography in the diagnosis of central spinal stenosis. J Bone Joint Surg 1985;67A:240.

286. Eisenstein S. The trefoil configuration of the lumbar vertebral canal. A study of South African skeletal material. J Bone Joint Surg 1980;62B:73.

287. Mikhael MA, Ciric I, Tarkington JA, et al. Neuroradiological evaluation of lateral recess syndrome. Radiology 1981;140:97.

288. Lee CK, Rauschning W, Glenn W. Lateral lumbar spinal canal stenosis: Classification, pathologic anatomy, and surgical decompression. Spine 1988;13:313.

289. Mikhael MA, Ciric I, Tarkington JA, et al. Neuroradiological evaluation of lateral recess syndrome. Radiology 1981;140:97.

290. Kirkaldy-Willis WH, Wedge JH, Yong-Hing K, et al. Lumbar spinal nerve lateral entrapment. Clin Orthop 1982;169:171.

291. Osborne DR, Heinz ER, Bullard D, et al. Role of computed tomography in the radiological evaluation of painful radiculopathy after negative myelography. Foraminal neural entrapment. Neurosurgery 1984;14:147.

292. Risius B, Modic MT, Hardy RW Jr, et al. Sector computed tomographic spine scanning in the diagnosis of lumbar nerve root entrapment. Radiology 1982;143:109.

293. Vanderlinden RG. Subarticular entrapment of the dorsal root ganglion as a cause of sciatic pain. Spine 1984;9:19.

294. Lee SH, Coleman PE, Hahn FJ. Magnetic resonance imaging of degenerative disc disease of the spine. Radiol Clin North Am 1988;26:949.

295. Mehalic TF, Pezzuti RT, Applebaum BI. Magnetic resonance imaging and cervical spondylitic myelopathy. Neurosurg 1990;26:216.

296. Kent DL, Haynor DR, Larson EB, et al. Diagnosis of lumbar spinal stenosis in adults: A metaanalysis of the accuracy of CT, MR, and myelography. AJR 1992;158:1135.

297. Deyo RA. Rethinking strategies for acute low back pain. Emerg Med 1995;11:38.

298. Borenstein D. Epidemiology, etiology, diagnostic evaluation, and treatment of low back pain. Curr Opin Rheumatol 1995;7:141.

299. Kallen B. You want to talk back pain? Forbes 1986;138:132.
300. Deyo RA, Loeser JD, Stanley JB. Herniated lumbar intervertebral disk. Ann Intern Med 1990;112:598.
301. Pope MH, Hansson TH. Vibration of the spine and low back pain. Clin Orthop 1992;279:49.
302. Maigne JY, Rime B, Deligne B. Computed tomographic follow-up study of forty-eight cases of nonoperatively treated lumbar intervertebral disc herniation. Spine 1992;17:1071.
303. Teplick JG, Haskin ME. Spontaneous regression of herniated nucleus pulposus. AJR 1985;145:371.
304. Modic MT, Brandt-Zawadzki M, Masaryk TJ. Imaging of low back pain in the 1990s. Presented at the Radiological Society of North America, Chicago, IL, November 29, 1994.
305. Fromeyer JW. Back pain and sciatica. N Engl J Med 1988;318:291.
306. Modic MT, Ross JS. Magnetic resonance imaging in the evaluation of low back pain. Orthop Clin North Am 1991;22:283.
307. Seidenwurm D, Russell EJ, Hambly M. Diagnostic accuracy, patient outcome, and economic factors in lumbar radiculopathy. Radiology 1994;190:21.
308. Boden SD, Davis DO, Dina TS, et al. Abnormal magnetic resonance scans of the lumbar spine in asymptomatic subjects. J Bone Joint Surg 1990;72A:403.
309. Berthelot JM, Maugars Y, Delecrin J, et al. Magnetic resonance imaging for lumbar disk pathology. Incidence of false negatives. [Editorial] Presse Med 1995;24:1329.
310. Russell EJ. Computed tomography and myelography in the evaluation of cervical degenerative disease. Neuroimaging Clin N Am 1995;5:329.

38

Neoplasms of the Spine*

ROLAND R. LEE, M.D.
ELIAS MELHEM, M.D.

The classic review article written by Nittner,[1] published in the *Handbook of Clinical Neurology*, estimated 1 in 5 central nervous system tumors to be in the spine. Kurland's study[2] evaluating the incidence of central nervous system tumors in the resident population of Rochester, Minnesota, estimated the yearly incidence of primary spinal tumors to be 2.5 per 100,000 people. Primarily because of the revolutionary improvement in spinal imaging afforded by magnetic resonance imaging (MRI), the diagnosis of these tumors is now much easier than when these classic articles were written in 1976 and 1958, respectively.

MRI is the best single modality for imaging spinal tumors. Its unsurpassed soft tissue differentiation (including the ability to differentiate between cerebrospinal fluid [CSF] and neural tissue without the use of intrathecal contrast material), absence of beam-hardening artifact from bone, and ability to directly image in multiple planes make it clearly superior to computed tomography (CT), myelography, plain film radiography, and ultrasonography in evaluating epidural and intradural disease. However, for characterizing bone disease and primary bone tumors, plain radiographs and CT are still essential.

TECHNIQUE

One screening MRI technique used for the evaluation of spinal tumors is sagittal TR 500 to 600, TE 11; this is followed by fast spin echo (FSE) sagittal TR 3000 to 4000, TE 102 to obtain a quick "myelogram" in about 4 minutes, with a better signal-to-noise ratio and resolution than obtainable with conventional spin-echo images.[3-6] Axial images are obtained through regions of interest only, *not* through the entire spine. The slice thickness should preferably be 3 mm on the sagittal images and 4 mm axially, with a 1-mm gap, in order to minimize partial-volume errors.

Phased-array coils, if available, are extremely valuable in obtaining a better signal-to-noise ratio and obviating the need to move the coil or patient when covering a large portion of the spine (as in screening for epidural cord compression).

Gadolinium enhancement (in sagittal and axial planes) is essential for evaluating intradural tumors.[7] Generally, intradural extramedullary tumors enhance significantly; enhancement of intramedullary tumors is more variable. However, in imaging vertebral metastases, gadolinium enhancement is actually detrimental, since T1-dark marrow metastases enhance and become isointense to normal marrow. This shortcoming can be circumvented with fat saturation, which allows visualization of enhancing metastases by suppressing the adjacent bright marrow fat.[8]

Inversion-recovery (and fat-saturated FSE inversion-recovery) sequences also demonstrate vertebral marrow metastases by nulling the bright normal marrow fat.[9, 10]

Coronal slices may be useful, as for example, in imaging cervicothoracic neurofibromas or in directly imaging the lumbosacral plexus.

Gradient-recalled echo images are generally not useful in the imaging of spinal tumors. The differentiation between CSF and soft tissue or tumor is often worse than on true T2- or FSE T2-weighted images. The main utility of gradient-recalled echo images would be to detect small amounts of hemosiderin or calcium, which would be missed on FSE images and may be missed on spin-echo T2-weighted images.

Good MRI technique is particularly important in imaging vertebral marrow metastases, which are the most common malignant tumors involving the spine encountered in everyday practice. The typical scenario facing the radiologist is a patient with known primary cancer presenting with severe back pain and acute arm or leg weakness: "Rule out cord compression!" Often the site of spinal disease cannot be accurately localized clinically. Hence, it is important to quickly and efficiently screen the entire spine in these patients. It is impractical and unnecessary to obtain sagittal and axial T1- and T2-weighted images, and sagittal and axial postgadolinium images, through all levels of the spine in these patients, who often suffer excruciating pain and who are unable to lie motionless for even moderate lengths of time. Instead, the screening examination should first consist of a *single* T1-weighted sagittal sequence using a large field of view (48 to 50 cm) with a large matrix (512 ×

---

*Portions of this chapter were previously published in Lee RR (ed). Spine: State of the Art Reviews, Vol. 9, Spinal Imaging, pp. 261–286. Philadelphia, Hanley & Belfus, 1995.

512 or 512 × 384), which covers essentially the entire spine in a single acquisition of about 6 minutes or less. An FSE sagittal T2-weighted screening sequence can give a myelogram-effect scan in another few minutes, pointing out regions of CSF effacement by tumor. Then, 4-mm axial images (either T1- or FSE T2-weighted) may be obtained *only* through the levels of cord compression, to better delineate the degree of compression. Gadolinium is generally not needed to diagnose and evaluate cord compression from bony vertebral metastases. Thus, a complete MRI examination can be obtained in about 20 minutes, which can be tolerated by almost all patients.

Good analgesia (e.g., morphine) is important to ensure patient comfort, while preventing image degradation by involuntary patient motion owing to pain. Anxiolytics such as diazepam (Valium) or midazolam are not as effective, since these patients move in the scanner more from pain than from claustrophobia or anxiety.

If available, phased-array coils give a superb signal-to-noise ratio and enable complete spinal coverage without moving the patient or the coil. However, lacking a phased-array coil, one should use the body coil to screen the entire spine using the single large–field-of-view T1-weighted sagittal sequence. The use of the conventional "license plate" surface coil to separately screen the cervical spine, the thoracic spine, and the lumbar spine—using both T1- and T2-weighted sequences in the axial and sagittal planes, followed by postgadolinium sagittal and axial images of the cervical, thoracic, and lumbar regions—takes hours and results in extreme patient discomfort and a completely nondiagnostic motion-degraded study.

TUMOR CATEGORIZATION

Spinal tumors are generally classified according to anatomic location as extradural; intradural, extramedullary; and intramedullary.

EXTRADURAL SPINAL TUMORS

Extradural spinal tumors account for approximately 30% of all spinal neoplasms. They have been classically categorized into primary spinal tumors, the vast majority of which arise from the bony component, and secondary extradural spinal tumors, which involve the osseous or epidural compartments via the hematogenous route or direct extension. Spinal tumors may be asymptomatic (e.g., hemangioma); however, the majority present with localized pain and tenderness corresponding to the site of the lesion. Signs and symptoms of myelopathy and radiculopathy occasionally may be present in cases of cord and nerve root compression by the spinal mass.

Both CT and MRI play an important role in the evaluation of extradural spinal tumors. MRI helps to identify subtle bone marrow and epidural involvement as well as to separate the extraosseous soft tissue component of the neoplasm from the normal paraspinal structures. Also, MRI (especially T2-weighted images) is invaluable in detecting secondary signal abnormalities in the cord resulting from the spinal tumor. On the other hand, CT

aids in the definition of the tumor's transition zone and the integrity of cortical bone, in the characterization of the tumor matrix (calcified or ossified), and in the identification of reactive sclerosis surrounding the osseous spinal tumor.

Finally, bone scintigraphy (^{99m}Tc–methylene diphosphonate [MDP]) is an important component of the imaging armamentarium for osseous spinal tumors. It is routinely used in screening for spinal metastases and is occasionally used for intraoperative separation of an avid osseous nidus from surrounding reactive changes (e.g., osteoid osteoma).

This section focuses on common extradural spinal tumors with emphasis on imaging characteristics. Pertinent demographic and histologic data are reviewed.

Primary Osseous Spinal Tumors

Benign

Hemangioma

Vertebral hemangiomas are the most common neoplasms affecting the spinal column. These benign vascular tumors have been detected in 11% of spines at autopsy.[11] Multiple lesions occur in 25% to 30% of cases and have a predilection for the thoracic spine (60%), followed by the lumbar spine (29%).[12] They are rarely symptomatic and are usually discovered incidentally. The symptomatic lesions tend to occur in the thoracic spine, predominantly between T3 and T9.[13] These present with localized pain and tenderness and rarely signs of radiculopathy and myelopathy secondary to bony expansion, epidural extension, pathologic fractures, or epidural hematoma. They are slightly more common in females and have been reported to grow and become symptomatic during pregnancy.[14] The vast majority of hemangiomas are confined to the vertebral body; however, they may extend into the posterior elements, paraspinal, and epidural spaces (Fig. 38–1).

Pathologically, hemangiomas are composed of endothelium-lined capillary and cavernous sinuses interspersed among bony trabeculae and adipose tissue, causing destruction of some trabeculae with compensatory thickening of the remaining vertical trabeculae.[12]

On plain films, hemangiomas give the appearance of thick parallel vertical densities in the vertebra simulating a jail-bar or a corduroy pattern (Fig. 38–2) corresponding to the thickened trabeculae.[15] Compression fractures through the involved vertebrae are rare. On CT, the remaining thickened trabeculae surrounded by low-attenuation fat give a typical spotted appearance (Fig. 38–3). MRI is very sensitive in the detection of vertebral hemangiomas and in the definition of their extent, especially into the epidural space. On T1- and T2-weighted images, the intraosseous component typically demonstrates high signal intensity, corresponding to the fatty and vascular components, interrupted by vertical bars of low signal intensity of bony trabeculae (Fig. 38–3).[11] The intraosseous lesions may occasionally be hypointense on T1-weighted images because of paucity of the fatty stroma. The signal intensity of the extraosseous component of the tumor usually approximates that of the cord on T1-

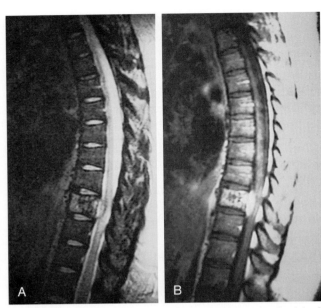

FIGURE 38–1 Hemangioma of a lower thoracic vertebral body with an extraosseous component extending into the epidural space, causing cord compression. The intraosseous component demonstrates mottled high signal intensity on the sagittal T2-weighted magnetic resonance imaging (MRI) study (*A*) and marked heterogeneous enhancement on the sagittal postgadolinium T1-weighted MRI study (*B*).

weighted images and demonstrates high signal on T2-weighted images (see Fig. 38–1).

Hemangiomas enhance vividly with gadolinium (see Fig. 38–1). On T2-weighted FSE images, both fat islands and small intravertebral hemangiomas may demonstrate high signal intensity, which may cause difficulties in differentiating between the two lesions.

Osteochondroma

Osteochondromas occur in bones that develop through endochondral ossification; they result in a bonelike outgrowth capped by cartilage, and their cortex and medullary cavity are continuous with those of the native bone.[16] Despite the high prevalence of these tumors, only 3% of solitary and 7% of multiple osteochondromas (multiple hereditary exostosis) occur in the spine. They arise exclusively from the posterior elements with a predilection for the spinous process.[17] Most osteochondromas are detected within the second decade of life, and there is a male predilection (approximately 2 to 1).[16] Spinal osteochondromas present with localized pain and tenderness and an associated overlying soft tissue mass. Rarely, signs of compressive radiculopathy and myelopathy can occur, especially as a result of growth spurts during the teenage years. Malignant degeneration occurs in 1% of solitary osteochondromas and in up to 25% of patients with multiple hereditary exostosis.

Pathologically, osteochondromas are composed of cancellous bone surrounded by cortical bone, both continuous with the bone of origin. A thin hyaline cartilage cap covers the tumor.

Plain films and CT often reveal a pedunculated or

sessile projection of bone arising from the posterior elements of a vertebra (Fig. 38–4). The cartilaginous cap may contain calcific foci. On MRI, these tumors have a heterogeneous appearance (Fig. 38–4).[17] The bone marrow within the cancellous bone has high signal intensity on T1-weighted images, and the cartilaginous cap demonstrates increased signal intensity on T2-weighted images. The ossified and calcified portions of the lesion have low signal intensity on all conventional pulse sequences.

The exact site of attachment, as well as spinal and neural foraminal extension of these lesions, is better delineated by CT and MRI compared with conventional plain films. Also, MRI and CT can be helpful in defining the thickness of the cartilaginous cap, a possible predictor of the malignant potential of these tumors.

Giant Cell Tumor (Osteoclastoma)

Giant cell tumors are the second most common benign bone tumors affecting the spinal column.[18] Only 3% to 7% of giant cell tumors occur in the spine, predominantly in the sacrum.[19] They present between the ages of 20 and 40 years and are rarely encountered before the closure of the epiphyseal plate. There is no sex predilection.[19]

Pathologically, these tumors are characterized by nonspecific multinucleated giant cells scattered in a background of mononuclear, round or spindle-shaped, fibroblast-like cells. The degree of anaplastic changes in mononuclear fibroblast-like cells determines the biologic behavior of these lesions.[20] Malignant transformation occurs in approximately 10% of cases.

On plain film radiographs and CT, giant cell tumors

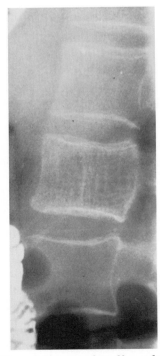

FIGURE 38–2 Hemangioma. A plain film radiograph of a lumbar vertebral body demonstrates thick parallel vertical densities corresponding to the thickened trabeculae, simulating a jail-bar or corduroy pattern.

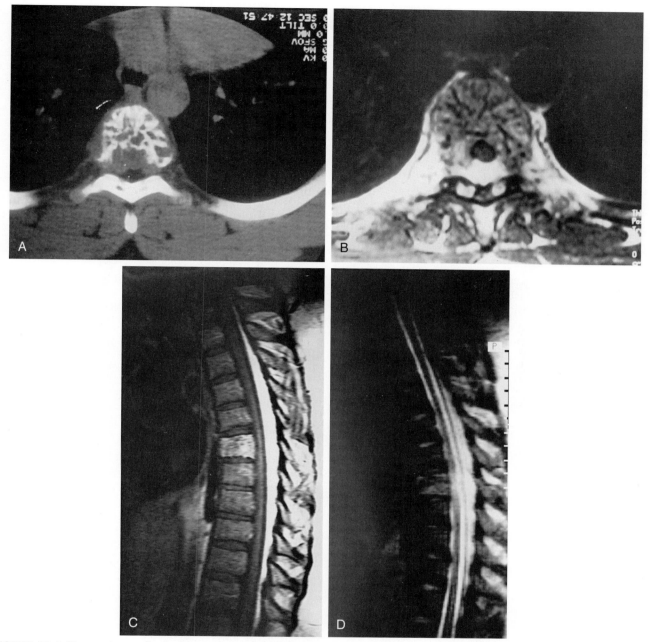

FIGURE 38–3 Hemangioma of a midthoracic vertebral body, demonstrating thickened trabeculae interspersed by low-attenuation fat, giving the typical spotted appearance on the axial computed tomography (CT) image (*A*). On MRI, the thickened trabeculae have a linear and spotted pattern of very low signal intensity, whereas the interspersed adipose tissue exhibits high signal intensity on axial and sagittal T1-weighted images (*B* and *C*). On the sagittal T2-weighted MRI study, the hemangioma exhibits high signal intensity (*D*). Note the extensive epidural lipomatosis dorsal to the cord.

typically present as well-defined lytic, expansile lesions with characteristic lack of sclerotic margins.[21] On MRI, the signal characteristics are nonspecific and heterogeneous on T1- and T2-weighted sequences, with the occasional presence of a blood-fluid level.[22] These tumors are commonly hypervascular and demonstrate heterogeneous enhancement with gadolinium (Fig. 38–5). Other sacral lesions that can mimic giant cell tumors include metastatic disease, plasmacytoma, chordoma, "brown tumor" in hyperparathyroidism, and malignant nerve sheath tumors (Fig. 38–6).

Aneurysmal Bone Cyst

Aneurysmal bone cysts are benign lesions of bone of uncertain cause and are not usually considered true neoplasms.[23] Twenty percent of all aneurysmal bone cysts occur in the spine, particularly the posterior elements (60%); approximately 40% arise from the vertebral body.[24] Involvement of contiguous vertebrae may occur. The thoracic and cervical regions are the most common locations. Eighty percent occur within the first 2 decades of life, with a mild female predominance.[25] From 30% to 50% are associated with other osseous lesions such as giant cell

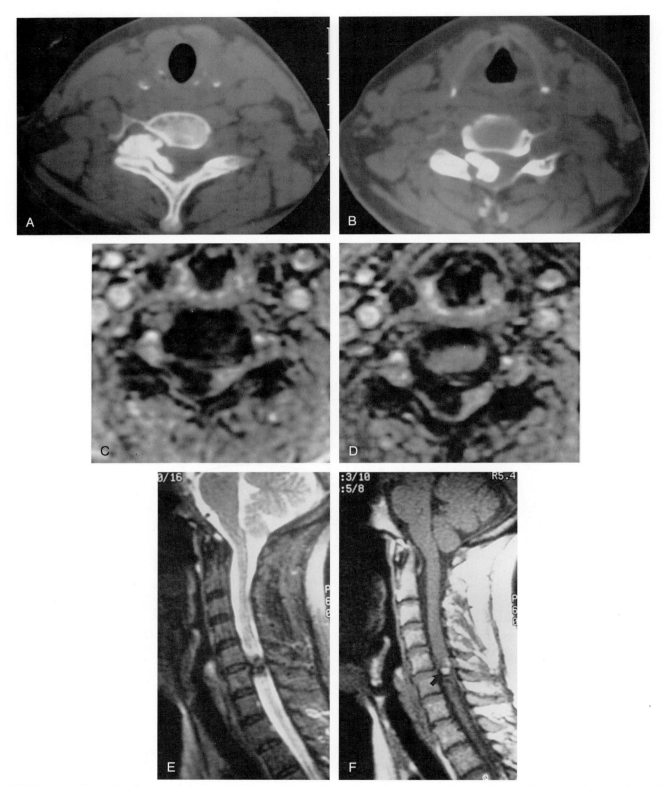

FIGURE 38–4 Osteochondroma of the cervical spine arising from the right superior facet and extending into the spinal canal, causing cord compression. A pedunculated projection of bone is noted on the axial CT images *(A and B)*, resulting in a very low signal mass on the axial T2°-weighted gradient-recalled echo MRI studies *(C and D)* and the sagittal T2-weighted MRI study *(E)*. The osteochondroma demonstrates heterogeneous signal intensities on the sagittal T1-weighted MRI study with central high signal *(arrow)* corresponding to bone marrow within the cancellous bone *(F)*.

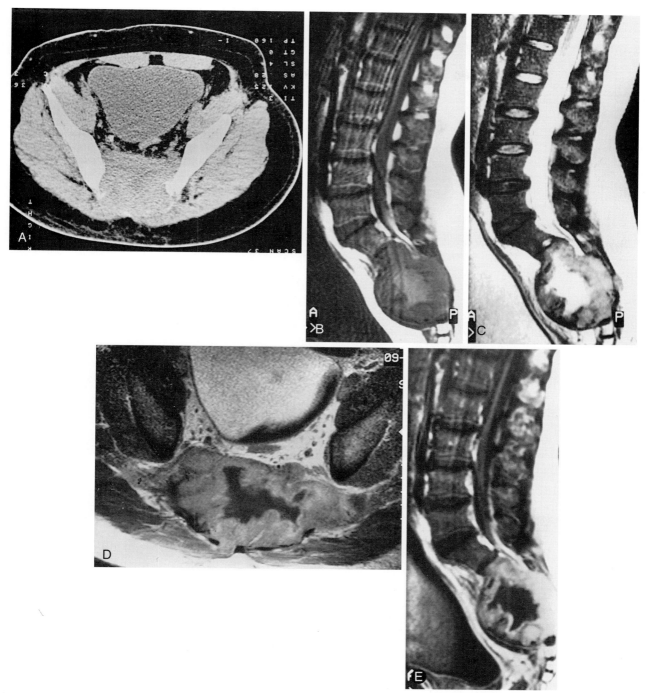

FIGURE 38–5 Giant cell tumor affecting the sacrum. An axial CT image demonstrates a large destructive soft tissue–density mass extending into the presacral space (*A*). The mass exhibits heterogeneous signal intensities on the sagittal T1- and T2-weighted images (*B* and *C*) and heterogeneous thick peripheral enhancement on the axial and sagittal postgadolinium T1-weighted images (*D* and *E*), suggesting central necrosis.

tumor, osteoblastoma, chondroblastoma, fibrous dysplasia, and nonossifying fibroma.[26] The remainder arise de novo in unaffected bone.

Pathologically, aneurysmal bone cysts are multiloculated, anastomosing, thin-walled, blood-filled pseudocysts. These blood-filled cavernous spaces are interspersed with a highly vascular solid component composed of a collage-

nous matrix containing benign spindle cells and multinucleated giant cells.[24]

On plain film radiographs and CT, aneurysmal bone cysts demonstrate a well-defined expansile lytic lesion (Fig. 38–7) with an occasional soft tissue component. On MRI, they exhibit a lobulated multiseptated lesion with occasional blood-fluid levels (Fig. 38–7). The signal inten-

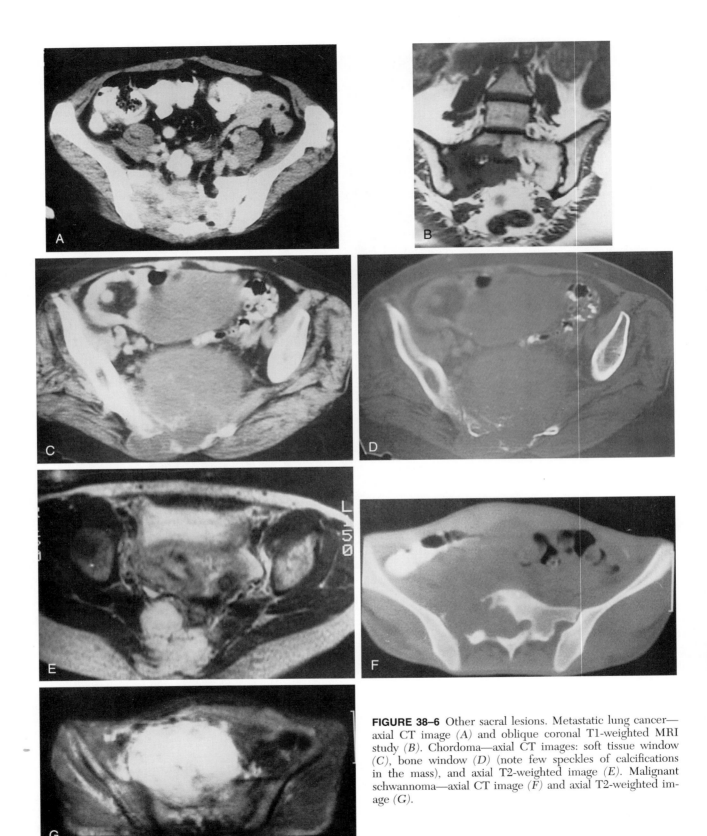

FIGURE 38–6 Other sacral lesions. Metastatic lung cancer—axial CT image (*A*) and oblique coronal T1-weighted MRI study (*B*). Chordoma—axial CT images: soft tissue window (*C*), bone window (*D*) (note few speckles of calcifications in the mass), and axial T2-weighted image (*E*). Malignant schwannoma—axial CT image (*F*) and axial T2-weighted image (*G*).

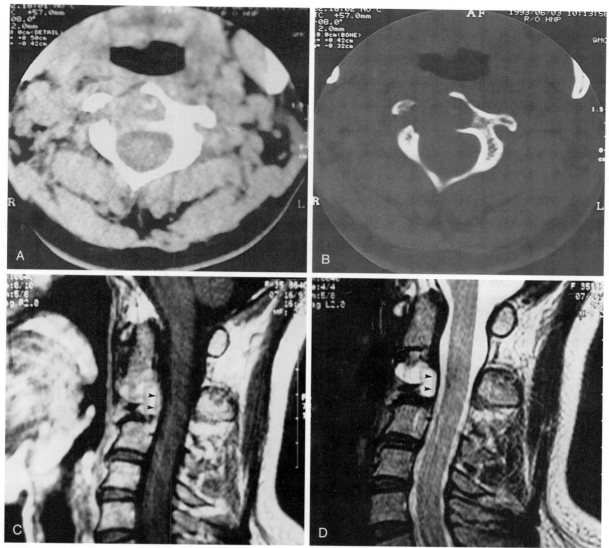

FIGURE 38–7 Aneurysmal bone cyst of the C2 vertebral body, demonstrating a well-defined expansile lytic lesion on axial CT images: soft tissue window (A) and bone window (B). The MRI T1-weighted (C) and T2-weighted (D) studies exhibit a lobulated multiseptated lesion with blood-fluid levels (arrowheads).

sity is variable on T1- and T2-weighted images depending on the state of the blood content.[27, 28] Blood-fluid levels, once thought to be specific for aneurysmal bone cysts, have been reported in other spinal tumors including telangiectatic osteosarcoma and giant cell tumors.[29]

Osteoid Osteoma and Osteoblastoma

Osteoid osteoma and osteoblastoma are histologically similar benign neoplasms of bone with the distinction made on the basis of the greatest diameter of the nidus: if it is less than 1.5 cm, the lesion is classified as an osteoid osteoma.[30] Ten percent of osteoid osteomas and 40% of osteoblastomas occur in the spine, with a predilection for the posterior elements.[31, 32] Extension into the vertebral body and the epidural and paraspinal spaces is more common with osteoblastomas. Most cases of osteoid osteomas present between the ages of 5 and 25 years with a typical complaint of intermittent pain that worsens at

night and is characteristically relieved by aspirin.[33] In contrast, osteoblastomas occasionally present beyond the third decade and the associated pain does not respond dramatically to aspirin therapy. There is a definite male predilection with both lesions.[33]

Pathologically, the nidus is composed of a tangled array of branching and anastomosing partially mineralized osteoid trabeculae separated by richly vascularized connective tissue stroma. Osteoblasts are often seen at the margins of the osteoid trabeculae. Surrounding the nidus is a dense sclerotic reaction that is more prominent with osteoid osteomas and occasionally may be absent with osteoblastomas.[34, 35]

On plain film radiographs and CT, osteoid osteomas demonstrate a lucent nidus occasionally containing punctate calcifications surrounded by dense bony sclerosis.[36] An associated scoliotic curve is commonly present. Often the nidus is better visualized with CT. ^{99m}Tc-MDP nuclear scans may play an important role in the intraoperative localization of the nidus.[37] On MRI, osteoid osteomas are heterogeneous with low signal intensity on T1- and T2-weighted images corresponding to the calcifications within the nidus and surrounding sclerosis. The noncalcified portion of the nidus demonstrates hyperintensity on T2-weighted images and enhancement with gadolinium.[38] Occasionally, hyperintensity on T2-weighted images is noted within adjacent cancellous bone and soft tissue beyond the sclerotic reaction, thought to be secondary to an inflammatory response.[39]

Osteoblastomas present with an expansile lytic lesion

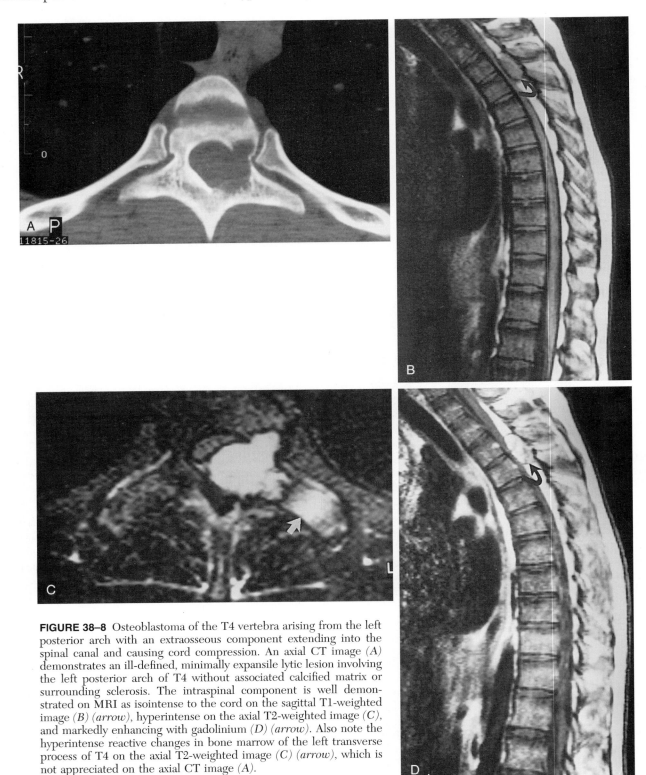

FIGURE 38–8 Osteoblastoma of the T4 vertebra arising from the left posterior arch with an extraosseous component extending into the spinal canal and causing cord compression. An axial CT image (A) demonstrates an ill-defined, minimally expansile lytic lesion involving the left posterior arch of T4 without associated calcified matrix or surrounding sclerosis. The intraspinal component is well demonstrated on MRI as isointense to the cord on the sagittal T1-weighted image (B) (arrow), hyperintense on the axial T2-weighted image (C), and markedly enhancing with gadolinium (D) (arrow). Also note the hyperintense reactive changes in bone marrow of the left transverse process of T4 on the axial T2-weighted image (C) (arrow), which is not appreciated on the axial CT image (A).

with associated soft tissue mass best defined on CT and MRI (Figs. 38–8 and 38–9). Their signal intensities may be quite heterogeneous on T1- and T2-weighted images, depending on the amount and distribution of calcifications and blood products within these lesions.[40] There is marked enhancement with gadolinium.

Eosinophilic Granuloma

Eosinophilic granulomas are benign conditions of uncertain cause.[41] They often present during the first 2 decades of life as solitary or multiple lesions of bone affecting the skull and ribs most commonly, followed by pelvis, spine, and proximal long bones.[42] These lesions rarely affect bones distal to the elbow and knee joints. In the spine, they most often involve the vertebral body, causing collapse (vertebra plana). There is a male predilection.[43] In addition to focal pain and tenderness corresponding to the osseous lesions, patients with eosinophilic granuloma may present with nonspecific systemic complaints (fever and weight loss), shortness of breath due to diffuse interstitial lung infiltrates, and deformities in the alignment of the spine.[41]

Pathologically, these lesions consist of foamy and vacuolated histiocytes usually within the medullary cavity of bone, variably admixed with eosinophils, lymphocytes, plasma cells, and neutrophils.[44] Rod-shaped HX bodies are occasionally seen within the histiocytes. In some cases, spontaneous healing of these lesions occurs, usually over the span of 2 years. During the recovery process, the inflammatory cells are replaced by connective tissue and bone.[45]

On plain film radiographs and CT, eosinophilic granulomas are seen as well-defined lytic lesions without surrounding sclerosis.[45] In the spine, they classically cause severe vertebral collapse (Fig. 38–10). On MRI, the signal characteristics are nonspecific with low signal on T1-weighted images compared with normal fatty marrow, and high signal on T2-weighted sequences.[46]

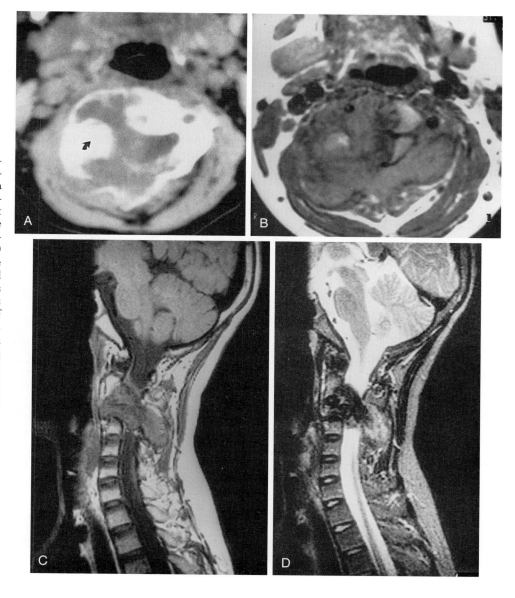

FIGURE 38–9 Large osteoblastoma arising from the right posterior arch of the C2 vertebra with an extraosseous component extending into the right paraspinal region and into the spinal canal, causing cord compression. An axial CT image *(A)* demonstrates a large expansile lytic mass with epidural and paraspinal extension, as well as associated marked sclerosis *(arrow)* in the lateral mass of C2, which is characteristic of osteoblastomas. MRI exhibits a large heterogeneous mass that is mildly hypointense compared with the cord on the axial *(B)* and sagittal *(C)* T1-weighted images and markedly hypointense on the sagittal T2-weighted image *(D)*.

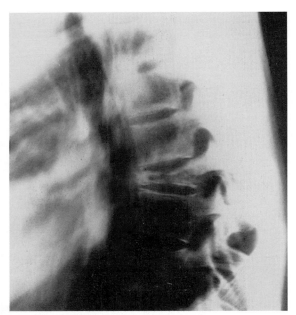

FIGURE 38–10 Eosinophilic granuloma. A lateral plain film radiograph of the thoracic spine demonstrates severe collapse of a vertebral body (vertebra plana).

Intermediate

Chordoma

Chordomas originate from notochordal remnants and therefore can involve any segment of the craniospinal axis extending from the sphenoid bone to the coccyx, favoring the two ends of the axis.[47] Chordomas arise predominantly in the sacrococcygeal area (50%), followed by the clivus (30% to 40%). Only 15% involve the rest of the spine, with the cervical region the most common.[48] They typically present in middle-aged adults, with a 2 to 1 male preponderance.[49] In the spine, this tumor exclusively af-

fects the vertebral body with common extension through the disk to involve the adjacent vertebra.[49] Metastases to lymph nodes, liver, and lungs have been reported in less than 10% of cases.[50]

Pathologically, there are two subtypes: typical chordomas consist of vacuolated physaliphorous cells embedded in a mucinous matrix; in chondroid chordoma, the matrix contains cartilaginous foci.[51] The physaliphorous cells are usually arranged in cords within the matrix, and their cytoplasm contains abundant glycogen.

On plain film radiographs and CT, chordomas typically appear as poorly marginated destructive lesions containing amorphous calcifications in 50% to 70% of cases (Fig. 38–11).[49] An extraosseous soft tissue component is often present in the paraspinal and epidural spaces. On MRI, these lesions are often heterogeneous, hypo- to isointense on T1-weighted images, and hyperintense on T2-weighted images (Fig. 38–12; see also Fig. 38–11).[52, 53] Enhancement with gadolinium is variable.

Malignant

Osteosarcoma

Osteosarcomas are the second most common primary malignancy of bone, predominantly occurring between the ages of 10 and 25 years.[54] A second smaller peak incidence during the fifth and sixth decades of life has been reported, often arising in pagetoid bone, postirradiated bone, and osteochondromas.[55] The ratio of involvement of males to females is 2 to 1. Primary involvement of the spine is rare, accounting for approximately 1% to 2% of all osteosarcomas[55]; metastatic osteosarcoma to the spine is relatively common, however.

Pathologically, osteosarcomas are subdivided into osteoblastic, chondroblastic, fibroblastic, and telangiectatic, depending on their dominant histomorphologic characteristics. Common to all subtypes are anaplastic mesenchymal tumor cells trapped in osteoid matrix.[56]

On plain film radiographs and CT, osteosarcomas pre-

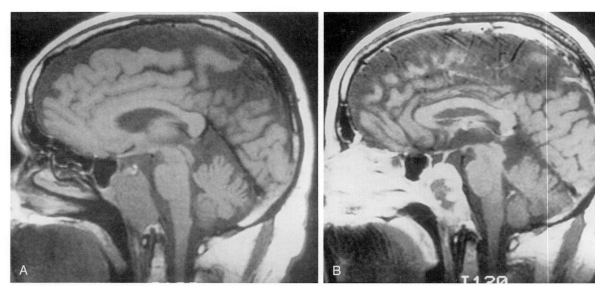

FIGURE 38–11 Clival chordoma that is minimally hypointense compared with the cord is seen on the sagittal T1-weighted image (*A*), with marked heterogeneous enhancement after administration of gadolinium, suggesting central necrosis (*B*).

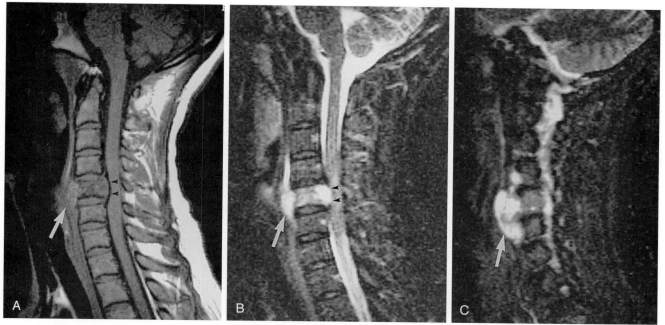

FIGURE 38–12 Chordoma involving the C5 vertebral body with prevertebral *(arrow)* and intraspinal *(arrowheads)* extension, causing cord compression. The osseous and extraosseous components of the mass demonstrate low signal intensity on the sagittal T1-weighted image *(A)* and high signal intensity on the sagittal T2-weighted images *(B and C)* compared with that of the cord.

sent as ill-defined destructive lesions that may be purely lytic, purely blastic, or mixed, depending on the distribution and amount of ossified matrix within the tumors.[57, 58] An associated soft tissue mass is often present. On MRI, these neoplasms are heterogeneous in signal intensity, again depending on the presence or absence of ossification, hemorrhage, or necrosis. The nonossified component of these tumors typically demonstrates low signal on T1-weighted images and high signal on T2-weighted images compared with bone marrow and paraspinal tissue (Fig. 38–13).[59]

Chondrosarcoma

Chondrosarcomas are cartilaginous tumors that account for approximately 20% of all primary malignant bone tumors.[60] Spinal involvement is rare, with a predilection for the vertebral body. They typically present in patients between 30 and 60 years of age, with a 2 to 1 male predominance.[61] These tumors may arise de novo or as secondary tumors from preexisting bone lesion such as enchondroma, osteochondroma, Paget's disease, irradiated bone, or unicameral bone cyst.[62, 63]

Pathologically, chondrosarcomas demonstrate anaplastic mesenchymal tumor cells trapped within cartilaginous lacunae. The degree of anaplasia correlates remarkably well with tumor behavior.[64] The majority of these tumors are slow-growing, nonaggressive lesions with good prognoses if treated adequately. Histologic variants include clear cell, mesenchymal, and dedifferentiated.[65–67]

On plain film radiographs and CT, chondrosarcomas present as ill-defined destructive lesions, often with a calcified matrix and an extraosseous soft tissue component.[68] The shape and distribution of the calcifications within the matrix may be a clue to the cartilaginous

origin of these tumors. On MRI, these tumors exhibit heterogeneous signal intensity on T1- and T2-weighted images because of a mixture of soft tissue, calcium, cartilage, and occasional hemorrhage.[69]

Ewing's Sarcoma

Ewing's sarcomas are highly malignant primary bone tumors of uncertain origin, possibly derived from primitive mesenchymal cells.[70] Most patients present between the ages of 5 and 30 years, with a slight male predominance; African Americans are rarely affected.[71] Ewing's sarcomas account for 7% to 15% of primary osseous malignancies.[72] Ewing's sarcomas frequently metastasize to the spine, but the spine is only uncommonly the site of origin of these tumors.[73] In addition to having focal pain and tenderness corresponding to the osseous lesions, patients with Ewing's sarcoma may present with nonspecific systemic complaints (fever, malaise, and weight loss), anemia, and an elevated erythrocyte sedimentation rate.

Pathologically, Ewing's sarcomas are composed of sheets of extremely undifferentiated, small round or oval cells having prominent nuclei and scant cytoplasm. The presence of periodic acid–Schiff–positive cytoplasmic granules in the tumor cells helps distinguish Ewing's sarcomas from other small round cell malignancies.[74]

On plain film radiographs and CT, Ewing's sarcomas present as ill-defined destructive bony lesions with extraosseous soft tissue components (Fig. 38–14).[75] The characteristic periosteal reaction seen in long bones affected by this tumor is often absent in the spine. On MRI, these tumors are hypointense on T1-weighted images and hyperintense on T2-weighted images compared with bone marrow and paraspinal soft tissue signal (Fig. 38–15).[76]

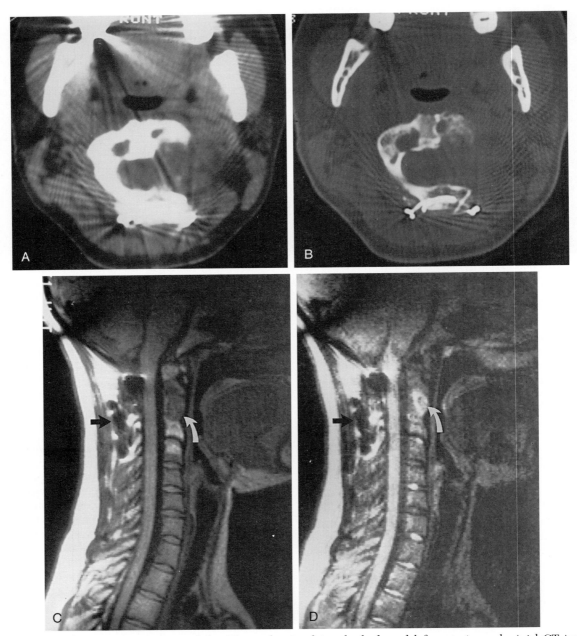

FIGURE 38–13 Telangiectatic osteosarcoma of the C2 vertebra involving the body and left posterior arch. Axial CT images (soft tissue window *[A]* and bone window *[B]*) demonstrate an ill-defined, purely lytic, destructive lesion with an associated extraosseous soft tissue mass. In the posterior elements, note the metal hardware used for posterior fusion. The osseous component of the mass demonstrates low signal intensity on the sagittal T1-weighted image *(C) (curved arrow)* and high signal intensity on the sagittal T2-weighted image *(D) (curved arrow)* compared with that of the cord. Note the signal void in *C* and *D* corresponding to the location of the metal hardware *(straight arrows).*

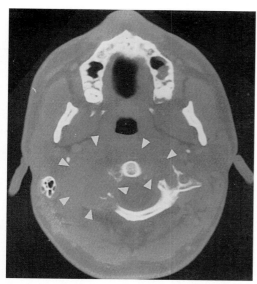

FIGURE 38–14 Primary Ewing's sarcoma of the C1 vertebra. An axial CT image demonstrates an ill-defined destructive lesion with a large extraosseous soft tissue component (*arrowheads*).

Lymphoma

Primary non-Hodgkin's lymphoma of bone is rare, and most often the skeleton is involved secondarily as part of a systemic disease.[77] The vast majority of patients present between the ages of 20 and 40 years, with a 2 to 1 male predominance.[78] Primary spinal involvement is uncommon, whereas metastases to the bony and epidural compartments of the spine are relatively common, especially in immunocompromised (human immunodeficiency vi-

rus–positive) individuals. Hodgkin's disease likewise only rarely originates in bone.

Pathologically, primary non-Hodgkin's lymphoma of bone demonstrates sheets of undifferentiated, small round or oval cells. This lesion tends to be highly vascular. For Hodgkin's disease, the presence of the Reed-Sternberg cells (neoplastic giant cells) admixed with other nonneoplastic inflammatory cells is characteristic.[79]

On plain film radiographs and CT, primary non-Hodgkin's lymphoma demonstrates an ill-defined destructive bone lesion, often with an extraosseous soft tissue component. Hodgkin's disease, on the other hand, can induce a lytic or sclerotic process in bone, hence the "ivory vertebra" (Fig. 38–16).[80] On MRI, the involved vertebra demonstrates low signal on T1-weighted and high signal on T2-weighted images.[81] In the case of an ivory vertebra, the sclerosis leads to loss of signal on T2-weighted images.

Secondary Extradural Tumors

Metastatic Disease to the Osseous Spine and Extradural Space

Metastatic disease is quite common in the spine, causing neurologic deficit in approximately 5% to 10% of cancer patients.[82] Hematogenous spread of tumor cell emboli, whether arterial or venous (Batson's plexus), is the usual route for spinal metastasis. In adults, 75% of spinal metastases are from carcinoma of the breast, lung, prostate, kidney, and thyroid and from myeloma, lymphoma, and leukemia (Figs. 38–17 through 38–21).[83] Metastatic osseous lesions from thyroid and renal carcinomas tend to be expansile and hypervascular (Fig. 38–19). The vertebral body is typically involved first, with the neural arch involved only one-seventh as often.

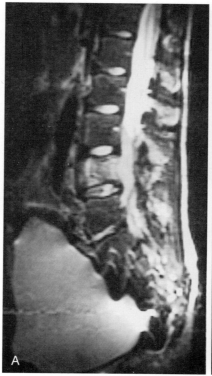
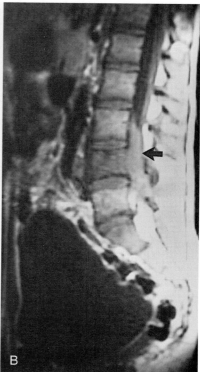

FIGURE 38–15 Metastatic Ewing's sarcoma to the L4 vertebral body with extensive epidural involvement, causing marked spinal stenosis. The affected vertebra demonstrates high signal intensity on the sagittal T2-weighted image (*A*) and low signal intensity on the gadolinium-enhanced sagittal T1-weighted image (*B*) compared with that of bone marrow. The epidural component exhibits modest enhancement (*arrow*). Note the marked distention of the urinary bladder.

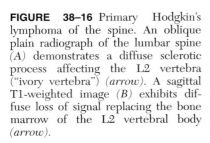

FIGURE 38–16 Primary Hodgkin's lymphoma of the spine. An oblique plain radiograph of the lumbar spine *(A)* demonstrates a diffuse sclerotic process affecting the L2 vertebra ("ivory vertebra") *(arrow)*. A sagittal T1-weighted image *(B)* exhibits diffuse loss of signal replacing the bone marrow of the L2 vertebral body *(arrow)*.

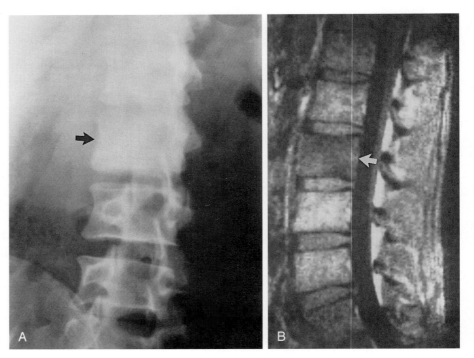

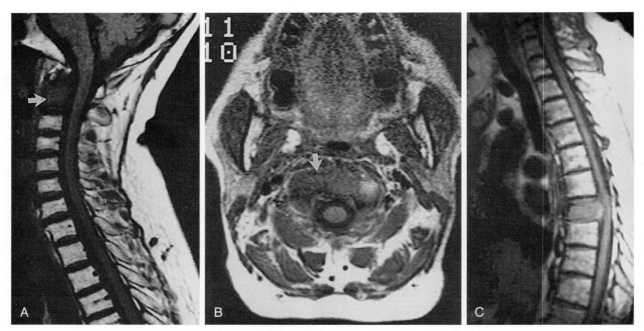

FIGURE 38–17 Metastatic breast cancer to the C2 vertebral body *(arrow)*, demonstrating low signal intensity on sagittal and axial T1-weighted images *(A and B)* compared with that of normal bone marrow. Another patient with metastatic breast cancer to a midthoracic vertebral body demonstrates epidural extension and cord compression on the sagittal T1-weighted image *(C)*.

In the pediatric age group, spinal metastases are often secondary to neuroblastoma, Ewing's sarcoma, osteogenic sarcoma, leukemia, Wilms' tumor (clear cell type), and medulloblastoma. Cerebellar medulloblastoma may demonstrate osteoblastic metastases.[84]

Only 5% of spinal metastases are purely epidural, with "small, blue, round cell" neoplasms (lymphoma, neuroblastoma, Ewing's sarcoma, rhabdomyosarcoma) and leukemias (Fig. 38–22) accounting for the majority of them. Ten percent of spinal metastases are purely osseous, and the remainder are complex.[85]

On plain film radiographs and CT, metastatic osseous lesions are often destructive and lytic (see Fig. 38–19A) but may be blastic, particularly in prostate cancer. There is commonly an associated extraosseous mass. Radionuclide bone scanning demonstrates regions of intense uptake of the radiotracer (^{99m}Tc-MDP) reflecting osteoblastic activity stimulated by malignant cells. Certain aggressive malignancies, such as myeloma, may not induce sufficient osteoblastic reaction to become apparent on the bone scan.[86]

MRI is the most sensitive method for detecting spinal metastases.[87] These lesions have low signal intensity on T1-weighted images compared with bone marrow (see Fig. 38–17). Osteolytic metastases typically demonstrate high signal intensity on T2-weighted images, whereas osteoblastic metastases show low signal intensity in the heavily sclerotic portions (see Fig. 38–18). The routine use of intravenous paramagnetic contrast material in screening for spinal metastatic disease is probably not warranted[88] and in fact may mask vertebral marrow involvement, with enhancing tumor becoming isointense to normal marrow. However, its use in evaluating malignancies that have a propensity for pure epidural metastases may aid in detection and definition of extent. Frequency-selective fat-saturation and short-tau inversion recovery techniques are other sensitive methods for the detection of spinal metastases, by suppressing neighboring marrow and epidural fat (Fig. 38–23).[9]

Direct Extension to the Spine and Epidural Space

Secondary involvement of the spine and epidural space can occasionally occur by direct extension of malignancies located in the pelvis, retroperitoneum, posterior mediastinum, lungs, and neck region. In the pediatric age group, neuroblastoma and ganglioneuroblastoma are the most common malignancies to present with direct spinal extension, occurring in approximately 13% of cases.[89] Neuroblastoma is a malignant tumor of primitive neuroblasts arising within the sympathetic neural system and adrenal medulla.[90] Eighty-five percent of patients present before 4 years of age, with approximately 60% of the tumors arising in the abdomen, 13% in the thorax, 5% in the neck, and 4% in the pelvis.[91] There is a slight male preponderance.[92]

Pathologically, neuroblastomas consist of small, round tumor cells arranged in rosettes. The presence of a delicate fibrillary background composed of neuroblastic processes is characteristic.[90] Immunohistochemistry and electron microscopy may be helpful in distinguishing neuroblastomas from other small, round cell tumors. Ganglioneuroblastomas arise from the same primitive neuroblasts but contain an abundance of mature ganglion cells.

On plain film radiographs and CT, neuroblastomas demonstrate a heterogeneous soft tissue mass with areas of necrosis and calcifications, displacing neighboring structures and occasionally extending to the spine.[93] MRI is, however, the best modality for evaluating epidural involvement and associated cord compression.[89] These malignancies tend to demonstrate heterogeneous signal intensities on T1- and T2-weighted images due to the presence of hemorrhage, necrosis, and calcification (Figs. 38–24 and 38–25).

In adults, spinal invasion may occur with aggressive lung and cervical carcinomas. Also, retroperitoneal and posterior mediastinal lymph nodes involved with lymphoma and genitourinary malignancies may be sources of direct spinal extension (Fig. 38–26).

INTRADURAL EXTRAMEDULLARY TUMORS

Nerve Sheath Tumors

The nerve sheath tumors are the *schwannomas* (Figs. 38–27 and 38–28) and *neurofibromas* (Fig. 38–29). These occur most often in the thoracic spine. Most are intradural extramedullary, although about 10% are both intra- and extradural; occasionally they are completely extradural.[1]

Schwannomas are usually solitary unless the patient

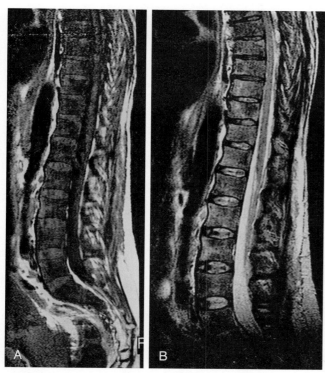

FIGURE 38–18 Diffuse blastic metastases from prostate cancer affecting the thoracolumbar spine and demonstrating many low signal intensity lesions on both the sagittal T1- and T2-weighted images (*A* and *B*).

Text continued on page 1354

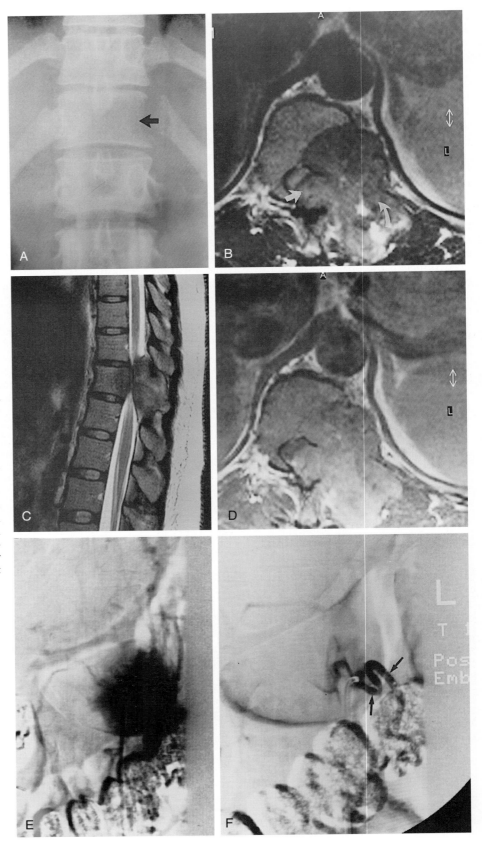

FIGURE 38–19 Large, hypervascular metastatic lesion from follicular thyroid carcinoma, centered in the left T12 pedicle. An anteroposterior (AP) plain film radiograph of the thoracic spine (A) demonstrates absence of the T12 pedicle on the left side (arrow). The axial T1-weighted and the sagittal T2-weighted images (B and C) exhibit a large low-signal-intensity mass that affects the left posterior elements of the T12 vertebra with extension into the vertebral body, paraspinal region (curved arrow), and epidural space (arrow). The mass homogeneously enhances after gadolinium administration (D). A pre-embolization AP digital subtraction spinal angiogram (E) demonstrates a hypervascular mass centered in the left T12 pedicle. A postembolization angiogram with polyvinyl alcohol foam (F) demonstrates a significant reduction in tumor vascularity and persistent enlargement of its feeding artery (arrows).

FIGURE 38–20 Systemic non-Hodgkin's lymphoma with secondary involvement of the L3 vertebral body *(arrow)* and adjacent epidural venous plexus *(arrowheads)*, demonstrated on the sagittal T1-weighted and the axial and sagittal T2-weighted images *(A–C)*. There is homogeneous enhancement of the osseous and epidural components on the postgadolinium sagittal T1-weighted image *(D)*.

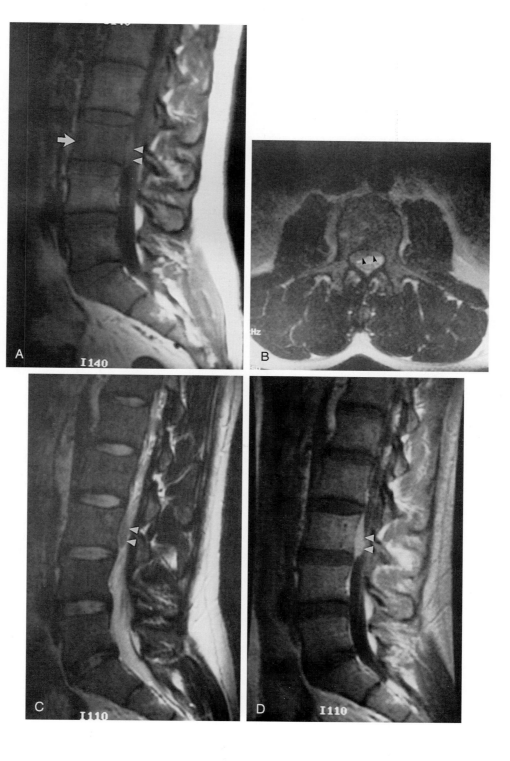

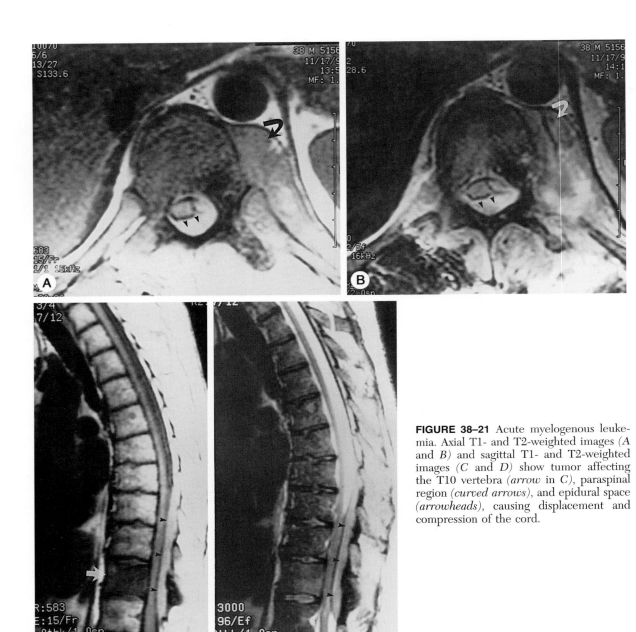

FIGURE 38–21 Acute myelogenous leukemia. Axial T1- and T2-weighted images (*A* and *B*) and sagittal T1- and T2-weighted images (*C* and *D*) show tumor affecting the T10 vertebra (*arrow* in *C*), paraspinal region (*curved arrows*), and epidural space (*arrowheads*), causing displacement and compression of the cord.

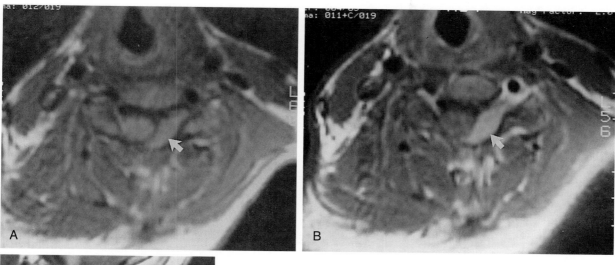

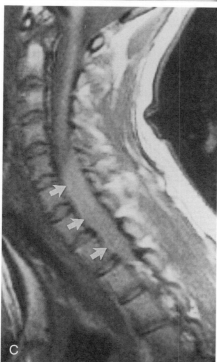

FIGURE 38–22 Axial T1-weighted image *(A)* and axial and sagittal postgadolinium T1-weighted images *(B* and *C)* of acute myelogenous leukemia with a purely epidural cervical metastasis *(arrows)*. Note the homogeneous enhancement of the epidural mass.

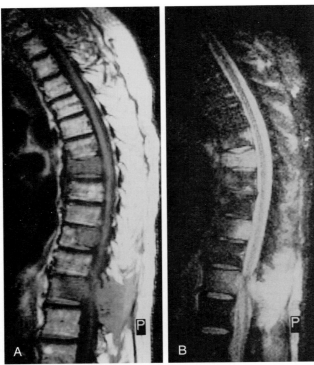

FIGURE 38–23 Metastatic screening examination of the thoracolumbar spine for a patient with lung cancer. T1 (*A*) and short-tau inversion recovery (STIR) (TR/TE/TI: 3000/20/160 msec) (*B*) techniques using the body coil, 512 × 256 matrix, field of view = 48 cm (rectangular field of view), and number of excitations = 4. There are multiple metastatic lesions affecting the thoracolumbar spine and demonstrating low signal intensity on the T1-weighted image and corresponding high signal intensity on the STIR image, compared with that of normal bone marrow. Note the suppression of normal marrow signal in the unaffected vertebrae on the STIR image.

has neurofibromatosis-2; along with meningiomas, they are the usual intradural extramedullary spinal neoplasm of neurofibromatosis-2 (Fig. 38–30). (The typical intramedullary tumor of neurofibromatosis-2 is the ependymoma [see Fig. 38–41]).[94] Most cases occur in young to middle-aged adults (males slightly younger than females); males and females are equally affected, which is not the case with meningiomas, which have a strong female predominance.[1, 95] In a large series of intraspinal tumors cited in the monograph by Slooff and colleagues,[96] schwannomas (29%) had a slightly higher prevalence than meningiomas or gliomas.

Schwannomas originate from Schwann cells, the myelin-investing analogue of the brain's oligodendrocytes. They may involve nerve roots at any level of the cord[97] and generally originate from sensory (posterior) nerve roots.[95] Most are completely intradural, although some may expand the neural foramina; rarely they are mostly intramedullary.

Pathologically, they are well-encapsulated tumors that splay rather than invade the parent nerve root.[95] Histologically, they are composed of dense bundles of spindle cells (Antoni A fibers), which unlike meningiomas, stain positive for S-100 protein. Antoni B fibers, less compact

collections of cells (perhaps degenerating), may also be seen. Cystic degeneration is not uncommon and may be a useful characteristic differentiating them from meningiomas or neurofibromas (see Fig. 38–28).

Intraspinal neurofibromas are rare and are almost always associated with neurofibromatosis-1. Grossly, they are glistening and often have a mucinous quality; they do not undergo cystic degeneration.[95] Histologically, neoplastic Schwann cells infiltrate the spinal nerve, insinuating between axon cylinders, in contrast to schwannomas.[95]

Schwannomas and neurofibromas have a similar radiographic appearance. They are well-circumscribed intradural extramedullary lesions, fairly isointense on T1-weighted images, and enhance with contrast material. In our experience, schwannomas may be bright or isointense on T2-weighted images; neurofibromas are almost always T2-bright. Sometimes schwannomas have a cystic component, unlike neurofibromas (see Fig. 38–28).[95] On post-gadolinium and T2-weighted images, neurofibromas may have a central nonenhancing, T2-dark focus (Fig. 38–31; see also Fig. 38–29).[98]

Meningioma

Spinal meningiomas constitute one-fourth to one-third of primary intraspinal masses and occur in middle-aged and older adults, with a marked (perhaps 10 to 1) female predominance, even more skewed than the known female predilection for intracranial meningiomas.[95] Eighty percent are located in the thoracic region.[1] About 6% are intradural and extradural, and an equivalent number are completely extradural.[1]

Grossly, these tumors are nodular and discrete, with dural attachment. Pathologically, meningiomas originate from meningothelial cells, which may be found in the spinal arachnoid membranes. Although these tumors are histologically heterogeneous, with multiple histologic subclassifications, most contain characteristic whorls of meningothelial cells and calcified psammoma bodies.[99] They stain positive for epithelial membrane antigen and are negative for S-100 protein, unlike the nerve sheath tumors described previously.[95]

Meningiomas have similar signal characteristics to schwannomas, being isointense to the cord on T1-weighted images[100] and isointense or dark on T2-weighted images. Calcification is not uncommon, found in the histologic psammoma bodies[95] and contributing to the T2-dark signal (Fig. 38–32). Meningiomas enhance brightly and homogeneously[101] and characteristically are dura-based, occasionally with a dural "tail" (see Fig. 38–32).

Paraganglioma

Spinal paragangliomas are rare tumors that are well circumscribed and are found in adults, generally attached to the filum terminale or cauda equina[95] (Fig. 38–33). They have the same histologic appearance (zellballen pattern and dense-core cytoplasmic granules)[95] as their more familiar counterparts elsewhere in the body, such as the adrenal medulla (pheochromocytoma) and carotid body. Their imaging characteristics are similar to those of other tumors in this region such as ependymoma. Paragangliomas are highly vascular and exhibit prominent contrast enhancement (Fig. 38–33).[102]

Text continued on page 1359

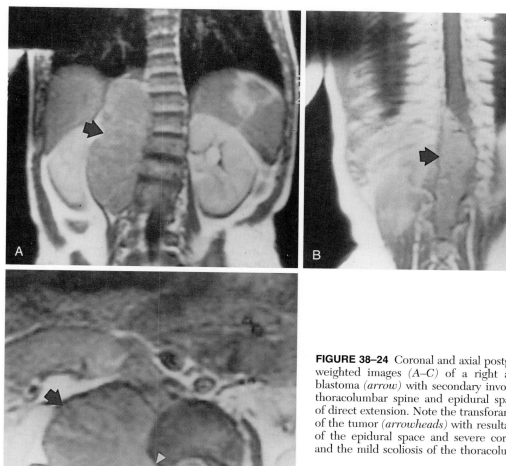

FIGURE 38–24 Coronal and axial postgadolinium T1-weighted images *(A–C)* of a right adrenal neuroblastoma *(arrow)* with secondary involvement of the thoracolumbar spine and epidural space as a result of direct extension. Note the transforaminal extension of the tumor *(arrowheads)* with resultant obliteration of the epidural space and severe cord compression and the mild scoliosis of the thoracolumbar spine.

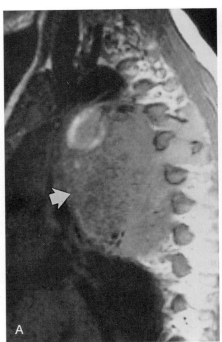

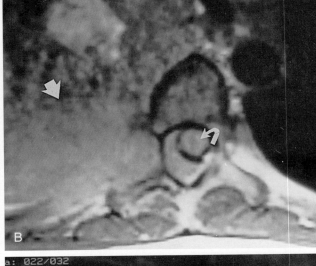

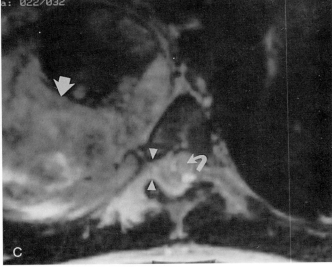

FIGURE 38–25 Sagittal and axial post-gadolinium T1-weighted images (*A* and *B*) and axial T2-weighted image (*C*) of a ganglioneuroblastoma (*arrows*) arising in the posterior mediastinum with direct transforaminal extension (*arrowheads*) into the epidural space, causing cord displacement and compression (*curved arrows*). Note the heterogeneous signal intensity of the mass on the T2-weighted image.

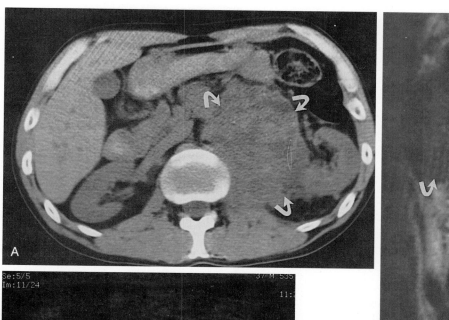

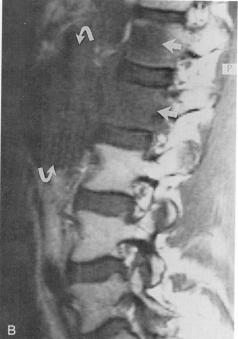

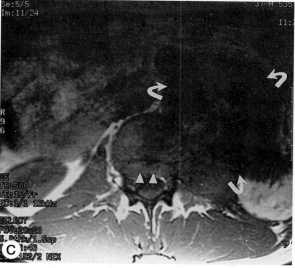

FIGURE 38–26 Noncontrast axial CT image of the abdomen at the level of the renal hila (A); sagittal and axial T1-weighted MRI studies (B and C) of a nonseminomatous testicular cancer metastasizing to the retroperitoneal lymph nodes (curved arrows) with secondary direct extension to the L1 and L2 vertebrae (straight arrows) as well as the epidural space (arrowheads).

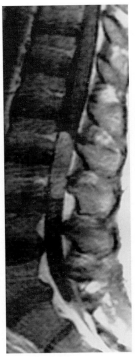

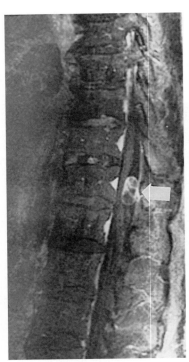

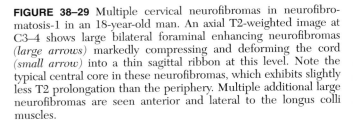

FIGURE 38–27 Schwannoma in a 14-year-old boy, who presented with low back pain and leg pain after a sports injury. Postgadolinium sagittal T1-weighted image shows a well-circumscribed oval intradural extramedullary, fairly uniformly enhancing mass extending from L2 to L3, which fills the spinal canal and displaces the cauda equina posteriorly.

FIGURE 38–28 Schwannoma in a 68-year-old man with chronic low back pain and new bilateral leg pain and weakness. Sagittal fat-saturated postgadolinium T1-weighted image shows a well-circumscribed oval intradural extramedullary enhancing mass at T12 (*arrow*), which contains darker cystic-appearing components; it compresses and displaces the cord anteriorly.

FIGURE 38–29 Multiple cervical neurofibromas in neurofibromatosis-1 in an 18-year-old man. An axial T2-weighted image at C3–4 shows large bilateral foraminal enhancing neurofibromas (*large arrows*) markedly compressing and deforming the cord (*small arrow*) into a thin sagittal ribbon at this level. Note the typical central core in these neurofibromas, which exhibits slightly less T2 prolongation than the periphery. Multiple additional large neurofibromas are seen anterior and lateral to the longus colli muscles.

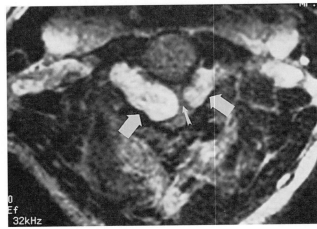

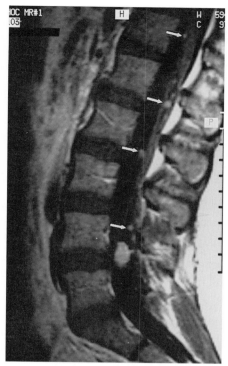

FIGURE 38–30 Multiple cauda equina schwannomas in neurofibromatosis-2 in an 18-year-old woman. A sagittal postgadolinium T1-weighted image shows multiple small nodular enhancing masses *(arrows)* adhering to the cauda equina, with a dominant mass at the L4–5 level.

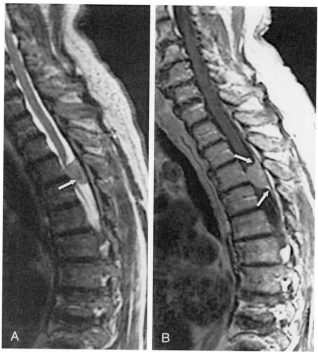

FIGURE 38–32 Meningioma in a 74-year-old woman with leg weakness and hyperreflexia. *A,* Sagittal T2-weighted image. The dark focus *(arrow)* represents calcification within the tumor, verified on pathologic examination after resection. *B,* Postgadolinium sagittal T1-weighted image shows uniform enhancement of the well-circumscribed intradural extramedullary mass, which markedly compresses the thoracic cord at the T3–4 level. Note the characteristic enhancing "dural tails" *(arrows).*

Embryonal Tumors

Developmental tumors (e.g., epidermoids, lipomas, dermoids, teratomas) have variable appearance on MRI, de-

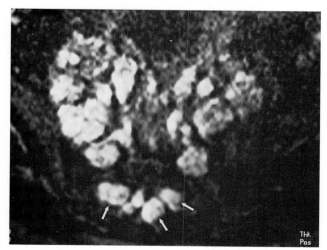

FIGURE 38–31 Multiple large sacral neurofibromas in neurofibromatosis-1 in an 8-year-old boy with leg cramps. An axial T2-weighted image through the pelvis shows multiple large bright neurofibromas affecting all the sacral nerve roots within the central spinal canal *(arrows)* and extending out along the sacral ala into the pelvis. Note the typical central core of darker signal in the tumors.

pending on the constituent components making up the tumor.

Spinal lipomas are usually located in the cervical and upper thoracic spine and are found at all ages.[95] Intradural spinal lipomas are typically subpial and intimately adherent to nerve roots.

Intradural epidermoid and dermoid tumors (also called epidermoid and dermoid *cysts*) are thought to arise from ectopic embryologic cell rests. This hypothesis is supported by association of these lesions with spinal dysraphism. It is also presumed that these lesions may result from direct inoculation of cutaneous epithelial cells into the intrathecal compartment, such as via lumbar puncture.[103, 104] They most commonly are located in the lumbosacral region.[103]

Grossly, epidermoid and dermoid cysts are white or light yellow, containing flaky or greasy material within a keratinizing squamous epithelium. The presence of sebaceous glands or hair makes the diagnosis of dermoid, rather than epidermoid, tumors.[95]

Lipomas and fatty components of embryonal tumors are easily and definitively diagnosed by imaging studies, using either fat-saturation techniques in MRI (Fig. 38–34) or CT (by fat's very low attenuation of approximately −100 Hounsfield units).

In the spine as in the brain, epidermoids may be difficult to detect on MRI, as they may be isointense to CSF on all pulse sequences[105] (Fig. 38–35).

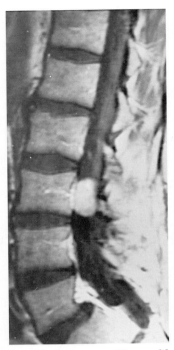

FIGURE 38–33 Paraganglioma in a 47-year-old man. A sagittal postgadolinium T1-weighted image shows a well-circumscribed, brightly enhancing mass adhering to the filum terminale at the L3 level. (Courtesy of Dr. P. Burger.)

As mentioned, abnormalities of spinal development such as meningomyeloceles or tethered cord are commonly accompanied by developmental tumors, especially lipomas (Fig. 38–36).

Metastases

Spinal subarachnoid metastases result from CSF seeding from intracranial primary tumors such as medulloblastoma (Fig. 38–37) or ependymoma, or from lung or breast cancer (Fig. 38–38), or lymphoma. These metastases are often isointense or slightly hyperintense on T1-weighted images, and somewhat hyperintense on T2-weighted images, although this may be masked by T2-bright CSF. Gadolinium enhancement is extremely helpful in increasing conspicuity of these intradural extramedullary lesions, which enhance fairly brightly.[101] Without the administration of intravenous gadolinium, these metastatic lesions may be missed, especially if they are localized to the nerve roots, where lesion conspicuity is low on T2-weighted images alone.

INTRAMEDULLARY TUMORS

Glioma

Gliomas are the predominant intramedullary tumor, notably ependymomas (especially at the conus and filum terminale) in adults and astrocytomas in children.[106]

Sixty percent of primary cord tumors are ependymomas (unlike the situation in the brain, where they are much less common than astrocytomas).[95] They occur predominantly in middle age.[96, 107] Ependymomas are most commonly located at the conus or filum, although any portion of the cord may be involved. Intramedullary ependymomas are most common in the cervical region[108] (Fig. 38–39).

Ependymomas are discrete lesions, usually solid, located centrally in the cord and expanding it. Histologically, they consist of cellular sheets of ependymal cells, interrupted by anuclear perivascular "pseudorosettes."[95]

The MRI appearance reflects their gross pathologic appearance: intramedullary tumors that may expand the cord. They are iso- or slightly hypointense on T1- and bright on T2-weighted images. Associated cysts or syrinx may be seen either caudal or rostral to ependymomas (see Fig. 38–39), which generally enhance with contrast material. Hemorrhage is not uncommonly associated with ependymomas, and this has been stressed by Nemoto and associates[109] in cervical ependymomas (see Fig. 38–39). They may also contain calcification. (Gradient-recalled echo sequences may be helpful in demonstrating hemosiderin and calcification, which may be missed on FSE imaging.)

The myxopapillary subtype of ependymoma warrants special mention.[95] These are well defined and almost exclusively found at the conus or filum terminale. Histologically, the tumor is distinctive, with fibrillated cells

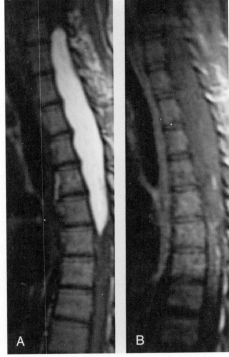

FIGURE 38–34 Intradural extramedullary subpial lipoma in a 20-year-old woman with a fairly acute onset of bilateral leg weakness. *A*, Sagittal T1-weighted image shows a very large well-circumscribed intradural extramedullary subpial T1-bright mass located posterior to, and markedly compressing, the upper thoracic cord. The spinal canal is widened and the posterior vertebral bodies are scalloped, indicating chronicity. *B*, Fat-saturated postgadolinium T1-weighted image shows complete suppression of the T1-bright signal, proving the presence of *fat* rather than T1-bright blood.

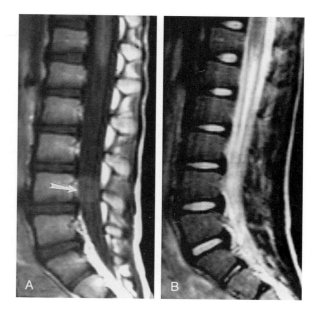

FIGURE 38–35 Epidermoid in a 6-year-old boy. *A*, Sagittal T1-weighted image shows a very subtle (nearly undetectable) round intradural mass *(arrow)* below the conus, at the L4 level. This lesion demonstrated *no* enhancement with gadolinium. *B*, Sagittal T2-weighted image shows the nearly imperceptible mass, which is almost isointense to cerebrospinal fluid.

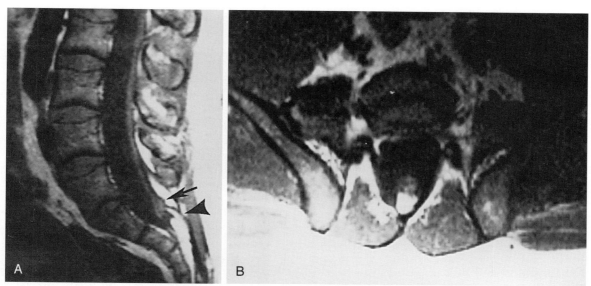

FIGURE 38–36 Tethered cord with conus lipomeningocele in a 35-year-old man with neurogenic bladder and no rectal tone. *A*, Sagittal T1-weighted image shows a tethered cord with a neural placode *(arrow)* at the S1 level, with a posteriorly adherent T1-bright intradural lipoma *(arrowhead)*. Note the absence of normal posterior elements and the wide spina bifida defect at the level of the arrow and arrowhead. *B*, Axial T1-weighted image shows the T1-bright lipoma adherent to the posterior aspect of the placode. Spina bifida is again demonstrated.

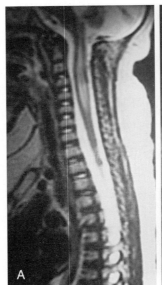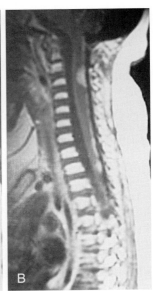

FIGURE 38–37 Intrathecal drop metastases from medulloblastoma in a 3-year-old boy. *A,* T2-weighted image shows expansion and edema of the cervical cord, extending up to the medulla. Note that cerebrospinal fluid occupies much of the midline posterior cranial fossa, because some cerebellum has been resected owing to involvement by medulloblastoma. *B,* Postgadolinium sagittal T1-weighted image shows multiple enhancing subarachnoid metastases coating the posterior aspect of the cord, with some larger deposits appearing to extend into the cord, accounting for the edema. (From Lee RR. Spinal tumors. In Lee RR [ed]. Spinal Imaging, pp. 261–286. Philadelphia, Hanley & Belfus, 1995.)

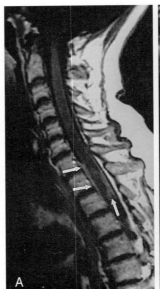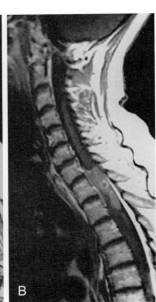

FIGURE 38–38 Intrathecal metastases from breast cancer in a 62-year-old woman presenting with right leg weakness and midthoracic pain. Consecutive sagittal postgadolinium T1-weighted images (*A* and *B*) show a diffuse, subtly enhancing tumor circumferentially coating the cord from C7 to T2 (*arrows*). Precontrast images showed no involvement of the vertebral body marrow at any level.

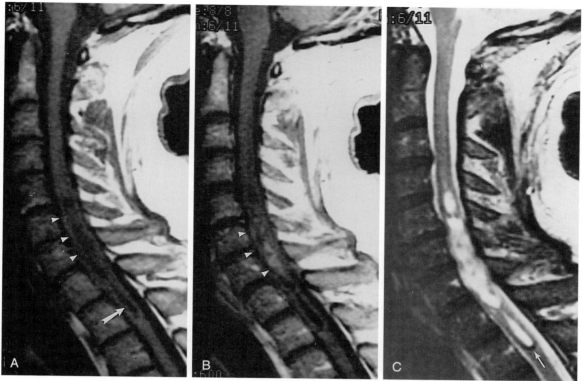

FIGURE 38–39 Cervicothoracic intramedullary ependymoma in a 52-year-old man. Sagittal precontrast (*A*) and postgadolinium (*B*) T1-weighted images show an ill-defined intramedullary mass at the C6 through the T1 levels, which demonstrates mild contrast enhancement (*arrowheads*). A small syrinx extends a few levels caudally (*arrow*), and there is also a small rostral syrinx at the C5 level. Sagittal T2-weighted image (*C*) clearly demonstrates the mass and syringes. The thin rim of T2-dark signal lining the caudal aspect of the syrinx (*arrow*) suggests the presence of hemosiderin (blood product), a useful clue favoring the diagnosis of ependymoma.

FIGURE 38–40 Myxopapillary ependymoma in a 42-year-old woman with weak, numb legs but no bowel or bladder dysfunction. Postgadolinium sagittal T1-weighted image (*A*) and T2-weighted image (*B*) show a large intradural mass extending from T11 through at least L3, filling the spinal canal and posteriorly displacing the cord, with rim enhancement around a mostly non-enhancing central region.

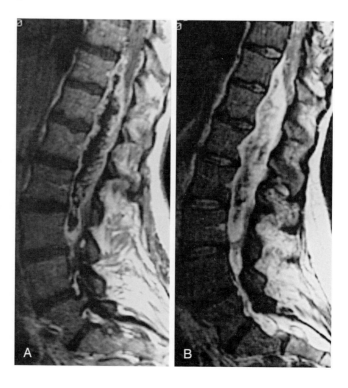

having both a glial and an epithelial appearance, forming glandlike structures and pseudopapillae.[95] Mucin is almost always present as well, hence the designation *myxopapillary*. The immunoperoxidase stain for glial fibrillary acidic protein is almost always positive.[95] These tumors may become very large, filling and occasionally expanding the lower thecal sac with enhancing soft tissue (Fig. 38–40). In our experience, the associated clinical symptoms are relatively mild and very nonspecific, allowing significant tumor growth before an imaging study (MRI) is ordered and the diagnosis made. The mean survival after complete resection is 19 years; after subtotal resection, about 14 years.[110]

As mentioned, ependymoma is the intramedullary tumor classically associated with neurofibromatosis-2[94] (Fig. 38–41).

Most astrocytomas are said to occur during the second through fifth decades of life;[95] they are also said to be the most common intramedullary spinal tumor of children.[106] Their relative incidence within the spine is proportional to the length of the spine, so in order of decreasing frequency, they appear in the thoracic, cervical, and lumbar regions.[95] Histologically, they fall into two groups:[95] (1) fibrillary, diffusely infiltrating, and (2) pilocytic, more circumscribed. The fibrillary diffuse form, which is more common, usually shows a fusiform expansion of the cord. Both forms exhibit a histologic appearance similar to that seen in their more common intracranial counterparts. Cysts may be present, either intrinsic to or at the edge of the tumor.

MRI of spinal astrocytomas reveals a fusiform expansion, associated with T2-prolongation (Figs. 38–42 and 38–43). The T1-image appearance is variable, but there is often hypointensity. Although it has been reported that virtually all spinal astrocytomas enhance,[111] in our

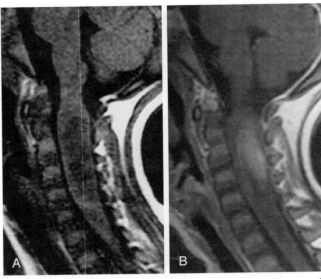

FIGURE 38–42 Astrocytoma in a 4-year-old girl who presented with a 10-day history of neck pain and spasm. A sagittal T1-weighted image (*A*) and a postgadolinium T1-weighted image (*B*) show fusiform expansion of the upper cervical cord, with mild partial enhancement, and some T1-dark edema extending up to the medulla and down to C6.

experience enhancement is variable and, when present, often subtle (Figs. 38–42 and 38–43). In particular, the fibrillary form does not generally enhance or does so very mildly, in contrast to the pilocytic form, which does enhance.

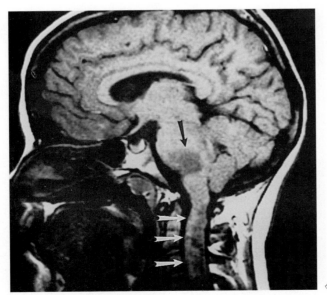

FIGURE 38–41 Cervical ependymoma in neurofibromatosis-2 in a 17-year-old woman. A sagittal T1-weighted image shows a diffuse mass expanding the upper cervical cord (*white arrows*). The black arrow indicates a large acoustic schwannoma, which is partially imaged on this midline slice.

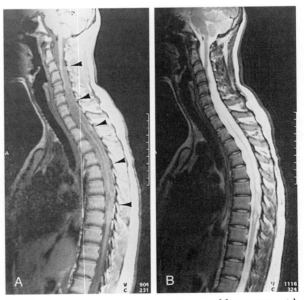

FIGURE 38–43 Astrocytoma in a 19-year-old woman with 2 years of left leg and arm weakness. A sagittal T1-weighted image (*A*) and a T2-weighted image (*B*) show a diffuse expansion of the cervicothoracic cord extending from C3–4 through T8 (*arrowheads*). This tumor demonstrated no contrast enhancement.

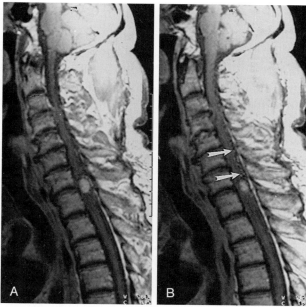

FIGURE 38–44 Hemangioblastoma in a 75-year-old man. Consecutive sagittal postgadolinium T1-weighted images (*A* and *B*) show an enhancing round mass within the spinal cord at the C7–T1 levels. Note the numerous small flow voids (*arrows*) immediately posterior to the cervical cord extending rostral from the mass, representing prominent associated vessels commonly associated with hemangioblastomas. The patient does not have von Hippel–Lindau syndrome.

Hemangioblastoma

Hemangioblastomas may occur sporadically but are often multiple and associated with cerebellar hemangioblastomas in von Hippel–Lindau syndrome. They present in the third to fifth decades of life[112] and are more common in men.

They often exhibit the typical cyst with associated mural nodule, which enhances brightly with gadolinium (Fig. 38–44). Almost all are intramedullary and abut the pial surface.[95] There is often associated edema. As in the brain, spinal hemangioblastomas are highly vascular and often have associated prominent draining veins or feeding arteries, which may initially be mistaken for the draining vein of a spinal arteriovenous dural fistula or some other

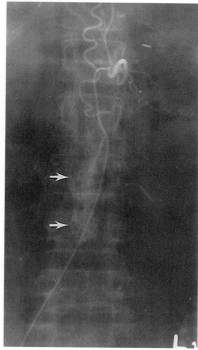

FIGURE 38–45 Hemangioblastoma in a 40-year-old woman with von Hippel–Lindau syndrome. An anteroposterior angiogram from left L1 injection shows a prominent tumor blush at L3 to L4 from the enhancing portion of the hemangioblastoma (*arrows*). Tortuous dilated feeding artery is noted superior to the tumor. (From Lee RR. Spinal tumors. In Lee RR [ed]. Spinal Imaging, pp. 261–286. Philadelphia, Hanley & Belfus, 1995.)

vascular malformation (Fig. 38–44).[95] Angiography sensitively demonstrates a tumor blush involving the enhancing nodular portion of the tumor (Fig. 38–45).

Embryonal Tumor

Embryonal tumors were discussed in the section on intradural extramedullary tumors but may also occur in an intramedullary location. As mentioned, embryonal tumors (especially lipomas) may be associated with spinal dysraphism. Dermoids and epidermoids have variable signal intensity, depending on their composition. Cystic teratomas may be found inside the cord substance (Fig. 38–46).

FIGURE 38–46 Recurrent intramedullary cystic teratoma in a 36-year-old woman. A sagittal T1-weighted image shows cystic expansion of the cord and spinal canal by proteinaceous fluid (*arrow*). There was essentially no enhancement. At surgery this tumor contained keratin, hair, and mucus.

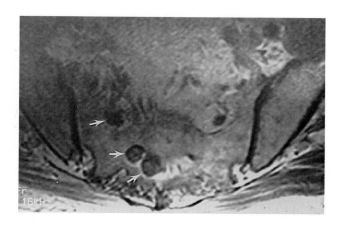

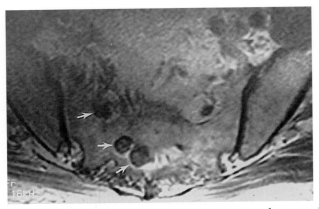

FIGURE 38–47 Metastatic prostate carcinoma invading sacral nerve roots in a 70-year-old man with right L5 and S1 radiculopathy. An axial postgadolinium T1-weighted image shows diffuse enlargement and subtle enhancement of the right-sided sacral nerve roots (*arrows*). At surgery, diffuse infiltration of the roots by prostate cancer was found. No involvement of the vertebral marrow was present.

Metastases

Rarely, metastases present as intramedullary lesions, with the primary site in the brain or outside the central nervous system. Signal intensity is low on T1- and bright on T2-weighted images; these usually enhance with gadolinium (Fig. 38–47).

References

1. Nittner K. Spinal meningiomas, neurinomas and neurofibromas and hourglass tumors. In Vinken PJ, Bruyn GW (eds). Handbook of Clinical Neurology, Vol. 20, pp. 177–322. New York, Elsevier North-Holland, 1976.
2. Kurland LT. The frequency of intraspinal neoplasms in the resident population of Rochester, Minnesota. J Neurosurg 1958;15:627–641.
3. Lee RR. Spinal tumors. In Lee RR (ed). Spinal Imaging, pp. 261–286. Philadelphia, Hanley & Belfus, 1995.
4. Hennig J, Nauerth A, Friedburg H. RARE imaging: A fast imaging method for clinical MR. Magn Reson Med 1986;3:823–833.
5. Mulkern RV, Wong STS, Winalski C, Jolesz FA. Contrast manipulation and artifact assessment of 2D and 3D RARE sequences. Magn Reson Imaging 1990;8:557–566.
6. Jones KM, Mulkern RV, Schwartz RB, et al. Fast spin-echo MR imaging of the brain and spine: Current concepts. AJR 1992;158:1313–1320.
7. Sze G, Abramson A, Krol G, et al. Gadolinium-DTPA in the evaluation of intradural extramedullary spinal disease. AJR 1988;150:911–921.
8. Georgy BA, Hesselink JR. Evaluation of fat suppression in contrast-enhanced MR of neoplastic and inflammatory spine disease. AJNR 1994;15:409–417.
9. Dwyer AJ, Frank JA, Sank VJ, et al. Short T1 inversion-recovery sequence: Analysis and initial experience in cancer imaging. Radiology 1988;168:837–841.
10. Jones KM, Schwartz RB, Mantello MT, et al. Fast spin-echo MR in the detection of vertebral metastases: Comparison of three sequences. AJNR 1994;15:401–407.
11. Ross JS, Masaryk TJ, Modic MT, et al. Vertebral hemangiomas. MR imaging. Radiology 1987;165:165–169.
12. Schmorl G, Junghanns H. The Human Spine in Health and Disease, 2nd ed., p. 325. New York, Grune & Stratton, 1971.
13. Fox MW, Onofrio BM. The natural history and management of symptomatic and asymptomatic vertebral hemangiomas. J Neurosurg 1993;78:36–45.
14. Tekkok IH, Acikgoz B, Saglams S, et al. Vertebral hemangioma symptomatic during pregnancy. Report of a case and review of the literature. Neurosurg 1993;32:302–306.
15. McAllister VL, Kendall BE, Bull JW. Symptomatic vertebral hemangiomas. Brain 1975;98:71–80.
16. Albrecht S, Crutchfield JS, SeGall GK. On spinal osteochondroma. J Neurosurg 1992;77:247–252.
17. Post MJD. Primary spine and cord neoplasms. In Categorical Course on Spine and Cord Imaging, pp. 58–70. American Society of Neuroradiology, Oak Brook, Il, 1988.
18. Dahlin DC. Giant cell tumor of bone: Highlights of 407 cases. Caldwell Lecture. AJR 1985;144:955–960.
19. McInerney DP, Middlemiss JH. Giant cell tumor of bone. Skeletal Radiol 1978; 2:195–204.
20. Yoshida H. Giant cell tumor of bone. Enzyme histochemical, biochemical, and tissue culture studies. Virchows Arch [Pathol Anat] 1982;395:319–330.
21. Aisen AM, Martel W, Braunstien EM, et al. MRI and CT evaluation of primary bone and soft tissue tumors. AJR 1986;146:749–756.
22. Aoki J, Moriya K, Yamashita K, et al. Giant cell tumors of bone containing large amounts of hemosiderin: MR-pathologic correlation. J Comput Assist Tomogr 1991;15:1024–1027.
23. Cory DA, Fritsch SA, Cohen MD, et al. Aneurysmal bone cysts: Imaging findings and embolotherapy. AJR 1989;153:369–373.
24. Tillman BP, Dalhin DC, Lipscomb PR, et al. Aneurysmal bone cyst: An analysis of 95 cases. Mayo Clin Proc 1968;43:478–495.
25. Biescker JL, Marcove RC, Huvos AG, et al. Aneurysmal bone cyst, a clinical pathologic study of 66 cases. Cancer 1970;26:615–625.
26. Dahlin DC, McLeod RA. Aneurysmal bone cyst and other nonneoplastic conditions. Skeletal Radiol 1982;8:243–250.
27. Munk PL, Helms CA, Holt RG, et al. MR imaging of aneurysmal bone cysts. AJR 1989;153:99–101.
28. Beltran J, Simon DC, Levy M, et al. Aneurysmal bone cyst: MR imaging at 1.5 T. Radiology 1986;158:689–690.
29. Tsai JC, Dalinka MK, Fallon MD, et al. Fluid-fluid level: A nonspecific finding in tumors of bone and soft tissue. Radiology 1990;175:779–782.
30. Jackson RP, Reckling FW, Mantz FA. Osteoid osteoma and osteoblastoma. Clin Orthop 1977;128:303–313.
31. Gamba JL, Martinez S, Apple J, et al. CT of axial skeletal osteoid osteoma. AJR 1984;142:769–772.
32. Nemoto O, Moser RP Jr, Van Dam BE, et al. Osteoblastoma of the spine: A review of 75 cases. Spine 1990;15:1272–1280.
33. MacLellan DI, Wilson FC. Osteoid osteoma of the spine. J Bone Joint Surg Am 1967;49:111–121.
34. Freiberger RH. Osteoid osteoma of the spine. Radiology 1960;75:232–235.
35. Steiner GC. Ultrastructure of osteoblastoma. Cancer 1977;39:2127–2136.
36. Kransdorf MJ, Stull MA, Gilkey FW, et al. Osteoid osteoma. Radiographics 1991;11:671–696.
37. Omojola MF, Cockshott P, Beatty EG. Osteoid osteoma: An evaluation of diagnostic modalities. Clin Radiol 1981;32:199–204.
38. Glass RB, Poznanski AK, Fisher MR, et al. Case report. MR imaging of osteoid osteoma. J Comput Assist Tomogr 1986;10:1065–1067.
39. Houang B, Grenier N, Greselle JF, et al. Osteoid osteoma of the cervical spine: Misleading features about a case involving the uncinate process. Neuroradiology 1990;31:549–551.
40. Syklawer R, Osborn RE, Kerber CW, et al. MR imaging of vertebral osteoblastoma: A report of two cases. Surg Neurol 1990;34:421–426.
41. McGavran MH, Spady HA. Eosinophilic granuloma of bone, a study of 28 cases. J Bone Joint Surg [Am] 1960;42:979–992.
42. Lieberman PH, Jones CR, Dargeon HW, et al. A reappraisal of eosinophilic granuloma of bone, Hand-Schüller-Christian syndrome and Letterer-Siwe syndrome. Medicine 1969;48:375–400.
43. Hamilton JB, Barner JL, Kennedy PC, et al. The osseous manifestations of eosinophilic granuloma: Report of nine cases. Radiology 1945;47:445–456.
44. Acromano JP, Barnett JC, Wunderlich HO. Histiocytosis. AJR 1961;85:663–679.
45. Ochsner SF. Eosinophilic granuloma of bone: Experience with 20 cases. AJR 1966;97:719–726.

46. De Schepper AMA, Ramon F, Van Mark E. MR imaging of eosinophilic granuloma: Report of 11 cases. Skeletal Radiol 1993;22:163–166.

47. Beaugie JM, Mann CV, Butler CB. Sacrococcygeal chordoma. Br J Surg 1969;56:586–588.

48. Heffelfinger MJ, Dahlin DC, McCarty CS, et al. Chordomas and cartilaginous tumors at the skull base. Cancer 1973;32:410–420.

49. Firooznia H, Pinto RS, Lin JP, et al. Chordoma: Radiologic evaluation of 20 cases. AJR 1976;127:797–805.

50. Fox JE, Batsakis JG, Owano LR. Unusual manifestations of chordoma. J Bone Joint Surg 1968;50A:1618–1628.

51. Sebag G, Dubois J, Beniaminovitz A, et al. Extraosseous spinal chordoma: Radiographic appearance. AJNR 1993;14:205–207.

52. Sze G, Uichanco LS, Brant-Zawadzki M, et al. Chordomas: MR imaging. Radiology 1988;166:187–191.

53. Yuh WTC, Flickinger FW, Barloon TJ, Montgomery WJ. MR imaging of unusual chordomas. J Comput Assist Tomogr 1988;12:30–35.

54. Dahlin DC, Unni KK. Osteosarcoma. In Bone Tumors: General Aspects and Data on 8,542 Cases, pp. 269–307. Springfield, IL, Charles C Thomas, 1986.

55. Dahlin DC, Coventry MB. Osteogenic sarcoma, a study of 600 cases. J Bone Joint Surg [Am] 1967;49:101–110.

56. Dahlin DC. Osteosarcoma of bone and a consideration of prognostic variables. Cancer Treat Rep 1978;62:189–192.

57. Patel DV, Hammer RA, Levin B, et al. Primary osteogenic sarcoma of the spine. Skeletal Radiol 1984;12:276–279.

58. Berger PE, Kuhn JP. Computed tomography of tumors of the musculoskeletal system in children. Radiology 1978;127:171–175.

59. Gillespy T III, Manfrini M, Ruggieri P, et al. Staging of intraosseous extent of osteosarcoma: Correlation of preoperative CT and MR imaging with pathologic macroslides. Radiology 1988;167:765–767.

60. Barnes R, Catto M. Chondrosarcoma of bone. J Bone Joint Surg [Br] 1966;48:729–764.

61. Henderson ED, Dahlin DC. Chondrosarcoma of bone. A study of 288 cases. J Bone Joint Surg 1963;45A:1450–1458.

62. Garrison RC, Unni KK, McLeod RA, et al. Chondrosarcoma arising in osteochondroma. Cancer 1982;49:1890–1897.

63. Grabias S, Mankin HJ. Chondrosarcoma arising in histologically proved unicameral bone cyst: A case report. J Bone Joint Surg 1974;56A:1501–1509.

64. Evans HL, Ayala AG, Romsdahl MM. Prognostic factors in chondrosarcoma of bone. A clinicopathologic analysis with emphasis on histologic grading. Cancer 1977;40:818–831.

65. Kumar R, David R, Cierney G, et al. Clear cell chondrosarcoma. Radiology 1985;154:45–48.

66. Pepe AJ, Kuhlmann RF, Miller DB. Mesenchymal chondrosarcoma. A case report. J Bone Joint Surg 1977;59A:256–258.

67. de Lange EE, Pope TL Jr, Fechner RE, et al. Dedifferentiated chondrosarcoma: Radiographic features. Radiology 1986;160:489–492.

68. Camins MB, Duncan AW, Smith J, et al. Chondrosarcoma of the spine. Spine 1978;3:202–209.

69. Cohen EK, Kressel HY, Frank TS, et al. Hyaline cartilage–origin bone and soft tissue neoplasm: MR appearance and histologic correlation. Radiology 1988;167:477–481.

70. Dickman PS, Liotta LA, Triche TJ, et al. Ewing's sarcoma. Characterization in established culture and evidence of its histogenesis. Lab Invest 1982;47:375–382.

71. Dahlin DC, Coventry MB, Scanlon PW. Ewing's sarcoma. A critical analysis of 165 cases. J Bone Joint Surg 1961;43A:185–192.

72. Kozlowski K, Beluffi G, Masel J, et al. Primary vertebral tumours in children. Report of 20 cases with brief review of the literature. Pediatr Radiol 1984;14:129–139.

73. Whitehouse GH, Griffith GJ. Roentgenologic aspects of spinal involvement by primary and metastatic Ewing's tumor. J Can Assoc Radiol 1976;27:290–297.

74. Mahoney JP, Alexander RW. Ewing's sarcoma. A light- and electron-microscopic study of 21 cases. Am J Surg Pathol 1978;2:283–298.

75. Ginaldi S, deSantos LA. Computed tomography in the evaluation of small round cell tumors of bone. Radiology 1980;134:441–446.

76. Frouge C, Vanel D, Coffre C, et al. The role of magnetic resonance imaging in the evaluation of Ewing sarcoma. Skeletal Radiol 1988;17:387–392.

77. Parker BR, Marglin S, Castellino RA. Skeletal manifestations of leukemia, Hodgkin disease, and non-Hodgkin lymphoma. Semin Roentgenol 1980;15:302–315.

78. Magnus HA, Wood LC. Primary reticulosarcoma of bone. J Bone Joint Surg [Br] 1956;38:258–278.

79. Rappaport H, Berard CW, Butler JJ, et al. Report of the committee on histopathologic criteria contributing to staging of Hodgkin's disease. Cancer Res 1971;31:1864–1865.

80. Daffner RH, Lupetin AR, Dash N, et al. MRI in the detection of malignant infiltration of bone marrow. AJR 1986;146:353–358.

81. Weaver GR, Sandler MP. Increased sensitivity of magnetic resonance imaging compared to radionuclide bone scintigraphy in the detection of lymphoma of the spine. Clin Nucl Med 1987;12:333–334.

82. Gilbert RW, Kim JH, Posner JB. Epidural spinal cord compression from metastatic tumour: Diagnosis and treatment. Ann Neurol 1978;3:40–51.

83. Harrington KD. Metastatic disease of the spine. J Bone Joint Surg [Am] 1986;68:1110–1115.

84. Debnam JW, Staple TW. Osseous metastases from cerebellar medulloblastoma. Radiology 1973;107:363–365.

85. Constans JP, de Divitiis E, Donzelli R, et al. Spinal metastases with neurologic manifestations: Review of 600 cases. J Neurosurg 1983;59:111–118.

86. Woolfenden JM, Pitt MJ, Durie BG, et al. Comparison of bone scintigraphy and radiography in multiple myeloma. Radiology 1980;134:723–728.

87. Smoker WRK, Godersky JC, Nutzon RK, et al. Role of MR imaging in evaluating metastatic spinal disease. AJNR 1987;8:901–908.

88. Sze G, Abramson A, Krol G, et al. Gadolinium-DTPA: Malignant extradural spinal tumors. Radiology 1988;67:217–233.

89. Siegel MJ, Jamroz GA, Glazer HS, et al. MR imaging of intraspinal extension of neuroblastoma. J Comput Assist Tomogr 1986;10:593–595.

90. Stowens D. Neuroblastoma and related tumors. Arch Pathol 1957;63:451–459.

91. Kirks DR, Merten DF, Grossman H, et al. Diagnostic imaging of pediatric abdominal masses: An overview. Radiol Clin North Am 1981;19:527–545.

92. Balakrishnan V, Rice MS, Simpson DA. Spinal neuroblastoma: Diagnosis, treatment, and prognosis. J Neurosurg 1974;40:431–438.

93. Kuhns LR. Computed tomography of the retroperitoneum in children. Radiol Clin North Am 1981;14:495–501.

94. Egelhoff JC, Bates DJ, Ross JS, et al. Spinal MR findings in neurofibromatosis types 1 and 2. AJNR 1992;13:1071–1077.

95. Burger PC, Scheithauer BW, Vogel FS. Spinal meninges, spinal nerve roots, and spinal cord. In Surgical Pathology of the Nervous System and Its Coverings, 3rd ed., pp. 605–660. New York, Churchill Livingstone, 1991.

96. Slooff JL, Kernohan JW, MacCarty CS. Primary Intramedullary Tumors of the Spinal Cord and Filum Terminale. Philadelphia, WB Saunders, 1964.

97. Levy WJ, Latchaw J, Hahn JF, et al. Spinal neurofibromas: A report of 66 cases and a comparison with meningiomas. Neurosurgery 1986;18:331–334.

98. Burk DL Jr, Brumberg JA, Kanal E, et al. Spinal and paraspinal neurofibromatosis: Surface coil MR imaging at 1.5 T. Radiology 1987;162:797–801.

99. Burger PC, Scheithauer BW, Vogel FS. Intracranial meninges. In Surgical Pathology of the Nervous System and Its Coverings, 3rd ed., pp. 67–142. New York, Churchill Livingstone, 1991.

100. Solero CL, Fornari N, Giombini S, et al. Spinal meningiomas: Review of 174 operated cases. Neurosurgery 1989;25:153–160.

101. Sze G, Abramson A, Krol G, et al. Gadolinium-DTPA in the evaluation of intradural extramedullary spinal disease. AJR 1988;150:911–921.

102. Levy RA. Paraganglioma of the filum terminale: MR findings. AJR 1993;160:851–852.

103. Manno NJ, Uihlein A, Kernohan JW. Intraspinal epidermoids. J Neurosurg 1962;19:754–765.

104. Machida T, Abe O, Sasaki Y, et al. Acquired epidermoid tumor in the thoracic spinal canal. Neuroradiology 1993;35:316–318.

105. Barkovich AJ, Edwards MSB, Cogen PH. MR evaluation of spinal dermal sinus tracts in children. AJNR 1991;12:123–129.

106. Epstein F, Epstein N. Intramedullary tumors of the spinal cord. In Shillito J Jr, Matson DD (eds): Pediatric Neurosurgery of the Developing Nervous System, pp. 529–539. New York, Grune & Stratton, 1982.

107. Barone BM, Elvidge AR. Ependymomas: A clinical survey. J Neurosurg 1970;33:428–438.

108. McCormick PC, Torres R, Post KD, et al. Intramedullary ependymoma of the spinal cord. J Neurosurg 1990;62:523–532.

109. Nemoto Y, Inoue Y, Tashiro T, et al. Intramedullary spinal cord tumors: Significance of associated hemorrhage at MR imaging. Radiology 1992;82:793–796.

110. Sonneland PRL, Scheithauer BW, Onofrio BM. Myxopapillary ependymoma. Cancer 1985;56:883–893.

111. Sze G, Stimac GK, Bartlett C, et al. Multicenter study of Gd-DTPA as an MR contrast agent: Evaluation in patients with spinal cord tumors. AJNR 1990;11:967–974.

112. Brown TR, Adams RD, Roberson GH. Hemangioblastoma of the spinal cord. Arch Neurol 1976;33:435–441.

39

Infectious and Inflammatory Diseases of the Spine*

A L E X A N D E R   S .   M A R K ,   M . D .

Magnetic resonance imaging (MRI) is the first imaging modality able to visualize the spinal cord directly, without contrast material. Its wide clinical use has enabled radiologists to demonstrate a number of inflammatory and infectious conditions that previously required the injection of intrathecal contrast material. This chapter includes infectious and inflammatory diseases of the spine and spinal cord. For each disease process, a brief discussion of the pathology of the disease precedes the description of the MRI findings.

TECHNICAL CONSIDERATIONS

The different techniques for spinal MRI have been described elsewhere in this book. This chapter only briefly emphasizes certain technical points pertinent to this subject.

Sagittal short-TR, short-TE images with a slice thickness of 3 mm or less and minimal or no interslice gaps are necessary for superior spatial resolution to the extent the signal-to-noise ratio can be maintained to acceptable levels within a reasonable examination time. If the patient is not perfectly aligned, the cord is imaged in a piecemeal fashion and the lesion may be difficult to see. Conversely, partial-volume artifacts may mimic disease. A coronal localizer followed by oblique sagittal images can alleviate this problem.

For the sagittal long-TR, long-TE sequences, flow compensation gradients or cardiac gating, or both, are very helpful. Gradient echoes have been very useful in the evaluation of cervical spondylosis, but their routine use in the evaluation of infectious and inflammatory diseases has not been fully evaluated. These sequences are helpful for intramedullary hemorrhagic or calcified lesions.

Gadolinium–diethylenetriaminepenta-acetic acid (DTPA) has been shown to be very helpful in the evaluation of infectious and inflammatory diseases and also for most

conditions discussed in this chapter, and it should be used routinely in all patients with myelopathy in whom the cause is not obvious on the unenhanced images. The use of fat-saturated T1-weighted sequences in conjunction with intravenous gadolinium-DTPA is useful for the evaluation of epidural and intradural infections.[1]

INFLAMMATORY AND DEMYELINATING LESIONS

Transverse Myelitis

Inflammatory and demyelinating lesions of the spine are usually considered under the clinical syndrome acute transverse myelitis. This syndrome is characterized by an acutely developing ascending or static spinal cord lesion affecting both halves of the cord in the absence of any known neurologic disease or cord compression. In the past, acute transverse myelitis was a diagnosis of exclusion after spinal cord compression was ruled out. Today, MRI may directly demonstrate an abnormal intramedullary signal, that is, low intensity on T1- and high intensity on T2-weighted images;[2] the cord may be of normal caliber or slightly expanded, occasionally suggesting a neoplasm. The disease may affect the cervical segment or thoracic segment (Fig. 39–1), or both segments (Figs. 39–1 and 39–2) of the cord. The abnormal signal may extend above the level of clinical deficit. After gadolinium administration, the abnormal areas may show enhancement (Fig. 39–3). Transverse myelitis may be associated with infections,[3] vaccination[4, 5] (Fig. 39–4), disorders of the immune system such as systemic lupus,[6–8] and multiple sclerosis (MS) or paraneoplastic syndromes.

The prognosis of transverse myelitis is variable, but recovery may occur over several weeks or months. Follow-up MRI in these patients may demonstrate resolution of the abnormal signal and return of the cord to a normal caliber or cord atrophy. The association of transverse myelitis and optic neuritis is called *Devic's syndrome*, or neuromyelitis optica.[9] Although MS is the most common cause of this condition, Devic's syndrome may be associated with viral infections,[10–12] tuberculosis,[13] and lupus.[14]

Although all the inflammatory and demyelinating dis-

*This chapter is adapted by permission from Mark AS. Infectious and inflammatory diseases of the spine. In Atlas SW (ed). Magnetic Resonance of the Brain and Spine, 2nd ed., pp. 1207–1264. Philadelphia, Lippincott-Raven, 1996.

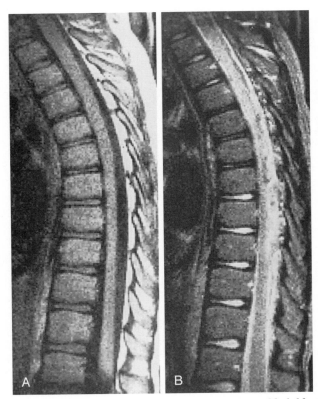

FIGURE 39–1 Acute transverse myelitis in a 9-year-old child. *A,* Sagittal T1-weighted image demonstrates mild expansion of the cord. *B,* Sagittal T2-weighted image demonstrates high signal intensity in the upper thoracic cord. (*A* and *B,* From Barakos JA, Mark AS, Dillon DW, Norman D. MR imaging of acute transverse myelitis and AIDS myelopathy. J Comput Assist Tomogr 1990;14:45–50.)

eases discussed in this section can produce a clinical picture of transverse myelitis, they are by no means the exclusive causes of this syndrome; in particular, venous ischemia secondary to radicullomedullary fistulas, spinal cord infarction due to occlusion of the anterior spinal artery, and the infectious myelitides should be excluded before the diagnosis of idiopathic transverse myelitis is made.

Multiple Sclerosis

Even though the earliest description of MS in 1849 involved lesions of the spinal cord, most of the initial literature about MRI in MS focused on the intracranial findings. Clinically it is estimated that one-third of MS patients exhibit spinal symptoms only, although it is most common that symptoms and signs indicate a mixed form of the disease, that is, involving cerebrum, cerebellum, optic nerves, brain stem, and spinal cord.[15]

On gross pathologic examination of the spinal cord in MS patients, the great majority show evidence of disease regardless of the clinical history, and indeed, the extent of involvement usually far exceeds that which would be suspected by the patient's history. The lesions in the cord demonstrate no particular functional correlation with topographic localization, except that it is generally recognized that the cervical spinal cord is twice as likely to be involved than the lower levels.[15] Lesions within the cord are usually firm and brittle, and there is often gross atrophy with disseminated superficial patches of disease along the entire length. Histologically, the early lesions are characterized by fragmentation of myelin, axonal preservation, and microglial proliferation. In the following weeks, the loss of myelin and oligodendrocytes becomes

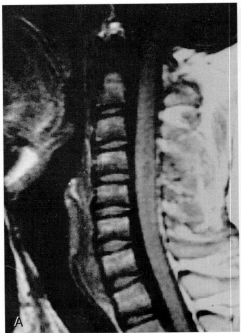
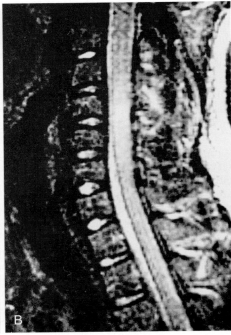

FIGURE 39–2 Acute transverse myelitis in a 30-year-old man. *A,* Sagittal T1-weighted image demonstrates an area of low intensity in the cervical cord. *B,* Sagittal T2-weighted image demonstrates diffuse high signal intensity in the cervical and upper thoracic cords.

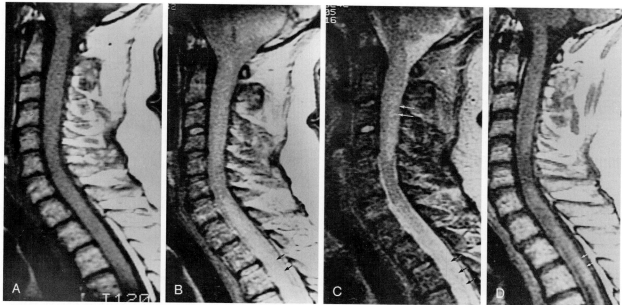

FIGURE 39–3 Inflammatory myelitis in 28-year-old woman with acutely progressive arm and truncal numbness, inability to walk, and urinary and fecal incontinence. *A,* Sagittal T1-weighted image demonstrates expansion of the cervical and upper thoracic cords. *B* and *C,* Sagittal proton and T2-weighted images demonstrate areas of high signal intensity in the cervical and upper thoracic cords *(arrows)* separated by an area of normal signal intensity at the C5 and C6 levels. *D,* Postgadolinium sagittal T1-weighted image demonstrates enhancement of the cervical and thoracic cords separated *(arrows)* by a nonenhancing area at the C6 level. Open biopsy demonstrates inflammatory myelitis without a syrinx. (*A–D,* From B Gero, G Sze, H Sharif. MR imaging of intradural inflammatory diseases of the spine. AJNR 1991;12[5]:1009–1019, © by American Society of Neuroradiology.)

total, neutral fat can be demonstrated free and within macrophages, and there is marked proliferation of astrocytes with perivascular inflammation. If the plaques involve the gray matter, there is a striking preservation of the neuronal cell bodies.

Several months later, fibrillary gliosis is established. In the very old plaques, there is evidence of wallerian degeneration, especially in the long tracts of the spinal cord. Iron deposition has been demonstrated at the edge of the plaques.[15] The significance of this histologic finding is uncertain in regard to its correlate on MRI, but it may explain some foci of low intensity on T2-weighted images.

The correlation between the clinical symptoms and the MS plaques is not fully understood. Experimental studies suggest that slowing of the nerve conduction after demyelination is probably the major factor in the symptoms of

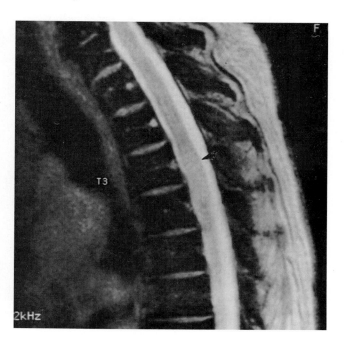

FIGURE 39–4 Transverse myelitis following flu vaccination. A 40-year-old woman developed an acute thoracic myelopathy 3 weeks after a flu vaccination. A sagittal T2-weighted image demonstrates mild cord swelling as an area of increased signal in the midthoracic cord *(arrow).* (Courtesy of Dr. W. Olane, Washington, DC.)

MS. Occasionally, MS is clinically silent and discovered unexpectedly at necropsy.[15]

MS lesions in the cord appear as areas of increased signal intensity on T2-weighted images[16, 17] with or without corresponding areas of low intensity on T1-weighted images (Fig. 39–5). These lesions may be seen in the absence of morphologic changes on T1-weighted images (Fig. 39–5) or be associated at the acute phase with swelling of the cord that can mimic an intramedullary neoplasm. In the late stages the cord may become atrophic (Fig. 39–6). Gadolinium enhancement seems to correlate with active disease.[16] One-third of patients with MS presenting clinically with myelopathy have no associated periventricular lesions on brain MRI (Fig. 39–7). Furthermore, a normal brain or spinal cord MRI does not exclude the diagnosis of MS, which is made clinically according to specific criteria,[18] requiring neurologic symptoms involving multiple areas of the nervous system or neurologic episodes at different separations in time, or both.

Acute Disseminated Encephalomyelitis

The term *acute disseminated encephalomyelitis* can be used to refer collectively to a group of inflammatory demyelinating diseases that share pathologic features and a clinical course. These entities show multiple foci of inflammation that involve perivenous regions of white matter and are accompanied by perivenous and subpial demyelination.[15] Clinically, these diseases are severe and sometimes fatal and usually relate to prior viral illness or vaccination. The basis of the inflammatory response and subsequent demyelination is thought to be an autoimmune phenomenon. When severe hemorrhagic necrosis is identified as a major component, the disease is referred to as *acute hemorrhagic leukoencephalopathy*, and a rapid progression to a fatal outcome is usual. The disease is clinically differentiated from MS by its clinical monophasic course, unlike MS, which classically has periods of exacerbation and remission. If the patients recover, there is usually no further neurologic deficit; however, there may be a fatal outcome.

MRI findings in cases of spinal involvement are nonspecific and indistinguishable from those of other myelitides. Hemorrhage may occur in the more severe forms, although it is not specific. In fact, the presence of a mass lesion in the spinal cord with hemorrhage in the absence of trauma would most likely represent an intramedullary neoplasm unless the classic history of a viral illness occurring 10 days to 2 weeks previously could be elicited.

Radiation Myelopathy

Radiation myelopathy is an uncommon complication of radiation therapy to lesions of the spine or adjacent tissues when the treatment plan does not allow protection of the spinal cord, such as radiation for nasopharyngeal carcinoma. The incidence of radiation myelopathy correlates positively with the total radiation dose, dose per fraction, and length of the spinal cord irradiated. The incidence of radiation myelopathy after radiotherapy for nasopharyngeal carcinoma is estimated to be between 1% and 10%. A 50% incidence of radiation myelopathy may be expected when the cord receives between 68 and 73 Gy and only 5% when the cord receives between 57 and 61 Gy.[19] The latent period of radiation myelopathy has two distinctive peaks, one at 12 to 14 months and the other at 24 to 28 months, and the latent periods decrease with an increasing dose.[20] The histopathologic appearance of radiation myelopathy can be classified as primarily white

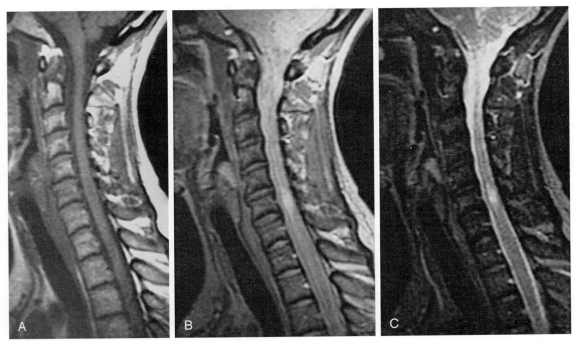

FIGURE 39–5 Multiple sclerosis. *A,* Sagittal T1-weighted image is normal. Notice the focal increase in the signal intensity of the cord at the C6 level in the sagittal proton density (*B*) and the T2-weighted (*C*) images.

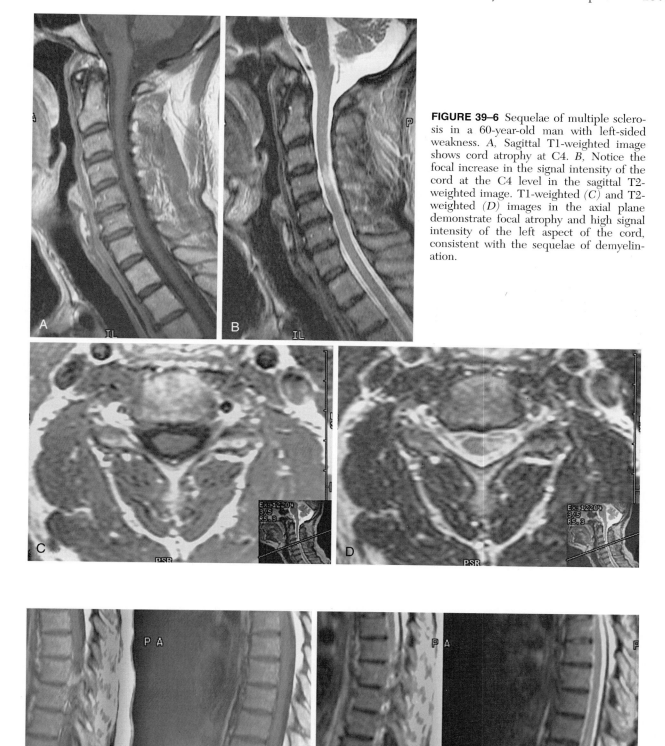

FIGURE 39–6 Sequelae of multiple sclerosis in a 60-year-old man with left-sided weakness. *A,* Sagittal T1-weighted image shows cord atrophy at C4. *B,* Notice the focal increase in the signal intensity of the cord at the C4 level in the sagittal T2-weighted image. T1-weighted *(C)* and T2-weighted *(D)* images in the axial plane demonstrate focal atrophy and high signal intensity of the left aspect of the cord, consistent with the sequelae of demyelination.

FIGURE 39–7 Multiple sclerosis in a 55-year-old woman with acute lower extremity weakness and numbness 30 years after an episode of optic neuritis. *A,* Sagittal T1-weighted image results are normal. *B,* Sagittal T2-weighted image. Notice the focal increase in the signal intensity of the lower thoracic cord. Brain magnetic resonance imaging (not shown) demonstrated optic atrophy correlating with the pallor of the optic nerve seen at funduscopic examination but no periventricular hyperintense lesions.

matter parenchymal lesions, primary vascular lesions, or a combination of vascular and white matter lesions. The white matter lesions and the combination of vascular and white matter lesions have the shorter latent period corresponding to the earliest peak at 12 to 14 months, whereas the vascular lesions are associated with a longer latent period corresponding to the second peak, 24 to 28 months. Pathologic studies in experimental rabbit models reveal demyelination, focal astrocytosis, erythrodiapedesis, and perineuronal edema. In autopsy studies the typical histopathologic finding associated with radiation myelopathy is leukomalacia. The gray matter is rarely involved, and never is it involved to the exclusion of the white matter.

Treatment for radiation myelopathy has been disappointing. Steroids have been helpful in some patients.

A spectrum of MRI findings has been described in patients with radiation myelopathy.[20, 21] There is no correlation between the MRI findings and the latency of radiation myelopathy; however, there appears to be a correlation between the time of MRI after the onset of symptoms and the MRI findings. Within less than 8 months after the onset of symptoms, MRI demonstrated low intensity on T1- and high intensity on T2-weighted images in a long segment of the cervical cord. Swelling of the cord or focal enhancement after contrast administration (Fig. 39–8) or both may also be seen. Imaging longer than 3 years after the onset of symptoms usually reveals atrophy of the cord. The diagnosis of radiation myelopathy remains a diagnosis of exclusion. MRI is extremely helpful in excluding tumor recurrence or carcino-

matous meningitis. Chemotherapy-induced myelitis should also be considered in the appropriate clinical context. Occasionally it may not be possible to ascribe a single cause to a treatment-related myelopathy in cancer patients.

Sarcoidosis

Sarcoidosis is a multisystem disease of unknown cause characterized by noncaseating granulomas. Young adults are most frequently affected, usually presenting with pulmonary symptoms. Bone involvement, seen in 1% to 13% of cases in various series, is usually late and commonly associated with cutaneous lesions. The tubular bones of the hand and feet are most often involved. Sarcoidosis of the vertebral bodies (Fig. 39–9) is rare, with only 20 cases reported in a recent review. The thoracolumbar spine region is affected most commonly. Typically, plain radiographs and computed tomographic scans reveal lytic lesions with variable regions of surrounding sclerosis involving single multiple bones.[22] Sclerotic lesions have also been reported.[23] An associated paraspinal mass may be present, and disk space involvement is rare. These findings usually suggest tuberculosis or a neoplasm. When the disk is involved,[24] pyogenic diskitis is the most common diagnosis. Biopsy is necessary for a definitive diagnosis.

Clinical involvement of the central nervous system occurs in 5% of patients with sarcoidosis. Primary involvement of the spinal cord is very rare, with only 72 cases reported in the literature in a recent review article.[25] In two-thirds of the cases, the diagnosis was not known before the onset of symptoms. Thirty-five percent of cases showed intramedullary (Fig. 39–10) and extramedullary involvement, respectively, and involvement of both was present in 23%. Gadolinium-MRI is extremely helpful and may actually suggest the diagnosis if, in addition to areas of intramedullary enhancement, pial enhancement is demonstrated. However, pial enhancement is not specific and may be seen in tuberculous, toxoplasmic, or human immunodeficiency–related meningitis,[26] leptomeningeal metastasis,[27] and postshunting meningeal fibrosis.

Behçet's Syndrome

Behçet's syndrome is characterized by recurrent ulcerations of the mouth and genitalia accompanied by uveitis or iridocyclitis, but 20% to 30% of the patients may have a disseminated central nervous system disease affecting the brain and spinal cord. Because of the diversity of the lesions, the condition may simulate MS. The neuropathology is that of multifocal necrotizing lesions with marked inflammatory cell reactions. In addition, necrosis may affect the gray and white matter, probably secondary to vasculitis.[28]

Necrotizing Myelopathy

Necrotizing myelopathy is a pathologic condition characterized by coagulative necrosis and thickening and hyalinization of the vascular walls.[29] The most common cause is

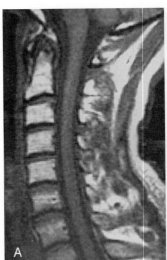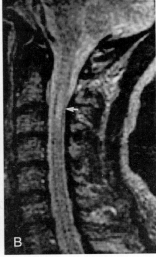

FIGURE 39–8 Radiation myelopathy. A 60-year-old man presented with cervical myelopathy 2 years after radiation therapy for laryngeal cancer. *A,* Sagittal T1-weighted image demonstrates increased signal intensity in the upper cervical vertebral bodies consistent with postradiation changes. No definite abnormalities are noted in the cord. *B,* Sagittal T2-weighted image demonstrates a focus of high signal intensity in the upper cervical cord at the C2–C3 level *(arrow).* (*A* and *B,* From Mark AS. Infectious and inflammatory diseases of the spine. In Atlas SW [ed]. Magnetic Resonance of the Brain and Spine, 2nd ed., p. 1216. Philadelphia, Lippincott-Raven, 1996.)

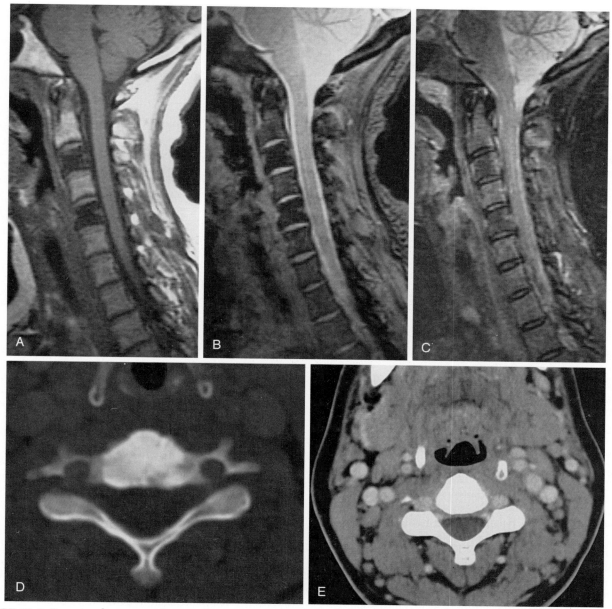

FIGURE 39–9 Bony involvement with sarcoidosis in a 30-year-old woman with neck pain and night sweats. Prior cervical node biopsy revealed sarcoidosis. Sagittal T1-weighted *(A),* T2°-weighted *(B),* and T2-weighted *(C)* images of the cervical spine demonstrate nonspecific homogeneous low signal intensity of the C3 and C5 vertebral bodies. *D,* Computed tomography (CT) through C3 demonstrates diffuse sclerosis of the vertebral body. *E,* Soft tissue windows demonstrate multiple small nodes. Computed tomography (CT)–guided biopsy of C5 revealed noncaseating granulomas compatible with sarcoidosis.

venous hypertension[30] in the medullary veins secondary to a dural arteriovenous fistula. Factors predisposed to its development include hypercoagulability, migratory thrombophlebitis, and polycythemia. The condition corresponds to the description by Foix and Alajouanine[31] and has been given a variety of names including *subacute necrotic myelitis.*

Although most commonly secondary to a dural fistula, necrotizing myelopathy is also associated with inflammatory and demyelinating conditions such as MS, acute disseminating encephalomyelitis, varicella-zoster mumps,[3] rubeola, infectious mononucleosis, systemic lupus erythe-

matosus,[7] pulmonary tuberculosis,[32] and clioquinol intoxication.[33]

In 15% to 20% of patients with systemic lupus erythematosus, the myelopathy is the presenting feature. Typically, the course of the illness is rapidly progressive and characterized by remissions and relapses. The most common segment of the spinal cord to be affected is the thoracic level,[34] but in one-quarter of the patients the cervical spine is involved. Pathologically, the lesions consist of one or more foci of subtle coagulative or liquefactive necrosis, although on occasion circumferentially distributed pallor of the white matter with ballooning

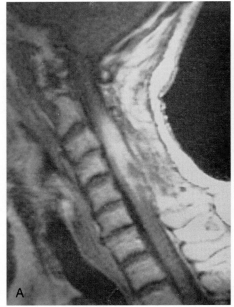
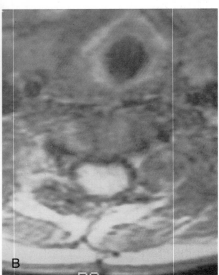

FIGURE 39–10 Intramedullary sarcoidosis in a 54-year-old woman with progressive myelopathy. Sagittal *(A)* and axial *(B)* T1-weighted postcontrast images demonstrate an enhancing intramedullary mass indistinguishable from a glioma. (*A* and *B*, From Mark AS. Infectious and inflammatory diseases of the spine. In Atlas SW [ed]. Magnetic Resonance of the Brain and Spine, 2nd ed., p. 1217. Philadelphia, Lippincott-Raven, 1996.)

degeneration of the myelin sheath and destruction of the axons has been described. The pathogenesis is not fully understood, but the presence of antiphospholipid antibodies has been implicated.[35] Lupus vasculitis is distinctly uncommon.[36]

A paraneoplastic necrotizing myelopathy not associated with radiation therapy, cord compression, or tumor infiltration has also been described.[37] The condition is associated with a variety of neoplasms, most commonly bronchopulmonary carcinoma and lymphoma.[38] It is characterized pathologically by massive or patchy multifocal areas of coagulative necrosis in both the gray and the white matter with a paucity of inflammatory cells. The pathogenesis is unknown, but two such cases have been associated with the presence of herpesvirus type II.[39] Finally, in a number of cases, no specific cause for the necrotic myelopathy can be determined. The MRI findings in patients with necrotic myelopathy have been described. As expected, the findings were nonspecific with diffuse areas of increased signal intensity on T2-weighted images and decreased signal intensity on T1-weighted images with variable enhancement on postcontrast studies.[41]

The similar MRI appearance of most inflammatory and demyelinating diseases of the spine probably reflects the limited number of responses to a variety of insults that the spinal cord can mount. Most of these responses macroscopically result in increased water concentration responsible for the increased signal intensity on T2-weighted images and occasionally disruption of the cord-blood barrier responsible for enhancement. The confusion caused by the noninflammatory necrotizing myelopathy is attributable to our lack of knowledge of the pathogenesis of most of the disorders and the difficulty of access to adequate amount of tissue for diagnostic purposes.

From a practical point of view, when enlargement of the cord and an increase in the signal intensity on T2-weighted images with or without enhancement is demonstrated on MRI in a patient with an acute or subacute myelopathy, it is incumbent on the neuroradiologist to consider foremost the treatable causes of such a condition. It is imperative to exclude a dural vascular malformation by scrutinizing the posterior subarachnoid space for dilated vessels. In difficult cases, myelography with the patient supine may be helpful in planning the site for spinal angiography. Treatable infectious myelitides such as bacterial, that is, pyogenic, syphilitic, or Lyme disease, should be excluded. Finally, noninfectious inflammatory conditions such as MS and lupus that may respond to steroid treatment should be considered. It has been suggested that the pattern of enhancement may be somewhat helpful in the differential diagnosis of various spinal cord lesions.[41] Focal nodular areas of enhancement have been associated with granulomatous conditions such as tuberculosis, toxoplasmosis, or other fungal infections. Diffuse areas of abnormal signal intensity or enhancement or both have been associated with viral infections or inflammatory or demyelinating processes or both.

INFECTIONS

Infections of the spine can be separated into infections of the vertebral bodies and disks, epidural spaces, intradural spaces, and the cord itself.

Pathophysiology of Spinal Infections

Hematogenous Spread

Hematogenous spread of infection to the vertebral body can occur by arterial or venous routes. The initial suggestion that Batson's plexus served as the principal route of infection has been refuted. It has been shown through selective retrograde injection in both human and rabbit cadavers that the bony vertebral tributaries of Batson's plexus are too small, and the injection could be achieved only with considerable pressure. Injection into the arterial nutrient vessels is much easier and demonstrates a rich vascular network. The lack of associated meningitis and extradural thrombophlebitis in patients with osteomyelitis suggests that the venous route of infection is very unlikely and hematogenous spread via the arterial route is the primary mechanism of osteomyelitis.[44]

In children, because of the richly vascularized end plate, the infection starts in the end plate and disk, resulting in "diskitis."[43] In adults, the blood supply to the intervertebral disk disappears and the primary site of infection becomes the vertebral body, particularly the metaphyseal area close to the anterior longitudinal ligament.[44] From there the infection can spread in a subligamentous fashion or extend to the disk and involve the adjacent vertebral body. Most disk space infections are limited to one interspace and adjacent vertebral body. Approximately 25% involve more than one level. A primary source of infection can be found in approximately 50% of patients, with the most common sources in the skin, upper respiratory tract, and genitourinary tract.

Contiguous Spread

Contiguous spread of vertebral and disk infection can result from soft tissue infection such as psoas abscess, decubitus ulcer, or paravertebral abscess. Tuberculous and fungal infections most frequently extend from the spine to the adjacent soft tissues and from there may extend in a subligamentous fashion to other vertebral bodies. Direct inoculation can result during surgical procedures or diagnostic invasive procedures such as diskograms or lumbar punctures. Postdisk surgery infections can also occur.

Infections Due to Specific Agents

Pyogenic Infections

Vertebral Osteomyelitis and Diskitis

Pyogenic infections of the spine involve primarily the disk space in children and the vertebral bodies in adults. Adults in the sixth and seventh decades are more frequently affected, and men are affected twice as often as women. The lumbar spine is most frequently involved. Most cases of juvenile diskitis occur in children younger than 2 years; they are more common in girls than in boys and are usually self-limited.[45] *Staphylococcus aureus* accounts for 60% of adult infection. *Escherichia coli,* *Pseudomonas aeruginosa,* and *Klebsiella* account for another 30%. *Salmonella* osteomyelitis is seen with increasing frequency in patients with sickle cell disease. The patient's symptoms often precede the radiographic findings by several weeks. Paraplegia develops in less than 1% of patients with osteomyelitis. Cultures of the disk material obtained by needle biopsy are negative in 50% to 70% of patients.

The MRI findings of diskitis and osteomyelitis closely match the pathologic findings.[46] The signal alterations reflect the early inflammatory response characterized by infiltration of polymorphonuclear leukocytes and fibrin deposition in the adjacent end plates. Bony destruction secondary to lytic enzymes and the associated increased

water content are reflected by the increased signal intensity on T2-weighted images and decreased signal intensity on T1-weighted images. The signal alterations often precede the destructive changes.[47–50]

The aim of any imaging modality is to make the diagnosis as early as possible.[51] Even though MRI is the most sensitive technique, the findings may lag behind the clinical symptoms of severe back pain. When the diagnosis is uncertain, a follow-up MRI in 1 week may be helpful to show the evolution of early changes.

In the same way the MRI findings lag behind the early signs of disk space infection, the MRI findings also lag in the healing phase of vertebral osteomyelitis. Once adequate antibiotic treatment has been instituted, the clinical symptoms improve dramatically, whereas the MRI findings evolve much more slowly (Fig. 39–11). The findings of healing osteomyelitis include persistent disk space narrowing, decreased signal intensity of the disk on T2-weighted images consistent with disk degeneration, fusion of the adjacent vertebral bodies, and resolution of the high signal intensity in the adjacent end plates corresponding to resolution of the edema. If an epidural abscess was present (see following section), the epidural space also returns to normal. Thus, in the early stages of treatment, laboratory findings such as sedimentation rate and white count are more helpful in monitoring the response to treatment than the MRI findings.

A number of conditions other than diskitis can produce similar changes and should be considered in the differential diagnosis. Modic and associates[52] have described three types of degenerative changes in the vertebral end plates secondary to degenerative changes. Type I changes are characterized by low signal intensity on T1-weighted images and high signal intensity on T2-weighted images that can mimic infection. The histologic correlation demonstrates fissures of the vertebral end plates with the presence of fibrous granulation tissue richly vascularized as confirmed by the increase in the signal intensity after gadolinium injection. A degenerated disk can also enhance even in its central portion or in the periphery adjacent to the vertebral end plates. However, the disk is usually of low signal intensity on T2-weighted images. A follow-up study in several weeks should demonstrate no change, in contrast to the changes of diskitis, which progresses. The type II and type III changes have signal characteristics that can easily be differentiated from diskitis and osteomyelitis.

Patients with osteomalacia secondary to renal osteodystrophy can present with noninfectious disk space erosions and partial collapse of the adjacent vertebral bodies mimicking an aggressive osteomyelitis. This condition is particularly worrisome since patients with renal osteodystrophy are at increased risk for infection. The disease most commonly affects the cervical spine. In dialysis-associated spondyloarthropathy, the vertebral bodies and end plates tend to be hypointense both on T1- and T2-weighted images, in contrast to the hyperintense end plates on T2-weighted images associated with diskitis.[53] In this setting, disk space aspiration or vertebral biopsy, or both, are often necessary to exclude infection. However, as mentioned, the yield of the aspiration is quite low.

Patients with ankylosing spondylitis may develop pseu-

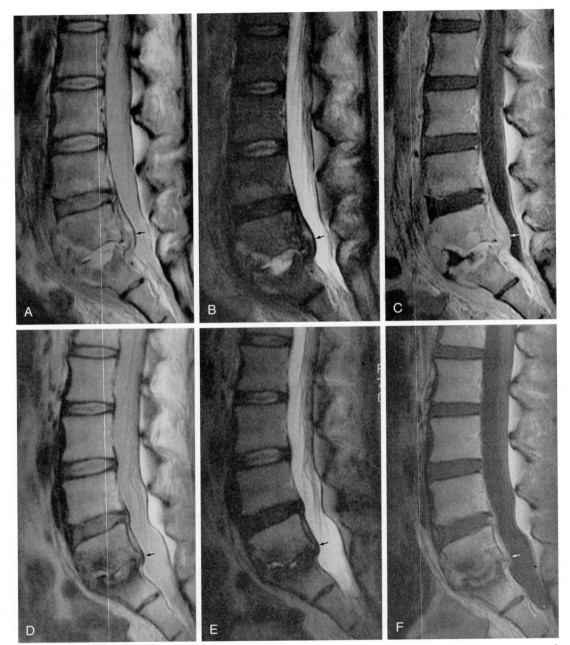

FIGURE 39–11 Evolution of diskitis following therapy. A 55-year-old woman with no infectious risk factors presented with severe low back pain. *A* and *B*, Sagittal proton density and T2-weighted images demonstrate typical findings of L5–S1 diskitis and a large epidural mass suggesting epidural abscess *(arrow)*. *C*, Postgadolinium T1-weighted image demonstrates no area of low intensity in the epidural mass to suggest pus. This appearance is more suggestive of granulation tissue. Sagittal proton density *(D)*, T2-weighted *(E)*, and sagittal postcontrast T1-weighted *(F)* images after antibiotic treatment demonstrate almost complete resolution of the disk infection and epidural granulation *(arrow)*. Notice the complete loss of disk height with fusion of the L4–L5 vertebral body. The patient was asymptomatic. *(A–F,* From Mark AS. Infectious and inflammatory diseases of the spine. In Atlas SW [ed]. Magnetic Resonance of the Brain and Spine, 2nd ed., p. 1224. Philadelphia, Lippincott-Raven, 1996.)

doarthrosis, which can mimic an infectious diskitis by MRI.[54] Again, follow-up MRI may help differentiate these two conditions.

Postoperative diskitis occurs in 0.75% to 2.8% of post-diskectomy patients in various series.[55, 56] The cause is assumed to be direct inoculation of the avascular disk space. *S. aureus* is the most frequent recovered pathogen,

but in many cases no organism is recovered, suggesting an alternative inflammatory disk process in some cases. When the postoperative findings in asymptomatic patients undergoing diskectomy are compared with those in patients who developed postoperative diskitis,[57] there is some overlap in the disk space abnormalities and adjacent bone marrow abnormalities between the normal and the abnormal groups, but the most reliable MRI finding of postoperative diskitis is the decrease in the signal intensity of adjacent vertebral bone marrow on T1-weighted images followed by enhancement of the same areas on postcontrast images. The marrow enhancement appears as a homogeneous horizontal band on either side of the disk space. Unenhanced T2-weighted sequences are less reliable since they are not present in the bone marrow of some patients with diskitis. Enhancement of the annulus fibrosus is an unreliable finding. High signal intensity on T2-weighted images developing in a previously dehydrated disk is also a useful finding suggesting diskitis.

Epidural Abscess

Acute epidural abscess is the result of direct hematogenous seeding of the epidural space from a cutaneous, pulmonary, or urinary tract source. The most common agent is *S. aureus*. Diabetes mellitus and immunosuppression are predisposing factors. The symptoms depend on the level of the infection. Epidural abscess may result in compression of the cord in the cervical and thoracic regions and thecal sac compression with cauda equina syndrome in the lumbar spine (Fig. 39–12). Thrombophlebitis of the epidural veins or adjacent arteries may lead to infarction of the cord (Fig. 39–13). At surgery, frank pus is often encountered.[46] Chronic epidural abscess is often the result of diskitis and contains granulation tissue rather than frank pus. MRI is very helpful in the diagnosis of epidural abscess by demonstrating an extradural mass.[58] It also visualizes the extent of involvement and the degree of cord compression. Gadolinium is usually not necessary for the diagnosis but may be helpful in subtle cases[59-61] to distinguish epidural granulation tissue from a frank abscess. Epidural granulation tissue enhances homogeneously, whereas an epidural abscess enhances in the periphery and contains nonenhancing

pus in its center (Fig. 39–14).[62] This differentiation may be very useful in surgical planning.[63] Areas of signal void within the epidural collection suggest a gas-forming organism.[64] The infection often extends over several levels and may extend in the paraspinous soft tissues (Fig. 39–15).

Subdural and Intramedullary Abscesses

Subdural and intramedullary abscesses are extremely rare conditions secondary to hematogenous spread of the organism to these structures. The clinical presentation of subdural abscesses is similar to that of epidural abscess (Fig. 39–16). Intramedullary abscesses can cause back pain and present clinically like a transverse myelitis type.

An intramedullary abscess has been reported on gadolinium-enhanced MRI, appearing as a ring-enhancing intramedullary lesion with a slightly enlarged cord.[64a] We have also encountered an intramedullary abscess involving the entire cord probably representing an infected syrinx (Fig. 39–17).

Brucellosis

Brucellosis is a worldwide infection, endemic in the Midwest of the United States. The infection in humans follows the ingestion of unpasteurized milk. The organism penetrates the lymphatics from the gastrointestinal tract and spreads to the reticuloendothelial system. The bone involvement is rare and involves the lumbar spine.[65]

Even though both tuberculosis and brucellosis induce a granulomatous inflammatory reaction in the spine, certain distinguishing features often allow differentiation of the two conditions by MRI. Brucellosis has a predilection for the lower lumbar spine, whereas tuberculosis tends to favor the lower thoracic spine. In brucellosis the height of the vertebral bodies is usually preserved even though signal abnormalities are noted consistent with osteomyelitis. In tuberculosis the vertebral bodies are severely dam-

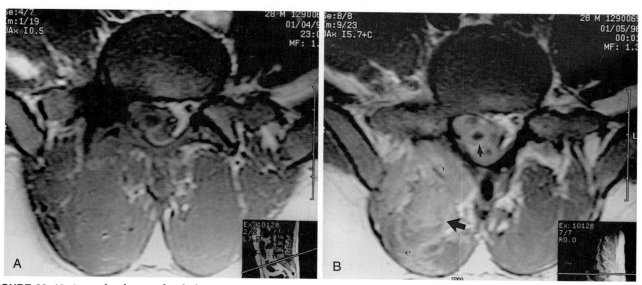

FIGURE 39–12 Acute lumbar epidural abscess in a man who is positive for the human immunodeficiency virus. Axial precontrast (*A*) and postcontrast (*B*) T1-weighted images demonstrate an anterior epidural collection (*small arrow*) in the lateral recess of S1 compressing the thecal sac and the right S1 root. Note the enhancement of the right paraspinous muscles (*large arrow*). Cultures of the aspirated material revealed *Staphylococcus aureus*.

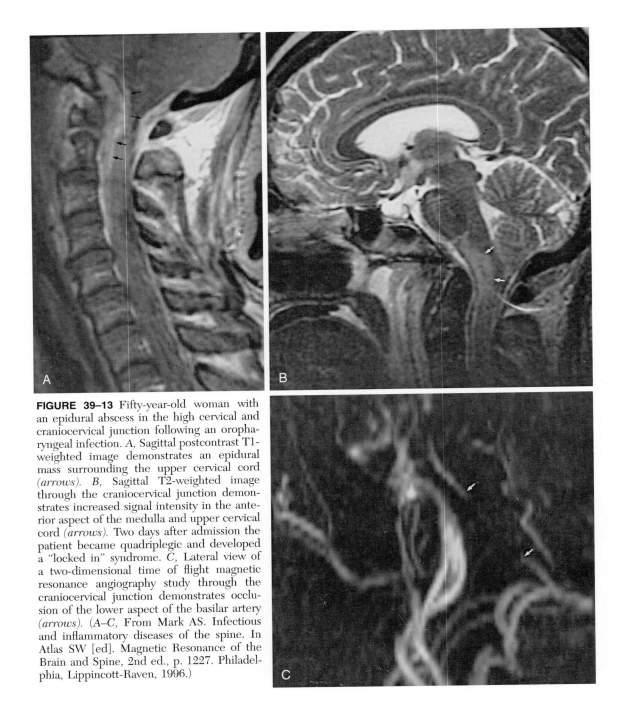

FIGURE 39–13 Fifty-year-old woman with an epidural abscess in the high cervical and craniocervical junction following an oropharyngeal infection. *A,* Sagittal postcontrast T1-weighted image demonstrates an epidural mass surrounding the upper cervical cord *(arrows). B,* Sagittal T2-weighted image through the craniocervical junction demonstrates increased signal intensity in the anterior aspect of the medulla and upper cervical cord *(arrows).* Two days after admission the patient became quadriplegic and developed a "locked in" syndrome. *C,* Lateral view of a two-dimensional time of flight magnetic resonance angiography study through the craniocervical junction demonstrates occlusion of the lower aspect of the basilar artery *(arrows). (A–C,* From Mark AS. Infectious and inflammatory diseases of the spine. In Atlas SW [ed]. Magnetic Resonance of the Brain and Spine, 2nd ed., p. 1227. Philadelphia, Lippincott-Raven, 1996.)

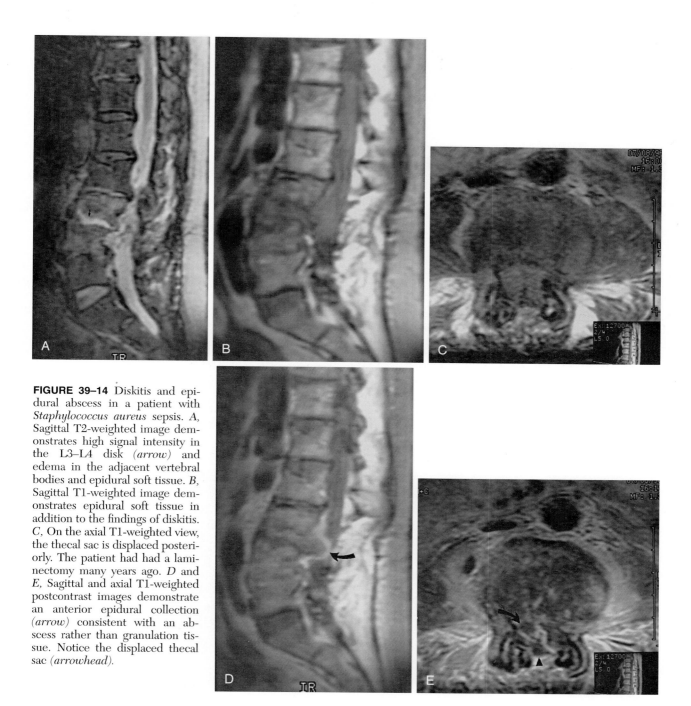

FIGURE 39–14 Diskitis and epidural abscess in a patient with *Staphylococcus aureus* sepsis. *A,* Sagittal T2-weighted image demonstrates high signal intensity in the L3–L4 disk *(arrow)* and edema in the adjacent vertebral bodies and epidural soft tissue. *B,* Sagittal T1-weighted image demonstrates epidural soft tissue in addition to the findings of diskitis. *C,* On the axial T1-weighted view, the thecal sac is displaced posteriorly. The patient had had a laminectomy many years ago. *D* and *E,* Sagittal and axial T1-weighted postcontrast images demonstrate an anterior epidural collection *(arrow)* consistent with an abscess rather than granulation tissue. Notice the displaced thecal sac *(arrowhead).*

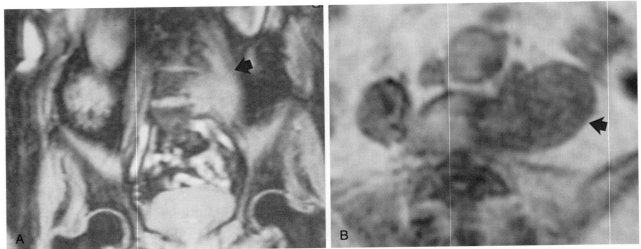

FIGURE 39–15 *Escherichia coli* osteomyelitis and psoas abscess. *A*, Coronal short-tau inversion recovery image demonstrates high signal intensity in the L3 and L4 vertebral bodies extending into a left psoas mass *(arrow)*. *B*, Axial T1-weighted image confirms these findings *(arrow)*.

aged with marked gibbus deformity. Brucellosis tends to spare the posterior elements, which may be affected by tuberculosis. The disk tends to be preserved in brucellosis, whereas it is severely destroyed by tuberculosis. Brucellosis rarely extends into the epidural space, whereas tuberculosis often extends to form epidural abscesses and involve the meninges. The paraspinous soft tissues are rarely affected by brucellosis and commonly affected by tuberculosis, which causes cold abscesses. Spinal deformities are very rare with brucellosis and common in tuberculosis. These radiographic findings enabled correct prediction of the type of infection in 94% of cases.[65] The imaging findings are important since the percutaneous

biopsy of the affected spinal region is of little use, because the organisms are very difficult to culture and the pathologic examination shows a nonspecific granulomatous reaction. The diagnosis is confirmed by positive serologic results or positive blood cultures or both.

Actinomycosis

Actinomycosis is caused by an anaerobic organism found normally in the mouth. It usually disseminates from the oral cavity in debilitated individuals. Osseous involvement results from contiguous extension of adjacent tissues, with the mandible and spine more commonly affected. The posterior elements of the spine and ribs can be affected,

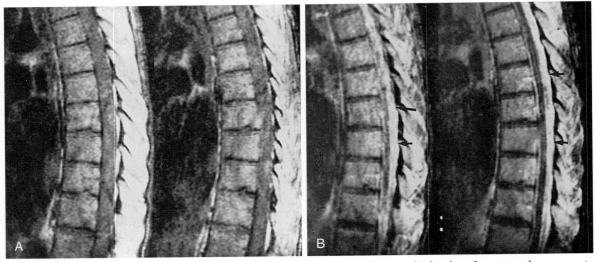

FIGURE 39–16 Enterococcal meningitis in a 26-year-old man with fever who subsequently developed sepsis and tetraparesis. Gram-positive cocci in the cerebrospinal fluid (CSF) smear and enterococci grown from blood confirmed enterococcal meningitis. Adjacent sagittal precontrast *(A)* and postcontrast *(B)* T1-weighted images of the thoracic spine. The precontrast image shows loss of the normal spinal cord–CSF interface and poor characterization of the type or location of the abnormality. On the postcontrast image, diffuse, thick, intradural enhancement *(arrows)* outlining the spinal cord locates the disease in the intradural extramedullary compartment. *(A* and *B,* From B Gero, G Sze, H Sharif. MR imaging of intradural inflammatory diseases of the spine. AJNR 1991;12[5]:1009–1019, © by American Society of Neuroradiology.)

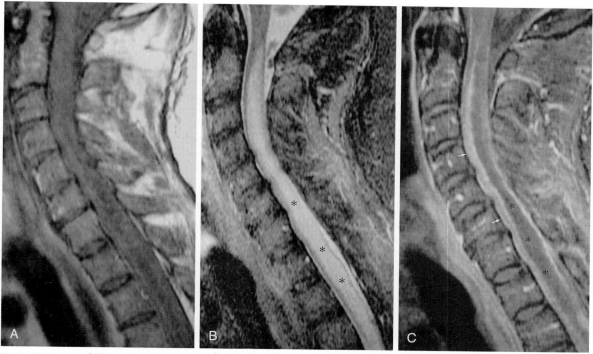

FIGURE 39–17 Intramedullary abscess in a 60-year-old man with long-standing paraplegia who became tetraplegic over 6 hours. *A,* Sagittal T1-weighted image demonstrates marked expansion of the cord. *B,* Sagittal T2-weighted view demonstrates diffuse hyperintensity of the cervical cord *(asterisks). C,* Postcontrast sagittal T1-weighted image demonstrates diffuse enhancement of the periphery of the cord *(arrows)* and a low-intensity center *(asterisks).* At surgery, the posterior columns were split open and pus was issuing from the central cavity. (*A–C,* From Mark AS. Infectious and inflammatory diseases of the spine. In Atlas SW [ed]. Magnetic Resonance of the Brain and Spine, 2nd ed., p. 1231. Philadelphia, Lippincott-Raven, 1996.)

and the association of such findings with sinus tracts should suggest the diagnosis.[44]

Syphilis

Syphilis caused by *Treponema pallidum* infection rarely affects the spine. Syphilitic transverse myelitis and polyradiculitis are rare manifestations of secondary syphilis. The disease is characterized pathologically by a plasmocytic infiltrate surrounding the vessels and affects primarily the meninges and the pia. The clinical manifestations are indistinguishable from those of transverse myelitis from any other cause.

MRI in patients with syphilitic myelitis has been reported.[41, 66] The precontrast images demonstrate a non-specific increase in the signal intensity of the cord on T2-weighted images. After contrast administration there is enhancement of the pia and of the spinal cord nerve roots. The lesions in one case resolved on follow-up imaging after adequate therapy with penicillin. The high-intensity area in the cord on T2-weighted images may reflect ischemic changes secondary to the severe vasculitis, which may lead to cord infarction.

Neuroborrelliosis (Lyme Disease)

Lyme disease is a tick-transmitted, spirochetal, infectious disease with multisystem inflammatory manifestations. It was first identified as a distinct entity in the United States in 1975[67] and is the most commonly reported vector-transmitted disease in the United States. The causative

organism, *Borrelia burgdorferi*, is transmitted by the nymph stage of infected ticks (*Ixodes dammini, Ixodes pacificus,* or *Ixodes ricinus*). These ticks are three-host organisms; in successive life stages, a tick may parasitize and infect a number of different animals, including mice, raccoons, and several other small mammals, in addition to deer, which is the preferred host and breeding ground for the adult ticks.

In most patients, the first evidence of Lyme disease is the appearance of a skin lesion, erythema chronicum migrans, at the site of a tick bite. Other signs and symptoms commonly associated with the early stage of Lyme disease include fever, chills, myalgias, arthralgias, headache, stiff neck, and exhaustion. Several weeks to a few months after the onset, most untreated patients have signs and symptoms of disseminated Lyme disease. In general, the sequence of organ involvement is predictable, but it can vary. Many patients do not seek treatment until late in the disease; therefore, initial clinical presentation with carditis, meningoencephalitis, or Lyme arthritis is not uncommon.

The neurologic manifestations of Lyme disease are variable[68] and may occur anytime from a few days after the onset of the disease to years later. In the United States, neurologic signs develop within the first few months of illness in 10% to 15% of persons not treated during the early stage of the disease. These include, in various combinations, meningitis, encephalitis, sensory and motor radiculoneuritis, and cranial neuritis. MRI may show enhancement of the leptomeninges and nerve roots as they exit the cord (Fig. 39–18). Lyme meningitis and encephalitis seem to be caused by direct borrelial infection of the central nervous system, and generally, appropriate antibiotic therapy is rapidly effective.

Listeriosis

Listeria monocytogenes commonly causes meningitis in the immunocompromised core host and less frequently brain or spinal cord abscesses. The disease may occur in individuals with occupational exposure to farm animals and occasionally in patients with no predisposing factors. The diagnosis is often difficult, and the organism is rarely identified from cerebrospinal fluid cultures but more commonly from blood cultures. In one case report,[69] an intramedullary *Listeria* abscess was demonstrated on MRI as an area of increased signal intensity on T2-weighted images and an elongated ring-enhancing lesion on postcontrast T1-weighted images.

Tuberculosis

Over the world, tuberculosis is the most common cause of vertebral body infection, in particular, in Third World countries. The current acquired immunodeficiency syndrome (AIDS) epidemic is responsible for a recrudescence of tuberculosis cases in the United States, particularly, spinal tuberculosis cases. Seventy-five percent of cases of tuberculous spondylitis occur in patients younger than 20 years. The involvement of the vertebral body occurs through hematogenous spread of *Mycobacterium tuberculosis* from a pulmonary source that may go unrecognized. Cord compression and neurologic deficit due to epidural extension occur in 10% to 20% of patients. These neurologic symptoms may be reversed more easily than in pyogenic infections. Infection usually starts anteriorly in the vertebral body and in 50% of cases spreads through the disk space to the adjacent vertebral body. Extension to distant vertebrae can occur secondary to subligamentous spread. The posterior elements are less frequently involved than in pyogenic or fungal infection. Massive bone destruction and severe gibbous deformity is characteristic

of this infection. Paraspinous masses that may calcify are also strongly suggestive of tuberculous abscess. Typical features on MRI include destruction of the anterior aspect of one or two vertebral bodies.[70] In the early stages, differentiation from pyogenic infection or a small neoplasm may be difficult (Figs. 39–19 and 39–20).

Tuberculous radiculomyelitis is most commonly a secondary tuberculous lesion, although it may rarely occur primarily. The disease may appear during the acute state of primary tuberculosis or in variable periods after the onset of the disease. Most patients with spinal radiculomyelitis secondary to tuberculosis are younger than 30 years, in contrast to those with the typical form of spinal arachnoiditis, which is usually seen in older patients. The clinical features of this condition include paraplegia and quadriplegia, pain, and other radicular symptoms depending on the site involved. The meninges of the cord show variable degrees of congestion and inflammatory exudates throughout their course. The spinal root and nerve roots are surrounded by gelatinous exudates and may be edematous. The tuberculoma may be located anywhere within the thecal sac. It is usually closely adherent to the inner aspect of the dura and may dig a crater in the cord, making it difficult to determine whether an intradural tuberculoma is extramedullary or intramedullary.[71] In the chronic stages, fibrin-covered roots stick to each other and to the thecal sac, forming dense collagen adhesions by proliferating fibrocytes.

Contrast-enhanced MRI is the imaging modality of choice. The study demonstrates enhancement of the dura arachnoid complex indicating the presence of active meningeal inflammation and may demonstrate the intramedullary tuberculoma as nodular areas of enhancement.[41, 72] Expansion of the cord with a diffuse increase in intensity on T2-weighted images may reflect cord edema without an intramedullary tuberculoma or infarction secondary to vasculitis or myelitis. During the chronic stages the roots and the thickened dura do not enhance, and these changes are difficult to distinguish from postsurgical or postpyogenic infectious arachnoiditis. *Mycobacterium avium-intracellulare* complex is a previously rare condi-

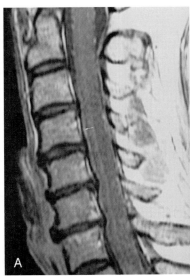
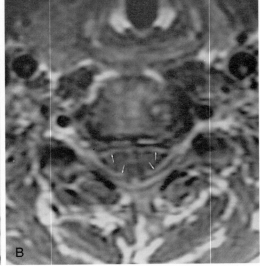

FIGURE 39–18 Lyme meningitis. *A,* Sagittal T1-weighted postcontrast image demonstrates pial enhancement *(arrow). B,* Axial postcontrast T1-weighted image demonstrates enhancement of the roots *(arrows). (A* and *B,* Courtesy of Dr. Monteferrante, Washington, DC.)

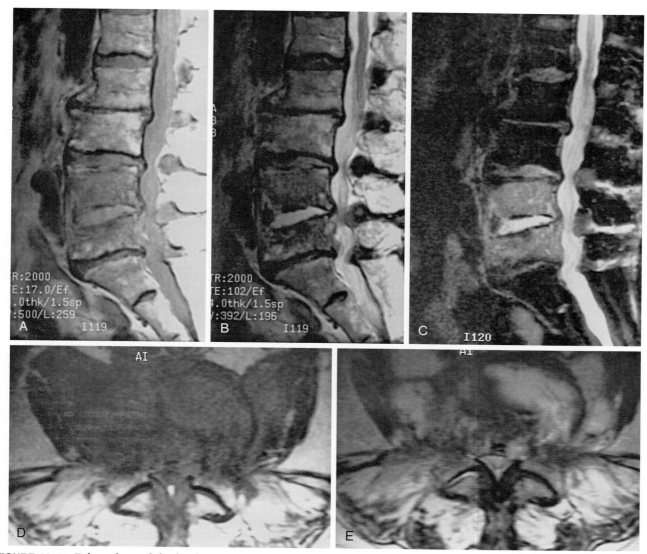

FIGURE 39–19 Tuberculosis of the lumbar spine. *A*, Sagittal T1-weighted image demonstrates widening of the L4–L5 disk that is due to the destruction of the adjacent endplates and decreased intensity of the adjacent vertebral body marrow. *B*, Sagittal T2-weighted image demonstrates increased signal intensity in the disk and adjacent vertebral bodies. *C*, Sagittal short-tau inversion recovery image demonstrates increased signal intensity in the disk and adjacent vertebral bodies to better advantage than the T2-weighted image. Axial T1-weighted (*D*) and T2-weighted (*E*) images at the L4–L5 level visualize bilateral psoas masses consistent with granulation tissue.

tion recently recognized with increased frequency among immunosuppressed patients, in particular patients infected with human immunodeficiency virus (HIV). The disease has been reported in up to 30% of patients infected with HIV and in 50% of patients who have AIDS. In addition to massive infiltration of the lymph nodes, the marrow may be diffusely infiltrated[73] with *Mycobacterium avium-intracellulare*, resulting in diffuse decreased intensity on T1-weighted images. This appearance is, however, nonspecific as it may be seen with any diffuse inflammatory or neoplastic process involving the marrow. Epidural extension of the *Mycobacterium avium-intracellulare* infection indistinguishable from other infections may be seen.

Fungal Infections

Fungal infections of the spine can be divided into two principal categories—those induced by pathogens, and those produced by saprophytes in patients who are immunosuppressed by conditions such as diabetes mellitus; leukemia; lymphoma; prolonged use of antibiotics or steroids; or HIV infection.[74] These infections are called *opportunistic* and include meningitis, the formation of abscesses and granulomas, and, because of the invasion of the walls of the vessels, thrombosis leading to cord infarction.

Blastomycosis

North American blastomycosis is caused by *Blastomyces dermatitides*. The disease is found in southern Africa, South America, and the southern, central, and mid-Atlantic states in the United States.[74] Disease is acquired by inhalation of spores, with bone involvement in about 50% of patients with systemic disease. The disease may both

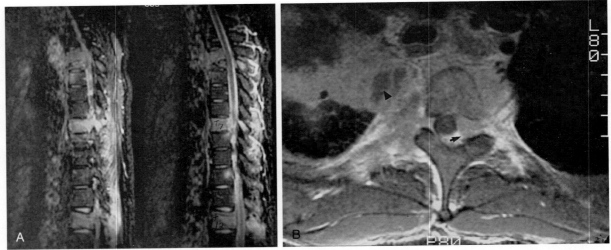

FIGURE 39–20 Tuberculosis involving multiple thoracic vertebral bodies. *A*, Sagittal T2-weighted image demonstrates multiple lesions of the thoracic vertebrae and posterior elements with a prevertebral soft tissue mass in the upper thoracic spine. *B*, Axial T1-weighted postcontrast image in the upper thoracic level confirms the prevertebral mass, which contains areas of low density *(arrowhead)* and a left epidural mass *(arrow)*. CT-guided biopsy confirmed the diagnosis. (Courtesy of Dr. J. Jelinek, Washington, DC.)

be a primary infection and occur as an opportunistic infection. In the nervous system, the disease can present as meningitis or as single or multiple abscesses. The meninges may be involved in the form of an extradural lesion that causes pachymeningitis leading to compression of the underlying cord. The fibropurulent exudates may result in obstruction of the cerebrospinal fluid flow of the foramen magnum and hydrocephalus. The prognosis is exceedingly poor.[74] The center of the abscess contains casseous necrotic material, neutrophils, and lymphocytes and is surrounded by epithelioid and multinucleated giant cells of the Langhans type. The fungus is identifiable in sections stained with hematoxylin and eosin.

The radiologic features are nonspecific and similar to those of tuberculosis.[75] The adjacent ribs are frequently involved.

Coccidioidomycosis

Coccidioidomycosis is caused by *Coccidioides immitis* and is endemic in the southwestern United States.[74] The primary focus is the lung. Osseous manifestation occurs in 10% to 50% of patients with disseminated disease.[76] The disease does not result in gibbous deformity. The MRI findings are nonspecific, and diagnosis is made by biopsy in a patient from an endemic area.

The disease is not an opportunistic infection. It usually causes a mild upper respiratory illness. In addition to the bone involvement, the central nervous system manifestation includes meningitis, primarily of the skull base, and granulomatous lesions may involve the spinal cord and the roots of the cauda.

Nocardiosis

Nocardia asteroides is the causative agent of this infection. It is an opportunistic parasite associated with patients who are immunosuppressed. The central nervous system is invaded from a primary pulmonary lesion. The disease results in an abscess or meningitis or both, and the spinal cord has been occasionally involved.[77]

Aspergillosis

Aspergillosis is ubiquitous, with over 350 species known, although the most common pathogen is *Aspergillus fumigatus*, consisting of branching septate hyphae with a diameter of 3 to 10 μm. It is estimated that 60% to 70% of patients with disseminated aspergillosis have neurologic lesions.[74] The disease may produce a granulomatous reaction but commonly results in abscess formation. The gross appearance is either that of a pale, soft area, sometimes with petechiae, or necrotic and hemorrhagic lesions with central cavitation. Histologically, the most striking feature is the intensity of the vascular invasion with thrombosis.

An aspergillus spinal cord abscess in an immunosuppressed patient has been described.[78] The lesion appeared as a nonspecific ring-enhancing medullary mass. An epidural abscess with cord compression secondary to aspergillosis has also been reported.[79]

Candidiasis

Candida albicans is a worldwide fungal opportunistic infection. The central nervous system is only occasionally involved by hematogenous dissemination, with primary focus in the respiratory gastrointestinal tract. The disease can occasionally occur in previously healthy individuals. The fungus usually produces a chain of elongated cylindric cells and oval buds. The early brain lesions described resemble hemorrhagic infarcts, with abscesses and granulomas without central foci of necrosis occurring later. The disease has been reported in the spinal cord[80] and may involve the disk space (Fig. 39–21).

Histoplasmosis

Histoplasmosis is caused by *Histoplasma capsulatum*, which can be isolated from soil contaminated by domestic

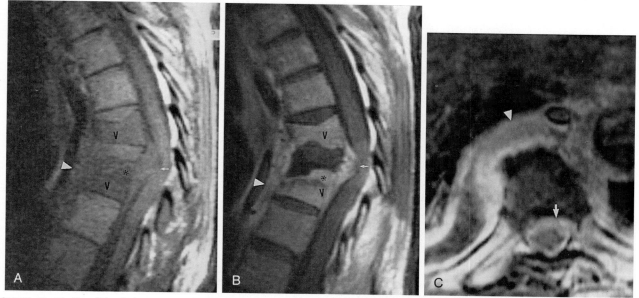

FIGURE 39–21 *Candida* diskitis in a 70-year-old diabetic man with back pain and paraplegia. *A,* Sagittal T1-weighted image demonstrates destruction of the disk, vertebral body *(asterisk),* and adjacent endplates (V) and a prevertebral mass *(arrowhead)* and an epidural mass compressing the cord *(arrow).* Postcontrast sagittal *(B)* and axial *(C)* T1-weighted images demonstrate the epidural mass to better advantage. (*A* and *B,* Courtesy of Dr. P. Baum, Sacramento, CA.)

and wild animals. Epidemics have occurred as a result of exposure to chicken, pigeon, and starling manure and bat guano. The disease is endemic in some regions of the United States such as the Ohio Valley and central Mississippi Valley. This disease may occur as an isolated benign infection or disseminated infection, which is usually due to reinfection involving the lungs. Involvement of the central nervous system is uncommon. A case of intramedullary *Histoplasma* granuloma has been reported.[81]

Parasitic Infections

Parasitic infections of the spine are uncommon but should be considered in endemic areas in patients with signs and symptoms of spine or spinal cord disease.

Cysticercosis

Cysticercosis is a worldwide disease particularly prevalent in South America and India. The disease has increased in frequency in the United States with an increase in the number of immigrants from these countries. The organism responsible for the disease is *Taenia solium,* a tapeworm. In the duodenum, the shells of the ova are dissolved and the embryos penetrate the wall of the intestine and are carried by the circulation to all organs, including occasionally the spine. In the central nervous system the cysts can take several forms. In most cases, they remain small and sequestered and eventually die. Less frequently, thin-walled racemose cysts develop in the subarachnoid space and basal cistern causing hydrocephalus in the brain or cord compression in the spine (Fig. 39–22).[82, 83] In the meninges the cysts appear as small, colorless structures adherent to the pia or floating freely in the subarachnoid space. Most subarachnoid racemose cysts are sterile. Intracerebral or intramedullary cysts[84, 85] are surrounded by a collagenous capsule produced by the host and elicit a

slight inflammatory reaction that becomes more evident after the death of the parasite.

Cryptococcosis

Cryptococcosis is caused by *Cryptococcus neoformans,* also known as *Torula histolytica,* which is harbored in fruit, milk, soil, and the manure of some birds. The disease has a worldwide distribution but is most commonly reported in southern parts of the United States and in Australia. The disease may develop in previously healthy individuals, but in 85% of patients it is an opportunistic infection. Although cryptococcal meningitis is extremely common in HIV-positive patients, cryptococcal spondylitis is a rare condition usually seen in immunosuppressed patients, occasionally reported in immunocompetent patients.[86] In a 1989 review of the literature, 11 documented cases were found up to 1989. In a report describing the MRI features of a case of cryptococcal spondylitis,[87] the findings were indistinguishable from those of tuberculous spondylitis with involvement of the vertebral body and extensive involvement of the posterior elements and paraspinous and perivertebral soft tissues with relative preservation of the disk (Fig. 39–23).

The central nervous system lesions consist primarily of meningitis involving the skull base and occasionally the spinal cord. In the acute cases, there is often very little inflammatory reaction with no meningeal enhancement.[74]

Schistosomiasis

Schistosoma mansoni and *Schistosoma haematobium* may rarely involve the spine. Four separate syndromes have been distinguished: medullary compression, acute transverse myelitis, granulomatous root involvement, and anterior spinal artery occlusion. Fifty-three histologically proven cases of spinal cord involvement by S. *mansoni*

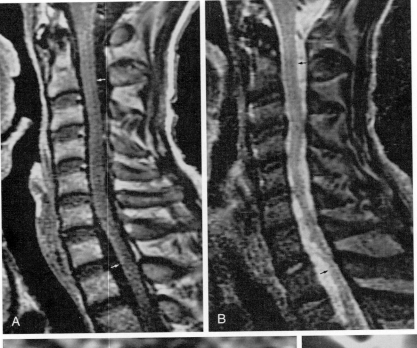

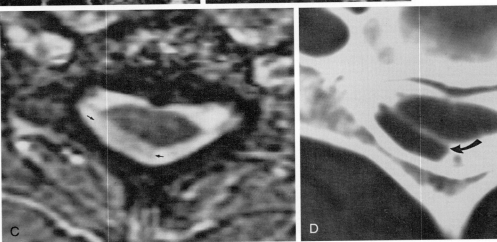

FIGURE 39–22 Extramedullary cervical spinal cysticercosis. Sagittal T1- *(A)* and T2-weighted *(B)* images demonstrate multiple subarachnoid lesions with signal intensity close to that of cerebrospinal fluid displacing the cord *(arrows)*. Axial T2-weighted image *(C)* demonstrates a subarachnoid mass *(arrows)*. Postmyelogram CT scan *(D)* shows the subarachnoid cysts to better advantage *(arrow)*. *(A–D, Courtesy of Dr. Sung Lee, Seoul, Korea.)*

and 15 cases involving *S. haematobium* have been reported.[88]

The disease involves the spine by extension from the inferior mesenteric venules or the perivesical venules. Host granulomatous reaction to the ova is the major factor in the pathogenesis of schistosomiasis. The importance of an early diagnosis is undermined by the relatively good response to praziquantel and steroids, which may reverse some of the symptoms early in the disease.

MRI reports of schistosomal myelitis secondary to *S. mansoni* infection revealed nonspecific enlargement of the lower thoracic spine and conus and increased signal intensity on the T2-weighted images (Fig. 39–24).[88, 89] After gadolinium administration, there was enhancement of the lower thoracic cord. Follow-up examination after treatment with praziquantel demonstrated resolution of these findings.

Granulomatous root involvement and medullary compression should also be easily demonstrated by MRI,

even though no reports have appeared. Occlusion of the anterior spinal artery may also result in enlargement of the spinal cord and increased signal intensity on long-TR sequences.

Echinococcosis

Hydatid disease in humans is caused by the larvae of *Echinococcus granulosus*. Humans may contract infection by direct contact with dogs or ingestion of food or drink containing the ova. After ingestion, the larvae have to penetrate through the liver barrier and then through the pulmonary capillaries to reach the systemic blood circulation, from which they can disseminate. Hydatid disease of the bone is, therefore, uncommon, encountered in between 0.5% and 4% of patients. The vertebrae are most commonly involved (44%), the long bones of the limbs in 28%, the pelvis and hip joints in 16%, the ribs and scapula in 8%, and the calvarium and phalanges in 4%. Unlike cysts in other parts of the body, hydatid

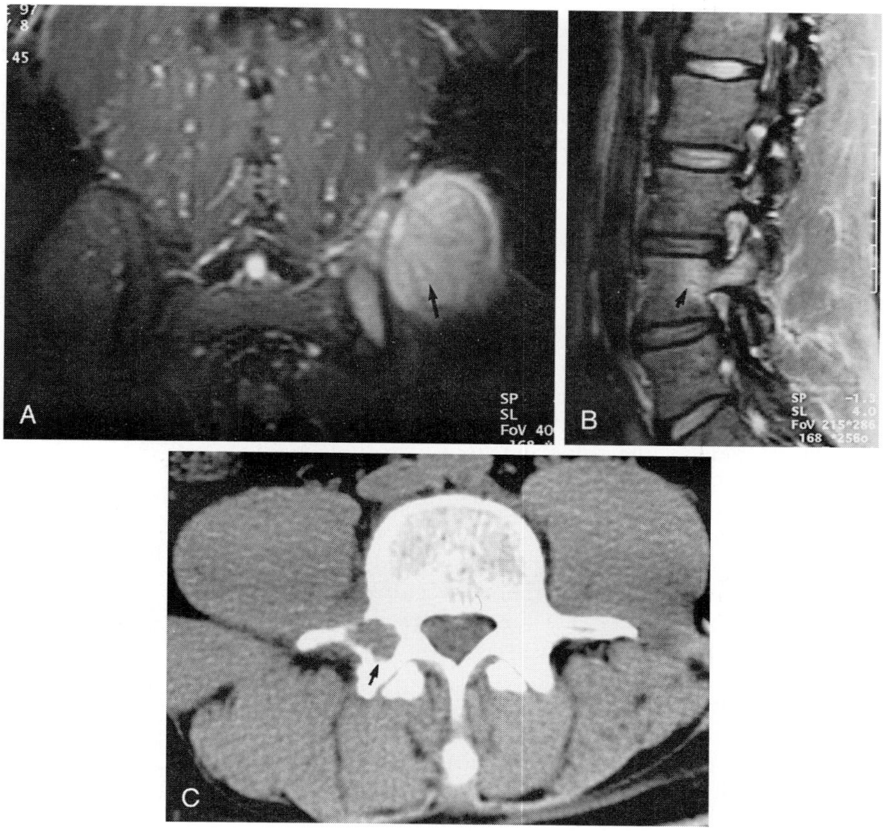

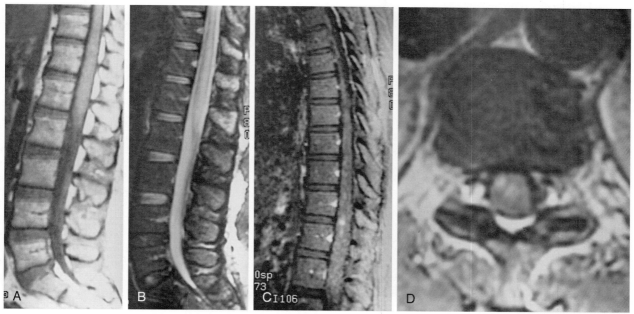

FIGURE 39–23 Cryptococcosis of the spine. *A,* Coronal short-tau inversion recovery image demonstrates a large left iliac soft tissue mass *(arrow)* extending into the left ilium. At surgery a Ewing sarcoma was found and the patient received chemotherapy. Several months later he complained of back pain. *B,* Sagittal T2-weighted image demonstrates abnormal signal in the L4 vertebral body and right pedicle *(arrow). C,* CT confirmed a lytic lesion *(arrow)* in the right L4 pedicle. Biopsy revealed *Cryptococcus.* (Courtesy of Dr. J. Jelinek, Washington, DC.)

disease is always multilocular. Within cancellous bone the parasite develops as multiple small cysts that grow along the path of least resistance and, with time, may destroy the cortex and extend into the adjacent soft tissues. The

differential diagnosis includes spinal tuberculosis, which may be difficult to distinguish preoperatively.

The plain radiographs show nonspecific bony destruction. MRI and computed tomography (CT) may demon-

FIGURE 39–24 Shistosomiasis due to *Shistosoma mansoni.* Sagittal T1- *(A)* and T2-weighted *(B)* precontrast images demonstrate nonspecific enlargement and hyperintensity in the conus. Postcontrast sagittal *(C)* and axial *(D)* T1-weighted images demonstrate enhancement of the conus. (Courtesy of Dr. S. Seltzer, Washington, DC.)

strate the massive bone destruction. The cysts on MRI demonstrate inhomogeneous low signal intensity on T1-weighted images and high intensity on T2-weighted images. The T2 measurements are not helpful in differentiating quiescent from active cysts. MRI may demonstrate the intradural extension to better advantage than CT (Fig. 39–25) without the need for subarachnoid contrast material.[90] CT is superior to MRI in demonstrating calcified lesions.

Sparganosis

Sparganosis is a rare infection caused by the migrating larvae of a tapeworm of the genus *Spirometra*. The majority of infections involve the subcutaneous soft tissues, and the organisms rarely invade the central nervous system. The involvement of the spine has been reported exceptionally.

In a case report,[91] the authors demonstrated effacement of the subarachnoid space on precontrast T1-weighted images and multiple subarachnoid enhancing nodules following the administration of contrast material. The diagnosis is made by a highly sensitive and specific enzyme-linked immunosorbent assay.

Toxoplasmosis

Toxoplasmosis is due to the infection with *Toxoplasma gondii* and is the most common focal infection of the brain in AIDS patients. Toxoplasmosis of the spinal cord is rare.[92] Two recent cases were reported by MRI.[93, 94] The lesions presented as a focally enhancing mass in the cord mimicking an intramedullary tumor. Pathologically, an eosinophilic and granulomatous reaction was noted on

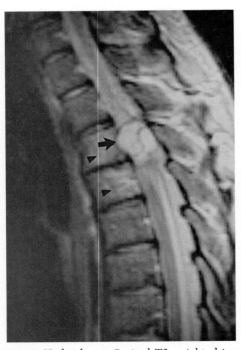

FIGURE 39–25 Hydatid cyst. Sagittal T2-weighted image demonstrates an extradural septated cystic mass (*arrow*) compressing the cord. Notice the reactive edema in the adjacent vertebral bodies (*arrowheads*). (Courtesy of Dr. Izet Rosanes, Istanbul.)

biopsy. The diagnosis may be considered in HIV-positive patients when the coexistence of an intramedullary mass and high serum *Toxoplasma* titers are noted. A therapeutic trial of anti-*Toxoplasma* medication may be warranted before biopsy.

Viral Diseases

Viruses may affect the spinal cord or the nerve roots. Some viral effects on the spinal cord were discussed in the sections on transverse myelitis and necrotic myelopathy. This section discusses some of the common viruses affecting the spine such as the herpes family of viruses and HIV.

Herpesvirus

The family of herpesviruses consists of a large group of double-stranded DNA viruses that includes herpes simplex virus type 1, herpes simplex virus type 2, cytomegalovirus, Epstein-Barr virus, varicella-zoster virus, B virus, herpesvirus 6, and herpesvirus 7. In addition to producing infection when the host initially acquires the virus, an important property shared by these viruses is the ability to produce latent infection and to be reactivated.

Although encephalitis is the most common manifestation, some herpesviruses may produce myelitis and polyradiculitis.

Myelitis associated with herpes zoster is an unusual complication.[95] The pathogenesis may involve a direct viral invasion of the spinal cord (Figs. 39–26 and 39–27),[96] a vasculitic process with ischemic necrosis, or an immunologic, parainfectious mechanism. The onset of the myelitis can occur weeks to months after an episode of herpes zoster. The lesions may regress after acyclovir treatment.[97]

Enhancement of the nerve roots may be seen in patients with herpes zoster radiculitis (Fig. 39–28).

Epstein-Barr Virus

Epstein-Barr virus is the cause of a common disease, infectious mononucleosis. Epstein-Barr virus has been associated with Guillain-Barré syndrome and transverse myelitis.[98]

Cytomegalovirus

Cytomegalovirus can cause HIV-related spinal polyradiculopathy (subacute progressive weakness, hyporeflexia, and mild sensory symptoms), which can be diagnosed with contrast-enhanced MRI. Enhancement of nerves and leptomeninges of the conus region can be identified (Fig. 39–29).[26, 99] Finally, cytomegalovirus infection has been incriminated as the cause of Guillain-Barré syndrome. Enhancement of the nerve roots of the cauda equina may also be seen in some patients with disk herniation.[100] It is commonly seen in normal patients when larger doses (0.3 mmol/kg) of Gd-DTPA are used. Some of the enhancing "roots" in the cauda equina may represent enhancement of radicular veins.[101] However, diffuse enhancement of the nerve roots is associated with inflammatory or neoplastic conditions and should be further evaluated by cerebrospinal fluid analysis.

Guillain-Barré Syndrome

Guillain-Barré syndrome, also known as *acute inflammatory demyelinating polyradiculoneuropathy*, is an ac-

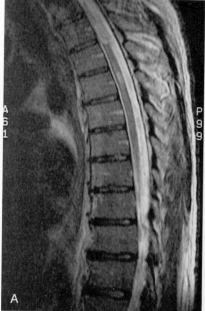
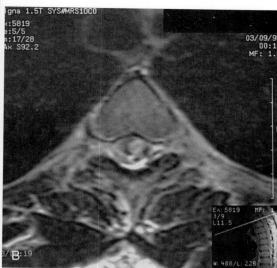

FIGURE 39–26 Herpes zoster myelitis in a 41-year-old man with progressive urinary retention and bilateral leg weakness. The patient had concomitant herpes zoster skin papules in some of the involved dermatomes. Sagittal *(A)* and axial T2-weighted *(B)* images demonstrate two foci of high intramedullary signal in the thoracic spine. Acyclovir therapy resulted in moderate clinical improvement. (*A* and *B*, From de Silva SM, Mark AS, Balish M, et al. Zoster myelitis: Improvement with antiviral therapy in two cases. Neurology 1996;47: 929–931.)

quired demyelinating neuropathy characterized by rapid-onset weakness, hyporeflexia or areflexia, and elevated levels of protein in the cerebrospinal fluid without pleocytosis. Weakness may progress for up to 4 weeks, is usually symmetric, and involves the lower extremities before spreading to the upper extremities and face. Involvement of cranial nerves and autonomic dysfunction are common. Although the cause of Guillain-Barré syndrome is unclear, most evidence now supports an immune-mediated phenomenon.

Cases of childhood and adult Guillain-Barré syndrome in which MRI studies showed marked enhancement of thickened nerve roots of the conus medullaris and cauda equina have been published.[102, 103]

Human Immunodeficiency Virus Infection

In addition to developing many cerebral neurologic complications, patients with AIDS may develop a vacuolar myelopathy[104] probably related to direct injury of the neurons by the HIV virus. In addition, there is demyelin-

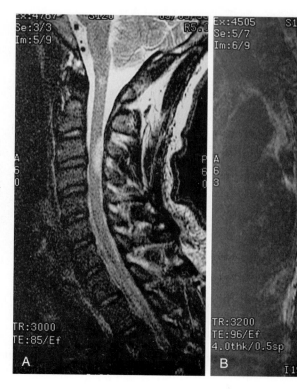

FIGURE 39–27 Herpes zoster myelitis in a man positive for the human immunodeficiency virus with progressive myelopathy. The patient had concomitant herpes zoster skin papules. Sagittal cervical *(A)* and thoracic T2-weighted *(B)* images demonstrate foci of high intramedullary signal. Acyclovir therapy resulted in clinical improvement. (*A* and *B*, From de Silva SM, Mark AS, Balish M, et al. Zoster myelitis: Improvement with antiviral therapy in two cases. Neurology 1996;47:929–931.)

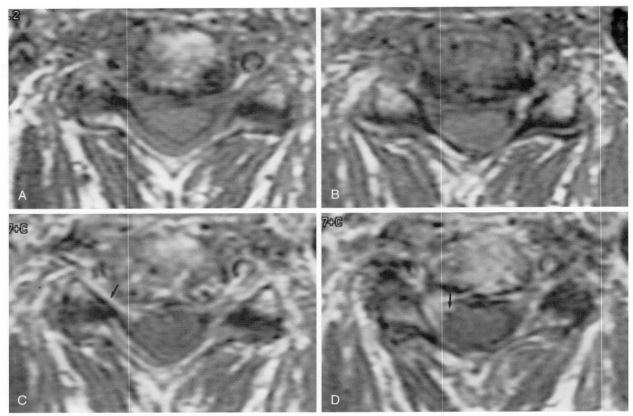

FIGURE 39–28 Herpes zoster radiculitis in a 74-year-old man with right shoulder weakness 1 week after a zoster infection over the right arm. *A* and *B*, Axial T1-weighted precontrast images at the level of C5 show normal results. *C* and *D*, Postcontrast axial T1-weighted images at the level of C5 reveal marked enhancement of the right C5 root *(arrows)*.

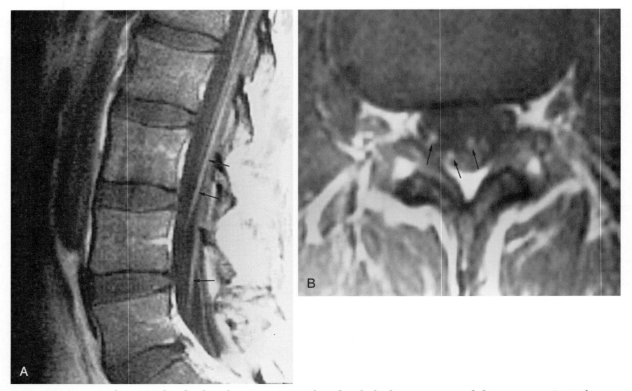

FIGURE 39–29 Cytomegalovirus polyradiculopathy in a patient infected with the human immunodeficiency virus. Sagittal precontrast T1-weighted images show normal results. Sagittal *(A)* and axial *(B)* postcontrast T1-weighted images demonstrate marked enhancement of the roots in the cauda equina *(arrows)*. (*A* and *B* Courtesy of Dr. Charles Lanzieri, Cleveland.)

ation of the posterior and lateral columns resembling subacute combined degeneration. MRI may be normal or demonstrate areas of increased signal intensity on T2-weighted images indistinguishable from transverse myelitis of other causes. The lesion may enhance after gadolinium administration (Fig. 39–30).

Tropical Spastic Paraparesis

Tropical spastic paraparesis is a neurologic disorder endemic in many tropical and subtropical countries, characterized by a progressive myelopathy associated with a human T-lymphotropic virus type I, which has been found in 68% of patients with tropical spastic paraparesis in Martinique.[105] Neuropathologic studies in these patients revealed an inflammatory myelopathy with focal spongiform demyelinating and necrotic lesions, perivascular and meningeal infiltrates, and focal gray matter destruction with a predilection for the posterior columns and corticospinal tracts. The spectrum of MRI findings includes nonspecific cord swelling and hyperintensity on T2-weighted images (Fig. 39–31) and cord atrophy in the late stages of the disease.

Arachnoiditis and Syringomyelia Secondary to Arachnoid Adhesions

Arachnoiditis (arachnoid adhesions) may develop secondary to infections such as syphilis (pachymeningitis cervicalis hypertrophica), tuberculosis (both Pott's disease and healed tuberculous meningitis), and pyogenic meningitis; or to trauma; surgery; nontraumatic subarachnoid hemorrhage; spinal anesthetic agents; reaction to radiopaque material, such as Pantopaque; and reactions to detergents in syringes used to introduce anesthetic or radiopaque substances. Finally, in a large group of patients, no cause can be found.[106–108] Surgery is probably the largest current cause because of the large number of operations for herniated disk and the decrease in the number of postinfectious arachnoiditis cases. Arachnoiditis may cause persistent symptoms following surgery in 6% to 16% of patients. The pathogenesis of postoperative arachnoiditis includes predominantly a fibrinous exudate with little cellular exudate. The fibrin-covered roots adhere to each other and to the thecal sac. Dense collagen adhesions are formed during the repair stage.[108]

The appearance of arachnoiditis has been described on myelography and postmyelogram CT.[109, 110] Two groups of patients have been described based on the myelographic findings. Group 1 patients present with symptoms caused by adhesions of the roots inside the meninges producing thickened "sleeveless" roots, and group 2 patients present with filling defects and narrowing of the thecal sac and myelographic block. On postmyelogram CT, the clumping of the roots can be directly visualized. The adherence of the roots to the thecal sac produces an empty sac appearance. The findings of postoperative arachnoiditis have also been described by MRI.[111] MRI is able to demonstrate the individual roots of the cauda equina in 78% of cases[112] and to detect moderate to

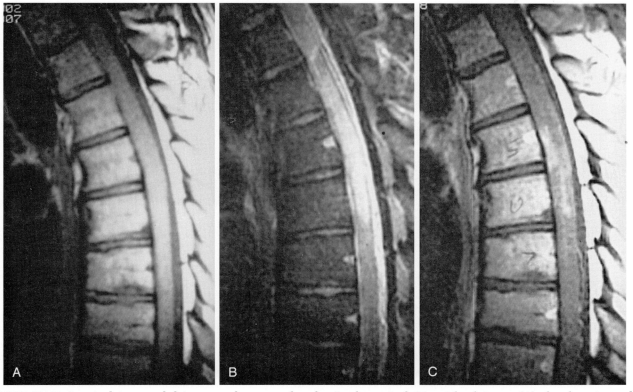

FIGURE 39–30 Acquired immunodeficiency syndrome myelopathy. In the sagittal T1-weighted image *(A)*, the thoracic cord is slightly swollen. The sagittal T2-weighted image *(B)* shows a high intramedullary signal in the same area. The postgadolinium sagittal T1-weighted image *(C)* shows patchy areas of intramedullary enhancement at the same level. *(A–C, From Barakos JA, Mark AS, Dillon DW, Norman D. MR imaging of acute transverse myelitis and AIDS myelopathy. J Comput Assist Tomogr 1990;14:45–50.)*

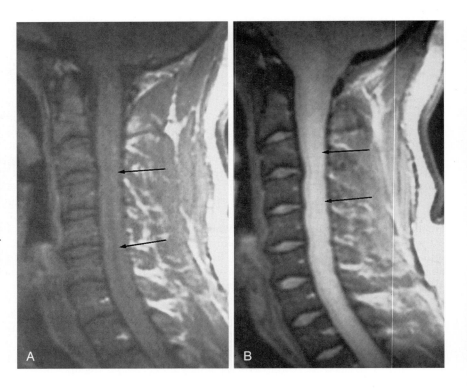

FIGURE 39–31 Tropical spastic paraparesis (HTLV-1 myelopathy) in a 34-year-old man from Barbados who presented with progressive quadraparesis. HTLV-1 infection was proved by cerebrospinal fluid titers. *A,* Sagittal precontrast T1-weighted image shows diffuse swelling of cervical spinal cord *(arrows)*. *B,* Sagittal postcontrast T1-weighted image shows peripheral enhancement of cord *(arrows)*. (*A* and *B,* From B Gero, G Sze, H Sharif. MR imaging of intradural inflammatory diseases of the spine. AJNR 1991;12[5]:1009–1019, © by American Society of Neuroradiology.)

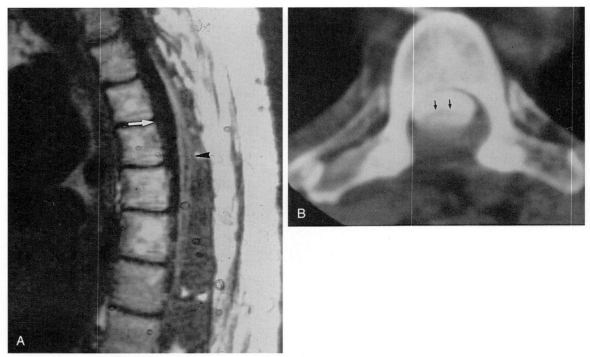

FIGURE 39–32 Syringomyelia secondary to arachnoid adhesions in a 30-year-old man with a history of trauma and previous midthoracic laminectomy. *A,* Sagittal T1-weighted image demonstrates an atrophic cord and a small syrinx *(arrowhead)*. The large anterior cerebrospinal fluid space *(arrow)* may suggest an arachnoid cyst. *B,* On a postmyelogram CT scan, the anterior aspect of the cord is convex anteriorly *(arrows)*, consistent with a posteriorly tethered cord and not an arachnoid cyst. (*A* and *B,* From Andrews BT, Weinstein PR, Rosenblum ML, Barbaro NM. Intradural arachnoid cysts of the spinal canal associated with intramedullary cysts. J Neurosurg 1988;688:544–549.)

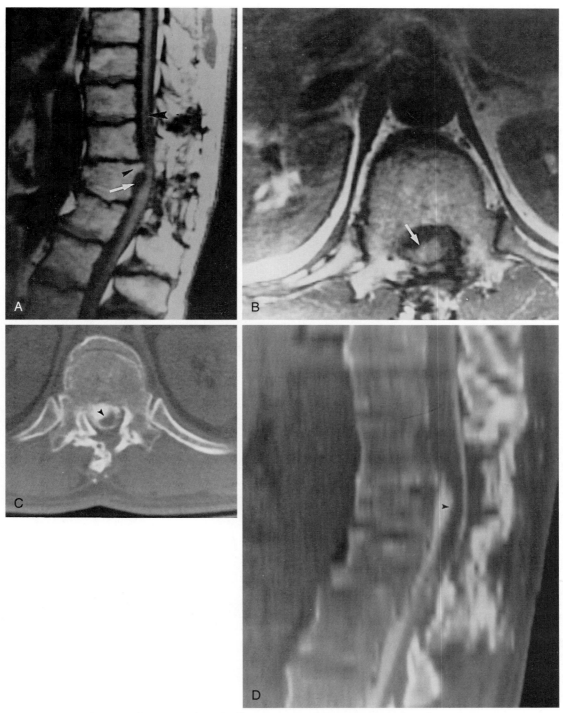

FIGURE 39–33 Syringomyelia secondary to arachnoid adhesions and subtle anterior arachnoid cyst better seen on postmyelogram computed tomography (CT) scan. *A,* Sagittal T1-weighted image shows an old compression fracture and osteophyte *(small arrowhead)* and a small central syrinx *(large arrowhead).* There is a large cerebrospinal fluid space anterior to the cord *(arrow). B,* Axial T1-weighted image below the osteophyte suggests mild cord flattening *(arrow). C,* Axial postmyelogram CT scan at the same level confirms the compression by an arachnoid cyst. *D,* Sagittal re-formations display the compression better *(arrowhead).* (A–D, From Andrews BT, Weinstein PR, Rosenblum ML, Barbaro NM. Intradural arachnoid cysts of the spinal canal associated with intramedullary cysts. J Neurosurg 1988;688:544–549.)

severe arachnoiditis, correlating well with the myelographic and postmyelogram CT findings. The axial T1-weighted images seemed the most helpful. The findings can be separated into three types: (1) type 1 shows conglomerates of adherent roots in the center of the sac, (2) type 2 demonstrates the roots adherent to the thecal sac peripherally (empty sac appearance), and (3) type 3 demonstrates soft tissue masses obliterating the subarachnoid space.[111]

Syringomyelia is defined as cavitation of the spinal cord extending over several vertebral levels. Syringomyelia secondary to Chiari's malformation and certain intramedullary neoplasms, in particular hemangioblastomas, is described in other chapters. This section discusses the MRI features of syringomyelia secondary to arachnoid adhesions (SSAA).

The pathogenesis of SSAA is still incompletely understood, but the obliteration of the subarachnoid space by the adhesions and secondary alteration in cerebrospinal fluid flow is thought to play a major role.[113–115]

In the late 19th century, SSAA was first reported as chronic meningitis or hypertrophic cervical pachymeningitis, and the cavitation was attributed to venous stasis and arterial thrombosis.

Compared with the incidences reported in earlier literature, in our experience the proportion of the cases secondary to infection was much smaller,[116] reflecting the marked decrease in the incidence of both syphilis and tuberculosis. The majority of the patients had arachnoid lesions secondary to trauma or previous spinal surgery.

Regardless of the origin of the adhesions, the clinical presentation is similar.[117] Symptoms develop months to years after the initial episode, and the condition that caused the adhesions may have been forgotten.

The majority of the syrinxes are located in the thoracic cord. Thoracic predilection for arachnoiditis has been described before in patients with arachnoiditis without cavitation. In one series, 68% of 41 cases was confined to the thoracic area.[114]

The MRI characteristics of this type of syrinx differ from the usual appearance of the syringomyelia secondary to Chiari's malformation. Loss of the sharp cord–cerebrospinal fluid interface seen in these patients results from obliteration of the subarachnoid space by arachnoid

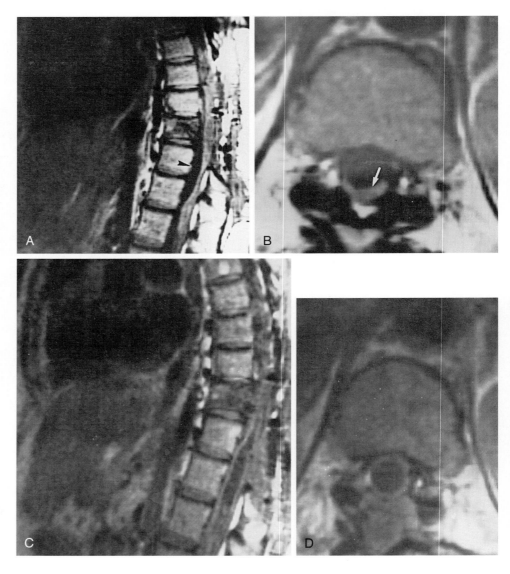

FIGURE 39–34 Syringomyelia secondary to arachnoid adhesions. An arachnoid cyst partially masking the syrinx in a middle-aged woman who had surgery for thoracic meningioma. The sagittal T1-weighted image (A) shows a large anterior subarachnoid space (arrowhead) in the lower thoracic spine that is compressing the cord. The axial T1-weighted image (B) shows that the cord is concave anteriorly (arrow), confirming the cord compression by an arachnoid cyst. The sagittal T1-weighted image (C) made after decompression of the cyst indicates a large visible syrinx, which is confirmed on the axial T1-weighted image (D). (A–D, From Andrews BT, Weinstein PR, Rosenblum ML, Barbaro NM. Intradural arachnoid cysts of the spinal canal associated with intramedullary cysts. J Neurosurg 1988;688: 544–549.)

adhesions. The metameric haustrations encountered within the syrinx on sagittal T1-weighted images in patients with Chiari's malformation are not present in patients with SSAA. The syrinx in patients with Chiari's malformation is usually central and smooth, most likely representing at least initially hydromyelia, rather than syringomyelia. In patients with SSAA, the syrinx may be septated on axial T1-weighted images, probably representing parallel areas of cavitation rather than septa within the same cavity.

The most striking finding in SSAA is the high incidence of associated extramedullary arachnoid cysts (arachnoid loculations).[116] Arachnoid adhesions containing cystic loculations were first described by Schwartz in 1897, and the condition was termed *meningitis serous spinalis* by Mendel and Adler in 1908.[114] These cysts have been encountered in 44% of patients operated on for arachnoiditis. In a review of 14 cases of syringomyelia secondary to arachnoiditis, 5 of the 14 patients had associated cysts.[116] The high incidence of arachnoid cysts noted on MRI probably reflects their better detection.

Most of the cysts are located at the upper aspect of the syrinx, suggesting they may play a role in the development of cord cavitation. These cysts are evenly distributed from the cervicothoracic junction to the lower thoracic region. Two-thirds of the cysts are ventral to the cord, and one-third predominantly dorsal. The diagnosis of an arachnoid cyst is made by demonstrating compression of the cord by a mass with cerebrospinal fluid signal characteristics. The anterior subarachnoid space may also appear enlarged when the cord is tethered posteriorly by adhesion, thus mimicking an arachnoid cyst. However, in this case, the anterior aspect of the cord is convex anteriorly and not concave as in the case of an arachnoid loculation (Fig. 39–32).

In difficult cases, delayed CT following subarachnoid injection of water-soluble contrast agents may be helpful (Fig. 39–33).[118] However, if extensive, the arachnoid adhesions may prevent the arrival of the contrast material to the area of arachnoid loculation. The arachnoid loculations may fill by diffusion of the contrast material through the arachnoid rather than direct communication of the cyst with the subarachnoid space. Thus, morphologic changes of the cord surface at the site of the arachnoid loculation rather than its filling with contrast material should be used as criteria for diagnosis. When all these signs are present in a patient with a history of a previous event that might have resulted in arachnoid adhesions, the MRI is virtually pathognomonic. However, the initial trauma might have been minor and overlooked; and if an arachnoid cyst is not present, SSAA may be difficult to differentiate from a tumor-related syrinx. A gadolinium-enhanced study is then indicated to exclude a neoplasm.

The recognition of the arachnoid loculations is important since in any given patient, the symptoms can be due to the arachnoiditis itself, to the underlying syrinx, or to the cystic loculation within the arachnoid leading to cord compression. Thus it is understandable that the patient's clinical presentation is often atypical and a long delay exists between the patient's clinical presentation and the correct diagnosis. The surgical treatment includes both shunting of the syrinx and fenestration of the cyst to relieve the cord compression.[119]

Occasionally the cyst masks the syrinx, which is revealed once the cyst is decompressed (Fig. 39–34). Post-traumatic arachnoid cysts may also occur in the absence of syringomyelia.[122, 123]

References

1. Georgy BA, Hesselink JR. Evaluation of fat supression in contrast-enhanced MR of neoplastic and inflammatory spine disease. AJNR 1994;15:409–417.
2. Barakos JA, Mark AS, Dillon DW, Norman D. MR imaging of acute transverse myelitis and AIDS myelopathy. J Comput Assist Tomogr 1990;14:45–50.
3. Friedman DP. Herpes zoster myelitis: MR appearance. AJNR 1992;13:1404.
4. Owen NL. Myelitis following type A2 influenza. JAMA 1971;215:1986–1987.
5. Harrington RB, Olin R. Incomplete transverse myelitis following rabies duck embryo vaccination. JAMA 1971;216:2137–2138.
6. Yamamoto M. Recurrent transverse myelitis associated with collagen disease. J Neurol 1986;233:185–187.
7. Johnson RT, Richardson EP. The neurological manifestations of systemic lupus erythematosus: A clinical-pathological study of 24 cases and review of the literature. Medicine 1968;47:337–369.
8. Al-Husaini A, Jamal GA. Myelopathy as the main presenting feature of systemic lupus erythematosus. Eur Neurol 1985;24:94–106.
9. Cloys DE, Netsky MG. Neuromyelitis optica. In Vinken PJ, Bruyn GW (eds). Multiple Sclerosis and Other Demyelinating Diseases, pp. 426–436. Handbook of Clinical Neurology, Vol. 9. Amsterdam, North-Holland, 1970.
10. Chusid MJ, Williamson SJ, Murphy JV, Ramey LS. Neuromyelitis optica (Devic disease) following varicella infection. J Pediatr 1979;95:737–738.
11. Williamson PM. Neuromyelitis optica following infectious mononucleosis. Proc Aust Assoc Neurol 1975;12:153–155.
12. McAlpine D, Kuroiwa Y, Toyokura Y, Araki S. Acute demyelinating disease complicating herpes zoster. J Neurol Neurosurg Psychiatry, 1959;22:120–123.
13. Silber MH, Wilcox PA, Bowen RM, Unger A. Neuromyelitis optica (Devic's syndrome) and pulmonary tuberculosis. Neurology 1990;40:934–938.
14. April RS, Vansonnenberg E. A case of neuromyelitis optica (Devic's syndrome) in systemic lupus erythematosus: Clinicopathologic report and review of the literature. Neurology 1976;26:1066–1070.
15. Allen IV. Demyelinating diseases. In Hume Adams J, Corsellis JAN, Duchen LW (eds). Greenfield's Neuropathology, 4th ed., pp. 337–339. New York, John Wiley, 1984.
16. Larsson E-M, Holtas S, Nilsson O. GD-DTPA-enhancement of suspected spinal multiple sclerosis. AJNR 1989;10:1071–1076.
17. Mark AS. Infectious and inflammatory diseases of the spine. In Atlas SW (ed). Magnetic Resonance of the Brain and Spine, 2nd ed., pp. 1207–1264. Philadelphia, Lippincott-Raven, 1996.
18. Poser CM, Paty DW, Scheinberg L, et al. New diagnostic criteria for multiple sclerosis: Guidelines for research protocols. Ann Neurol 1983;13:227–231.
19. Marcus RB Jr, Million RR. Incidence of myelitis after irradiation of the cervical spinal cord. Int J Radiat Oncol Biol Phys 1990;19:3.
20. Wang P-Y, Shen W-C, Jan J-S. MR imaging in radiation myelopathy. AJNR 1992;13:1049.
21. Sze G, Russell E, Lee D. MR imaging of chronic radiation myelopathy. Presented at the 75th Annual Meeting and Scientific Assembly of the RSNA, Chicago, 1989.
22. Dinerstein SL, Kovarsky J. Vertebral sarcoidosis: Demonstration of bone involvement by computerized axial tomography. South Med J 77:1060–1061, 1984.
23. Atanes A, Gomez N, de Toro FJ, et al. The bone manifestations in 94 cases of sarcoidosis. Ann Med Interna. 1991;8:481–486.
24. Kenney CM III, Goldstein SJ. MRI of sarcoid spondylodiskitis. J Comput Assist Tomogr 1992;16:660.
25. Nesbit GM, Miller GM, Baker HL, et al. Spinal cord sarcoidosis: A new finding at MR imaging with Gd-DTPA enhancement. Radiology 1989;173:839–843.
26. Grafe MR, Wiley CA. Spinal cord and peripheral nerve pathology

in AIDS: The roles of cytomegalovirus and human immunodeficiency virus. Ann Neurol 1989;25:561–566.

27. Lim V, Sobel DF, Zyroff J. Spinal cord pial metastasis: MR imaging with gadopentetate dimeglumine. AJNR 1990;11:975–982.

28. Morrissey SP, Miller DH, Hermaszewski R, et al. Magnetic resonance imaging MRI of the central nervous system in Behçet's disease. Eur Neurol 1993;33:287–293.

29. Kim RC. Necrotizing myelopathy. AJNR 1991;12:1084–1086.

30. Henderson FC, Crockard HA, Stevens JM, et al. Spinal cord oedema due to venous stasis. Neuroradiology 1993;35:312.

31. Foix C, Alajouanine T. La myelite necrotique subaigue. Rev Neurol 1926;33:1–42.

32. Hughes RAC, Mair WGP. Acute necrotic myelopathy with pulmonary tuberculosis. Brain 1977;100:223–238.

33. Tateishi J, Kuroda S, Saito A, Otsuki S. Experimental myeloptico neuropathy induced by clioquinol. Acta Neuropathol 1973;24:304–320.

34. Provenzale JM, Barboriak DP, Gensler EHL, et al. Lupus-related myelitis: Serial MR findings. AJNR 1994;15:1911–1917.

35. Lavalle C, Pizarro S, Drenkard C, et al. Transverse myelitis: A manifestation of systemic lupus erythematosus strongly associated with antiphospholipid antibodies. J Rheumatol 1990;17:34–37.

36. Devinsky O, Petito CK, Alonso DR. Clinical and neuropathological findings in systemic lupus erythematosus: The role of vasculitis, heart emboli, and thrombotic thrombocytopenic purpura. Ann Neurol 1988;23:380–384.

37. Norris FH Jr. Remote effects of cancer on the spinal cord. In Vinken PJ, Bruyn GW, Klawans HL (eds). Neurological Manifestations of Systemic Diseases, Part I, pp. 669–677. Handbook of Clinical Neurology, Vol. 38. Amsterdam, North-Holland, 1979.

38. Ojeda VJ. Necrotizing myelopathy associated with malignancy: A clinicopathologic study of two cases and literature review. Cancer 1984;53:1115–1123.

39. Iwamasa T, Utsumi Y, Sakuda H, et al. Two cases of necrotizing myelopathy associated with malignancy caused by herpes simplex virus type 2. Acta Neuropathol 1989;78:252–257.

40. Mirich DR, Kucharczyk W, Keller MA, et al. Subacute necrotizing myelopathy: MR imaging in four pathologically proved cases. AJNR 1991;12:1077.

41. Gero B, Sze G, Sharif H. MR imaging of intradural inflammatory diseases of the spine. AJNR 1991;12:1009.

42. Wiley AM, Trueta J. The vascular anatomy of the spine and its relationship to pyogenic vertebral osteomyelitis. J Bone Joint Surg 1959;41B:796–809.

43. Hossler O. The human intervertebral disc. Acta Orthop Scand 1969;40:765–772.

44. Resnick D, Niwayama G. Osteomyelitis, septic arthritis, and soft tissue infections: The axial skeleton. In Resnick D and Niwayama G (eds). Diagnosis of Bone and Joint Disorders, pp. 2130–2153. Philadelphia, WB Saunders, 1981.

45. Hensey OJ, Coad N, Carty HM, Sills JM. Juvenile discitis. Arch Dis Child 1983;58:983–987.

46. D'Angelo CM, Whisler WW. Bacterial infections of the spinal cord and its coverings. In Vinken PJ, Bruyn GW (eds). Infections of the Nervous System. Handbook of Clinical Neurology. Amsterdam, North-Holland, 1978.

47. Modic MT, Feiglin DH, Piraino DW, et al. Vertebral osteomyelitis: Assessment using MR. Radiology 1985;157:157–166.

48. Colombo N, Berry I, Norman D. Infections of the spine. In Manelfe C (ed). Imaging of the Spine and Spinal Cord, pp. 489–512. New York, Raven, 1992.

49. Thrush A, Enzmann D. MR imaging of infectious spondylitis. AJNR 1990;11:1171.

50. Smith AS, Blaser SI. Infectious and inflammatory processes of the spine. Radiol Clin North Am 1991;29:809.

51. Sharif HS. Role of MR imaging in the management of spinal infections. AJR 1992;158:1333.

52. Modic MT, Steinberg PM, Ross JS, et al. Degenerative disc disease: Assessment of changes in vertebral body marrow with MR imaging. Radiology 1988;166:193–199.

53. Cuffe MJ, Hadley MN, Herrera GA, Morawetz RB. Dialysis-associated spondylarthropathy: Report of 10 cases. J Neurosurg 1994;80:694–700.

54. Eschelman DJ, Beers GJ, Naimark A, et al. Pseudoarthrosis in ankylosing spondylitis mimicking infectious diskitis: MR appearance. AJNR 1991;12:1113.

55. Lindholm TS, Pylkkanen P. Diskitis following removal of intervertebral disk. Spine 1982;7:618–622.

56. Fernand R, Lee CK. Post-laminectomy disk space infection: A review of the literature and a report of three cases. Clin Orthop 1986;209:215–218.

57. Boden SD, Davis DO, Dina TS, et al. Postoperative diskitis: Distinguishing early MR imaging findings from normal postoperative disk space changes. Radiology 1992;184:765.

58. Angtuaco EJC, McConnell JR, Chadduck WM, Flanigan S. MR imaging of spinal epidural sepsis. AJNR 1987;8:879–883.

59. Sandhu FS, Dillon WP. Spinal epidural abscess: Evaluation with contrast-enhanced MR imaging. AJNR 1991;12:1087.

60. Martijn A, van der Vliet AM, van Waarde WM, et al. Gadolinium-DTPA enhanced MRI in neonatal osteomyelitis of the cervical spine. Br J Radiol 1992;65:720.

61. Shen WC, Lee SK, Ho YJ, et al. Acute spinal epidural abscess in the whole spine: Case report of a 2-year-old boy. Eur Radiol 1992;26:589.

62. Numaguchi Y, Rigamonti D, Rothman MI, et al. Spinal epidural abscess: Evaluation with gadolinium-enhanced MR imaging. Radiographics 1993;13:545–560.

63. Quencer RM. Spinal epidural abscess: Evaluation with gadolinium-enhanced MR imaging: Invited commentary. Radiographics 1993;13:559.

64. Kokes F, Iplikcioglu AC, Camurdanoglu M, et al. Epidural spinal abscess containing gas: MRI demonstration. Neuroradiology 1993;35:497.

64a. David C, Brasme L, Peruzzi P, et al. Intramedullary abscess of the spinal cord in a patient with right to left shunt: A case report. Clin Infect Dis 1997;24:89–90.

65. Sharif HS, Clark DC, Aabed MY, et al. Granulomatous spinal infections: MR imaging. Radiology 1990;177:101–107.

66. Nabatame H, Nakamura K, Matuda M, et al. MRI of syphilitic myelitis. Neuroradiology 1992;34:105.

67. Steere AC, Malawista SE, Snydman DR, et al. Lyme arthritis: An epidemic of oligoarticular arthritis in children and adults in three Connecticut communities. Arthritis Rheum 1977;20:7–17.

68. Coyle PK. Neurologic lyme disease. Semin Neurol 1992;12:200–208.

69. King SJ, Jeffree MA. MRI of an abscess of the cervical spinal cord in a case of *Listeria* meningoencephalomyelitis. Neuroradiology 1993;35:495.

70. Smith AS, Weinstein MA, Mizushima A, et al. MR imaging characteristics of tuberculous spondylitis vs vertebral osteomyelitis. AJNR 1989; AJNR 1989;10:619–625.

71. Golkap HZ, Ozkal E. Intradural tuberculoma of the spinal cord. Report of two cases. J Neurosurg 1981;55:289–292.

72. Chang KH, Han MH, Choi YW, et al. Tuberculous arachnoiditis of the spine: Findings on myelography, CT, and MR imaging. AJNR 1989;10:1255–1266.

73. Gorbach SL, Bartlett JG, Blacklow NR. Infectious Diseases, pp. 1254–1255. Philadelphia, WB Saunders, 1992.

74. Scaravilli F. Parasitic and fungal infections of the nervous system. In Hume Adams J, Corsellis JAN, Duchen LW (eds). Greenfield's Neuropathology, 4th ed., pp. 305–333. New York, John Wiley, 1984.

75. Gehweiler JA, Capp MP, Chick EW. Observation on the roentgen pattern in blastomycosis of bone. A review of cases from the blastomycosis cooperative study of the Veteran's Administration and Duke University Medical Center. AJR 1970;108:497–510.

76. McGahan JP, Graves DS, Palmer PES. Coccidioidal spondylosis; usual and unusual radiographic manifestations. Radiology 1980;136:5–9.

77. Welsh JD, Rhodes ER, Jacques W. Dissiminated nocardiosis involving the spinal cord. Case report. Arch Intern Med 1961; 108:73–79.

78. Parker SL, Laszewski MJ, Trigg ME, et al. Spinal cord aspergillosis in immunosuppressed patients. Pediatr Radiol 1990;20:351.

79. Reich JM. Aspergillus epidural abscess and cord compression in a patient with aspergilloma and empeyema. [Letter] Am Rev Respir Dis 1993;147:1322–1323.

80. Ho KC, Williams A, Gronseth G, Aldrich M. Spinal cord swelling and candidiasis. A case report. Neuroradiology 1982;2:117–118.

81. Voelker JL, Muller J, Worth RM. Intramedullary spinal histoplasma granuloma. Case report. J Neurosurg 1989;70:959–961.

82. Firemark HM. Spinal cysticercosis. Arch Neurol 1978;35:250–251.
83. Palasis S, Drevelengas A. Extramedullary spinal cysticercosis. Eur J Radiol 1991;12:216.
84. Akiguchi I, Fujiwara T, Matsuyama H, et al. Intramedullary spinal cysticercosis. Neurology 1979;29:1531–1534.
85. Castillo M, Quencer RM, Post MJD. MR of intramedullary spinal cysticercosis. AJNR 1988;9:393–395.
86. Lie KW, Yu YL, Cheng IKP, et al. Cryptococcal infection of the lumbar spine. J R Soc Med 1989;83:172–173.
87. Cure JK, Mirich DR. MR imaging in cryptococcal spondylisis. AJNR 1991;12:1111.
88. Dupuis MJM, Atrouni S, Dooms GC, et al. MR imaging of schistosomal myelitis. AJNR 1990;11:782.
89. Silbergleit R, Silbergleit R. Schistosomal granuloma of the spinal cord: Evaluation with MR imaging and intraoperative sonography. AJR 1992;158:1351.
90. Ogut AG, Kanberoglu K, Altug A, et al. CT and MRI in hydatid disease of cervical vertebrae. Neuroradiology 1992;34:430.
91. Cho YD, Huh JD, Hwang YS, et al. Sparganosis in the spinal canal with partial block: An uncommon infection. Neuroradiology 1992;34:241.
92. Nag S, Jackson AC. Myelopathy: An unusual presentation of toxoplasmosis. Can J Neurol Sci 1989;16:422–425.
93. Poon TP, Tchertkoff V, Pares GF, et al. Spinal cord toxoplasma lesion in AIDS: MR findings. J Comput Assist Tomogr 1992;16:817.
94. Mehren M, Burns PJ, Mamani F, et al. Toxoplasmic myelitis mimicking intramedullary spinal cord tumor. Neurology 1988;38:1648–1650.
95. Reichman RC. Neurological complications of varicella-zoster infections. In Dolin R (ed). Herpes-Zoster Varicella Infections. Ann Intern Med 1978;89:375–388.
96. Hogan EL, Krigman MR. Herpes zoster myelitis: Evidence for viral invasion of spinal cord. Arch Neurol 1973;29:309–313.
97. de Silva SM, Mark AS, Gilden DH, et al. Zoster myelitis: Improvement with antiviral therapy in two cases. Neurology 1996;47:929–931.
98. Silverstein A, Steinberg G, Nathanson M. Nervous system involvement in infectious mononucleosis: The heralding and/or major manifestation. Arch Neurol 1972;26:353–358.
99. Talpos D, Tien RD, Hesselink JR. Magnetic resonance imaging of AIDS related polyradiculopathy. Neurology 1991;41:1996–1997.
100. Jinkins JR. MR of enhancing nerve roots in the unoperated lumbar spine. AJNR 1993;14:193.
101. Lane JI, Koeller KK, Atkinson JLD. Enhanced lumbar nerve roots in the spine without prior surgery: Radiculitis or radicular veins? AJNR 1994;15:1317–1325.
102. Crino PB, Zimmerman R, Laskovitz D, et al. Magnetic resonance imaging of the cauda equina in Guillain-Barré syndrome. Neurology 1994;44:1334–1336.
103. Baran GA, Sowell MK, Sharp GB, Glasier CM. MR findings in a child with Guillain-Barré syndrome. AJR 1993;161:161–163.
104. Petito CK, Navia BA, Cho E-S, et al. Vacuolar myelopathy pathologically resembling subacute combined degeneration in patients with acquired immunodeficiency syndrome. N Engl J Med 1985;312:874–879.
105. Victor M, Adams RD. Tropical spastic paraparesis and HTLV1 infection. In Victor M, Adams RD (eds). Principles of Neurology, 5th ed., pp. 665, 1109. New York, McGraw-Hill, 1993.
106. Wolman L. The neuropathological effects resulting from the intrathecal injection of chemical substances. Paraplegia 1966;4:97–115.
107. Hoffman GS, Ellsworth CA, Wells EE, et al. Spinal arachnoiditis: What is the clinical spectrum? II. Arachnoiditis induced by Pantopaque/autologous blood in dogs, a possible model for human disease. Spine 1983;8:541–551.
108. Shaw DM, Russell JA, Grossart KW. The changing pattern of spinal arachnoiditis. J Neurol Neurosurg Psychiatry 1978;41:97–107.
109. Jorgensen J, Hansen PH, Steenskov V, Ovesen NA. Clinical and radiological study of lower spinal arachnoiditis. Neuroradiology 1975;9:139–144.
110. Simmons JD, Newton TH, Arachnoiditis. In Newton TH, Potts DG (eds). Computed Tomography of the Spine and Spinal Cord. San Anselmo, CA, Clavadel, 1983.
111. Ross JS, Masaryk TJ, Modic MT. MR imaging of lumbar arachnoiditis. AJR 1987;8:885–892.
112. Monajati A, Wayne WS, Rauschning W, Ekholm SE. MR of the cauda equina. AJNR 1987;8:893–900.
113. Barnett JHM, Foster JB, Hudgson P. Syringomyelia, pp. 179–220. Philadelphia, WB Saunders, 1973.
114. Barnett HJM. Syringomyelia associated with spinal arachnoiditis. In Syringomyelia, pp. 220–243. Philadelphia, WB Saunders, 1973.
115. Barnett HJM. The pathogenesis of syringomyelic cavitation associated with arachnoiditis localized to the spinal canal. In Syringomyelia, pp. 245–259. Philadelphia, WB Saunders, 1973.
116. Mark AS, Andrews BT, Sanchez J, et al. MRI of syringomyelia secondary to arachnoid adhesions (arachnoiditis) with emphasis on associated arachnoid cysts. In VIth Annual Meeting of the Society of Magnetic Resonance in Medicine, New York, August 1987, p. 251.
117. Savoiardo M. Syringomyelia associated with postmeningitic spinal arachnoiditis. Neurology 1975;26:551–554.
118. Andrews BT, Weinstein PR, Rosenblum ML, Barbaro NM. Intradural arachnoid cysts of the spinal canal associated with intramedullary cysts. J Neurosurg 1988;68:544–549.
119. Barbaro NM, Wilson CB, Gutin PH, Edwards MSB. Surgical treatment of syringomyelia: Favorable results with syringoperitoneal shunting. J Neurosurg 1984;61:531–538.
120. Cilluffo JM, Miller RH. Posttraumatic arachnoidal diverticula. Acta Neurochir 1980;54:77–87.
121. Palmer JJ. Spinal arachnoid cysts: Report of six cases. J Neurosurg 1974;41:728–735.

40

Spine Trauma

BLAINE L. HART, M.D.

JOHN A. BUTMAN, M.D., Ph.D.

EDWARD C. BENZEL, M.D.

Spine injuries are a significant cause of neurologic damage, disability, and pain. Many of the victims of spine injury are young or middle-aged adults, which compounds the social and economic costs of spine trauma. In fact, the estimated lifetime cost of injury for a 25-year-old rendered paraplegic is greater than $400,000, and his or her life span is reduced by 13 years.[1, 2] Diagnostic imaging plays an integral role in the evaluation of spine injuries. Radiography remains the mainstay of initial evaluation, but computed tomography (CT) and magnetic resonance imaging (MRI) are often required to complete the imaging evaluation. Because the consequences of missed injuries may be serious, careful attention to imaging studies is paramount.

Spine trauma is notable for the importance of both musculoskeletal and neural elements. Pain and limitations of movement may result from bone and joint injuries of the spine. Injuries to the spinal cord, nerve roots, and spinal nerves are the major cause of severe morbidity and mortality from spine injury, however. This neural injury may result from direct trauma at the time of injury or may be delayed as a consequence of mechanical instability. Acute intervention is aimed at halting the progression of neural injury. The emphasis in this chapter is on factors directly related to neural injury or to placing the patient at risk for such. Clinicians and radiologists should remember the importance of evaluating both musculoskeletal and neural elements of the spine in patients who have suffered trauma.

The spectrum of spinal injuries is as varied as the mechanisms by which such trauma occurs, although certain characteristic patterns have been recognized. Classification of fractures according to these patterns is helpful, not only in understanding prognosis and options for treatment but also in communicating the extent of injury and the radiographic findings in a clear, concise manner. These classification systems are to some extent ad hoc, and fractures may be described according to mechanisms, eponym, or anatomy. The analysis of probable mechanisms of injury, including combinations of flexion, extension, axial loading, rotation, and lateral bending, is helpful to understanding a spinal injury. For some fracture types, the usual mechanism of injury is well understood. For a

few injuries, a variety of mechanisms can result in similarly appearing fractures, but the extent of soft tissue injury varies depending on the mechanism. Fracture pattern, misalignment, evidence of soft tissue injury, clinical history, and concurrent injuries are all helpful in deducing the likely mechanism of injury.

EPIDEMIOLOGY

The incidence of spinal cord injury (SCI) in the United States is approximately 40 per 1 million, or 10,000 new cases per year. More than 200,000 people are thought to have SCI in the United States, or about 700 to 900 per 1 million population.[1] The level of SCI is fairly evenly distributed among complete paraplegia (29%), incomplete tetraplegia (29%), incomplete paraplegia (22%), and complete tetraplegia (18%).[2] Motor vehicle accidents account for 36% of SCI. Violent acts (primarily gunshot wounds) have increased in proportion. Falls and sporting injuries constitute most of the remainder (Fig. 40–1).

SCI affects young men disproportionately (Fig. 40–2). About 57% of injuries occur among 16- to 30-year-olds, and the average age at injury is 31 years. Eighty percent are male. African Americans and Hispanics are dispropor-

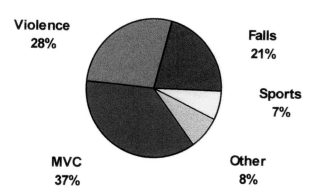

FIGURE 40–1 Causes of spinal cord injuries in the United States. MVC, motor vehicle collisions. (Data from NSCICS. Spinal Cord Injury Facts and Figures at a Glance. Birmingham, AL, National Spinal Cord Injury Statistical Center, 1998.)

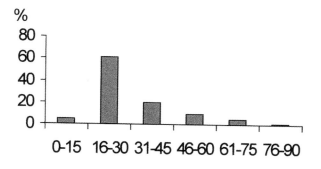

FIGURE 40–2 Age of spinal cord injury patients at injury. (Data from NSCICS. Spinal Cord Injury Facts and Figures at a Glance. Birmingham, AL, National SCI Statistical Center, 1998.)

tionately affected, and this disproportion has increased markedly in recent years. From 1970 to 1980, whites accounted for approximately 77% of SCI, African Americans, 13%; Hispanics, 6%; Native Americans, 2%; and Asian Americans, 0.8%. Since 1990, 56% were white; 29%, African American; 10%, Hispanic; 0.4%, Native American; and 2.1%, Asian American. Life expectancy is markedly affected by level of injury. For a 20-year-old surviving the first 24 hours after SCI, the life expectancy ranges from 15 years if the patient is ventilator dependent to 43 years if paraplegic.[2, 3]

PATHOPHYSIOLOGY

Neurologic complications of spinal trauma result primarily from injury to the spinal cord. Deformations of the spine, spinal canal, and spinal cord at the time of trauma are widely believed to be much greater than that imaged at the time of patient presentation. In cadaveric models, the posttraumatic canal diameter may be threefold the acute transient diameter measured at the instant of injury.[4] Therefore, the direct trauma to the spinal cord occurs by the initial transient force applied as well as residual compression if any.

After an acute injury, damage to the spinal cord occurs not only from the direct physical trauma but also from so-called secondary injury mechanisms, as pathologic deterioration may progress in the absence of persistent applied force.[5–8] The pathologic changes in the cord involve axonal damage and loss of myelination.[9] Petechial hemorrhage progresses to a coagulative necrosis over the first 4 hours, leading to hematomyelia and eventually syrinx formation. Secondary injury mechanisms are mediated by the generation of free radicals and lipid peroxidation;[8, 10, 11] vascular insult and subsequent ischemia;[12] pump failure with alteration of Na^+, Ca^{2+}, and K^+ concentrations;[13, 14] and initiation of apoptotic cell death mechanisms.[15]

These findings have led to the use of high-dose meth-

ylprednisolone as a spinal cord protectant in the acute stage.[8] At high doses, methylprednisolone acts as a free radical scavenger, preventing lipid peroxidation and breakdown of cell membranes. The glucocorticoid effects of methylprednisolone, seen with lower doses, do not appear to have a beneficial effect.[8, 16] In the subacute phase, the inflammatory response does appear to be beneficial because of the promotion of endogenous mechanisms of neural regeneration. In fact, high-dose steroids are detrimental in the subacute phase, presumably because of their anti-inflammatory (glucocorticoid) effects.[17] Much as with ischemic stroke, a limited time window may exist for reversibility of spinal cord damage. The duration of this window is unknown.

IMAGING TECHNIQUES IN SPINE TRAUMA

Imaging is necessary for (1) assessment of the extent of injury (if any), (2) determination of management strategies, and (3) prediction of long-term outcome. A wide range of imaging techniques is available for the evaluation of spine trauma, from simple radiography and motion studies to advanced techniques of CT and MRI. Invasive tests, such as myelography and angiography, are used infrequently for spinal trauma but have specific roles. Each technique has inherent advantages and disadvantages for spine trauma that are related both to the technique and to the anatomy of the region and as such may be particularly helpful in specific situations. Understanding the relative merits of the variety of techniques aids in developing appropriate utilization strategies.

Radiography

Radiographs have historically been the first and most widely used method of imaging the injured spine. They are relatively inexpensive and readily available. Alignment is well demonstrated with plain films. Alterations in bone contour are generally well seen. For all of these reasons, radiographs remain the initial imaging test of choice for acute spinal trauma.

There is no consensus on the most appropriate combination of views that should be obtained in the setting of acute cervical spine trauma. A cross-table lateral cervical spine view is nearly always obtained as part of the initial evaluation of a seriously injured patient. If the patient has been immobilized for transportation, this radiograph is performed without removing cervical spine restraints. Sensitivity of a single cross-table lateral view for fracture is approximately 85%.[18–20] In the seriously injured patient, especially with multisystem trauma, further radiographic evaluation is usually deferred until completion of the initial phase of rapid evaluation and resuscitation. During the secondary, more thorough evaluation after stabilization or during initial evaluation of a less seriously injured patient, additional views are usually obtained as part of a routine radiographic examination. Lateral, anteroposterior, and odontoid views constitute the most common combination used as a routine trauma cervical spine series. Oblique views and pillar views may also be useful. The limitations that arise from patient movement, or lack thereof, must be considered.

The limitations of plain films relate to overlapping structures and small structures. The posterior elements in particular are difficult to visualize well. Oblique views can be helpful, but the usual technique for oblique views involves turning the patient's head and neck. It is possible to obtain oblique views by angling the tube and not turning the patient. These are more technically challenging to obtain with good results, and the images may appear somewhat distorted. Several studies have indicated that plain films may miss up to 50% of cervical spine fractures, largely those of the dorsal elements.[21–27] This number represents a percentage of individual fractures missed, however—often when multiple fractures are present—not a percentage of patients with missed fractures. In addition, the significance of these missed fractures is not clear. The percentage of clinically significant fractures missed by plain films is not well defined but is certainly greater than zero.[23, 28] Radiographic evaluation of the acutely injured thoracic or lumbar spine is generally simpler. Lateral and anteroposterior views are adequate to detect most clinically significant fractures.

Computed Tomography

CT is sensitive for detection of cervical spine fractures, more so than plain radiographs. CT is particularly helpful for detection of dorsal element fractures and for the evaluation of the spinal canal when displaced fragments are present. Limitations of CT include cost, availability, and restriction (in spine trauma patients) to the axial plane. Fractures that are oriented primarily in the axial plane may be difficult to detect with CT. Abnormalities of alignment are more difficult to appreciate with CT than with radiographs.

Sagittal and coronal re-formation views from the axial views of CT are readily available with current CT scanners. The reconstructed views are not identical to radiographs regarding the information provided. There may be an additional advantage to CT in enabling oblique or tailored projections through an area of interest, such as the facet joints. The quality of such re-formatted projections depends on immobility of the patient during the acquisition and on quality and slice thickness of the original images.

Because of the cost, time, and greater difficulties in obtaining CT, it is often reserved for problem-solving situations. In this setting, only a designated portion of the spine is usually imaged by CT. The authors recommend slice thickness of no more than 3 mm for cervical spine CT. Thinner sections of 1.5 or 2 mm can be helpful at the craniocervical junction or when high-quality re-formation views are desired. Overlapping slices can also be helpful in improving quality of reconstruction in other than axial planes. Slice thickness of 3 mm is usually adequate for the thoracic and lumbar spines.

Helical or spiral CT provides some additional options. When spiral CT is available, rapid scanning of the entire spine becomes more feasible. Lower-pitch ratios are desirable for better detail. In the authors' experience, a pitch of 1.0 is usually optimal for imaging spine trauma.

Patient motion is also likely to be minimized with more rapid techniques, leading to better reconstructions. If tube heat allows, screening with spiral CT for spine fractures may be efficient for high-risk patients who already are to undergo CT of the head or abdomen.

Magnetic Resonance Imaging

MRI is widely used for evaluation of spinal cord compromise and complications of spine trauma. The use of MRI for the evaluation of acute injuries has been increasing. Understanding the strengths and weaknesses of MRI helps to plan its effective use.

Advantages of MRI relate primarily to its sensitivity to soft tissue injury.[29–37] In a blinded evaluation of 113 trauma patients who had plain films, CT, and MRI of the cervical spine, MRI had greater sensitivity, with statistical significance, in the detection of ligamentous injury, spinal canal compromise, epidural hematoma, and disk protrusion.[27] Other authors have also clearly demonstrated the sensitivity of MRI for disk herniation.[38] SCI was one of the earliest and most clearly demonstrated uses of MRI in trauma patients. Finally, MRI provides a noninvasive method for evaluation of arterial damage, such as traumatic vertebral artery occlusion.

Limitations of MRI include the practical considerations of cost, time of acquisition, and availability. More rapid pulse sequences help limit the time of scanning. Patient access is restricted, which can be a problem for severely injured patients. MRI-compatible ventilators and monitoring equipment are available. Coil placement can be a problem for trauma patients, who often have spine immobilization precautions. Standard posterior neck coils therefore may not be feasible, unless spine collars or other immobilization devices are removed and the patient is moved with appropriate care. Alternatively, other coils, such as flexible coils, may be used with immobilization devices in place. Strategies for spine MRI depend, in part, on the urgency for such an examination.

Optimal sequences have not been defined, but usually at least two pulse sequences are used, with T1 weighting and with T2 weighting. The sagittal plane is used routinely. Axial images are helpful for the evaluation of disk protrusion and spinal cord compression from disk or bone fragments. A potentially limiting factor with fast spin echo techniques is the persistent bright appearance of fat. Even with conventional spin echo techniques, fat near the coil may be bright on T2-weighted images. The bright fat signal can make it more difficult to detect hemorrhage or edema in the dorsal soft tissues. This difficulty can be countered by using fat-suppression or inversion recovery sequences, which suppress fat and highlight edema.

Tomography

Conventional tomography is less used than in the past because of CT. Spatial resolution with tomography is excellent, and tomography may be helpful in a few selected situations.

Dynamic Radiography

Motion or dynamic studies can also be used in selected situations. The most common such study is the lateral flexion and extension view. Flexion-extension radiographs are the standard for the evaluation of instability. There are significant limitations, however, in the setting of acute trauma. Optimal flexion and extension views are performed with the patient in an upright position and under patient control. The acutely injured patient may not be able to cooperate for such an examination. The most serious risk is that of exacerbating or causing an injury if instability, in fact, exists. Although such instances are uncommon, they have occurred.

An additional limitation of flexion and extension radiographs in the acutely injured patient is poor movement because of guarding or spasm. In patients who undergo flexion-extension radiography for acute trauma, approximately one-quarter to one-third of patients can be expected to show little actual movement with attempted flexion and extension.[39, 40] Such a finding should be viewed as a suspicious but nondiagnostic result. Lack of movement may be due to involuntary spasm or guarding related to significant injury or may be caused by guarding because of pain without instability or fracture.[41] Such patients must be considered at risk of instability. A common course is to place patients with worrisome or nondiagnostic flexion-extension views in a cervical collar and repeat the examination in 2 or more weeks. There is also a small risk of a false-negative examination if involuntary guarding initially protects an injured segment enough to prevent movement.[39, 42] Delayed instability may then occur after the protection of muscle contraction has passed.

For the aforementioned reasons, flexion-extension radiographs are most useful on a delayed basis after an injury but of limited value in the acute setting. MRI offers a method of assessing ligament damage acutely without requiring patient movement and should be considered as an alternative if urgent assessment of soft tissue integrity is needed.

ANATOMIC CONSIDERATIONS

Regional differences in spinal anatomy are important in understanding the consequences of trauma to the spine. Obviously, the higher the level, the greater the significance of the injury. It is also important to recognize the differential response of the relatively mobile cervical spine as compared with the more anatomically constrained thoracolumbar spine.

Craniocervical Junction and Upper Cervical Spine

The craniocervical junction is different from every other region of spine. Complex articulations and ligamentous attachments enable rotation and tilt (lateral bending) of the head relative to the spine. The region can be difficult to image because of overlapping structures of spine, skull, and face. The occipital condyles are rounded, convex surfaces that articulate with the lateral masses of C1 (the atlas). The atlas has a unique shape among the vertebrae, with ventral and dorsal arches, two lateral masses, and no centrum or body. Rather, the odontoid process of C2 articulates with the dorsal margin of the ventral arch.

This relationship is maintained by the transverse ligament, which takes a broad V-shaped course posterior to the odontoid process. The transverse ligament attaches to tubercles on the medial aspect of the lateral masses of C2. There are synovial spaces both ventral and dorsal to the odontoid process. The lateral masses of C1 articulate, also by synovial joints, caudally with the rostral surface of the lateral masses of C2 adjacent to the odontoid process.

C2, or the axis, also has a unique shape and function. The dens or odontoid process projects rostrally from the body and maintains a relationship with the atlas as described earlier. In addition, the dorsal elements also differ from all lower vertebrae. The pedicle is a broad region that projects more laterally than in most vertebrae, and the lateral masses provide support for the lateral masses of C1 in rotation. The pars interarticularis projects from the lateral mass to the lamina. Most of the normal rotation of the head as it is turned actually takes place between C1 and C2 (mean of about 40 degrees to each side). Lesser degrees of rotation take place through the lower cervical spine, only a few degrees at each level.[43]

Subaxial Cervical Spine

The lower cervical vertebrae from C3 through C7 closely resemble one another in shape. Each vertebra consists of a body with transverse processes and a dorsal neural arch. The bodies sustain most of the supporting forces of the spine. The uncinate process projects from the rostral, dorsolateral aspect of the vertebral body and articulates with the vertebral body above, allowing for rotation of the vertebral bodies not possible in the thoracolumbar spine. The transverse processes project laterally from the body and provide sites for attachment of paraspinous muscles. The vertebral arteries pass through the foramen transversarium in the transverse processes, usually of the upper six cervical vertebral bodies. Fractures of the transverse processes carry some risk of vertebral artery injury.

The neural arch is formed by the pedicles, articular masses, and lamina, with spinous processes projecting dorsally. The articular masses have articular surfaces or facets rostrally and caudally. The facet or apophyseal joints are synovial joints. They are angled approximately 35 degrees from vertical, with the facet of the superior articular mass lying dorsal and superior to the facet of the inferior articular mass. The spinal cord lies within the canal created by the bodies ventrally and the neural arch dorsally. The nerves exit between the pedicles. In the cervical spine, the nerves lie just above the pedicles.

Thoracic and Lumbar Spine

The thoracic and lumbar vertebra are more massive and, in general, less mobile than their cervical counterparts. The shape in axial cross-section is roughly square in the lumbar spine and slightly triangular (narrower anteriorly) in the thoracic spine. There is a progressive increase in size of the vertebral bodies in a more caudal direction of the spine. Both transverse and anteroposterior dimensions of the vertebral bodies increase in a more caudal direction down the spine. Height normally increases from the upper thoracic spine to the L2 level; below this level, there is usually a slight decrease in height. There is no uncinate process below the cervical spine. The facets have a more nearly sagittal orientation than in the cervical spine, with a change to more oblique orientation in the lower lumbar levels.

Soft Tissues (Ligaments and Disks)

The intervertebral disks absorb shock between the bodies and allow movement. A hydrated nucleus pulposus provides this hydrostatic cushion. The disk can be disrupted by acute injury, but there is a higher incidence of chronic, degenerative disk changes. There is therefore a significant chance of detecting preexisting disk disease in older patients who undergo MRI for acute spine trauma. Fibers of the annulus fibrosus attach firmly to the adjacent vertebral bodies (Sharpey's fibers) and cartilaginous endplates (inner fibers). Disruptive forces transmitted through a disk space may therefore result in avulsions of the vertebral body or endplate, especially with hyperextension injuries.[44]

Spinal ligaments are important contributors to spinal stability. The anterior and posterior longitudinal ligaments run along the ventral and dorsal margins of the vertebral bodies. The anterior longitudinal ligament runs from the clivus to the sacrum and is firmly attached to the vertebral bodies. The anterior longitudinal ligament is more adherent to the vertebral body than to the disk. The posterior longitudinal ligament runs along the posterior aspect of the vertebral bodies and is less strong than the anterior longitudinal ligament. The posterior longitudinal ligament is attached more firmly to the annulus fibrosus at the disk level than to the vertebral body. An epidural venous plexus often lies between the posterior longitudinal ligament and the dorsal margin of the vertebral bodies. The ligamentum flavum extends dorsolaterally between adjacent lamina and is separated at the midline. The interspinous ligaments extend between the spinous processes. Although they are not as strong as other ligaments, the relative distance from the axis of rotation in flexion allows them to provide greater tension than might be expected. Capsular ligaments span the facet joints and are relatively strong.

The complex motion allowed at the craniocervical junction by the atlantoaxial and atlanto-occipital joints necessitates a more complex ligamentous arrangement. The transverse ligament is dense and strong. As mentioned earlier, it maintains the normal relationship between the dens and the ventral arch of the atlas. The alar ligaments extend between the occipital condyles and the tip of the dens and are also strong. The tectorial membrane is a dense band that extends from the occipital bone to the dorsal surface of the C2 body. The atlanto-occipital membrane or ligament extends between the ventral margin of the foramen magnum and the ventral arch of C1. The apical dental ligament is a thin ligament extending from the ventral margin of the foramen magnum to the tip of the dens. Because the entire complex of ligaments at the craniocervical junction is strong, injuries that result in damage to these ligaments usually require major force. Such injuries, affecting the high spinal cord and associated with great force and, often, concur-

rent brain injuries, frequently result in death or serious neurologic deficit.

Spine Trauma in Children: Special Considerations

Children have greater mobility in joints and ligaments than adults. Particularly in the upper cervical spine, this greater mobility can create difficulties. The well-known entity of pseudosubluxation is a common example. Up to the age of 8 years, physiologic ventral translation of the body of C2 relative to C3 or of C3 relative to C4 is commonly seen (24% and 14% at these two levels).[45] In physiologic pseudosubluxation (i.e., normal childhood spine), the spinolaminar line of C2 should lie within 1 to 2 mm of a line drawn between the spinolaminar margins of C1 and C3 (Fig. 40–3).[46, 47]

It is also important in children to recognize the normal appearance of multiple separate ossification centers that eventually fuse. Failure of the fusion of the posterior arch of C1 is a common variant (about 4% of the population), and failure of fusion of the anterior C1 arch is much less common. Differential growth of C1 relative to C2 creates a "pseudospread" appearance on an anteroposterior view in most children from about 3 months to 4 years (see later). A fracture unique to children is fracture through the subdental synchondrosis of C2 (see later).

Children are much more prone than adults to have injuries of the upper cervical spine and craniocervical

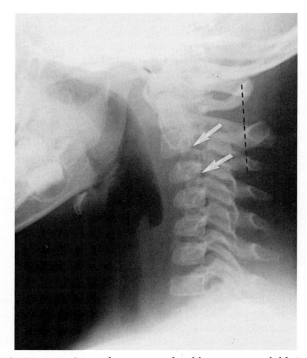

FIGURE 40–3 Cervical spine pseudosubluxation in a child. Lateral radiograph in an infant shows apparent subluxation of the C2 body anterior to the C3 vertebral body (*arrows*). The spinolaminar line (*dashed line*) is normal, and the appearance is normal for a child of this age. (From Hart BL, Benzel EC, Ford CC. Fundamentals of Neuroimaging, p. 149. Philadelphia, WB Saunders, 1997.)

junction. In children younger than 9 years, fractures below the level of C3 are uncommon.[48, 49] Both bone and ligament injuries in young children occur primarily from the occiput to C3.[50]

APPROACH TO IMAGING ACUTE SPINAL INJURY

A wide variety of protocols have been proposed and used for imaging suspected acute spine injuries, and large population studies to support a specific protocol are still lacking. Probably the most important principle in imaging spine trauma is to establish and consistently use an ordered approach. As with any diagnostic test in medicine, a given imaging test or combination of tests is not perfectly accurate for detection of spine injuries. Careful clinical evaluation and follow-up are essential in evaluating spine trauma. Because the incidence of noncontiguous spine fractures in trauma patients is 4.5% to 9%, evaluation must be thorough and cannot be limited to a region identified on an initially abnormal but incomplete radiograph.[51, 52]

Plain films are nearly always the first imaging test obtained and are often sufficient. Lateral views are obtained first, often followed by anteroposterior views and, in the cervical spine, an odontoid view. With the growing availability of helical or spiral CT, CT of the cervical spine is an alternative in some patients. For example, it may be time-effective to perform a spiral CT of the cervical spine in a multisystem trauma patient who is to receive a CT scan of the head or abdomen. Adequate plain films are often time-consuming and difficult to obtain in intubated

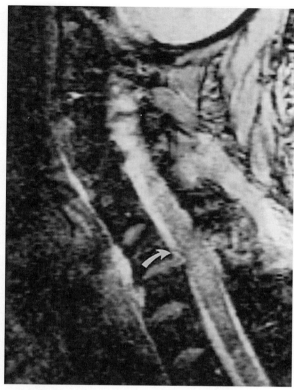

FIGURE 40–5 Traumatic disk herniation, hyperextension dislocation. On sagittal inversion recovery MRI study of a patient who had a central cord syndrome after hyperextension injury, both prevertebral and dorsal soft tissue edema are present, and the disk margin is distorted, with elevation of the posterior longitudinal ligament (*arrow*). The spinal cord is swollen and edematous. There were no fractures.

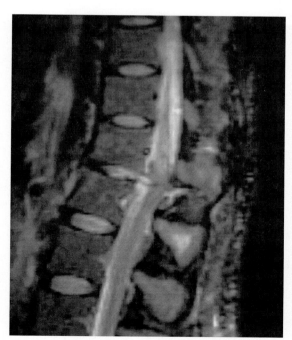

FIGURE 40–4 Traumatic T12–L1 herniated nucleus pulposus. Sagittal inversion recovery magnetic resonance imaging (MRI) study of a pedestrian hit by a car demonstrates traumatic disk herniation and spinal cord compression and edema.

patients. Spiral CT can be a rapid method of assessing the cervical spine in critically injured patients.

Both plain films and CT remain limited with respect to soft tissue evaluation, and MRI is clearly superior for this purpose. Patients with neurologic deficit are obvious candidates for MRI. MRI can play an important role in multiple other clinical settings of acute spine trauma. Several examples of these are as follows:

Detecting herniated nucleus pulposus. Injuries of the cervical spine in which the annulus fibrosus and posterior longitudinal ligament are damaged are likely to result in protrusion of disk material. If this occurs, closed reduction of a fracture or dislocation may result in a new or worse neurologic deficit as the spinal cord is compressed.[53, 54] Thus, the surgeon may modify operative plans if a disk protrusion is known to be present (Figs. 40–4 and 40–5).

Evaluating vertebral artery injury. Although angiography is more sensitive to intimal injury, MRI provides a noninvasive method of evaluating vertebral artery flow (Fig. 40–6).

Evaluating radiographic abnormalities of uncertain age. MRI can be particularly helpful in patients with extensive degenerative changes, old trauma,

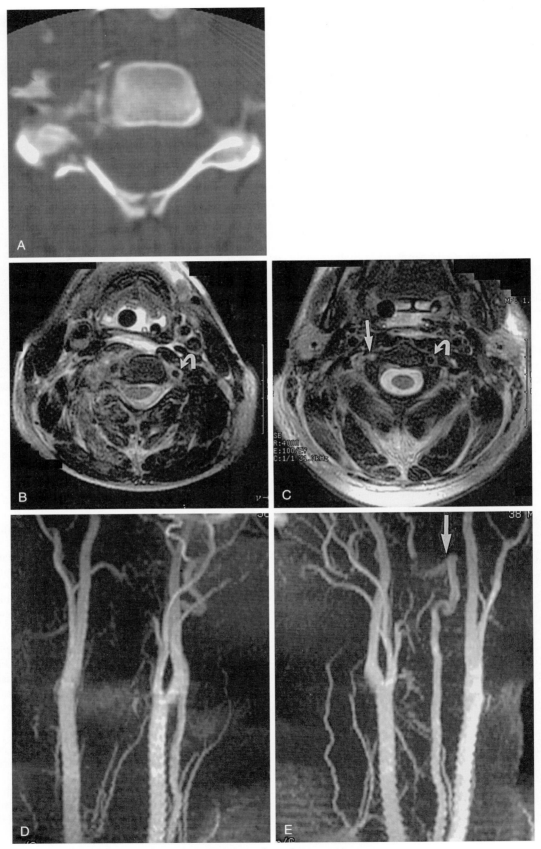

FIGURE 40–6 *See legend on opposite page*

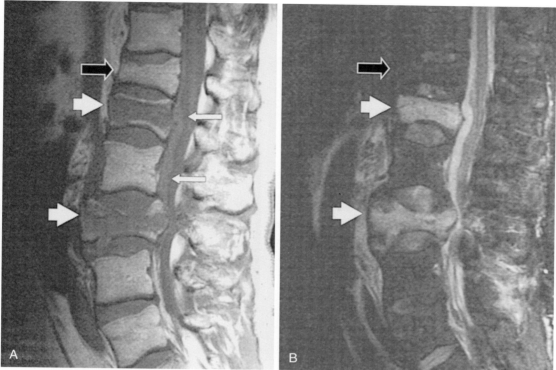

FIGURE 40–7 Acute versus old fractures. Plain films (not shown) of a patient who fell from a height of about 20 feet demonstrated fractures of T12, L1, and L3. MRI study shows the same injuries. There is severe narrowing of the canal at L3. Sagittal T1-weighted (*A*) and T2-weighted (*B*) images show edema within the L1 and L3 acute fractures (*thick white arrows*). Marrow signal intensity of T12 (*black arrow*) is normal, and this compression fracture is old. Epidural hematoma is visible (*thin white arrows*).

or congenital anomalies. In such cases, it is difficult to determine by radiographic methods alone whether a new abnormality is present (Fig. 40–7). Normal MRI, especially with no evidence of significant soft tissue injury, significantly decreases the likelihood of an acute injury being present.

Evaluating the patient with limited clinical examination. Patients who are comatose, intubated, or otherwise limited in their ability to respond to clinical examination pose a dilemma to the trauma physician and radiologist. Normal MRI is also helpful in this group and can facilitate nursing care by permitting early removal of stabilization collars.[55] Although uncommon, major ligamentous injury or occult fracture combined with ligamentous injury poses a threat to patients with normal radiographs and no ability to communicate pain or sensory deficits.

MRI can be helpful in many other clinical situations. Thoughtful use of the various imaging modalities available for spine trauma patients and understanding the specific strengths and limitations of each should lead to cost-effective management of these potentially devastating injuries.

INTERPRETATION OF SPINAL IMAGING STUDIES

Plain Radiography

Evaluation of the lateral radiograph begins with an assessment of adequacy, particularly as to the visualization of the cervical spine in its entirety and the relation of C7 to T1. Swimmer's views are often necessary to establish this

FIGURE 40–6 Lateral mass fractures and occluded vertebral artery. The patient had fractures of C4, C5, and C6, including fractures through the lateral masses at all levels, with extension into the foramen transversarium at the latter two levels. *A,* Computed tomography (CT) scan shows comminuted fractures of the right lateral mass, pedicle, lamina, and spinous process, with foramen transversarium involvement. *B,* Axial T2-weighted MRI study with fat suppression at a comparable level shows extensive edema around the right side of the posterior elements as well as in the prevertebral soft tissues and supraspinous region. There is flow void in the left vertebral artery (*arrow*) but none in the right. *C,* Axial T2-weighted MRI study at C2, above the fracture level, demonstrates abnormal high signal intensity in the occluded right vertebral artery (*straight arrow*) and flow void in the left (*curved arrow*). *D* and *E,* Paired images from magnetic resonance angiography obtained with two-dimensional time-of-flight technique, oblique projections, show symmetric appearance of the carotid bifurcation, normal appearance of the left vertebral artery (*arrow in E*), but no flow in the right vertebral artery.

relationship. Alignment is evaluated along the normally lordotic curves of the anterior and posterior vertebral body margins, facet joints, spinolaminar line, and spinous processes (Fig. 40–8).

The soft tissues are assessed for abnormal widening of the prevertebral soft tissues and for splaying of the spinous processes. Soft tissue thickness ventral to C3 using 1-m target-film distance should not exceed 4 mm in a normal adult. Criteria for normal measurements of the prevertebral soft tissues lower in the cervical spine have been proposed[56, 57] but appear to be unreliable for practical use.[58]

The bony elements are examined for cortical disruption, with particular attention paid to the integrity of the *ring of Harris*. The ring appearance is formed by the pedicles of C2, the base of the odontoid process, and dorsal cortex of the C2 body (Figs. 40–9 and 40–10). Measurements between the spine and the skull base are discussed later.

Anteroposterior imaging evaluation of the odontoid (open-mouth view) is primarily to assess for horizontal fractures of the odontoid as well as to assess for Jefferson's fracture by the relation of the lateral masses of C1 to the odontoid (see earlier) (Fig. 40–11). Evaluation of the anteroposterior view is directed to bony integrity as well as to alignment, particularly of the spinous processes. An abrupt change in the position of the spinous processes suggests the presence of unilateral facet dislocation or other alignment abnormality (see Figs. 40–33 and 40–40).

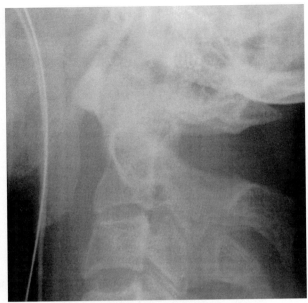

FIGURE 40–9 Odontoid fracture (type II Anderson and D'Alonzo). A lateral radiograph shows prevertebral soft tissue swelling and slight anterior displacement of the odontoid process relative to the body of C2. The fracture plane itself is not visualized, but the alignment is abnormal. The ring of Harris remains intact, indicating this is a type II not type III fracture.

Oblique views, if obtained, provide an additional plane to identify fractures. Normal imbrication (shingling) of the laminae is well appreciated. The neural foramina are also well assessed. Obscuration of the lower cervical spine by the shoulders is much less marked than on the lateral view. Pillar views are not commonly performed in the setting of acute cervical spine trauma because the usual technique for obtaining this projection involves moving the patient's head. Pillar views can be helpful in cases of suspected articular mass fractures,[59] but CT is more accurate.

Computed Tomography

CT allows one to perform the same assessment as for plain radiographs. Sagittal reconstructions allow alignment of the central canal and the facets to be assessed without overlap. Identification of subluxations or facet dislocations may be made on the axial images if attention is paid to the endplates and to the normal "hamburger bun" appearance of the facets, as opposed to the "naked facet" observed with facet dislocation. The paraspinal soft tissues should be evaluated for edema, which suggests ligamentous injury. Occasionally, an epidural or subdural hematoma may be identified within the spinal canal, but beam-hardening artifact usually precludes this. Prevertebral tissues should also be evaluated.

Fractures are readily identified by CT. Pitfalls include basivertebral veins, usually seen at the dorsal midline and ventrolateral aspects of the vertebral body, as well as the occasional unfused neural arch. Fractures of the foramina transversaria raise the concern for vertebral artery injury (see Fig. 40–6).

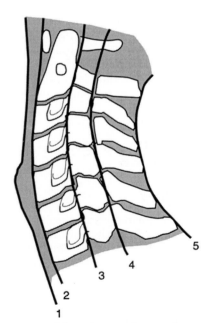

FIGURE 40–8 Normal lateral cervical spine alignment. Diagram of lines to evaluate alignment of the lateral cervical spine. There should be a smooth curve as illustrated, without focal angulation (kyphosis) or step-off. Indicated at 1 is the anterior margin of the prevertebral soft tissues; at 2 is the anterior spinal line (anterior margin of the vertebral bodies); at 3 is the posterior spinal line (posterior margin of the vertebral bodies); at 4 is the spinolaminar line; and at 5 is the spinous process line. (From Hart BL, Benzel EC, Ford CC. Fundamentals of Neuroimaging, p. 149. Philadelphia, WB Saunders, 1997.)

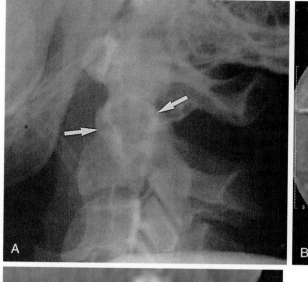

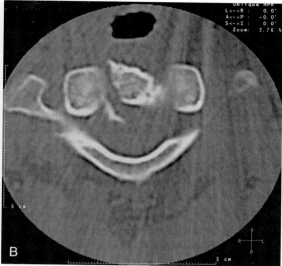

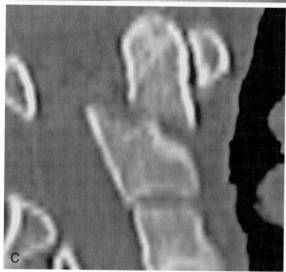

FIGURE 40–10 Type 3 C2 body (low odontoid or Anderson and D'Alonzo type III odontoid) fracture. The patient was in a motorcycle accident and hit his head, with loss of consciousness. *A*, Lateral radiograph shows disruption of ring of Harris (*arrows*), even though displacement is not otherwise visible. *B*, Part of the fracture line is visible on an axial CT scan. *C*, Two-dimensional sagittal CT reconstruction view shows displacement of the dens at this time.

Magnetic Resonance Imaging

The limited trauma cervical spine MRI used by the authors consists of sagittal T1-weighted and fast short-tau inversion recovery (STIR) sequences, followed by axial fast spin echo T2-weighted sequences, usually with fat saturation. The sagittal fast STIR is particularly important because the nulling of fat signal allows for evaluation of marrow and ligamentous edema (Fig. 40–12). Because spinal cord hematoma provides prognostic information, a gradient-echo sequence may be added if cord contusion is suspected.

As with CT and plain radiographs, alignment is assessed. The ligamentous structures are evaluated for edema or disruption. Esophageal and pharyngeal fluid, particularly in intubated patients, may be confused with prevertebral edema. Attention to the prevertebral region on the axial images often resolves this issue. The anterior longitudinal ligament and posterior longitudinal ligament may be difficult to identify discretely. Evidence of fluid in their expected location suggests injury or disruption. The dense ligaments normally have low signal intensity

on MRI, and disruption of the dark line of the ligament can sometimes be directly visualized.

Dorsal to the spinal canal, the ligamenta flava and interspinous and supraspinous ligaments are assessed similarly. Although fluid signal in the anterior longitudinal ligament, posterior longitudinal ligament, or ligamentum flavum strongly suggests injury, edema in the interspinous ligaments may represent true ligamentous injury or simply edema related to rupture of neighboring vessels or generalized edema. Veins may be seen in the interspinous region. A pixel size on the order of about 1 mm² is helpful with a high-field scanner to distinguish veins confidently from interspinous edema in many cases. The confluent contour of soft tissue edema can also often be distinguished from curvilinear veins. The capsular ligaments are difficult to assess directly. Fluid in the facet joints and significant subluxation of the facets should be signs to suggest capsular disruption, with possible accompanying facet fracture. The sagittal images must include the facets so that the integrity of the capsular ligaments may be assessed. The supraodontoid bursa normally is dominated

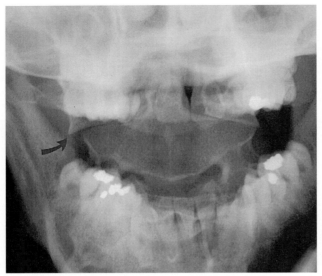

FIGURE 40–11 Jefferson's burst fracture. Odontoid view of a patient with Jefferson's burst fracture. The right lateral mass of C1 is laterally displaced (*arrow*).

paucity of marrow within and the small size of the neural arches as well as of C1 results in relatively minimal edema related to fractures. Thus, MRI is relatively insensitive in these regions. Avulsion injuries also result in relatively less edema, compared with compression or burst-type fractures. For example, the teardrop fragment in a flexion injury is associated with a large amount of marrow edema, whereas a similar fragment in a distraction injury may show appreciably less edema. Contusions of superior endplates may be observed at multiple levels.

The sagittal images should include the facets so that assessment of the facet joints, capsular ligaments, alignment, and vertebral artery flow may be adequately assessed. Intervertebral disks are evaluated for abnormal high T2 signal suggesting shear as well as for traumatic herniation. The spinal canal is evaluated for the presence of hematoma. The cord is evaluated for the presence or absence of contusion or hemorrhage as well as the extent of compression (percent decrease in canal diameter) (Fig. 40–13).

ASSESSMENT OF THE SPINAL CORD INJURY PATIENT

Imaging Evaluation of Neurologic Injury

MRI is the test of choice for evaluation of SCI. CT-myelography can be used when MRI cannot be performed, but it shows only the outline of the spinal cord.

on MRI by fat signal intensity and minimal fluid signal. Edema in the supraodontoid bursa should be a clue to craniocervical or upper cervical injuries.

Marrow is assessed for edema, which is suggestive of bone contusion or fracture (see Fig. 40–7). The relative

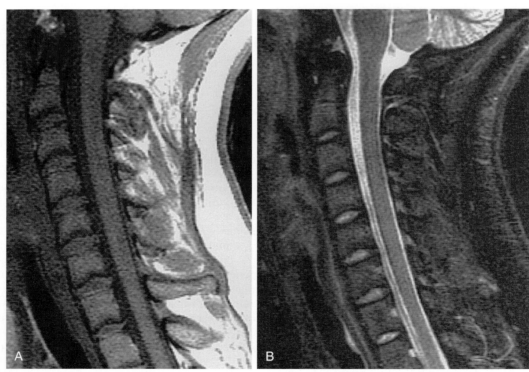

FIGURE 40–12 Normal MRI study of trauma patient. Sagittal T1-weighted (*A*) and T2-weighted inversion recovery (*B*) images show normal marrow signal intensity, contour, and signal intensity of the cervical spinal cord and no signal abnormality in prevertebral or dorsal soft tissues. *B*, The fast inversion recovery sequence suppresses fat in the subcutaneous and deeper soft tissues that would otherwise remain bright on a fast spin echo sequence. Marrow signal intensity is also low except for the basivertebral veins, making it easier to recognize edema.

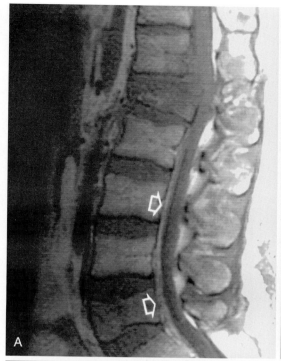

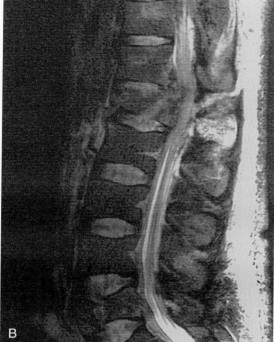

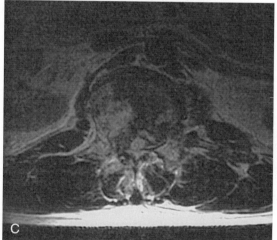

FIGURE 40–13 Burst fracture of L1 with cord compression and epidural hematoma. MRI study of a patient who fell from a height, resulting in axial loading injury. There are burst fractures at separate levels, both L1 and L5. The fracture and loss of height are obvious at L5, but there is only mild narrowing of the spinal canal. Greater dispersion of fracture fragments at L1, heterogeneous marrow signal intensity, and cord compression at L1 are visible on both sagittal T1 (*A*) and fast inversion recovery (*B*) images. Edema is present within the spinal cord. A band of intermediate signal intensity on *A* (*arrows*) and low signal intensity on *B* represents epidural blood. *C*, Axial fast spin echo T1-weighted image confirms the circumferential narrowing of the spinal canal. Low signal intensity anterolateral to the spinal cord represents bone fragments or epidural blood, or a combination of both.

MRI not only directly shows the size and position of the spinal cord and evidence of impingement but also gives information about the substance of the cord itself (see Figs. 40–5, 40–13, 40–35, 40–38, 40–39, 40–45, 40–51, and 40–52). Several investigators have shown that edema and spinal cord hemorrhage detected on MRI correlate with outcome.[60–64] Prognosis for recovery is worse for patients with worse spinal cord swelling and edema and is worst for those with MRI evidence of intramedullary hemorrhage.[60–62]

Late sequelae of SCI are also best assessed with MRI (Figs. 40–14 and 40–15). Syrinx is common and appears as a region of fluid signal intensity on all pulse sequences within the cord (Fig. 40–16). Signal intensity may differ slightly from cerebrospinal fluid outside the cord because of pulsatile flow in the latter location. MRI can be used to follow a syrinx, once detected, for possible growth,

and to detect loculations that may complicate attempted treatment.[63] If MRI is not possible, postmyelography CT may be helpful. Delayed images (several hours after intrathecal contrast injection) occasionally demonstrate slow filling of a syrinx cavity with contrast medium.

Scarring or adhesions can occasionally effectively result in spinal cord tethering. Posttraumatic adhesions can also result in localized, extramedullary cerebrospinal fluid collections. Either of these conditions may act to further limit an already compromised spinal cord. Some patients may benefit from surgical relief of these conditions. MRI is the simplest and best method of demonstrating these conditions, but CT-myelography may be helpful in some cases to assess possible loculations.

MRI and CT can both demonstrate compromise of neural foramina in cases of nerve root damage. CT is superior for the evaluation of bone, and MRI is better

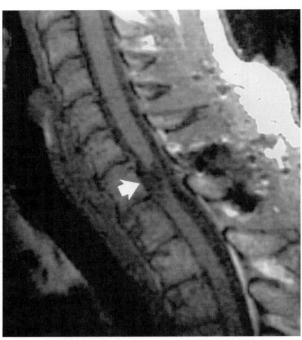

FIGURE 40–14 Late sequela of spinal cord injury. Sagittal T1-weighted MRI study shows severe myelomalacia (*arrow*) at C7 3 months after a C7–T1 bilateral facet dislocation that caused severe spinal cord compression. The spinal cord was nearly transected. There is metal artifact posteriorly from instrumentation.

for the demonstration of disk protrusion. Techniques for the evaluation of nerve root avulsion are discussed later.

Vascular damage resulting from spinal injury can cause brain damage, most often secondary to vertebral artery injury. Up to 50% of patients with fractures that involve the foramen transversarium have angiographic evidence of vertebral artery injury.[65] Many of these patients do not manifest any clinical evidence of posterior fossa damage, however, presumably because of adequate supply from the contralateral vertebral artery in most cases of unilateral vertebral occlusion. Posterior fossa ischemic changes are best visualized by MRI. Angiography is the most

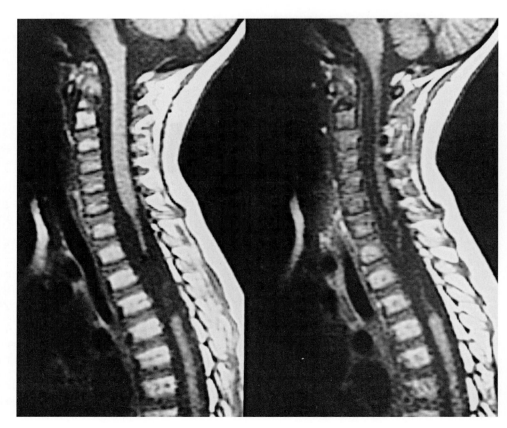

FIGURE 40–15 Spinal cord atrophy after trauma. MRI study (cervical T1-weighted image, two adjacent slices) of a 1-year-old infant who had been in an automobile accident 2 months previously and was now paraplegic. Radiographs of the cervical spine were normal. There is severe atrophy of the lower cervical and upper thoracic spinal cord. There were no fractures. (From Hart BL, Benzel EC, Ford CC. Fundamentals of Neuroimaging, p. 159. Philadelphia, WB Saunders, 1997.)

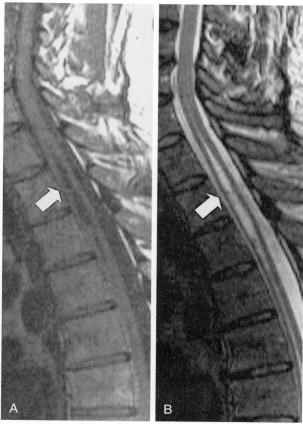

FIGURE 40–16 Syrinx. Sagittal T1-weighted (*A*) and T2-weighted (*B*) MRI studies of a patient with a history of previous trauma shows central fluid signal intensity within the spinal cord (*arrows*) on both sequences. Presumed posttraumatic syrinx.

sensitive technique for evaluation of possible vertebral artery damage, including dissection and pseudoaneurysm formation. In view of the low frequency of clinical adverse outcome from vertebral artery damage, however, noninvasive screening techniques are desirable. Doppler ultrasound is of more limited value for the cervical vertebral artery than for the carotid artery. Magnetic resonance angiography has the advantage of relative insensitivity to bone and is a reasonable screening test for vertebral artery injury. Axial MRI studies should be inspected for the presence of normal flow in the vertebral arteries (see Fig. 40–6). Dissection can sometimes produce an eccentric crescent of altered flow or thrombus in the region of the arterial wall. Carotid dissection is less commonly a result of spine trauma but can also be assessed with MRI and magnetic resonance angiography.

Clinical Assessment of the Spinal Cord Injury Patient

Classification Systems of Spinal Cord Injury

SCI is generally classified as complete or incomplete, based on the presence or absence of sensory and motor function below the level of injury, with particular regard to the sacral segments. Frankel and colleagues[66] devised a basic classification of SCI that is easily applied in clinical

practice. This classification has been subsequently modified (American Spinal Injury Association [ASIA] impairment score) to emphasize sacral function (bowel and bladder control) and to define the level of injury rigorously (Table 40–1). The international standards classification of SCI is a comprehensive assessment, including not only the injury grade but also the neurologic level, the sensory and motor scores, and the disability scores. As with many detailed ranking systems, training is required to use this system accurately, and it is designed for clinical outcome research. The Frankel/ASIA score is satisfactory for clinical assessment.[67]

Incomplete injuries are further characterized according to the following syndromes:

Central cord syndrome results from a diffuse lesion in the central cord, typically in the cervical enlargement. Weakness in the upper limbs is greater than that in the lower limbs, and sacral sensation is preserved. This is an incomplete lesion, which typically exhibits a better prognosis than other cord lesions. It is most commonly observed in patients with cervical spondylosis and may be present in the absence of spine fracture (see later).

Anterior cord syndrome (or *anterior spinal artery syndrome*) results from disruption of the anterior spinal artery supplying the anterior two-thirds of the spinal cord, typically in the upper thoracic cord. Direct trauma localized to the anterior spinal cord can produce the same deficits. The lesion produces variable loss of motor function and of pain and temperature sensation, while preserving proprioception and light touch.

Brown-Séquard syndrome is caused by a functional

TABLE 40–1 ASIA Impairment Scale*

A	Complete	No motor or sensory function is preserved in the sacral segments S4–S5
B	Incomplete	Sensory but not motor function is preserved below the neurologic level. This extends through the sacral segment S4–S5
C	Incomplete	Motor function is preserved below the neurologic level, and more than half of key muscles below the neurologic level have a muscle grade < 3
D	Incomplete	Motor function is preserved below the neurologic level, and at least half of key muscles below the neurologic level have a muscle grade ≥ 3
E	Normal	Sensory and motor function are normal

Definitions

Neurologic level	The most caudal segment of the spinal cord with normal sensory and motor function on both sides of the body.
Sensory level	The most caudal segment of the spinal cord with normal sensory function on both sides of the body.
Motor level	The most caudal segment of the spinal cord with normal motor function on both sides of the body.

*By permission from the American Spinal Injury Association.
Abbreviation: ASIA, American Spinal Injury Association.

hemisection of the spinal cord. This hemisection results in ipsilateral motor loss and contralateral sensory loss. This syndrome is often associated with fairly normal bowel and bladder function.

Conus medullaris syndrome reflects injury of the sacral cord (conus) and lumbar nerve roots within the neural canal. Such injury usually results in an areflexic bladder, bowel, and lower limbs. Sacral segments may occasionally show preserved reflexes with higher lesions. With lower lesions, sacral function is lost, whereas lumbar nerve root function is preserved.

Cauda equina syndrome results from canal compromise below the conus medullaris. Signs include a flaccid paralysis of the lower extremities as well as bowel and bladder incontinence.

Complications of Spinal Cord Injury

Complications of SCI include skin breakdown (decubitus ulcers), fractures, pneumonia, heterotopic ossification, spasticity, autonomic dysreflexia, deep vein thrombosis, cardiovascular disease, syringomyelia, and neuropathic pain. Evaluation of most of these complications of SCI typically falls outside the purview of neuroradiology.

Syringomyelia refers to the posttraumatic enlargement of the central canal occurring in approximately 1% to 3% of all SCI patients. The primary risk of syringomyelia is a loss of function above the level of the original SCI. For example, a patient with a thoracic-level SCI may complain of numbness and weakness involving the extremities. The condition usually progresses with time and usually needs to be surgically treated. Often, patients with early evidence of a syrinx are followed to evaluate the progression of the condition.

PATTERNS OF SPINE INJURY

Craniocervical Junction

Occipital Condyle Fractures

Occipital condyle fractures are uncommon injuries that result from significant forces to the head and neck.[68, 69] Associated cranial injuries are common. The true incidence is unknown because the fractures are often difficult to detect without CT. Reported clinical and plain film findings include prevertebral swelling, torticollis, atlanto-occipital distraction, and pain. Plain films may be normal or may demonstrate displaced condylar fragments. Palsies of cranial nerves IX through XII are reported in a minority of cases, probably on the basis of damage at the level of the nearby jugular and hypoglossal foramina. Three types of condylar fractures have been described. Compression fractures from axial loading are termed *type I fractures*. The ipsilateral alar ligament may be damaged, but the other ligaments usually remain intact. Skull fractures of the basilar occiput that extend into the condyles are termed *type II fractures*. *Type III fractures* result from avulsion and are most likely to be unstable. The mechanism is lateral bending and forced rotation. There is avulsion of a fragment from the condyle and often ligamentous injury involving the contralateral alar liga-

ment and tectorial ligament. CT is the best method for the demonstration of these fractures (Fig. 40–17), and thin or overlapping sections are especially helpful to allow coronal and parasagittal reconstructions. MRI demonstrates abnormal signal intensity around the region of the craniocervical junction.

Atlanto-Occipital Dissociation

Atlanto-occipital dissociation is usually a fatal injury. The ligament complex attaching the skull to the cervical spine is strong, and severe forces are required to disrupt this complex (Fig. 40–18).[70, 71] Survival is rare but can occur, although often with major neurologic deficit.[72] Recognition is important, in cases with mild displacement, to avoid further injury.

Radiographic diagnosis of atlanto-occipital dissociation is not always simple (Fig. 40–19; see also Fig. 40–18). Displacement can take place in several directions. A variety of methods of measuring the normal relation at the occiput and C1 have been proposed, including those of Powers.[73, 74] Most of these methods have limitations. They rely on the accurate visualization of the opisthion and are much more reliable for ventral than dorsal dislocations. The Powers ratio is determined by measuring the distance from basion (B) to the dorsal arch of the atlas (midpoint of the ventral aspect of the dorsal arch, C) and the distance from opisthion (dorsal margin of the foramen magnum, O) to the midpoint of the dorsal surface of the ventral arch (A). The ratio BC/OA is normally less than 1. With ventral dislocation, the ratio increases. Harris and colleagues[75, 76] have described two measurements that are easier to perform, more accurate, and less sensitive to flexion, extension, or dorsal versus ventral dislocation. The first measurement is between a dorsal axial line (upward extension from the posterior vertebral body of C2) and the basion. This basion-axial interval should be no less

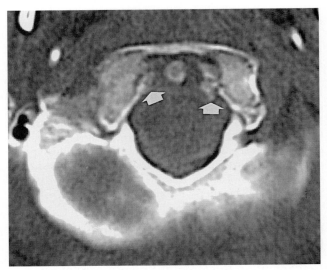

FIGURE 40–17 Occipital condyle fractures. Axial CT scan at the cervicocranial junction shows bilateral fractures at the medial aspects of the occipital condyles (*arrows*). Plain films were remarkable only for significant prevertebral soft tissue swelling.

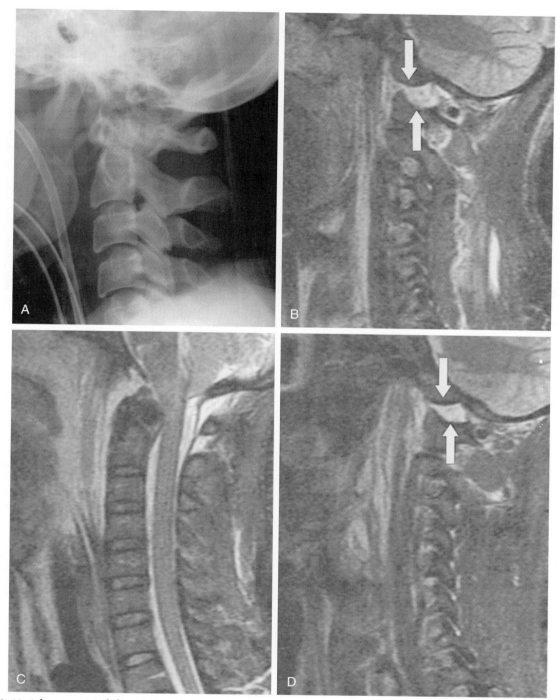

FIGURE 40–18 Atlanto-occipital dissociation. *A,* Lateral radiograph shows abnormal distraction of the skull base on the spine, with mild anterior translation of the occiput. There is prevertebral soft tissue swelling. *B–D,* Sagittal inversion recovery MRI studies, including midline and both right and left parasagittal images, show prevertebral and suboccipital edema, fluid in the supraodontoid bursa, and disruption of the tectorial membrane and atlanto-occipital ligament. The parasagittal images demonstrate the occipital condyles displaced from their normal articular surface of C1, with a widened, fluid-filled joint space (*arrows* in *B* and *D*).

than 6 mm or more than 12 mm in adults or children (Fig. 40–19*B*). The second measurement is the basion-dens interval, the distance between the basion and the tip of the dens. This interval should not be more than 12 mm. The basion-dens measurement is predicated on

complete ossification of the dens and is therefore not accurate in children younger than 13 years of age. The techniques described by Harris and colleagues appear to be the most accurate and reproducible measurements for assessment of atlanto-occipital dissociation.[76]

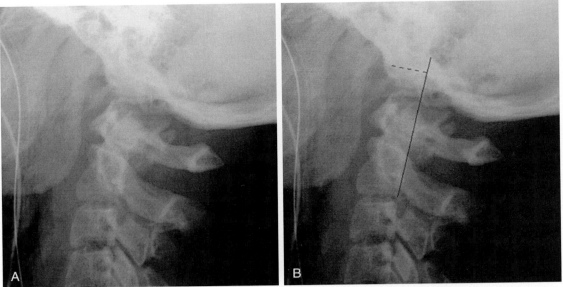

FIGURE 40–19 Atlanto-occipital dissociation. *A,* Lateral radiograph shows severe prevertebral soft tissue swelling and distraction and anterior translation of the occiput relative to the cervical spine. *B,* The posterior axial line is illustrated with a *solid line* extending superiorly from the posterior cortical margin of the body of C2. The distance to the basion (*dashed line*) normally should not exceed 12 mm. In this case, both the basion-axial interval and the basion-dental interval were greater than 12 mm.

Atlantoaxial Rotatory Fixation

Rotation of C1 on C2 may be physiologic or a manifestation of trauma or torticollis from other causes (Fig. 40–20). Therefore, the demonstration of fixation requires a high index of suspicion. It is more common in children than in adults and presents as torticollis after trivial trauma, surgical procedures, or upper respiratory infections.[77, 78]

Rotation of C1 on C2, whether resulting from physiologic rotation or traumatic subluxation, changes the shape and position of the C1 lateral masses with respect to the odontoid. On the open-mouth anteroposterior view, the C1 lateral mass displaced anteriorly appears larger and is displaced medially, and the opposite lateral mass may appear to be displaced slightly laterally.[77, 79] On CT, the relative rotation of C1 and C2 may be measured directly (see Fig. 40–20).[80]

Frank dislocation occurs with rotations of 65 degrees with an intact transverse ligament or greater than 45 degrees with a disrupted transverse ligament.[81] Normally, about 40 to 45 degrees of the rotation of the head on the torso occurs at the C1–C2 facets, with the remainder of the rotation distributed throughout the C2–T1 facets.[43] Because of this, apparent subluxation of C1 on C2 may be seen as a result of normal head rotation. Therefore, if a rotatory subluxation is present, it should be reducible by rotating the patient's head. Observation of the relative motion of C1 on C2 with the head rotated 15 degrees in either direction by anteroposterior radiography[77, 79] or CT[80] has been suggested. Reduction of the abnormal intervals indicates physiologic motion, whereas no reduction indicates fixation. In fixation, cineradiography of the lateral neck demonstrates the posterior elements of C1 and C2 moving as a unit, rather than their normal independent motion.[79]

The term *atlantoaxial rotatory fixation* is applied to these irreducible subluxations or dislocations of C1 on C2. Fielding and Hawkins[79] have classified these injuries in terms of progressive severity. *Type I* rotatory fixation occurs about the odontoid within the normal range of C1–C2 motion. The atlantodental interval is normal (<3 mm) indicating that the transverse ligament remains intact. These injuries require motion studies to confirm fixation of C1–C2 movement. *Type II* rotatory fixation occurs with an axis of rotation around one of the lateral masses. The contralateral mass is displaced anteriorly. The atlantodental interval is 3 to 5 mm, indicating that there has been disruption of the transverse ligament. *Type III* injuries occur when the atlantodental interval is greater than 5 mm, with anterior subluxation of both lateral masses in addition to the rotatory component. *Type IV* is similar to type II except that the lateral mass rotates posteriorly. This injury can occur only if the odontoid process is deficient.[77]

Fractures of C1

Axial loading injuries can lead to a Jefferson burst fracture of C1.[82] Force transmitted axially through the occipital condyles to the lateral masses of C1 causes outward pressure on both lateral masses. Although the Jefferson fracture was initially described with bilateral fractures in the ring of C1, involving both ventral and dorsal arches, numerous variations are possible.

Imaging findings depend on the extent of displacement. Prevertebral soft tissue swelling is nearly always visible on the lateral radiograph. A fracture line through the dorsal arch of C1 may also be visible on the lateral view. On the odontoid view, lateral displacement of the lateral masses can be identified. The outer margins of the lateral masses of C1 and the underlying articular processes of C2 should normally align in adults. Separation of fracture fragments leads to lateral displacement of the lateral masses of C1 on the open-mouth odontoid view (see Fig. 40–11). Minimally displaced fractures can be difficult to identify on plain radiographs. In such instances, prevertebral soft tissue swelling can be an important clue to the presence of occult fractures.

The significance of lateral displacement on the odontoid view can be more difficult to assess in children. From approximately 3 months of age to at least 4 years of age, the lateral masses of C1 frequently project lateral to the margins of C2 on an anteroposterior view. This projection appears to be due to differential growth of the two vertebrae. The appearance may be seen with decreasing frequency up to 7 years of age.[83] Children are in general more tolerant of axial loading injuries than adults, perhaps because of lighter weight and more flexible spine and skull, and Jefferson's fractures are rare in children.[83]

CT is effective in demonstrating the specific sites involved in a Jefferson fracture and the degree of displacement (Fig. 40–21). MRI can also demonstrate fractures, but it is far more useful in demonstrating the extent of ligamentous injury. In the authors' experience, MRI findings in a Jefferson fracture are variable and may occasionally include only minimal edema. CT is therefore particularly useful in evaluation of suspected Jefferson fractures.

Although the typical outward displacement of bone leads to decompression rather than compromise of the spinal canal, instability can result. This is particularly true if the transverse ligament is disrupted. It has been suggested that if the sum of lateral displacement of C1 relative to C2 on the odontoid view, adding right and left, is greater than 7 mm, transverse ligament injury is likely.[84] This guideline can be useful to alert one to such a risk, but direct visualization of the ligament is possible with MRI.[85] Transverse atlantal ligament injury associated with odontoid fractures is less likely to heal nonoperatively.[86]

In addition to the Jefferson burst fracture, another common fracture of C1, which involves the dorsal arch only, can occur. This fracture is the result of hyperextension, with compressive force directed to the dorsal arch. The fracture can be observed on a lateral radiograph or

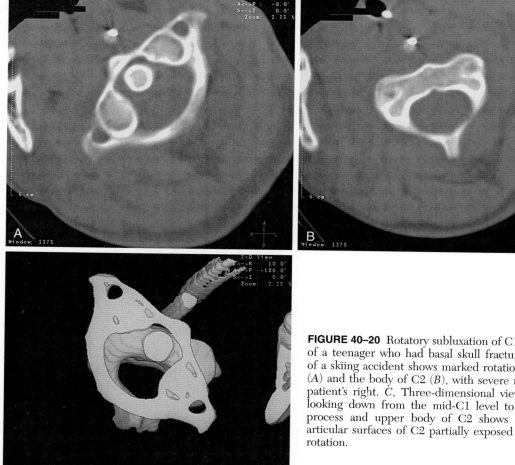

FIGURE 40–20 Rotatory subluxation of C1–C2. CT scan of a teenager who had basal skull fractures as a result of a skiing accident shows marked rotation between C1 (*A*) and the body of C2 (*B*), with severe rotation to the patient's right. *C,* Three-dimensional view from above looking down from the mid-C1 level to the odontoid process and upper body of C2 shows both superior articular surfaces of C2 partially exposed by the severe rotation.

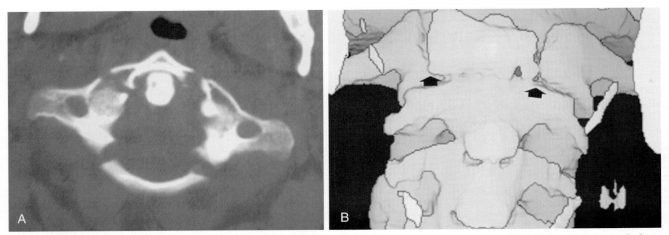

FIGURE 40–21 Jefferson's burst fracture. *A,* Axial CT scan demonstrates four fractures of the ring of C1. *B,* Coronal three-dimensional re-formation of the same case shows the anterior fractures *(arrows)* and mild displacement of the fragments of C1.

on CT. In the absence of other injuries, there is no prevertebral soft tissue swelling. The fracture is usually of little significance in itself, but it serves as a sign of an extension injury and often accompanies fractures at other levels.

Hyperextension can cause an avulsion fracture of the ventral arch of C1 at the inferior aspect, where the anterior atlantoaxial ligament attaches. Imaging findings include local prevertebral swelling as well as visualization of the fracture itself on lateral views. The fracture may be combined with other hyperextension injuries. It usually heals well.

Fractures of C2

Odontoid Fractures

The odontoid process of C2 is subject to fracture from a variety of forces because of its unique shape and position. The transverse atlantal ligament, part of the cruciate ligament, maintains the appropriate relationship of the dens

to the ventral arch of C1. Other ligamentous attachments include the dental ligament at the apex of the dens and the nearby alar ligaments, which extend dorsally and laterally. Three patterns of fractures are often described by the numbering system (I, II, and III) devised by Anderson and D'Alonzo.[87] The third type is actually a fracture of the C2 body itself and is described in the following section. As noted subsequently, a designation of *high* and *low* fractures of the odontoid process may be more accurate.

An oblique fracture near the apex of the dens is extremely uncommon and was postulated by Anderson and D'Alonzo to result from avulsion at the site of the alar ligament. Subsequent authors have reviewed the literature extensively and concluded that a type I odontoid fracture under the Anderson and D'Alonzo scheme has not been clearly demonstrated and either does not exist or is so rare that it does not warrant separate consideration as a distinct fracture type.[88]

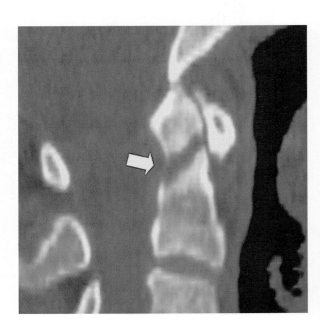

FIGURE 40–22 Nonhealing dens fracture. Sagittal two-dimensional reconstruction from an axial CT scan of a patient who had a dens fracture (type II Anderson and D'Alonzo) 3 months earlier. There is now distraction and widening of the fracture line *(arrow)* as well as sclerosis at the margins of the fracture. High (type II) odontoid fractures are less likely to heal with good bone union than low odontoid (type III, or type 3 C2 body, fractures).

The high (type II) odontoid fracture extends transversely in the lower third of the dens; this is a true dens fracture (Fig. 40–22; see also Fig. 40–9). The mechanism of injury is variable. Hyperflexion, hyperextension, lateral flexion, and combinations have all been described as causes of high dens fractures.[89-92] This type of fracture has a relatively high risk of nonunion (Fig. 40–22).[93] As with any of the odontoid fractures, prevertebral soft tissue swelling is usually present. Minimally displaced fractures may be quite difficult to diagnose by plain film (see Fig. 40–9), and axially oriented fractures represent a particular pitfall for CT. The axial dens fracture is often visible on an anteroposterior open-mouth (dens view) radiograph. Mach lines from overlying structures, especially the teeth and the ring of C1, are common and must be distinguished from fractures. The fractures may also be visible on the lateral view. If CT is performed, thin slices or overlapping slices are critical for the attainment of a high-quality reconstruction view.

Fractures through the subdental synchondrosis before ossification are unique to children. The entire dens ossification center separates from the centrum of C2 below, resulting in unusually sharp, geometric margins at the fracture site (Fig. 40–23).

C2 Body Fractures

Although they have received relatively little attention in the past, fractures that primarily involve the body of C2 are not uncommon. Three distinct patterns occur: coronally oriented fractures through the dorsal aspect of the C2 body, obliquely sagittally oriented fractures that result from axial loads, and horizontally oriented fractures through the rostral portion of the body.[94]

The coronal fracture of C2, termed *type 1* by Benzel and colleagues,[94] involves the dorsal aspect of the C2 body and the contiguous pedicles. In some respects, this fracture is similar to a more ventrally positioned "hangman's" fracture, and lateral plain film findings can be similar. More than one mechanism can result in this type of fracture, including extension with axial load, hyperextension with axial load, flexion–axial load, and flexion-distraction. Important observations on lateral radiographs include widening or narrowing of the C2–C3 disk space, presence of an accompanying fracture of the anterior-inferior corner of C2, and lucent fracture line in the posterior portion of the C2 body. CT accurately reveals the extent of C2 body involvement and possible posterior element involvement (Fig. 40–24). A combination variant of traumatic spondylolisthesis on one side and fracture

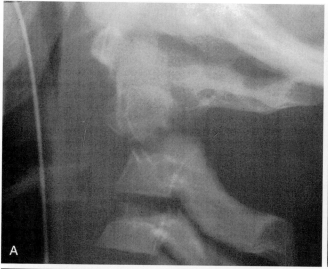
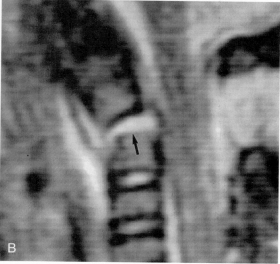
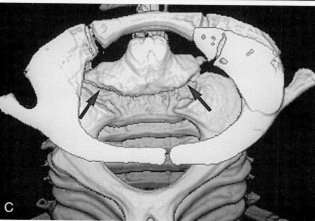

FIGURE 40–23 Fracture through the C2 subdental synchondrosis. *A,* Lateral radiograph shows anteriorly displaced fracture through the synchondrosis below the dens, with prominent prevertebral soft tissue swelling. *B,* Sagittal inversion recovery MRI study demonstrates the fracture through the synchondrosis (*arrow*) and both prevertebral and dorsal soft tissue edema. *C,* Three-dimensional CT reconstruction of another child with a similar fracture, looking from above and behind through the ring of C1, shows the displaced odontoid process (*arrows*). The gaps in the ring of C1 are due to incomplete ossification because of the patient's young age, not fractures.

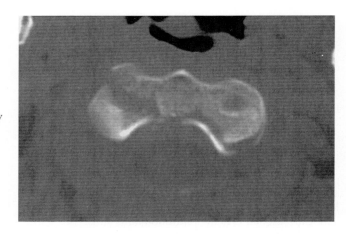

FIGURE 40–24 Type 1 C2 body fracture. CT scan shows coronally oriented fracture through the body of C2.

extending into the C2 body on the other side is common. In the authors' experience, prognosis for healing is good with this fracture, and neurologic deficit is uncommon.

The type 2 fracture of the C2 body results from force transmitted downward through a lateral mass of C1. Although this resembles a burst-type fracture of the lower cervical spine, the mechanism is different because the force is not transmitted through an intervertebral disk. The resultant fracture is usually roughly sagittal in orientation (Fig. 40–25). Because some obliquity is common, direct visualization on plain film may be difficult. Prevertebral hematoma usually occurs. CT is best for demonstration of the fracture and the extent of displacement. A variation can occur in which the fracture is more laterally positioned, toward or into the lateral mass. These patients often have a significant associated head injury.

A fracture below the base of the odontoid process, termed a *low odontoid fracture* or *type III odontoid fracture* of Anderson and D'Alonzo, is actually a horizontally oriented fracture through the rostral aspect of the body of C2. On the lateral view, these type 3 C2 body fractures create a break in the apparent ring that projects over the upper body of C2 (see Fig. 40–10). This ring appearance is due to a superimposition of densities from the junction of pedicle and body, dens and body, and dorsal cortex of the C2 body.[95] On an anteroposterior view in the open-mouth projection, there is a characteristic appearance of an inferiorly convex fracture, an appearance that has been compared with a draped cape or mantle.[96] This fracture, which involves cancellous bone, has a much better chance of bony healing than the high dens (type II odontoid) fracture. It is an unstable type of fracture, however.

The extension teardrop fracture is an avulsion injury of the anterior-inferior corner of C2.[97] It is the result of hyperextension and avulsion at the site of attachment of the anterior longitudinal ligament. There is a characteristic triangular shape of the fragment, in which the vertical height equals or exceeds the width (Figs. 40–26 and 40–27). Prevertebral swelling varies and is often prominent in otherwise normal individuals but minimal in osteoporotic, elderly patients.[96] Lower cervical vertebrae less commonly suffer extension teardrop fractures, also from avulsion at attachments of the anterior longitudinal ligament.

Posterior Element Fractures

Traumatic spondylolisthesis, commonly referred to as the *hangman's fracture*, consists of bilateral fractures through the pars interarticularis (not the pedicles) (see Fig. 40–27).[98–103] Despite the common name, the injury is not the result of hanging but of a combination of hyperextension followed by flexion, most commonly a whiplash injury that occurred during a motor vehicle accident. Limited information about judicial hanging indicates entirely different injuries.[104] Variable degrees of displacement can

FIGURE 40–25 Type 2 C2 body fracture. Axial CT scan shows oblique, roughly sagittally oriented, displaced fractures of C2 body.

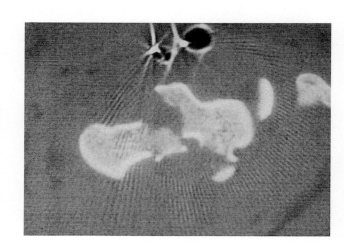

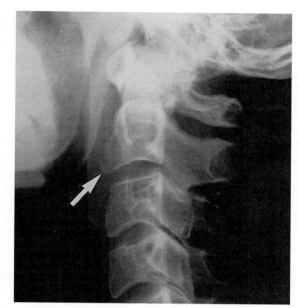

FIGURE 40–26 Extension teardrop fracture of C2 (*arrow*).

TABLE 40–2 Effendi Classification of Traumatic Spondylolisthesis (Hangman's Fracture)

Type I	Minimal displacement of the body of C2, disk space intact
Type II	Anterior segment displacement and abnormal C2–C3 disk
Type III	Anterior displacement of body of C2 in flexion, bilateral facet dislocation of C2–C3

From Effendi B, Roy D, Cornish B, et al: Fractures of the ring of the axis: A classification based on the analysis of 131 cases. J Bone Joint Surg Br 1981;63:319–327.

decompress the spinal canal. Traumatic spondylolisthesis, however, is generally considered an unstable injury, and significant neurologic injury can occur with significant displacement. Plain film findings include lucency through the pars interarticularis, variable displacement, and prevertebral hematoma in many cases. CT is helpful to confirm the fractures in cases with minimal displacement and to evaluate other possible fractures. The fractures are readily visible on CT. A combination fracture through the dorsal body of C2 on one side is a fairly common variant.[107] Fractures through the lamina are usually the result of hyperextension injuries and are similar to laminar fractures of the lower cervical spine (Fig. 40–28).

Lower Cervical Spine Injuries

Axial Loading Injuries

Axial loading to failure of the lower cervical spine results in a burst fracture (Fig. 40–29).[91, 96, 108] Force is transmitted through the intervertebral disk into the centrum of the vertebra below. The extent of fracture is quite variable. There is nearly always a prominent sagittal component, visible on anteroposterior radiographs as well as on

occur. Effendi and associates[105] have classified traumatic spondylolisthesis into three types according the amount of displacement (Table 40–2). The Effendi classification has been modified by Levine and Edwards.[106] Patients with mild-to-moderate displacement often suffer little to no neurologic injury because the fractures often tend to

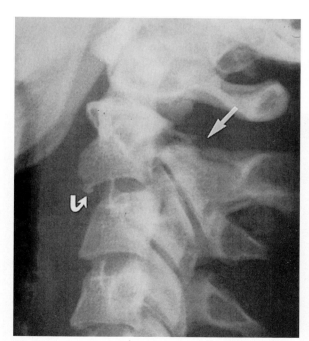

FIGURE 40–27 Traumatic spondylolisthesis (hangman's fracture). Lateral radiograph demonstrates mild anterior translation of C2 on C3, prevertebral soft tissue swelling, and fractures through the pars interarticularis (*straight arrow*). A tiny extension teardrop fracture is also present at the ventral inferior corner of C2 (*curved arrow*); both fractures result from a hyperextension mechanism.

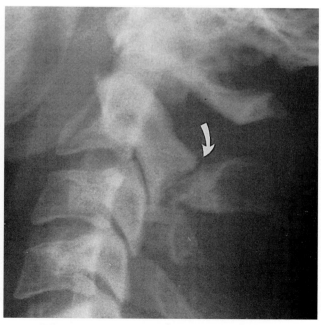

FIGURE 40–28 Laminar fractures of C2 (*arrow*).

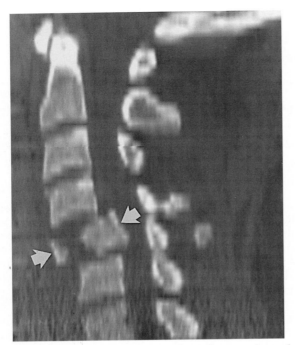

FIGURE 40–29 Lower cervical spine burst fracture. Sagittal reformation view from a CT scan of a patient who suffered a burst fracture of C5 after an axial-loading mechanism injury. There is major displacement of the fragments of the vertebral body (*arrows*). (From Hart BL, Benzel EC, Ford CC. Fundamentals of Neuroimaging, p. 152. Philadelphia, WB Saunders, 1997.)

CT (Fig. 40–30). The overall alignment of the cervical spine generally remains straightened. This fact is helpful in differentiating the burst fracture from a flexion teardrop fracture, in which there is focal kyphosis at the

fracture level. The burst fracture is frequently comminuted, and displacement of the dorsal cortex into the spinal canal can cause significant spinal cord compromise. Dorsal element fractures are also common. In the authors' experience, the extent of ligamentous and other soft tissue injury revealed by MRI is related to the extent of bone displacement. This fracture should be considered unstable even if immediate neurologic injury has not occurred. Plain film findings should be recognized, but CT is superior for the demonstration of dorsal element fractures and the degree of spinal canal compromise. MRI is helpful in some cases for evaluation of the spinal cord and possible associated disk herniation.

Flexion Injuries of the Lower Cervical Spine

A variety of flexion injuries occur in the lower cervical spine, ranging from avulsion fractures of minimal clinical significance to catastrophic flexion teardrop fractures. Alignment of the cervical spine on the lateral radiograph is often indicative of the mechanism in these cases.

Disruption of the interspinous and other dorsal ligaments results in segmental fanning of the adjacent facets and widening of the space between the spinous processes. Focal kyphosis can also be observed between adjacent vertebral bodies, especially at the dorsal cortical margin (Fig. 40–31). These findings alone accompany a hyperflexion sprain, a soft tissue injury that can lead to a risk of delayed instability (Fig. 40–32).[97, 109–112] Disruption of the dorsal ligament complex also occurs with some of the flexion-mechanism fractures described subsequently (Fig. 40–33).

Avulsion fracture of the spinous process occurs most commonly at C7, C6, and T1, with other levels occurring less frequently. This is sometimes referred to as a *clay-shoveler's* fracture and results from sudden flexion, with the ligaments remaining intact. The fracture is best visual-

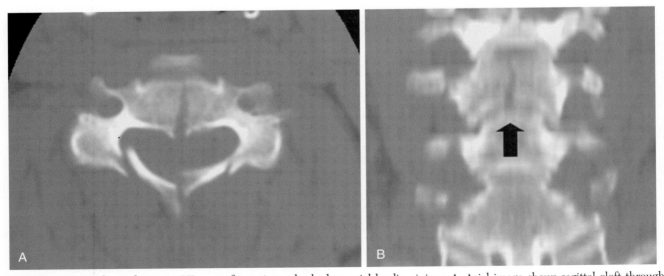

FIGURE 40–30 C4 burst fracture. CT scan of a patient who had an axial loading injury. *A,* Axial image shows sagittal cleft through the vertebral body and bilateral laminar fractures and fracture through the spinous process. *B,* Coronal two-dimensional reconstruction view also shows the prominent sagittal component of the vertebral fracture (*arrow*), common in burst fractures.

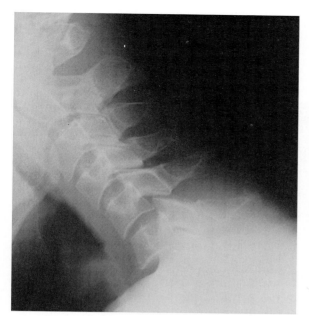

FIGURE 40–31 Flexion sprain with instability. Lateral radiograph several weeks after a flexion injury shows focal kyphosis and widening between the posterior elements at C5–C6.

ized on the lateral radiograph, although a swimmer's view may also be necessary (Fig. 40–34). Sagittal reconstruction views may be necessary to accurately detect this fracture on CT because the space between spinous processes may simulate the false appearance of fracture. In the authors' experience, MRI of patients with a clay-shoveler's fracture often shows the fracture itself as a linear area of high signal intensity on T2-weighted images, but nearby soft tissue signal abnormality may be limited,

presumably because the primary injury is of bone rather than of ligaments. A fracture of the spinous process alone is of little clinical significance, other than as evidence of trauma to the neck and often severe pain; the detection of one fracture of the spine should always suggest the possibility of others. Occasionally, the fracture can extend more deeply and involve the lamina, in which case bone stability is of more concern.

Flexion leading to ventral compressive forces on a vertebral body causes a wedge or compression fracture (see Fig. 40–33). The fracture is usually well demonstrated on the lateral radiograph. There is loss of ventral height, and the ventral cortical margin or superior endplate, or both, are usually buckled. The anterior-superior corner of the fractured body may be a separate fragment in cases with greater force. Although dorsal element fracture does not usually accompany a simple wedge fracture, soft tissue injury of a flexion sprain is common. In some cases, however, the dorsal ligament complex remains intact. As described earlier, these features include widening of the facets and interspinous space. MRI can demonstrate the extent of soft tissue injury. Focal interspinous signal abnormality (high signal intensity on T2-weighted images) is typical. More extensive soft tissue injury results in a pattern in which a band of high signal intensity extends from the level of flexion sprain rostrally, with the lower margin of the band at the level of injury. Optimal demonstration by CT usually requires thin enough slices or overlap to obtain good sagittal reconstructions because the fracture may lie substantially in the axial plane. A simple wedge fracture alone does not require CT visualization.

Greater flexion forces can cause bilateral facet dislocation (Figs. 40–35 and 40–36). The spine exhibits a flexed alignment in the sagittal or lateral view. Dorsal distraction greater than in the flexion sprain causes actual dislocation

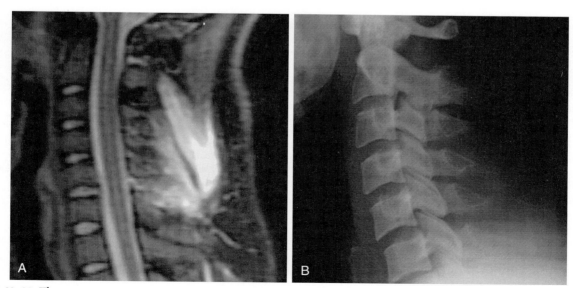

FIGURE 40–32 Flexion injury on MRI. *A,* Sagittal inversion recovery image shows supraspinous edema from C2 to C6 and deep, interspinous injury at C5–C6. *B,* Initial lateral radiograph showed only minimal kyphosis at C5–C6. MRI can identify ligamentous injury when radiographs are minimally abnormal.

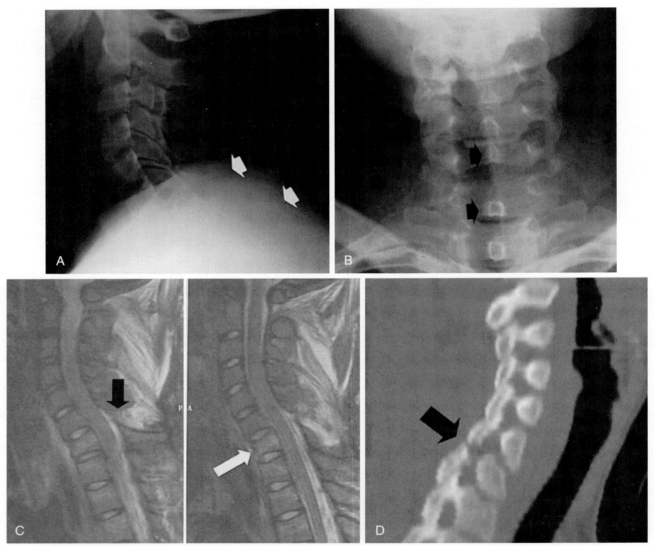

FIGURE 40–33 Flexion injury with compression fracture and posterior subluxation. *A,* Lateral radiograph shows posterior widening between the spinous process of C6 and C7 (*arrows*). Compression of C7 is difficult to visualize. *B,* Anteroposterior view of the same patient confirms the posterior interspinous widening; there is abnormal space between the spinous process of C6 and C7 (*arrows*). *C,* Sagittal inversion recovery sequence, two adjacent images, shows mild anterior compression of the C7 vertebral body (*white arrow*); a broad region of dorsal soft tissue edema extending from C7 to the occiput; posterior widening of the spinous processes at C6–C7; and deep interspinous edema at C6–C7 that extends to the level of the spinal canal, through the ligamentum flavum (*black arrow*). *D,* Parasagittal two-dimensional CT reconstruction of the same patient demonstrates "perched" facets at C6–C7 (*arrow*).

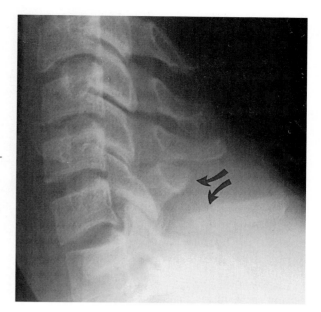

FIGURE 40–34 Spinous process (clay-shoveler's) fracture. Lateral radiograph shows fracture of the spinous process of C7 (*arrows*).

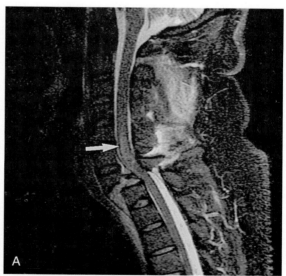

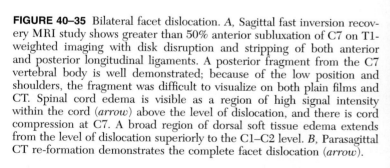

FIGURE 40–35 Bilateral facet dislocation. *A*, Sagittal fast inversion recovery MRI study shows greater than 50% anterior subluxation of C7 on T1-weighted imaging with disk disruption and stripping of both anterior and posterior longitudinal ligaments. A posterior fragment from the C7 vertebral body is well demonstrated; because of the low position and shoulders, the fragment was difficult to visualize on both plain films and CT. Spinal cord edema is visible as a region of high signal intensity within the cord (*arrow*) above the level of dislocation, and there is cord compression at C7. A broad region of dorsal soft tissue edema extends from the level of dislocation superiorly to the C1–C2 level. *B*, Parasagittal CT re-formation demonstrates the complete facet dislocation (*arrow*).

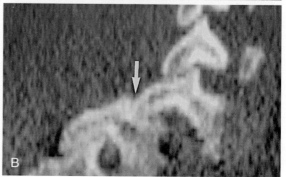

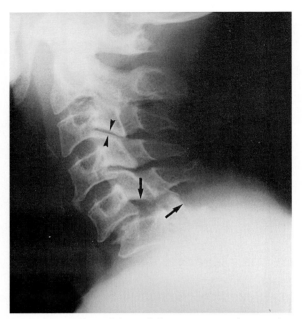

FIGURE 40–36 Bilateral facet dislocation. Lateral cervical spine radiograph of a man who fell off a bridge shows bilateral facet dislocation at C5–C6. There is greater than 50% anterior displacement of C5 on C6. Space between the posterior elements is widened at that level. The normal relationship of the facets (e.g., *arrowheads* at C3–C4) is disrupted at C5–C6 (*arrows* point to facets that should articulate). (From Hart BL, Benzel EC, Ford CC. Fundamentals of Neuroimaging, p. 155. Philadelphia, WB Saunders, 1997.)

of both facet joints and disruption of the normal "shingle" appearance on the lateral radiograph. The vertebral body above the level of dislocation is ventrally displaced more than 50% relative to the vertebral body below in the case of complete dislocation. Partial dislocation results in less than 50% ventral subluxation. Severe ligamentous injury is always part of this injury, and bilateral facet dislocation is considered unstable.[113–116] Minor impaction fractures are common.[117]

MRI reveals the extent of soft tissue edema and hemorrhage at the dislocation level and often in a broad band of abnormal signal intensity extending rostrally from the level of injury. Sagittal MRI also can show the anterior and posterior longitudinal ligaments (see Fig. 40–35). They may be disrupted but often appear avulsed from the vertebral bodies, stretched, and taut because of the displacement of bones, appearing as a parallelogram.

The normal appearance of a facet joint on axial CT is similar to a clamshell, with the flat surfaces of two semilunar shapes adjoining one another. In the case of facet dislocation, this relationship is reversed. Dorsal element fractures may be present. These are best demonstrated by CT. Significant facet fractures may affect the likelihood of reduction and the surgeon's choice of approach. Although axial CT shows the diameter of the spinal canal, re-formatted images are helpful to evaluate the relationship of the facets and vertebral bodies. The diagnosis of bilateral facet dislocation can usually be made on plain films, however. CT has a supplementary role.

Severe flexion forces can cause the flexion teardrop

fracture, often accompanied by a devastating clinical outcome.[118] The lateral radiograph shows a large, triangular fragment at the anterior-inferior corner of the vertebral body (Fig. 40–37). The cervical spine is flexed at the level of injury.[119] The usual clinical outcome is an anterior cord syndrome, in which there is quadriplegia with preservation of dorsal column sensation only.[120, 121] As with other serious disruptions of the spine, MRI can be of benefit to evaluate the severity of cord compression, presence or extent of intramedullary edema or hemorrhage, and presence of disk herniation or epidural hematoma.

Extension Injuries

A variety of cervical spine injuries can result from extension forces, in varying combination with axial loading, rotational, or flexion forces. Several distinct patterns exist; upper cervical spine extension injuries of C1 ventral arch avulsion, extension teardrop fracture, and hangman's fracture have already been described.

Laminar fractures through the cervical spine can result from hyperextension. Lateral or oblique radiographs can demonstrate laminar fractures, and CT is more sensitive (see Fig. 40–28). Although extension teardrop fractures occur most frequently at C2 at the attachment of the anterior longitudinal ligament, similar fractures can occur less commonly in the lower cervical spine.

The hyperextension dislocation is important to recognize; radiographic findings may be subtle, and significant clinical impairment can occur. The mechanism is hyperextension and dislocation through a disk level. Transient compression of the spinal cord may result. The anterior longitudinal ligament is torn, and the intervertebral disk is disrupted (see Fig. 40–5).[44, 122, 123] The usual clinical outcome is a central cord syndrome, in which upper extremity symptoms exceed those of the lower extremities. Fibers to the upper extremities within the pyramidal tract in the spinal cord lie more centrally than those to

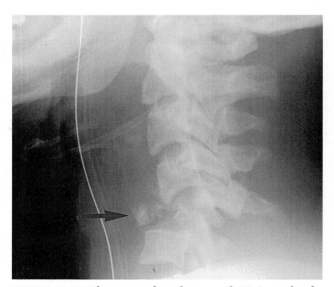

FIGURE 40–37 Flexion teardrop fracture of C5. Lateral radiograph shows flexed position of the cervical spine, posterior disruption and widening, and teardrop fragment at the level of injury (*arrow*).

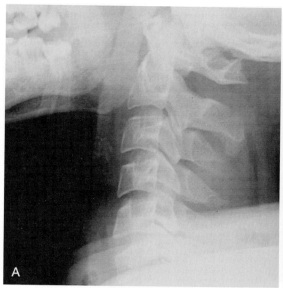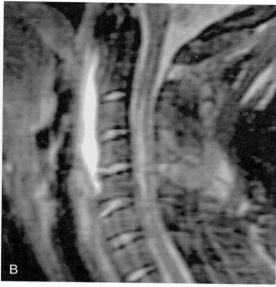

FIGURE 40–38 Hyperextension dislocation. *A,* Lateral radiograph of a patient with a central cord syndrome after a motor vehicle accident shows diffuse prevertebral soft tissue swelling. There is slight widening of the C5–C6 disk space. *B,* Sagittal inversion recovery MRI study shows prevertebral edema, posterior interspinous and supraspinous edema, and spinal cord edema. There were no fractures. Contrast to Figure 40–39, which shows central cord syndrome from Taylor mechanism, also from hyperextension.

the lower extremities, explaining the differential findings in central cord syndrome. The most common radiographic appearance is that of a straight cervical spine with diffuse prevertebral soft tissue swelling (Fig. 40–38).[112, 124, 125] In about 65% of cases, there is an avulsion fracture of the inferior endplate above the level of dislocation. This fracture fragment is wider than it is tall, in distinction to the extension teardrop fragment. In the latter case, the height of the fragment equals or exceeds its width in the lateral view. Gas within the disk space and disk space widening are less common findings in hyperextension dislocation.

The central cord syndrome can also result from hyperextension injury in patients with severe spinal canal narrowing from osteophytes (Taylor mechanism).[126, 127] In contradistinction to patients with hyperextension dislocation, the prevertebral soft tissues are normal (Fig. 40–39).[96]

MRI can directly demonstrate the ligament injury and disk disruption, in addition to the edema within the spinal cord (see Figs. 40–5 and 40–38). Hemorrhage within the spinal cord is uncommon.[128] MRI of hyperextension dislocation shows extensive dorsal soft tissue as well as

FIGURE 40–39 Central cord injury related to degenerative changes (Taylor mechanism). Sagittal inversion recovery MRI study of a patient who had a central cord syndrome after a motor vehicle accident. The spinal canal is narrow, there is mild prevertebral and posterior soft tissue edema, and there is focal high signal intensity within the spinal cord (*arrow*). There were no fractures on CT. This represents central cord injury resulting from hyperextension in a patient with preexisting degenerative changes, the mechanism described by Taylor.

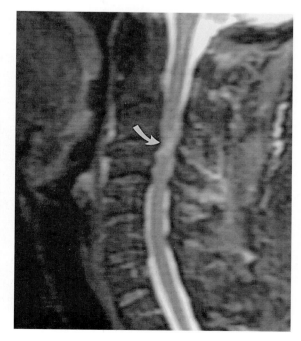

prevertebral edema, reflecting a combination of both extension and flexion forces. Despite the frequent lack of fractures, significant instability in extension accompanies this injury.

Combined Rotational Injuries

Unilateral facet dislocation results from a combination of flexion and rotation. At the level of dislocation, there is ventral subluxation of the rostral vertebra, with dislocation of the upper articular process over the lower.[129] Milder degrees of displacement may result in a "perched" facet, in which the upper facet lies just above the lower facet, disrupting the normal shingle arrangement, but without

the further movement that results in a "locked" appearance and reversal of the arrangement of the facets. The capsule of the facet joints both on the dislocated side and on the contralateral side is disrupted, and the annulus fibrosus is also stretched or torn.

Plain film findings in unilateral facet dislocation are usually characteristic (Fig. 40–40). On the lateral view, the spine above the level of dislocation appears rotated, presenting an appearance similar to that normally observed on an oblique view. A normal lateral appearance is seen below the level of dislocation. The vertebral body above the dislocation level is displaced ventrally less than half of the width of the vertebral body. The disrupted

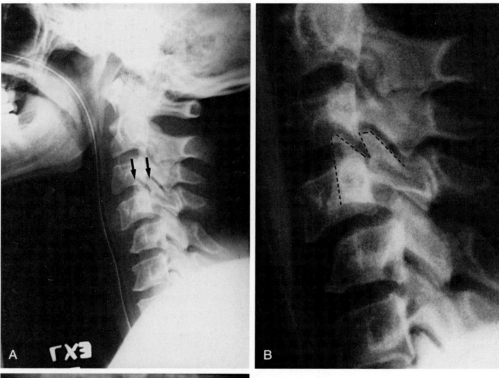

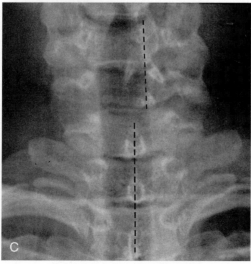

FIGURE 40–40 Unilateral facet dislocation. *A,* Lateral view of the cervical spine. The C4 vertebral body is displaced anteriorly less than one-half of its width relative to C5. The upper cervical spine has a rotated or oblique orientation, and the lower cervical spine has a straight lateral orientation. At C4, both facets are visible (*arrows*). The more anterior facet is dislocated on C5. *B,* The "bow-tie" appearance at the level of dislocation is visible on a magnified view (*dotted lines*). *C,* Anteroposterior view of another patient with unilateral facet dislocation shows rotation above C6–C7, which is manifested by an abrupt change in the alignment of the spinous processes (*dashed lines*). (*A–C,* From Hart BL, Benzel EC, Ford CC. Fundamentals of Neuroimaging, p. 156. Philadelphia, WB Saunders, 1997.)

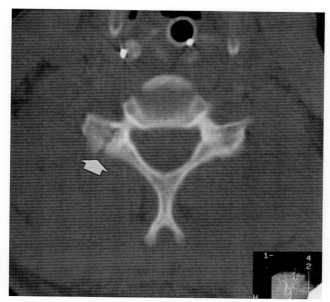

FIGURE 40–41 Lateral mass fracture at C6 on CT (*arrow*).

articular processes can be directly visualized; a "bow-tie" configuration results from the facet displacement. Abrupt change in distance between the spinolaminar line and the dorsal margins of the articular masses can also be a clue on the lateral radiograph.[130] On the anteroposterior view, there is an abrupt change in position of the spinous processes at the level of the dislocation.

CT of unilateral facet dislocation reveals disruption of the normal facet relationship. On the side of the dislocation, the "clamshell" or "hamburger bun" appearance is absent. It may be reversed, or the tips of the facets may be adjacent if the dislocation is incomplete. CT can be valuable to assess for fractures of the articular processes, which are common and may complicate reduction. Although tiny fractures are common, larger fractures involving the articular facet are more likely to result in instability. Re-formatted views are helpful to assess sagittal alignment and diameter of the spinal canal.[131] The disrupted facet joint and vertebral body subluxation can be visualized directly on sagittal MRI. Dorsal soft tissue injury is demonstrated, and disk fragments may be visible.[38, 132]

A combination of extension and rotation can result in fracture of the pillar or articular mass (Fig. 40–41).[96, 133] These fractures can be difficult to identify on routine plain films. Slight irregularity of the margins of the pillar on lateral or anteroposterior views may be the only finding on these views. If there is displacement of fracture fragments, facet joint spaces may become visible on the affected side on the anteroposterior view. Oblique or, especially, pillar views are often helpful. These fractures are much more readily demonstrated by CT.

The extent of soft tissue injury associated with pillar fractures is variable, and MRI is helpful to assess the extent of ligamentous injury. Anterior or posterior longitudinal ligament injury is common with rotatory injuries and probably indicates a greater risk of instability (Fig. 40–42).[134]

Hyperextension and rotation is also the presumed mechanism for combined fractures of the pedicle and lamina on the same side. These fractures separate the articular mass from the remainder of the vertebral body, with a significant risk of instability (Fig. 40–43). Various names have been used for this injury, including *pedicolaminar fracture-separation*.[96, 135] Four subtypes have been described. The first three are unilateral: *Type I* has minimal displacement and may be difficult to identify without CT. *Type II* pedicolaminar fracture-separation demonstrates greater displacement of the articular mass and ventral translation of the vertebra without disk space narrowing. The presence of disk space narrowing identifies a *type III* separation.[96]

The combination of rotation and mild ventral subluxation may simulate a unilateral facet dislocation on plain films, but careful inspection of radiographic features, especially on CT, enables identification of these hyperextension injuries. MRI demonstrates more directly the extent of soft tissue injury. Fracture into or isolating the articular mass, both prevertebral and dorsal soft tissue injury and focal injury around the facet joint or pillar, is associated with a greater risk of instability.

Type IV pedicolaminar fracture-separation is also known as *hyperextension fracture-dislocation*. The mechanism has been described by Forsyth[123] as a force to the upper face or forehead that forces the head and upper cervical spine backward and down. Circular movement ensues as the articular masses are fractured, and the forward component at the level of injury results in ventral translation of the vertebral body. Typically, there is an articular mass fracture on one side and facet dislocation on the other side. The anterior longitudinal ligament is disrupted. Despite the seemingly paradoxical ventral translation that occurs, it is important to recognize that this unstable injury results from a hyperextension injury.

Thoracic and Lumbar Spine

Denis[136] described a three-column model of the thoracolumbar spine by which stability is maintained. Each column consists of osseous and ligamentous elements. The *anterior column* is defined as the anterior half of the vertebral body and includes the anterior longitudinal ligament and anterior annulus fibrosus. The *middle column* consists of the posterior half of the vertebral body and pedicles, including the posterior annulus fibrosus and the posterior longitudinal ligament. The osseous elements of the *posterior column* are the facets, laminae, and spinous processes. The ligamentous elements are the facet joint capsules, the ligamenta flava, and the interspinous and supraspinous ligaments. As originally proposed, disruption of two of the three columns indicated a potentially unstable spine. The mechanisms of each of the four fracture types described next with respect to the three columns are summarized in Table 40–3. As in the cervical spine, MRI of the thoracic and lumbar spine can be used to evaluate injury to the posterior ligament complex, which is especially likely to be damaged in patients with burst fractures and fracture-dislocation.[137, 138]

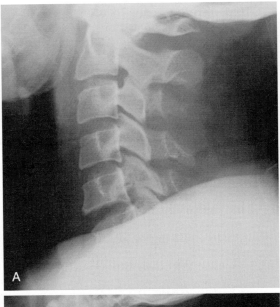

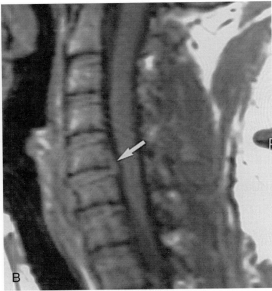

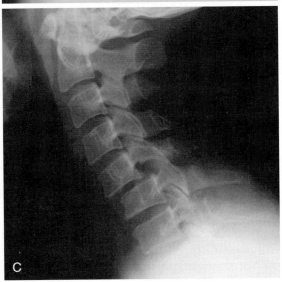

FIGURE 40–42 Value of MRI for identifying ligamentous injury. *A,* Initial lateral radiograph of a patient who was in a motor vehicle accident shows only minimal kyphosis and posterior widening at C5–C6. The patient had significant pain. *B,* Sagittal T1-weighted MRI was performed on the same day and revealed posterior disk disruption with extension of disk material or blood superior to the level of injury (*arrow*). Anterior and posterior longitudinal ligament injury was present, and there was dorsal interspinous injury (not shown). Unilateral articular mass fractures identified on CT were not significantly displaced. *C,* Despite treatment with rigid immobilization, the patient returned 13 days later with evidence of instability on a lateral radiograph. There is anterior subluxation, posterior widening, and evidence of rotational instability.

Compression Fractures

Ventral compression fractures from flexion are common in the thoracic and lumbar spines. Loss of ventral height of the vertebral body can be identified on the lateral view (Figs. 40–44 and 40–45). Mild fractures often involve only the ventral portion of the vertebral body (anterior column injury), but greater forces may cause buckling of the dorsal cortex (middle column injury) or, less commonly, fractures of the posterior elements (posterior column injury).

Burst Fractures

As with the cervical spine, axial loading injuries can produce burst-type fractures in the thoracic and lumbar spine. Fractures involve ventral and dorsal portions of the vertebral body and the posterior elements. Displaced bone often narrows the spinal canal (Fig. 40–46). There is a significant risk of SCI. Displaced fragments are readily recognized on plain films, and CT is best for evaluation

of the spinal canal itself. MRI is more sensitive for the demonstration of traumatic disk herniation and epidural hematoma and for the direct visualization of the spinal cord (see Figs. 40–7 and 40–13).

TABLE 40–3 Failure Mechanisms of Columns in Thoracolumbar Fractures

Fracture Type	Anterior Column	Middle Column	Posterior Column
Compression	Compression	None	None or severe distraction
Burst	Compression	Compression	None
Chance	None or compression	Distraction	Distraction
Fracture-dislocation	Compression rotation shear	Distraction rotation shear	Distraction rotation shear

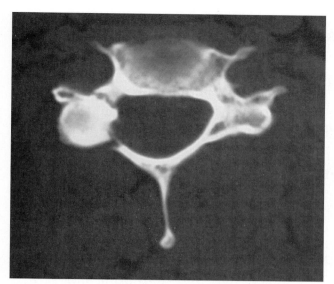

FIGURE 40–43 Pedicolaminar fracture, separation. Axial CT scan shows fractures of both pedicle and lamina on the patient's right.

Thoracolumbar Flexion-Distraction Injuries

Chance[139] originally described a pattern of horizontal fracture through the spine and neural arch associated with flexion. This occurs most often at the thoracolumbar junction or upper lumbar spine. Later investigators recognized the importance of flexion over an anterior fulcrum, commonly in the setting of an automobile accident in which the victim is wearing a lap belt but not a shoulder belt. The mechanism has been attributed to flexion over an anterior fulcrum combined with distraction, but other factors have also been suggested, including flexion followed by axial loading with higher-speed accidents.[140–143]

Involvement of the vertebral body is variable in Chance fractures, and there is often a mild loss of ventral

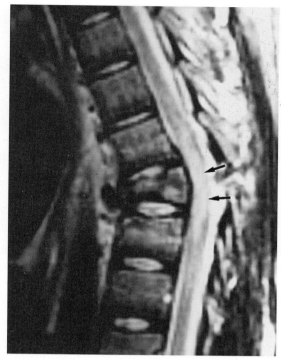

FIGURE 40–45 Thoracic compression fracture and spinal cord edema. MRI study of an 18-year-old who was in a motor vehicle accident. Sagittal T2-weighted image shows compression fracture of a midthoracic vertebral body, narrowing of the spinal canal, and high signal intensity within the spinal cord (*arrows*). The patient was paraplegic. (From Hart BL, Benzel EC, Ford CC. Fundamentals of Neuroimaging, p. 157. Philadelphia, WB Saunders, 1997.)

height. Altered alignment and the ventral fracture can be identified on the lateral plain film. Distraction of the posterior elements may also be demonstrated. The horizontal fractures through the pedicles are usually visible

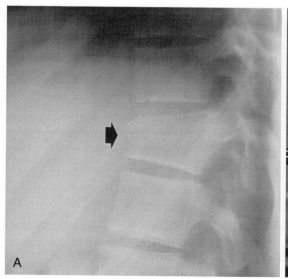 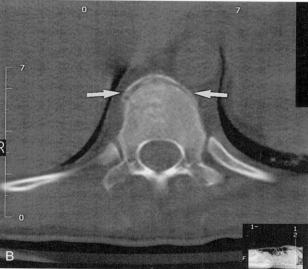

FIGURE 40–44 T11 compression fracture. *A,* Lateral radiograph shows typical features of compression fracture, with anterior loss of height and slight irregularity of the anterior cortex (*arrow*). *B,* On axial CT scan, the findings may be limited to an apparent double cortical margin (*arrows*) resulting from the anterior cortical fracture in mild cases.

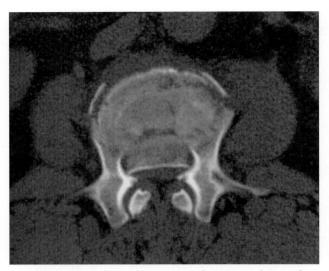

FIGURE 40–46 L2 burst fracture. Axial CT scan shows a burst fracture, with comminution of the vertebral body and widening of the facet joints. A fragment from the posterior aspect of the body narrows the spinal canal.

on the anteroposterior view. Because the fracture lies in the transaxial plane, the Chance fracture may be difficult to visualize on axial CT. Therefore, re-formatted views are necessary (Fig. 40–47). MRI demonstrates the dorsal soft tissue injury that accompanies this injury.

Other related injury patterns can also result from flexion-distraction (or similar mechanisms).[140, 142–144] Rather than fracturing through the midvertebral body, the distraction may occur primarily through the intervertebral

disk level. The disk space is disrupted, and there is usually disruption of the facet joints, often with posterior element fractures as well (Fig. 40–48). A variation also occurs with more oblique involvement of posterior elements on one side than the other. A combination of imaging studies is helpful to demonstrate the exact distribution of complex injuries.[137, 138]

In patients with seatbelt-type injuries, seatbelt contusion on the anterior abdominal wall is common. Abdominal organ lacerations or perforations are seen in up to 50% of patients.[143, 144] Neurologic deficits are present in 17% to 27% of patients.[140, 143] The levels of injury are typically T12–L4.

Thoracic and Lumbar Fracture-Dislocation

Severe forces on the thoracic and lumbar spine may cause major dislocations, nearly always resulting in paraplegia. Plain radiographs usually show the dislocation, and CT is more helpful to define the fractures and assist in planning stabilization strategies (Figs. 40–49 and 40–50). The status of the spinal cord and the presence of epidural hematoma and disk herniation are best visualized with MRI. MRI also reveals the extent of ligamentous injury.[137, 138]

Soft Tissue Injuries with and Without Fracture

Spinal Cord Injury Without Radiographic Abnormality

The entity of SCI without radiographic abnormality (SCIWORA) poses a difficult clinical problem. SCIWORA is more common in children than in adults. The term *spinal cord injury without radiographic abnormality*

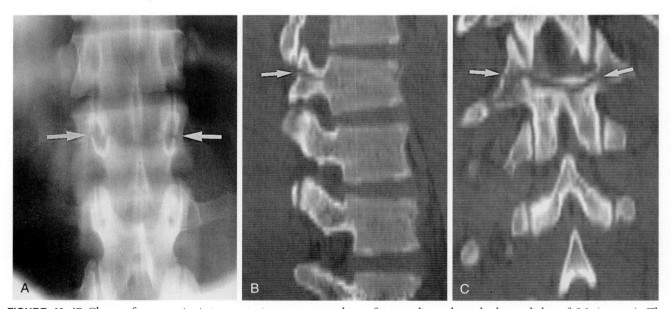

FIGURE 40–47 Chance fracture. *A,* Anteroposterior tomogram shows fracture lines through the pedicles of L1 (*arrows*). The fracture line is difficult to identify on axial CT, but parasagittal (*B*) and coronal (*C*) reconstructions from CT scans of a different patient with a similar fracture show the fracture extending through the posterior elements (*arrows*). There is anterior loss of height of L1 and a mild compression fracture of L3.

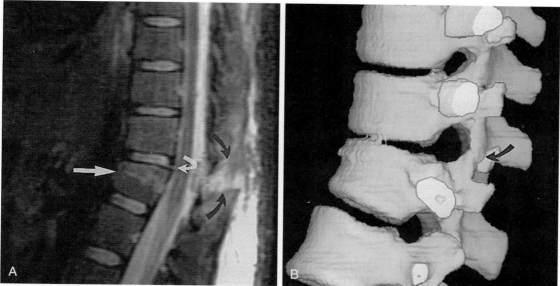

FIGURE 40–48 Flexion-distraction injury between posterior elements. *A,* Sagittal inversion recovery MRI study of a patient who had a flexion-distraction injury (seat-belt–type injury) shows not only edema and loss of height of a lower thoracic vertebral body (*straight white arrow*), but also disruption through the posterior margin of the disk space (*curved white arrow*). The plane of injury is easily visible extending through the posterior elements and soft tissues (*black arrows*). *B,* Three-dimensional CT reconstruction from a lateral view demonstrates the anterior compression fracture, widening of the disk space, and subluxation of the facet joints (*arrow*).

has been objected to because it is a nonspecific description that covers a variety of mechanisms. Most of these cases do have demonstrable abnormalities on MRI (Figs. 40–51 and 40–52; see also Fig. 40–13).[28, 145] Postulated mechanisms include transient distraction, flexion, or compression of the spinal cord and ischemia. Neurologic abnormalities without obvious radiographic findings are an indication for spinal MRI.

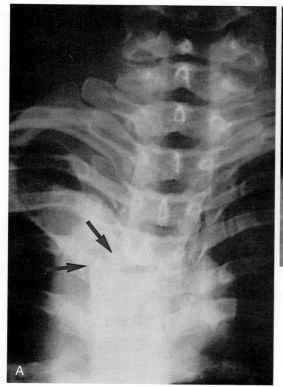

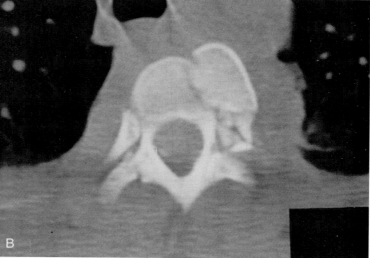

FIGURE 40–49 Thoracic fracture-dislocation. *A,* Anteroposterior radiograph of a young adult who was in an automobile accident shows fracture-dislocation in the upper thoracic spine, with lateral translation of the spine at the level of dislocation (*arrows*). *B,* Axial CT scan reveals comminuted fractures and lateral translation that results in visualization of parts of two vertebral bodies. The patient remained neurologically intact.

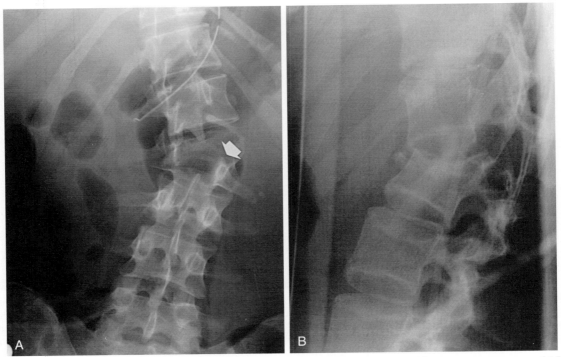

FIGURE 40–50 Upper lumbar fracture-dislocation. Anteroposterior (*A*) and lateral (*B*) views of a patient in a motor vehicle accident. There is a lateral compression of L2 and distraction, resulting in facet dislocation. The "empty" left superior articular facet of L2 is visible (*arrow* in *A*).

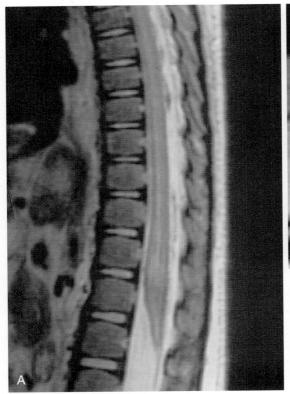

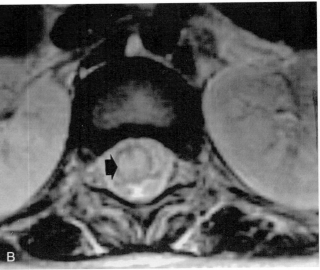

FIGURE 40–51 Spinal cord injury without fracture. MRI study of a 2-year-old child who was not moving the lower extremities after a motor vehicle accident. There were no fractures. Sagittal (*A*) and axial (*B*) T2-weighted images show a lengthy region of edema within the distal spinal cord (*arrow* in *B*). The most likely cause is ischemia.

FIGURE 40–52 Central cord and cervicocranial injury. The patient was a child who had a central cord syndrome after a motor vehicle accident. A seat-belt mark was present on the anterior neck. *A,* Sagittal inversion recovery MRI study shows extensive dorsal soft tissue injury and edema within the spinal cord (*straight arrow*). High-signal-intensity blood is present dorsal to the clivus, elevating the dura and tectorial membrane (*curved arrow*). *B,* Axial CT scan at the level of the foramen magnum confirms the presence of epidural blood (*arrow*). The injury is presumed to have resulted from a distraction mechanism.

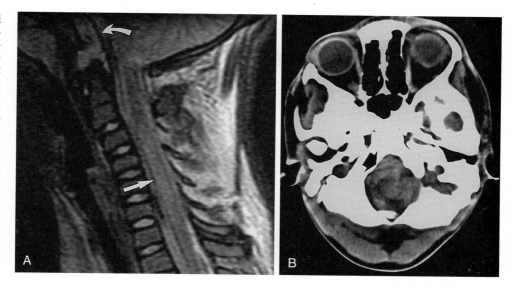

Ligamentous Injury

Significant spine injury and instability can result from soft tissue injury without fracture. Examples have been discussed earlier of atlanto-occipital dissociation, rotatory subluxation or dislocation, hyperextension dislocation or sprain, and flexion sprain. Minor fractures may accompany these, but the major damage is to the supporting ligaments of the cervical spine. Major neurologic damage can occur without any fractures (see Figs. 40–5, 40–15, 40–38, 40–39, 40–51, and 40–52).

Transverse ligament rupture is usually observed in association with Jefferson's or other upper cervical spine fractures, but it can infrequently occur as an isolated injury. Two patterns have been described: rupture of the ligament in its midportion and unilateral avulsion of the ligament at its attachment. The latter often results in a small bone fragment avulsed from the tubercle of C1, which can be visible on CT. The identification of fractures involving the tubercle of C1 on CT suggests the possibility of transverse ligament disruption. Loss of the ligament integrity can cause widening of the anterior atlantodental space on the lateral radiograph or on CT. Flexion views to elicit this sign are potentially dangerous, however, and should rarely be obtained in the setting of acute trauma. MRI can directly demonstrate the transverse ligament as a low-signal-intensity structure in the axial plane and is the technique of choice for evaluation of suspected transverse ligament disruption. In such choices, MRI demonstrates lack of continuity of the ligament and higher signal intensity than expected in the region of the rupture. Thin slice thickness is most effective for demonstration of the transverse ligament.

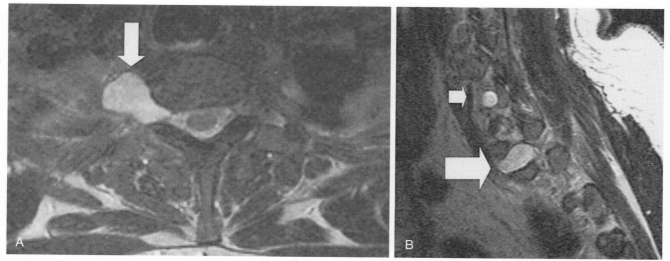

FIGURE 40–53 Nerve root avulsion. *A,* T2-weighted axial MRI study shows a pseudomeningocele extending anterolaterally from the right neural foramen (*arrow*). Ten days after major trauma, the patient had difficulty moving the right upper extremity. *B,* Parasagittal T2-weighted image shows an oval fluid collection at the same level (*large arrow*) and a smaller fluid collection superior to that level (*small arrow*) that represents a second pseudomeningocele from nerve root avulsion.

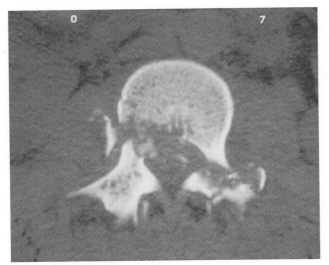

FIGURE 40–54 Gunshot injury of the upper lumbar spine. The trajectory of the bullet is clearly visible on the CT scan, passing through the posterior body of C2 on the patient's right, displacing fragments into the spinal canal, and passing through the posterior elements on the left.

Brachial Plexus and Nerve Root Injuries

Traction injuries on the shoulder and upper extremity can lead to brachial plexus injury. Clinical deficits can result from stretching of the plexus or from outright tearing or avulsion of some components of the plexus. Avulsion of nerve roots can occur as they exit the spinal canal, often resulting in pseudomeningocele at the levels involved. Such pseudomeningoceles can be demonstrated by myelography, postmyelography CT, or MRI (Fig. 40–53).

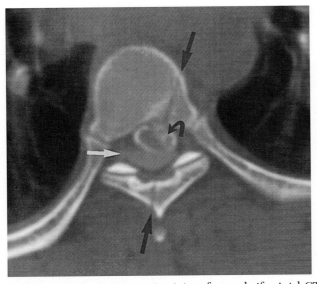

FIGURE 40–55 Penetrating spine injury from a knife. Axial CT scan after thoracic myelogram shows fractures involving the right lamina and left side of the vertebral body (*straight black arrows*). Contrast material has leaked into the posterior right epidural space (*white arrow*), and the spinal cord has been disrupted on the patient's left side (*curved black arrow*).

T2-weighted sequences are especially helpful, and coronal images in addition to more routine axial and sagittal images are beneficial if nerve root avulsion is suspected. MRI is the only imaging technique appropriate for evaluation of more peripheral brachial plexus injuries. In the lower neck, the course of the brachial plexus lies between the anterior and the middle scalene muscles.

PENETRATING INJURIES

Penetrating injuries of the spine are as varied as the combination of their velocity, mass, and trajectory allows. Although spinal instability can result, it is relatively uncommon. Neural element injury results from direct transection or from energy transmitted via a concussion wave effect.

Missile injuries are usually most devastating in nature (Fig. 40–54). High-velocity missiles have a tendency to disrupt stability and cause neural element injury. Stability is usually disrupted only if the anterior and middle columns of Denis are disrupted. SCI results if the missile passes through or close to the spinal canal.

Spinal cord stab wounds (usually knives) are uncommon. They most commonly result from dorsal penetration (Fig. 40–55). The pathway of a penetrating knife is usually lateral to midline. This is so because of the bony confines created by the spinous processes medially and the facet complex laterally. These confines direct a horizontally oriented knife between the lamina lateral to midline. This penetrating knife wound often results in a Brown-Séquard syndrome. Although uncommon, cerebrospinal fluid leakage may occur after penetrating spine injury.

References

1. DeVivo MJ, Rutt RD, Black KJ, et al. Trends in SCI demographics and treatment outcomes between 1973 and 1986. Arch Phys Med Rehabil 1992;73:424–430.
2. NSCICS. Spinal Cord Injury Facts and Figures at a Glance. Birmingham, AL, National Spinal Cord Injury Statistical Center, 1998.
3. Stover SL, Whiteneck GG, DeLisa JA. Spinal Cord Injury: Clinical Outcome from the Model Systems. Gaithersburg, MD, Aspen, 1995.
4. Chang DG, Tencer AF, Ching RP, et al. Geometric changes in the cervical spine canal during impact. Spine 1994;19:973–980.
5. Young W. Secondary injury mechanisms in acute SCI. J Emerg Med 1993;11(Suppl 1):13–22.
6. Coen SD. Spinal cord injury: Preventing secondary injury. Neurol Res 1991;13:138–159.
7. Brodkey JS, Miller CF Jr, Harmody RM. The syndrome of acute central cervical SCI revisited. Surg Neurol 1980;14:251–257.
8. Bracken MB, Shepard MJ, Collins WF, et al. A randomized, controlled trial of methylprednisolone or naloxone in the treatment of acute spinal-cord injury: Results of the Second National Acute Spinal Cord Injury Study. N Engl J Med 1990;322:1405–1411.
9. Anthes DL, Theriault E, Tator CH. Characterization of axonal ultrastructural pathology following experimental spinal cord compression injury. Brain Res 1995;702:1–16.
10. Demopolous HB, Flamm ES, Seligman ML, et al. Further studies on free-radical pathology in the major central nervous system disorders: Effects of very high doses of methylprednisolone on the functional outcome, morphology, and chemistry of experimental SCI. Can J Physiol Pharmacol 1982;60:1415–1424.
11. Hall ED. The neuroprotective pharmacology of methylprednisolone. J Neurosurg 1992;6:13–22.
12. Tator CH, Koyanagi I. Vascular mechanisms in the pathophysiology of human SCI. J Neurotrauma 1997;14:507–515.
13. Agrawal SK, Fehlings MG. Mechanisms of secondary injury to

spinal cord axons in vitro: Role of Na+, Na(+)-K(+)-ATPase, the Na(+)-H+ exchanger, and the Na(+)-Ca2+ exchanger. J Neurosci 1996;16:545–552.

14. Fehlings MG, Agrawal S. Role of sodium in the pathophysiology of secondary SCI. Spine 1995;20:2187–2191.

15. Hayashi T, Sakurai M, Abe K, et al. Apoptosis of motor neurons with induction of caspases in the spinal cord after ischemia. Stroke 1998;29:1007–1012.

16. Hall ED, Yonkers PA, Taylor BM, Sun FF. Lack of effect of postinjury treatment with methylprednisolone or tirilazad mesylate on the increase in eicosanoid levels in the acutely injured cat spinal cord. J Neurotrauma 1995;12:245–256.

17. Bracken MB, Shepard MJ, Collins WF Jr, et al. Methylprednisolone or naloxone treatment after acute SCI: 1-year follow-up data. Results of the Second National Acute Spinal Cord Injury Study. J Neurosurg 1992;76:23–31.

18. Shaffer MA, Doris PE. Limitation of the cross table lateral view in detecting cervical spine injuries: A retrospective analysis. Ann Emerg Med 1981;10:508–513.

19. Streitweiser DR, Knopp R, Wales LR, et al. Accuracy of standard radiographic views in detecting cervical spine fractures. Ann Emerg Med 1983;12:538–542.

20. Ross SE, Schwab CW, David ET, et al. Clearing the cervical spine: Initial radiologic evaluation. J Trauma 1987;27:1055–1060.

21. Acheson MD, Livingston RR, Richardson ML, Stimac GK. High-resolution CT in the evaluation of cervical spine fractures: Comparison with plain film examinations. AJR 1987;148:1179–1185.

22. Woodring JH, Lee C. The role and limitations of computed tomographic scanning in the evaluation of cervical trauma. J Trauma 1992;33:698–708.

23. Woodring JH, Lee C. Limitations of cervical radiography in the evaluation of acute cervical trauma. J Trauma 1993;34:32–39.

24. Blacksin MF, Lee HJ. Frequency and significance of fractures of the upper cervical spine detected by CT in patients with severe neck trauma. AJR 1995;165:1201–1204.

25. Borock EC, Gabram SG, Jacobs LM, et al. A prospective analysis of a two-year experience using CT as an adjunct for cervical spine clearance. J Trauma 1991;31:1001–1006.

26. Nunez DB, Zuluaga A, Fuentes-Bernardo DA, et al. Cervical spine trauma: How much more do we learn by routinely using helical CT? Radiographics 1996;16:1307–1318.

27. Orrison WW, Benzel EC, Willis BK, et al. Magnetic resonance imaging evaluation of acute spine trauma. Emerg Radiol 1995;2:120–128.

28. Davis JW, Phreaner DL, Hoyt DB, Mackersie RC. The etiology of missed cervical spine injuries. J Trauma 1993;34:342–346.

29. Beers GJ, Raque GH, Wagner GG, et al. MR imaging in acute cervical spine trauma. J Comput Assist Tomogr 1988;12:755–761.

30. Chakeres DW, Flickinger F, Bresnahan JC, et al. MR imaging of acute spinal cord trauma. AJNR 1987;8:5–10.

31. Goldberg AL, Rothfus WE, Deeb ZL, et al. The impact of magnetic resonance on the diagnostic evaluation of acute cervicothoracic spinal trauma. Skeletal Radiol 1988;17:89–95.

32. Hackney DB, Asato R, Joseph PM, et al. Hemorrhage and edema in acute spinal canal compression: Demonstration by MR imaging. Radiology 1986;161:387–390.

33. McArdle CB, Crofford MJ, Mirjakhraee M, et al. Surface coil MR of spinal trauma: Preliminary experience. AJNR 1986;7:886–893.

34. Mirvis SE, Geisler FH, Jelinek JJ, et al. Acute cervical spine trauma: Evaluation with 1.5T MR imaging. Radiology 1988;166:807–816.

35. Tarr RW, Drolshagen LF, Kerner TC, et al. MR imaging of recent spinal trauma. J Comput Assist Tomogr 1987;11:412–417.

36. Warner J, Shanmuganathan K, Mirvis SE, Cerva D. Magnetic resonance imaging of ligamentous injury of the cervical spine. Emerg Radiol 1996;3:9–15.

37. Benzel EC, Hart BL, Ball PA, et al. Magnetic resonance imaging for the evaluation of patients with occult cervical spine injury. J Neurosurg 1996;85:824–829.

38. Rizzolo SJ, Piazza MR, Cotler JM, et al. Intervertebral disk injury complicating cervical spine trauma. Spine 1991;16:S187–S189.

39. Lewis LM, Docherty M, Ruoff BE, et al. Flexion-extension views in the evaluation of cervical-spine injuries. Ann Emerg Med 1991;20:117–121.

40. Bohrer SP, Chen YM, Sayers DG. Cervical spine flexion patterns. Skeletal Radiol 1990;19:521–525.

41. Juhl JH, Miller SM, Roberts GW. Roentgenographic variations in the normal cervical spine. Radiology 1962;78:591–597.

42. Webb JK, Broughton RBK, McSween T, et al. Hidden flexion injury of the cervical spine. J Bone Joint Surg Br 1976;68:322–327.

43. Penning L, Wilmink JT. Rotation of the cervical spine: A CT study in normal subjects. Spine 1987;12:732–738.

44. Taylor AR, Blackwood W. Paraplegia in cervical injuries with normal radiographic appearance. J Bone Joint Surg Br 1948;30:245–248.

45. Cattell HS, Filtzer DL. Pseudosubluxation and other normal variations in the cervical spine in children. J Bone Joint Surg Am 1965;47:1295–1309.

46. Silverman FN, Kuhn JP. Caffey's Pediatric X-Ray Diagnosis: An Integrated Imaging Approach, 9th ed. Chicago, Mosby, 1995.

47. Swischuk LE. Anterior dislocation of C2 in children: Physiologic or pathologic? Radiology 1977;122:759–763.

48. Hill SA, Miller CA, Kosnik EJ, Hunt WE. Pediatric neck injuries. J Neurosurg 1984;60:700–706.

49. McGrory BJ, Klassen RA, Chao EYS, et al. Acute fractures and dislocations of the cervical spine in children and adolescents. J Bone Joint Surg Am 1993;75:988–995.

50. Kuhns LR. Imaging of Spinal Trauma in Children. Hamilton, Ont., BC Decker, 1998.

51. Calenoff L, Chessare JW, Rogers LF, et al. Multiple level spinal injuries: Importance of early recognition. AJR 1978;130:665–669.

52. Shear P, Hugenholtz H, Richard MT, et al. Multiple noncontiguous fractures of the cervical spine. J Trauma 1988;28:655–669.

53. Olerud C, Jonsson H. Compression of the cervical spine cord after reduction of fracture dislocation: Report of 2 cases. Acta Orthop Scand 1991;62:599–601.

54. Robertson PA, Ryan MD. Neurological deterioration after reduction of cervical subluxation: Mechanical compression by disk tissue. J Bone Joint Surg Br 1992;74:224–227.

55. Keiper MD, Zimmerman RZ, Bilaniuk LT. MRI in the assessment of the supportive soft tissues of the cervical spine in acute trauma in children. Neuroradiology 1998;40:359–363.

56. Penning L. Roentgenographic evaluation: Obtaining and interpreting plain films in cervical spine injury. In Bailey RW (ed): The Cervical Spine, pp. 62–95. The Cervical Spine Research Society. Philadelphia, JB Lippincott, 1983.

57. Hay PD. Measurement of the soft tissues of the neck. In Lusted LB, Keats TE (eds): Atlas of Roentgenographic Measurement, 3rd ed., pp. 23–27. Chicago, Year Book Medical, 1972.

58. Harris JH Jr. Abnormal craniocervical retropharyngeal soft-tissue contour in the detection of subtle acute craniocervical injuries. Emerg Radiol 1994;1:15–23.

59. Miller MO, Gehweiler JA, Martinez S, et al. Significant new observations on cervical spine trauma. AJR 1978;130:659–663.

60. Kulkarni MV, McArdle CB, Kopanicky D, et al. Acute SCI: MR imaging at 1.5T. Radiology 1987;164:837–843.

61. Schaefer DM, Flanders AE, Osterhold JL, Northrup BE. Prognostic significance of magnetic resonance imaging in the acute phase of cervical spine injury. J Neurosurg 1992;76:218–223.

62. Flanders AE, Schaefer DM, Doan HT, et al. Acute cervical spine trauma: Correlation of MR imaging findings with degree of neurologic deficit. Radiology 1990;177:25–33.

63. Silberstein M, Tress BM, Hennessy O. Prediction of neurologic outcome in acute SCI: The role of CT and MR. AJNR 1992;13:1597–1608.

64. Yamashita Y, Takahashi M, Matsuno Y, et al. Acute SCI: Magnetic resonance imaging correlated with myelopathy. Br J Radiol 1991;64:201–209.

65. Willis BK, Greiner F, Orrison WW, Benzel EC. The incidence of vertebral artery injury after midcervical spine fracture or subluxation. Neurosurgery 1994;34:435–441.

66. Frankel HL, Hancock DO, Hyslop G, et al. The value of postural reduction in the initial management of closed injuries of the spine with paraplegia and tetraplegia: I. Source. Paraplegia 1969;3:179–192.

67. Ditunno JF Jr, Graziani V, Tessler A. Neurological assessment in SCI. Adv Neurol 1997;72:325–333.

68. Clayman DA, Sykes CH, Vines FS. Occipital condyle fractures: Clinical presentation and radiologic detection. AJNR 1994;15:1309–1315.

69. Bettini N, Malaguti MC, Sintinti M, et al. Fractures of the occipital

70. Werne S. Studies in spontaneous atlas dislocation. Acta Orthop Scand 1957;23(Suppl):1–159.

71. Bucholz RW, Burkhead WZ. The pathological anatomy of fatal atlanto-occipital dislocations. J Bone Joint Surg Am 1979;61:248–250.

72. Kaufman RA, Dunbar JS, Botsford JA, et al. Traumatic longitudinal atlanto-occipital distraction injuries in children. AJNR 1982;3:415–419.

73. Powers B, Miller MD, Kramer RS, et al. Traumatic anterior atlanto-occipital dislocation. Neurosurgery 1979;4:12–17.

74. Lee C, Woodring JH, Goldstein SJ, et al. Evaluation of traumatic atlantooccipital dislocations. AJNR 1987;8:19–26.

75. Harris JH Jr, Carson GC, Wagner LK. Radiologic diagnosis of traumatic occipitovertebral dissociation: 1. Normal occipitovertebral relationships on lateral radiographs of supine subjects. AJR 1994;162:881–886.

76. Harris JH Jr, Carson GC, Wagner LK, et al. Radiologic diagnosis of traumatic occipitovertebral dissociation: 2. Comparison of three methods of detecting occipitovertebral relationships on lateral radiographs of supine subjects. AJR 1994;162:887–892.

77. Wortzmann G, Dewar FP. Rotatory fixation of the atlantoaxial joint: Rotational atlantoaxial subluxation. Radiology 1968;90:479–487.

78. Van Holsbeeck EM, MacKay NN. Diagnosis of acute atlanto-axial rotatory fixation. J Bone Joint Surg Br 1989;71:90–91.

79. Fielding JW, Hawkins RJ. Atlanto-axial rotatory fixation. J Bone Joint Surg Am 1977;59:37–44.

80. Murray JB, Ziervogel M. The value of computed tomography in the diagnosis of atlanto-axial rotatory fixation. Br J Radiol 1990;63:894–694.

81. Coutts MB. Rotary dislocations of the atlas. Ann Surg 1934;29:297–311.

82. Jefferson G. Fracture of the atlas vertebra: Report of four cases, and a review of those previously recorded. Br J Surg 1920;7:407–422.

83. Suss RA, Zimmerman RD, Leeds NE. Pseudospread of the atlas: False sign of Jefferson fracture in young children. AJR 1983;140:1079–1082.

84. Spence KF, Decker S, Sell KW. Bursting atlantal fracture associated with rupture of the transverse ligament. J Bone Joint Surg Am 1970;52:542–549.

85. Dickman CA, Mamourian A, Sonntag VK, Drayer BP. Magnetic resonance imaging of the transverse atlantal ligament for the evaluation of atlantoaxial instability. J Neurosurg 1991;75:221–227.

86. Green KA, Dickman CA, Marciano FF, et al. Transverse atlantal ligament disruption associated with odontoid fractures. Spine 1994;19:2307–2314.

87. Anderson LD, D'Alonzo RT. Fractures of the odontoid process of the axis. J Bone Joint Surg Am 1974;56:1663–1674.

88. Burke JT, Harris JH Jr. Acute injuries of the axis vertebra. Skeletal Radiol 1989;18:335–346.

89. Gehweiler JA Jr, Clark WM, Schaaf RE, et al. Cervical spine trauma: The common combined conditions. Radiology 1979;130:77–86.

90. Gehweiler JA Jr, Duff DE, Martinez S, et al. Fractures of the atlas vertebra. Skeletal Radiol 1976;1:97–102.

91. Kazarian L. Injuries to the human spinal column: Biomechanics and injury classification. Exerc Sport Sci Rev 1981;9:297–352.

92. Wilson TAS Jr, McWhorter JM. Atlantoaxial injuries. In Caminas MB, O'Leary PF (eds). Disorders of the Cervical Spine, pp. 288–289. Baltimore, Williams & Wilkins, 1992.

93. Schatzker J, Rorabeck CH, Waddell JP. Fractures of the dens (odontoid process): An analysis of thirty seven cases. J Bone J Surg Br 1971;53:392–405.

94. Benzel EC, Hart BL, Ball PA, et al. Fractures of the C-2 vertebral body. J Neurosurg 1994;81:206–212.

95. Harris JH Jr, Burke JT, Ray RD, et al: Low (type III) odontoid fracture: A new radiologic sign. Radiology 1984;153:353–356.

96. Harris JH Jr, Mirvis SE. The Radiology of Acute Cervical Spine Trauma. Baltimore, Williams & Wilkins, 1996.

97. Holdsworth F. Fractures, dislocations and fracture-dislocations of the spine. J Bone Joint Surg Am 1970;52:1534–1551.

98. Cornish BL. Traumatic spondylolisthesis of the axis. J Bone Joint Surg Br 1968;50:31–43.

99. Francis WR, Fielding JW. Traumatic spondylolisthesis of the axis. Orthop Clin North Am 1978;9:1011–1027.

100. Sherk HH, Howard T. Clinical and pathologic correlations in traumatic spondylolisthesis of the axis. Clin Orthop 1983;174:122–126.

101. Francis WR Jr, Fielding JW, Hawkins RJ, et al. Traumatic spondylolisthesis of the axis. J Bone Joint Surg Br 1981;63:313–318.

102. Schneider RC, Livingston KE, Cave AJE, Hamilton G. "Hangman's fracture" of the cervical spine. J Neurosurg 1965;22:141–154.

103. Brashear HR Jr, Venters GC, Preston ET. Fractures of the neural arch of the axis. J Bone Joint Surg Am 1975;57:879–887.

104. Wallace SK, Cohen WA, Stern EJ, Reay DT. Judicial hanging: Post mortem radiographic, CT, and MR imaging features with autopsy confirmation. Radiology 1994;193:263–267.

105. Effendi B, Roy D, Cornish B, et al. Fractures of the ring of the axis: A classification based on the analysis of 131 cases. J Bone Joint Surg Br 1981;63:319–327.

106. Levine AM, Edwards CC. The management of traumatic spondylolisthesis of the axis. J Bone Joint Surg Am 1985;67:217–226.

107. Starr JK, Eismont FJ. Atypical hangman's fractures. Spine 1993;18:1954–1957.

108. Allen BL Jr, Ferguson RL, Lehmann TR, O'Brien RP. A mechanistic classification of closed, indirect fractures and dislocations of the lower cervical spine. Spine 1982;7:1–27.

109. Braakman R, Penning L. The hyperflexion sprain of the cervical spine. Radiol Clin Biol 1968;37:309–320.

110. Green JD, Harle TS, Harris JH Jr. Anterior subluxation of the cervical spine: Hyperflexion sprain. AJNR 1981;2:243–250.

111. Scher AT. Anterior cervical subluxation: An unstable position. AJR 1979;133:275–280.

112. Harris JH Jr, Yeakley JS. Radiographically subtle soft tissue injuries of the cervical spine. Curr Probl Diagn Radiol 1989;18:161–190.

113. Beatson F. Fractures, dislocations and fracture-dislocations of the spine. J Bone Joint Surg Am 1970;52:1534–1551.

114. White AA, Johnson RM, Panjabi MD, et al. Biomedical analysis of clinical stability in the cervical spine. Clin Orthop 1975;109:85–96.

115. Taylor RG, Gleave JRW. Injuries to the cervical spine. Proc R Soc Med 1962;55:1053–1058.

116. King DM. Fractures and dislocations of the cervical part of the spine. Aust N Z J Surg 1967;37:57–64.

117. Bedbrook GM. Stability of spinal fractures and fracture dislocations. Paraplegia 1971;9:23–32.

118. Schneider RC, Kahn EA. Chronic neurological sequelae of acute trauma to the spine and spinal cord: Part 1. The significance of the acute-flexion or "teardrop" fracture-dislocation of the cervical spine. J Bone Joint Surg Am 1956;38:985–997.

119. Kim KS, Chen HH, Russell EJ, Roger LF. Flexion tear-drop fracture of the cervical spine: Radiographic characteristics. AJR 1989;152:319–326.

120. Schneider RC. A syndrome in acute cervical spine injuries for which early operation is indicated. J Neurosurg 1951;8:360–367.

121. Schneider RC. The syndrome of acute anterior SCI. J Neurosurg 1955;12:95–122.

122. Marar BC. Hyperextension injuries of the cervical spine: The pathogenesis of damage to the spinal cord. J Bone Joint Surg Am 1974;56:1655–1662.

123. Forsyth HF. Extension injuries of the cervical spine. J Bone Joint Surg Am 1964;46:1792–1797.

124. Edeiken-Monroe B, Wagner LK, Harris JH Jr. Hyperextension dislocation of the cervical spine. AJR 1986;146:803–808.

125. Harris JH Jr, Yeakley JW. Hyperextension-dislocation of the cervical spine. J Bone Joint Surg Br 1992;74:567–570.

126. Taylor AR. The mechanism of injury to the spinal cord in the neck without damage to the vertebral column. J Bone Joint Surg Br 1951;33:543–547.

127. Borovich B, Peyser E, Gruskiewicz J. Acute central and intermediate cervical cord injury (case V). Neurochirurgia 1978;21:77–84.

128. Quencer RM, Bunge RP, Egnor M, et al. Acute traumatic central cord syndrome: MRI pathological correlations. Neuroradiology 1992;34:85–94.

129. Braakman R, Vinken PJ. Unilateral facet interlocking in the lower cervical spine. J Bone Joint Surg Br 1967;49:249–257.

130. Young JWR, Resnick CS, DeCandido P, Mirvis SE. The laminar space in the diagnosis of rotational flexion injuries of the cervical spine. AJR 1989;152:103–107.

131. Shanmuganathan K, Mirvis SE, Levine AM. Rotational injury of cervical facets: CT analysis of fractures patterns with implications for management and neurologic outcome. AJR 1994;163:1165–1169.

132. Doran SE, Papadopoulos SM, Ducker T, Lillehei KO. Magnetic resonance imaging documentation of coexistent traumatic locked facets of the cervical spine and disk herniation. J Neurosurg 1993;79:341–345.

133. Smith GR, Beckly DE, Abel MS. Articular mass fracture: A neglected cause of post-traumatic neck pain? Clin Radiol 1976;27:335–340.

134. Halliday AL, Henderson BR, Hart BL, Benzel EC. The management of unilateral lateral mass/facet fractures of the subaxial cervical spine. Spine 1997;22:2614–2621.

135. Fuentes JM, Benezech J, Lusszie B, Bloncourt J. Fracture-separation of the articular process of the inferior cervical vertebrae: A comprehensive review of 13 cases. In Kehr P, Weidner A (eds). Cervical Spine I, pp. 227–231. New York, Springer-Verlag, 1987.

136. Denis F. The three-column spine and its significance in the classification of acute thoracolumbar spine injuries. Spine 1983;8:817–831.

137. Terk MR, Hume-Neal M, Fraipont M, et al. Injury of the posterior ligament complex in patients with acute spinal trauma: Evaluation by MR imaging. AJR 1997;168:1481–1486.

138. Petersilge CA, Pathria MN, Emery SE, Masaryk TJ. Thoracolumbar burst fractures: Evaluation with MR imaging. Radiology 1995;194:49–54.

139. Chance GQ. Note on a type of flexion fracture of the spine. Br J Radiol 1948;21:452–453.

140. Smith WS, Kaufer H. Patterns and mechanisms of lumbar injuries associated with lap seat belts. J Bone Joint Surg Am 1969;51:239–254.

141. Rennie W, Mitchell N. Flexion distraction fractures of the thoracolumbar spine. J Bone Joint Surg Am 1973;55:386–390.

142. Bucholz RW, Gill K. Classification of injuries to the thoracolumbar spine. Orthop Clin North Am 1986;17:67–73.

143. Gertzbein SD, Court-Brown CM. Flexion-distraction injuries of the lumbar spine: Mechanisms of injury and classification. Clin Orthop 1988;227:52–60.

144. Gumley G, Taylor TKF, Ryan MD. Distraction fractures of the lumbar spine. J Bone Joint Surg Br 1982;64:520–525.

145. Matsumura A, Meguro K, Tsurushima H, et al. Magnetic resonance imaging of SCI without radiologic abnormality. Surg Neurol 1990;33:281–283.

41

The Larynx

SURESH K. MUKHERJI, M.D.
MAURICIO CASTILLO, M.D.

ANATOMY

The Endolarynx

The larynx is divided into endolaryngeal and exolaryngeal regions.[1] Many otolaryngologists consider the larynx to be a compartment comprising a mucosal surface and a supporting cartilaginous skeleton.[2] The endolarynx is divided by the true vocal cords into supraglottic, glottic, and subglottic compartments.[3] The supraglottic larynx extends from the tongue base and valleculae inferiorly to the laryngeal ventricle. The contents of the supraglottic larynx include the epiglottis, aryepiglottic folds, false vocal cords, laryngeal ventricle, and arytenoid processes of the arytenoid cartilages.[4] The epiglottis attaches inferiorly to the thyroid cartilage via the thyroepiglottic ligament and anteriorly to the hyoid bone via the thyrohyoid ligament. The superior portion of the epiglottis, which is situated posterior to the hyoid bone and vallecula, is called the *free margin*. The aryepiglottic folds are formed by mucosal reflections extending from the inferior and lateral aspects of the epiglottis to the tip of the arytenoid cartilages. The false vocal cords are the inferior continuation of the aryepiglottic folds and form the superior border of the laryngeal ventricle.[2, 3]

The Exolarynx

The exolarynx is formed by the supporting structures, mainly the thyroid and cricoid cartilages.[2] The thyroid cartilage, the largest, is composed of two alae that fuse anteriorly in the midline. Its superior cornua are the attachments for the thyrohyoid ligament, and its inferior cornua articulate with the cricoid cartilage. The cricoid cartilage is shaped like a signet ring and is the only complete cartilaginous ring of the larynx. The arytenoid cartilages articulate with the superior and posterior margins of the cricoid cartilage. The intrinsic laryngeal muscles include the thyroarytenoid, vocalis, cricoarytenoid, and cricothyroid.[1] The latter are innervated by the superior laryngeal nerves, whereas the rest are mostly innervated by the recurrent inferior laryngeal nerves.[5] The extrinsic strap muscles are innervated by the hypoglossal nerves.[6]

IMAGING STRATEGIES

Computed Tomography

The imaging area should extend from the vertebral body of C1 to the thoracic inlet. We recommend the following protocol for routine laryngeal imaging:

Three-millimeter-thick sections obtained at 5-mm increments from C1 to the hyoid bone

Contiguous 3-mm-thick sections from the hyoid bone to the base of the cricoid cartilage

Three-millimeter-thick sections obtained at 5-mm increments from the base of the cricoid cartilage to the thoracic inlet

The studies should be reconstructed utilizing soft tissue algorithms. High-resolution bone algorithms should also be used to evaluate the laryngeal cartilages for tumor invasion. "Lung windows" should be obtained for evaluation of images that extend inferiorly to include the lung apex. This is especially important in patients with recurrent tumors, who have a higher incidence of lung metastases. The field of view should be optimized to include the region of interest with a general standard field of view to range from 16 to 18 cm.

For false vocal cord, true vocal cord, and primary subglottic carcinomas, we perform an additional spiral computed tomography (SCT) sequence using the following parameters:

Slice thickness = 2 mm; table feed = 2 mm (pitch = 1) performed from the false vocal cords to the base of the cricoid cartilage

Reconstructed images using 2-mm contiguous sections with magnification over the region of interest

All studies should be performed after iodinated contrast administration, as this emphasizes subtle differences between tumor and adjacent normal tissue. Opacification of the vascular structures also makes it easier to distinguish lymph nodes in the neck from blood vessels. The technique utilized at our institution consists of an initial bolus of 50 ml administered at 2 ml/sec. The total amount of contrast used is approximately 150 ml. Properly performed, this technique ensures excellent vascular opacification and allows easy separation of vessels from the adjacent cervical nodes.

Patients should be instructed to breathe quietly and refrain from talking, swallowing, and coughing. Even with rapid (1- to 2-second) scan times, motion can thoroughly degrade an image. At the current time, we prefer dynamic computed tomography (DCT) over SCT. Because the tube heating capabilities of DCT are superior to those obtained with SCT, the use of DCT allows imaging with greater milliampere-second and better overall image resolution than is possible with SCT. SCT does have several benefits over DCT. However, recent advances in tube heating capabilities will eventually result in SCT being the technique of choice for laryngeal imaging with CT.

Magnetic Resonance Imaging

Advances in magnetic resonance imaging (MRI) technology since the mid-1980s have significantly improved the image quality attainable for laryngeal imaging. MRI has several advantages over CT that may be helpful for presurgical planning. The multiplanar capabilities of MRI are superior to the re-formations available with CT. Coronal imaging is helpful for determining involvement of the laryngeal ventricle and transglottic spread. Sagittal midline images are helpful for demonstrating the relationship between the tumor and the anterior commissure. MRI is also superior to CT for specific tissue characterization.

However, despite the development of more rapid imaging techniques, a greater proportion of laryngeal studies performed with MRI are degraded by motion artifact compared with CT. The continued development of new pulse sequences that allow rapid T1-weighted and T2-weighted image acquisition may reduce the amount of motion artifact and improve overall image quality.

MRI for laryngeal and hypopharyngeal carcinoma should extend from the vertebral body of C1 to the thoracic inlet. Imaging should be performed in the sagittal, axial, and coronal planes, thereby maximizing the multiplanar capabilities of MRI. The study should be performed using a surface coil as a receiver to ensure maximal resolution. The phase-encoded gradients should be placed in the anteroposterior direction, thereby reducing the amount of image degradation by pulsation artifact from the great vessels of the neck.

Unlike CT, portions of the MRI examination should be performed before and after contrast administration. Tumor on nonenhanced studies is of intermediate signal and easily separable from adjacent fat. However, enhanced tumor on the T1-weighted sequence is often difficult to separate from adjacent fat. Additionally, enhanced tumor may be indistinguishable from the marrow-containing laryngeal cartilages normally seen in older patients. Therefore, the sensitivity of MRI for detecting cartilage invasion may be decreased if MRI imaging is performed only after contrast administration.

BENIGN DISORDERS

Developmental Disorders

Benign disorders of the upper aerodigestive tract are classified as developmental and acquired. Developmental lesions include stenosis of the subglottis, laryngeal atresia, laryngeal webs, laryngotrachealesophageal cleft, laryngomalacia, laryngeal cysts, and congenital vocal cord paralysis.[7] Most developmental anomalies in this region are evaluated clinically with the use of endoscopy. Plain radiographs and fluoroscopy are helpful in initially assessing the patency of the airway. Occasionally, CT with three-dimensional re-formations is helpful in depicting the lesions. This is particularly true of stenoses. In our opinion, MRI does not play a significant role in the evaluation of these lesions. Trauma to the larynx is most often found in adults and is discussed in a separate section.[8] Initially, these patients may be evaluated with plain radiographs and, in selected cases, with CT. Because significant airway compromise may be present in these patients, we do not perform MRI. After chronic intubation, strictures may develop at the level of the anterior and posterior commissures and the immediate subglottic region.[9] Although MRI may have a limited role in demonstrating these strictures, we prefer to utilize CT with three-dimensional re-formations (Fig. 41–1). Infectious processes such as epiglottitis and croup are also better evaluated with plain radiographs and CT rather than MRI. The most common benign laryngeal tumors in children are squamous papillomas[7] (Fig. 41–2). When multiple, this entity is referred to as *laryngeal papillomatosis*. It is commonly found before 3 years of age. Again, these patients are better evaluated with plain radiographs and CT. Benign lesions of the hypopharynx and larynx in which MRI may be helpful include neurofibromas, vascular malformations, and other less-common masses. MRI may also have a role in the diagnosis of retropharyngeal infections.

Acquired Disorders

Neurofibromas

Isolated neurofibromas involving the airway are almost always seen in the context of neurofibromatosis type 1 (NF-1).[10] This disorder occurs in approximately 1 in 5000 live births and is related to an anomaly in chromosome 17. There is no gender predilection, and the penetrance of the trait is variable. In the airway, most neurofibromas involve the regions of the arytenoid cartilages and the aryepiglottic folds (Fig. 41–3). However, the lesions may be extensive and involve the entire airway (Fig. 41–4). Degeneration into sarcomas is extremely rare. These slow-growing lesions are commonly treated with local resection and the patients are prone to recurrences. Extensive recurrences may necessitate securing the airway with a tracheostomy and partial or total laryngectomy. Neurofibromas have a nonspecific MRI appearance. They are of intermediate signal intensity on precontrast T1-weighted images and iso- to hyperintense on T2-weighted sequences, and most show marked enhancement after contrast administration. Reduced T2 signal intensity may correlate with increased cellularity or fibrous components. They may contain nonenhancing areas, which may be related to cyst formation or necrosis. Coronal MRI studies help in demonstrating the extent of airway compromise. Laryngeal paragangliomas may also occur in patients with neurofibromatosis type 1 as well as those patients with the von Hippel–Lindau syndrome.[11] These lesions typi-

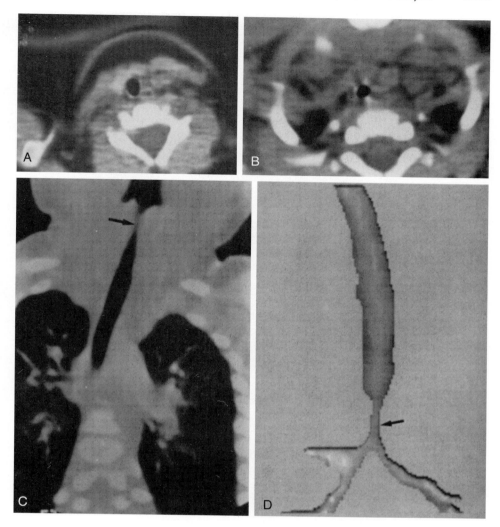

FIGURE 41-1 Segmental tracheal stenosis. *A,* Axial computed tomography (CT) scan shows a normal tracheal lumen. *B,* Axial CT slice below *A* shows reduction of the tracheal lumen compatible with stenosis, which in this case was secondary to a complete tracheal ring. Note that the rings are not calcified and therefore not visible. *C,* Direct coronal CT scan shows a focal glottic/subglottic stenosis *(arrow).* *D,* Three-dimensional re-formation from magnetic resonance imaging (MRI) data set in a child with a low vascular ring shows a focal stenosis *(arrow)* of the distal trachea. (*A* and *B,* Courtesy of D. Merten, University of North Carolina, Chapel Hill. *C,* Courtesy of J. Lucaya, M.D., Institut Catala de la Salut, Hospital Universitari Materno-infantil Vall d'Hebron, Barcelona. *D,* Courtesy of E.R. Bank, M.D., Egleston Children's Hospital, Atlanta.)

cally arise from the paired inferior paraganglia at the level between the inferior horns of the thyroid cartilage and the cricoid cartilages. Although their MRI features are nonspecific, the lesions tend to be hypervascular and may demonstrate internal flow voids as they do in other regions of the head and neck.

Hemangiomas

Airway hemangiomas are usually found in children, particularly during the first year of life. Over 85% of them present during the initial 6 months of life.[12] Subglottic hemangiomas are more common in females and have a slight left-sided predominance. Overlying cutaneous stigmata are present in approximately half of these patients. Clinically, patients present with progressive respiratory obstruction that is aggravated by excitement, crying, and upper respiratory tract infections. Histologically, most lesions are of the capillary type. Most hemangiomas are diagnosed by endoscopy and treated with laser excision and therefore do not require imaging. Occasionally, these lesions are large and infiltrative, and imaging is required to define them before resection. By MRI, hemangiomas have a nonspecific appearance and are mostly of low signal intensity on T1-weighted images.[13] Involuting hem-

angiomas may show areas of hyperintensity that represent fat. On T2-weighted sequences, hemangiomas are iso- to hyperintense and of heterogeneous appearance. They may contain areas of flow void related to large vessels or calcified phleboliths. Satellite lesions are common. Hemangiomas enhance after contrast administration. Lymphangiomas typically show large cystic spaces that may contain blood-fluid levels. Venous malformations may show large blood lakes with scattered calcified phleboliths. High-flow lesions (arteriovenous malformations) show serpiginous, tortuous vessels containing flow voids and, rarely, accompanying solid infiltrative masses.

Other Less-Common Masses

Laryngeal cysts commonly arise at the level of the ventricle[14] (Fig. 41–5). They are seen in all ages and are a well-known cause of respiratory stridor in infants and children. There is no gender predilection. Internal laryngoceles are confined to the endolarynx. External laryngoceles extend outwardly via the thyrohyoid membrane.[15] Laryngoceles with both internal and external components may be considered mixed (Fig. 41–6). In children, laryngoceles are generally congenital and due to simple atresia of the saccular orifice. In adults, they should be considered

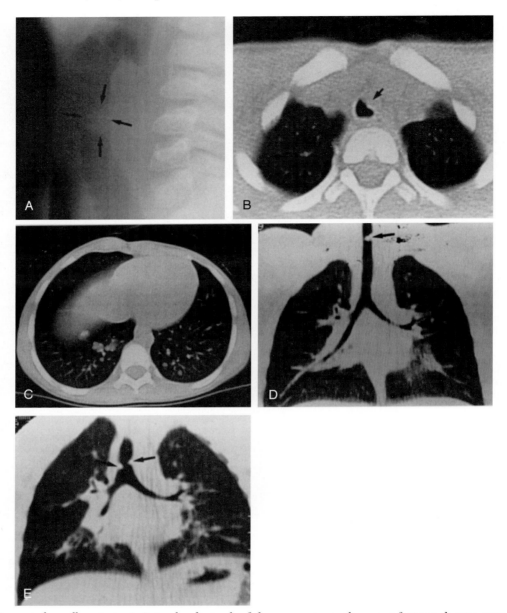

FIGURE 41–2 Laryngeal papillomatosis. *A,* Lateral radiograph of the upper airway shows a soft tissue density mass *(arrows)* in the subglottic region. *B,* Axial CT scan shows a mass *(arrow)* in the right lateral and anterior tracheal wall. *C,* Axial CT scan at the lung bases shows multiple nodules posteriorly caused by distal airway papillomas. *D,* Direct coronal CT scan shows a nodular soft tissue mass *(arrow)* in the left tracheal wall. *E,* Direct coronal CT scan shows papillomas *(arrows)* from the tracheal walls just above the carina. (*A–C,* Courtesy of D. Frush, M.D., Duke University, Durham, NC. *D* and *E,* Courtesy of J. Lucaya, M.D., Institut Catala de la Salut, Hospital Universitari Materno-infantil Vall d'Hebron, Barcelona.)

secondary to a lesion obstructing the ventricle until proved otherwise. These lesions may be infectious, inflammatory, neoplastic, or traumatic. Laryngoceles may become infected in the presence of concomitant upper respiratory tract infections. By MRI, these lesions are smoothly marginated and can have internal characteristics of fluid.[7] Because this fluid may be proteinaceous, increased T1 signal intensity may be present. Enhancement of their rim can occur with infection. Areas of nodular enhancement may be related to underlying tumor.

Benign lesions arising from minor salivary glands are most commonly pleomorphic adenomas.[7] These lesions

tend to occur in adults. Other benign lesions arising in the hypopharynx and larynx include fibromas, fibromatosis, rhabdoid tumors, epidermoids, dermoids, and angiomas.[16] Leiomyomas involving the upper esophagus may also project into the airway. All of these lesions have a nonspecific MRI appearance, and the correct diagnosis may be reached only by biopsy. Occasionally, these lesions have an aggressive appearance, and by MRI, they may be indistinguishable from true malignant masses.

Although thyroglossal duct cysts most commonly involve the extralaryngeal soft tissues, they are briefly mentioned here because they may protrude into the airway.

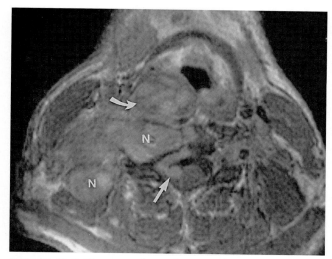

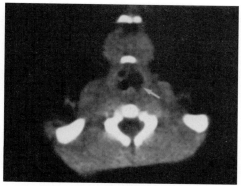

FIGURE 41–5 Saccular laryngeal cyst. Axial CT scan shows a cyst (*arrow*) in the left supraglottic larynx, probably arising at the level of the vallecula. (Courtesy of W. Nemzek, M.D., University of California, Davis.)

FIGURE 41–3 Contrast-enhanced T1-weighted image shows a neurofibroma involving the right aryepiglottic fold (*curved arrow*) in a patient with neurofibromatosis type I. Note other multiple neurofibromas in the neck (N) and spinal canal (*straight arrow*).

These lesions result from fluid accumulation in the remnants of the thyroid anlage.[17] They are midline masses most commonly found in children. The thyroid migrates from the base of the tongue to the inferior neck. Lack of obliteration of the thyroglossal duct results in the formation of cysts. Approximately 20% of these cysts are located in the suprahyoid region and 15% at the level of the hyoid bone. They commonly measure 2 to 4 cm in diameter at diagnosis and can enlarge rapidly in the presence of infection. Carcinomas arise in less than 1% of these cysts. On MRI, thyroglossal duct cysts are of fluid intensity[7] (Fig. 41–7). Soft tissue intensity on precontrast MRI T1-weighted study and intense enhancement after contrast administration should raise the suspicion of intracystic tumor.

Sarcoidosis has been reported to involve the larynx.

The radiographic findings demonstrate abnormal nodular or circumferential soft tissue throughout the larynx. These findings are nonspecific and the diagnoses are typically made on the basis of clinical history or biopsy.[2]

Collagen vascular diseases have also been reported to involve the larynx. Manifestations of rheumatoid arthritis (RA) may occur in the larynx owing to the presence of the cricothyroid and cricoarytenoid joints, which are true synovial joints. The inflammatory reaction caused by rheumatoid arthritis results in swelling and hoarseness, with long-standing cases resulting in cord fixation. Reported CT findings are of erosions and sclerosis situated within the cricoarytenoid joint.[18]

Relapsing polychondritis is a rare, episodic, multiple-system inflammatory process that affects the cartilages and special sense organs. The cause is unknown. Relapsing polychondritis is most commonly seen in men in their 40s, although all age groups can be involved. Characteristic sites of involvement include the cartilages that make up the ear, nasal septum, and trachea. Laryngeal findings on imaging studies include sclerosis and enlargement of the affected laryngeal cartilages.[2, 19]

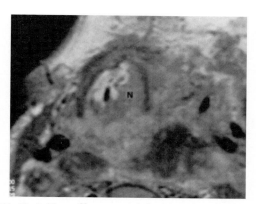

FIGURE 41–4 Neurofibroma. Axial postcontrast T1-weighted image in a patient with neurofibromatosis type I shows a neurofibroma (N) involving the left true vocal cord. Note the extensive plexiform neurofibromas in the neck. (From Castillo M, Mukherji SK [eds]. Imaging of the Pediatric Head, Neck, and Spine. Philadelphia, Lippincott-Raven, 1996.)

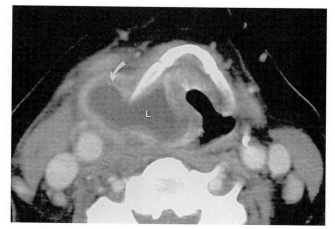

FIGURE 41–6 Contrast-enhanced CT scan shows a characteristic appearance of a mixed laryngocele (L) that extends through the thyrohyoid membrane and into the soft tissues of the neck (*arrow*).

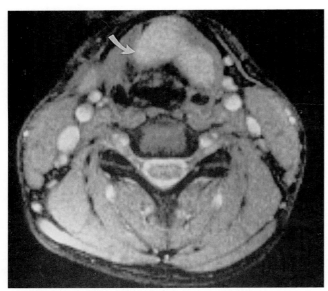

FIGURE 41–7 Axial gradient-echo T1-weighted image demonstrates a fluid signal mass deep to the strap muscles in the anterior neck *(arrow)*, consistent with a thyroglossal duct cyst.

Croup (Laryngotracheitis)

Croup (laryngotracheitis) is a viral upper respiratory tract infection believed to be caused by parainfluenza types 1 and 2, and it is most often seen in young children between the ages of 1 and 3 years. This disease frequently occurs in winter and is more common in males than in females. Croup usually lasts between 3 and 7 days. Croup may be called atypical if it lasts more than 7 days, occurs in an infant less than 1 year of age, or is unresponsive to antibiotics. Patients characteristically present with a characteristic barking cough and stridor. The infection results in diffuse edema of the mucosa of the subglottic region and trachea.[20]

The imaging method of choice for evaluating patients suspected of having croup is anteroposterior and lateral plain films of the neck. CT and MRI have no role in the initial diagnosis. Imaging is done to confirm the clinical diagnosis of croup and exclude other causes of stridor, such as a foreign body.[2] The characteristic plain film finding is of loss of the normal subglottic angles resulting in a "steeple-shaped" or "wine-bottle" appearance of the subglottic region on the anteroposterior films (Fig. 41–8). The lateral films reveal indistinctness of the normal soft tissue structures of the glottic region. Instead of the distinct soft tissue–air interphase between the glottic and the subglottic regions, in croup there is an ill-defined haziness between these structures. There is often dilatation of the piriform sinuses and ballooning of the pharynx resulting from airway obstruction below the level of the glottis.[2]

Epiglottitis

Epiglottitis is an acute infection involving the supraglottic region, especially the epiglottis. Epiglottitis is, in fact, a systemic disease, with supraglottic involvement being a major feature of the process. The most common organism causing epiglottitis is *Haemophilus influenzae* type B. This disease usually occurs in children between the ages of 2 and 4 years, although recent reports suggest that its incidence is increasing in patients less than 2 years of age. The newborn is felt to be protected from developing this disease because of immunity to the capsular antigen acquired from the mother. This passive immunity is believed to resolve by 3 months of age. The child's own immune system does not appear to produce significant amount of similar antibody until 3 to 4 years after birth. This window of diminished antibody levels is believed to partly explain the high incidence of *H. influenzae* in this age group. There is no reported gender predilection. Fortunately, the incidence in children has dramatically decreased. This is likely related to immunization of the pediatric population with *H. influenzae* vaccine, which began in April 1985.[21]

Patients with epiglottitis characteristically present with high fever and signs of respiratory obstruction. Blood

FIGURE 41–8 Croup. *A,* Frontal radiograph shows smooth tapering *(arrows)* of the subglottic region secondary to mucosal edema. *B,* In a different patient with croup, frontal radiograph shows a tapered *(arrows)* subglottic region, also known as the *steeple* or *wine-bottle* sign. (*A* and *B,* Courtesy of D. Merten, University of North Carolina, Chapel Hill.)

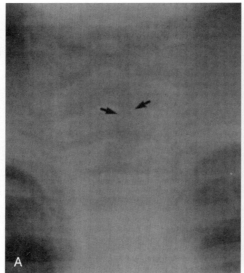

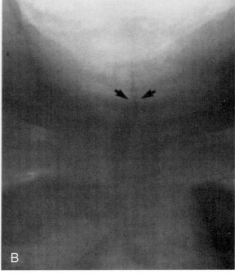

cultures are frequently positive in these patients. Affected children are often sitting upright and drooling. These individuals have greater inspiratory than expiratory stridor. The onset of symptoms is often acute and may occur over a 2- to 6-hour period.[20]

On examination, the epiglottis is swollen and cherry-red in appearance. The aryepiglottic folds are usually swollen with resultant narrowing of the supraglottic airway. The secretions in patients with epiglottitis are often thick and tenacious, and sudden respiratory arrest may be caused by mucus plugging of an already compromised airway.[21]

On initial presentation, the anesthesiologist and otolaryngologist should be notified. Because the airway in these individuals is susceptible to acute laryngospasm and prone to obstruction during forced inspiration, every attempt should be made not to excite the child during initial evaluation. Initial examination should be kept to a minimum. Initial radiographic evaluation should be a lateral plain film of the neck performed in the emergency room. Affected children will require nasotracheal or orotracheal intubation under anesthesia. Tracheostomy is not currently recommended for achieving airway control. The treatment of epiglottitis is antibiotic therapy with cephalosporins, which are now believed to be the drug of choice at many institutions.[21]

A lateral plain film of the soft tissues of the neck should be performed in patients suspected of having epiglottitis. Plain films should be performed in the emergency department. Patients must be accompanied by the otolaryngologist or anesthesiologist if imaging has to be performed in the radiology department. There is no role for CT and MRI in imaging such patients at initial presentation, and in fact, these studies may be life-threatening, as placing the patient in the supine position will further reduce the caliber of an already narrowed airway.[2]

The findings on plain radiography are those of a diffusely thickened epiglottis that is often two to three times the size of a normal epiglottis. (Fig. 41–9). The aryepiglottic folds of the false vocal cord are also thickened. There may be dilatation of the oropharynx if the supraglottic larynx is narrowed as a result of diffuse edema caused by infection.[2]

Other Infections

Rhinoscleroma is a chronic and progressive disorder of the respiratory passages believed to be caused by the organism *Klebsiella rhinoscleromatis*. This infection is found mainly in Latin America, Eastern Europe, and northern Africa.[22] Individuals between 20 and 40 years of age are most commonly affected. Clinically, patients typically complain of nonspecific symptoms such as nasal discharge or obstruction, cough, stridor, and dyspnea. On direct endoscopy, the lesions simulate carcinoma and usually present as multilobulated infiltrative masses. The overlying mucosa is hyperplastic and shows marked inflammation. In the chronic stage, scarring is prominent. Scarring of the airway may produce dyspnea even when the lesion is inactive. On histologic examination, there is squamous metaplasia, inflammatory and granulation tissues, and foamy histiocytes containing the microorganism (Mikulicz' bodies).[22] Treatment is with tetracyclines and

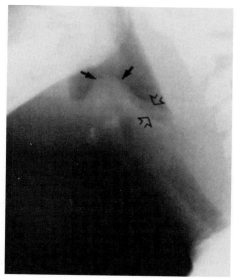

FIGURE 41–9 Epiglottis. Lateral radiograph shows a thickened ("thumblike") epiglottis *(solid arrows)* and edema of the aryepiglottic folds *(open arrows)*. (Courtesy of D. Merten, University of North Carolina, Chapel Hill.)

typically requires a prolonged course. Radiographically, these lesions may present as a focal mass that may mimic a carcinoma (Fig. 41–10). These masses may be associated with reticulation of the adjacent fat planes. Because of the nonspecific imaging features, biopsy is required to reach a definitive diagnosis.

Other less-common infections that have been reported

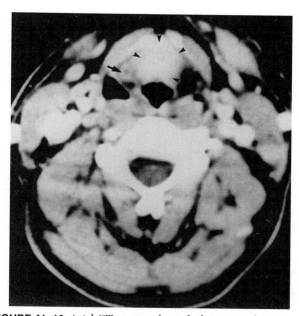

FIGURE 41–10 Axial CT section through the preepiglottic space shows the mass *(arrowheads)* as well as the soft tissue density replacing the normal fat in the right paralaryngeal space *(arrow)*, probably representing inflammatory changes or a small internal fluid-filled laryngocele. (From Castillo M. CT findings in a case of rhinoscleroma. AJNR 14:770, 1993.)

to involve the larynx include aspergillus, cytomegalovirus, and tuberculosis. The latter two processes have been described in patients who are positive for the human immunodeficiency virus. Tuberculosis rarely involves the larynx but, when present, is typically associated with pulmonary manifestations. Radiographically, the findings are nonspecific. Thickening of the epiglottis and fixation of the cricoarytenoid joint owing to direct involvement have been reported.[2]

MALIGNANT LESIONS

Squamous Cell Carcinoma

Squamous cell carcinoma (SCCA) is the most common malignancy of the larynx and one of the most frequent indications for laryngeal imaging. Laryngeal carcinoma (LC) accounts for between 2% and 5% of all malignancies annually. There are about 11,000 new cases reported annually, with an overall incidence of 3 to 8 per 100,000. In 1991, over 3500 deaths were due to LC.[23–25]

LC is more common in males than in females, with most patients presenting between the ages of 50 and 80 years. A number of risk factors have been associated with SCCA of the larynx, the most important being cigarette smoking. Other forms of smoking, including cigar, pipe, and marijuana, are also felt to increase the likelihood of developing LC. Fortunately, the risk of tobacco-related cancers appears to be reversible; the risk of developing LC for exsmokers abstaining for over 10 years is nearly equal to that for nonsmokers. Other risk factors include alcohol consumption, prior irradiation, and viruses (herpes simplex, papillomavirus).[6]

Histologically, SCCA is classified as well, moderately, and poorly differentiated. On microscopic examination, SCCA is manifested as anaplastic-appearing cells found below the basement membrane with a variable degree of keratin production and intracellular bridges. Besides SCCA, other squamous cell aberrations that may arise in the larynx include: benign hyperplasia, benign keratosis, atypical hyperplasia, keratosis with atypical epithelial atypia, intraepithelial carcinoma, and microinvasive SCCA.[24, 26] These lesions cannot be distinguished by cross-sectional imaging.

Because of the differences in embryogenesis, lymphatic drainage, and anatomic boundaries, a topographic classification of the larynx carcinomas based on their anatomic origin is routinely used by otolaryngologists and radiation oncologists and is the basis for the tumor-nodes-metastasis (TNM) staging of laryngeal carcinoma. The following discussion focuses on this commonly used classification system.

Supraglottic Carcinoma

Aryepiglottic Fold Carcinomas

Aryepiglottic fold tumors are typically exophytic lesions that, when detected early, are confined laterally along the aryepiglottic fold (Fig. 41–11). Such tumors have been termed *marginal lesions. Advanced lesions* may extend laterally to involve the adjacent wall of the piriform sinus or medially to invade the epiglottis. These malignancies

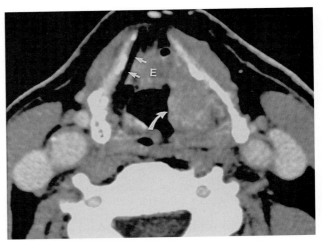

FIGURE 41–11 Contrast-enhanced CT scan shows an aggressive mass arising from the left aryepiglottic fold *(curved arrow)* invading the left paralaryngeal fat planes. Note the normal appearance of the epiglottis (E) and the paralaryngeal fat plane *(straight arrows)* on the uninvolved side.

may also grow superiorly to involve the pharyngoepiglottic fold and eventually the suprahyoid portion of the epiglottis. Inferiorly, these lesions may involve the false vocal cords and ventricle. *Very advanced lesions* may extend to involve the cricoarytenoid joint (resulting in fixation of the true vocal cord), invade the laryngeal cartilages, and extend into the tongue base and pharyngeal wall. The signal characteristics of aryepiglottic fold tumors are similar to other SCCAs. The diagnosis of such a carcinoma is based on the location and the known spread pattern of these tumors. Radiographically, early lesions are identified as lobulated masses arising from the aryepiglottic fold. Very early mucosal lesions may not be detected by MRI.[27]

False Vocal Cord Carcinomas

SCCAs that arise from the false vocal cords and laryngeal ventricle tend to be ulcerative and infiltrative with little exophytic component. Deep invasion by such tumors results in access of these tumors to the paraglottic space and may lead to fixation of the supraglottic larynx. Because of the close proximity, these tumors may extend inferiorly to involve the true vocal cords. Such submucosal spread is often clinically occult and may lead to understaging of the lesion if this extension is undetected before surgery. False vocal cord tumors may extend laterally to involve the medial wall of the piriform sinus and medially to the inferior portion of the epiglottis, thereby increasing the likelihood of invasion of the preepiglottic space. Cartilage invasion by false vocal cord tumors is less common than is seen with glottic carcinomas and, when present, is typically found with advanced lesions. MRI is well suited for imaging false vocal cord carcinomas. Coronal imaging is beneficial for evaluating the superior and inferior extent of these lesions and for evaluating for the presence of transglottic spread.[27]

Epiglottic Carcinomas

The epiglottis is the most common location of cancers that arise in the supraglottic larynx. Tumors may arise from either the suprahyoid or the infrahyoid epiglottis. Radiographically, these lesions are often exophytic, circumferential masses that, when detected early, are confined to the midline of the supraglottis (Fig. 41–12). On MRI, these lesions are of intermediate signal and homogeneously enhance with contrast. Advanced lesions may extend superiorly to invade the vallecula and tongue base and laterally to involve the aryepiglottic folds, false vocal cords, and paralaryngeal space. Direct inferior extension to involve the anterior commissure and subglottis is seen only in very advanced lesions.[27]

Tumors arising from the epiglottis may extend anteriorly to involve the preepiglottic space. This form of spread is facilitated by the presence of numerous foramina that provide access for tumor invasion. Invasion of the preepiglottic space is often difficult to detect clinically, and when present, it alters the tumor stage (T3). Invasion of the preepiglottic space is readily seen on MRI and best evaluated with noncontrast T1-weighted sequences by replacement of normal high-signal fat with intermediate-signal tumor. Because tumor normally enhances, postgadolinium MRI has the potential of underestimating the amount of preepiglottic space invasion.

Glottic Carcinomas

The true vocal cords are the most common site of laryngeal carcinomas, with the ratio of glottic carcinomas to supraglottic carcinomas being approximately 3 to 1. The anterior portion of the true vocal cord is the most common location of SCCA, with the majority of lesions occurring along the free margin of the vocal cord.[27] As the tumor enlarges, it may extend in all directions. Anterior tumor spread can involve the anterior commissure. From the anterior commissure, lesions may grow to involve the contralateral true vocal cord (Fig. 41–13). Lesions can also extend along the tendon of the anterior commissure (Broyles' ligament). This ligament inserts directly into the thyroid cartilage and may facilitate invasion of the carti-

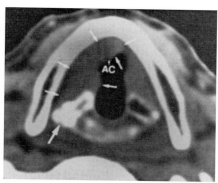

FIGURE 41–13 CT scan of a 1.74-cm³ T2 gliottic tumor that was successfully controlled with radiation therapy alone. Axial image at the level of the cricoarytenoid joint shows an infiltrating lesion involving the right true cord, which spreads across the anterior commissure (AC) to involve the contralateral true cord (*small arrows*). There is associated sclerosis of the right arytenoid cartilage (*large arrow*). (From Mukherji SK, Mancuso AA, Mendenhall W, et al. Can pretreatment CT predict local control of T2 glottic carcinomas treated with radiation therapy alone? AJNR 1995;16:655–662.)

lage by tumor. Occasionally, tumors may arise from the anterior commissure region, and these are generally associated with a poorer prognosis, believed to be due to early anterior extension along Broyles' ligament. Advanced lesions arising within the anterior aspect of the vocal cord or those tumors arising along the posterior third of the cord may extend posteriorly to involve the cricoarytenoid joint and interarytenoid region. Tumors can extend inferiorly either mucosally or submucosally to involve the subglottic region.

Cartilage invasion can be detected with both CT and MRI and is more common in glottic tumors than in supraglottic carcinomas. On noncontrast T1-weighted MRI, replacement of the high signal within the cartilage by adjacent intermediate-signal tumor is suggestive of cartilage invasion (Fig. 41–14). On T2-weighted sequences, increased signal within the cartilage is indicative of neoplastic invasion. Recent reports suggest that MRI

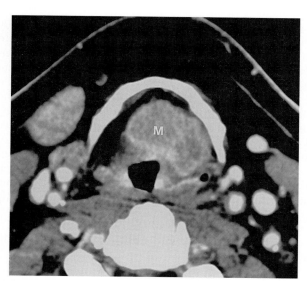

FIGURE 41–12 Contrast-enhanced CT scan shows an aggressive mass (M) arising from the epiglottis. The tumor extends anteriorly and laterally to invade the preepiglottic space.

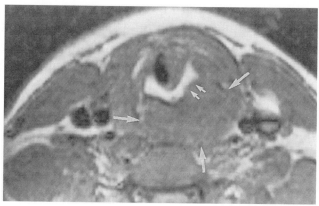

FIGURE 41–14 Noncontrast T1-weighted MRI shows a hypopharyngeal mass (*large arrows*) that has replaced the high-signal marrow in the posterior aspect of the cricoid cartilage (*small arrows*) consistent with cartilage invasion.

appears to be more sensitive than CT for detecting invasion (89% vs. 66%, respectively); however, MRI is less specific than CT (84% vs. 94%).[28]

Subglottic Larynx Carcinomas

Carcinomas arising primarily within the subglottic larynx are rare. When present, the lesions are characteristically circumferential and have often extended to involve the undersurface of the true vocal cords. These lesions have a tendency for early invasion of the cricoid cartilage and extension through the cricothyroid membrane. Radiographically, these lesions have similar characteristics to other more-common forms of laryngeal carcinomas (Fig. 41–15). MRI obtained in the coronal plane is helpful for determining the full extent of the lesion and its relationship to the undersurface of the true vocal cords. Unlike supraglottic and glottic tumors, which characteristically drain to the internal jugular chain of nodes, primary subglottic carcinomas have a propensity to drain to the paratracheal nodes. The reported incidence of clinically positive nodes in patients with subglottic carcinoma is 10%.[29]

Other Malignant Lesions

Kaposi's sarcoma is an unusual malignancy that has become more prevalent with the increasing incidence of the acquired immunodeficiency syndrome. Histologically, these lesions comprise a mixture of spindle cells, vascular slits, and branching channels. The origin of the lesion is believed to be from vascular endothelium.[30] Laryngeal involvement is rare but has been reported. When present, it is usually associated with other lesions involving the trachea or pharynx. Laryngeal involvement usually occurs in the presence of cutaneous lesions. Clinically, patients with laryngeal involvement present with stridor, persistent voice changes, or hoarseness.[31] On cross-sectional imaging, the lesions present as lobulated or circumferential soft tissue masses that enhance with contrast. Because

the radiographic findings are nonspecific, biopsy is necessary for diagnosis.

Primary sarcomas of the larynx account for only 0.3% to 1% of laryngeal malignancies. These lesions do not appear to be associated with the typical risk factors for SCCA such as smoking and alcohol abuse. Previous reports have suggested an association between prior irradiation and osteogenic sarcomas, fibrosarcomas, and spindle cell sarcomas. Additionally, prior exposure to Thorotrast and polyvinyl chloride has been associated with an increased likelihood of developing angiosarcomas. Grossly, sarcomas appear as firm, lobulated, polypoid masses that are usually pink, gray, or white. Multiple biopsies are usually required to establish the final diagnosis. Sarcomas that have been reported to occur within the larynx include fibrosarcoma, rhabdomyosarcoma, malignant fibrous histiocytoma, leiomyosarcoma, osteogenic sarcoma, liposarcoma, angiosarcoma, hemangiopericytoma, malignant schwannoma, synovial sarcoma, malignant mesenchymoma, and chondrosarcoma. The radiographic appearance of the majority of these lesions is nonspecific and mimics that of SCCA.

The one main exception is chondrosarcomas.[32] Chondrosarcomas are the most common sarcoma of the larynx, accounting for 48% of all laryngeal sarcomas. Both benign and malignant chondroid lesions most commonly arise from the posterior lamina of the cricoid cartilage, with a small number arising from the thyroid cartilage. Patients typically present with signs of airway obstruction owing to endophytic growth of tumor.[30] Radiographically, these lesions are best visualized by CT and appear as an expanded cartilage that contains multiple calcifications that at times resemble rings and circles. The presence of these calcifications may be suggested on MRI by the presences of focal areas of signal loss within the affected cartilage. The presence of a distinct soft tissue mass is variable. Unfortunately, it may be difficult by imaging studies alone to differentiate between benign and malignant chondroid lesions.[2]

Malignant tumors originating from the seromucinous glands within the larynx are in the form of adenoid cystic carcinomas and adenocarcinomas. These malignancies are rare and believed to constitute less than 1% of all laryngeal neoplasms. These lesions are believed to originate from the epithelium of the larynx, which contains the seromucinous glands. When they arise in the larynx, the subglottis is the most common location for both adenocarcinomas and adenoid cystic carcinomas. Up to one-third of adenoid cystic carcinomas, however, have been reported in the supraglottic larynx. Adenoid cystic carcinomas have a predilection for perineural invasion and, when arising from the supraglottis, may invade and extend along the superior laryngeal nerve. These lesions are slightly more common in females and typically seen in patients over 50 years of age. Radiographically, the appearance is nonspecific and they cannot be differentiated from SCCA by imaging studies alone.

Like adenoid cystic carcinoma, lymphoma may be identical to SCCA on imaging studies. It is important to make the diagnosis (usually by biopsy), since lymphoma is treated not surgically but with radiation therapy.

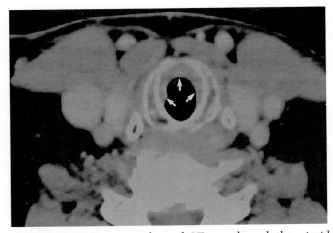

FIGURE 41–15 Contrast-enhanced CT scan through the cricoid cartilage shows a soft tissue mass (*arrows*) involving the anterior aspect of the subglottis. Although biopsy of the mass revealed Wegener's granulomatosis, these radiographic findings are indistinguishable from those of a primary subglottic carcinoma.

POSTTREATMENT NECK

The current treatment for SCCA of the upper aerodigestive tract includes surgery or radiation therapy (RT), or a combination of both.[33] The exact treatment depends in part on the location and extent of the tumor and institutional preference. Both radiotherapy and surgery alter the underlying normal anatomic structures, thereby making interpretation of posttreatment imaging challenging. Familiarization with the expected imaging changes after therapy allows accurate evaluation of imaging studies and may prevent misinterpretation of posttreatment changes as recurrent disease.

Radiation Therapy

Control with RT allows the patient to retain a functioning larynx in cases where surgical cure may require laryngectomy. Because of this advantage and the dispersion of centers capable of modern treatment planning and delivery, a growing number of patients are treated with RT alone.[33] The effects of RT occur within all areas of the larynx, hypopharynx, and superficial soft tissues of the neck included within the radiation port. The histologic changes and the associated radiographic changes that occur as a result of radiation have been described previously and result mainly from edema and fibrosis.[34] Therefore, the radiographic appearance of the irradiated neck is significantly altered from that on pretreatment baseline imaging studies.[35, 36]

Histologically, RT results in an acute inflammatory reaction within the deep connective tissues characterized by leukocytic infiltration, histiocyte formation, necrosis, and hemorrhage. Microscopic examination of the small arteries, veins, and lymphatics demonstrates detachment of the lining endothelial cells causing increased permeability, resulting in interstitial edema. Within 1 to 4 months, there is deposition of rich collagenous fibers with sclerosis and hyalinosis of connective tissues. This inflammatory process eventually results in obstruction in the small arteries, veins, and lymphatics. By 8 months, there is advanced sclerosis, hyalinosis, and fragmentation of the collagen fibers within connective tissues. Eventually, there may be a reduction in interstitial fluid resulting from the formation of collateral neocapillary and lymphatic channels.[34] The extent of the observed changes in the area included within the radiation port is mainly dependent on the total dose. More advanced and persistent changes may be seen in patients who continue to smoke after RT.

RT results in radiographic changes involving both the exolaryngeal and the endolaryngeal regions. Within 4 months after the completion of RT, reactive changes can be visualized within the skin and subcutaneous tissues in the majority of patients. These changes include thickening of the skin and platysma muscle, as well as reticulation of the subcutaneous and deep investing fat (Fig. 41–16). Resolution of these changes occurs in about half of treated patients. Pharyngeal changes include increased enhancement of the pharyngeal mucosa, thickening of the posterior pharyngeal wall, and retropharyngeal space edema (Figs. 41–16 and 41–17). These changes occur in over half of treated patients.

Irradiation initially results in acute sialadenitis of the submandibular glands within 12 hours after delivery of treatment. The acute effects are transient and usually resolve within 1 to 2 days.[37] Increased size and enhancement of the gland may be seen if imaging is performed within 1 week after the completion of RT. Because imaging is usually performed at least 2 months after completion of RT, the radiographic changes most commonly

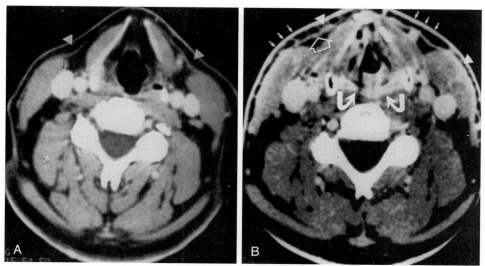

FIGURE 41–16 *A*, Pretreatment CT study illustrates the normal appearance of the superficial cervical structures and the pharyngeal mucosa. Note the homogeneous, low attenuation of the subcutaneous fat (*arrowheads*). *B*, Study obtained 3 months after completion of radiation therapy reveals extensive thickening of the skin (*straight arrows*) and the platysma (*open arrow*). Subcutaneous fat (*arrowheads*) is reticulated on the posttreatment scan. Note increased pharyngeal mucosal enhancement (*curved arrows*). (*A* and *B*, From Mukherji SK, Mancuso AA, Kotzur IM, et al. Radiologic appearance of the irradiated larynx. Part I. Expected changes. Radiology 1994;193:141–148.)

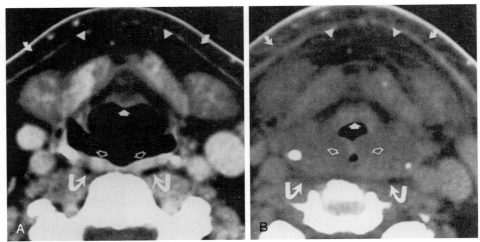

FIGURE 41–17 *A,* Pretreatment CT study demonstrates normal-appearing subcutaneous fat *(small curved arrows),* deep fat *(arrowheads),* infrahyoid epiglottis *(solid arrow),* posterior pharyngeal wall *(open arrows),* and retropharyngeal space *(large curved arrows). B,* CT study obtained 7.5 months after completion of radiation therapy shows extensive reticulation of the subcutaneous fat *(small curved arrows)* and fat deep to the platysma *(arrowheads).* Note diffuse thickening of the infrahyoid epiglottis *(solid arrow)* and the posterior pharyngeal wall *(open arrows)* associated with the internal development of edema within the retropharyngeal space *(large curved arrows). (A* and *B,* From Mukherji SK, Mancuso AA, Kotzur IM, et al. Radiologic appearance of the irradiated larynx. Part I. Expected changes. Radiology 1994;193:141–148.)

observed are those of chronic sialadenitis, including increased enhancement and atrophy of the submandibular glands (Fig. 41–18).

Lymph node atrophy occurs in the vast majority of pretreatment CT-negative nodes. Treated nodes involute to about 25% of their original pretreatment size (Fig. 41–19). Consequently, enlarging lymph nodes after RT are an ominous sign in patients treated with definitive RT for SCCA of the upper aerodigestive tract.

RT also results in thickening of the suprahyoid (Fig. 41–20) and infrahyoid epiglottis (Fig. 41–21). This is usually detected by CT within 3 months after completion

of RT. Almost all patients will have thickening and infiltration of the fat within the aryepiglottic folds as well as thickening of the false vocal cords and increased attenuation of the paralaryngeal fat (Fig. 41–22). These changes are initially seen within 2.5 months after conclusion of treatment and are usually irreversible.

Early changes at the glottic level include increased attenuation on CT of the paraglottic fat planes, which is usually seen within 2 months after RT.[38] Symmetric subglottic thickening is expected and seen in about 80% of patients. Late changes at the glottic level include thickening of the anterior and posterior commissure (Fig.

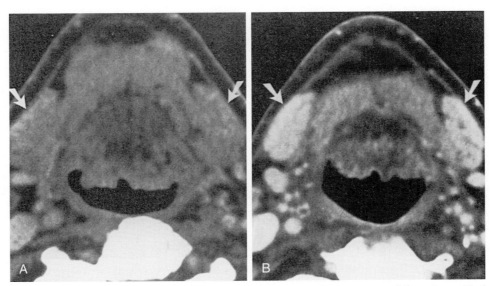

FIGURE 41–18 *A,* Pretreatment contrast-enhanced CT scan demonstrates normal appearance of the submandibular glands *(arrows). B,* Study obtained 15 months after completion of radiation therapy reveals interval reduction in size and increased enhancement of the submandibular glands *(arrows). (A* and *B,* From Mukherji SK, Mancuso AA, Kotzur IM, et al. Radiologic appearance of the irradiated larynx. Part I. Expected changes. Radiology 1994;193:141–148.)

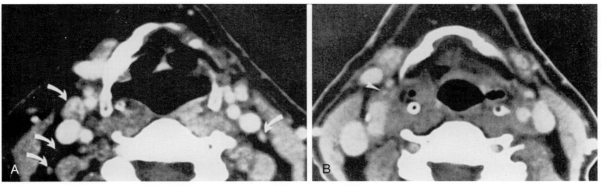

FIGURE 41–19 *A*, Pretreatment CT study demonstrates multiple normal-appearing group II and group V lymph nodes *(arrows)*. *B*, Fifteen months after completion of radiation therapy, there is complete shrinkage of the bilateral group V and the left-sided group II lymph nodes. Right-sided group II lymph node *(arrowhead)* shows an approximately 75% reduction in size. (*A* and *B*, From Mukherji SK, Mancuso AA, Kotzur IM, et al. Radiologic appearance of the irradiated larynx. Part I. Expected changes. Radiology 1994;193:141–148.)

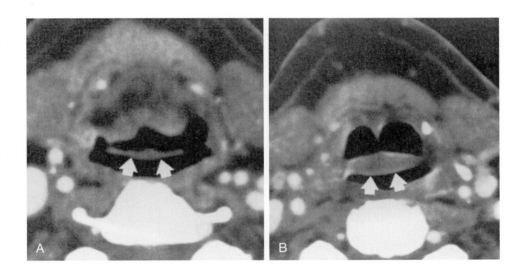

FIGURE 41–20 *A*, Pretreatment CT scan illustrates the normal appearance of the suprahyoid epiglottis *(arrows)*. *B*, Two and one-half months after the conclusion of radiation therapy, the suprahyoid epiglottis *(arrows)* is markedly thicker (compare with *A*). Diffuse epiglottis thickening is one of the early radiologic findings present after radiation therapy. (*A* and *B*, From Mukherji SK, Mancuso AA, Kotzur IM, et al. Radiologic appearance of the irradiated larynx. Part I. Expected changes. Radiology 1994;193:141–148.)

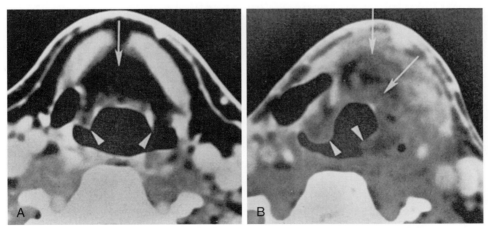

FIGURE 41–21 *A*, Pretreatment CT study demonstrates the normal appearance of the aryepiglottic folds *(arrowheads)* and the preepiglottic fat *(arrow)*. *B*, Follow-up scan obtained 14 months after conclusion of treatment reveals diffuse increased attenuation of the preepiglottic fat *(arrows)*. This is an inconstant finding after radiation therapy. Aryepiglottic folds *(arrowheads)* are markedly thickened, with obliteration of the adjacent paralaryngeal fat planes bilaterally. (*A* and *B*, From Mukherji SK, Mancuso AA, Kotzur IM, et al. Radiologic appearance of the irradiated larynx. Part I. Expected changes. Radiology 1994;193:141–148.)

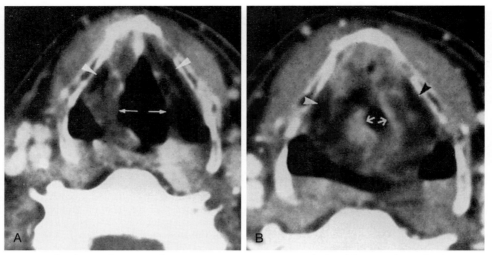

FIGURE 41–22 *A,* CT study shows the normal pretreatment appearance of the false vocal cords *(arrows)* and the adjacent paralaryngeal fat planes *(arrowheads)*. *B,* Posttreatment scan obtained 5 months after radiation therapy reveals symmetric thickening of the false vocal cords bilaterally *(arrows)*. Comparison with the pretreatment study *(A)* demonstrates diffuse, increased attenuation of the paralaryngeal fat planes *(arrowheads)*. These findings are present in the majority of patients after radiation therapy. (*A* and *B,* From Mukherji SK, Mancuso AA, Kotzur IM, et al. Radiologic appearance of the irradiated larynx. Part I. Expected changes. Radiology 1994;193:141–148.)

41–23). These changes occur within 7 and 14 months, respectively, and are persistent.[35]

Primary Site

Imaging plays an important role in helping to identify patients who are successfully treated with RT from those in whom treatment fails.[36] Imaging should be performed before treatment and approximately 3 to 4 months after the completion of treatment in patients with tumors of the upper aerodigestive tract who are to be treated with

definitive RT. Complete resolution of the lesion on the posttreatment study strongly suggests a successfully controlled primary site (Fig. 41–24). Patients with a persistent mass at the primary site that is unchanged in radiographic appearance correlates with treatment failure (Fig. 41–25). Partial resolution of a mass on the posttreatment CT study is an indeterminate finding. These patients require further imaging and close clinical observation. Interval enlargement of a focal mass is suggestive of recurrent disease or laryngeal necrosis.[36] Regardless of

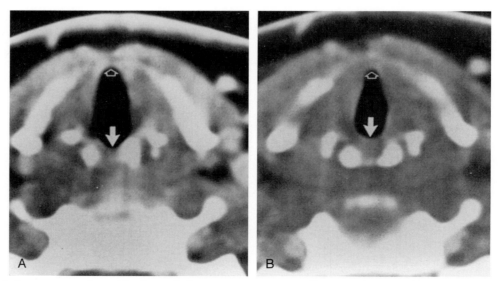

FIGURE 41–23 *A,* Pretreatment CT study obtained during quiet respiration illustrates the normal-appearing anterior *(open arrow)* and posterior *(solid arrow)* commissures. Adequate evaluation of the commissures is possible only when the true vocal cords are abducted. *B,* CT scan obtained 13 months after completion of radiation therapy demonstrates thickening of the anterior *(open arrow)* and posterior *(solid arrow)* commissures. Typically, these changes can be seen on average 7.7 and 14 months, respectively, after treatment. (*A* and *B,* From Mukherji SK, Mancuso AA, Kotzur IM, et al. Radiologic appearance of the irradiated larynx. Part I. Expected changes. Radiology 1994;193:141–148.)

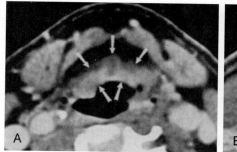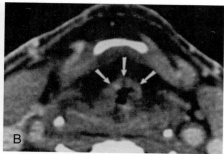

FIGURE 41–24 *A*, Pretreatment CT study shows the infrahyoid epiglottis thickened as a result of involvement by a superficial carcinoma *(arrows)*. Note minimal invasion of the preepiglottic space on the left and some thickening of both aryepiglottic folds. *B*, Posttreatment CT scan obtained 8 months after conclusion of radiation therapy demonstrates complete resolution of the tumor at the primary site *(arrows)*. This case typifies the expected radiologic appearance of the primary site for laryngeal tumors successfully treated by radiation therapy alone. Forty-eight months after completion of treatment, the patient had no evidence of recurrent disease. (*A* and *B*, From Mukherji SK, Mancuso AA, Kotzur IM, et al. Radiologic appearance of the irradiated larynx. Part II. Primary site response. Radiology 1994;193:149–154.)

these potential benefits, differentiation between recurrent tumor and laryngeal necrosis is often not possible by CT or MRI alone. Imaging modalities aimed at measuring metabolic activity may prove beneficial for aiding in this differentiation. The value of metabolic imaging agents such as ^{18}F–fluoro-2-deoxy-D-glucose and thallium-201[39, 40] for differentiating recurrent disease from radiation changes is currently under investigation.

Changes in cartilage sclerosis may be used to help predict outcome in patients treated with RT.[36] Progressive sclerosis of laryngeal cartilages is associated with an increased likelihood of local tumor recurrence, whereas resolution of pretreatment cartilage sclerosis is indicative of successful control.

Postsurgical Appearance

Historically, the treatment of choice for laryngeal cancers has been surgical resection. The exact type of procedure that is performed depends on the location and extent of the primary lesion, the presence and extent of nodal

metastases, and the preference of the otolaryngologist. An understanding of the more commonly performed procedures is essential for adequate evaluation of the postoperative CT studies.

Laryngectomy

Total laryngectomy is the surgical procedure of choice for treating advanced laryngeal cancers. This procedure entails complete resection of all endolaryngeal structures, including the epiglottis, aryepiglottic folds, true and false vocal cords, and subglottis. The entire thyroid and cricoid cartilages and the hyoid bone are removed. After total laryngectomy, the pharynx has a typical appearance, which should be familiar to radiologists interpreting postoperative studies. Because the larynx is removed and there are no firm anterior structures compressing the pharynx, the esophagus has a more anterior location and is located just deep to the subcutaneous fat of the neck.[41] Thus, the pharynx is more anteriorly located and more prominent in appearance (Fig. 41–26). The walls of the pharynx are typically not thickened and usually 2 to 3 mm in diameter.

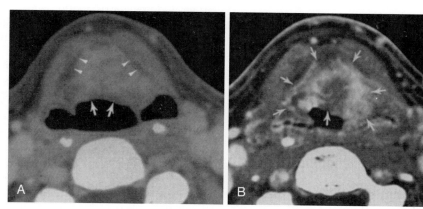

FIGURE 41–25 *A*, Pretreatment CT scan demonstrates a high-volume carcinoma involving the infrahyoid epiglottis *(arrows)* with extension into the preepiglottic space *(arrowheads)*. *B*, Four months after the completion of radiation therapy, CT study shows a persistent heterogeneously enhancing mass *(arrows)* at the primary site. This was interpreted as highly suspicious for persistent tumor. Subsequent biopsy findings confirmed the presence of malignancy. The patient underwent salvage supraglottic laryngectomy and is currently without evidence of recurrent disease. (*A* and *B*, From Mukherji SK, Mancuso AA, Kotzur IM, et al. Radiologic appearance of the irradiated larynx. Part II. Primary site response. Radiology 1994;193:149–154.)

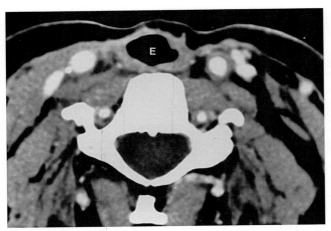

FIGURE 41–26 Contrast-enhanced CT scan shows the characteristic appearance after total laryngectomy. Because the larynx has been resected, the esophagus (E) is anteriorly situated.

Supraglottic laryngectomy is performed for low-volume tumors arising from the supraglottic larynx. Primary sites that may be suitable for treatment with this form of partial laryngectomy include the epiglottis, aryepiglottic fold, and false vocal cord. This procedure involves resection of endolaryngeal structures above the laryngeal ventricle, including the aryepiglottic folds, false vocal cords, and epiglottis. The ipsilateral thyroid cartilage is also excised. The hyoid bone may need to be resected for those tumors that invade the preepiglottic space.[42] Radiographically, the postoperative appearance of the supraglottic region of the larynx is often air-filled and dilated owing to resection of the normal structures. The glottic and subglottic structures appear normal, as they are not involved in the primary resection.

Early glottic cancers may be successfully treated with *hemilaryngectomy*. This procedure involves resection of the affected true vocal cord along with the ipsilateral arytenoid cartilage. The overlying thyroid ala and its external perichondrium are included in the resection.[43]

TRAUMA

Laryngotracheal trauma (LTT) is an uncommon occurrence, but if undiagnosed, may be life-threatening. LTT can involve the supraglottic, glottic, and infraglottic (subglottis and trachea) regions of the airway. Most cases of LTT involve the subglottic and upper tracheal regions. The glottic region, which includes the true vocal cords and the arytenoid and thyroid cartilages, is the second most common location. Injuries of the supraglottic structures, including the false vocal cords, aryepiglottic folds, epiglottis, and hyoid bone, are rare in children. This is due to the fact that in infants and young children, the larynx is in a higher position than in adults and the mandible acts as a protective agent against crush injuries involving the anterior neck. With age, the larynx descends in the neck and the incidence of supraglottic injuries increases in older children.[8]

LTT has been classified into two types of injury: internal and external. The causative factors and demographics are different for each type of injury. The remainder of the discussion focuses on clinical and imaging findings of these injuries.

Internal Injuries

Internal LTT most commonly occurs in children less than 12 years of age. The majority of such injuries are caused by inciting agents that affect the endolaryngeal surface of the lumen of the trachea and larynx. The most common cause is prolonged endotracheal intubation. Injury results from denuding of the laryngeal mucosa, chronic irritation, or pressure necrosis. Traumatic intubation may also cause dislocation of the arytenoid cartilages. Other causes of internal injury include ingestion of caustic substances (toxic chemical, smoke inhalation) and aspiration of foreign bodies. Healing and re-epithelialization of the injured laryngeal mucosa results in scarring and fibrosis. Severe scarring may narrow the airway and reduce vocal cord mobility.[8, 44]

The damage caused by prolonged intubation may localize to the area of the posterior commissure and subglottic region or may result in diffuse fibrosis involving the larynx and trachea. Stenosis caused by tracheotomy is normally seen 1 to 2 cm distal to the tracheostomy stoma. Ingestion of a toxic substance may result in diffuse edema of the larynx and trachea and also involve the esophagus and lower gastroesophageal junction, resulting in stricture formation. Affected patients typically present with stridor, hoarseness, cough, dyspnea, and difficulty clearing secretions. Stenosis caused by prolonged intubation may develop immediately after extubation or may be delayed by as much as 90 days. Treatment of the injuries occurring from internal trauma is dependent on the extent of the damaged segment. Localized granulomas may be resected using laser excision. Partial or circumferential subglottic and tracheal stenosis may require more aggressive treatment. Patients who are unresponsive to repeated dilatations may require open surgical repair.[8, 44]

External Injuries

The most common cause of external injuries involving the larynx and trachea is motor vehicle accidents. Tracheal injuries account for 1% of traffic fatalities, with 30% of injured patients succumbing within the first hour after the accident. Three percent to 11% of motor vehicle accident victims have injuries found at autopsy. Other causes of external injuries to the larynx and trachea include various forms of penetrating injuries such as gunshot wounds, metallic fragment injuries, and stab wounds. Such injuries are more common in older children owing in part to the fact that the larynx is in a lower position and less likely to be protected by the mandible.[8, 44]

External trauma may result in different types of injuries including tracheal tear or transection, complete laryngotracheal disruption, fracture or dislocation of various laryngeal cartilages (thyroid, arytenoid, cricoid), and hematomas. Severe forms of trauma are often associated with injuries to one or both recurrent laryngeal nerves or esophageal lacerations. Tracheal trauma may be accompanied by injuries affecting other organs including the esophagus, cervical spine, and brachiocephalic vessels.[8, 44]

Several mechanisms have been proposed for this form

of LTT. In cases of blunt trauma, the larynx is crushed between the inciting force and the rigid spine, resulting in fracture of the cartilages or rupture of the membranous tracheal wall. Tracheal injury may also result from severe hyperextension of the cervical spine causing a marked increase in intraluminal pressure, which, if severe enough, may result in laceration or transection.[8]

Patients with LTT injuries resulting from blunt or penetrating trauma present with signs and symptoms of pending respiratory obstruction, including respiratory difficulties (stridor, wheezing, retractions), hoarse or muffled voice, deglutition, and subcutaneous emphysema. Patients may also present with hemoptysis and odynophagia. Physical examination may reveal neck or chest contusions or lacerations and loss of the normal prominence of the cricoid and thyroid cartilages.

Treatment of such injuries is initially directed at stabilizing the airway. Emergent intubation may be necessary in patients with significant trauma. Laryngeal injuries consisting primarily of hematomas may be managed conservatively. Extensive injuries with disruption of the laryngeal architecture can require open surgical intervention. Some investigators report good functional results if acute laryngeal fractures are reduced within 3 to 7 days after the injury. Continued delays in surgery may increase the likelihood of scarring and chronic laryngeal stenosis.[8]

The preferred imaging of patients with LTT is dependent on whether the trauma is due to internal or external causes. Infants and young children believed to have internal injuries are best imaged with CT. Granulation tissue or scarring resulting from prolonged intubation produces characteristic findings of partial or circumferential soft tissue thickening involving the subglottis or trachea. Cross-section capabilities of both CT and MRI provide important information on the caliber of the residual lumen and the extent of the involvement. Deformity of the air column or dystrophic calcification of the cricoid cartilage or tracheal rings is suggestive of associated laryngomalacia or tracheomalacia[2] (Fig. 41–27).

In the acute setting of external trauma, plain film radiography may provide important evidence of underly-

ing LTT. Findings suggestive of acute LTT include diffuse soft tissue swelling, subcutaneous air, fracture or displacement of the hyoid bone, and opacification of the lung parenchyma. The films should also be evaluated for the presence of foreign bodies. Complete laryngotracheal separation may be suggested by malalignment or step-off of the tracheal air column. However, the majority of these cases are not imaged owing to the high mortality of this injury and associated abnormalities.[2, 4]

Imaging should be performed in all cases for evaluation before surgical intervention. Multiplanar capabilities of MRI permit direct coronal and sagittal imaging. Characteristic findings of soft tissue injuries caused by trauma include diffuse swelling and edema of the endo- and exolaryngeal structures. Focal or diffuse hemorrhage may be present throughout the area of injury. Cross-sectional imaging provides valuable information regarding the degree of airway compromise due to soft tissue edema or hematoma (Fig. 41–28). Severe trauma may cause disruption of the thyroepiglottic ligaments, resulting in subluxation of the epiglottis. The presence of subcutaneous air is indicative of airway laceration and resultant communication (Fig. 41–29). Severe trauma may also be associated with subluxation or fracture and dislocation of the hyoid bone. The normal segmentation of the hyoid bone should not be mistaken for fractures.[4]

Severe laryngeal trauma may result in fracture and dislocation of the thyroid cartilage. Thyroid cartilage fractures are typically horizontally or vertically oriented. Vertical fractures are best detected with CT, as they are perpendicular to the acquisition plane of CT (Fig. 41–30). Comminuted and displaced fractures of the thyroid cartilage provide no support for the true and false vocal cords, resulting in reduced vocal function.[4]

The cricoid cartilage is the foundation of the larynx and its status after severe trauma is one of the most important prognostic factors regarding function in the posttraumatic larynx. Fractures of the cricoid cartilage are generally associated with a reduced likelihood of regaining normal laryngeal function. Cricoid fractures result in deformity and collapse of the cricoid ring, which is

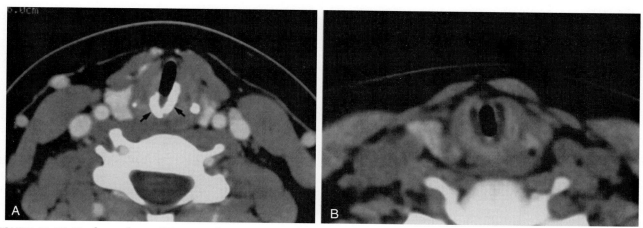

FIGURE 41–27 Tracheomalacia, CT. *A,* Axial postcontrast CT scan shows marked reduction of the lateral tracheal diameter. The cricoid cartilage *(arrows)* has dystrophic calcification and has assumed a V shape because of collapse. *B,* Axial CT scan in a different patient with tracheomalacia shows reduced lateral tracheal diameter and slight flattening of posterior tracheal wall. In this case, there are no dystrophic calcifications. (*A* and *B,* Courtesy of D. Marten, University of North Carolina, Chapel Hill.)

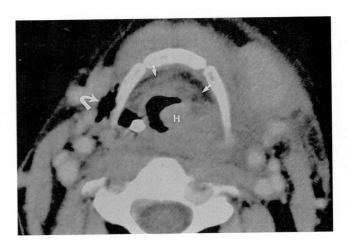

FIGURE 41–28 Contrast-enhanced CT scan performed in a patient involved in a severe motor vehicle accident shows thickening of the left aryepiglottic fold due to hematoma (H). There is also reticulation of the preepiglottic fat (*straight arrows*) and air lateral to the hyoid bone (*curved arrow*).

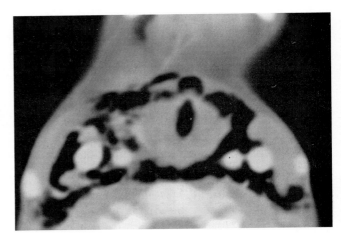

FIGURE 41–29 Contrast-enhanced CT scan performed in a patient with pharyngeal perforation demonstrates diffuse air tracking along the fascial neck planes with anterior displacement of the airway.

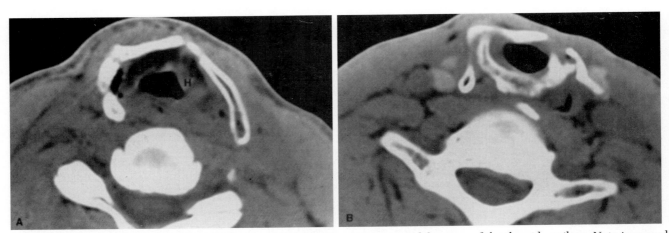

FIGURE 41–30 Tracheal injury with fractures. *A*, Axial CT scan shows comminuted fractures of the thyroid cartilage. Note increased and localized density in the left paraglottic fat (H), indicating hematoma. *B*, Axial CT scan (below *A*) in the same patient shows collapse of thyroid cartilage due to fractures and irregularly shaped left cricoid, also secondary to fracture. The tracheal air column has lost its normal shape and is flat in its anteroposterior diameter. (*A* and *B*, From Castillo M, Mukherki SK [eds]. Imaging of the Pediatric Head, Neck, and Spine. Philadelphia, Lippincott-Raven, 1996.)

manifested as a deformity of the airway. Severe crush injury may result in comminution of the anterior and posterior portions of the cricoid ring causing the two halves to "spring" apart. Resultant migration of fragments into the airway may cause respiratory compromise.[4]

Lack of calcification of the cartilages may make these structures difficult to evaluate with CT in young children. With age, progressive calcification and fatty replacement of marrow make these structures more readily evaluated with both CT and MRI, making these modalities more useful with older patients. Further diagnostic studies should be performed in patients suspected of having associated injuries. Esophagography may be necessary in patients suspected of having esophageal perforation. Aortography may be indicated in patients with an external injury associated with severe chest trauma or in selected individuals with stab wounds.[2, 4]

References

1. Hanafee WN, Ward PH. The Larynx, pp. 13–20. New York, Thieme, 1990.
2. Curtin HC. The larynx. In Som PM, Bergeron RT (eds). Head and Neck Imaging, 2nd ed., pp. 593–692. St. Louis, Mosby–Year Book, 1991.
3. Harnsberger HR. Handbook of Head and Neck Imaging, 2nd ed, pp. 224–260. St. Louis, Mosby–Year Book, 1995.
4. Mancuso AA, Hanafee WN. Larynx and hypopharynx. In Computed Tomography and Magnetic Resonance Imaging of the Head and Neck, 2nd ed., pp. 241–357. Baltimore, Williams & Wilkins, 1985.
5. Hiatt JL, Gartner LP. Textbook of Head and Neck Anatomy, pp. 225–260. Stamford, CT, Appleton-Century-Crofts, 1982.
6. Hast MH. Developmental anatomy of the larynx. In Gardner J (ed): Scientific Foundations of Otolaryngology, p. 369. London, Heineman Medical, 1976.
7. Castillo M, Mukherji SK. Imaging of the Pediatric Head, Neck, and Spine, pp. 517–616. Philadelphia, Lippincott-Raven, 1996.
8. Alonso WA. Injuries to the lower respiratory tract. In Bluestone CD, Stool SE, Scheetz MD (eds). Pediatric Otolaryngology, Vol. 2, pp. 1178–1182. Philadelphia, WB Saunders, 1990.
9. Cotton RT, Andrews TM. Laryngeal stenosis. In Johnson JT, Kohut RI, Pillsbury HC, Tardy ME (eds). Head and Neck Surgery, Otolaryngology, Vol. 1, pp. 658–660. Philadelphia, Lippincott-Raven, 1993.
10. Pransky SM, Seid AB. Tumors of the larynx, trachea and bronchi. In Bluestone CD, Stool SE, Scheetz MD (eds). Pediatric Otolaryngology, Vol. 2, pp. 1220–1222. Philadelphia, WB Saunders, 1990.
11. Thawley S. Cysts and tumors of the larynx. In Paparella MM, Shumrick DA, Gluckman JL, Meyerhoff WL (eds). Otolaryngology, Vol. 3, 3rd ed., pp. 2310–2312. Philadelphia, WB Saunders, 1991.
12. Vasquez E, Enriquez G, Castellote A, et al. US, CT, and MR imaging of neck lesions in children. Radiographic 1995;15:105–122.
13. Baker LL, Dillon WP, Hieshima GB, et al. Hemangiomas and vascular malformations of the head and neck: MR characterization. AJNR 1993;14:307–314.
14. Doengan JO, Strife JL, Seid AB, et al. Internal laryngocele and saccular cysts in children. Ann Otol 1980;89:408–410.
15. Lewis CS, Castillo M, Patrick E. Symptomatic external laryngocele in a newborn: Findings on plain radiographs and CT scans. AJNR 1990;11:1002.
16. Chen PC, Ball WS, Towbin RB. Aggressive fibromatosis of the tongue: MR demonstration. J Comput Assist Tomogr 1989;13:343–345.
17. Reede DL, Bergeron RT, Som PM. CT of thyroglossal duct cysts. Radiology 1985;157:121–125.
18. Brazeau-Lamontagne L, Charlin B, Levesque RY, Lussier A. Crico-arytenoiditis: CT assessment in rheumatoid arthritis. Radiology 1986;158:463–466.
19. Casselman JW, Lemahieu SF, Peene P, Stoffels G. Polychondritis affecting the laryngeal cartilages: CT findings. AJR 1988;150:355.
20. Jones KR, Pillsbury HC. Infections and manifestations of systemic disease of the larynx. In Cummings CW, Fredrickson JM, Harker LA, et al. (eds). Otolaryngology and Head and Neck Surgery, Vol. 3, pp. 1854–1857. St. Louis, Mosby–Year Book, 1993.
21. MayoSmith MF, Hirsch PJ, Wodzinski SF, Schiffman FJ. Acute epiglottitis in adults: An eight-year experience in the state of Rhode Island. N Engl J Med 1986;314:1133–1139.
22. Becker TS, Shum TK, Waller TS. Radiological aspects of rhinoscleroma. Radiology 1981;141:433–438.
23. Lawson W, Biller HF, Suen JV. Cancer of the larynx. In Myers EN, Suen JV (eds). Cancer of the Head and Neck, pp. 533–580. New York, Churchill Livingstone, 1989.
24. Boyd JH, Johnson JT, Curtin H. Carcinoma of the supraglottic larynx. In Self Instructional Package, pp. 1–20. Rochester, MN, Custom Printing, 1993.
25. Leach JL, Schaefer SD. Diagnosis and treatment of cancer of the glottis and subglottis. In Self Instructional Package, pp. 1–25. Rochester, MN, Custom Printing, 1993.
26. Batsakis JF. Tumours of the Head and Neck: Clinical and Pathological Considerations, 2nd ed., p. 203. Baltimore, Williams & Wilkins, 1979.
27. Million RR, Cassisi NJ, Mancuso AA. Larynx. In Million RR, Cassisi NJ (eds). Management of Head and Neck Cancer: A Multidisciplinary Approach, pp. 431–497. Philadelphia, Lippincott-Raven, 1994.
28. Becker M, Zbaren P, Laeng H, et al. Neoplastic invasion of the laryngeal cartilage: Comparison of MR imaging and CT with histopathologic correlation. Radiology 1995;194:661–669.
29. Lederman M. Place de la radiotherapie dans le traitement du cancer. Ann Radiol (Paris) 1961;4:433–454.
30. Michaels L. Ear, Nose and Throat Histopathology, p. 440. Heidelberg, Springer-Verlag, 1987.
31. Ognibene FP. Upper and lower airway manifestations of human immunodeficiency virus infection. Ear Nose Throat J 1990;69:424–431.
32. Barnes L, Gnepp DR. Diseases of the larynx, hypopharynx, and esophagus. In Barnes L (ed). Surgical Pathology of the Head and Neck, p. 188. New York, Marcel Dekker, 1985.
33. Amdur RJ, Parsons JT, Mendenhall WM, et al. Postoperative irradiation for squamous cell carcinoma of the head and neck: An analysis of treatment results and complications. Int J Radiat Oncol Biol Phys 1989;16:25–36.
34. Manara M. Histological changes of the human larynx irradiated with various technical therapeutic methods. Arch Ital Otol 1966;79:596–635.
35. Mukherji SK, Mancuso AA, Kotzur I, et al. Radiologic appearance of the irradiated larynx. Part I: Expected changes. Radiology 1994;193:141–148.
36. Mukherji SK, Mancuso AA, Kotzur I, et al. Radiologic appearance of the irradiated larynx. Part II: Primary site response. Radiology 1994;193:149–154.
37. Parsons JT. The effect of radiation on normal tissues of the head and neck. In Million RR, Cassisi NJ (eds). Management of Head and Neck Cancer: A Multidisciplinary Approach, 2nd ed., pp. 173–205. Philadelphia, JB Lippincott, 1984.
38. Calcaterra TC, Stern F, Ward PH. Dilemma of delayed radiation injury of the larynx. Ann Otol Rhinol Laryngol 1972;81:501–507.
39. Mukherji SK, Drane WE, Tart RP, Mancuso AA. Comparison of SPECT FDG and SPECT thallium-201 for imaging of squamous cell carcinoma of the head and neck. AJNR 1994;15:1837–1842.
40. Mukherji SK, Buejenovich S, Weeks S, Castillo M. Initial experience using thallium-201 SPECT for imaging patients with squamous cell carcinoma of the upper aerodigestive tract. [Abstract] American Society of Head and Neck Radiology, Conference Proceedings, 1995.
41. Fried MP, Girdhar-Gopal HV. Advanced cancer of the larynx. In Bailey BJ (ed). Head and Neck Surgery, pp. 1347–1359. Philadelphia, JB Lippincott, 1993.
42. Desanto LW. Supraglottic laryngectomy. In Bailey BJ (ed). Head and Neck Surgery, pp. 1334–1345. Philadelphia, JB Lippincott, 1993.
43. Bailey BJ. Early glottic cancers. In Bailey BJ (ed). Head and Neck Surgery, pp. 1313–1333. Philadelphia, JB Lippincott, 1993.
44. Stark P. Congenital anomalies of the trachea. In Radiology of the Trachea, pp. 13–15. Stuttgart, Georg Thieme, 1991.

42

The Hypopharynx

JAMES N. SUOJANEN, M.D.

The hypopharynx is the caudal extension of the pharyngeal mucosal space located between the hyoid bone and the lower edge of the cricoid cartilage and cricopharyngeus muscle. Its external boundary is the middle layer of the deep cervical fascia that encompasses the visceral space of the infrahyoid neck. Anteriorly and superiorly, this facial plane arises from the hyoid bone; posteriorly and superiorly, it arises from the skull base. Inferiorly, it extends into the upper mediastinum.[1] Three areas comprise the hypopharynx: the piriform sinuses, the posterior pharyngeal wall, and the postcricoid region. Some authors also include a fourth region, *the marginal area,* comprising the lateral surfaces of the aryepiglottic folds, which form the medial walls of the piriform sinuses. However, lesions in this area are more properly included in the discussion of the other major component of the visceral space, the larynx, and are classified as marginal supraglottic lesions.[2]

The piriform (pear-shaped) sinuses lie on either side of the hypopharynx (Fig. 42–1A). Superiorly and anteriorly, they abut the paraglottic fat; inferiorly, their apices extend to approximately the level of the vocal cords. The thyrohyoid membrane and thyroid cartilage form their membranous and cartilaginous lateral boundaries, with the aryepiglottic folds forming their medial margins (Fig. 42–1B). Posteriorly, they are contiguous with the posterior hypopharyngeal wall (Fig. 42–1C).

The posterior hypopharyngeal wall is also inseparable from the posterior oropharyngeal wall but, by convention, begins at the level of the valleculae, continuing caudally where it becomes contiguous with the anterior wall of the cricopharyngeus muscle (Fig. 42–2). The inferior constrictor muscle forms a large portion of the posterior hypopharyngeal wall lying just deep to the mucosa and submucosa but just anterior to the deep cervical fascia. Superiorly, its fibers arise from a midline posterior raphe and insert on the thyroid cartilage (Figs. 42–2 and 42–3). Inferiorly, its fibers run obliquely, so that between it and the cricopharyngeus is a triangular area of potential muscular insufficiency called *Killian's dehiscence* (Fig. 42–2A).[3, 4]

The most inferior portions of this muscle then blend with the upper circular muscle of the cervical esophagus. The lateral edges of the cricoid cartilage provide the origins for the cricopharyngeus and also the lateral boundaries for the postcricoid region. This latter region

extends from the mucosal surfaces posterior to the arytenoid cartilages to the inferior edge of the cricoid cartilage, forming the anterior surface of the hypopharynx in its most caudal portion (see Fig. 42–2B).

Embryologically, the hypopharynx develops from portions of the third, fourth, and sixth pharyngeal arches as well as their associated clefts and pouches.[5, 6] As such, it receives innervation from both the glossopharyngeal nerve (derived from the third arch) and the superior laryngeal branch of the vagus nerve (arising from the fourth arch) (see Fig. 42–2A). Both nerves provide sensory input, and the vagal branch supplies motor innervation to the constrictor muscle and cricopharyngeus. The sympathetic innervation to the mucosa derives mainly from the superior cervical ganglia. During deglutition, the pharyngeal constrictors act in a coordinated fashion to propel the bolus inferiorly. The cricopharyngeus relaxes, permitting passage of the bolus, then closes by returning to its normal constricted state, thus preventing reflux.[7–9]

Arterial and venous supplies derive principally from the superior and inferior thyroidal arteries and veins, with some direct venous drainage into the internal jugular veins. The lymphatics generally parallel these vessels, draining mostly to jugular nodes, although the posterior wall lymphatics drain via retropharyngeal nodes.[3, 6]

IMAGING STUDIES

Fluoroscopic Studies

Although often ignored in neuroradiologic discussions of upper aerodigestive disease, fluoroscopic barium swallowing studies are an important modality for evaluating the hypopharynx. After clinician-performed endoscopy, a barium swallow is commonly the first imaging procedure performed in patients with dysphasia or odynophagia.[8–10]

Protocols for fluoroscopic studies vary depending on the nature of each patient's problems. Generally, our examinations include posteroanterior (PA) views of the larynx and hypopharynx in quiet respiration, with phonation ("e") and with puffed cheeks, and lateral views obtained in quiet respiration and with puffed cheeks. PA and lateral views taken after several swallows of thick barium suspension permit views of the hypopharyngeal mucosal surfaces (Fig. 42–4). Although these views can detect mucosal abnormalities including tumors (Fig. 42–

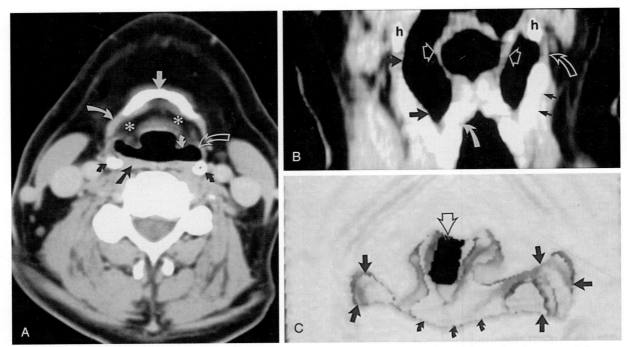

FIGURE 42–1 *A,* Axial computed tomography (CT) scan obtained at the level of the hyoid bone *(straight white arrow)* demonstrates quite nicely the preepiglottic fat *(asterisks)* as well as the piriform sinuses *(open curved arrow)* and the lateral surface of the aryepiglottic folds *(small white curved arrow).* The thyrohyoid membrane *(large white curved arrow)* is also well demonstrated, as is the posterior boundary of the hypopharynx, the inferior constrictor *(straight black arrow),* which passes between the superior cornu of the thyroid cartilage *(small black curved arrows).* *B,* Coronal reconstruction of the hypopharynx from spiral CT data. Three-millimeter-thick CT sections were reconstructed at 1-mm increments and have been reconstructed coronally to show the piriform sinuses *(large black arrows)* with the apex of the piriform sinus at the level of the cricoarytenoid articulation *(curved white arrow)* that represents approximately the level of the true cords as noted in the text. The *straight open arrows* point to the aryepiglottic folds, which form the medial wall of the sinus, the *curved open arrow* points to the thyrohyoid membrane, and the *small black arrows* point to the thyroid cartilage, which forms the lateral wall. The hyoid bone (h) is also well depicted. *C,* Three-dimensional reconstruction of normal hypopharynx. This view is from the top looking down on a three-dimensional reconstruction derived from an axial spiral CT data set and threshold set to show the mucosal surfaces of the piriform sinuses *(straight solid arrows)* and the posterior hypopharyngeal wall *(curved arrows).* The laryngeal airway *(open arrow)* is well demonstrated, as are the mucosal surfaces of the false cords forming its lateral margins.

5), most mucosal masses are detected by endoscopy before study. The real advantage of barium studies over computed tomography (CT) or magnetic resonance imaging (MRI) is the former's ability to study the physiologic action of swallowing (Figs. 42–6 and 42–7). Typically, this examination begins with thin barium suspension, although various substances of different texture and consistency can also be used to evaluate a patient's deglutition. More complete discussions of these techniques can be found in standard gastrointestinal radiology texts.

Cross-Sectional Techniques

Both CT and MRI can be used to evaluate hypopharyngeal disease and are necessary for accurate preoperative staging.[11] Much has been written extolling the virtues of MRI,[11–17] but both modalities offer advantages and disadvantages.[18] Our preference is to use helical (spiral) CT scanning.

For CT studies, the patient is placed supine on the table and instructed to breath quietly and to not swallow during the scan. Administration of intravenous iodinated contrast material begins before imaging and continues during the scan. Spiral (helical) scanning begins at the skull base using 5-mm scan collimation and continues to the thoracic inlet. If the patient has multiple dental fillings, two scans are performed and angled so as to avoid the beam-hardening artifacts from the amalgams. If the larynx and hypopharynx are the areas of interest, another scan utilizing 3-mm-section collimation is obtained, reviewed at 1-mm increments, and studied using three-dimensional (see Fig. 42–1C) and multiplanar reconstructions (see Fig. 42–1B).[19, 20]

For MRI examination, we use a neck coil, although some authors advocate surface coils.[11] However, the neck coil permits evaluation of the entire neck from the skull base to the thoracic inlet and is more acceptable to patients. Our standard sequences include coronal and axial T1-weighted spin-echo and axial T2-weighted short-tau inversion recovery images. Magnetization transfer may help differentiate benign from malignant disease,[16] although usually this is known before imaging. Contrast enhancement may help in detecting tumor extent and cartilage invasion,[14] and some authors advocate contrast administration with most studies.[13, 15, 21] However, we reserve the use of contrast material on our MRI examina-

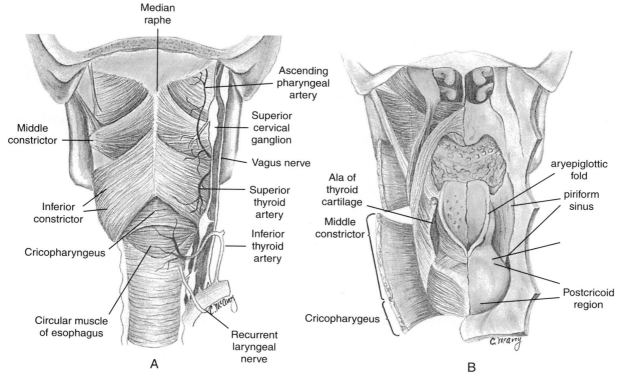

FIGURE 42–2 *A,* A view of the pharynx from behind shows the muscles, nerves, and vascular supply to this region, as noted in the text. The cricopharyngeus marker points to the triangular region where there may be a muscular deficiency known as *Killian's dehiscence. B,* View of the pharynx from behind with the constrictor muscles reflected. On the left, the mucosa has been removed to show some of the underlying muscular and cartilagenous anatomy. This shows well the lateral portion of the thyroid cartilage (the ala), which forms the lateral cartilagenous wall of the piriform sinus. This also shows how the cricopharyngeus muscle inserts on the lower portion the cricoid cartilage. On the right, the aryepiglottic fold forms the medial border of the piriform sinus. The postcricoid region is well depicted. (*A* and *B,* Courtesy of Caitlin McAvoy.)

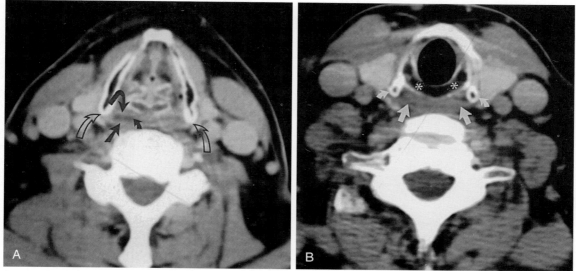

FIGURE 42–3 *A,* Axial CT section obtained at the level of the thyroarytenoid articulations shows the inferior constrictor *(straight arrow)* running between the most posterior aspects of the laryngeal cartilage *(open arrows).* Between this muscle and the anterior mucosal surface of the hypopharynx *(large solid curved arrow)* are the mucosal and the submucosal portions of the hypopharynx *(small solid curved arrow). B,* Axial CT section obtained at the most distal portion of the hypopharynx—that at the level of the cricoid cartilage *(asterisks).* This again shows the inferior constrictor muscle passing between the inferior cornu of the thyroid cartilage *(curved arrows)* as well as the mucosal and submucosal portions of the pharyngeal tube *(straight arrows).*

FIGURE 42–4 *A,* A lateral view from a double-contrast barium swallow study. This "puffed-cheek" view well demonstrates the contours of the piriform sinuses *(solid arrows).* The posterior hypopharyngeal wall *(curved open arrows)* and the anatomic landmarks defining the upper and lower extent of the hypopharynx are also well demonstrated. An *asterisk* shows the hyoid bone, and a *straight open arrow* indicates the level of the cricopharyngeus muscle. *B,* An anteroposterior (AP) view from the same study also well demonstrates the contour of the piriform sinuses *(straight arrows).* Astute observers will also note the reflux into the left eustachian tube *(curved arrow).*

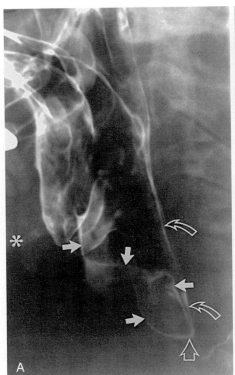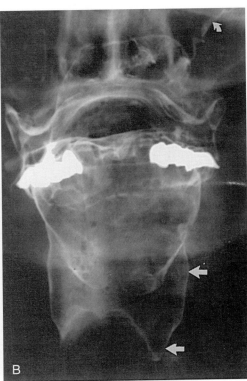

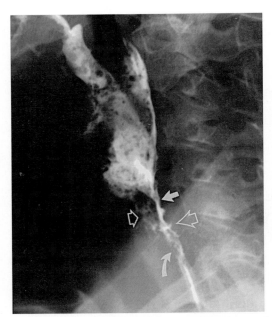

FIGURE 42–5 Squamous cell carcinoma. Lateral view from a barium swallow shows an irregularly narrowed distal hypopharynx *(straight solid arrow).* The mucosal irregularity continues below the level of the pharyngoesophageal junction *(large open arrow)* into the upper cervical esophagus *(curved arrow).* The barium is somewhat flocculated in this case, giving the most inferior portion of the piriform sinuses a somewhat irregular appearance *(small open arrow).*

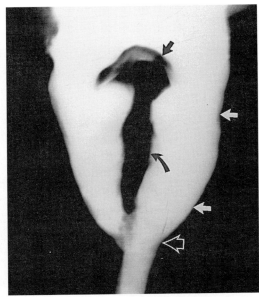

FIGURE 42–6 An AP view obtained during the swallowing phase of a barium study shows a well-distended hypopharynx *(white arrows)* and demonstrates the junction with the esophagus *(open arrow).* The epiglottis *(straight black arrow)* and the posterior wall of the larynx *(curved black arrow)* can produce a filling defect.

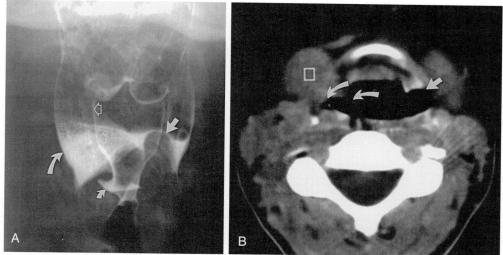

FIGURE 42–7 *A,* An AP view from a double-contrast barium swallow shows an apparent mass in the left piriform sinus *(straight white arrow)* and a fairly normal-appearing distended right piriform sinus *(large curved arrow).* However, note that the right laryngeal ventricle is enlarged *(small curved arrow)* compared with the left and that the false cord above and the true cord below are thickened and rounded, indicative of vocal cord paralysis on this side produced by a skull-base tumor in this patient. Therefore, the left piriform sinus is normal, with an appearance produced by incomplete distention of a normal piriform sinus. The patient also had a swallowing abnormality owing to cranial nerve dysfunction that allows barium to coat the inner surface of the aryepiglottic folds *(open arrows),* which as noted in the text, is considered part of the larynx. *B,* Axial CT section of the same patient confirms that the left piriform sinus is normal *(straight arrow).* Note the flattened right sinus and the thinned aryepiglottic fold *(curved arrows)* produced by the cranial nerve paralysis. The *box* should be disregarded.

tions to those cases of suspected cartilage invasion. Sections are typically 5-mm-thick with 1-mm gaps, although thin-section T1-weighted images using 3 mm of thickness with 0.3-mm gaps or using interleaved contiguous 3-mm sections can be very helpful for larynx and hypopharynx evaluation.

MRI offers the advantage of superior contrast resolution to CT and does not require intravenous contrast administration in most instances. It also has multiplanar capabilities, although spirally acquired CT data can also provide these. CT offers better anatomic resolution, improved nodal staging capability, and very fast scanning times. This rapid, high-resolution scanning can be performed while patients puff their cheeks, allowing even better evaluation of the piriform sinuses (Fig. 42–8).[19, 22] Positron-emission tomography scanning may be helpful when attempting to differentiate recurrent tumor from changes produced by surgery or radiation therapy, or both.[23]

PATHOLOGY

Hypopharyngeal diseases can be separated practically into masses and functional disorders. An important anatomic point to keep in mind when evaluating patients with

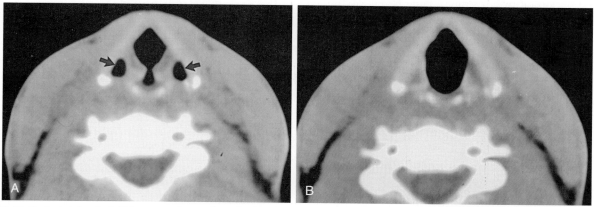

FIGURE 42–8 *A,* Axial spiral CT image obtained at the level of the true vocal cords while the patient performs a "puffed-cheek" maneuver allows very good distention of the piriform sinuses, including their most distal extent *(arrows).* *B,* Spiral CT image from the same patient as in Figure 42–1A obtained while the patient was breathing quietly. Note that the most distal portion of the piriform sinuses is not seen by this examination.

TABLE 42–1 Masses of the Hypopharynx

Neoplastic: Malignant

Squamous cell carcinoma
Minor salivary gland neoplasms
Lymphoma
Kaposi's sarcoma
Sarcomas

Neoplastic: Benign

Minor salivary gland tumors
Lipomas
Retention cyst
Neurofibroma

Infectious

Granulomatous disease
Rhinoscleroma

Inflammatory

Postradiation edema
Inhalational injury

Traumatic

Hematoma
Granulation tissue

Congenital

Branchial cleft cyst (III and IV)
Aberrant carotid

Miscellaneous

Zenker's diverticulum
Pharyngocele

proven or suspected hypopharyngeal disease relates to sensory enervation. The internal branch of the superior laryngeal nerve (a branch of the vagus nerve) provides sensation to portions of the hypopharynx. This nerve is closely associated with another vagal sensory branch—the auricular (Arnold's) nerve. Commonly, hypopharyngeal disease causes otalgia, and otic disease can also present as a sore throat, odynophagia, and other conditions.[2]

Hypopharyngeal Masses

Hypopharyngeal masses have many causes (Table 42–1). The most important by far is the squamous cell carcinoma (SCCA). Table 42–2 summarizes the primary tumor staging of these masses. The piriform sinus is the most common site of carcinoma in the hypopharynx (60%), followed by the postcricoid region (25%), and the posterior pharyngeal wall (15%). Early symptoms are usually vague

TABLE 42–2 Primary Tumor Staging Criteria—Hypopharyngeal Carcinoma

T1	Tumor limited to one subsite°
T2	Tumor involves more than one subsite or an adjacent site; no fixation of hemilarynx
T3	T2 criteria with hemilarynx fixation
T4	Tumor invades adjacent structures—thyroid or cricoid cartilage; soft tissues of neck

Abbreviation: T, tumor.
°Subsites: piriform sinus, posterior pharyngeal wall, postcricoid area.

and include sore throat or intolerance to hot and cold liquids. Dysphagia, odynophagia, otalgia, and weight loss usually occur with more advanced disease. Because of this paucity of early signs and symptoms, most hypopharyngeal carcinomas are T3 or T4 at diagnosis, and 50% have nodal metastases. The prognosis is poor. Twenty percent to 40% of patients have or develop distant metastases or second primary tumors, or both. Postcricoid carcinomas have 5-year survival rates of less than 25%. Most patients are male with significant smoking and ethanol abuse histories.[2, 3, 24, 25] When a woman presents with hypopharyngeal SCCA, the Plummer-Vinson syndrome should be suspected. This syndrome is characterized by hypopharyngeal and esophageal webs, atrophic mucosa, achlorhydria, and iron-deficiency anemia, with hypopharyngeal carcinoma being a well-known complication (Fig. 42–9).[2, 26]

The imaging features of SCCA are quite variable. On barium swallow, there may be mucosal irregularity (see Fig. 42–5) or perhaps simply poor motility. There may be subtle asymmetry of normal structures (Fig. 42–10) or gross deformity (Fig. 42–11). Piriform sinus tumors, when small and near the apex, may escape detection on clinical examination. Therefore, this area must be inspected carefully when studying a patient with an "unknown" head

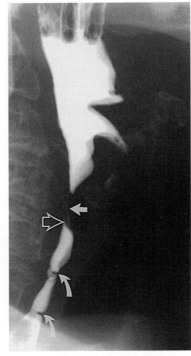

FIGURE 42–9 Lateral view from a barium swallow shows narrowing of the distal hypopharynx (*straight white arrow*) just above the pharyngoesophageal junction (*open arrow*). This area was not distensible during any portion of this swallowing examination. The mucosa is not well visualized, although it does not appear irregular, and indeed the mucosa in the upper cervical esophagus adjacent to this narrowing is rather featureless with multiple webs (*curved arrows*). This upper cervical esophagus is also nondistensible. This was all due to membranous pemphigoid, although Plummer-Vinson webs are similar.

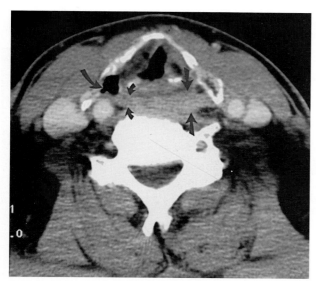

FIGURE 42–10 Posterior pharyngeal wall carcinoma. Axial CT section in the midportion of the hypopharynx shows slightly irregular thickening of the left hypopharyngeal wall *(straight arrows)* in this patient with dysphagia. Compare this thickness with the normal right hypopharynx *(small curved arrows)*. The right piriform sinus is normal *(large curved arrow)*, whereas the mass on the left causes effacement of the left sinus.

and neck primary tumor.[27] Piriform sinus carcinomas typically spread posterolaterally and initially spare the thyroid cartilage (Fig. 42–11), although the cartilage must be studied carefully. MRI may be more accurate than CT for assessing cartilage invasion,[14] although it can be misleading. The decision to remove any pharyngeal cartilage surgically usually takes place in the operating room, and the diagnosis of cartilage invasion can be made definitively only by microscopic examination of the surgical specimen.[28] Similar problems occur in the radiographic staging of postcricoid tumors. Because the posterior hypopharynx abuts the pharyngobasilar fascia and the retropharyngeal spaces, tumors here can spread infiltratively superiorly into the oro- and nasopharynx or inferiorly into the upper mediastinum.[29] These tumors can also have retropharyngeal as well as jugular nodal metastases.[30]

Minor salivary glands occupy the hypopharyngeal submucosa. All varieties of benign and malignant salivary gland tumors can occur in the hypopharynx. Here, as elsewhere, these tumors are radiographically indistinguishable from SCCA. Salivary gland retention cysts, however, have the characteristic CT and MRI features of a cyst. Most other neoplasms, such as hemangioma, of the hypopharynx are exceedingly rare. Lipomas and fibrolipomas may have the characteristic imaging features of fat to aid in their identification, but malignant lymphomas and sarcomas appear identical to SCCA.[31–33]

Nonneoplastic Masses

Hypopharyngeal hematomas commonly occur after ingestion of a fish or chicken bone, or after instrumentation such as a traumatic intubation.[34, 35] Impacted foreign bodies can also lead to abscess formation, as can various

primary infections. In immunocompromised patients, fungal and viral infections may produce marked hypopharyngeal swelling. Burns produced by inhalation of very hot gases (from fire or crack cocaine) and radiation therapy mucositis can produce striking imaging findings (Fig. 42–12).[3]

Although rare, third or fourth branchial cleft cysts can arise in the hypopharynx owing to its previously described embryologic origin. Third branchial clefts or fistulas have origins similar to second cleft anomalies, but their courses are posterior to the carotid arteries and connect to the upper piriform sinuses. Fourth branchial cleft cysts arise from the apex of the piriform sinus and pass inferior to the superior laryngeal nerve (a fourth arch derivative) and superior to the recurrent laryngeal nerve (a sixth arch derivative). Most of these cysts are on the left side and can be associated with recurrent thyroid infections (Fig. 42–13).[5]

Extrahypopharyngeal masses can also produce marked distortion of the hypopharynx. Most important is an aberrant carotid (Fig. 42–14). Retropharyngeal tumors and abscesses commonly deform the hypopharynx, as can vertebral osteophytes, infections, or metastases. Similarly, laryngeal masses such as neoplasms or laryngoceles (Fig. 42–15) may also cause marked hypopharyngeal distortion and can make anatomic delineation of tumor origin difficult.

Functional Disorders and Masses

The functional disorders include swallowing abnormalities[8, 9] and sleep apnea[36, 37] and are largely beyond the

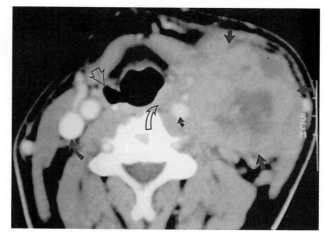

FIGURE 42–11 Piriform sinus squamous cell carcinoma with nodal metastases. Axial CT section obtained in the upper portion of the hypopharynx shows a large heterogeneous left neck mass *(straight black arrows)* with an indistinct medial margin. The left internal jugular vein is obstructed (compared with the normal right *[large curved solid arrow]*). The left internal carotid artery *(small curved solid arrow)* is smaller than the right artery, and the fat surrounding it is effaced. All of this suggests an infiltrative or inflammatory lesion. However, given the size and lack of fatty infiltration surrounding the mass laterally, a large metastatic nodal mass is more likely. The primary tumor is shown as an area of enhancement, at the tip of the *curved open arrow,* that effaces the left piriform sinus. The right piriform sinus *(straight open arrow)* is normal.

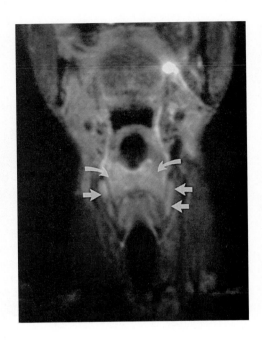

FIGURE 42–12 Radiation therapy mucositis. Coronal T2-weighted short-tau inversion recovery (STIR) image of the neck reveals thickened high-signal soft tissue in the piriform sinuses *(straight arrows)* and in the postcricoid region *(curved arrows)*. Other mucosal surfaces are also involved. The diffuse nature of the abnormalities and the history of recent completion of radiation therapy suggest the correct diagnosis.

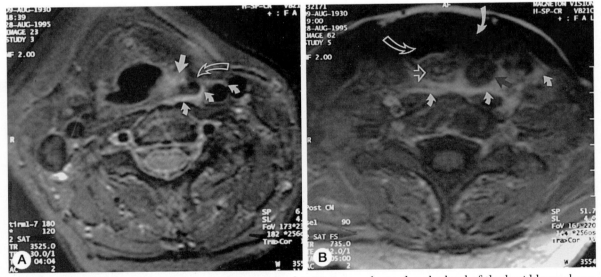

FIGURE 42–13 *A,* Fourth branchial cleft cyst. Axial T2-weighted STIR image obtained at the level of the hyoid bone shows an area of high signal intensity *(straight arrow)* effacing the left piriform sinus. Associated with this is high signal intensity in the adjacent vascular and retroperitoneal spaces *(curved solid arrows)*, which may be connected by a thin fistula through the thyrohyoid membrane *(curved open arrow)*. Note the excellent fat suppression obtained by this technique, which permits the identification of edema or infiltration in the other soft tissue spaces. *B,* Axial T1-weighted spin-echo image with fat saturation obtained after intravenous gadolinium administration. Just behind the left lobe of the thyroid *(large curved white arrow)* and contiguous with the high signal intensity seen in *A* is a rounded hypointense mass *(black arrow)* surrounded by an infiltrative pattern of enhancement *(small curved white arrows)*. The mass abuts the esophagus *(straight open arrow)* and appears to displace the trachea *(curved open arrow)*. At operation, this mass was found to contain fluid, blood products, and parathyroid tissue.

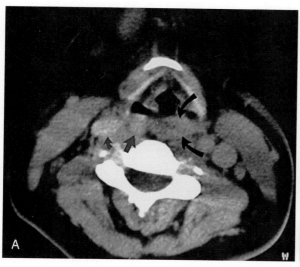

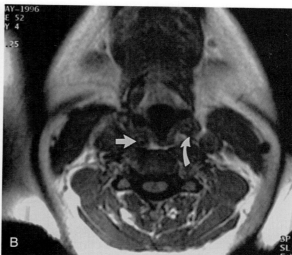

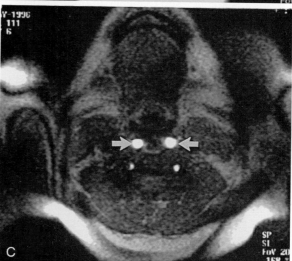

FIGURE 42–14 *A*, Aberrant carotid. Axial CT image obtained at the upper level of the hypopharynx shows an area of enhancement posterior to the right hypopharynx *(straight arrow)* with some apparent thickening of the left hypopharyngeal wall *(large curved arrows)*. However, communication with the referring clinician confirmed concern regarding the right hypopharyngeal posterior wall. The image shows some enhancement medial to the right internal jugular vein *(small curved arrow)*, suggesting that it was an aberrent common carotid. *B*, Axial T1-weighted spin-echo image shows a mass within the right retropharyngeal region *(straight arrow)* similar in appearance to the left common carotid artery *(curved arrow)*. This image clearly shows a normal posterior hypopharyngeal wall, piriform sinuses, and aryepiglottic folds as well as normal preepiglottic fat. This suggests that the thickening along the left posterior hypopharyngeal wall was probably an artifact. *C*, Axial flow-sensitive gradient-echo image confirms that the common carotid arteries *(arrows)* do follow an aberrant course and are responsible for the deformity of the posterior hypopharyngeal wall seen by the endoscopist, who is grateful that she did not biopsy this lesion.

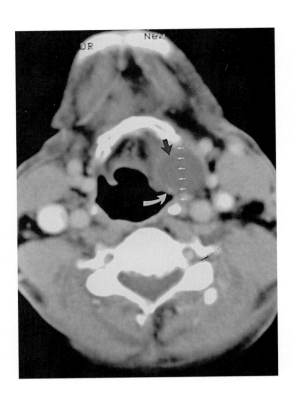

FIGURE 42–15 Axial CT section taken at the upper portion of the hypopharynx shows a fairly well-defined cystic lesion *(black arrow)* in the lateral portion of the pharynx. Note, however, that the mass extends beyond the confines of the thyrohyoid membrane *(small white arrows* define where the membrane should be). The mass effaces the left piriform sinus *(curved arrow)* and flattens the aryepiglottic fold. This is a mixed laryngocele, not a hypopharyngeal lesion but a laryngeal lesion. However, it does cause distortion of hypopharyngeal anatomy and can resemble a fourth branchial cleft cyst, a congenital anomaly of the hypopharynx (see Fig. 42–13).

scope of this chapter. However, a few do merit mention because of their frequency and tendency to produce mass effect. The cricopharyngeus muscle acts as a sphincter at the pharyngoesophageal junction to help prevent reflux. When it fails to relax fully during deglutition, the poste-

rior pharyngeal wall retains a marked fullness. This cricopharyngeal prominence is a common finding in dysphagic patients and has a characteristic appearance on barium swallow (Fig. 42–16A). It may be an isolated finding. This can also be produced by neurologic disease (e.g.,

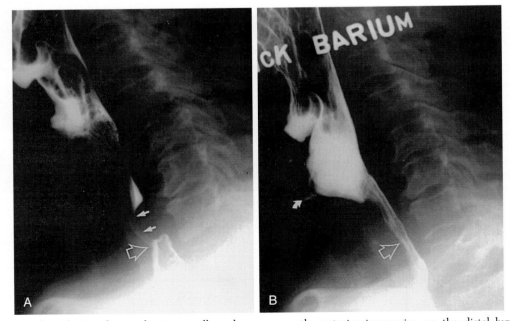

FIGURE 42–16 *A,* A lateral view from a barium swallow shows a smooth posterior impression on the distal hypopharynx *(solid arrows)* just above the pharyngoesophageal junction *(open arrow).* The mucosa adjacent to this impression is quite smooth and normal. *B,* A lateral view from a barium swallow on the patient after cricopharyngeal myotomy. The larger posterior impression is now absent, and the pharyngoesophageal junction *(open arrow)* is quite normal with normal mucosa and a smooth transition. Astute observers will note a small amount of barium penetrating the false cords with some pooling in the laryngeal ventricle *(curved arrow).*

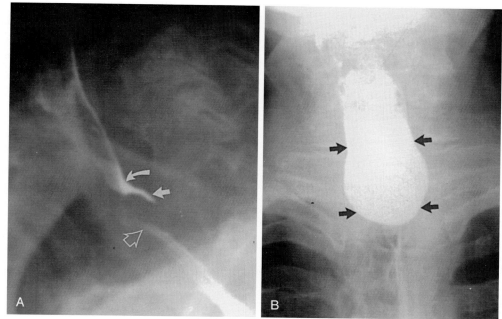

FIGURE 42–17 *A,* Lateral view from a barium swallow shows an extraluminal penetration of barium posteriorly *(straight solid arrow)* through a defect in the posterior wall of the hypopharynx *(curved arrow)* just above the pharyngoesophageal junction *(open arrow).* This is the classic appearance of a Zenker diverticulum. This represents herniation of mucosa and submucosa through a dehiscence between the oblique and the circular fibers of the cricopharyngeus muscle. Without exception, the diverticular neck is in the midline and usually fills with barium before the thoracic esophagus. *B,* An AP view of a barium swallow in a different patient from *A* shows a very large Zenker diverticulum *(arrows),* which remains filled long after the passage of the barium column.

Parkinson's disease) and is frequently associated with significant esophageal diseases.[9] This can be successfully treated by operation (Fig. 42–16*B*).[7]

Associated with cricopharyngeal prominence but also occurring independently of it are herniations of the hypopharyngeal mucosa and submucosa through a muscular

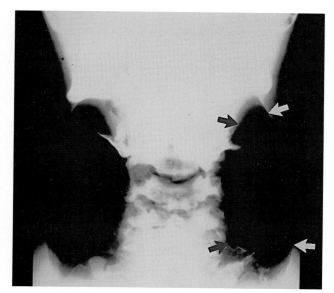

FIGURE 42–18 AP, puffed-cheek view from a pharyngogram in a trumpet player shows large distended and air-filled extensions of the piriform sinuses *(arrows)* with very smooth walls. This is the classic appearance of pharyngoceles.

deficiency that commonly exists at Killian's dehiscence (see Fig. 42–2*A*). This pulsion-type, or Zenker's, diverticulum begins centrally and posteriorly and may extend laterally to the left (Fig. 42–17).[38] These are usually detected on barium swallow but may produce retropharyngeal masses on CT or MRI. Because they may contain air, they should not be confused with gas-containing abscesses, which typically incite adjacent fatty infiltration. Increased pharyngeal pressures from playing musical instruments or from cricopharyngeal and esophageal motility disorders can also give rise to mucosal outpouchings from the piriform sinuses.[38] These pharyngoceles can appear as broad-based, air-filled masses best seen during a Valsalva maneuver on barium swallow (Fig. 42–18), although they may be visible on CT. These air-filled masses should not be confused with abscesses, as they lack adjacent inflammatory change. If any question arises, a spiral or helical CT scan acquired during a Valsalva maneuver may prove helpful.[19, 22, 39] Ultrafast CT or MRI may be of use in studying patients with obstructive sleep apnea, which can arise from hypopharyngeal pathology.[36, 37]

In the hypopharynx as elsewhere in the upper aerodigestive tract, the imager must work closely with referring clinicians to optimize imaging protocols and the diagnostic accuracy of the subsequent studies. In this way, radiologists can contribute significantly to the treatment of those patients entrusted to their care.

References

1. Smoker W, Harnsberger R. Differential diagnosis of head and neck lesions based on their space of origin. 2. The infrahyoid portion of the neck. AJR 1991;157:155–159.

2. Harnsberger R. Head and Neck Imaging. Osborn AG, Bragg DG (ser. eds). Handbooks in Radiology. Chicago, Year Book Medical, 1990.

3. Weissman JL, Holliday RA. Hypopharynx. In Som PM, Curtin HD (eds). Head and Neck Imaging, Vol. 1, pp. 472–487. St. Louis, CV Mosby, 1996.

4. Bosma JF, Bartner H. Ligaments of the larynx and the adjacent pharynx and esophagus. Dysphagia 1993;8:23–28.

5. Benson M, Dalen K, Mancuso A, et al. Congenital anomalies of the branchial apparatus: Embryology and pathologic anatomy. Radiographics 1992;12:943–960.

6. Crafts R. A Textbook of Human Anatomy. New York, Ronald Press, 1966.

7. Gates GA. Upper esophageal sphincter: Pre- and post-laryngectomy—A normative study. Laryngoscope 1980;90:454–464.

8. Donner M, Bosma J, Robertson D. Anatomy and physiology of the pharynx. Gastrointest Radiol 1985;10:196–212.

9. Jones B, Raivch W, Donner M, et al. Pharyngoesophageal interrelationships: Observations and working concepts. Gastrointest Radiol 1985;10:225–233.

10. Ekberg O, Nylander G. Double-contrast examination of the pharynx. Gastrointest Radiol 1985;10:263–271.

11. Lufkin RB, Hanafee WN, Wortham D, Hoover L. Larynx and hypopharynx: MR imaging with surface coils. Radiology 1986;158:747–754.

12. Panush D, Fulbright R, Sze G, et al. Inversion-recovery fast spin-echo MR imaging: Efficacy in the evaluation of head and neck lesions. Radiology 1993;187:421–426.

13. Ross M, Schomer D, Chappell P, Enzmann D. MR imaging of head and neck tumors: Comparison of T1-weighted contrast-enhanced fat-suppressed images with conventional T2-weighted and fast spin-echo T2-weighted images. AJR 1994;163:173–178.

14. Sakai F, Sone S, Kiyono K, et al. MR evaluation of laryngohypopharyngeal cancer: Value of gadopentetate dimeglumine enhancement. AJNR 1993;14:1059–1069.

15. Vogl T, Mack M, Juergens M, et al. MR diagnosis of head and neck tumors: Comparison of contrast enhancement with triple-dose gadodiamide and standard-dose gadopentetate dimeglumine in the same patients. AJR 1994;163:425–432.

16. Yousem D, Montone K, Sheppard L, et al. Head and neck neoplasms: Magnetization transfer analysis. Radiology 1994;192:703–707.

17. Held P, Rupp N. [Tumors of the oropharynx, hypopharynx and larynx—Diagnosis with magnetic resonance imaging]. [German with English abstract] Bildgebung 1991;58(3):132–140.

18. Silverman PM, Bossen EH, Fisher SR, et al. Carcinoma of the larynx and hypopharynx: Computed tomographic–histopathologic correlations. Radiology 1984;151:697–702.

19. Suojanen JN, Mukherji SK, Dupuy DE, et al. Spiral CT in evaluation of head and neck lesions: Work in progress. Radiology 1992;183:281–283.

20. Suojanen JN, Mukherji SK, Wippold FJ. Spiral CT of the larynx. AJNR 1994;15:1579–1582.

21. Tien R, Hesselink J, Chu P, Szumowski J. Improved detection and delineation of head and neck lesions with fat suppression spin-echo MR imaging. AJNR 1991;12:19–24.

22. Hillel AD, Schwartz AN. Trumpet maneuver for visual and CT examination of the pyriform sinus and retrocricoid area. Head Neck 1989;11:231–236.

23. Lapela M, Grenman R, Kurki T, et al. Head and neck cancer: Detection of recurrence with PET and 2-[F-18] fluor-2-deoxy-D-glucose. Radiology 1995;197:205–211.

24. Mansfield EL, Cote DN. Hypopharyngeal carcinoma. J La State Med Soc 1995;147:489–492.

25. Sulfaro S, Barzan L, Querin F, et al. T staging of the laryngohypopharyngeal carcinoma. A 7-year multidisciplinary experience. Arch Otolaryngol Head Neck Surg 1989;115:613–620.

26. Ekberg O, Nylander G. Webs and web-like formations in the pharynx and cervical esophagus. Diagn Imaging 1983;52:10–18.

27. Mancuso AA, Hanafee WN. Elusive head and neck carcinomas beneath intact mucosa. Laryngoscope 1983;93:133–139.

28. Guerrier Y. [The anatomic bases of the surgical treatment of pharyngo-laryngeal cancers]. [French with English abstract] J Otolaryngol 1983;12:146–150.

29. Lamprecht J, Lamprecht A, Kurten-Rothes R. [Mediastinal involvement in cancers of the subglottis, hypopharynx and cervical esophagus]. [German with English abstract] Laryngol Rhinol Otol (Stuttg) 1987;66:88–90.

30. Hasegawa Y, Matsuura H. Retropharyngeal node dissection in cancer of the oropharynx and hypopharynx. Head Neck 1994;16:173–180.

31. Lamoral Y, Lemahieu SF, Fossion E, Baert AL. Rhabdomyoma of the hypopharynx. Rofo Fortschr Geb Rontgenstr Neuen Bildgeb Verfahr 1990;152:727–728.

32. Tan KK, Abraham KA, Yeoh KH. Lipoma of hypopharynx. Singapore Med J 1994;35:219–221.

33. Amano Y, Tamai J, Katayama N, et al. [Hemangioma of the hypopharynx: A case report and value of MRI]. [Japanese with English abstract] Rinsho Hoshasen 1990;35:1427–1430.

34. Kiukaanniemi H, Pirila T, Jokinen K. Perforation in hypopharynx and deep cervical emphysema caused by blunt external trauma. Mil Med 1995;160:479–481.

35. Ward MP, Glazer HS, Heiken JP, Spector JG. Traumatic perforation of the pyriform sinus: CT demonstration. J Comput Assist Tomogr 1985;9:982–984.

36. Shellock F, Schatz C, Julien P, et al. Occlusion and narrowing of the pharyngeal airway in obstructive sleep apnea: Evaluation by ultrafast spoiled GRASS MR imaging. AJR 1992;158:1019–1024.

37. Shepard JW Jr, Stanson AW, Sheedy PF, Westbrook PR. Fast-CT evaluation of the upper airway during wakefulness in patients with obstructive sleep apnea. Prog Clin Biol Res 1990;345:273–279; discussion 280–282.

38. Norris CW. Pharyngoceles of the hypopharynx. Laryngoscope 1979;89:1788–1807.

39. Lenz M, Ozdoba C, Bongers H, Skalej M. [CT functional images of the larynx and hypopharynx]. [German with English abstract] Rofo Fortschr Geb Rontgenstr Nuklearmed 1989;150:509–515.

Pediatrics

43

Normal Development of the Neonate's, Infant's, and Young Child's Brain

SHARON E. BYRD, M.D.
CRYSTAL F. DARLING, M.D.

In the early and mid-1970s, the "gold standard" for imaging the pediatric brain was computed tomography (CT). With the advent of high-resolution real-time ultrasonography (US) in the mid- and late 1970s, US became an important modality in imaging the neonate's and infant's brain. However, by the 1980s, magnetic resonance imaging (MRI) was rapidly becoming the modality of choice to evaluate the pediatric brain. There is a role for each of these three modalities (CT, US, and MRI) in the evaluation of the young child's brain. The brain develops continually throughout childhood, with a number of important changes occurring during the first 2 years of life such as myelination; water content of the gray and white matter; brain weight, size, and shape; and configuration of the ventricles and subarachnoid spaces. It is important to understand how and where these changes are normally manifested on these modalities.

COMPUTED TOMOGRAPHY

CT continues to be the most widely used modality in the evaluation of the pediatric brain for all ages. CT uses ionizing radiation to produce an image of the brain, and it is still the best modality to evaluate head trauma, infarction (in children under 2 years of age), and calcification. CT scanners are more readily available than MRI scanners across the United States, and a CT scan will be the first modality for the majority of children who require a brain imaging study. CT's spatial resolution and anatomic detail are superior to those of any other current imaging modality except MRI.

On CT, the brain of a premature infant (30- to 34-week gestational age) has large sylvian fissures, basal cisterns, and cerebral subarachnoid spaces, with a thin cortex; prominent frontal, periventricular, and parietal white matter; and limited gyration (Fig. 43–1).[1, 2] The ventricles in the premature infant vary from slitlike to well seen (Fig. 43–2). At birth, the brain of a full-term infant (36- to 41-week gestational age) on CT demonstrates small

slitlike ventricles that become more prominent in appearance after the first week of life (Figs. 43–3 and 43–4). The white matter continues to be more prominent at the periventricular and frontal lobe areas; the basal cisterns

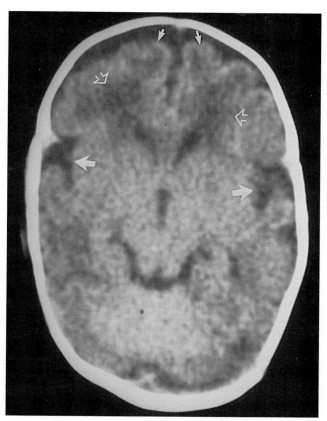

FIGURE 43–1 Computed tomography (CT) scan of a 32-week premature newborn. Prominent sylvian fissures *(large closed arrows)*, anterior frontal subarachnoid spaces, thin frontal cortex *(small closed arrows)*, and prominent frontal periventricular white matter *(open arrows)*.

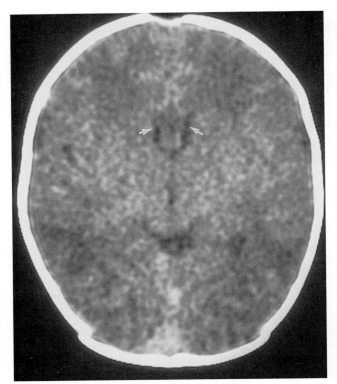

FIGURE 43–2 CT scan of a 32-week premature newborn. Small frontal horns (*arrows*) of the lateral ventricles.

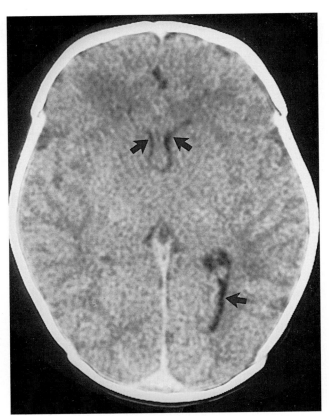

FIGURE 43–4 CT scan of an 11-day-old full-term neonate. Lateral ventricles (*arrows*) are more prominent and asymmetric in size.

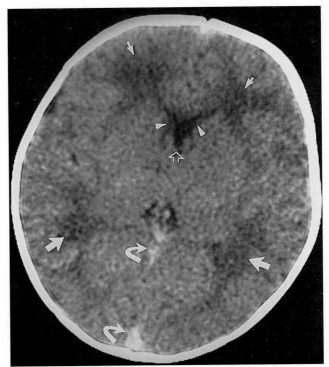

FIGURE 43–3 CT scan of a full-term newborn. Prominent frontal (*small straight arrows*) and atrial periventricular (*large straight arrows*) white matter, small slitlike frontal horns of the lateral ventricles (*arrowheads*), normal cavum septum pellucidum (*open arrow*), and normal increased density of flowing blood in deep veins and dural venous sinuses (*curved arrows*).

and sylvian fissures are still prominent; and all of the secondary and tertiary sulci have developed, with more sulci seen in the full-term than in the premature brain (Figs. 43–4 and 43–5).[1–3] The prominent areas of white matter continue during the first month of life, and the frontal lobe white matter prominence may continue up to 2 to 3 months of age.[2] In the premature and full-term infant, a normally high hematocrit of the flowing blood can be seen in the deep veins and dural venous sinuses (Figs. 43–3 and 43–4).[1] On CT, the white matter will always be more lucent than gray matter. These findings are related to the water content of gray and white matter and the myelination of the white matter. The changing water content of the gray and white matter and the process of myelination are better defined and elucidated on MRI (see Figs. 43–51 through 43–73). The overall density of the neonatal premature brain is less than the full-term brain because of greater water content, especially of the white matter.[4, 5] The weight of the brain of a full-term infant at birth is approximately 330 gm; by 6 months of age, it weighs 660 gm (50% of the adult weight); and by 2 years of age, 1000 gm (80% of adult weight).[4]

The brain continues to grow and develop after birth. At birth, the frontal and anterior portions of the temporal lobes are less developed than the other parts of the lobes.[3, 5] During the first year of life, there is marked growth of all lobes of the brain but with greater growth

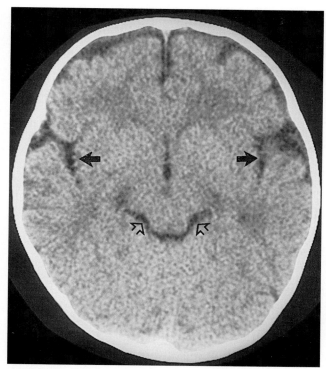

FIGURE 43–5 CT scan of a full-term newborn. Normal variant of asymmetry in size of the sylvian fissures *(closed arrows)* and prominent perimesencephalic cistern *(open arrows)*.

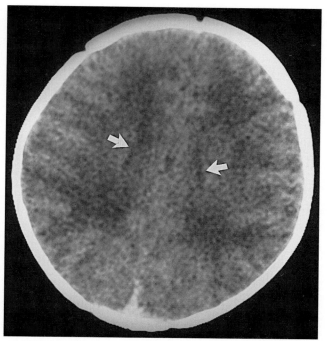

FIGURE 43–6 CT scan of a full-term newborn. Normal small slitlike lateral ventricles *(arrows)*.

of the frontal lobes.[6] In the neonate's brain, the insula may not be completely covered by the prominent sylvian fissure. The cerebellum (posterior fossa) is larger and the third ventricle and tentorium cerebelli are higher in the infant than in the older child.[3, 4, 6] This is due to the level of functioning of the neonate's and infant's brain on primitive and vital reflexes in the brain stem and cerebellum before the more selective and sophisticated higher functioning of the cerebrum takes over. At birth and extending into late childhood, the cerebrum increases in size, growing toward the third ventricle. The cerebellum decreases in size, growing away from the third ventricle. During this time, the course of the sylvian fissures changes from steep to parallel with the base of the skull.[3, 7, 8]

The ventricular system consists of the lateral ventricles (one in each cerebral hemisphere), the third ventricle between the halves of the thalamus, and the fourth ventricle in the posterior fossa (with the brain stem, pons, and medulla anteriorly and the cerebellum posteriorly). There is a greater degree of variation in size of the lateral ventricles in comparison to the third and fourth ventricles during the first 2 years of life (Figs. 43–6 through 43–10). The lateral ventricles are usually slitlike at birth. They become prominent after the first week of life. Although there are numerous studies for the normal variation in size of the ventricular system, especially the lateral ventricles, most imagers "eyeball" the ventricular system to estimate size. If it is necessary to measure the size of the ventricles, some of the accepted measurements follow:[9–14]

The Evans index is the ratio between the greatest width of the anterior horns of the lateral ventricles and the internal transverse diameter of the skull (Fig. 43–11).[3, 14] A ratio of 0.3 or greater indicates abnormal dilatation of the anterior horns. The anterior horns of the lateral ventricles should normally be semilunar.

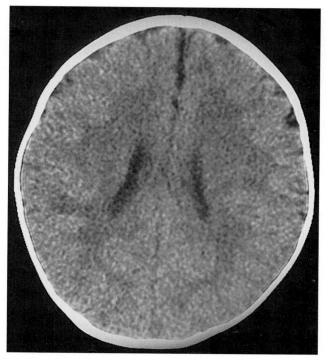

FIGURE 43–7 CT scan of a 4-month-old infant. Normal lateral ventricles and sulci.

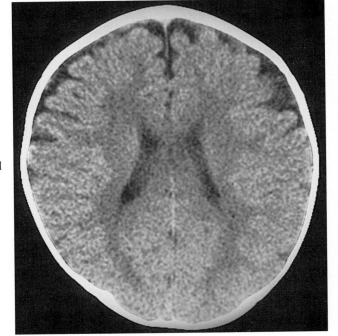

FIGURE 43–8 CT scan of a 6-month-old infant. Normal lateral ventricles and normal prominent anterior sulci.

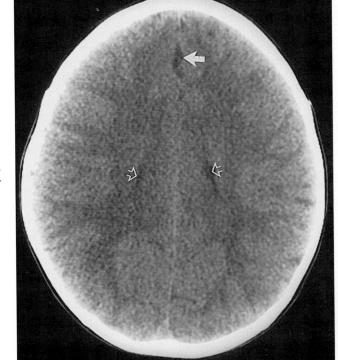

FIGURE 43–9 CT scan of a 1-year-old. Normal small lateral ventricles *(open arrows)*, small sulci, and normal prominent anterior interhemispheric fissure *(closed arrow)*.

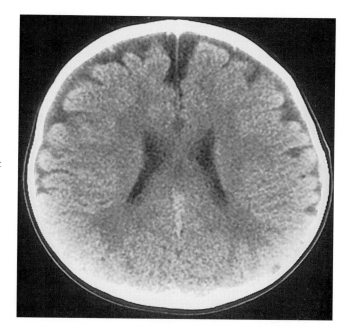

FIGURE 43–10 CT scan of a 3-month-old infant. Prominent but normal lateral ventricles and sulci.

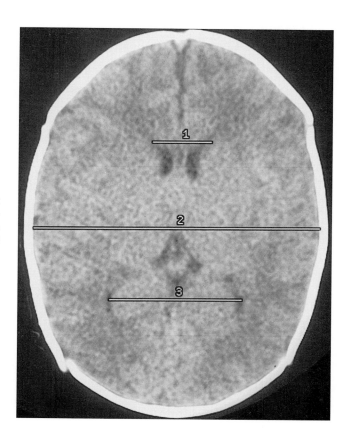

FIGURE 43–11 The Evans index is the ratio between the greatest width of the anterior horns (1) and the internal transverse diameter of the skull (2). The ventricular index is the distance between the choroid plexi of the atria (3) divided by the greatest distance between the anterior horns (1).

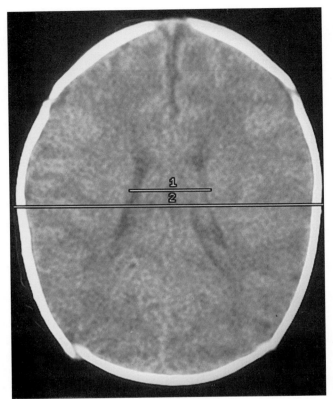

FIGURE 43–12 The Schiersmann index is the biparietal distance of the outer table (2) divided by the distance between the bodies of the lateral ventricles (1).

For the atrial region of the lateral ventricles, the ventricular index is used. The ventricular index is the distance between the choroid plexi at the atria divided by the greatest distance between the anterior horns (see Fig. 43–11). The ventricular index should be greater than 1.6.[3]

The size of the bodies of the lateral ventricles is calculated by the Schiersmann index (Fig. 43–12). This index is calculated at the parietal area of the bodies of the lateral ventricle, with the biparietal distance of the outer table of the calvarium divided by the distance between the bodies of the lateral ventricles. The index is abnormal when it is less than 4.[3, 9, 13]

Slight variation in size of the lateral ventricles is a common normal variation. The temporal horns of the lateral ventricles are normally not seen at birth and may not be visible during the first year of life. The occipital horns of the lateral ventricles commonly vary in size and shape and may not be visible during the first month of life. The third ventricle is slitlike or almost invisible at birth. It becomes prominent after 7 days of life and may normally appear slightly enlarged during the first 2 years of life. The normal width of the third ventricle in children is 3.5 to 6.5 mm; 6.0 to 8.0 mm suggests a mild dilatation, and 8.0 mm or greater indicates definite dilatation.[3] The fourth ventricle is triangular or rectangular, and the size varies from very small at birth to very prominent during the first 2 years of life (Figs. 43–13 through 43–15). Parts of the posterior fossa, even in the neonate, can be obscured by the beam-hardening artifacts of the mastoid

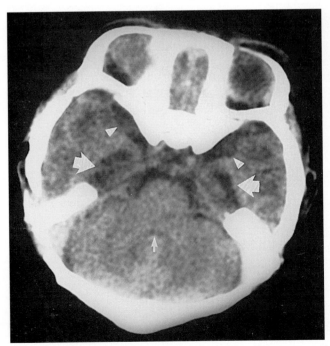

FIGURE 43–13 CT scan of a full-term newborn. Normal small fourth ventricle *(small arrow)*, beam-hardening artifacts *(large arrows)* from the petrous bones, and prominent basal cisterns *(arrowheads)*.

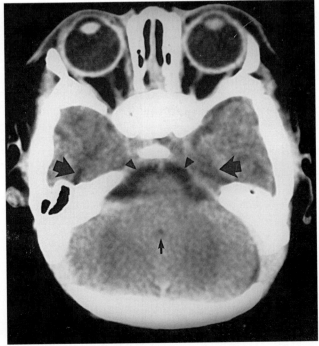

FIGURE 43–14 CT scan of an 11-day-old full-term newborn. Normal small fourth ventricle *(small arrow)*, beam-hardening artifacts from the petrous bones *(large arrows)*, and prominent prepontine cisterns *(arrowheads)*.

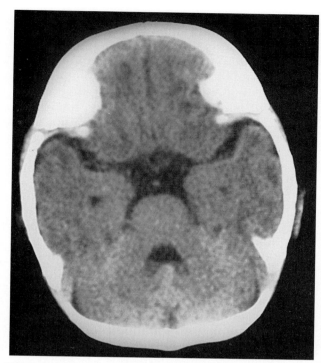

FIGURE 43–15 CT scan of a 6-week-old infant. Normal fourth ventricle and basal cisterns.

and petrous parts of the temporal bone (Figs. 43–13 and 43–14).[3, 4] The choroid plexus of the fourth and third ventricles are not well seen at birth and during the neonatal period. Intravenous iodinated contrast material is usually necessary to see them on CT during this period. However, the choroid plexi of the lateral ventricles appear very prominent in the premature infant and prominent in the full-term infant (Figs. 43–16 and 43–17). The choroid plexi are more readily seen on US during the neonatal period.

The anatomy of the normal subarachnoid spaces in the posterior fossa, base of the brain, and convexity areas varies during the first 2 years of life. The cisterna magna can vary considerably in size and shape. It may be extremely small or invisible to very large, and it may extend upward beyond the torcular Herophili. As long as there is no mass effect on the vermis, cerebellar hemispheres, or fourth ventricle, the cisterna magna is considered normal.[3, 4] The superior vermian cistern may be quite prominent in the neonatal and infancy periods (Fig. 43–18).

The primary sulci and fissures of the brain begin to appear from the 8th to the 25th week of gestation, with the secondary and tertiary sulci continuing to form until the 36th week of gestation.[3, 15, 16] Sulci and gyri are better developed and therefore better seen in the full-term brain. The normal interdigitation of the white matter U-fibers in the gyri are seen at birth. The interhemispheric fissure begins to develop by the 8th week, the sylvian fissures by the 14th week, and the rolandic or central sulci by the 20th week of gestation.[16] At birth, the interhemispheric fissure is small, but it may become quite prominent during the first 2 years of life. The basal

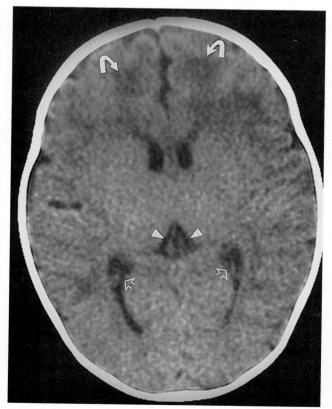

FIGURE 43–16 CT scan of a 4-week-old neonate. Normal prominent frontal lobes, white matter *(curved arrows)*, prominent choroid plexi of lateral ventricles *(open arrows)*, and normal cavum velum interpositum *(arrowheads)*.

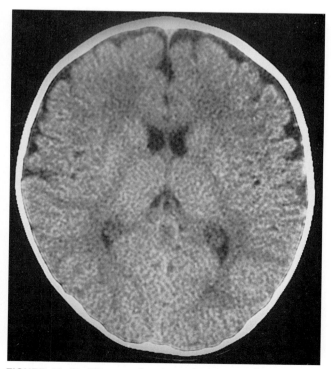

FIGURE 43–17 CT scan of a 5-month-old infant. Normal choroid plexi of the atria of the lateral ventricles, normal ventricles, and sulci.

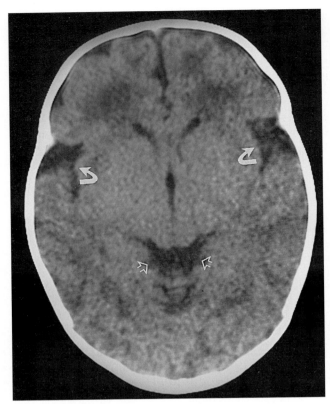

FIGURE 43–18 CT scan of a 4-week-old neonate. Prominent superior vermian cistern *(open arrows)*, sylvian fissures *(curved arrows)*, and third ventricle.

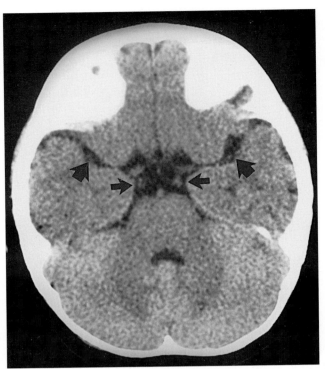

FIGURE 43–20 CT scan of a 6-month-old infant. Normal basal cisterns suprasellar—chiasmatic cistern *(small arrows)* and inferior aspect of sylvian fissures *(large arrows)*.

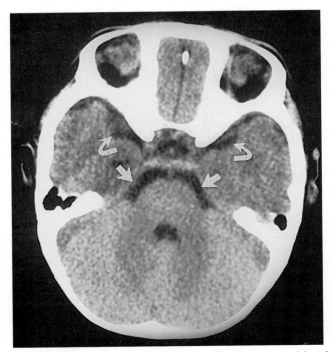

FIGURE 43–19 CT scan of a 4-month-old infant. Normal basal cisterns—inferior aspect of sylvian fissures *(curved arrows)* and prepontine *(straight arrows)*.

cisterns and sylvian fissures are prominent in the neonate. The basal cisterns consist of the cisterns anterior to the brain stem (anterior medullary, prepontine, and interpeduncular), chiasmatic, inferior temporal (middle cranial fossa), and inferior aspect of the sylvian fissures (Figs. 43–19 and 43–20). The subarachnoid spaces of the convexity areas of the brain are small or barely visible in the newborn. The cortical sulci of the convexity subarachnoid spaces are normally maximally dilated at 3 to 6 months of age, although these spaces may be prominent anywhere from 1 month to 2 years of age (Fig. 43–21).[3, 4, 17] It is not unusual and even very common to see a normal variation in which the lateral ventricles appear mildly dilated, with mild dilatation of the subarachnoid spaces anterior to temporal and frontal lobes, basal cisterns, and anterior one-third of the interhemispheric fissure (Figs. 43–22 and 43–23).[18] This normal variation of dilatation of the lateral ventricles and anterior subarachnoid spaces can be seen from 1 month of age to 2 years.[3, 4, 18]

ULTRASOUND

US is a good noninvasive imaging technique that uses nonionizing sonic energy to evaluate the neonate and infant brain.[19] Its major advantage is its portability that allows the examination to be performed at the bedside in critically ill and premature infants. It provides excellent delineation of ventricular size and hemorrhage. However, its detailed resolution of the overall brain is considerably less than that of CT or MRI. There are relative blind areas on the routine US scans (frontal and occipital poles

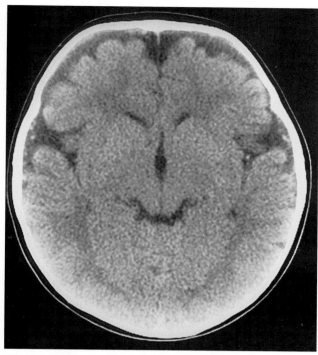

FIGURE 43–21 CT scan of a 3-month-old infant. Prominent sylvian fissures and anterior frontal sulci.

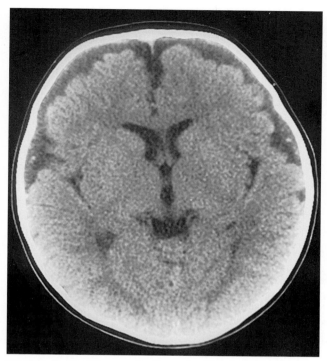

FIGURE 43–23 CT scan of a 5-month-old infant. Normal variation of prominence of the ventricles, sulci, and anterior interhemispheric fissure.

and high-convexity regions of the brain). The need for a US window limits performing US after 1 year of age (because the anterior fontanelle is usually closed).[1, 2, 19–24]

The overall echogenicity on US of the premature brain is less, but the white matter echogenicity greater, in comparison to the full-term brain (Figs. 43–24 and 43–25). There are more gyri and sulci present and demonstrated in the full-term brain (Figs. 43–26 through 43–28). The hyperechogenicity of the sulci is related to the vascu-

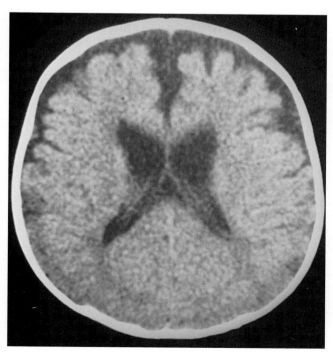

FIGURE 43–22 CT scan of a 6-month-old infant. Normal variation—prominent anterior frontal sulci, lateral ventricles, and anterior interhemispheric fissure.

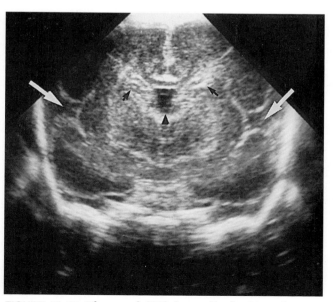

FIGURE 43–24 Ultrasound (US) (coronal) of a 30-week gestational age newborn. Prominent sylvian fissures (*large arrows*), decreased sulcation; the bodies of the lateral ventricles are small and not visualized, but prominent periventricular white matter (*small arrows*) is seen and normal cavum vergae (*arrowhead*).

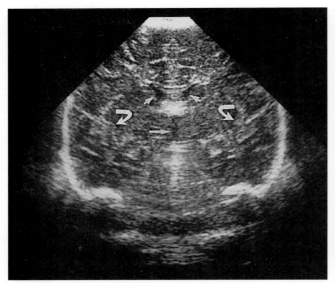

FIGURE 43–25 US (coronal) of a 2-week-old full-term newborn. Normal bodies of the lateral ventricles *(small straight arrows)* and third ventricle *(large straight arrow)*. The *curved arrows* outline the sylvian fissures bilaterally.

lar structures. The suprasellar cisterns and sylvian fissures are prominent in size, with greater prominence in the premature brain. Increased echogenicity is present in the suprasellar cisterns and sylvian fissures secondary to the vascular pulsations of the circle of Willis and middle cerebral arterial branches. The cisterna magna and superior vermian cistern may normally vary from small to large in both premature and full-term brains. The convex subarachnoid spaces are not prominent in the newborn

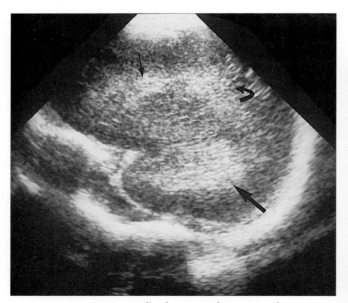

FIGURE 43–26 US (sagittal) of a 30-week gestational age newborn. Decreased sulcation and shallow sylvian fissure but increased echogenicity of white matter of the temporal *(large straight arrow)*, frontal *(small straight arrow)*, and parietal *(curved arrow)* lobes.

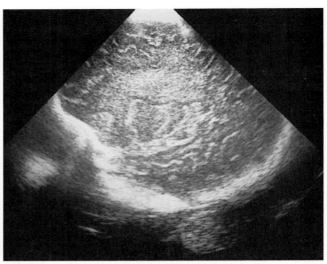

FIGURE 43–27 US (sagittal) of a 40-week gestational age newborn. Normal sulcation with less prominent sylvian fissure.

premature or full-term brain, but they tend to increase in size after 1 month of age and may be very prominent especially at the high-convexity areas during the first year of life on US. The cisterns anterior to the brain stem (interpeduncular, prepontine, and anteriorly medullary) are usually not well seen because of increased echogenicity from the clivus and the pulsation of the vertebrobasilar arterial complex (Fig. 43–29). At times in the premature more often than in the full-term brain, there may be prominence in size of the inferior temporal (middle cranial fossa) cisterns. The basal cisterns and sylvian fissures usually decrease in size after the neonatal period but may continue to be prominent on US during the first year of life.

The ventricles are usually small in the brains of prema-

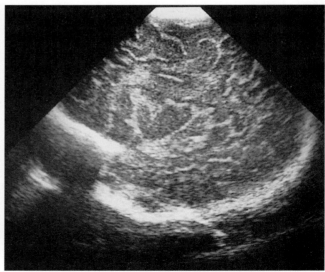

FIGURE 43–28 US (sagittal) of a 2-week-old full-term neonate. Normal sulcation and gyration and less prominent sylvian fissure.

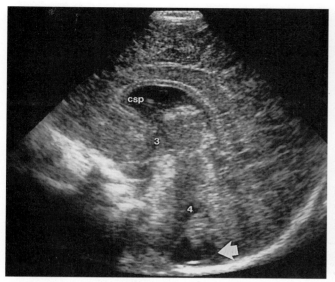

FIGURE 43–29 US (sagittal midline) of a 40-week gestational age newborn. Cavum septum pellucidum (csp), third ventricle (3), fourth ventricle (4), and cisterna magna *(arrow)*.

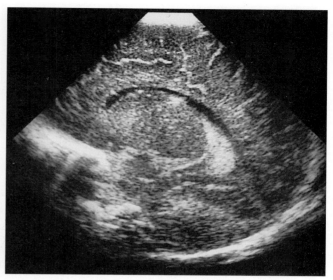

FIGURE 43–31 US (sagittal) of a 2-week-old full-term neonate. Normal left lateral ventricle.

ture and full-term newborns during the first week of life (Fig. 43–30). The lateral ventricles become more visible after the first week of life (Fig. 43–31). The third ventricle may not be readily visible on the coronal views during the first week, but its outline can be seen on the sagittal midline images (see Fig. 43–29). After the first week, the slitlike appearance of the third ventricle is visible on the coronal view at the level of the anterior bodies of the lateral ventricles (see Fig. 43–25). The normal fourth ventricle is always better visualized on the midline sagittal images (see Fig. 43–29). The ventricular and subarachnoid cerebrospinal fluid (CSF) spaces follow a similar appearance and course as on CT. The lateral ventricles

can normally be slightly asymmetric in size and appearance and can vary in size from small to very prominent where their appearance may even suggest mild dilatation.[1, 2, 6, 20, 22–24] The size of the ventricular system is usually estimated from routine visual inspection by the sonographer or radiologist. However, if necessary, there are some routine measurements used from the coronal and sagittal views (Fig. 43–32). On the coronal images at the level of the third ventricle and bodies of the lateral ventricles, the width (right to left measurement) of the third ventricle should not exceed 2 mm and the longest width (oblique superior to inferior measurement) of the bodies of the lateral ventricle should not exceed 3 mm (Fig. 43–32A). On the sagittal view, measurement of the occipital horn (from its tip to the glomus) should not exceed 16 mm (Fig. 43–32B).[24] It must be remembered that these measurements are rough guides and that "eyeballing" the size is an accepted and valid form of interpretation. A normal variant on US is the appearance of the ventricles, especially the lateral ventricles and anterior convexity subarachnoid spaces, as very prominent with the suggestion of mild enlargement (Fig. 43–33). This finding can normally be seen in some infants (after the first month to the end of infancy on US).

Increased echogenicity is commonly seen in the periventricular white matter of the premature brain and, to a lesser extent, in the full-term infant (Figs. 43–34 through 43–37). This area of increased echogenicity decreases by the end of the first month of life. Anatomic structures of the brain can be delineated using a detailed high-resolution real-time US technique. However, the resolution of brain structures, gray-white matter, and myelination on US can never compare with that of MRI. Even so, US is a good modality and extremely important and useful in imaging the premature and full-term newborn and infant brain.

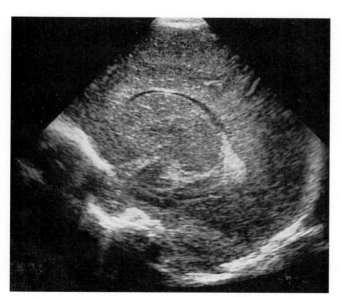

FIGURE 43–30 US (sagittal) of a 40-week gestational age newborn. Normal left lateral ventricle.

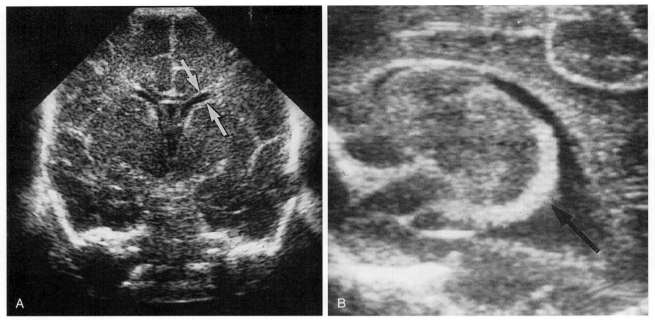

FIGURE 43–32 *A,* US (coronal) of a 42-week gestational age newborn. Measurement for size of the body of the lateral ventricle *(arrows). B,* US (sagittal) of a 42-week gestational age newborn. Measurement for size of the occipital horn of the lateral ventricle *(arrow* indicates the measurement used for the occipital horn from the posterior aspect of the tip of the occipital horn to the glomus of the choroid plexus).

MAGNETIC RESONANCE IMAGING

MRI is the best modality to evaluate the pediatric brain. It provides the exquisite detail and resolution necessary to visualize all of the important structures in the neonate, infant, and young child's brain. If the newborn, infant, or young child is medically stable to undergo an MRI study, the best imaging information of the brain will be ob-

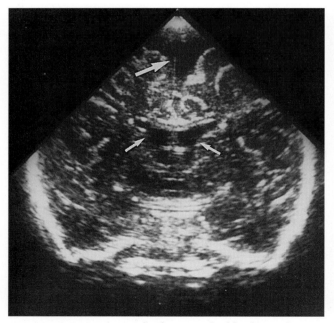

FIGURE 43–33 US (coronal) of a 6-month-old infant with prominence of the ventricles *(small arrows),* sulci, and interhemispheric fissure *(large arrow).*

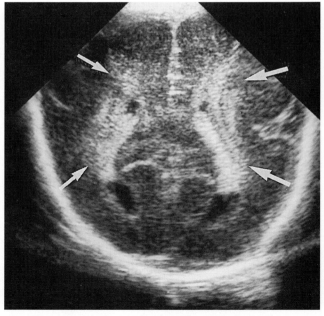

FIGURE 43–34 US (coronal) of a 30-week gestational age newborn. Prominent periventricular white matter *(arrows)* and choroid plexi of the lateral ventricles.

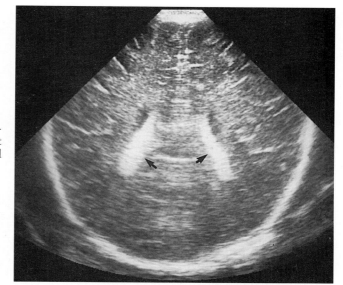

FIGURE 43–35 US (coronal) of a 40-week gestational age newborn. Less-prominent periventricular white matter but prominent choroid plexi of the lateral ventricles *(arrows* on left choroid plexus).

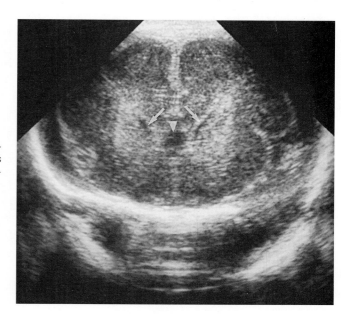

FIGURE 43–36 US (coronal) of a 30-week gestational age newborn. Prominent white matter of the frontal lobes, frontal horns of lateral ventricles *(arrows),* and cavum septum pellucidum *(arrowhead).*

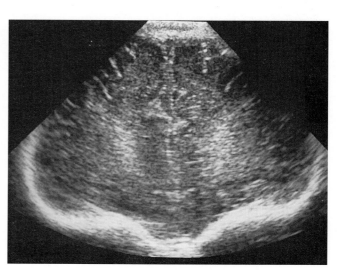

FIGURE 43–37 US (coronal) of a 40-week gestational age newborn. Less-prominent white matter of the frontal lobes.

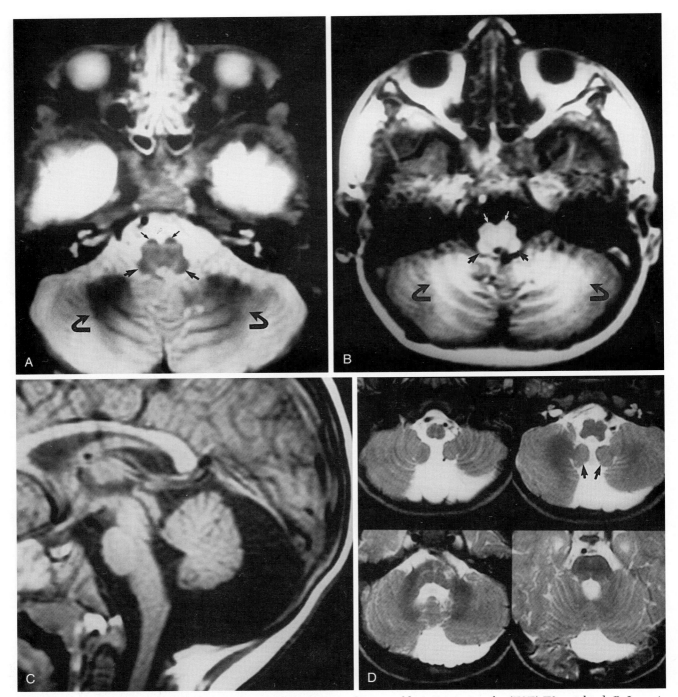

FIGURE 43–38 Axial magnetic resonance imaging (MRI) of a normal 2-year-old. *A,* Fast spin echo (FSE) T2-weighted. *B,* Inversion recovery (IR) T1-weighted. Medulla with myelination in the pyramids *(small straight arrows),* inferior cerebellar peduncles *(large straight arrows),* and cerebellar hemispheric white matter *(curved arrows). C,* Sagittal MRI spin-echo (SE) T1-weighted of a normal large cisterna magna. *D,* Axial MRI SE T2-weighted of a normal large cisterna magna with prominent vallecula and cerebellar tonsils *(arrows).*

tained. Although the brain continues to grow, develop, and mature into early adulthood, for practical purposes, the brain of a 2-year-old child can be used as the norm for the pediatric brain. A basic understanding of the normal 2-year-old brain will set the foundation for an understanding of the development of the pediatric brain during the first 2 years of life.

Normal MRI Anatomy of the Young Child's Brain

Infratentorial (Posterior Fossa)

Beginning inferiorly within the posterior fossa at the level of the medulla oblongata, anteriorly the ventral median sulcus separates the pyramids containing the corticospinal

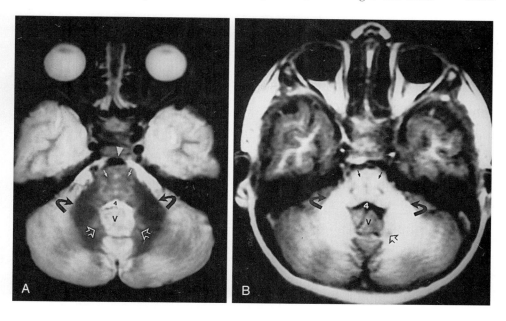

FIGURE 43–39 Axial MRI of a normal 2-year-old. *A*, FSE T2-weighted. *B*, IR T1-weighted. Pons with myelinated white matter tract *(small arrows)*, middle cerebral peduncles *(curved arrows)*, vermis (V), fourth ventricle (4), vertebrobasilar artery complex *(arrowhead)*, dentate nucleus *(open arrows)*.

tracts (motor fibers) (Fig. 43–38A and B). The anterolateral eminences are the olives, and the inferior cerebellar peduncles form the dorsolateral lobulations of the medulla (Fig. 43–38A and B). The inferior extent of the fourth ventricle separates the medulla from the inferior vermis and tonsils. The vallecula is a CSF pathway extending from the midline outlet of the fourth ventricle (Magendie) to the cisterna magna. The lateral outlets of the fourth ventricles are Luschka. The outlets of the fourth ventricle are normally not visible on MRI unless they are abnormally dilated from an obstruction. The cerebellar tonsils form the lateral walls of the vallecula (which should not be greater than 2 mm in diameter). The vallecula leads to the cisterna magna, which can vary considerably in size in children. A mega or large cisterna magna is considered normal in children, as long as there is no associated mass effect on the cerebellum (Fig. 43–38C and D). The flow void of the vertebral arteries is normally seen anterior to the medulla within the anterior medullary cistern (Fig. 43–36A and B).[25–33]

At the level of the pons, the middle cerebellar peduncles expand its anterior border and course dorsolaterally into the cerebellar hemispheres (Figs. 43–39 through 43–41). The major portion of the fourth ventricle is between the tegmentum of the pons (anteriorly) and the cerebellar vermis (posteriorly). The fourth ventricle is triangular or rectangular on the axial view, triangular on the sagittal view, and rectangular on the coronal view. It

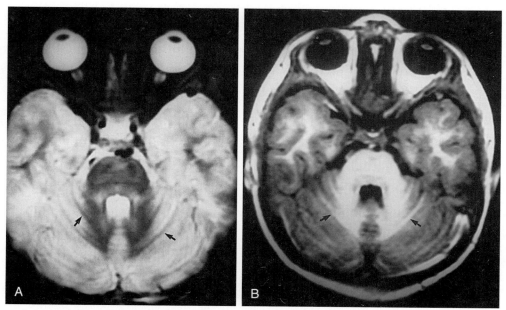

FIGURE 43–40 Axial MRI of a normal 2-year-old. *A*, FSE T2-weighted. *B*, IR T1-weighted. Myelinated white matter tracts in the pons, folia *(arrows)*, and temporal lobes.

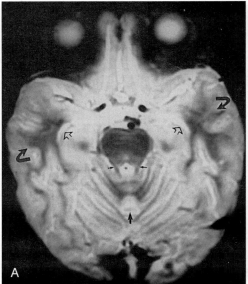
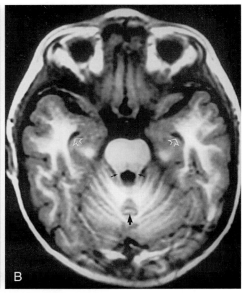

FIGURE 43–41 Axial MRI of a normal 2-year-old. *A,* FSE T2-weighted. *B,* IR T1-weighted. Myelinated white matter of the superior cerebellar peduncles *(small solid arrows),* superior vermis *(large solid arrows),* temporal lobes *(curved arrows),* temporal horns *(open arrows).*

can vary in size from small to very prominent. If the fourth ventricle becomes rounded, this is an early sign of hydrocephalus with entrapment or outlet obstruction. The flow void of the basilar artery is seen anterior to the belly of the pons in the prepontine cistern (Figs. 43–39 through 43–41).[25–33]

At the level of the mesencephalon or midbrain, the cerebral peduncles containing the corticospinal tracts form its anterolateral borders (Figs. 43–42 through 43–43). The substantia nigra is deep to these tracts and isointense to gray matter on T1- and T2-weighted images. The iron deposition in the substantia nigra is histologically visible at 9 to 12 months but not visible on T2-weighted MRI studies until around 10 years of age. The paired red nuclei are dorsomedial to the substantia nigra. The red nuclei are similar in intensity to the substantia nigra in the young child's brain because iron is not demonstrated

histologically until 18 to 24 months of age and not demonstrated on MRI T2-weighted studies until 10 years of age. The decussation of the superior cerebellar peduncles arch across the midportion of the midbrain. The CSF flow void of the cerebral aqueduct (aqueduct of Sylvius) is present within the middle of the posterior aspect of the midbrain on the axial view. The midline sagittal projection allows its full length to be evaluated. The superior and inferior colliculi flank the cerebral aqueduct and form the posterior part of the midbrain, the quadrigeminal (collicular) plate or tectum. At the axial level of the midbrain, the flow voids of the arteries of the circle of Willis can be seen in the suprasellar cisterns, and the posterior cerebral artery can be seen coursing laterally around the midbrain (Figs. 43–43 and 43–44).[25–36]

The brain stem is best evaluated on axial and sagittal images, with the sagittal midline and paramidline images

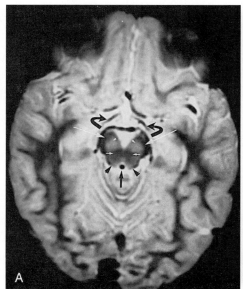
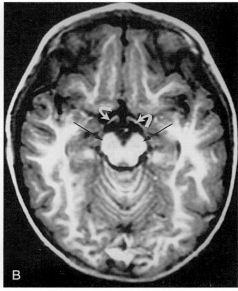

FIGURE 43–42 Axial MRI of a normal 2-year-old. *A,* FSE T2-weighted. *B,* IR T1-weighted. Myelinated corticospinal tracts of the cerebral peduncles *(long arrows),* decussation of the superior cerebellar peduncles *(short white arrows),* and optic tracts *(curved arrows);* substantia nigra *(small arrowheads);* inferior colliculi *(large arrowheads);* flow void of aqueduct *(large black arrow in A).*

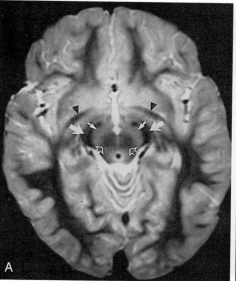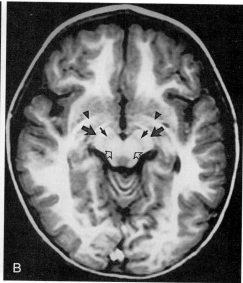

FIGURE 43–43 Axial MRI of a normal 2-year-old. *A,* FSE T2-weighted. *B,* IR T1-weighted. Anterior commissures *(arrowheads),* cerebral peduncles *(large solid arrows),* substantia nigra *(small solid arrows),* and decussation of the superior cerebellar peduncles *(open arrows).*

providing better evaluation of the full extent of its length. All parts of the brain stem are clearly visible at birth on MRI. The cranial nerves of the brain stem including the seventh and eighth but not the fifth are never clearly seen on a routine brain MRI in the newborn, infant, or young child's brain. The cisterns around the brain stem can vary in size from small to very prominent in a child 2 years of age and younger. The cisterns always appear

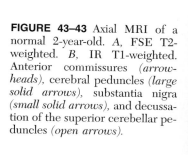

FIGURE 43–44 Axial MRI FSE T2-weighted. Normal full-term newborn at the level of the dentate nuclei *(arrows).*

more prominent on the T2-weighted MRI studies than on the US or CT scans in the same child.[25–45]

The cerebellum is composed of the midline vermis and two cerebellar hemispheres (Fig. 43–45; see also Figs. 43–38 through 43–44). The gray-white matter of the cerebellum can be delineated on MRI from as early as the newborn period. But the cortical surface of the cerebellar hemispheres, which is composed of folia and sulci, may not be as readily visible on MRI in the newborn. The vermis with lobules is readily visible on MRI, best seen on a midline sagittal projection in the newborn. The cerebellar tonsils are readily visible at birth and better seen on the sagittal views just off midline. The tonsils normally do not extend below the foramen magnum, but in some children, they may extend from 1 to 5 mm below the foramen. As long as the tonsils maintain their rounded inferior border (they are not "beaked" in appearance), this extension is considered a normal variation. The superior and inferior vermian cisterns can vary in size similar to the cisterns anterior to the brain stem (see Figs. 43–38 through 43–45).[25–33, 44, 45]

The dentate nucleus in the cerebellum, although composed of gray matter, may change with signal intensity on MRI owing to iron deposition. Histologic staining demonstrates iron at 3 years of age, but MRI changes with hypointensity on T2-weighted images may not be seen in children. If hypointensity is demonstrated on the T2-weighted images, it is not seen until 15 to 25 years of age and is only demonstrated in one-third of these patients (see Figs. 43–39 and 43–44).[33–35]

Supratentorial

On the midline sagittal MRI study at the level of the cerebral hemisphere and its deep gray matter, the limits and recesses of the third ventricle can be identified (see Fig. 43–45). The third ventricle is normally slitlike on axial images but well seen on the midline sagittal image. The anteroinferior recesses of the third ventricle are supraoptic and infundibular. They may be separated by

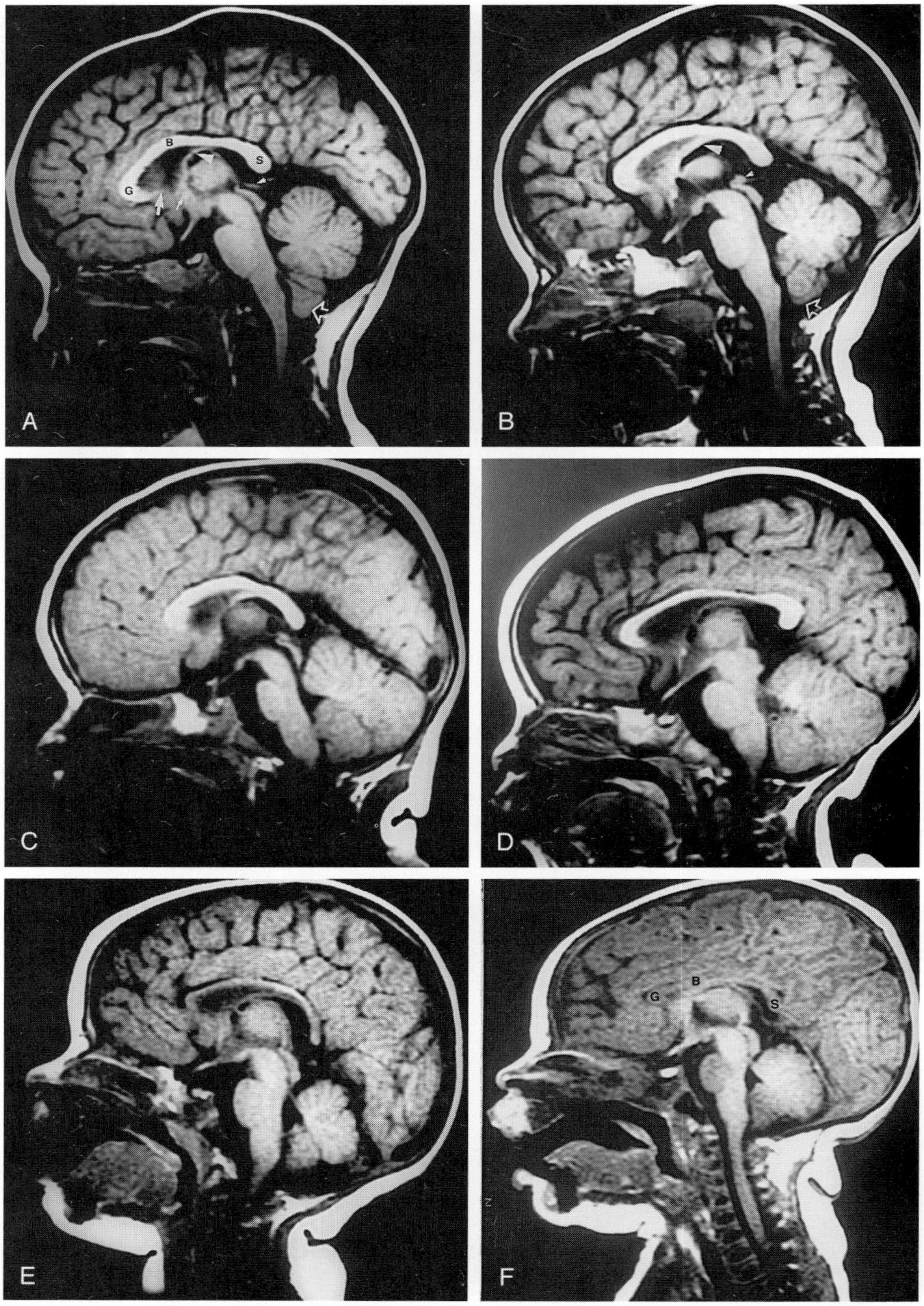

FIGURE 43–45 Sagittal SE T1-weighted. Normal appearance of the corpus callosum consisting of the rostrum *(large solid arrow)*, genu (G), body (B), and splenium (S) at 2 years (A), 16 months (B), 13 months (C), 7 months (D), 3 months (E), and newborn (F). Also demonstrated are the pineal gland *(small arrowhead)*, body of fornix *(large arrowhead)*, anterior commissure *(small solid arrow)*, and cerebellar tonsils *(open arrow)*.

the optic chiasm. The anterior wall of the third ventricle is composed of the lamina terminalis and anterior commissure. The choroid plexus of the third ventricle occupies its roof and is covered by its superior wall above which lies the cavum velum interpositum and the body of the fornix. The thalamus forms its lateral walls. The massa intermedia (gray matter connecting the two halves of the thalamus) extends through the midline of the third ventricle. The posterior wall of the third ventricle consists of recesses and commissures. From superior to inferior, the posterior wall is composed of suprapineal recess,

habenular commissure, pineal recess, and posterior commissure. The anterior and posterior recesses of the third ventricle are not well delineated in the infant and young child's brain unless the third ventricle is mildly to moderately dilated from hydrocephalus. The anterior, posterior, and habenular commissures are white matter fibers, and the myelination in these structures as well as the other white matter structures is discussed in the last part of this chapter under Myelination.[25–33, 44–50]

The corpus callosum, the largest white matter commissure, connects the two cerebral hemispheres and forms

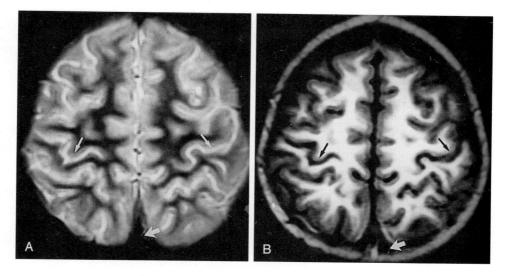

FIGURE 43–46 Axial MRI of a normal 2-year-old. FSE T2-weighted (A) and IR T1-weighted (B) with myelination in all of the major white matter fibers and tracts. Central sulcus (small arrows) and flow void of the superior sagittal sinus (large arrow).

the roof of the frontal horns and bodies of the lateral ventricles. There are four parts from anteroinferior to posterior (rostrum, genu, body, and splenium) (see Fig. 43–45). At birth, the neonatal corpus callosum has a uniformly thin appearance with a signal intensity similar to or slightly greater than that of the centrum semiovale. During the ensuing 6 to 8 months, the corpus callosum grows into its adult configuration. The genu becomes more prominent, and the splenium acquires its rounded, bulbous appearance. The body of the corpus callosum enlarges more slowly, and focal thinning can be a normal variant (see Fig. 43–45).[51–53] The pineal gland lies within the quadrigeminal cistern between the splenium of the corpus callosum and the collicular plate of the midbrain (see Fig. 43–45). The pineal gland is just posterior to the pineal recess and is attached to the posterior wall of the third ventricle by a stalk. It has a signal intensity of intermediate strength. Pineal calcification is common in adults but rare in children under 10 years of age, and its presence suggests neoplasm. Gradient-echo acquisition

using a partial flip angle appears to be more sensitive than routine spin-echo (SE) sequences for the detection of intracranial calcifications, but it may not be sensitive enough to detect subtle punctate calcifications within the pineal gland. CT is still the best modality to evaluate pineal calcification.[54–57]

Beginning from the superior high-convexity areas to the inferior deep gray matter of both cerebral hemispheres, MRI superbly delineates the gray and white matter structures with the interdigitation of white matter projecting into each cortical gyrus forming the white matter U-fibers. At the superior margins of both cerebral hemispheres, on the axial images, the interhemispheric fissure divides the hemispheres into roughly equal anterior and posterior halves (frontal and parietal lobes) (Figs. 43–46 and 43–47).

The precentral gyrus is immediately anterior to the central sulcus and is the primary motor region of the brain. The postcentral gyrus, representing the primary sensory region of the brain, lies immediately posterior to

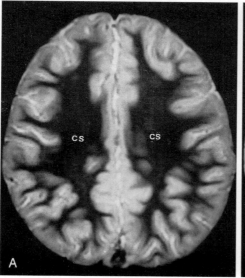
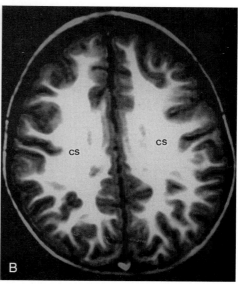

FIGURE 43–47 Axial MRI of a normal 2-year-old. FSE T2-weighted (A) and IR T1-weighted (B) with myelination in all of the major white matter fibers and tracts. Centrum semiovale (CS).

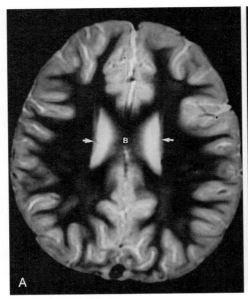
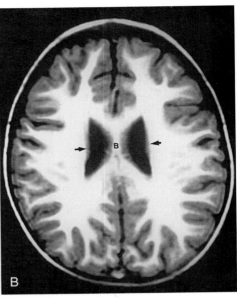

FIGURE 43–48 Axial MRI of a normal 2-year-old. FSE T2-weighted *(A)* and IR T1-weighted *(B)* with myelination in all of the major white matter fibers and tracts. Bodies of the lateral ventricles *(arrows)* and body of the corpus callosum (B).

the central sulcus. Both of these major gyri and the central sulcus extend from the level of the sylvian fissures over the convexities onto the medial surface of each hemisphere. Therefore, the precentral and postcentral gyri are seen on both the lateral and the medial surfaces of the hemisphere. A flow void representing the superior sagittal sinus may be seen at the anterior and posterior extent of the interhemispheric fissure (see Figs. 43–46 and 43–47).

The large white matter region of the centrum semiovale of the parietal and frontal lobes is seen at a slightly inferior level (see Fig. 43–47). At the next inferior level just above the bodies of the lateral ventricles, the interhemispheric fissure is not continuous from anterior to posterior but, rather, is interrupted in the midline by the body of the corpus callosum (Fig. 43–48). The depth of the interhemispheric fissure reaches the cingulate gyrus

anteriorly and posteriorly, since this gyrus curves around the corpus callosum deep within the medial surface of each hemisphere.

At the levels of the lateral ventricles, the bodies have a lateral concave configuration lying medial to the bodies of the caudate nuclei (Figs. 43–49 through 43–51; see also Fig. 43–48). The frontal horns are semilunear, indented by the heads of the caudate nuclei. The atria with the most prominent choroid plexi are always well seen. The temporal horns may not be well seen on the axial views, but the full extent is better seen on the sagittal views. The occipital horns commonly may be asymmetric in size and shape (Figs. 43–48 through 43–51).

The low ventricular axial section reveals a more complex array of deep gray and white matter structures (see Figs. 43–50 and 43–51). The thalamus forms the lateral wall of the thin midline third ventricle. At the anterior

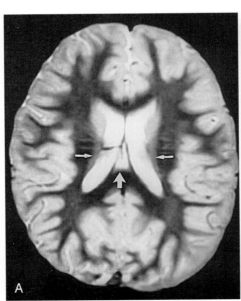
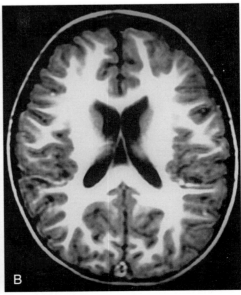

FIGURE 43–49 Axial MRI of a normal 2-year-old. FSE T2-weighted *(A)* and IR T1-weighted *(B)* with myelination in all of the major white matter fibers and tracts. Bodies of the lateral ventricles, superior extension of a prominent cavum velum interpositum *(large arrow)*, and body of the caudate nuclei *(small arrows)*.

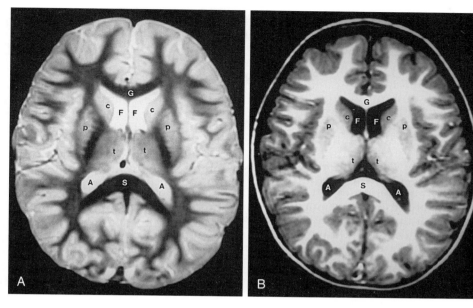

FIGURE 43–50 Axial MRI of a normal 2-year-old. FSE T2-weighted (A) and IR T1-weighted (B) with myelination in all of the major white matter fibers and tracts. Frontal horns (F) and atria (A) of the lateral ventricles, head of the caudate (c), putamen (p), thalamus (t), genu (G), and splenium (S) of the corpus callosum.

aspect of the third ventricle, CSF continuity can often be seen between the third ventricle and the lateral ventricles, via the Y-shaped foramina of Monro. Numerous quantitative methods have been described to evaluate the size of the ventricles, especially the lateral ventricles, and thereby determine whether ventriculomegaly exists. In daily practice, however, ventricular size is estimated by visual inspection of the axial MRI studies. In children under 2 years of age, mild enlargement of the ventricles and subarachnoid spaces is a frequent finding and considered normal. Minimal asymmetry of the brain, including the ventricles, is also a normal finding.

The septum pellucidum is seen as a thin midline structure separating the frontal horns and bodies of the lateral ventricles posterior to the genu of the corpus callosum. The septum pellucidum is created during the embryologic fusion of the cerebral hemispheres. Before complete fu-

sion, there is a cavity. The portion of the cavity anterior to the columns of the fornix is called the *cavum septum pellucidum;* the cavity posterior to the columns is the *cavum vergae.* Fusion begins posteriorly and progresses anteriorly. Thus, the cavum vergae is the first space to be obliterated. Fusion is usually complete during the first months of life, but 15% of children have a persistent cavum septum pellucidum with or without a cavum vergae (see Figs. 43–52D, 43–64A, and 43–65A).

The anterior and posterior limbs of the internal capsule meet at an obtuse angle or genu. Anteromedial to the anterior limb is the head of the caudate nucleus. Posteromedial to the posterior limb is the thalamus. Lateral to each internal capsule is the wedge-shaped lentiform nucleus, composed of a medial globus pallidus and a lateral putamen. The external capsule defines the lateral extent of the putamen. A barely visible claustrum and an

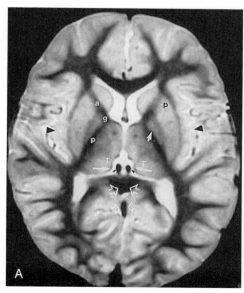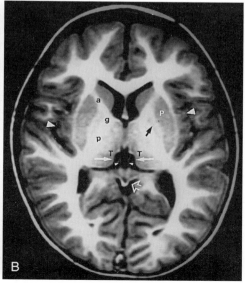

FIGURE 43–51 Axial MRI of a normal 2-year-old. FSE T2-weighted (A) and IR T1-weighted (B) with myelination in all of the major white matter fibers and tracts. Anterior (a), genu (g), and posterior (p) limbs of the internal capsule, thalamus (T), globus pallidus (*small solid arrow*), putamen (P), insular cortex (*large arrowheads*), internal cerebral veins (*small arrowheads*) in the quadrigeminal cistern–cavum velum interpositum (*large solid arrows*), vein of Galen (*large open arrows*), and straight sinus (*small open arrows*).

extreme capsule complete the outward progression to the cortical gray matter of the insula. The signal intensities of these deep gray matter structures (thalamus, caudate nucleus, globus pallidus, putamen, and claustrum) parallel that of the cortical gray matter, except for the globus pallidus owing to iron deposition. Histologic staining demonstrates involvement of the globus pallidus at 6 months of age. But the hypointensity on the T2-weighted MRI studies may not be visible until 10 to 15 years of age. The internal capsule's signal intensity varies with the extent of myelination, eventually becoming similar to that of cortical white matter (see Figs. 43–49 through 43–51).

Anterior to the frontal horns of the lateral ventricles, the genu of the corpus callosum limits the depth of the anterior aspect of the interhemispheric fissure. Posterior to the thalamus, the splenium of the corpus callosum similarly limits the depth of the posterior aspect of the interhemispheric fissure. Posterior to the splenium in the midline, the flow void of the vein of Galen is imaged, and it is not unusual to see the midline linear flow voids created by the internal cerebral veins within the cistern of the velum interpositum. At this axial level, the lateral ventricles consist of frontal horns anteriorly and the atria and occipital horns posteriorly. The deep extent of the sylvian fissure is the prominent feature of the lateral cortical surface. The infolded cortical tissue is the frontal, parietal, and temporal opercula. The frontal lobe and a small portion of the parietal lobe lie anterior to the sylvian fissure in this plane, and the temporal and occipital lobes are posterior (see Figs. 43–45 and 43–49 through 43–51).

On the sagittal midline images, anterior to the genu of the corpus callosum, along the medial surface of the cortex, the cingulate and superior frontal gyri are seen. Posterior to the splenium of the corpus callosum, the medial surface of the cortex is more extensive, and it is possible to see the posterior extent of the cingulate gyrus. A prominent landmark, the parieto-occipital sulcus, is seen in cross section separating the parietal lobe from the more posterior occipital lobe (see Fig. 43–45).

Axial images at the infraventricular level section the inferior aspects of each frontal and temporal lobe (see Figs. 43–41 through 43–43 and 43–45). Anteriorly, the interhemispheric fissure separates the gyrus recti and is contiguous posteriorly with the stellate-appearing suprasellar cistern. The anterior aspect of the suprasellar cistern, the chiasmatic cistern, contains the optic chiasm. Depending on the angulation of the axial image at this level, it may demonstrate the distal optic nerves extending anterior into the optic chiasm and the optic tracts extending posteriorly out from the chiasm. These structures maintain the same signal intensity as white matter. The sylvian fissure extends laterally between the frontal and the temporal lobes. The temporal horns of the lateral ventricles may be seen as curvilinear CSF structures in the medial aspects of each temporal lobe. The mammillary bodies and optic tract may be seen in the suprasellar cistern, anterior to the midbrain. At this level, the tentorium is also sectioned. Because of its configuration, structures lateral to the cut surface of the tentorium are supratentorial, and those structures medial to the cut surface are infratentorial. Thus, the superior vermis of the cerebellum is seen posteriorly in the midline at this axial level (see Figs. 43–41 through 43–43 and 43–45).[32, 33, 44]

There is considerable variation in size and shape of the ventricular system; the sizes of the cisterns and other subarachnoid spaces in the newborn, infant, and young child are similar to the variation seen on CT and US scans. The CSF pathways always appear more prominent on MRI in comparison to the CT and US scans, even in the same child. The CSF pathways can be very prominent in the child during the first 2 years of life and can simulate dilatation (mild hydrocephalus or atrophy). This is a normal finding in young children. It may be more common around 6 months of age, but should not be present after 2 years of life (Fig. 43–52A and B).

White Matter

The last process to understand in the development of the pediatric brain during the first 2 years of life is maturation and myelination of the white matter fibers. During fetal gestation, the white matter of the cerebral hemispheres first appears at the seventh week as an intermediate zone between the subventricular germinal matrix and the developing cortical plate of the fetal brain. At this stage, the white matter consists primarily of a radial glial guide network of fibers with primitive neural cells migrating on this network to form the cortex of the brain. At the end of this stage of neuronal migration (which occurs from the 7th to the 15th week of fetal gestation), axongenesis begins. Axongenesis starts with the formation of a growth cone at the end of the axon. This growth cone helps to generate and guide the developing axon in the continued formation of the white matter.[58–60]

The white matter fibers begin to myelinate at about the 16th week of fetal gestation with myelin seen histologically in the column of Burdach. By the 20th week, myelin can be seen in the cerebellar tracts. After birth, myelination progresses rapidly with 90% of this process completed by 2 years of life. The remainder of the process of myelination, however, continues into adulthood. In the child over 2 years of age and in the adult, the white matter is mostly myelinated and consists of myelinated axons with neuroglial cells and some nonmyelinated axons. Astrocytes and oligodendrocytes are the neuroglial cells.[46–50]

MYELIN

Myelin is an important material whose functions are to act as an insulator of the axons and to facilitate the transmission of impulses. Because the conduction velocity of impulses is faster in myelinated as opposed to nonmyelinated white matter, this results in improved functioning of the brain. Myelin is produced by the oligodendrocytes. The role of the oligodendrocyte in the formation of myelin was elucidated by Bunge. Myelin is a multilayered membranous structure composed of protein and lipid that enwraps the axon in a spiral fashion. Virchow suggested the name *myelin* to describe the sheaths around the nerve fibers. Myelin is produced by the oligodendrocyte extending its cell membrane to enwrap the axon in layers. One oligodendrocyte may myelinate as many as 50 axons.[58–61]

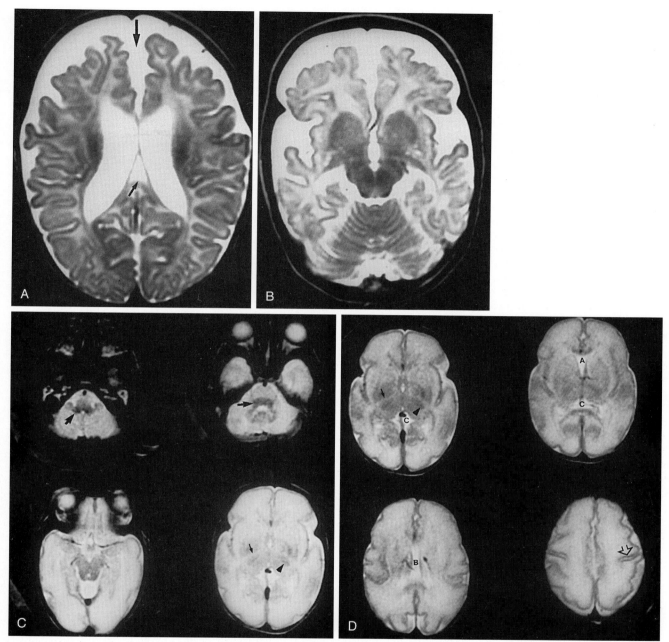

FIGURE 43–52 *A,* Axial MRI FSE T2-weighted of a normal 3-month-old infant with prominence of the anterior cerebrospinal fluid spaces, the anterior aspect of the interhemispheric fissure *(large arrow),* and bodies of the lateral ventricles with superior extension of the cavum velum interpositum *(small arrow). B,* Axial MRI FSE T2-weighted of a normal 3-month-old infant with prominence of the anterior cerebrospinal subarachnoid spaces, sylvian fissures, and anterior interhemispheric fissure. *C* and *D,* Axial MRI FSE T2-weighted of a normal 32-week gestational age newborn with myelination in the dorsal aspect of the brain stem *(large solid arrows),* dorsal thalamus *(arrowheads),* posterior limb of the internal capsule *(small solid arrows);* central sulcus *(open arrow);* cavum septum pellucidum (A); cavum vergae (B); and cavum velum interpositum (C). Almost all of the white matter is not myelinated.

Myelin is a molecular bilayer with the unique feature of having a very high ratio of lipid to protein. This predominantly lipid molecular bilayer with both hydrophilic and hydrophobic components gives myelin its stability. Myelin is only 40% hydrated, but it contains 70% to 80% lipid and 20% to 30% protein. The lipid composition of mature myelin, in the adult, consists of 25% to 28% cholesterol, 27% to 30% galactolipid, and 40% to 45%

phospholipid. The protein composition of mature myelin in the adult consists of 70% to 80% proteolipid protein and basic protein with the remainder as glycoprotein and Wolfgram protein. The composition of myelin in the immature brain differs from that of the myelin in the adult brain. This immature myelin, called *transitional* or *early myelin,* consists of an increase in galactolipids and a decrease in the phospholipids. Although there is a chemical difference between the myelin in the immature brain and that in the adult brain, these differences are minimal. The consensus in the medical literature is that the major differences between myelin in early life and that in early adulthood is "quantity and not quality." This raises the question of what is "mature myelin." It must be remembered that myelin is laid down in a lamellar configuration around the axon. In a mature myelin sheath, the cell membranes are condensed into a compact structure in which each membrane unit is closely opposed to the adjacent one. There is a great deal of variation in the number of myelin lamellae in the sheaths surrounding different axons. The larger the diameter of the axon, the thicker its myelin sheath. We use the term *myelin* to refer to the formation of a complete, compact myelin sheath.[58, 61–66]

Myelination

Myelination of the brain proceeds in an orderly temporal fashion in a caudocranial direction, with the paleontologically older structures myelinating earlier and the newer structures later. The myelination process can be seen extending from posterior fossa structures (brain stem and cerebellum) into thalamus and cerebrum. Within the cerebrum, myelination is seen in the occipital and parietal lobes before the temporal and frontal lobes. The myelination process is seen earlier within the sensory input fibers before proceeding into those output (motor) fiber tracts that mediate the sensory data into movement. The sensory tracts in the dorsal brain stem contain the medial lemniscus and medial longitudinal fasciculus, which transmit vestibular, acoustic, tactile, and proprioception sensation. These tracts are myelinated at birth. The sensory tracts of the calcarine (visual), postcentral (somesthetic), and precentral (propriokinesthetic) areas of the cerebrum are myelinated at birth or shortly thereafter.[59, 67–71]

The relationship between the progress of myelination and the functional maturity of the brain has been a controversial subject debated in the neurology and pathology literature. When Fleichsig[72, 73] demonstrated that the white matter tracts of the human nervous system become myelinated in a very definite sequence, this led to the assumption that tracts become myelinated at the time they become functional. Keene and Huwer[72, 73] disagreed with this theory because reflexes can occur while nerve fibers are still unmyelinated. Tilney and Casamajor, Langworthy, Yakovlev, and Lecours[72, 73] modified this theory of Flechsig and concluded that apart from the movements observed in early fetal life, there is a close correlation between myelination of tracts in the nervous system and acquisition of function.[72, 73]

MRI of Myelination

MRI is the best noninvasive modality to assess the process of myelination in vivo. However, MRI has certain limitations. The normal progression of myelination in the neuropathologic studies by Yakovlev and Lecours[47, 74–80] and Brody and colleagues[48, 74–80] can be used only as a rough guide to identify the structures on MRI. These neuropathologic studies are based on the histology of tissue specimens specially stained for myelin, and the resolution on MRI lags far behind these histologic specimens. The MRI timetables for the visualization of myelination are dependent on the field strength of the MRI magnet used and the pulse sequences employed. Most of the timetables published in the United States were developed on high-field-strength magnets using an SE pulse sequence with short-TR and -TE T1-weighted or long-TR/TE T2-weighted series. McArdle and associates,[77–81] Dietrich and coworkers,[69, 77–81] and Barkovich[68, 77–81] have published myelination timetables based on SE. In England, the Hammersmith group advocated using inversion-recovery (IR) pulse sequences to evaluate myelination. In the last few years, many of the MRI manufacturers have developed fast T2-weighted pulse sequences to decrease the amount of scan time. Routinely, these fast T2-weighted pulse sequences are used to evaluate the pediatric brain. Although there is some slight decrease in the resolution with these fast T2-weighted pulse sequences in comparison to the conventional sequences, for the most part there is no noticeable interference with evaluating the myelination process on these fast T2-weighted SE and IR sequences. Our timetable for the myelination process is based on the radiologic and pathologic literature using a 1.5-Tesla MRI scanner with T1-weighted SE and IR and T2-weighted conventional spin echo (CSE) and fast spin echo (FSE) and IR pulse sequences.[47, 48, 68, 69, 74–82]

An understanding of the changes in the pediatric brain during the first 2 years of life when myelination is rapidly developing is necessary in order to understand the MRI. The MRI appearance is due to the changing water content of the gray and white matter and to the myelination of the white matter structures. The brain of a child 2 years of age and older can be used as the norm for the pediatric brain and is similar in appearance to the young adult brain. In the adult and pediatric brain over 2 years of age, the majority of the white matter fibers are myelinated with a water content of 72% for the white matter and 82% for the gray matter. At birth, the water content of the white matter is 87% and that of gray matter is 89%. There is a higher water content of white matter in the newborn brain in comparison to the young adult brain.[83]

The signal intensities of the myelinated and nonmyelinated white matter are (1) on T2-weighted SE and IR pulse sequences, the myelinated white matter is hypointense (because myelin is predominantly a lipid) and the nonmyelinated white matter is hyperintense; and (2) on T1-weighted SE and IR pulse sequences, the myelinated white matter is hyperintense and the nonmyelinated white matter is hypointense.

Myelination on T2-Weighted SE Images

The T2-weighted SE pulse sequence more closely reflects the neuropathologic timetables for myelination. The exact reason for this is not known. The neuropathologic timetables are based on 75% of a structure being mature myelin. The long-TR/TE SE pulse sequence may be more sensitive to delineating mature myelin. This pulse sequence may correspond more closely with the formation of the complete myelin sheath, and it probably reflects the changes in water distribution of an intact myelin sheath.

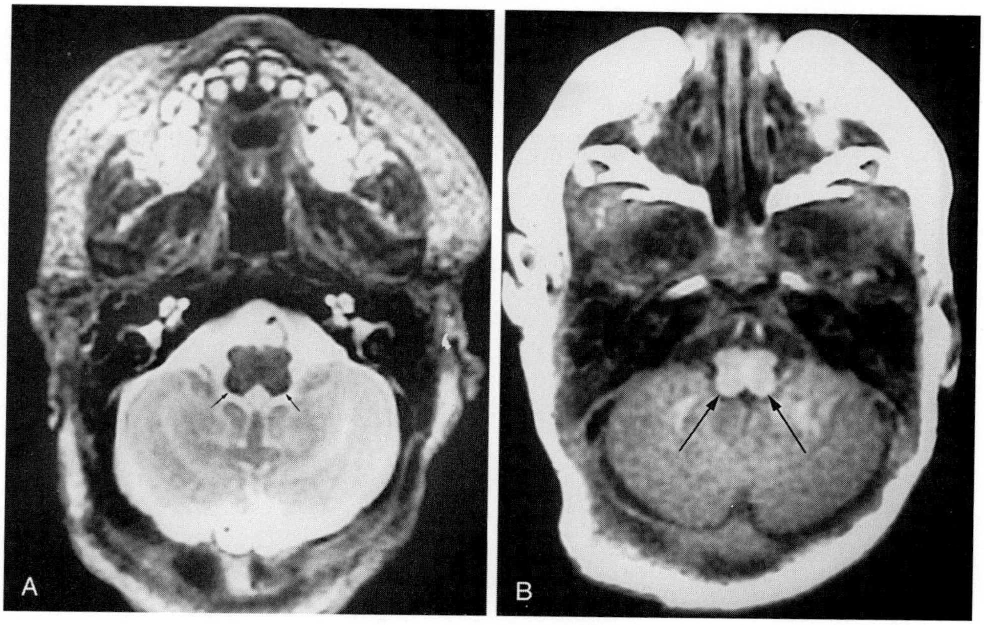

FIGURE 43–53 Axial MRI of normal myelination in a full-term newborn. *A,* FSE T2-weighted. *B,* SE T1-weighted. Myelination in the inferior cerebellar peduncles *(arrows).*

The parameters used for evaluating myelination on the CSE pulse sequence are: TR 3000 to 4000 msec; TE 100 to 120 msec; number of excitation (NEX) 2; matrix 192 × 256 or 256 × 256; slice thickness 4 to 5 mm with a 0.5- to 1-mm interslice gap in the axial projection. The parameters used for the FSE are TR 3000 to 4000 msec; TE 102 msec; echo train length (ETL) 8; NEX 2; matrix 256 × 256; slice thickness same as for CSE. It is important to use a TR of 3000 msec or greater to evaluate the myelination stages on this pulse sequence. The TE should be lengthened in order to avoid obtaining a proton-density pulse sequence that is useless for adequately evaluating myelination.

The white matter changes on MRI can be divided into four stages: neonatal (first month of life) (Figs. 43–52C and D through 43–60), early infancy (after 1 month to 6 months of life) (Figs. 43–61 through 43–64), late infancy (after 6 months to 1 year of life) (Figs. 43–65 through 43–69), and early childhood (after 1 year to 3 years of life) (Figs. 43–70 through 43–75). The MRI findings of the white matter on the T2-weighted images during the neonatal and early infancy periods are due primarily to the water content of the gray and white matter and the relative paucity of myelinated structures. The nonmyelinated white matter fibers predominate and demonstrate a hyperintensity on the T2-weighted images. The brain structures that are myelinated at birth are (1) in the posterior fossa, the dorsal white matter tracts of the brain

Text continued on page 1510

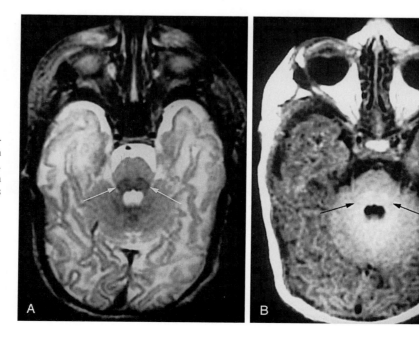

FIGURE 43–54 Axial MRI of normal myelination in a full-term newborn. *A,* FSE T2-weighted. *B,* SE T1-weighted. Myelination in the dorsal aspect of the pons *(arrows).*

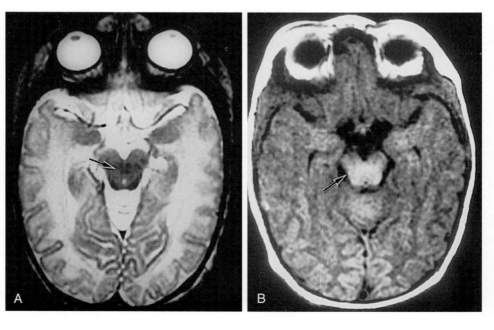

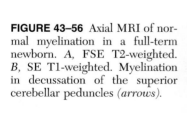

FIGURE 43–55 Axial MRI of normal myelination in a full-term newborn. *A,* FSE T2-weighted. *B,* SE T1-weighted. Myelination in the dorsal aspect of the pons and superior vermis *(arrows)* and the temporal horns *(arrowheads).*

FIGURE 43–56 Axial MRI of normal myelination in a full-term newborn. *A,* FSE T2-weighted. *B,* SE T1-weighted. Myelination in decussation of the superior cerebellar peduncles *(arrows).*

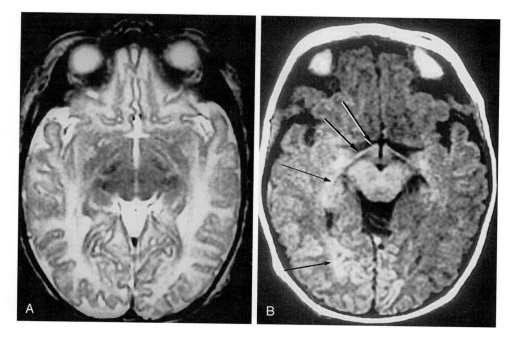

FIGURE 43–57 Axial MRI of normal myelination in a full-term newborn. *A*, FSE T2-weighted. *B*, SE T1-weighted. Myelination in the optic chiasm, optic tracts, and optic radiations (*arrows* in *B*).

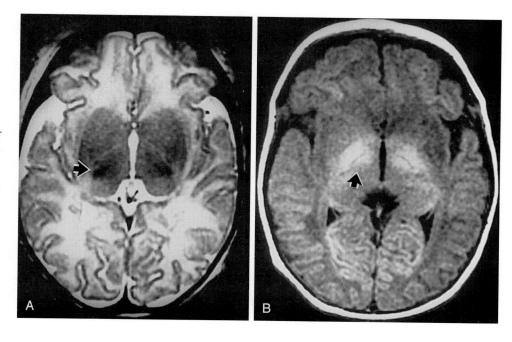

FIGURE 43–58 Axial MRI of normal myelination in a full-term newborn. *A*, FSE T2-weighted. *B*, SE T1-weighted. Myelination in the dorsal thalamus (*arrows*).

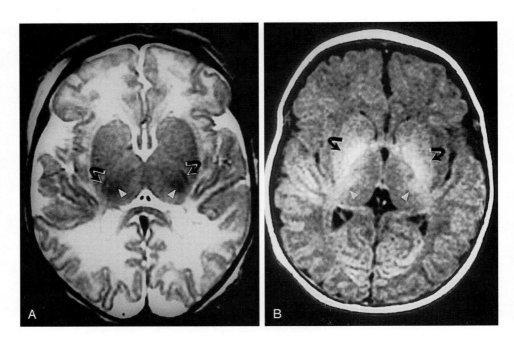

FIGURE 43–59 Axial MRI of normal myelination in a full-term newborn. *A,* FSE T2-weighted. *B,* SE T1-weighted. Myelination in the posterior limb of the internal capsule *(curved arrows)* and the dorsolateral thalamus *(arrowheads).*

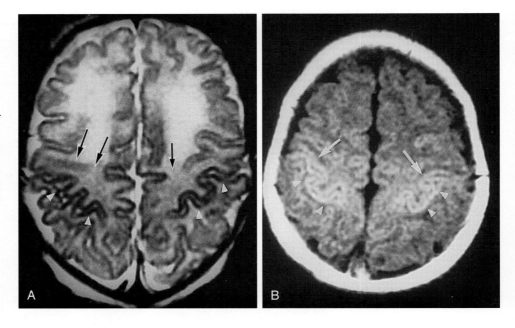

FIGURE 43–60 Axial MRI of normal myelination in a full-term newborn. *A,* FSE T2-weighted. *B,* SE T1-weighted. Central sulcus *(arrowheads)* and myelination in the white matter of the precentral gyrus *(arrows).*

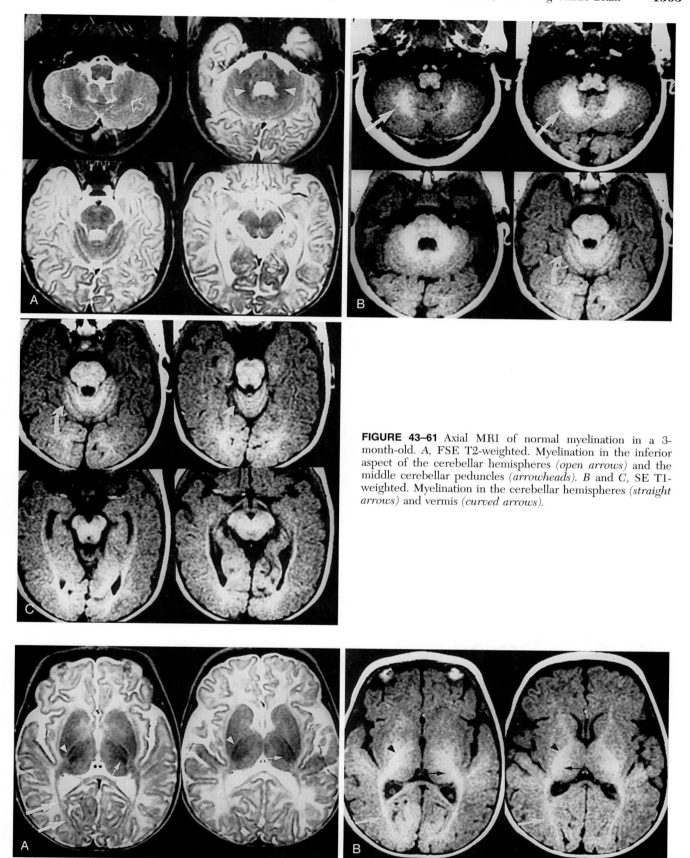

FIGURE 43–61 Axial MRI of normal myelination in a 3-month-old. *A*, FSE T2-weighted. Myelination in the inferior aspect of the cerebellar hemispheres *(open arrows)* and the middle cerebellar peduncles *(arrowheads)*. *B* and *C*, SE T1-weighted. Myelination in the cerebellar hemispheres *(straight arrows)* and vermis *(curved arrows)*.

FIGURE 43–62 Axial MRI of normal myelination in a 3-month-old. *A*, FSE T2-weighted. *B*, T1-weighted. Myelination in the posterior limb of the internal capsule *(arrowheads)*, dorsolateral thalamus *(small arrows)*, and optic radiations *(large arrows)*.

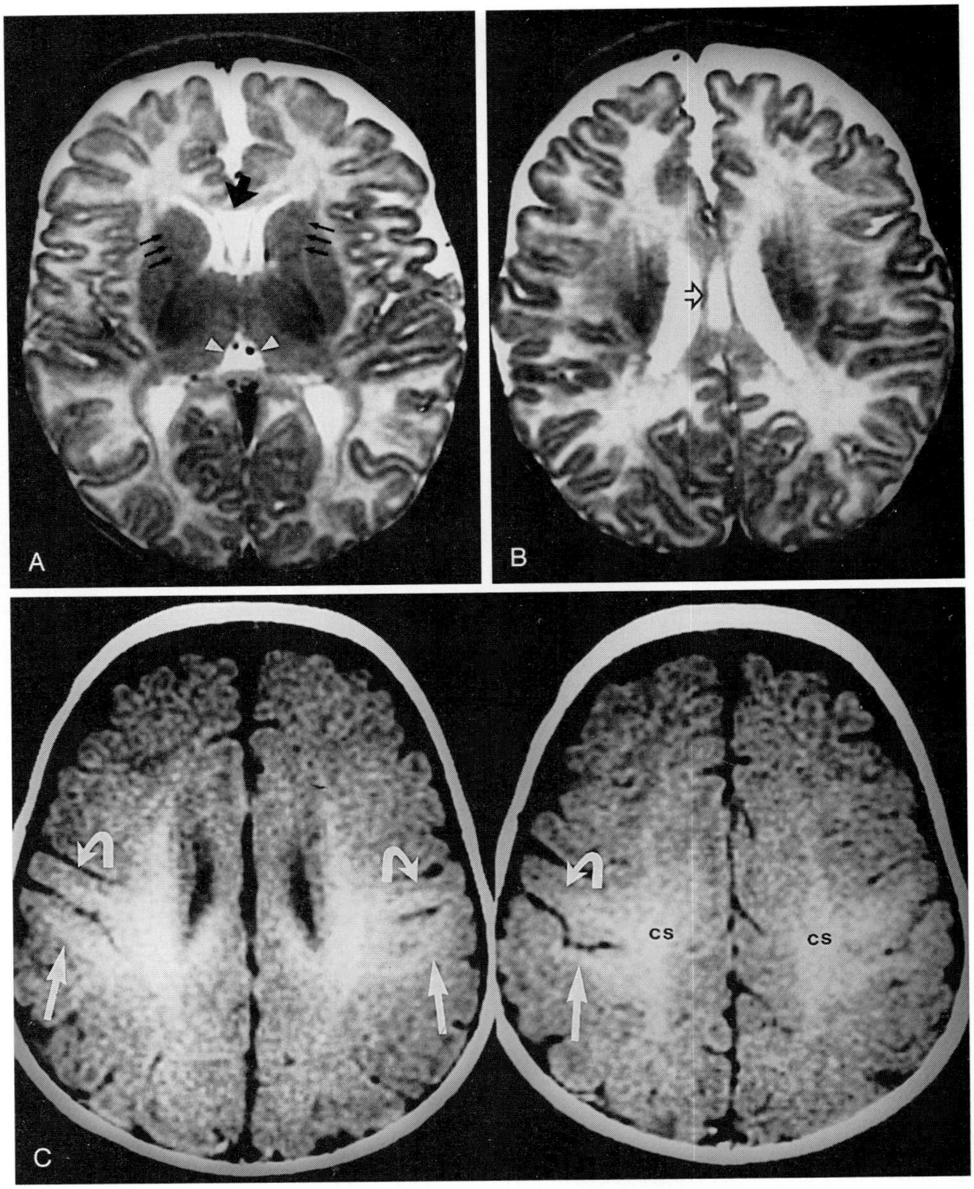

FIGURE 43–63 Axial MRI of normal myelination in a 3-month-old. *A,* FSE T2-weighted. *B,* T1-weighted. *A* and *B,* A normal 3-month-old infant with myelination in the anterior limb *(small arrows)* of the internal capsule; normal cavum septum pellucidum *(large solid arrow),* cavum velum interpositum *(arrowheads),* and cavum vergae *(open arrow). C,* Axial MRI T1-weighted in a normal 3-month-old infant with myelination in the centrum semiovale (CS) and precentral *(curved arrows)* and postcentral *(straight arrows)* gyral white matter.

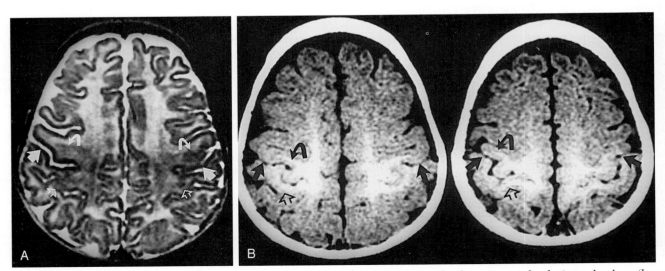

FIGURE 43–64 Axial MRI of normal myelination in a 3-month-old. *A,* FSE T2-weighted. *B,* T1-weighted. Central sulcus *(large straight arrows)* with myelination in the white matter of the precentral *(curved arrows)* and postcentral *(open arrows)* gyri.

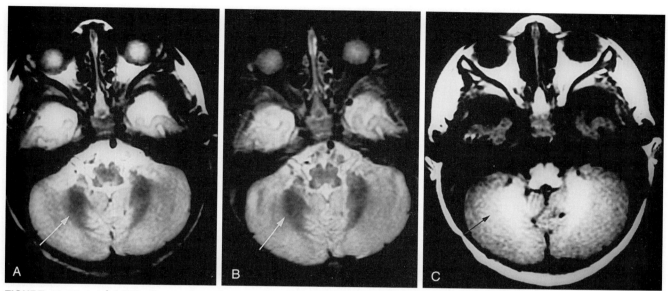

FIGURE 43–65 Axial MRI of normal myelination in a 7-month-old. *A*, FSE T2-weighted. *B*, Fast inversion recovery (FIR) T2-weighted. *C*, SE T1-weighted. Increase in myelination in the medulla and cerebellar hemispheres *(arrows)*.

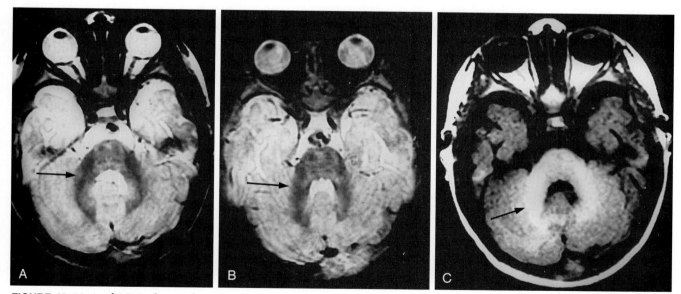

FIGURE 43–66 Axial MRI of normal myelination in a 7-month-old. *A*, FSE T2-weighted. *B*, FIR T2-weighted. *C*, SE T1-weighted. Increase in myelination in the pons and middle cerebellar peduncles *(arrows)*.

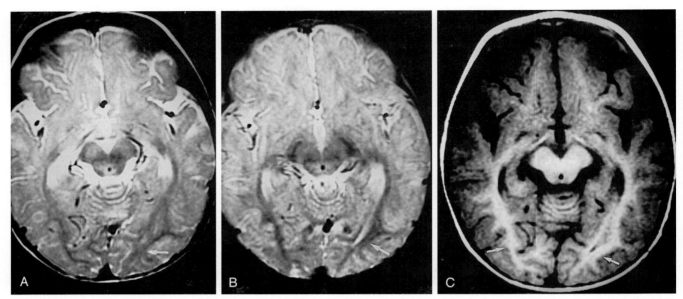

FIGURE 43–67 Axial MRI of normal myelination in a 7-month-old. *A,* FSE T2-weighted. *B,* FIR T2-weighted. *C,* SE T1-weighted. Increase in myelination in occipital white matter *(arrows).*

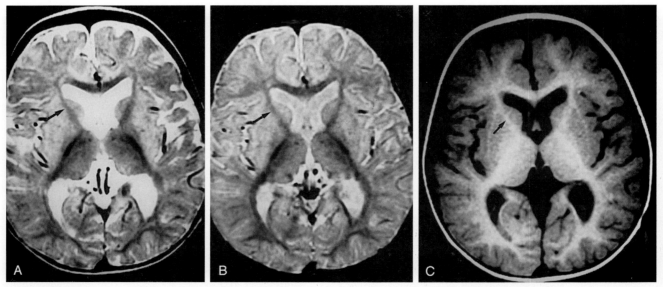

FIGURE 43–68 Axial MRI of normal myelination in a 7-month-old. *A,* FSE T2-weighted. *B,* FIR T2-weighted. *C,* SE T1-weighted. Myelination in all parts of the internal capsule but less in the anterior limb *(arrows).*

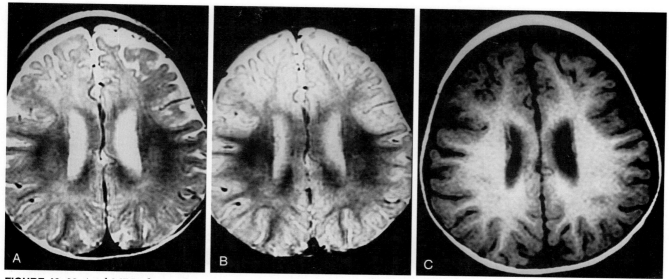

FIGURE 43–69 Axial MRI of normal myelination in a 7-month-old. *A,* FSE T2-weighted. *B,* FIR T2-weighted. *C,* SE T1-weighted. Greater myelination of the periventricular and occipital lobes' white matter than in the frontal lobes.

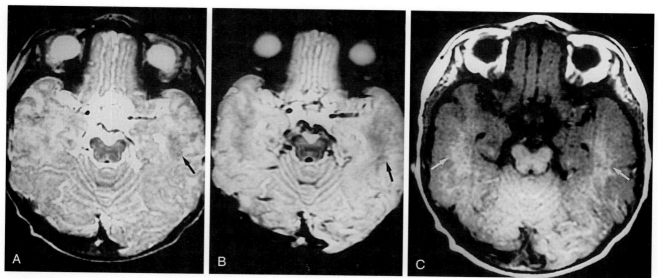

FIGURE 43–70 Axial MRI of normal myelination in a 13-month-old. *A,* FSE T2-weighted. *B,* FIR T2-weighted. *C,* SE T1-weighted. Increase in myelination of the white matter of the temporal lobes *(arrows)* is better demonstrated on FIR *(B).*

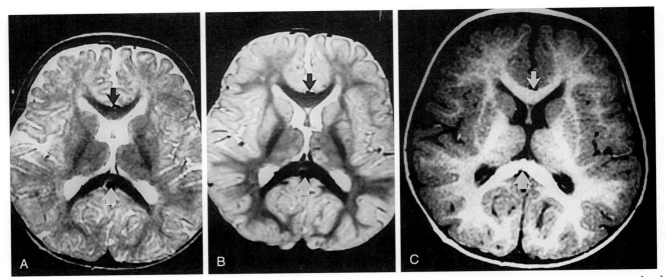

FIGURE 43–71 Axial MRI of normal myelination in a 13-month-old. *A*, FSE T2-weighted. *B*, FIR T2-weighted. *C*, SE T1-weighted. Greater myelination in the internal capsule with complete myelination of the corpus callosum—genu *(small arrows)* and splenium *(large arrows)*; greater myelination is found in the posterior than in the anterior white matter of the cerebral hemispheres.

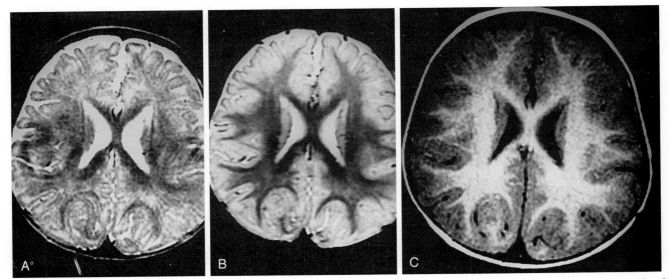

FIGURE 43–72 Axial MRI of normal myelination in a 13-month-old. *A*, FSE T2-weighted. *B*, FIR T2-weighted. *C*, SE T1-weighted. Greater myelination in the mid- and posterior white matter of the cerebral hemispheres with less myelination in the frontal lobes.

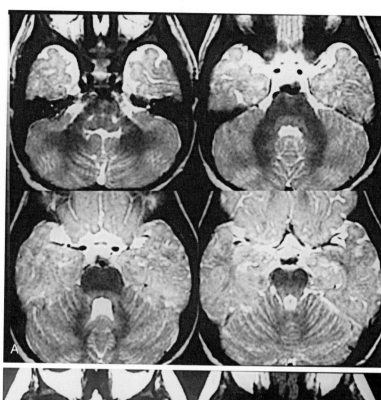

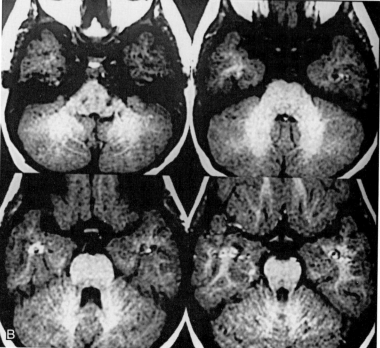

FIGURE 43–73 Axial MRI of normal myelination in an 18-month-old. *A*, FSE T2-weighted. *B*, SE T1-weighted. Further increase in myelination of the white matter fibers of the brain stem and cerebellum.

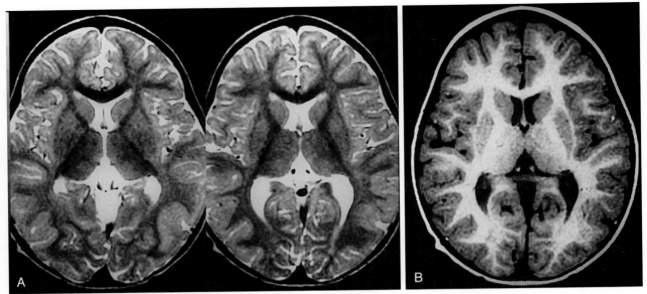

FIGURE 43–74 Axial MRI of normal myelination in an 18-month-old. *A*, FSE T2-weighted. *B*, SE T1-weighted. Further increase in myelination of the white matter fibers but less mature myelination in the frontal lobes.

stem, superior and inferior cerebellar peduncles; (2) in the diencephalon, the medial-dorsal white matter tracts; (3) in the supratentorial region, the posterior limb of the internal capsule and the postcentral gyrus white matter. All of the myelinated structures demonstrate hypointensity on the T2-weighted images.

As the myelination process continues during the neonatal and early infancy period, additional structures are seen to myelinate, such as small portions of the deep white matter of the cerebellar hemispheres seen by 1 month with further extension to involve more of the central portion at 3 months; the middle cerebellar peduncles at 3 months; optic radiation by 1 to 2 months; precentral gyrus white matter by 2 to 3 weeks; anterior limb of the internal capsule at 4 months; splenium of the corpus callosum by 4 months; cingulum gyrus white matter by 2 months; and calcarine gyrus white matter by 3 months.

During this time, several structures have mature myelin (when 75% of the structure is completely myelinated). By 6 months of age, the brain stem and cerebellar peduncles have mature myelin.

The MRI findings of the white matter on the T2-weighted images during the late infancy period are due primarily to the rapidly changing water content of the gray and white matter and the continued progress of the myelination process. The white matter fibers lose water faster than the gray matter during the first year of life. At late infancy, an isointense stage is seen on MRI between the nonmyelinated white matter and the nonmyelinated gray matter fibers (Fig. 43–76). The myelination process at this stage demonstrates further myelination of the cerebellar hemispheres, with extension into the white matter of the cerebellar folia by 8 months. All parts of the internal capsule are myelinated by 8 months, with mature

FIGURE 43–75 Axial MRI of normal myelination in an 18-month-old. *A*, FSE T2-weighted. *B*, SE T1-weighted. Less mature myelination in the anterior aspect of the frontal lobes (*arrows* in *A*).

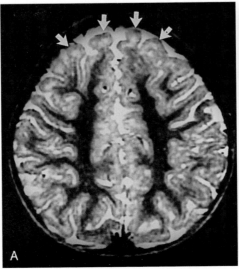
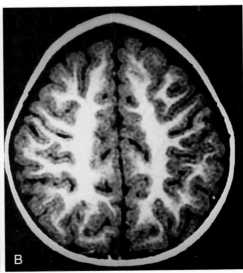

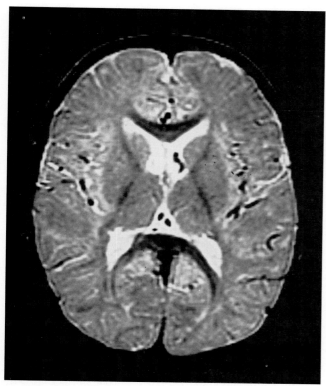

FIGURE 43–76 Axial MRI conventional SE T2-weighted of the isointense stage of most of the nonmyelinated white matter in a 1-year-old.

myelin in this structure by 1 year. Additional portions of the lobes of the cerebrum (occipital, posterior parietal, and posterior frontal) begin to show myelin by 7 months.

By early childhood, the myelination process predominates on the T2-weighted MRI studies with mature myelin seen in the cerebellum by 18 months and in the occipital, posterior parietal, and posterior frontal portions by 15 months. By 2 years, myelin should be seen in major portions of the temporal lobe, temporal pole, and frontal pole; these areas should be mature by 3 years of age (Table 43–1). However, it is not unusual to have a normal area of slow myelination involving the periventricular white matter at the posterior aspect of the bodies of the lateral ventricles (Fig. 43–77). This area may not myelinate until 9 to 10 years of age.

Myelination on T1-Weighted SE Images

The T1-weighted SE pulse sequence does not reflect the neuropathologic timetable for myelination as closely as T2-weighted SE. It is postulated that the differences in timing of the brain myelination on T2-weighted SE and T1-weighted SE are due to these neuropathologic timetables being based on the percentage of mature myelin. It is felt that the T1-weighted SE images are more sensitive to demonstrating immature as well as mature myelin.

The parameters used for evaluating myelination on this pulse sequence are TR 400 to 800 msec; TE 6 to 20 msec; NEX 2; matrix 192 × 256 or 256 × 256; slice thickness 4 to 5 mm with a 0.5- to 1-mm interslice gap in the axial plane. The progression of myelination seen

with T1-weighted SE sequences parallels that seen on T2-weighted SE except that the presence of myelin in any specific structure is seen earlier on the T1-weighted SE images (Table 43–2).

The MRI findings of the white matter on T1-weighted images during the neonatal period are again due primarily to the water content of the gray and white matter and less to the small amount of myelinated white matter structures. The nonmyelinated white matter is hypointense to gray matter, and the myelinated white matter is hyperintense. Although the water content of neonatal gray and nonmyelinated white matter (89% and 87% ± 1%, respectively) is similar, the tissues are different. Their MRI profiles (relaxation rates) are different, which accounts for their different appearance on the T1-weighted images.

At birth, myelin can be seen in the dorsal brain stem, all three cerebellar peduncles, the thalamus, posterior

TABLE 43–1 Myelination Timetable on T2-Weighted Spin-Echo Conventional and Fast Spin Echo

Brain Structure	Myelination	
Posterior Fossa		
Brain stem (dorsal)	Birth	Mature by 6 mo
Cerebellar peduncles		
Superior and inferior	Birth	Mature by 6 mo
Middle	2–3 mo	
Cerebellar hemisphere		
Deep inferior portion	1 mo	Mature by 18 mo
Central portion	3 mo	
Peripheral extension into folia	8 mo	
Diencephalon		
Thalamus (medial-dorsal)	Birth	
Supratentorial		
Optic		
Radiations	2 mo	
Tract	1 mo	
Internal capsule		
Posterior limb	Birth	
Anterior limb	4 mo	
All parts	8–12 mo	
Corpus callosum		
Splenium	4 mo	
Genu	8 mo	
All parts	12 mo	
Postcentral gyrus	Birth	
Calcarine gyrus	3 mo	
Precentral gyrus	2–3 wk	
Centrum semiovale (central)	Birth–2 mo	
Cingulum	2 mo	
Lobes of Brain		
Calcarine cortex		
Heschl's gyrus		
Postcentral gyrus		
Precentral gyrus	Mature by 6.5–15 mo	
Posterior frontal		
Posterior parietal		
Occipital pole		
Subcortical White Matter Association Fibers of		
Temporal lobe		
Temporal pole	Mature by 21–26.5 mo	
Frontal pole		

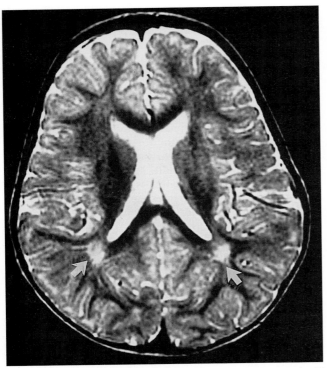

FIGURE 43–77 Axial MRI FSE T2-weighted of a 16-month-old child with a normal area of nonmyelinated white matter (*arrows*).

limb of the internal capsule, optic nerves, tracts, chiasm, and radiations as well as the precentral and postcentral gyri white matter. Myelin can be seen earlier involving the splenium of the corpus callosum at 3 months and the lobes of the brain at 6 months (see Table 43–2).

An isointense stage between gray and nonmyelinated white matter can be seen usually at 6 to 8 months of age on this pulse sequence (Fig. 43–78). The myelination process appears to take over earlier on the T1-weighted SE pulse sequence at around 10 to 12 months, whereas myelination appears to predominate after 1 year of age (around 15 to 18 months) on the T2-weighted SE sequences.

Myelination on CSE and FSE T2-Weighted and T1-Weighted IR Studies

The IR pulse sequences provide better resolution of the brain with both the T2- and the T1-weighted pulse sequences in comparison to SE. IR T2- and T1-weighted pulse sequences demonstrate a slight difference in the time of appearance of myelination when compared with their SE counterparts (Tables 43–3 and 43–4). The parameters used for the conventional T2-weighted IR (CIR) sequence are TR 2500 to 3000 msec; time to inversion (TI) 300 to 500 msec; TE 40 msec; NEX 2; matrix 192 × 256 or 256 × 256; 4- to 5-mm slice thickness with a 0.5- to 1-mm interslice gap in the axial projection. The parameters used for the fast T1-weighted IR pulse sequence are TR 2500–3000 msec; TI 165 msec; TE 20

TABLE 43–2 Myelination Timetable on T1-Weighted Spin-Echo

Brain Structure	Myelination
Posterior Fossa	
Brain stem (dorsal)	Birth
Cerebellar peduncles	Birth
Cerebellar hemispheric (deep white matter)	1 mo
Folia	3 mo
Diencephalon	
Thalamus (medial-dorsal)	Birth
Supratentorial	
Optic nerves, chiasm, tracts, radiations	Birth
Internal capsule	
Posterior limb	Birth
Anterior limb	3 mo
Corpus callosum	
Splenium	3 mo
Genu	6 mo
Postcentral gyrus	Birth
Precentral gyrus	Birth
Lobes of Brain	
Occipital	
Posterior parietal	
Posterior temporal	6 months
Posterior frontal	
Anterior parietal	
Anterior frontal	8 months
Midtemporal	
Frontal pole	
Temporal pole	12 months

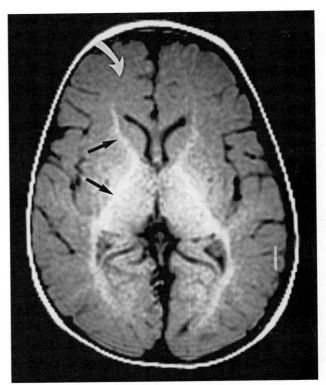

FIGURE 43–78 Axial MRI SE T1-weighted of the isointense stage of most of the nonmyelinated white matter (*curved arrow*) in a 6-month-old infant. Myelination is seen in the internal capsule (*straight arrows*) and corpus callosum.

msec; ETL 8; NEX 2; matrix 256 × 256 or 192 × 256; with the same slice thickness as for CIR.

The parameters used for the T1-weighted IR pulse sequence are TR 2500 to 3000 msec; TI 900 to 1200 msec; and TE 30 msec; with the remaining parameters the same as for the T2-weighted IR. The IR pulse sequences take a longer time to perform than SE. Because the majority of children have to be sedated for their MRI examination, this may pose a problem in obtaining a complete examination if IR pulse sequences are employed.

An excellent evaluation of the myelination process in a child can be obtained using T2- and T1-weighted SE pulse sequence. Both T2- and T1-weighted SE sequences should be employed. It is important to remember that the demonstration of myelin on MRI is dependent on a host of variable factors such as field strength of the MRI

TABLE 43–3 Myelination Timetable on T2-Weighted Inversion Recovery

Brain Structure		Myelination
Posterior Fossa		
Brain stem (dorsal)	Birth	Mature by 6 mo
Cerebellar peduncles		
Superior and inferior	Birth	Mature by 6 mo
Middle	1 mo	
Cerebellar hemisphere		
Deep inferior portion	1 mo	
Central portion	3 mo	Mature by 18 mo
Peripheral extension into folia	8 mo	
Diencephalon		
Thalamus (medial-dorsal)	Birth	
Supratentorial		
Optic		
Radiations	1 mo	
Tract	1 mo	
Internal capsule		
Posterior limb	Birth	
Anterior limb	2 mo	
All parts	6–8 mo	
Corpus callosum		
Splenium	3 mo	
Genu	6–8 mo	
All parts	8–10 mo	
Postcentral gyrus	Birth	
Calcarine gyrus	1–2 mo	
Precentral gyrus	Birth–2 wk	
Centrum semiovale (central)	Birth–1 mo	
Cingulum	1 mo	
Lobes of Brain		
Calcarine cortex		
Heschl's gyrus		
Postcentral gyrus		
Precentral gyrus		Mature by 6–10 mo
Posterior frontal		
Posterior parietal		
Occipital pole		
Subcortical White Matter Association Fibers of		
Temporal lobe		
Temporal pole		Mature by 12–15 mo
Frontal pole		

TABLE 43–4 Myelination Timetable on T1-Weighted Inversion Recovery

Brain Structure	Myelination
Posterior Fossa	
Brain stem (dorsal)	Birth
Cerebellar peduncles	Birth
Central deep white matter of cerebellar hemispheres	1 mo
Extension into white matter of folia of cerebellar hemisphere	3 mo
Diencephalon	
Thalamus (medial-dorsal)	Birth
Supratentorial	
Optic nerves, chiasm, tracts, radiations	Birth
Internal capsule posterior limb	Birth
Internal capsule anterior limb	2 mo
Corpus callosum	
Splenium	3 mo
Genu	6 mo
Postcentral gyrus	Birth
Precentral gyrus	Birth
Calcarine	1 mo
Lobes of Brain	
Occipital	
Posterior parietal	
Posterior temporal	6 mo
Posterior frontal	
Anterior parietal	
Anterior frontal	8 mo
Midtemporal	
Frontal pole	
Temporal pole	10 mo

magnet and the pulse sequences employed. The myelination tables developed are only a rough guide to aid in the assessment of the degree of myelination with the various pulse sequences frequently employed.

References

1. Fitz CR. The brain and spinal cord. In Silverman FN, Kuhn JP (eds). Essentials of Caffey's Pediatric X-Ray Diagnosis, pp. 106–174. Chicago, Year Book Medical, 1990.
2. Rumack CM, Johnson ML. Perinatal and Infant Brain Imaging. Chicago, Year Book Medical, 1984.
3. Yamada H. Pediatric Cranial Computed Tomography, pp. 3–15. Tokyo, Igaku-Shoin, 1983.
4. Hammock MK, Milhorat TH. Cranial Computed Tomography. Infancy and Childhood, pp. 1–46. Baltimore, Williams & Wilkins, 1981.
5. Maravilla KR, Pastel MS, Kirkpatrick JB. White matter of the cerebellum demonstrated by computed tomography. Normal anatomy and physical principles. J Comput Asst Tomogr 1978;2:156–161.
6. Hardwood-Nash DC, Fitz CR. Neuroradiology in Infants and Children. St. Louis, CV Mosby, 1976.
7. Meese W, Kluge W, Grumme T, Hopefemaller W. CT evaluation of the CSF spaces of healthy persons. Neuroradiology 1980;19:131–136.
8. Matsui T. Anatomical correlation of CT scan in infants and children.

[Japanese with English abstract] Child's Brain (Tokyo) 1977;2:151–160.

9. Meese W, Lanksch W, Wende S. Diagnosis and postoperative follow-up studies of infantile hydrocephalus using computerized tomography. In Lanksch W, Kaznet E (eds). Cranial Computerized Tomography, pp. 424–429. Berlin, Springer-Verlag, 1976.

10. Pedersen H, Gyldensted M, Gyldensted C. Measurement of the normal ventricular system and supratentorial subarachnoid space in children with computed tomography. Neuroradiology 1979;17:231–237.

11. Pellici LJ, Bedrick AD, Cruse RP, Vannucci RC. Frontal ventricular dimensions of the brain in infants and children. Arch Neurol 1979;36:852–853.

12. Penn RD, Belanger MG, Yasnoff WA. Ventricular volume in man computed from CAT scans. Ann Neurol 1978;3:216–223.

13. Schiersmann O. Einfuhrung in die Encephalographie. Leipzig, Georg Thieme, 1942.

14. Synek V, Reuben JR, du Boulay GH. Comparing Evans' index and computerized axial tomography in assessing relationship of ventricular size to brain size. Neurology 1976;26:231–233.

15. Dorovini-Zis K, Dolman C. Gestational development of brain. Arch Pathol Lab Med 1977;101:192.

16. Chi JG, Dooling EC, Gilles FN. Gyral development of the human brain. Ann Neurol 1977;1:86–93.

17. Fukuyama Y, Miyan M, Ishizu T, Maruyama H. Developmental changes in normal cranial measurements by computed tomography. Dev Med Child Neurol 1979;21:425–432.

18. Faerber E. Cranial Computed Tomography in Infants and Children. New York, Springer-Verlag, 1986.

19. Kirks DR. Practical Pediatric Imaging: Diagnostic Radiology of Infants and Children, 2nd ed. Boston, Little, Brown, 1991.

20. Fischer AQ, Anderson JC, Shuman RM, Stinson W. Pediatric Neurosonography—Clinical, Tomographic and Neuropathologic Correlates. New York, John Wiley, 1985.

21. Naidich TP, Quencer RM. Clinical Neurosonography. Ultrasound of the Central Nervous System. Berlin, Springer-Verlag, 1987.

22. Babcock DS, Han BK. Cranial Ultrasonography of Infants. Baltimore, Williams & Wilkins, 1981.

23. Grant EG. Neurosonography of the Pre-Term Neonate. New York, Springer-Verlag, 1986.

24. Sanders RC. Clinical Sonography—A Practical Guide, 2nd ed. Boston, Little, Brown, 1991.

25. Daniels DL, Haughton VM, Naidich TP. Cranial and Spinal Magnetic Resonance Imaging—An Atlas and Guide. New York, Raven, 1987.

26. Brant-Zawadzki M. MR imaging of the brain. Radiology 1988;166:1–10.

27. Newton TH, Ports DG (eds). Radiology of the Skull and Brain. St. Louis, CV Mosby, 1977.

28. Starke DD, Bradley WG. Magnetic Resonance Imaging. St. Louis, CV Mosby, 1988.

29. Barkovich AJ, Wippold FJ, Sherman H, Citrin CM. Significance of cerebellar tonsillar position on MR. AJNR 1986;7:795–799.

30. Daniels DL, Williams AL, Haughton VM. Computed tomography of the medulla. Radiology 1982;145:63–69.

31. Atlas SW. Magnetic Resonance Imaging of the Brain and Spine. New York, Raven, 1991.

32. Faerber EN. Magnetic Resonance Imaging in Infants and Children. London, MacKeith, 1995.

33. Barkovich AJ. Pediatric Neuroimaging, 2nd ed. New York, Raven, 1995.

34. Aoki S, Okada Y, Nishimura K, et al. Normal deposition of brain iron in childhood and adolescence. MR imaging at 1.5T. Radiology 1989;172:381–385.

35. Drayer B, Burger P, Darwin R, et al. Magnetic resonance imaging of brain iron. AJNR 1986;7:373–380; and AJR 1986;147:103–110.

36. Citrin CM, Sherman JL, Gangarosa RE, Stanlon D. Physiology of the CSF flow-void sign: Modification by cardiac gating. AJNR 1986;7:1021–1024; and AJR 1987;148:205–208.

37. Kleinman PK, Zito JL, Davidson RI, Raptopoulos V. The subarachnoid spaces in children: Normal variations in size. Radiology 1983;147:455–457.

38. McArdle CB, Richardson CJ, Nicholas DA, et al. Developmental features of the neonatal brain: MR imaging. Part II. Ventricular size and extracerebral space. Radiology 1987;162:230–234.

39. Shapiro R, Galloway SJ, Shapiro MD. Minimal asymmetry of the brain: A normal variant. AJR 1986;147:753–756.

40. Brant-Zawadzki M, Kelly W, Kjos B, et al. Magnetic resonance imaging and characterization of normal and abnormal intra-cranial cerebrospinal fluid (CSF) spaces: Initial observations. Neuroradiology 1985;27:3–8.

41. Han JS, Bonstelle CT, Kaufman B, et al. Magnetic resonance imaging in the evaluation of the brainstem. Radiology 1984;150:705–712.

42. Flannigan BD, Bradley WG, Mazziotta JC, et al. Magnetic resonance imaging of the brainstem: Normal structure and basic functional anatomy. Radiology 1985;154:375–385.

43. Press GA, Hesselink JR. MR imaging of cerebellopontine angle and internal auditory canal lesions at 1.5T. AJNR 1988;9:241–252; and AJR 1988;150:1371–1381.

44. Kretschmann HJ, Weinrich W. Cranial Neuroimaging and Clinical Neuroanatomy. Magnetic Resonance Imaging and Computed Tomography. New York, Georg Thieme, 1992.

45. Leblanc A. Anatomy and Imaging of the Cranial Nerves. Berlin, Springer-Verlag, 1992.

46. Norton WT. Formation, structure, and biochemistry of myelin. In Siegel GJ, Alberts RW, Agranoff BW, Katzman R (eds). Basic Neurochemistry, pp. 63–69. Boston, Little, Brown, 1981.

47. Yakovlev PI, Lecours AR. The myelogenetic cycles of regional maturation of the brain. In Minkowski A (ed). Regional Development of the Brain in Early Life, pp. 3–79. Oxford, Blackwell Scientific, 1967.

48. Brody BA, Kinney HC, Kloman AS, Giles FH. Sequence of central nervous system myelination in human infancy. I. An autopsy study of myelination. J Neuropathol Exp Neurol 1987;46:283–301.

49. Homes GI. Morphological and physiological maturation of the brain in the neonate and young child. J Clin Neurophysiol 1986;3:209–238.

50. Kinney HC, Brody BA, Kloman AS, Gilles FH. Sequence of central nervous system myelination in human infancy. II. Patterns of myelination in autopsied infants. J Neuropathol Exp Neurol 1988;47:217–234.

51. Reinarz SJ, Coffman CE, Smoker WRK, Godersky JC. MR imaging of the corpus callosum. Normal and pathologic findings and correlation with CT. AJNR 188;9:649–656; and AJR 1988;151:791–798.

52. Barkovich AJ, Kjos BO. Normal postnatal development of the corpus callosum as demonstrated by MR imaging. AJNR 1988;9:487–491.

53. Curnes JT, Laster DW, Koubek TD, et al. MRI of corpus callosal syndromes. AJNR 1986;7:617–622.

54. Atlas SW, Grossman RI, Gomori IM, et al. Calcified intra-cranial lesions: Detection with gradient-echo acquisition rapid MRI imaging. AJR 1988;150:1383–1389.

55. Kilgore DP, Strother CM, Stanslak RJ, Haughton VM. Pineal germinoma: MR imaging. Radiology 1986;158:435–438.

56. Ganti SR, Hilal SK, Stein BM, et al. CT of pineal region tumors. AJNR 1986;7:97–104; and AJR 1986;158:435–438.

57. Grant EG, Williams AL, Schellinger D, Slovis TL. Intracranial calcification in the infant and neonate: Evaluation by sonography and CT. Radiology 1985;157:63–68.

58. Barkovich AJ, Lyon G, Evrard P. Formation, maturation, and disorders of white matter. AJNR 1992;10:731–740.

59. Norris CR. Morphology and cellular interactions of growth cones in the developing corpus callosum. J Comp Neurol 1990;293:268–281.

60. Smith SJ. Neuronal cytomechanics: The actin-based motility of growth cones. Science 1988;242:708–715.

61. Valk J, Van der Knaap MS. Magnetic Resonance of Myelin, Myelination, and Myelin Disorders. New York, Springer-Verlag, 1989.

62. Holmes GL. Morphological and physiological maturation of the brain in the neonate and young child. J Clin Neurophysiol 1986;3:209–238.

63. Koenig SH. Cholesterol of myelin is the determinant of gray-white contrast in MRI of brain. Magn Reson Med 1991;20:285–291.

64. Lee BC. Hypoxic/ischemic events in the infant's brain: Normal myelination as seen on MRI. Presented at the 35th Annual Meeting of the Society for Pediatric Radiology, Orlando, FL, 1992.

65. O'Brien JS. Lipids and myelination. In Hinwich WA (ed). Developmental Neurobiology, pp. 262–286. Springfield, IL, Charles C Thomas, 1970.

66. Wiggins RC. Myelin development and nutritional insufficiency. Brain Res Rev 1982;4:151–175.

67. Baierl P, Forster CH, Fendel H, et al: Magnetic resonance imaging of normal and pathological white matter maturation. Pediatr Radiol 1988;18:183–189.
68. Barkovich AJ, Kjos BO, Jackson Jr DH, Norman D. Normal maturation of the neonatal and infant brain: MR imaging at 1.5T. Radiology 1988;166:173–180.
69. Dietrich RB, Bradley WG Jr. Normal and abnormal white matter maturation. Semin Ultrasound CT MR 1988;9:192–200.
70. Johnson MA, Pennock JM, Bydder GM, et al. Clinical NMR imaging of the brain in children. Normal and neurological disease. AJR 1983;141:1005–1018.
71. Martin C, Kikinis R, Zuerrer M. Developmental stages of human brain. An MR study. J Comput Assist Tomogr 1988;12:917–922.
72. Harbord MG, Finn JP, Hall-Craggs MA, et al. Myelination patterns on magnetic resonance of children with developmental delay. Dev Med Child Neurol 1990;32:295–303.
73. Van der Knaap MS, Valk J, Bakker J, et al. Myelination as an expression of the functional maturity of the brain. Dev Med Child Neurol 1991;33:849–857.
74. Bird CR, Hedberg M, Draye B. MR assessment of myelination in infants and children: Usefulness of marker sites. AJNR 1990;10:731–740.
75. Christophe C, Muller MF, Baleriaux D, et al. Mapping of normal brain maturation in infants on phase-sensitive inversion-recovery MR image. Neuroradiology 1990;32:173–178.
76. Curnes JT, Burger PC, Djang WT. MR imaging of compact white matter pathways. AJNR 1988;9:1061–1068.
77. Dietrich RB, Bradley WG, Zaragoza EJ IV, et al. MR evaluation of early myelination patterns in normal and developmentally delayed infants. AJR 1988;150:889–896.
78. Hayakawa K, Konishi Y, Kuriyama M, et al. Normal brain maturation in MRI. Eur J Radiol 1991;12:208–215.
79. Holland BA, Haas DK, Norman D. MRI of normal brain maturation. AJNR 1986;7:201–208.
80. Kinney HC, Brody BA, Kloman AS, Gilles FH. Sequence of central nervous system myelin in human infancy. II. Patterns of myelination in autopsied infants. J Neuropathol Exp Neurol 1988;47:217–234.
81. McArdle CB, Richardson CJ, Nicholas DA, et al. Developmental features of the neonatal brain: MR imaging. Part I. Gray-white matter differentiation and myelination. Radiology 1987;162:223–229.
82. Van der Knapp MS, Valk J. MR imaging of the various stages of normal myelination during the first year of life. Neuroradiology 1990;31:459–470.
83. Koenig SH, Brown RD III, Spiller M, Lundbom N. Relaxometry of brain: Why white matter appears bright in MRI. Magn Reson Med 1990;14:482–495.

44

Imaging of Congenital Malformations of the Brain

MAURICIO CASTILLO, M.D.

SURESH K. MUKHERJI, M.D.

This chapter addresses the imaging features of classic congenital malformations of the brain. Since most of these patients have anomalies of the corpus callosum, its development and abnormalities are discussed first. The imaging features addressed here refer to those seen by magnetic resonance imaging (MRI) unless otherwise stated. MRI is the imaging method of choice in patients suspected of harboring congenital brain anomalies.

THE CORPUS CALLOSUM

Development

The formation of the corpus callosum progresses from anterior to posterior with the exception that the rostrum is the last of the four callosal structures to form. The sequence of formation is thus: (1) genu, (2) body, (3) splenium, and (4) rostrum. The vesicles, which will form the telencephalon, are bridged rostrally by the lamina terminalis. During the seventh week of fetal life, the rostrally located lamina terminalis thickens and becomes the lamina reuniens.[1] The lamina reuniens develops a ventral sulcus filled with meninx primitiva (the precursor of the subarachnoid space). This sulcus is bridged superiorly by glial cells that will guide axons across it and give origin to three transcerebral structures: the corpus callosum, the anterior commissure, and the posterior commissure. The formation of these three structures begins anteriorly and progresses posteriorly. Therefore, the genu of the corpus callosum forms first and is followed by the body and splenium. The rostrum, although the anteriormost aspect of the corpus callosum, forms last. This order of development helps explain the absence of the body and splenium with preservation of the genu in most cases of dysgenesis of the corpus callosum, since the genu is the earliest corpus callosal structure to form.[2]

The corpus callosum may be completely absent (agenesis) or partially formed (hypogenesis). Hypogenesis generally is related to malformation of portions of the corpus callosum that develops late (posterior body, splenium, and rostrum). The corpus callosum may also be defective (dysgenesis). Absence of the anterior portion of the cor-

pus callosum occurs in only two instances: holoprosencephaly and secondary destructive processes such as ischemia.[3]

The formation of the corpus callosum culminates at about the 20th week of life.[1] Maturation of myelin in this structure occurs after birth and may be assessed by MRI. At birth, the corpus callosum is not myelinated and its signal intensity is low to intermediate on T1-weighted images and intermediate to high on T2-weighted images.[4] These appearances reflect a high content of water and the presence of hydrophilic myelin. At approximately 4 to 6 months of life, T1-weighted images show increased signal intensity in the genu. The splenium of the corpus callosum becomes relatively hyperintense on T1-weighted images at 3 to 4 months of life and relatively hypointense on T2-weighted at 4 to 6 months of age. The genu becomes relatively hypointense on T2-weighted images at 5 to 8 months of life. *Therefore, the two generally accepted rules for the development of the corpus callosum are that it develops from front to back and that it myelinates from back to front.*

Although these rules apply to the majority of abnormalities, the presence of an intact interhemispheric fissure is also an important factor in the normal formation of the corpus callosum. Masses of any sort within the fissure may prevent normal development of the corpus callosum. Most congenital malformations of the brain are accompanied by abnormal formation of the corpus callosum.

The Abnormal Corpus Callosum

Agenesis of the corpus callosum occurs in approximately 1 in 1000 live births.[5] It is associated with posterior fossa malformations (Dandy-Walker complex and Chiari malformations), encephaloceles, midline facial clefts, and more than 25 genetic syndromes. Clinically, these patients may have profound developmental delay but, on rare occasions, may be near normal. The presence of gray matter heterotopias may lead to epilepsy.[6]

Midsagittal MRI or sonographic studies show complete absence of the corpus callosum with a "spoke-wheel"

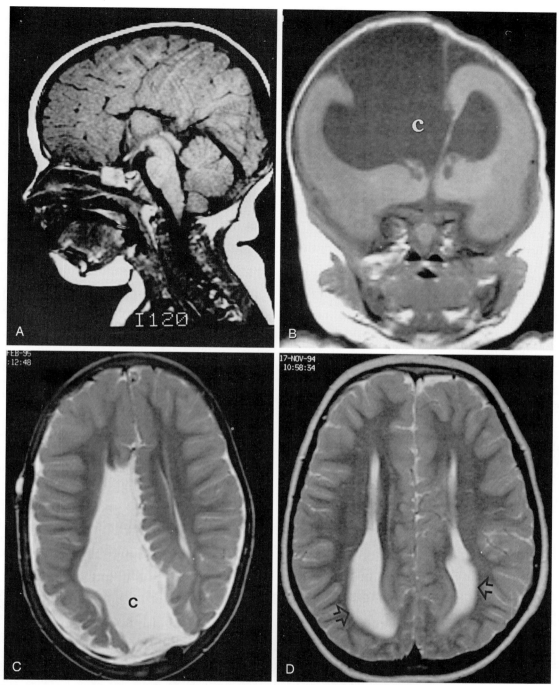

FIGURE 44–1 Agenesis of the corpus callosum. *A,* Midsagittal magnetic resonance imaging (MRI) T1-weighted shows complete absence of the corpus callosum. The massa intermedia is prominent and the position of the third ventricle is slightly high. *B,* Coronal MRI T1-weighted in a different patient shows agenesis of the corpus callosum with a large interhemispheric cyst (c), which communicates with the right lateral ventricle. This term newborn has lissencephaly. *C,* Axial MRI T2-weighted shows absence of the corpus callosum in a different patient. A dorsal interhemispheric cyst (c) is present. *D,* Axial MRI T2-weighted in a different patient with agenesis of the corpus callosum shows that the lateral ventricles are parallel with each other and that their posterior aspects *(arrows)* are prominent (colpocephaly).

arrangement of the medial hemispheric sulci that radiate outwardly[3] (Fig. 44–1*A*). The cingulate sulci are absent. On coronal images, the frontal horns of the lateral ventricles acquire a crescentic configuration and are indented medially by the bundles of Probst. The cingulate gyri and

fornices form the medial roof of the lateral ventricles and are everted. The third ventricle is high riding and may communicate posteriorly with a dorsal cerebrospinal fluid (CSF)–filled interhemispheric cyst (Fig. 44–1*B* and *C*). On axial MRI or CT studies, the atria and occipital horns of the lateral ventricles balloon out, giving rise to what is referred to as *colpocephaly* (Fig. 44–1D). The presence of colpocephaly implies malformation of the white matter in the posterior regions of the cerebral hemispheres. The lateral ventricles lose their medial concavities and assume a parallel configuration. Both the lateral and the third ventricles may communicate posteriorly with the dorsal cyst. Interhemispheric lipomas may be present and may contain calcifications.[7]

THE HEMISPHERIC WHITE AND GRAY MATTER

Development

At 4 weeks of fetal life, the rostral end of the neuropore closes and, between 4 and 7 weeks of life, undergoes a process termed *ventral induction.* During this period, three segments arise: the rhombencephalon or hindbrain, the mesencephalon or midbrain, and the prosencephalon or forebrain.[1] This last segment further subdivides into the diencephalon that will produce the thalami and hypothalamus, and the telencephalon that will produce the cerebral hemispheres. Once these segments are present, the stages of cellular proliferation and differentiation begin.

The lateral margins of the ventricular system contain the germinal matrix. The primitive cells in this structure evolve to neuroblasts, which then migrate and establish the cortex. These neuroblasts migrate along radial-glial fibers that guide them. Neuronal migration begins during the early second trimester of intrauterine life and is mostly completed by the end of this period. There is a one-to-one correspondence between the site of origin and the eventual resting place in the cortex for these young neurons. The most recent neurons reside in the deeper layers of the cortex. The radial-glial fibers involute and eventually become astrocytes. The germinal matrix fragments and involutes. The caudothalamic region is the last to contain the germinal matrix, but by term birth this has also disappeared.

Myelination is briefly addressed here and only as it pertains to its evaluation with MRI. The T1 shortening produced by mature myelin is probably related to the presence of cholesterol and glycolipids. These compounds are hydrophobic. Accumulation of cholesterol and glycolipids accompanies the formation of myelin by the oligodendrocytes. The T2 shortening associated with mature myelin is probably a reflection of tightening of the myelin sheaths around their axons. As a general rule, maturation of myelin begins caudally and posteriorly and extends superiorly and rostrally.[8] Therefore, in all term newborns, MRI T1-weighted studies show increased signal intensity in the brain stem, dorsal midbrain, middle cerebellar peduncles, and posterior limbs of the internal capsules. The T2 shortening always lags 1 to 2 months behind the T1 shortening of mature myelin. The anterior limb of the internal capsules myelinates by 2 to 3 months. The occipital white matter myelinates centrally at 3 to 5 months and peripherally at 4 to 7 months of age. The frontal white matter myelinates centrally at 3 to 6 months and peripherally at 7 to 11 months. The centrum semiovale myelinates at 2 to 6 months of age. All these dates are given for T1-weighted images. Also, myelination during the initial 6 months of life is more easily appreciated on T1-weighted images, whereas after that age T2-weighted images are useful.[1] Myelin milestones for the corpus callosum are described earlier.

Abnormalities of Neuronal Migration

The most severe abnormality of neuronal migration is probably *lissencephaly* (smooth brain)[9] (Fig. 44–2A). Its incidence is not known, but this abnormality is rare. Maternal infection with cytomegalovirus may play a role in the genesis of this malformation, as this virus exhibits tropism for the germinal matrix and may destroy it. On MRI studies, the appearance of the brain is that of a fetal

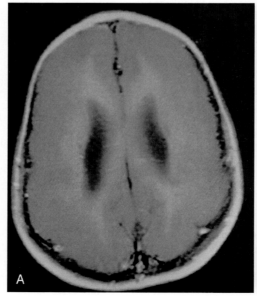 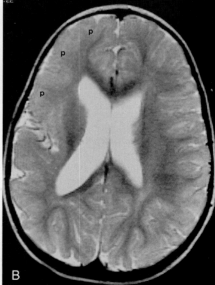

FIGURE 44–2 Anomalies of neuronal migration. *A,* Axial MRI T1-weighted shows complete absence of the cortical gyri and sulci compatible with lissencephaly (argyria). Note the increased thickness of the cortex. *B,* Axial MRI T2-weighted in a different patient shows pachygyria (p) involving the right frontotemporal region. (*A,* From Castillo M. Neuroradiology Companion. Philadelphia, Lippincott-Raven, 1995.)

brain before the 25th week of life.[10] There are no cortical sulci, and the temporal operculae are open, resulting in a "figure-of-8" appearance. The cortex is thick and initially may contain a deep zone of T2 signal hyperintensity reflecting the sparse neuronal layer. On MRI studies, this appearance may be initially indistinguishable from a diffuse band heterotopia. The cortex is formed by only four layers. Type 1 lissencephaly is associated with the Miller-Dieker and Norman-Roberts syndromes. Type 2 lissencephaly is associated with Fukuyama's congenital muscular dystrophy and the Walker-Warburg syndrome.[11] These children have eye abnormalities, hypotonia, hydrocephalus, and posterior encephaloceles. True microencephaly, radial microbrain, and diffuse polymicrogyria may be part of the spectrum of lissencephalies.

Pachygyria refers to incomplete lissencephaly.[3] MRI shows a smooth brain devoid of cortical sulci, particularly in the frontotemporal regions (see Fig. 44–2B). The occipitoparietal regions are less affected.

Polymicrogyria or non-lissencephalic cortical dysplasia is not a true anomaly of migration. In these patients, the cortex contains all six neuronal layers, but they are disorganized.[12] This abnormality probably results from ischemia or infection with cytomegalovirus. It commonly involves the perisylvian regions and may be bilateral (Fig. 44–3A). However, any part of the brain may be affected. Patients present with varying degrees of hemiplegia, pseudobulbar palsy, and seizures.[5] On MRI studies, the appearance is that of a zone of smooth brain and thickened cortex (identical to focal pachygyria). The posterior aspect of a sylvian fissure may be prominent and continue superiorly and posteriorly more than might be expected. The cortex of this sylvian continuation may be thickened and appear as polymicrogyria. On gross examination, the abnormal cortex contains many minute gyri resembling the surface of a cauliflower. These small gyri are not

resolved on MRI. Occasionally, the dysplastic cortex may be calcified. Also, since the cortex does not form normally, condensation of the superficial veins does not occur and large draining veins may overlie the zone of pachygyria.[13] It is important not to confuse these vessels with a true arteriovenous malformation. In approximately 20% of patients, T2-weighted images will demonstrate hyperintensity of the underlying white matter that may be related to gliosis from a prior ischemic insult (Fig. 44–3B).

Gray matter *heterotopias* may account for up to 10% of cases of medically intractable seizures.[14] These are the result of aberrations in the normal migration of neurons from the germinal matrix to the cortex. Therefore, gray matter heterotopias may be located anywhere from the walls of the ventricles to the cortex (Fig. 44–4). Nodular subependymal gray matter rests are commonly located along the outer walls of the lateral ventricles. Focal subcortical heterotopias may trap CSF spaces and vessels and, if large, may have a masslike configuration (Fig. 44–5). Heterotopias follow the MRI signal intensity of gray matter in all imaging sequences and do not enhance.[15] The most severe form of heterotopic gray matter is called a *band heterotopia*. In these cases, a circumferential band of gray matter is "sandwiched" within the white matter, creating the impression of a double cortex[16] (Fig. 44–6). Band heterotopias may be diffuse and bilateral but occasionally are localized.

The last form of anomaly that contains multiple errors of neuronal migration is *unilateral megaencephaly*. In this disorder, hamartomatous overgrowth of one cerebral hemisphere or a portion of it occurs.[17] Patients may have corporal hemihypertrophy and seizures. MRI is the imaging method of choice and shows an enlarged cerebral hemisphere that contains multiple zones of pachygyria (Fig. 44–7A). The underlying white matter may be hyperintense on T2-weighted images, reflecting the presence

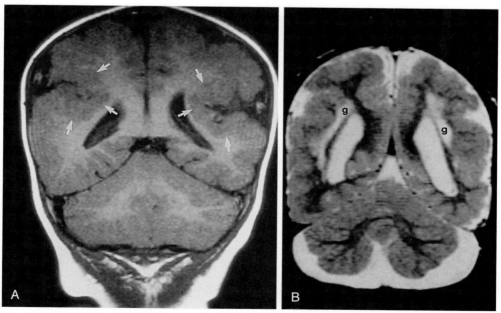

FIGURE 44–3 Polymicrogyria. *A*, Coronal MRI T1-weighted shows deep posterior clefts lined with thickened gray matter *(arrows)*. *B*, Coronal MRI T2-weighted shows dysplastic cortex in the posterior parietal regions with underlying high signal intensity (g) related to gliosis.

SECTION **IV** Pediatrics

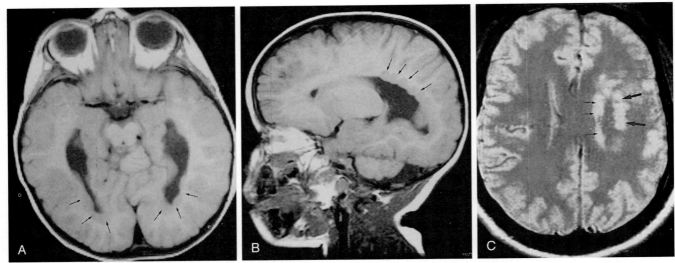

FIGURE 44–4 Heterotopias. *A,* Axial noncontrast MRI T1-weighted in a child with intractable seizures shows nodular subependymal gray matter heterotopias *(arrows)* lining both occipital horns of the lateral ventricles. *B,* Parasagittal T1-weighted image in the same child confirms the presence of the heterotopias *(arrows).* Note that they have signal intensity equal to that of the cortex. *C,* In a different child, MRI proton density shows subependymal left gray matter heterotopias *(thin arrows)* as well as gray matter *(thick arrows)* arrested within the white matter of the centrum semiovale. Note that all heterotopias have signal intensity similar to that of the cortex.

of gliosis (Fig. 44–7*B*). The frontal horn of the lateral ventricle on the same side as the malformation is coapted (anteriorly and superiorly narrowed). The involved hemisphere is usually nonfunctioning, and these patients may benefit from a functional hemispherectomy.

Schizencephalies

A *schizencephaly* is a CSF-filled cleft extending from the surface of the cortex to the lining of a ventricle.[18] Histologically, the pia forms a contiguous seam with the ventricular ependyma. It is discussed here because, although schizencephaly is probably related to destruction of the brain by ischemia, it is intimately associated with neuronal migration aberrations. Its incidence is unknown, and it may be familial or sporadic. Maternal carbon monoxide intoxication and fetal ischemia are known to be predisposing factors. Fetal ischemia between 12 and 17 weeks of life may be responsible for schizencephaly. The severity of clinical signs and symptoms is directly related to the size, bilaterality, and location of the clefts. In approximately 35% of cases, these clefts are bilateral.[19] Most clefts involve the frontal and perisylvian regions. Some patients are blind secondary to optic nerve hypoplasia and may be categorized as having septo-optic dysplasia. Pathologically and on MRI, schizencephalies may be divided into two types: open- and closed-lip. In the former, CSF fills the cleft; in the latter, there is no CSF and the lips of the cleft are in apposition to each other (Fig. 44–8*A*). Most schizencephalies communicate with a lateral ventricle. This ventricle tends to be more prominent than that in the normal side. The ipsilateral cerebral hemisphere is smaller than that on the uninvolved side. The lips of the cleft are lined by polymicrogyric gray matter. As such, anomalies of venous drainage may also be seen with schizencephalies (Fig. 44–8*B*). The overlying

subarachnoid spaces are prominent, and occasionally a CSF-filled cyst is present adjacent to the outer opening of the cleft. This cyst may produce scalloping of the overlying calvarium, presumably owing to fluid pulsations. Occasionally these cysts need to be shunted. The septum pellucidum is usually absent in cases of open-lip schizencephalies (Fig. 44–8*C*). In the closed-lip type, there is a band of smooth gray matter from which a nipple projects into the ventricle. In these cases, the clinical manifestations are less severe than in those patients with the open-lip type of schizencephaly.

When large bilateral open-lip schizencephalies are found, the findings are identical to those of hydranencephaly (Fig. 44–9). Both entities presumably originate from severe vascular insults with destruction of large zones of brain parenchyma. The differential diagnosis is that of severe hydrocephalus. For practical purposes, these patients need to be shunted to prevent inordinate head growth and to facilitate their daily management.

Holoprosencephalies

The *holoprosencephalies* are a group of disorders in which the forebrain has failed in its diverticulation and midline cleavage.[20] Abnormalities in midline differentiation of the face accompany the most severe types of holoprosencephaly (Fig. 44–10*A*). Also, the premaxillary segments of the face are hypoplastic. The brain abnormalities range from mild (lobar type), to intermediate (semilobar type), to severe (alobar). At times, differentiating them may be impossible. Therefore, it is better to consider them as a spectrum of the same disorder. Holoprosencephaly is found in approximately 1 in 16,000 live births and occurs in association with maternal diabetes mellitus, dizygotic twinning, bleeding during early stages of pregnancy, toxo-

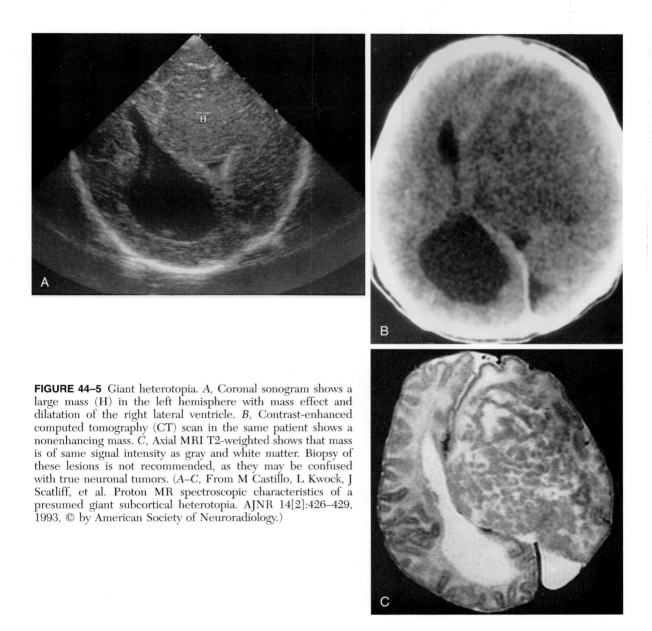

FIGURE 44–5 Giant heterotopia. *A,* Coronal sonogram shows a large mass (H) in the left hemisphere with mass effect and dilatation of the right lateral ventricle. *B,* Contrast-enhanced computed tomography (CT) scan in the same patient shows a nonenhancing mass. *C,* Axial MRI T2-weighted shows that mass is of same signal intensity as gray and white matter. Biopsy of these lesions is not recommended, as they may be confused with true neuronal tumors. (*A–C,* From M Castillo, L Kwock, J Scatliff, et al. Proton MR spectroscopic characteristics of a presumed giant subcortical heterotopia. AJNR 14[2]:426–429, 1993, © by American Society of Neuroradiology.)

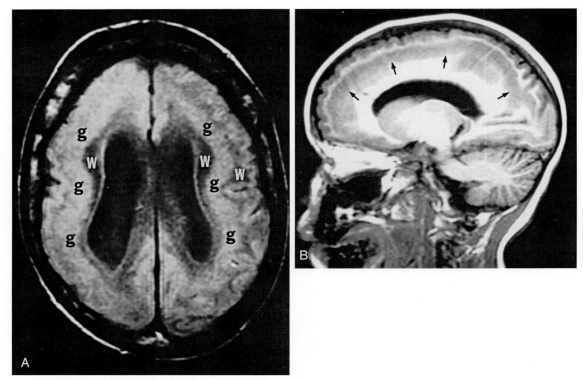

FIGURE 44–6 Band heterotopia. *A,* Axial MRI proton density shows a band of gray matter (g) between the white matter (W). *B,* Parasagittal MRI T1-weighted in a different case shows an ectopic band of gray matter *(arrows)* in the white matter and overlying pachygyria. (*A,* From Castillo M. Neuroradiology Companion. Philadelphia, Lippincott-Raven, 1995. *B,* Courtesy of S. Birchansky, M.D., Miami Children's Hospital, Miami, FL.)

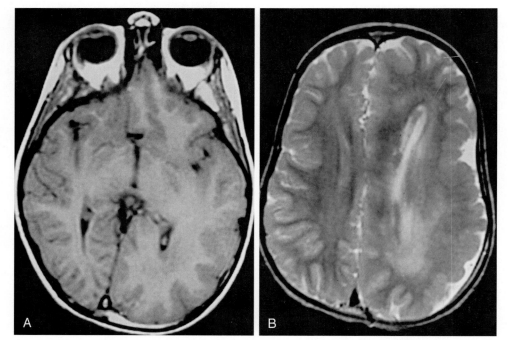

FIGURE 44–7 Hemimegaencephaly. *A,* Axial MRI T1-weighted shows an enlarged left cerebral hemisphere, which contains a thick cortex and pachygyria. *B,* In the same patient, axial MRI T2-weighted shows a pachygyric left cerebral hemisphere with underlying increased signal intensity from white matter. (*A* and *B,* Courtesy of S. Birchansky, M.D., Miami Children's Hospital, Miami, FL.)

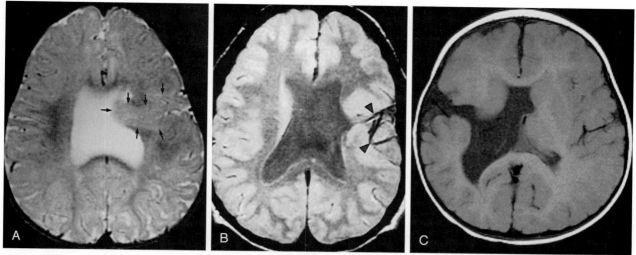

FIGURE 44–8 Schizencephaly. *A,* MRI T2-weighted shows closed-lip schizencephaly as a band of gray matter *(arrows)* extending from the cortex to the lateral ventricle, into which it projects as a nipple-like protrusion. *B,* MRI proton density shows multiple anomalous veins *(arrowheads)* associated with a closed-lip defect. *C,* Axial MRI T1-weighted shows right temporal open-lip schizencephaly. The septum pellucidum is absent, and the right lateral ventricle is enlarged. There is right frontal pachygyria. (*A* and *B,* From Castillo M. Neuroradiology Companion. Philadelphia, Lippincott-Raven, 1995.)

plasmosis, syphilis, fetal alcohol syndrome, and several chromosomal aberrations.

Alobar holoprosencephaly is the most severe type of this disorder. The face harbors defects involving its pre-maxillary segments (hypotelorism, flat nose, single nostril, central proboscis) (see Fig. 44–10*A*). Cyclopia is extremely rare, and these patients are stillborn. Microcephaly is always present. These children show failure to thrive, developmental delay, poor temperature control, seizures, and spasticity. The prognosis is uniformly poor, with death occurring before 1 year of age. On MRI

studies, the third ventricle, interhemispheric fissure, falx cerebri, septum pellucidum, and corpus callosum are absent (Fig. 44–10*B* and *C*). The thalami are fused in the midline (Fig. 44–10*D* and *E*). The brain is crescent-shaped and located mostly anteriorly (Fig. 44–10*F*). There is gray-white midline continuation. There is a single horseshoe-shaped ventricle that may communicate posteriorly with a cyst. A single anterior cerebral artery is present. The venous sinuses may be ectopic, and MRI venography aids in assessing their location before the insertion of a shunt.

The intermediate form of the disease is *semilobar holoprosencephaly.* The abnormalities are less marked than in the alobar type. There is some differentiation of the brain, particularly posteriorly (Fig. 44–11*A* and *B*). The thalami are only partially fused, and there may be a small third ventricle (Fig. 44–11*C*). The temporal and occipital horns of the lateral ventricles may be partially insinuated. The hippocampi are hypoplastic. The posterior aspects of the corpus callosum, interhemispheric fissure, and falx cerebri may be present. The septum pellucidum is absent. Patients have only mild facial anomalies, and on occasion, the face may be normal.

The mildest type of the disease is *lobar holo-prosencephaly.* In these children, the brain is nearly normal and the face is normal. The third ventricle is present, and the thalami are not fused. Rudimentary frontal horns of the lateral ventricles are present (Fig. 44–12). However, the septum pellucidum is absent. The interhemispheric fissure is well formed, but the anterior falx cerebri may be absent or hypoplastic. Some patients may have hypoplastic optic nerves and may be classified as having septo-optic dysplasia.

Septo-Optic Dysplasia

This syndrome shares imaging features with both schizencephaly and holoprosencephaly. Its main features

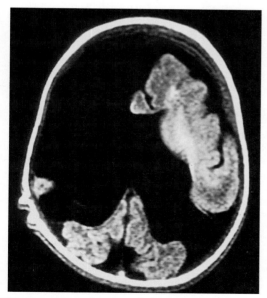

FIGURE 44–9 Bilateral open clefts versus hydranencephaly. Axial MRI T1-weighted shows large bilateral open-lip schizencephalies that are so extensive they may be considered as hydranencephaly.

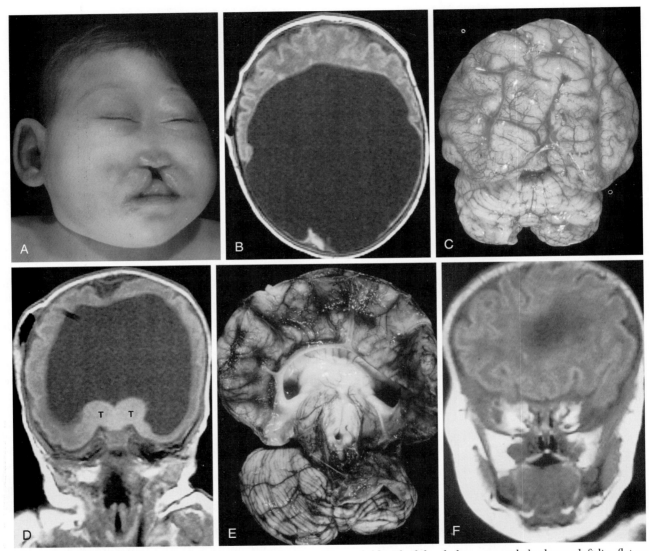

FIGURE 44–10 Alobar holoprosencephaly. *A,* Photograph of a stillborn child with alobar holoprosencephaly shows cleft lip, flat nose, hypotelorism, and microcephaly. *B,* Axial MRI T1-weighted in a different child shows a crescent-shaped brain anterior with no midline structures and a large monoventricle that communicates dorsally with a cyst. *C,* Gross specimen in a different child shows a small brain with absent midline structures. *D,* Coronal MRI T1-weighted in a different child shows a large monoventricle with fused thalami (T). *E,* Gross specimen from a different child shows a monoventricle and fused thalami. *F,* Coronal T1-weighted image in a different child shows no anterior interhemispheric fissure and absence of olfactory bulbs. (*A,* From Castillo M, Boulding TW, Scatliff JH, Suzuki K. Radiologic-pathologic correlation. Alobar holoprosencephaly. AJNR 1993;14:1151–1156.)

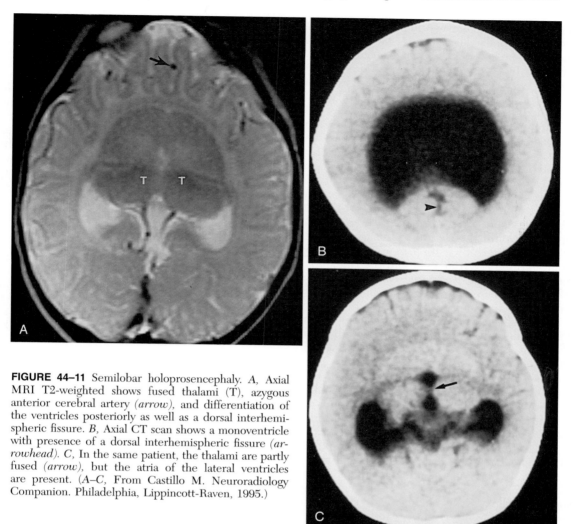

FIGURE 44-11 Semilobar holoprosencephaly. *A,* Axial MRI T2-weighted shows fused thalami (T), azygous anterior cerebral artery *(arrow),* and differentiation of the ventricles posteriorly as well as a dorsal interhemispheric fissure. *B,* Axial CT scan shows a monoventricle with presence of a dorsal interhemispheric fissure *(arrowhead). C,* In the same patient, the thalami are partly fused *(arrow),* but the atria of the lateral ventricles are present. *(A–C,* From Castillo M. Neuroradiology Companion. Philadelphia, Lippincott-Raven, 1995.)

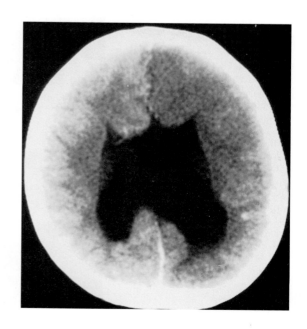

FIGURE 44-12 Lobar holoprosencephaly. Axial CT scan shows near-normal lateral ventricles with absence of the septum pellucidum. The interhemispheric fissure is present.

are hypoplasia of the optic nerves and partial or complete absence of the septum pellucidum. Its incidence is not known, and it may be inherited as an autosomal dominant or recessive trait. It is more common in firstborns. *Septo-optic dysplasia* has been linked to maternal ingestion of quinidine, anticonvulsant medications, cocaine use, diabetes mellitus, and infection of the fetus by cytomegalovirus. Clinical features include nystagmus, decreased visual acuity, hypotelorism, color blindness, hypotonia or spasticity, microcephaly, anosmia, and hyposmia.[5] The latter two may be related to an association between septo-optic dysplasia and Kallmann's syndrome. Hypoplasia of the optic nerves is better evaluated clinically (it is seen as small optic discs on funduscopy), as it is difficult to detect reliably on MRI. Septo-optic dysplasia may be divided into two groups according to clinical and imaging characteristics.[21] Approximately 65% of patients will develop hypothalamic-pituitary dysfunction, and the remainder will present with seizures. Endocrine dysfunction often consists of deficient secretion of a growth hormone, low adrenocorticotropic hormone, low thyroid-stimulating hormone, diabetes insipidus, and rarely, hyperprolactinemia and precocious puberty. In those patients with endocrine dysfunction, the septum pellucidum is partially or completely absent. The roof of the frontal horns of the lateral ventricles is flat, giving them a boxlike configuration. The optic nerves and chiasm are small in a symmetric or an asymmetric fashion. The intrasellar pituitary gland is absent, and there is translocation of the posterior lobe to the hypothalamus (Fig. 44–13). Abnormalities of the corpus callosum and hypoplasia of the hemispheric white matter may also be present. In the second group of patients, schizencephaly and neuronal migration anomalies are present. An association has been noticed by the authors of midline facial clefting with septo-optic dysplasia.

THE POSTERIOR FOSSA

Development of the Cerebellum

Early in embryonic life the cerebellum is contained inside the fourth ventricle.[22] At about 5 weeks of life, the lateral aspects of the alar plate of the rhombencephalon become thick and form the rhombic lips that will later develop into the cerebellar hemispheres. The hemispheres continue to grow; at approximately 9 weeks of life, they come in contact with each other in the midline and induce formation of the cerebellar vermis. The superior portion of the vermis is formed first, and the inferior portion last. Therefore, agenesis of the cerebellar vermis may coexist with developed hemispheres, but the reverse is not possible. Formation of the fourth ventricle also occurs simultaneously. The choroid plexus within the fourth ventricle separates the posterior and anterior membranous regions. The posterior membranous region cavitates, giving origin to the midline foramen of Magendie. The anterior membranous region normally incorporates itself into the choroid plexus. If the posterior membranous region fails to cavitate, the anterior membranous region will balloon outward as the fourth ventricle becomes fluid-filled, giving origin to the Dandy-Walker complex of malformations. The germinal matrix that surrounds the fourth ventricle generates neurons that migrate to the cerebellar cortex between 9 and 13 weeks of life. Neuronal migration continues until the end of the first year of extrauterine life.

Chiari Malformations

The *Chiari malformations* are a group of disorders involving mainly the posterior fossa.[23] In our opinion, the type I malformation is not related to the other two, but types

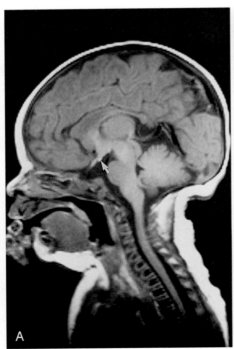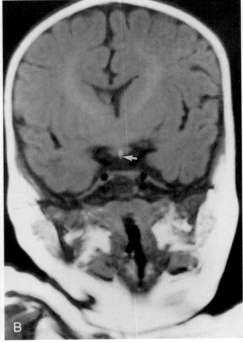

FIGURE 44–13 Septo-optic dysplasia. *A,* Midsagittal MRI T2-weighted in a child with hypoplastic optic disks on funduscopy shows absence of the pituitary stalk and translocation of the posterior lobe *(arrow)* to the hypothalamus. The corpus callosum is small. *B,* Coronal MRI T1-weighted in the same patient shows the ectopic posterior pituitary lobe *(arrow),* small optic chiasm, absent septum pellucidum, and thin corpus callosum.

II and III are likely related to each other. The so-called Chiari type IV most likely does not exist as a distinct entity and probably represents a variation of cerebellar hypoplasia.

The normal position of the cerebellar tonsils varies according to the age of the patient. The cerebellar tonsils may be located slightly inferiorly in newborns and young children but in elderly adults are commonly above the level of the foramen magnum. The position of the cerebellar tonsils is easily assessed with MRI sagittal studies slightly off the midline. Cerebellar tonsils located less than 3 mm below the foramen magnum may be considered a normal variant, and this has been called *benign tonsillar ectopia*. Tonsils located inferior to the foramen magnum by 3 to 6 mm are indeterminate, and their significance needs to be correlated with clinical symptoms. If asymptomatic, they are probably also an extreme variation of normal. Tonsils herniated inferiorly by more than 6 mm are definitely abnormal and are compatible with a Chiari type I malformation.

The *Chiari type I malformation* is the most common cerebellar anomaly identified on MRI.[24] The location of the tonsils may be determined by drawing a line between the basion and the opisthion. In this malformation, most tonsils assume a triangular configuration with their apex pointing caudally (Fig. 44–14A). Most patients with herniations over 10 mm will be symptomatic. The Chiari type I malformation is more common in females. The most common symptoms include recurrent occipital or frontal headaches, neck pain, gait abnormalities, progressive ataxia, and difficulty swallowing. Hydrocephalus is present in 25% of cases.[5] Dilatation of the central spinal cord canal (hydromyelia) is found in 20% to 80% of patients and may result in a myelopathy (Fig. 44–14B). Spinal cord cysts are more common in the upper and midcervical regions but may involve any portion of the spinal cord.

A different group of patients is defined when the cerebellar tonsillar herniation is associated with abnormalities of the base of the skull. In approximately 25% of cases, basilar invagination is present. Patients with Klippel-Feil syndrome may also have herniation of the cerebellar tonsils. Other anomalies associated with Chiari type I malformation are occipital encephaloceles and craniosynostosis.

The *Chiari type II malformation* is a complex set of anomalies involving the spinal cord, cerebellum, and cerebrum.[25] For practical purposes, all patients with this malformation have a myelomeningocele. This open spinal dysraphism is commonly located in the lumbosacral region but may involve any part of the spine. When the dysraphism involves the craniocervical junction, it may be considered a Chiari type III malformation (discussed later). Spinal cord cysts, usually in the form of syringomyelia (cysts outside the central canal), are present in approximately 50% of patients.[3] These cysts commonly involve the lower cervical and thoracic regions but may occur anywhere. Intracranially, most anomalies may be traced to the presence of a small posterior fossa. The foramen magnum is wide, the tentorial incisura is hypoplastic, and scalloping of the posterior surface of the petrous bones and clivus occurs. All of these findings are related to a mesodermal dysplasia. Although the cerebellum may appear enlarged on MRI, it is more commonly pathologically small. The cerebellar tonsils and vermis herniate inferiorly through the foramen magnum (Fig. 44–15A). Occasionally they may extend into the thoracic spine. The choroid plexus is also displaced inferiorly and should not be confused with a true enhancing tumor on postcontrast MRI studies. The upper medulla is also dragged inferiorly and kinks at its attachments with the dentate ligaments (so-called cervicomedullary kink). Anomalies of cervical vertebral segmentation are present in about 10% of patients, and the posterior arch of C1 may be absent. In an attempt to accommodate themselves

FIGURE 44–14 Chiari type I malformation. *A,* Midsagittal MRI T1-weighted shows cerebellar tonsillar herniation (T) 10 mm below the foramen magnum. *B,* In a different case of Chiari type I malformation, midsagittal MRI T1-weighted shows multiseptated syringomyelia in the cervical and upper thoracic spinal cord.

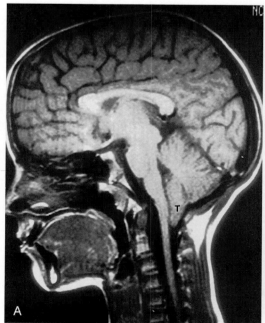
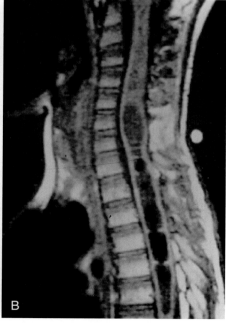

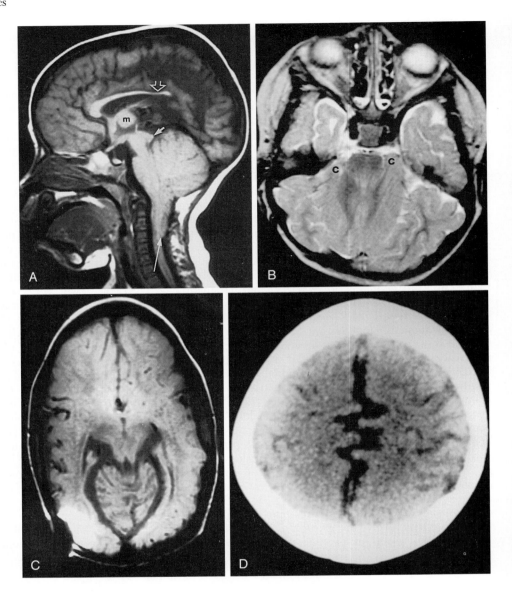

FIGURE 44–15 Chiari type II malformation. *A,* Midsagittal MRI T1-weighted shows herniation of the vermis *(long arrow)* below the foramen magnum, absent fourth ventricle, smooth cerebellar vermis, beaked tectum *(short arrow),* large massa intermedia (m), small third ventricle, and dysplastic corpus callosum *(open arrow). B,* Axial MRI T2-weighted in a different patient shows the cerebellar hemispheres (c) wrapping laterally and anteriorly to the brain stem. *C,* Axial MRI proton density in a different case of Chiari type II malformation shows incompetent tentorial incisura with upward projection of the heart-shaped cerebellum. *D,* Axial CT scan shows absent falx cerebri with midline interdigitation of the gyri. (*D,* From Castillo M. Neuroradiology Companion. Philadelphia, Lippincott-Raven, 1995.)

within the small posterior fossa, the cerebellar hemispheres grow anteriorly, filling the cerebellopontine angle cisterns and may even wrap around the brain stem (Fig. 44–15B). They should not be confused with true masses in these regions. The vermis is smooth and the fourth ventricle should be barely present or not visible. In patients with Chiari type II malformations who have been shunted, the presence of a "normal"-appearing fourth ventricle should be considered abnormal and possibly indicative of shunt malfunction. The dorsal midbrain is disorganized, with fusion of the superior and inferior colliculi giving it a "beaked" appearance. Within the brain stem, its nuclei are disorganized. The cerebellum may tower superiorly via an incompetent tentorial incisura and, on axial images, assumes a heart-shaped configuration (Fig. 44–15C). Supratentorially, the corpus callosum may be absent. In these cases, the white matter in the forceps major is deficient and results in dilatation of the atria and occipital horns of the lateral ventricles (colpocephaly). Gray matter heterotopias may be present. The

falx cerebri may be absent, hypoplastic, or fenestrated, and this leads to midline interdigitation of gyri (Fig. 44–15D). The third ventricle is small, and the massa intermedia of the thalami appears enlarged on midsagittal MRI T1-weighted studies. Hydrocephalus is common and at times may be due to stenosis of the aqueduct of Sylvius. The cortical sulci in the parieto-occipital regions are numerous but histologically normal (stenogyria).

The *Chiari type III malformation* comprises anomalies similar to those of the type II malformation in addition to a high cervical and low occipital encephalocele[26] (Fig. 44–16). All of the anomalies described earlier for the Chiari type II malformation may be present in these patients. The encephalocele involves the cerebellum and upper cervical spinal cord but may also include the occipital and posterior parietal lobes. The brain stem may be dragged posteriorly. The herniated tissues may contain brain, cisterns, the fourth ventricle, and commonly, venous structures. The intracranial dural venous sinuses are commonly aberrant in position, and MRI venography

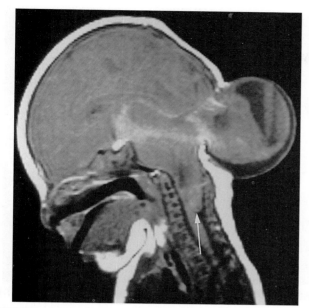

FIGURE 44–16 Chiari type III malformation. Midsagittal MRI T1-weighted shows an occipital encephalocele and inferiorly displaced cerebellar vermis (*arrow*).

helps to verify their location before surgery. The contents of the herniated sac are composed of disorganized and nonfunctioning brain, which may be safely resected. Therefore, prognosis is directly related to the size of the encephalocele and to the number of anomalies harbored by the intracranial brain. Syringomyelia may also be present in the cervical spinal cord.

The cause of these three malformations is uncertain.

Types II and III are probably the result of anomalous closure of the neural tube that results in the chronic escape of CSF during intrauterine life.[27] This leads to intracranial hypotension with inferior displacement of the brain stem and cerebellum. A second contributing factor is related to the altered expression of surface molecules in the developing surface of the brain.[27] These molecules are a requirement for normal closure of the neural tube and for the formation of cavities within the brain.

Dandy-Walker Anomalies

The *Dandy-Walker complex of malformations* includes the classic syndrome, the variant, and the megacisterna magna. Precise differentiation between them may not be possible by MRI; therefore, the term *Dandy-Walker complex* has been suggested.[28] The genesis of the most severe *Dandy-Walker syndrome* is probably related to incomplete opening of the foramina of the fourth ventricle with massive dilatation. The insult also involves the developing cerebellar hemispheres. In the *Dandy-Walker variant*, the insult is primarily to the developing cerebellar hemisphere. Lastly, in the *megacisterna magna*, the insult is probably isolated to the fourth ventricle. Dandy-Walker syndrome occurs in approximately 1 in 30,000 live births.[5] Most cases are sporadic, but familial instances are known to occur. Systemic associations include polycystic kidneys, cataracts, and retinal abnormalities. Most patients show development delay. In the full Dandy-Walker syndrome, the fourth ventricle balloons out and fills the posterior fossa (Fig. 44–17A). The cerebellar hemispheres are hypoplastic (Fig. 44–17B). The vermis is hypoplastic, and only its superior lobules are present. The posterior fossa is large, and the tentorium inserts higher than nor-

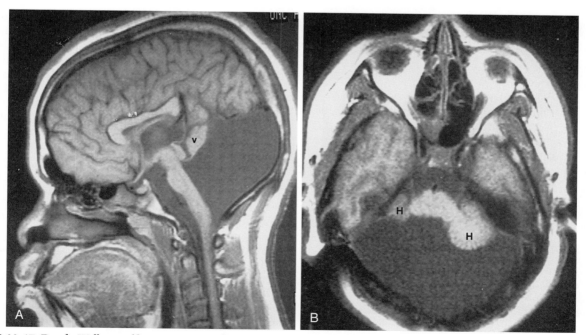

FIGURE 44–17 Dandy-Walker malformation. *A*, Midsagittal MRI T1-weighted shows a very large fourth ventricle and a hypoplastic vermis (v), which is rotated superiorly. The corpus callosum is also dysplastic. *B*, Axial MRI T1-weighted shows a large cerebrospinal fluid cyst in the posterior fossa and hypoplastic cerebellar hemispheres (H).

mal. The venous torcular is also therefore higher than the straight sinus, and this is referred to as *torcular inversion*. All of these patients will eventually develop hydrocephalus. The corpus callosum is dysgenetic in approximately one-third of the cases.[29] Gray matter heterotopias are present in 10% of patients. Occipital cephaloceles may be seen but, in our experience, are rare in the presence of a Dandy-Walker syndrome.

In the Dandy-Walker variant, the anomalies are generally confined to the posterior fossa with the cerebral hemispheres having a normal appearance on MRI. The fourth ventricle is dilated but may be less prominent than it is in the full syndrome. The cerebellar vallecula is wide. The posterior fossa is normal in size. The vermis is hypoplastic, but its dorsal lobules may be present in addition to its superior lobules. In the megacisterna magna, a large CSF-filled structure is located inferior and posterior to the cerebellum (Fig. 44–18). The vermis is normal or near normal but may be rotated superiorly. The cerebellar vallecula is enlarged, and the fourth ventricle may be mildly prominent. The inferior aspect of the posterior fossa may be expanded presumably owing to pulsations of CSF within the large cistern. Supratentorially, there are no abnormalities.

Arachnoid Cyst

Although *arachnoid cysts* are not always classified as congenital abnormalities of the posterior fossa, they are discussed here because they should be considered in the differential diagnosis of cerebellar cystic lesions. The

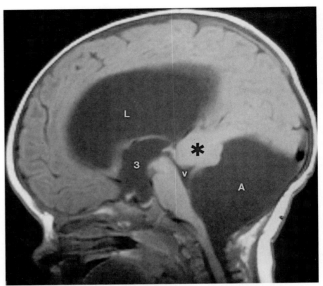

FIGURE 44–19 Posterior fossa arachnoid cyst. Midsagittal MRI T1-weighted shows a large posterior fossa arachnoid cyst (A) with compression of the fourth ventricle (v) and a superiorly displaced and compressed cerebellar vermis *(asterisk)*. The third (3) and lateral (L) ventricles are dilated. (From Castillo M, Mukherji SK. Imaging of the Pediatric Head, Neck, and Spine. Philadelphia, Lippincott-Raven, 1996.)

cause of these cysts is uncertain, but they appear to represent an anomalous development of the subarachnoid space. The walls of these cysts are formed by arachnoid cells that secrete fluid.[30] Some cysts, however, may fill with CSF by action of a "ball-valve"–like mechanism. Those within the posterior fossa account for 10% of all intracranial arachnoid cysts. In the posterior fossa, they commonly occupy the region of the cisterna magna, but they may also be located in the cerebellopontine angle regions (Fig. 44–19). Arachnoid cysts classically compress the fourth ventricle and result in hydrocephalus. The calvarium may be expanded. Arachnoid cysts may be differentiated from a megacisterna magna because they are not crossed by veins and they displace the falx cerebelli. Also, in patients with a megacisterna magna, the configuration and position of the fourth ventricle are normal.

Joubert's Syndrome

This syndrome is usually inherited as an autosomal recessive trait and occurs more commonly in males. Its incidence is unknown. It may be associated with the Dandy-Walker malformation, occipital encephaloceles, and Werdnig-Hoffman disease. Clinically, these patients present with neonatal hyperpnea, apnea, abnormal eye movements, ataxia, and mental retardation.[31] Some of these children fall into the category of oculomotor apraxia.[32] In patients with Joubert's syndrome, the cerebellar vermis is nearly or completely absent. The cerebellar hemispheres are dysplastic and may harbor neuronal migration anomalies. Histologically, the pyramidal decussations, inferior olivary nuclei, descending trigeminal tracts, solitary fasci-

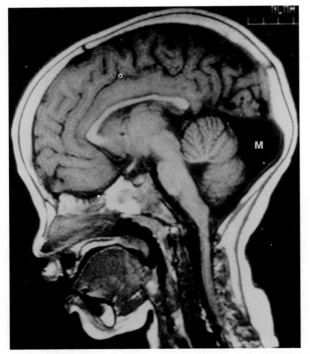

FIGURE 44–18 Megacisterna magna. Midsagittal MRI T1-weighted shows a large cisterna magna (M). The vermis is well formed, and there is no mass effect on the fourth ventricle. The calvarium is scalloped dorsal to this cistern.

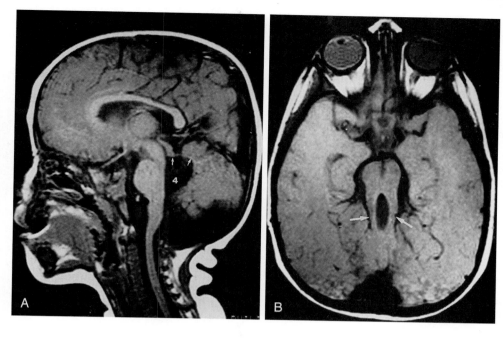

FIGURE 44–20 Joubert's syndrome. *A*, Midsagittal MRI T1-weighted shows a large fourth ventricle (4), which is bulbous superiorly *(arrows)*. *B*, Axial MRI T1-weighted shows that the superior cerebellar peduncles are parallel with each other and elongated *(arrows)*. The vermis is absent.

cles, and dorsal column nuclei may be absent. MRI sagittal studies show an absent vermis and horizontally oriented superior cerebellar peduncles (Fig. 44–20*A*). Axial images show that the fourth ventricle has a "bat-wing" configuration and is bulbous superiorly. The superior cerebellar peduncles are parallel to each other on axial MRI studies (Fig. 44–20*B*). The cerebellar hemispheres are separated in the midline. The tectum may be dysplastic.

Rhombencephalosynapsis

In this extremely rare malformation, the vermis is absent and the cerebellar hemispheres are fused across the midline.[33] Its incidence is not known. Clinical symptoms include mental retardation, abnormal equilibrium, seizures, convergent strabismus, optic nerve atrophy, spasticity, behavioral disorders, dysarthria, and apraxia. In many instances, the symptoms are related to the degree and number of supratentorial anomalies rather than to the cerebellar malformation. The majority of patients die in infancy. Pathologically, there is fusion of the cerebellar hemispheres, dentate nuclei, superior cerebellar peduncles, and thalami. The septum pellucidum may be absent, and hydrocephalus may be present. On axial MRI studies, there is midline continuation of the cerebellar white matter and also of the surface folia and sulci (Fig. 44–21*A*). The fourth ventricle assumes a "keyhole" configuration. The quadrigeminal plate is dysplastic. The brain stem is small, and the tentorial incisura may be incompetent. Often, the corpus callosum is dysgenetic (Fig. 44–21*B*). In some patients, findings similar to those of septo-optic dysplasia may be present. The hippocampi may also be hypoplastic.

THE SUBARACHNOID SPACE
Development

The brain is surrounded by a sheath of mesenchyme called the *meninx primitiva*.[7] This meninx primitiva will differentiate into the pia and the subarachnoid spaces. Anomalous differentiation of pluripotential cells in the immature subarachnoid spaces results in the formation of lipomas. As such, lipomas are not tumors but rather congenital lesions. Arachnoid cysts may also be considered as congenital lesions of the subarachnoid space. Arachnoid cysts arising in the posterior fossa have been discussed previously. In this section, supratentorial arachnoid cysts are addressed.

Lipomas

Because they arise within the subarachnoid space, lipomas will encase normal structures such as cranial nerves and blood vessels. Almost one-half of all intracranial lipomas occur in the region of the interhemispheric fissure and are commonly associated with dysgenesis of the corpus callosum (Fig. 44–22*A*). Intracranial lipomas may also be associated with median facial cleft syndromes, cephaloceles, and scalp lipomas. Other locations are the peritectal region, suprasellar region, cerebellopontine angle cisterns, and the sylvian fissures[7] (Fig. 44–22*B*). Computed tomography (CT) shows calcifications within or in the periphery of the fatty mass. On MRI, these lipomas follow the signal intensity of fat on all sequences, and their signal may be decreased with the use of fat-suppression techniques.

Arachnoid Cysts

As discussed earlier, arachnoid cysts are focal expansions of the subarachnoid space. The cells lining their walls secrete CSF.[30] The most common location is the middle cranial fossa, where they tend to expand posteriorly, following the course of the sylvian fissure (Fig. 44–23). Other supratentorial locations include the suprasellar cistern, quadrigeminal plate cistern, interhemispheric fissure, and cerebral convexities.[30] They may produce sei-

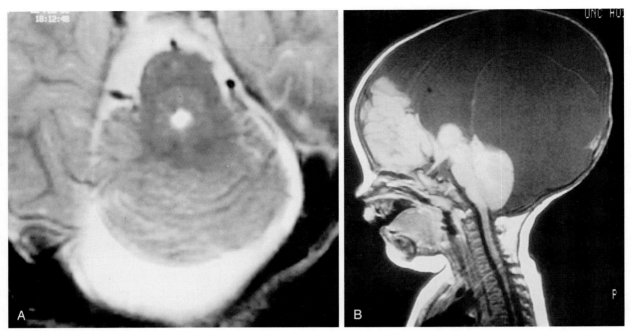

FIGURE 44–21 Rhombencephalosynapsis. *A,* Axial MRI T2-weighted shows an absent cerebellar vermis with midline fusion of the cerebellar hemispheres. *B,* Midsagittal MRI T1-weighted in the same patient shows an absent fourth ventricle, large posterior fossa cyst, absent corpus callosum, and large supratentorial cyst. (*A* and *B,* From Castillo M, Mukherji SK. Imaging of the Pediatric Head, Neck, and Spine. Philadelphia, Lippincott-Raven, 1996.)

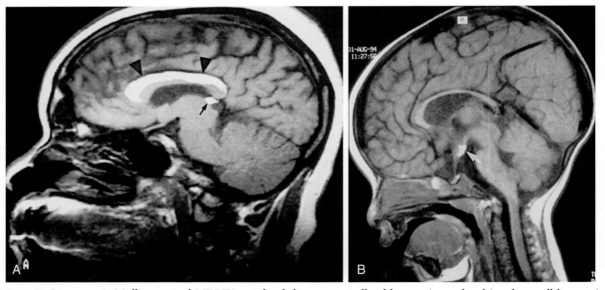

FIGURE 44–22 Lipomas. *A,* Midline sagittal MRI T1-weighted shows a pericallosal lipoma *(arrowheads)* and a small lipoma *(arrow)* in the quadrigeminal plate region. *B,* Midsagittal MRI T1-weighted in a different child shows a lipoma *(arrow)* in the suprasellar region. (*A* and *B,* From Castillo M. Neuroradiology Companion. Philadelphia, Lippincott-Raven, 1995.)

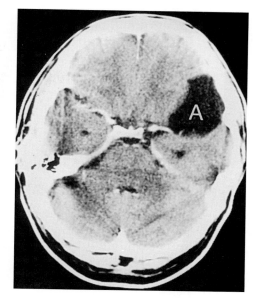

FIGURE 44–23 Arachnoid cyst. Axial postcontrast CT scan shows a cerebrospinal fluid density cyst (A) in the left middle cranial fossa splaying the sylvian fissure. (From Castillo M. Neuroradiology Companion. Philadelphia, Lippincott-Raven, 1995.)

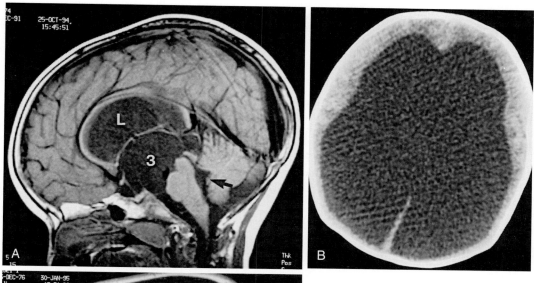

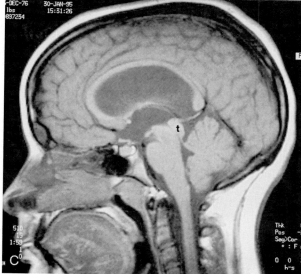

FIGURE 44–24 Aqueductal stenosis. *A,* Midsagittal MRI T1-weighted shows a normal size fourth ventricle *(arrow)* and enlarged third (3) and lateral (L) ventricles due to a web in the superior aspect of aqueduct of Sylvius. *B,* Axial CT scan in a different patient with aqueductal stenosis shows severe dilatation of the lateral ventricles. *C,* Midsagittal MRI T1-weighted shows dilatation of the third and lateral ventricles with a normal size fourth ventricle. The tectum (t) is deformed and appears bulbous and was of high T2 signal intensity but did not enhance after gadolinium administration. The possibility of tumor at this level cannot be excluded.

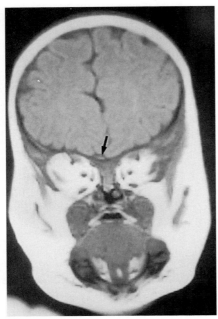

FIGURE 44–25 Kallmann's syndrome. Coronal MRI T1-weighted in a child with hypogonadism shows an absent left olfactory bulb and a normal right olfactory bulb *(arrow)*. (From Castillo M, Mukherji SK. Imaging of the Pediatric Head, Neck, and Spine. Philadelphia, Lippincott-Raven, 1996.)

zures, headaches, hemiparesis, and hydrocephalus but are usually asymptomatic. When they occur in the middle cranial fossa, the underlying temporal lobe may be hypoplastic and the sphenoid bone deformed. Arachnoid cysts are of CSF density on CT and isointense to CSF on all MRI sequences. They do not enhance after contrast administration. They may produce scalloping of the overlying calvarium. Occasionally, they may contain blood, and they can bleed spontaneously.

OTHER CONGENITAL ANOMALIES

Aqueductal Stenosis

Embryologically, the aqueduct of Sylvius is formed by compression of the primitive ventricular system by the growing midbrain. Aqueductal stenosis occurs in 1 in 1000 live births and accounts for approximately 20% of all cases of hydrocephalus. Although it is more commonly diagnosed during childhood, it may present in adults. Anatomically, the aqueduct may be absent, may contain a membrane or web, may be segmentally hypoplastic, or may be forked[34] (Fig. 44–24A). The overlying tectum may be intrinsically deformed and extrinsically compressed by dilated ventricles. Aqueductal stenosis may also be secondary to gliosis and secondary to prior infections or hemorrhage. The onset of hydrocephalus is clinically insidious and characterized by chronic headaches and other signs of increased intracranial pressure. By imaging studies, the classic appearance is that of dilatation of the lateral and third ventricles with a normally sized fourth ventricle (Fig. 44–24B). MRI should be performed to

rule out a small tectal neoplasm (such as astrocytoma) that may initially result in hydrocephalus (Fig. 44–24C).

Kallmann's Syndrome

This syndrome is clinically characterized by anosmia and hyposmia and hypogonadism owing to low levels of gonadotropin hormone and testosterone. In addition, secretion of luteinizing and follicle-stimulating hormones is markedly decreased.[35] Embryologically, Kallmann's syndrome results from a failure of genetic expression of protein cell markers that guide the migration of cells from the olfactory placodes to the hypothalamus. On MRI, the olfactory bulbs are dysplastic, hypoplastic, or absent (Fig. 44–25). They may appear as masses *(neuromatous masses)*.[35] On the undersurface of the frontal lobes, the olfactory sulci are not present. The anterior lobe of the pituitary gland may be small or absent, and the neurohypophysis may be translocated to the hypothalamus.

References

1. Barkovich AJ. Normal development of the neonatal and infant brain, skull, and spine. In Barkovich AJ (ed). Pediatric Neuroimaging, 2nd ed., pp. 9–38. New York, Raven, 1995.
2. Barkovich AJ, Lyon G, Evrard P. Formation, maturation, and disorders of the white matter. AJNR 1992;13:447–461.
3. Castillo M, Dominguez R. Imaging of common congenital anomalies of the brain and spine. Clin Imaging 1992;16:73–88.
4. Barkovich AJ, Kjos BO. Normal postnatal development of the corpus callosum as demonstrated by MR imaging. AJNR 1988;9:487–491.
5. Castillo M, Mukherji SK (eds). Imaging of the Pediatric Head, Neck, and Spine. Philadelphia, JB Lippincott, 1996.
6. Barkovich AJ, Norman D. Anomalies of the corpus callosum: Correlation with further anomalies of the brain. AJNR 1988;9:493–501.
7. Truwit CL, Barkovich AJ. Pathogenesis of intracranial lipomas: An MR study in 42 patients. AJNR 1990;11:665–674.
8. McArdle CB, Richardson CJ, Nicholas DA, et al. Developmental features of the neonatal brain: MR imaging. Part 1. Gray-white matter differentiation and myelination. Radiology 1987;162:223–229.
9. Barkovich AJ, Gressens P, Evrard P. Formation, maturation, and disorders of the brain neocortex. AJNR 1992;13:423–446.
10. Barkovich AJ, Koch TK, Carrol CL. The spectrum of lissencephaly: Report of ten cases analyzed by magnetic resonance imaging. Ann Neurol 1991;30:139–146.
11. Dobyns WB, Kirkpatrick JB, Hittner HM, et al. Syndromes with lissencephaly. 2: Walker-Warburg and cerebral ocular muscular syndromes and a new syndrome with type 2 lissencephaly. Am J Med Genet 1985;22:157–195.
12. Barkovich AJ, Kjos BO. Non-lissencephalic cortical dysplasia: Correlation of imaging findings with developmental and neurological manifestations. Radiology 1992;182:493–499.
13. Barkovich AJ. Abnormal vascular drainage in anomalies of neuronal migration. AJNR 1988;9:939–942.
14. Smith AS, Weinstein MA, Quencer RM, et al. Association of heterotopic gray matter with seizures: MR imaging. Radiology 1988;168:195–198.
15. Barkovich AJ, Kjos BO. Gray matter heterotopias: MR characteristics and correlation with developmental and neurological manifestations. Radiology 1992;182:493–499.
16. Barkovich AJ, Jackson DE, Boyer RS. Band heterotopias: A newly recognized neuronal migration anomaly. Radiology 1989;171:455–458.
17. Barkovich AJ, Chuang SH. Unilateral megalencephaly: Correlation of MR imaging and pathologic characteristics. AJNR 1990;11:523–531.
18. Castillo M. MRI of schizencephaly. MRI Decis 1992;6:22–26.
19. Barkovich AJ, Kjos BO. Schizencephaly: Correlation of clinical findings and MR characteristics. AJNR 1992;13:85–94.

20. Castillo M, Boulding TW, Scatliff JH, Suzuki K. Radiologic-pathologic correlation. Alobar holoprosencephaly. AJNR 1993;14:1151–1156.
21. Barkovich AJ, Fram EK, Norman D. MR of septo-optic dysplasia. Radiology 1989;171:189–192.
22. Barkovich AJ. Congenital malformations. In Barkovich AJ (ed). Pediatric Neuroimaging, pp. 246–248. New York, Raven, 1995.
23. Castillo M. Imaging of Chiari malformations. Appl Radiol 1992;21:31–37.
24. Elster AD, Chen MYM. Chiari 1 malformations: Clinical and radiologic reappraisal. Radiology 1992;183:347–353.
25. Wolpert SM, Anderson M, Scott RM, et al. The Chiari II malformation: MR imaging evaluation. AJNR 1987;8:783–791.
26. Castillo M, Quencer RM, Dominguez R. Chiari III malformation: Imaging features. AJNR 1992;13:107–113.
27. McClone DG, Naidich TP. Developmental morphology of the subarachnoid space, brain vasculature and contiguous structures, and the cause of the Chiari II malformation. AJNR 1992;13:463–482.
28. Barkovich AJ, Kjos BO, Norman D, Edwards MSB. Revised classification of posterior fossa cysts and cyst-like malformations based on results of multiplanar MR imaging. AJNR 1989;10:977–988.
29. Altman NR, Naidich TP, Braffman BH. Posterior fossa malformations. AJNR 1992;13:691–724.
30. Barkovich AJ. Hydrocephalus. In Barkovich AJ (ed). Pediatric Neuroimaging, pp. 448–453. New York, Raven, 1995.
31. Kendall B, Kingsley D, Lambert SR, et al. Joubert syndrome: A clinico-radiological study. Neuroradiology 1990;31:502–506.
32. Whitsel EA, Castillo M, D'Cruz O. Cerebellar vermis and midbrain dysgenesis in oculomotor apraxia: MR findings. AJNR 1995;16:831–834.
33. Truwit CL, Barkovich AJ, Shanahan R, Maroldo TV. MR imaging of rhombencephalosynapsis: Report of three cases and review of the literature. AJNR 1991;12:957–965.
34. Barkovich AJ, Edwards MSB. Applications of neuroimaging in hydrocephalus. Pediatr Neurosurg 1992;18:65–83.
35. Truwit CL, Barkovich AJ, Grumbach MM, Martini JJ. MR imaging of Kallmann's syndrome: A genetic disorder of neuronal migration affecting the olfactory and genital systems. AJNR 1993;14:827–838.

45

Imaging of Congenital Abnormalities of the Spine and Spinal Cord

M A U R I C I O   C A S T I L L O, M.D.

S U R E S H   K.   M U K H E R J I, M.D.

Congenital defects of the spine and spinal cord require magnetic resonance imaging (MRI) for optimal evaluation, and the findings addressed in this chapter refer to MRI unless otherwise stated. Knowledge of the embryology of this region is indispensable for understanding its different anomalies. Here, for purposes of discussion, we have grouped these anomalies according to their embryology.

EMBRYOLOGY OF THE SPINE

Between 12 and 14 days of life, ectodermal cells located in the cephalic portion of the embryonic disk migrate to establish the notochord.[1] The notochord is located anterior to a depression (the primitive streak) on the dorsal aspect of the embryonic disk. This depression deepens and becomes the neural groove (Fig. 45–1A). On both sides of the neural groove are the neural crests that undergo progressive infolding until the neural tube is completely closed (Fig. 45–1B). The closure of the neural tube begins in its midportion and progresses *both caudad and cephalad*. The neural tube contains communications between the notochord and the yolk sac and amnion. These communications are referred to as the *canals of Kovalevsky* and normally involute about the 17th day of life.[2] At 25 days, the closure of the neural tube is complete. At this time, the neural tube separates from the overlying ectoderm. The mesenchyme, which surrounds the tube, will produce the bones of the spine (sclerotome) and the paraspinal muscles (myotome). The notochord induces the formation of all of the structures listed and later involutes, leaving behind only the nucleus pulposus of the intervertebral disks.

The formation of the distal spine is, however, incomplete at this stage. A blending of the distal notochord and the neural tube results in the caudal cell mass (see Fig. 45–1C). This mass is canalized by multiple vacuoles that coalesce to form a central cavity. When this central cavity is formed, the caudal cell mass begins to differentiate into the neural structures that will give rise to the conus medullaris. The distalmost part of the caudal cell mass involutes, leaving behind the filum terminale. This process is termed *canalization of retrogressive differentiation*. The embryology of the vertebral bodies is discussed separately (see later).

According to this sequence of events, congenital disorders of the spine may be divided into

1. Disorders of abnormal notochordal development: diastematomyelia, diplomyelia, and neurenteric cysts and fistulas
2. Disorders of closure (neurulation) of the tube: myeloceles and myelomeningoceles
3. Disorders of abnormal separation (nondisjunction or premature disjunction) of the neural tube from the mesoderm and ectoderm: lipomyeloceles, lipomyelomeningoceles, epidermoids, dermoids, dermal sinuses, and lipomas
4. Disorders of canalization and retrogressive differentiation: lipomas of the filum terminale, tight filum terminale syndrome, caudal regression syndrome, myelocystocele, terminal myelocystocele, teratoma, and anterior sacral meningoceles.
5. Disorders of vertebral segmentation and notochordal resorption: hemivertebrae, block vertebrae, and butterfly vertebrae
6. Spinal cord cysts

These congenital disorders of the spine are optimally studied with MRI. Contrast administration is not routinely needed.

DISORDERS ARISING FROM ABNORMAL NOTOCHORDAL DEVELOPMENT

Diastematomyelia

Diastematomyelia is a sagittal splitting of the spinal cord. Embryologically, it is possible that a persistent canal of

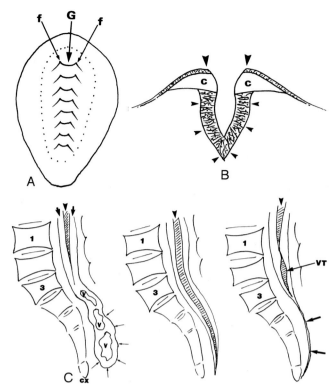

FIGURE 45–1 Development of the spine. *A,* Diagram showing the embryonic disk. On its dorsal surface is a midline depression called the neural groove (G), which is flanked on each side by the neural folds (f). *B,* With progressive development, the neural groove deepens and differentiates into neuroectoderm (*small arrowheads*). The neural crests (c) are composed of mesodermal elements and superficial ectoderm (*large arrowheads*). *C, Left:* Formation of the distal spine involves vacuolization (v) of the caudal cell mass (*thin arrows*). 1, first lumbar vertebra; 3, third lumbar vertebra; cx, coccyx; *thick* arrows, spinal cord; *arrowhead,* central spinal canal. *Middle:* The caudal cell mass differentiates and is now thinner and continuous with the spinal cord. The vacuoles have merged into a single cavity that communicates with the central spinal canal. *Right:* The caudal cell mass differentiates into the filum terminale (*arrows*), and its central cavity is obliterated. The distal spinal canal (*arrowhead*) narrows, but the superior extent of the caudal cell mass vacuoles may remain patent at the ventriculus terminalis (VT). (*A–C,* From Castillo M, Mukherji SK. Imaging of the Pediatric Head, Neck, and Spine. Philadelphia, Lippincott-Raven, 1996.)

Kovalevsky acts as a physical barrier to the migrating notochord.[2] Therefore, the notochord is forced to migrate around this obstruction, dividing itself and inducing the formation of two hemicords.

Clinically, these patients often have a cutaneous abnormality overlying the site of diastematomyelia. These abnormalities include hairy patches, nevi, lipomas, dimples, or hemangiomas.[3] The patients may also have difficulty in controlling bowels and bladder; club feet or dislocated hips or both; myelopathy; and impotence later in life. Diastematomyelia is more common in girls. It may be found in 5% of patients with scoliosis and in up to one-third of patients with myelomeningocele.[3] Pathologically,

diastematomyelia may be divided into external and internal types. In external diastematomyelia there is a septum that spits the spinal cord, and each hemicord is contained within its own subarachnoid space and meningeal sheath (Fig. 45–2A).[4] The septum may be fibrous, bony, cartilaginous, fatty, or any combination of these. The septum arises from the posterior elements and joins the vertebral body, which is always abnormal. In about 5% of cases, multiple spurs may be present. The conus medullaris is low lying, and the spinal cord is tethered at the site of the spur in all patients. Bony spurs are well seen by computed tomography (CT), but fibrous spurs need to be imaged with postmyelogram CT or gradient-echo axial and coronal T2-weighted MRI. This latter technique takes advantage of magnetic susceptibility artifacts induced by the spurs against the background of bright cerebrospinal fluid (CSF). When a patient with a myelomeningocele, de novo or previously repaired, is evaluated, the entire spine should be imaged with MRI to exclude a diastem.

In internal diastematomyelia, there is no spur (see Fig. 45–2B and C). The cord is divided into hemicords that are contained within the same thecal sac. This combination accounts for approximately 50% of cases of diastematomyelia.[3] Rarely, intraspinal epidermoids or dermoids may be found in association with diastematomyelia. Screening of this abnormality may be performed with sonography (see Fig. 45–2B), but definitive imaging requires MRI (see Fig. 45–2C).

Diplomyelia

Diplomyelia is a complete duplication of the spinal cord, that is, by definition each hemicord must contain one pair of ventral nerve rootlets and one pair of dorsal nerve rootlets. In order for this to occur, duplication of the spinal column is required. In this extremely rare malformation, it is possible that the persistence of a canal of Kovalevsky leads to complete duplication of the notochord, neural tube, and overlying mesoderm and ectoderm.[5] Another plausible hypothesis is that the migration of mesodermal cells along sides of the primitive streak results in duplication of the caudal cell mass and in the formation of double distal spines.[5] Gastrointestinal and genitourinary anomalies are common in patients with diplomyelia.[6] CT and MRI show complete duplication of the bony spine, but the accessory spine may be dysmorphic and have little resemblance to a normal one. The spinal cord is duplicated, and each spine contains individual sets of neural foramina (Fig. 45–3). The spinal cord may contain fluid-filled cysts and there may be diastems.

Neurenteric Cysts and Fistulas

Neurenteric cysts and fistulas may be obvious at birth due to severe vertebral anomalies but may also present later in life. In the latter group of patients, the cysts and fistulas are small and intraspinal and present with local pain and myelopathy. Cysts and fistulas commonly tend to involve the lower cervical and upper thoracic regions but may be found anywhere in the spine (Fig. 45–4).[1] Neurenteric cysts are located in the intradural compart-

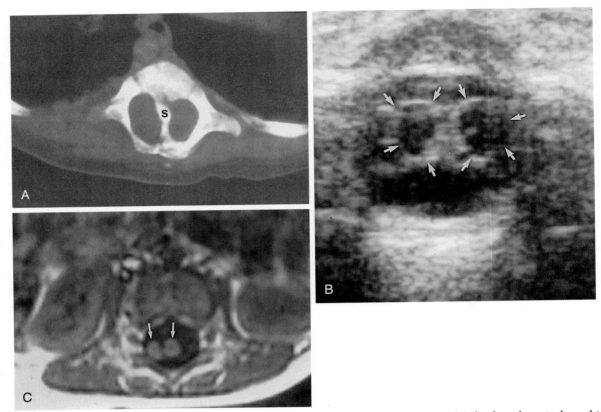

FIGURE 45–2 Diastematomyelia. *A*, Axial computed tomography (CT) scan shows a bony spur (S) dividing the spinal canal into two compartments in a case of external diastematomyelia. *B*, Axial sonogram shows two hemicords *(arrows)*. *C*, Axial T1-weighted magnetic resonance imaging (MRI) study in the same patient and at the same level shows two hemicords *(arrows)*. Note the absence of a spur in this case of internal diastematomyelia. Note a central canal in each hemicord.

FIGURE 45–3 Diplomyelia. *A*, Coronal T1-weighted MRI study shows two coni medullaris *(small arrows)* and a distal spinal cord cyst *(large arrow)*. *B*, In the same patient, this section shows duplication of the sacrum *(asterisks)*. Each sacrum has two sets of neural foramina with duplicated nerve roots *(arrowheads)*, implying complete duplication of neural elements. (*A* and *B*, Reprinted from Magn Reson Imaging, vol. 10. Castillo M, Hankins L, Kramer L, Wilson BA. MR imaging of diplomyelia, pp. 699–703, ©1992, with kind permission from Elsevier Science Ltd, The Boulevard, Langford Lane, Kidlington 0X5 1GB, UK.)

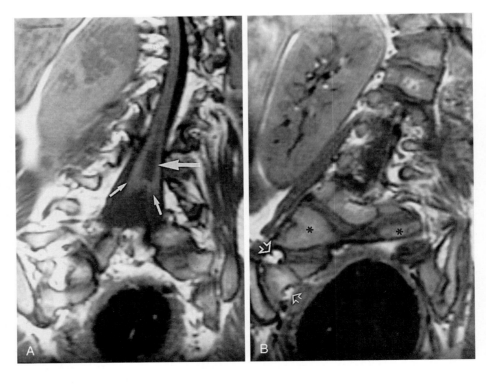

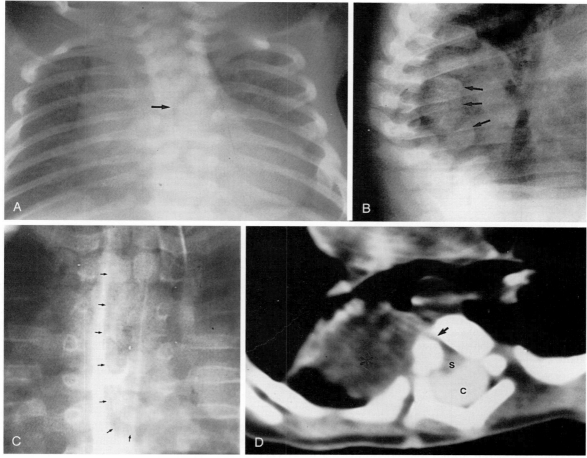

FIGURE 45–4 Neurenteric fistula and cyst. *A,* Frontal chest radiograph in a newborn shows anomalies of vertebral segmentation *(arrow)* in the midthoracic spine. *B,* Lateral radiograph also shows segmentation anomalies *(arrows).* *C,* Frontal view from myelogram suggests the presence of an intraspinal cyst *(arrows).* *D,* Postmyelogram computed tomography scan shows that the dorsal cyst (C) has filled with contrast material. The spinal cord (S) lies in the anterior of the canal and is tethered by the fistula *(arrow),* which traverses the segmentation defect in the vertebral body. The fistula communicates with a gastrointestinal tract duplication cyst *(asterisk).*

ment but outside the spinal cord. These cysts are more common in a ventral location, but they may be lateral and occasionally dorsal. If dorsal, they usually result in a vertical split of the spinal cord (diastematomyelia). As a general rule, all neurenteric cysts and fistulas are accompanied by bony abnormalities that include segmentation defects, intervertebral body fusions, scoliosis, and widening of the spinal canal. The cysts or fistulas are commonly located at or above the level of the vertebral abnormalities. The cyst usually contains fluid and is hard to see by CT unless myelographic contrast material has previously been introduced into the thecal sac. By MRI, these cysts may be isointense to CSF or of high T1-signal intensity, a finding that may be related to proteins or blood within the cyst.[1] There may be associated fistulas with the gastrointestinal tract that may tether the spinal cord. Gastrointestinal duplication cysts may also be present.

DISORDERS OF NEURULATION
Myeloceles

In patients with myelocele (as in those with myelomeningoceles), the neural tube does not close and the unfolded

spinal cord (neural placode) is visible through a defect in the skin. Since the migration of the mesenchyme and ectoderm posteriorly does not occur, there are no muscles, bones, or skin dorsal to the neural placode. The vertebral bodies at this level usually harbor multiple segmentation anomalies that may give rise to scoliosis. Myeloceles are most commonly located in the lumbosacral region. The neural placode is continuous with the skin laterally, and therefore, the spinal cord is always tethered inferiorly (Fig. 45–5). In a myelocele, the neural placode is flush with the surface of the surrounding skin and does not project outwardly. Since these defects are clinically obvious at birth, the therapeutic goal is to protect the neural placode by closing the dysraphism. This prevents drying up of the placode and subsequent infection and ulceration. Therefore, imaging during the acute period is not indicated in these patients. Patients are commonly imaged later in life when new symptoms develop and the possibility of retethering is of concern.

Myelomeningoceles

Open spinal dysraphism occurs in 1:1000 live births.[7] More than 75% of these patients develop hydrocephalus

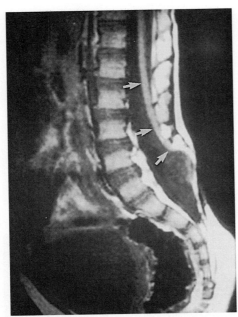

FIGURE 45–5 Repaired myelocele. Midsagittal T1-weighted MRI study shows a low-lying spinal cord (*arrows*) that is inseparable from the dysraphic defect posteriorly. Note the dilated rectum and bladder.

and require shunting. Without treatment, 50% to 80% of these children would die. A myelomeningocele is similar to a myelocele, but in the former, the neural placode is pushed outward by a large CSF-filled compartment ventral to it. As with myeloceles, the goal is to close them as early as possible. Surgery involves untethering the placode by resecting it free from its skin boundaries. The placode is then folded on itself to create a tube. Theoretically, this may avoid the formation of scar and tethering of the newly folded spinal cord at the surgical site. In the majority of patients, there is redundant skin surrounding the defect, the margins of which may be approximated to close the gap. Ventricular shunting is generally performed concomitantly if the patient has hydrocephalus. Because scar tissue develops between the neural placode and the overlying graft, all patients may be considered as having tethering. Therefore, the role of imaging in these patients is not only to visualize the dysraphic site but to explore the remainder of the spine in search of diastematomyelia, arachnoid cysts, dermoids, epidermoids, lipomas, and syringomyelia (Fig. 45–6). Ischemia of the spinal cord may also occur, particularly near or at the surgical bed, where scarring may constrict the newly folded neural placode. Spinal cord fluid–filled cysts are found in 30% to 80% of all patients with open spinal dysraphism (Fig. 45–6B). An important point is the difference between clinical and histologic or radiologic retethering in patients who have undergone prior closure of an open dysraphic state. Although histologically and by MRI practically all patients have tethering, clinically only 30% show deterioration compatible with retethering.

DISORDERS OF DISJUNCTION

Lipomyeloceles and Lipomyelomeningoceles

Lipomyeloceles and lipomyelomeningoceles are considered closed defects because the dysraphic site is covered by skin and subcutaneous fat.[8] In these patients, the subcutaneous fat is continuous with the neural placode. The subcutaneous fat may be extremely prominent and present as a mass in the lower lumbar region (lipoma). As in the open defects, most patients are female. Symptoms include motor and sensory deficits, bowel and bladder problems, dislocated hips, and club feet. Most lipomyeloceles and lipomyelomeningoceles occur in the lumbosacral region.

In lipomyeloceles, the subarachnoid space ventral to the neural placode is of nearly normal size and there is a skin-covered lipoma protruding in the back of the patient.[9] The neural placode is rounded anteriorly and flat dorsally where it is contiguous with the subcutaneous fat. In lipomyelomeningoceles, the subarachnoid space ventral to the neural placode is enlarged.[9] Therefore, the placode and subarachnoid space herniate dorsally through the bony defect (Fig. 45–7). A lipoma (and overlying skin) covers this site. The neural placode is a flat structure whose posterior surface is contiguous with subcutaneous fat. Resection of these lipomas involves liquefaction with laser. If any lipoma remains within the newly folded neural placode, growth or recurrence is likely. Complete resection of these lipomas is difficult as they may contain viable neural elements. The lipoma may enter the spinal canal in both lipomyeloceles and lipomyelomeningoceles. It may extend superiorly and inferiorly on the dorsal surface of the spinal cord or in the extradural spaces. Associated vertebral anomalies, namely segmentation defects and sacral agenesis, are found in half of these patients.

Epidermoids and Dermoids

Epidermoids and dermoids, which are intraspinal tumors, arise from embryologic cell rests within the spinal canal secondary to incomplete disjunction of the neural tube from the mesoderm and ectoderm. Also, they may occasionally be iatrogenically induced after surgery and on rare occasions after needle insertions.[10] They may be considered a hamartomatous malformation as they are formed by normal tissues in ectopic locations. They constitute 1% to 2% of all intradural tumors and 10% of intradural tumors in children 10 years of age or younger.[11] A small number of patients harbor multiple tumors. Dermal sinuses are present in 20% of patients with intraspinal epidermoids and dermoids (Fig. 45–8). Patients may present with a dermal sinus orifice (usually above the level of the intergluteal fold), hairy patch, cutis aplasia, or hemangioma. Over one-half of all patients with dermal sinuses have an intraspinal epidermoid or dermoid. The conus medullaris, cauda equina, or filum terminale may be tethered by these masses. Surgery is the treatment of choice and consists of removal of the tumor contents with

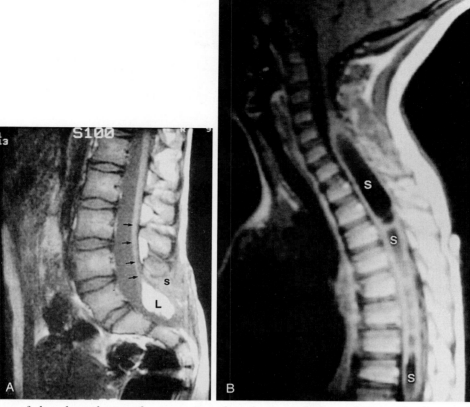

FIGURE 45–6 Causes of clinical retethering after correction of myelocele. *A*, Midsagittal T1-weighted MRI study shows the low-lying spinal cord *(arrows)* extending into a bright intraspinal mass (L), which could be a lipoma or a dermoid. This mass is contiguous posteriorly with scar (s) at the site of prior repair. *B*, Midsagittal T1-weighted MRI study in a different patient with repaired dysraphism and a Chiari type II malformation (note the low position of the cerebellar tonsils). There is a large, expansile, multiseptated cyst (s) in the spinal cord.

preservation of the capsule. The capsule is usually left in place in order to avoid complications secondary to damaging viable neural structures during its removal. Epidermoids are difficult to visualize by either CT or MRI as their density and signal intensity are very similar to those of CSF. Dermoids are commonly fatty and easy to identify but occasionally are difficult to visualize. Over 50% of dermoids are extradural. If a dermoid ruptures, droplets of fat may be present in the subarachnoid space.[12] Contrast administration may be indicated if the mass is suspected to be infected.

Dermal Sinuses

Dermal sinuses arise from incomplete disjunction of the surface ectoderm from the neural tube as it closes. The result is a tract that extends from the surface of the skin to the spinal canal (Fig. 45–8A) This tract may be contiguous with the spinal cord and tether it. Dermal sinuses are more common in the lumbar region and less common in the cervical spine. Unlike other forms of dysraphism, these dermal tracts occur with equal frequency in both sexes.[1] In the lumbar region, they present as tiny paramedian ostia, generally above the intergluteal folds. These ostia are commonly associated with hairy

patches, nevi, or hemangiomata. Over 50% of dermal sinuses terminate in intraspinal epidermoids or dermoids.[1] Dermoids are more common when the ostia are midline, whereas epidermoids are more common with paramedian ostia. Because there is communication with the skin surface, infections (including meningitis and abscesses) may occur. Since the tract courses through the extraspinal, extradural, and subarachnoid compartments, masses may occur at each of these levels. Bony defects are commonly minor and include spina bifida occulta and hypoplastic or bifid spinous processes. Sinus tracts should be imaged with MRI to exclude the presence of intraspinal abnormalities. Approximately 30% of all sinus dermal tracts terminate blindly. Ostia (pilonidal sinuses) occurring below the level of the intergluteal line tend to be isolated; if these patients are asymptomatic, imaging may not be indicated. Contrast administration is needed only if superimposed infection is suspected or present.

Lipomas

Lipomyeloceles and lipomyelomeningoceles have been previously discussed and are not addressed here. Other fatty masses in the spine include intradural lipomas (which are true masses) and lipomas of the filum termi-

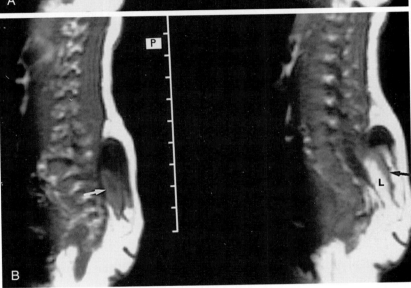

FIGURE 45–7 Lipomyelomeningocele. *A,* Sagittal T1-weighted MRI studies show a low lumbar lipoma (L) that is contiguous with a low-lying spinal cord *(arrows). B,* Parasagittal images in the same patient show posterior herniation of a fluid-filled meningocele that contains portions of the lipoma (L) intermingled with a tethered spinal cord *(arrows).*

nale. Intradural lipomas arise from premature disjunction of the neural tube from mesoderm and ectoderm. Mesenchymal cells are then trapped within the folding spinal cord and prevent its closure, giving origin to a placode. These pluripotential mesenchymal cells then differentiate into fatty cells. These lipomas tend to be completely intradural. They are more common in females and may present at any age. Lipomas are most common in the cervical spine, followed by the thoracic region and the lumbar regions (Fig. 45–9A). The overlying bones tend to be normal, but occasionally a spina bifida occulta may be present (Fig. 45–9B). Most intradural lipomas occur in the posterior aspect of the spinal canal. By both CT and MRI, they have the characteristics of fat (Fig. 45–9B–D).

DISORDERS OF CANALIZATION AND RETROGRESSIVE DIFFERENTIATION

Filar Lipomas

Linear lipomas of the filum terminale are incidentally found in approximately 6% of the general population.[13]

They are commonly asymptomatic, and if MRI shows the conus medullaris is at a normal level, they can be ignored (Fig. 45–10). Filar lipomas are, however, more commonly seen in patients with myelomeningoceles and may also result in thickening of the filum terminale and tethering of the spinal cord.

Tight Filum Terminale Syndrome

In tight filum terminale syndrome there is incomplete retrogressive differentiation of the distal caudal cell mass into the filum terminale. This results in a low-lying conus medullaris and a short and thick filum terminale, which tethers the spinal cord inferiorly. There is no gender predilection, and symptoms may commence at any time during the life of the patient. The symptomatology is complex and includes motor and sensory abnormalities in the lower extremities, abnormal reflexes, bowel and bladder dysfunction, scoliosis, and pain.[14] Pain may be more severe after exercise as repeated traction on the spinal cord may result in ischemia. In these patients, MRI shows

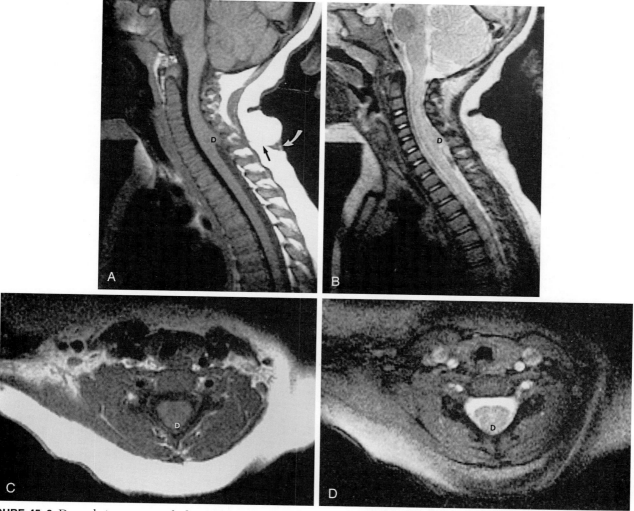

FIGURE 45–8 Dermal sinus tract with dermoid. *A,* Midsagittal T1-weighted MRI study shows a defect in the skin *(curved arrow)* continuing through the subcutaneous fat as a tract *(arrow).* On the dorsal aspect of the cervical spinal cord there is a dermoid (D) that is isointense to the spinal cord. *B,* Corresponding T2-weighted MRI study shows again that the dermoid (D) is isointense to the spinal cord. *C,* Axial T1-weighted MRI study in the same case shows that the dermoid (D) is inseparable from the spinal cord. *D,* Corresponding T2-weighted MRI study shows the dermoid (D) to be isointense to and inseparable from the spinal cord. *(A–D,* From Castillo M, Mukherji SK. Imaging of the Pediatric Head, Neck, and Spine. Philadelphia, Lippincott-Raven, 1996.)

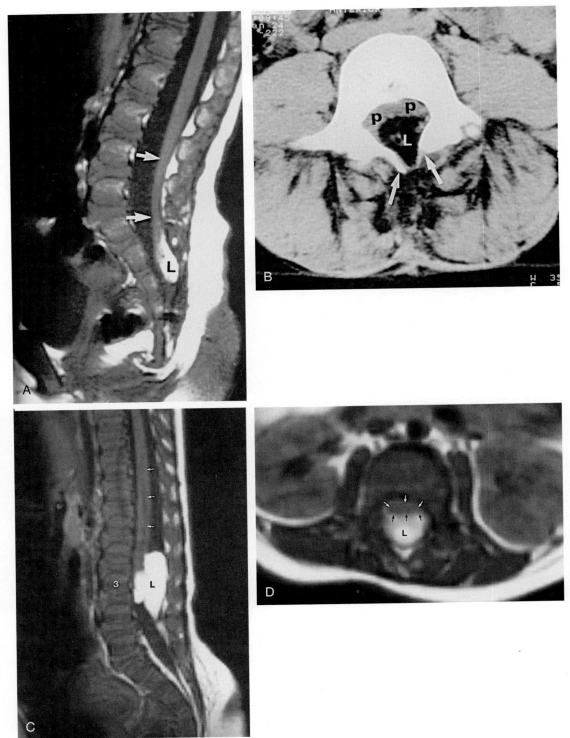

FIGURE 45–9 Intraspinal lipomas. *A*, Midsagittal T1-weighted MRI study shows the low-lying spinal cord *(arrows)* tethered inferiorly by a lipoma (L). *B*, Axial CT scan in a different patient shows the intraspinal lipoma (L) and neural placode (p) anteriorly located. Note the posterior spina bifida occulta defect *(arrows)*. *C*, Midsagittal T1-weighted MRI study in a different patient shows an intraspinal lipoma (L) that tethers a low-lying spinal cord (3, third lumbar vertebra). Note the suggestion of syringomyelia *(arrows)*. *D*, Axial T1-weighted MRI study in the same patient as in *C* shows an intraspinal lipoma (L) and an anteriorly located neural placode *(arrows)*. Note the similarity to the findings shown in *B*.

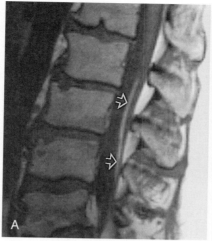
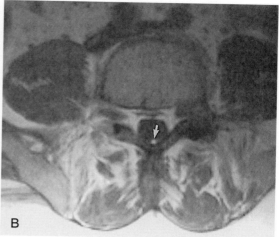

FIGURE 45–10 Filar lipoma. *A*, Midsagittal T1-weighted MRI study in an adult shows an incidental and asymptomatic segmental lipoma (*arrows*) of the filum terminale. Note the normal position of the conus medullaris. *B*, Axial T1-weighted MRI study in the same patient shows a dorsally located lipoma (*arrow*) in the expected location of the filum terminale.

the filum terminale to be thicker (greater than 2 mm in diameter) than the adjacent nerve roots. The diagnosis may be made with confidence if, in addition, at the thick filum terminale the conus medullaris terminates below the L2–3 disk space (Fig. 45–11). Approximately one-fourth of these patients may show abnormal increased T2-signal intensity within the spinal cord related to either fluid-filled cysts or myelomalacia probably secondary to ischemia.[1]

Caudal Regression Syndrome

In caudal regression syndrome, the sacrum and distal lumbar spine may be absent and accompanied by abnor-

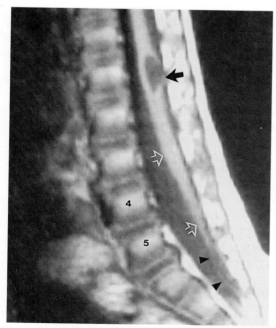

FIGURE 45–11 Tight filum terminale syndrome. Midsagittal T1-weighted MRI study in a child with bladder difficulties and club feet. Note that the spinal cord (*open arrows*) is low lying and extends inferiorly to the level of the fourth (4) and fifth (5) lumbar vertebrae. The filum terminale (*arrowheads*) is short and thick. The spinal cord contains a cyst (*black arrow*).

malities of the conus medullaris, cauda equina, genitourinary system, rectum, and anus.[15] The syndrome is rare and occurs in 1:7500 to 25,000 live births. Maternal diabetes mellitus is an important predisposing factor. Symptoms include severe motor deficits, sensory abnormalities, scoliosis, club feet, hip dislocation, renal anomalies, neurogenic bladder, exstrophy of the bladder, congenital heart disease, and pulmonary hypoplasia. The malformed distal spinal cord may be inferiorly tethered, and these patients may benefit from surgery.

The initial diagnosis is rapidly confirmed with plain radiographs (Fig. 45–12*A*). In the so-called scimitar sacrum, one-half of it is absent. Isolated coccygeal agenesis is probably a normal variant. The vertebrae above the level of the agenesis may be fused.[1] The spine terminates at T11–12 in 35% of patients, at L1–4 in 40% of patients, and below L5 in 27% of patients.[15] Segmentation anomalies and dysraphic states are also common. By MRI, these patients may be classified into two distinct groups. In group 1, the conus medullaris terminates abruptly and is wedge shaped (Fig. 45–12*B*).[16] Some nerve roots of the cauda equina are absent. In group 2, the conus medullaris is of normal configuration but extends inferiorly to the level of the agenesis. In these patients, the distal spinal cord is commonly tethered inferiorly.[15]

Myelocystocele and Terminal Myelocystocele

Myelocystocele and terminal myelocystocele are the least common types of spinal dysraphisms. They occur when a dilated and fluid-filled intramedullary cyst herniates through a spina bifida defect into the subcutaneous tissues.[17] The most common of these defects is the so-called terminal myelocystocele, which occurs in the lumbosacral region and is generally accompanied by abnormalities of the lower gastrointestinal tract and the genitourinary tract. Only the terminal myelocystocele may be considered a true anomaly of canalization and retrogressive differentiation.[1] In this anomaly, a pial-lined cyst is present in the distal aspect of a low-lying spinal cord and protrudes dorsally. The inner surface of the cyst is ependyma-lined and continuous with the central canal of the dysplastic spinal cord.

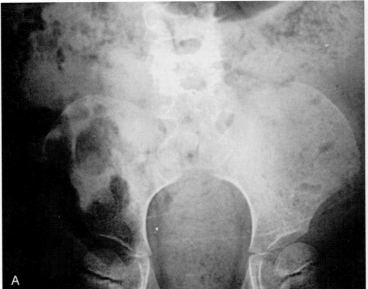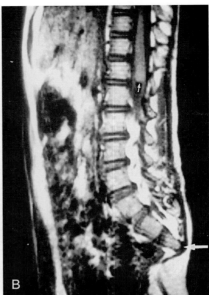

FIGURE 45–12 Caudal regression syndrome. *A,* Frontal radiograph of the pelvis shows the absence of the sacrum. *B,* Midsagittal T1-weighted MRI study in a different patient shows that only the first sacral segment *(large arrow)* is present. Note the truncation *(small arrow)* of the tip of the conus medullaris and the absence of a well-defined cauda equina, probably secondary to the absence of some of the nerve rootlets. (*A,* Case courtesy of David Merten, M.D., Chapel Hill, NC. *B,* From Castillo M. Neuroradiology Companion. Philadelphia, JB Lippincott, 1995.)

Teratoma

In this section, only sacrococcygeal teratoma is addressed. These rare tumors probably arise from pluripotential cell rests from the caudal cell mass. They are more common in females. Although most present in the early years of life, they may become symptomatic at any time. Patients may complain of constipation, urinary frequency, and pain. These symptoms are probably related to the mass effect exerted on the pelvic organs by the teratoma. The majority of these teratomas are histologically mature, but up to one-third of them may be immature and malignant.[18] By imaging, all teratomas are characterized by their inhomogeneous nature. They contain zones of fat and soft tissue; the latter may enhance after contrast administration. Unilocular or multilocular cysts may also be present. Immature teratomas are less well differentiated and therefore may have a more homogeneous imaging appearance. All teratomas may produce bone erosion. Occasionally, purely intraspinal teratomas are associated with overt or occult dysraphic states.

Anterior Sacral Meningoceles

Anterior sacral meningoceles are CSF-filled meningeal sacs protruding into the pelvis via a hypogenetic sacrum and as such may be considered a disorder of canalization and retrogressive differentiation. Both sexes are equally affected, and this disorder is usually diagnosed during the second or third decade of life.[19] Symptoms are related to a mass effect on the pelvic organs by the meningocele and include bladder and bowel difficulties, menstrual irregularities, painful sexual intercourse, and rarely radiculopathies (Fig. 45–13A). On plain radiographs, the sacrum is hypoplastic, bifid, or scalloped. MRI shows the

fluid-filled sac to be continuous with the thecal sac (Fig. 45–13B). If nerve roots are present within the sac, its resection may be contraindicated. Occasionally, there are associated intraspinal dermoids, epidermoids, or lipomas that may tether the spinal cord inside the meningocele.

Persistent Ventriculus Terminalis

Persistent ventriculus terminalis is a fluid-filled cyst located in the conus medullaris. This anomaly is probably related to persistent vacuoles in the distal aspect of the conus medullaris. It is a rare anomaly whose incidence is not known. Patients are generally asymptomatic, and the cyst is incidentally discovered at MRI. However, patients occasionally have back pain, radiculopathy, and bladder dysfunction. In symptomatic patients, shunting of the cyst may be indicated. These cysts may produce an expansion of the cord but are smooth, contain no septations, and show no enhancement after contrast administration (Fig. 45–14).[20]

DISORDERS OF VERTEBRAL SEGMENTATION AND NOTOCHORD RESORPTION

Embryology

At approximately 3 weeks of life, paired cellular groups appear along both sides of the notochord. The mesodermal groups are called *somites.*[21] The notochord stimulates the differentiation and growth of the somites. The outer portion of the somites gives origin to the skin and subcutaneous tissues and is called a *dermatome.* The inner component separates into a dorsolateral one (myotome)

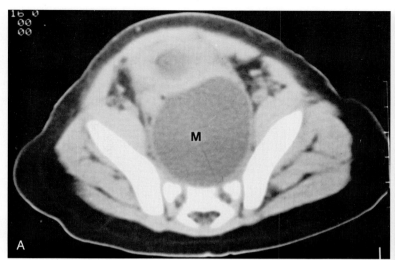

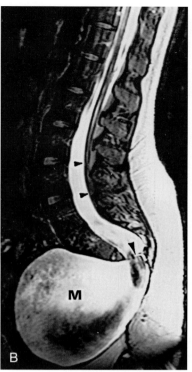

FIGURE 45–13 Anterior sacral meningocele. *A*, Axial CT scan shows a cystic mass (M) in the presacral region. *B*, Midsagittal T2-weighted MRI study in a different patient shows a large anterior sacral meningocele (M), which communicates *(large arrowhead)* with the distal thecal sac. The distal spinal canal is wide. The spinal cord *(small arrowheads)* is low lying and contains increased signal intensity, suggesting a syrinx. (*A* and *B*, Cases courtesy of S. Birchansky, M.D., and N. Altman, Miami Children's Hospital, Miami, FL.)

that produces the paraspinal muscles, and a ventromedial one (sclerotome) that produces the vertebrae. On each side of the notochord, a segment that includes the lower one-half of a vertebral body, inferior end plate, and one-

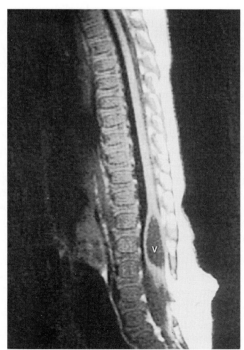

FIGURE 45–14 Ventriculus terminalis. Midsagittal T1-weighted MRI study shows the cystic structure (V) in the conus medullaris. (From Castillo M, Mukherji SK. Imaging of the Pediatric Head, Neck, and Spine. Philadelphia, Lippincott-Raven, 1996.)

half of the disk (to the level of the internuclear cleft) will fuse with the adjacent segment that includes the upper one-half of a disk, superior end plate, and superior one-half of a vertebral body (to the level of the basivertebral vein canal). These will form one vertebral body. Anomalies in segmentation lead to formation of hemivertebrae and fused (block) vertebrae. Kinking of the notochord may also contribute to the formation of hemivertebrae.[21] Incomplete resorption of the notochord may result in midline clefts and butterfly vertebrae. Because the formation of the posterior elements is under a different influence, they may be normal in patients with vertebral body anomalies.

Hemivertebrae, Block Vertebrae, and Butterfly Vertebrae

Hemivertebrae occur secondary to the absence of one side of the sclerotome. In this condition, only one of the lateral ossification centers of the vertebral body develops. This may lead to fusion of one-half of a vertebral body with adjacent ones. Hemivertebrae may result in scoliosis and lack of stability. Pain is a prominent complaint. Hemivertebrae are usually isolated but may occur in a variety of congenital syndromes. Plain radiographs are diagnostic, and spiral CT with three-dimensional reformations beautifully depicts these anomalies (Fig. 45–15).

If the intervertebral sclerotomes fail to develop bilaterally, the adjacent vertebrae are fused, resulting in blocks of vertebrae rather than discrete ones.[21] Block vertebrae may be complete or incomplete (unilateral unsegmented bar). In the latter, the disk space and facet joints are fused on only one side. Ipsilateral rib fusion and scoliosis are generally present. When a unilateral unsegmented

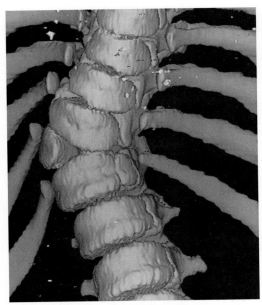

FIGURE 45–15 Hemivertebra. A three-dimensional computed tomography scan shows the right T11 hemivertebra with fusion of T10 and T12 on the left. Note the scoliosis.

bar occurs in association with a contralateral hemivertebra, rapidly progressing scoliosis is the rule. Bilateral failure of segmentation at multiple levels results in fused (block) vertebrae. Commonly, there is a thin residual disk between the fused vertebrae. This block of vertebrae grows slower and to a lesser extent than normal vertebrae, resulting in a shortening of the spine.[22] Scoliosis may develop. Block vertebrae are classically seen in the Klippel-Feil syndrome (Fig. 45–16).

A butterfly vertebra is a midline cleft that is secondary to incomplete resorption of the notochord. This results in a defect that generally is confined to only the anterior

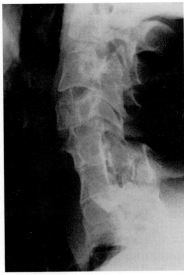

FIGURE 45–16 Block vertebrae. Lateral radiograph in a patient with Klippel-Feil syndrome shows fusion of C4–T1.

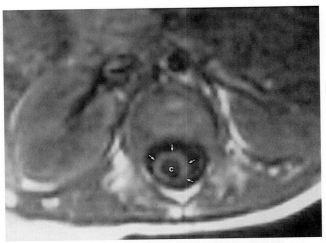

FIGURE 45–17 Spinal cord fluid-filled cyst. Axial T1-weighted MRI study shows a cyst (c) expanding the spinal cord (*arrows*). This patient had a myelomeningocele repaired at birth.

two-thirds of a vertebra on CT and MRI axial images. It is generally asymptomatic, but rarely patients may complain of pain and kyphosis. It should not be confused with a fracture.

SPINAL CORD CYSTS

Syringomyelia is a fluid-filled cavity lying outside the central canal of the spinal cord. Hydromyelia is a dilated and fluid-filled central spinal canal. Histologically, hydromyelia is lined by ependyma, whereas the walls of a syringomyelic cavity are composed of glioses. Distinguishing them by imaging studies is not feasible, and therefore, we prefer to refer to them simply as *spinal cord fluid-filled cysts.*

Spinal cord cysts are associated with Chiari's malformations and spinal dysraphism. Although the causes of these cysts are many, only the previously mentioned ones are addressed here. Spinal cord cysts occur in 20% to 60% of patients with Chiari's type I malformation, most often in the cervical and high thoracic regions.[23] Up to 80% of patients with Chiari's type II malformation develop spinal cord cysts.[23] In this group of patients, these cysts commonly occur in the thoracic region. From 20% to 80% of patients with open spinal dysraphism also develop spinal cord cysts. Optimal evaluation of these cysts requires MRI (Fig. 45–17). If no abnormalities of the posterior fossa or dysraphism is present, contrast administration is mandatory to exclude underlying tumor.

References

1. Barkovich AJ. Congenital anomalies of the spine. In Barkovich AJ (ed). Pediatric Neuroimaging, 2nd ed., pp. 477–537. Philadelphia, Lippincott-Raven, 1995.
2. Naidich TP, McLone DG. Growth and development. In Kricun ME (ed). Imaging Modalities in Spinal Disorders, pp. 1–19. Philadelphia, WB Saunders, 1988.
3. Castillo M. MRI of diastematomyelia. MRI Decisions 1991; 5:12–17.
4. Naidich TP, Harwood-Nash DC. Diastematomyelia: Hemicord and meningeal sheaths; single and double arachnoid and dural tubes. AJNR 1983;4:633–637.

5. Castillo M, Hankins L, Kramer L, Wilson BA. MR imaging of diplomyelia. Magn Reson Imaging 1992;10:699–703.
6. Dominguez R, Rott J, Castillo M, et al. Caudal duplication syndrome. Am J Dis Child 1993;147:1048–1052.
7. Naidich TP, Zimmerman RA, McLone DG, et al. Congenital anomalies of the spine and spinal cord. In Atlas SW (ed). Magnetic Resonance Imaging of the Brain, pp. 865–875. Philadelphia, Lippincott-Raven, 1991.
8. Naidich TP, McLone DG, Mutleur S. A new understanding of dorsal dysraphism with lipoma: Radiological evaluation with surgical correction. AJNR 1983;4:103–116.
9. McLone DG, Mutleur S, Naidich TP. Lipomeningoceles of the conus medullaris. In American Society for Pediatric Neurosurgeons (eds). Concepts in Pediatric Neurosurgery, pp. 170–177. Basel, Karger, 1983.
10. Machida T, Abe O, Sasaki Y, et al. Acquired epidermoid tumor in the thoracic spinal canal. Neuroradiology 1993;35:316–318.
11. Castillo M, Mukherji SK. Imaging of the Pediatric Head, Neck, and Spine. Philadelphia, JB Lippincott, 1996.
12. Barsi P, Kenéz J, Várallyay G, Gergely L. Unusual origin of free subarachnoid fat drops: A ruptured spinal dermoid tumour. Neuroradiology 1992;34:343–344.
13. Uchino A, Mori T, Ohno M. Thickened fatty filum terminale: MR imaging. Neuroradiology 1991;33:331–333.
14. Raghavan N, Barkovich AJ, Edwards MS, Norman D. MR imaging in the tethered cord syndrome. AJNR 1989;10:27–36.
15. Nievelstein RAJ, Valk J, Smith LME, Vermeij-Keers C. MR of the caudal regression syndrome: Embryologic implications. AJNR 1994;15:1021–1029.
16. Barkovich AJ, Raghavan N, Chuang S. MR of lumbosacral agenesis. AJNR 1989;10:1223–1231.
17. McLone DG, Naidich TP. Terminal myelocystocele. Neurosurgery 1985;16:36–43.
18. Schey WL, Shkolnick A, White H. Clinical and radiographic considerations of sacrococcygeal teratomas. Analysis of 26 new cases and review of the literature. Radiology 1977;125:189–195.
19. Lee K, Gower DJ, McWhorter JM, Albertson DA. The role of MR imaging in the diagnosis and treatment of anterior sacral meningoceles. J Neurosurg 1988;69:628–631.
20. Sigal R, Denys A, Halimi P, et al. Ventriculus terminalis of the conus medullaris: MR imaging in four patients with congenital dilatation. AJNR 1991;12:733–737.
21. Ogden JA, Ganey TM, Sasse J, et al. Development and maturation of the axial skeleton. In Weinstein SL (ed). The Pediatric Spine. Principles and Practice, Vol. 1, pp. 3–70. Philadelphia, Lippincott-Raven, 1994.
22. McMaster MJ. Congenital scoliosis. In Weinstein SL (ed). The Pediatric Spine. Principles and Practice, Vol. 1, pp. 227–235. Philadelphia, Lippincott-Raven, 1994.
23. Castillo M, Dominguez R. Imaging of common congenital anomalies of the brain and spine. Clin Imaging 1992;16:73–88.

46

Pediatric Brain Tumors

MARK H. DEPPER, M.D.

BLAINE L. HART, M.D.

The focus of this section is the neuroimaging of primary brain neoplasms of children. Neoplasms of the spine, spinal cord, skull base, and coverings of the brain as well as the orbits are more fully addressed in other sections.

Pediatric brain neoplasms constitute the largest group of solid neoplasms in children (22% of childhood cancers), second only to leukemia (30%) in overall frequency during childhood.[1] The annual incidence is about 2.5 cases per 100,000 children per year.[2]

Most pediatric brain tumors are primary tumors, as intracranial metastatic disease, although well described and common in the adult, is rare in children. Most observations in children are limited to case reports of metastatic disease from primary tumors of the central nervous system such as medulloblastoma and ependymoma[3] and metastasis from extracranial neuroblastoma.[4] A more recent review of 31 children with metastatic disease found the most common location of primary tumors to be primary to the central nervous system itself (medulloblastoma, astrocytoma, and ependymoma) followed by peripheral neuroblastomas and sarcomas. The diagnosis of malignancy is usually made before the discovery of intracranial metastatic disease.[5]

Overall, cancer is the second most frequent cause of death among children aged 1 to 14 years.[6] The peak incidence of pediatric brain tumors is around 5 to 9 years, with a slightly higher rate among whites compared with blacks. Incidence rates also show international variation, which may in part be due to differences in medical care and cancer reporting, but range from 1.1 per 100,000 in Japan to 3.5 per 100,000 in Sweden.[7]

The 5-year survival rate for children with brain tumors is about 58%, accounting for about 24% of the mortality from childhood cancer.[8] The advances in survival seen with childhood leukemia have unfortunately not been seen with primary pediatric brain neoplasms. Evidence has accumulated that the incidence of brain tumors in children has increased,[9–11] making diagnosis of these diseases important, especially in view of the increasing complexity of treatment and increasing survival of patients into adulthood.[12]

An increasing rate of brain tumors in adults has been noted and seems to correlate with the quality and availability of health care, health care technology, and socioeconomic status.[13–15] Although the incidence of pediatric brain neoplasms is not decreasing overall, recent evidence supports a decline in the incidence of medulloblastoma,[16] possibly due to prenatal folate, multivitamin, and iron supplementation.

Familial risk factors for childhood brain tumors suggest a modest increase in the risk of childhood brain tumors associated with a maternal family history of birth defects, especially in female patients, but a family history of tumors does not appreciably increase this risk.[17] A family history of epilepsy does not appear to impart an increased risk of childhood brain tumors either,[17] although a previous report suggested such a link.[18]

Epidemiologic studies of risk factors for childhood brain tumors are frequently inconsistent. An increased risk of childhood brain tumors is seen with therapeutic cranial irradiation,[19] but the low doses of current diagnostic radiographic techniques probably do not increase the risk to a fetus or child.[8] A slight increase in risk has also been associated with proximity to nuclear testing sites in the (former) Soviet republic of Kazakhstan, but exposure data from this region may be confounded by industrial and chemical exposure as well as differences in ethnicity and urban versus rural location.[20] Most data on parental occupational exposure are inconsistent, but recent evidence suggests some increased risk of childhood brain tumors from antenatal maternal consumption of cured meats (containing N-nitroso compounds with potential carcinogenic properties) and exposure to second-hand tobacco smoke, but no increased risk from maternal antihistamine, barbiturate, or diuretic use despite previous reports suggesting an association.[21] Despite the biologic plausibility of a link between smoking and brain malignancy as well as the well-known association of smoking and some adult cancers, no definite association between parental smoking, by either the mother or the father, from 2 years before childbirth through the child's first year, was found in a large population-based study.[22] Studies exist supporting[23] and refuting[24] an association of maternal smoking, or cigarette exposure during pregnancy, and the development of pediatric brain tumors.

Associations with some types of parental occupational exposures including farming as well as employment in the paper-manufacturing industry, aerospace industry, and Air

Force have also been noted.[7] Contact with organic solvents has been implicated in some of these industries.

Several conflicting reports have implicated exposure to electromagnetic fields, including those originating from power lines and in homes, with an increased risk of pediatric cancer.[25, 26] Some research implicates prenatal maternal exposure to magnetic fields,[27] whereas studies of paternal electromagnetic field exposure have both supported[28] and refuted[29] such an association. For childhood exposure, the literature also varies in support of an association,[30–32] and attempts to compile reliable data free of confounding variables are difficult.[33] Additional complications arise from associations with proximity to power lines, including household wiring configurations, but not with measured fields.[34] An association of residential electric consumption and childhood brain cancer has been noted.[35]

A lack of a biologic mechanism further complicates this issue although altered (reduced) melatonin production[36] and interaction with cellular ferritin[37] have been proposed. These two mechanisms are not completely understood or proved in experimental studies. DNA itself does not appear to be directly altered by electromagnetic fields, and if in fact electromagnetic fields are tumor promoters, no site or mechanism has been found.[38] Specifically, agents associated with cancer are expected to affect DNA in an adverse manner, and in vitro studies of human cells exposed to electromagnetic fields do not appear to have DNA-strand breaks. Electromagnetic fields also do not appear to potentiate DNA damage produced by oxidative stress.[39]

At the present time the association between exposure to electromagnetic fields and the subsequent development of cancer cannot be supported but remains of interest for radiologists and patients who use magnetic resonance imaging (MRI). The reader is referred to a recent review[26] for more information.

CLINICAL PRESENTATION

The initial signs and symptoms of brain tumors vary with the patient's age as well as the location of the tumor. Hemispheric tumors may present with increased head circumference, split sutures, and bulging fontanelles in young infants.[40] Diplopia, vomiting, papilledema, and strabismus from sixth cranial nerve palsy may be present. Older children may complain of headaches that are worse on awakening.[41]

Hemispheric masses may also present with focal neurologic deficits including facial weakness, hemi- or monoparesis, visual-field defects, language deficits, and sensory loss. Personality changes may be associated with larger tumors and elevated intracranial pressure. Hemispheric masses, especially low-grade neoplasms, may present with seizures in 50% to 90% of patients.[40]

Posterior fossa neoplasms often present with nonspecific signs and symptoms. In younger children, symptoms may be confined to those of increased intracranial pressure including vomiting, cranial nerve palsies, increasing head circumference, and lethargy.[42] Older children may have complaints that localize to the posterior fossa including ataxia and cranial nerve palsies.

Headaches are not an uncommon complaint in childhood, having been reported in up to 59% of school-aged children, although frequent headaches were seen in only 10%.[43] A more recent study revealed that 28% of children experienced headache at least once a month.[44] Determining the utility of brain imaging in children with headaches is thus made difficult by the high prevalence of headache in this population, the often nonspecific signs and symptoms of brain tumors in children, and the proliferation of brain-imaging centers with widespread availability of computed tomography (CT) and MRI. Few studies of the value of brain imaging in children are available.[45, 46] Although limited in size, or to children younger than 7 years, one study identified only a single patient with a brain tumor (choroid plexus papilloma) who also had downward gaze preference,[45] and the other found only incidental findings and no brain neoplasms.[46] A more recent study of children with headaches found no neoplasms in the group of children studied.[47] It seems likely that when children with headaches are evaluated, brain imaging should be reserved for those with atypical patterns of headaches, or focal neurologic signs and symptoms, when there is clinical suspicion of an underlying structural lesion, and in very young patients or when a reliable history cannot be obtained. Imaging should be performed when children present with headaches associated with neurologic abnormality, ocular findings including papilledema or loss of vision, vomiting, a change in the character of the headache, and headaches that repeatedly awaken the child or occur in the morning.[48]

APPROACH TO IMAGING

Computed Tomography and Magnetic Resonance Imaging

When the decision to study a child with a known or suspected brain neoplasm is made, a variety of methods are currently available. CT is often the first imaging study used. It is readily available in most hospitals and is less expensive than MRI and is commonly used for the initial diagnosis of brain neoplasms. Unlike MRI, CT can sometimes provide some specific information for the prediction of histologic type, narrowing the differential diagnosis of a brain neoplasm. CT can more readily detect the calcifications that are seen in 20% of cerebellar astrocytomas, about 50% of ependymomas, 90% of craniopharyngiomas, and many of the more well differentiated glial tumors such as gangliogliomas and oligodendrogliomas. CT can also unequivocally identify the fluid found within the large cysts typically associated with juvenile pilocytic astrocytomas and the fat and calcifications of teratomas.[49] The density of the cellular components of the tumor on CT images is also helpful. Astrocytomas in children are usually hypodense when compared with brain parenchyma, whereas tumors composed of small round cells with high nucleus to cytoplasm ratios such as primitive neuroectodermal tumor (PNET), medulloblastomas, and germinomas are often isodense or hyperdense.[50]

When CT is used and MRI is unavailable or noncontrast images demonstrate a mass, scans should be obtained both before and after the intravenous administration of an iodinated contrast agent. The specific type of contrast agent given will not affect the image quality (for a given dose and concentration of iodine); however, nonionic or low-osmolality agents would be expected to be better tolerated and associated with a lower incidence of contrast reactions. The typical recommended dose of contrast material, with an iodine concentration of 300 mg/mL, is 3 mL/kg of body weight, up to a maximal dose of 120 mL. Images are acquired immediately after the administration of the contrast material as a single bolus. For older children, axial slices are acquired in the same manner as for adults, aligned parallel to the canthomeatal line. Infants and younger children should have the slice thickness reduced to 5 mm. Coronal images are helpful for evaluation of small lesions near the dura or bone and evaluating masses near the foramen magnum or tentorium. Sagittal (reformatted) images allow better evaluation of the midline structures and the relationship of the mass to adjacent structures of the posterior fossa. Photographing bone windows and measuring the density of a region of interest are useful in distinguishing hemorrhage from calcification.

MRI has become the primary method of tumor imaging in both adults and children. MRI has multiplanar capability, excellent sensitivity to hemorrhage, and better soft tissue discrimination in the posterior fossa than CT, which is hindered by beam-hardening artifact from the adjacent dense bone of the skull base. MRI can also be utilized for detection of the spread of tumor through the cerebrospinal fluid (CSF) of the entire neuroaxis, which may be seen with pediatric brain tumors (discussed later).

Typical pulse sequences consist of a spin-echo (SE) T1-weighted sagittal sequence with repetition time (TR) of 500 to 600 msec, echo time (TE) of 11 to 20 msec, and slice thickness of 3 to 5 mm with 1-mm gaps, with enough slices to cover the entire brain. After this, axial T1- and T2-weighted sequences are obtained, with the T2 sequences using a TR of 2500 to 3000 msec, a TE of 30 to 60 msec for the first-echo "proton-density (PD)" or intermediate-weighted image, and a TE of 70 to 120 msec for the second echo. The slice thickness for the T2-weighted images can be 4 to 5 mm with a gap of 2 to 2.5 mm. Fast spin echo (FSE) is readily available in most clinical MRI units and is frequently used in adult neuroimaging. The technique allows decreased scan times and the acquisition of images with greater spatial resolution (larger matrix size). For imaging of pediatric brain tumors and children and infants with focal neurologic findings, and for evaluating congenital anomalies, FSE sequences provide satisfactory evaluation and may be utilized in pediatric neuroimaging.[51] Currently available FSE sequences are, however, less sensitive to subtle abnormalities of the white matter and to hemosiderin deposition. Although a single white matter lesion is frequently an insignificant finding in an adult brain, a solitary lesion may be the only abnormality found in a pediatric brain study, and some authors recommend that FSE not be used for the evaluation of children with developmental delay or other nonspecific symptoms.[52] Typical FSE parameters include a TR of 2500 to 3000 msec, a TE (effective) of 17 to 100 msec, and an echo-train length of 8.

Three-dimensional gradient-echo sequences with pulses to reduce residual transverse magnetization (spoiled gradient-recalled acquisition—in the steady state [GRASS] [SPGR]; field echo [FE]; fast field echo [FFE]) and other fast sequences that produce a volume of contiguous images (three-dimensional multiplanar rapidly acquired gradient echo [MP-RAGE]; fast GRASS; three-dimensional [3-D]) are also useful for tumor evaluation. These sequences produce thin (1- to 1.5-mm) T1-weighted sections of the entire brain that may be reformatted into any plane desired on an independent workstation, requiring only single T1-weighted acquisition. Three-dimensional images may also be reformatted from these sequences, which are useful for preoperative planning and functional mapping of the cortex.

The use of paramagnetic MRI contrast agents has become routine in the evaluation of primary (and metastatic) brain tumors as well as central nervous system infectious and inflammatory diseases, and neoplasms of the spinal cord and canal.[53, 54] These agents increase contrast on conventional MRI studies by shortening the T1 relaxation time of adjacent water molecules. This effect is only seen in blood vessels; normal structures lacking an intact blood-brain barrier such as the pituitary gland, dura, and choroid plexus; and areas of pathologic blood-brain barrier breakdown, including intracerebral tumors. These agents do not cross the intact blood-brain barrier,[55, 56] allowing improved contrast between tumor and adjacent normal structures. The actual interaction is between the unpaired electrons of the paramagnetic ion (gadolinium in the currently available MRI contrast agents) and water protons.[57] Paramagnetic agents also produce decreased T2 signal but at the typical, low concentrations used clinically and present within the brain during postcontrast MRI studies, the T1 effect predominates. No significant differences among the commercially available gadolinium chelates in the degree of enhancement produced have been seen. These agents are given intravenously at a dose of 0.1 mmol/kg. When children with brain tumors are imaged and it is anticipated that follow-up imaging will be performed, it is important that these agents be administered at a consistent time in relation to the acquisition of images during subsequent studies. The gadolinium chelates can diffuse through the extracellular space, and delayed images may demonstrate larger areas of enhancement, resulting in a false interpretation of tumor growth.

Currently three gadolinium-based MRI contrast agents are available for clinical use in the United States: gadopentetate dimeglumine (Magnevist, Berlex Laboratories, Wayne, NJ), gadoteridol (ProHance, Squibb Diagnostics, Princeton, NJ), and gadodiamide (Omniscan Nycomed, Princeton, NJ). All three agents are safe and efficacious for imaging of the central nervous system in adults and children.[58–62] All three agents have far fewer side effects than iodinated contrast agents used in other radiographic procedures. The safety and efficacy of using gadolinium-based contrast material in infants (children younger than 2 years) have not been clearly established, and no controlled scientific studies of side effects of these agents have been performed in these young patients. Experience suggests that the rate of adverse reactions and indications of these agents in infants are comparable to those in adults,[63] and it is likely that the use of gadolinium contrast material is justified in infants with a clear indication, for example, evaluation of a central nervous system tumor, or possible leptomeningeal metastasis.

Contrast in conventional MRI depends on differences in T1 and T2 relaxation times. Another technique, magnetization transfer contrast (MTC), relies on differences in the relaxation properties of free and bound water molecules.[64, 65] Although the physics of MRI is discussed in detail elsewhere in this book, a brief review of the mechanism of MTC is given here. Water molecules that are bound to macromolecules, especially myelin in the brain, have very short T1 and T2 relaxation times and do not contribute much signal to the image in conventional MRI. A constant exchange of free and bound water molecules takes place; molecules that are bound at the initial radiofrequency pulse of the MRI sequence that then separate from their macromolecules have shorter T1 and T2 relaxation times than the molecules that were free at the start of the pulse. The effect is to shorten the relaxation time of the entire pool of free water molecules. Application of a radiofrequency pulse slightly off the peak resonance of free water saturates the bound water protons (which have a broad absorption peak) but has a minimal effect on the free pool of protons. Thus this additional pulse has the effect of negating the contribution of bound water molecules to the T1 relaxation time of the free pool of protons. The decline in the MRI signal seen with MTC does not affect the T2 relaxation time, and the decline in brain tissue signal is usually greater in nonenhanced tissues than in gadolinium-enhanced structures, improving the contrast on postgadolinium images in patients with brain tumors.[66] The effect on enhancement with gadolinium and MTC is synergistic and has been used in clinical imaging of brain tumors.[67] Further development and application of MTC-image techniques may allow the earlier detection of subtle enhancement from recurrent brain tumors in children.

Evaluation of the Postoperative Patient

Craniotomy and surgical incision into the brain parenchyma can produce significant changes in the appearance of the brain on postoperative MRI studies. It is important to recognize the appearance of these changes and to appropriately use gadolinium contrast agents in evaluating pediatric patients after surgery.

Postoperative studies of the brain should include both T2-weighted images and pre- and postgadolinium T1-weighted sequences. The precontrast images are needed to visualize any subacute hemorrhage, in the form of methemoglobin, during the early postoperative period. Early experience with postoperative pediatric brain tumor patients demonstrated that gadolinium improved the detection of tumor when compared with images without contrast, including T2-weighted images, and was useful for distinguishing tumor from edema and ischemic changes. Gadolinium images also allow detection of subtle disease not seen on noncontrast images.[68] Care must be taken to distinguish recurrent tumor from the normal postoperative changes seen with enhanced MRI studies. In a large series of postoperative adults and children,

some degree of enhancement of the operative site was seen in 64%.[69] Dural enhancement was seen in every patient during the first year after surgery and in 50% of patients 1 to 2 years later. The dural enhancement can persist for an extremely long time, up to 40 years in this series. The typical postoperative dural enhancement is smooth and thin, measuring up to 2 mm thick. The enhancement can involve the cerebral convexities and the tentorium. When large craniectomies are performed, some surgeons elect to suture the dural margins to the adjacent bony defect or to the overlying galea, producing a layer called the *meningogaleal complex*[70] rather than using dural allograft or other exogenous materials. This complex is thicker than simple dura mater and may measure up to 3 mm thick; however, its edges are typically smooth. Enhancement of the operative site in the brain itself can be noted within 24 hours after surgery; this enhancement is smooth and thin and begins to resolve within 6 weeks with resolution within 1 year (Figs. 46–1 and 46–2).

Because of this early enhancement, if postoperative MRI to detect residual tumor is desired, the imaging should be performed in the first 72 hours after surgery.[50] Steroid administration can diminish this enhancement in the early stages by stabilizing the blood-brain barrier.[71] The early formation of methemoglobin at tumor resection sites has been reported during the first 4 days after surgery, visible as high signal intensity on unenhanced T1-weighted images. This finding may confound interpretation of postoperative MRI studies and may be due to accelerated formation of methemoglobin from local application of peroxide during surgery.[72]

A study of the normal postoperative MRI meningeal findings in children has been reported.[73] The authors noted that the enhancement patterns of the meninges were similar for different types of surgical procedures (craniotomy versus ventriculostomy placement) and that no specific patterns of enhancement correlate with a given type of surgical procedure. T1-weighted images should be obtained before the administration of contrast material to rule out hemorrhage or unusual metallic artifact adjacent to the dura, arising from metal fragments or devices used to reconstruct the skull at the operative site, as a source of hyperintense signal. Overall, about three-fifths of patients demonstrate no or mild diffuse dural enhancement, which is a normal postoperative finding. Normal dura lacks a functional blood-brain barrier but is relatively avascular, explaining the small amount of variable dural enhancement seen in postoperative patients. The pia and arachnoid have capillaries with walls composed of endothelial cells with tight junctions, which in part produce the intact blood-brain barrier in these layers, and any postoperative enhancement of these structures as well as nodular dural enhancement should be considered abnormal in the postoperative patient. The causes of this abnormal enhancement include leptomeningeal metastatic disease, hemorrhage, and meningitis, including infectious and chemical in one case that was produced by spill of fluid from a ruptured, cystic craniopharyngioma.[73] Radiation therapy may produce breakdown of the blood-brain barrier, but this effect may be delayed[74] and not seen on studies obtained early in the treatment of chil-

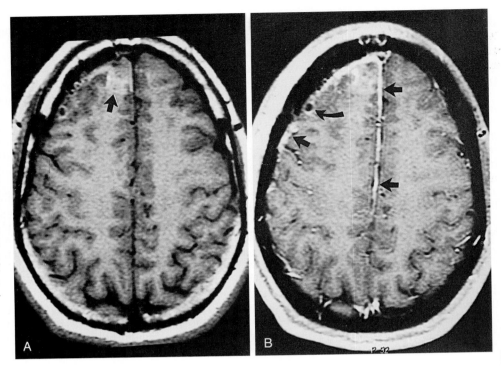

FIGURE 46-1 Magnetic resonance imaging (MRI) studies obtained 3 days after biopsy of a low-grade frontal lobe glioma. *A*, T1-weighted image demonstrates some hyperintensity consistent with early subacute hemorrhage at the biopsy site *(arrow)*. *B*, Gadolinium-enhanced image demonstrates no significant enhancement of the operative site but does show smooth, thin dural enhancement along the falx and dura over the right frontal lobe *(straight arrows)*. Note the small focal hypointensities *(curved arrow)* produced by subdural air. These are normal early postoperative findings.

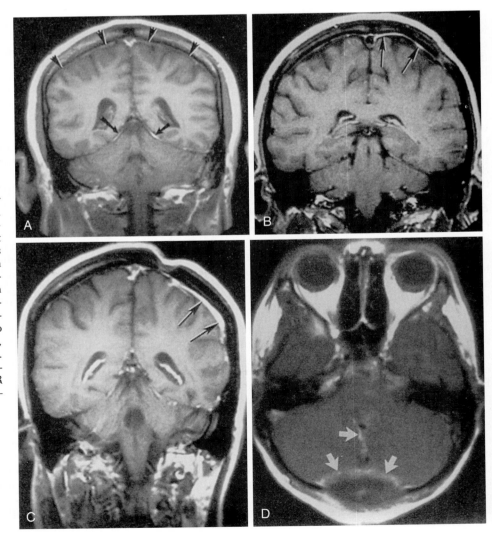

FIGURE 46-2 Patterns of meningeal contrast enhancement after surgery. *A*, Grade 0: Normal enhancement of the dura. Thin, symmetric enhancement is visible over the convexities *(arrowheads)* and tentorium *(arrows)*. *B*, Grade 1: Focal, asymmetric dural enhancement at the craniotomy site *(arrows)*, less than 2 mm thick, with no brain involvement. *C*, Grade 2: More extensive enhancement, greater than 2 mm in thickness *(arrows)*. *D*, Enhancement of the brain at the surgical site *(arrows)* in addition to meningogaleal enhancement. (*A–D*, From Elster AD, DiPersio DA. Cranial postoperative site: Assessment with contrast-enhanced MR imaging. Radiology 1990; 174:93–98.)

dren with brain tumors. Corticosteroids are often given in conjunction with radiation therapy and are known to stabilize the blood-brain barrier.[75] The net result is that changes in the degree of contrast enhancement of the meninges after radiation therapy may be subclinical or below the threshold for visualization with MRI, and meningeal enhancement should not be ascribed to radiation therapy until other causes have been ruled out.

Benign subdural fluid collections are a frequent finding after craniotomy in children and may demonstrate peripheral enhancement. Typically, the enhancement is more prominent around the superficial portion of the collection[76] due to permeation of capillaries into the outer dural aspect of the collection, forming a relatively vascular membrane compared with the inner avascular membrane on the arachnoid side.

Compared with CT, MRI is significantly better at the detection of meningeal lesions[76] and is likely to detect subtle breakdown of the blood-brain barrier earlier.[77]

Disseminated CSF metastases from central nervous system malignant tumors are well known. From 4% to 32% of children with central nervous system tumors have CSF metastases when diagnosed primarily or at the time of tumor recurrence, and up to half of all patients with disseminated tumor are diagnosed at or before the time of diagnosis of their primary brain tumor.[78] These leptomeningeal metastases usually spread from primary PNET, medulloblastomas, germ cell tumors, ependymomas, and malignant gliomas.[79–81] The most common locations for intracranial leptomeningeal metastases include the vermian and basilar cisterns, subependymal region of the lateral ventricles, and subfrontal area. Survival after the diagnosis of leptomeningeal metastatic disease is typically 6 months, and treatment (including both radiation therapy and intra-CSF chemotherapy) is palliative. However, therapy can offer stabilization and protection from further neurologic deterioration in children with leptomeningeal metastases who succumb to progressive systemic or parenchymal brain disease.[82] Leptomeningeal involvement by acute lymphoblastic leukemia is also common in children; however, survival from this disease is affected by prophylactic chemotherapy treatment of the CSF. Leptomeningeal metastasis can potentially affect any part of the central nervous system, and in compilations of patients with CSF dissemination, a variety of clinical signs and symptoms have been found.[83–85] It should be noted that most published data reflect findings in adults with metastatic disease, usually from primary tumors outside the central nervous system. Involvement of the cerebral hemispheres themselves produces headache, mental status changes, seizures, and focal weakness. Papilledema and hemiparesis may be present. The cranial nerves may also be involved, producing diplopia, hearing loss, loss of vision, and numbness. Ophthalmoplegia can be due to involvement of any of the cranial nerves innervating the oculomotor muscles, most frequently the abducens, followed by the oculomotor and trochlear nerves.

Symptoms referable to the spine include extremity weakness, dermatomal sensory changes, bowel or bladder dysfunction, and nuchal rigidity. Extremity weakness may be produced by lower motor neuron involvement at the cauda equina, with decreased deep tendon reflexes, or

involvement at the upper motor neuron level with a myelopathy or conus medullaris disease, with increased deep tendon reflexes.

The presence of malignant cells in the CSF is frequently used as the "gold standard" for the diagnosis of leptomeningeal metastasis, although negative CSF cytologic findings do not exclude the presence of leptomeningeal disease; a postmortem study (of adults) found that 41% of patients with autopsy-proven leptomeningeal metastases had negative antemortem CSF cytologic findings and that the false-negative rate is likely to be higher with focal, masslike tumor deposits compared with diffuse CSF spread of tumor.[86] The exact number of CSF samples needed to detect tumor is not well defined. In one adult series, little benefit was seen in performing additional lumbar punctures after two collections, with 75% of patients with CSF disease detected after the second collection.[87] Another study, also of adults, noted a much higher positive yield (>90%) after two lumbar punctures.[88] The exact protocol followed for children with brain tumors is likely to vary, with some support for requiring two lumbar punctures and (if both lumbar punctures are negative for malignant cells) a cisternal or ventricular sample obtained from a ventriculostomy to determine the presence or absence of malignant cells in the CSF.[82]

Leptomeningeal metastasis, although a histologic diagnosis, may be identified with imaging in children at risk for spread of their primary brain tumors through the CSF. Contrast-enhanced CT (CECT) studies of patients (not limited to children) with leptomeningeal metastasis found abnormalities in 26% to 56%. Abnormalities include ependymal, subependymal, sulcal, and cisternal enhancement, nodular subarachnoid or intraventricular enhancement, nodular or irregular tentorial enhancement, and communicating hydrocephalus.[89–91] Initial experience with MRI compared with CECT found much better sensitivity for leptomeningeal disease with CECT, as the areas of enhancement seen with CT were frequently isointense with noncontrast MRI.[92, 93] In view of the superior sensitivity of postcontrast (gadolinium) MRI in the detection of normal and abnormal postoperative meningeal enhancement, it is not surprising that comparison of CECT and postgadolinium MRI found MRI studies to be more sensitive.[94, 95] It should be noted that contrast-enhanced MRI can be diagnostic of intracranial leptomeningeal metastasis even in the absence of positive CSF cytologic results, and that both CECT and postgadolinium MRI may produce false-negative results (58% and 30%, respectively, in a comparison study[95]). Currently, postgadolinium MRI is the imaging study of choice for the detection of leptomeningeal disease in brain tumor patients (Figs. 46–3 and 46–4).

Previously, CT myelography had been the accepted imaging method for the evaluation of suspected spinal leptomeningeal disease.[96] These metastatic lesions, sometimes referred to as *drop metastases,* are most commonly found about the dorsal thoracic cord and in the lumbosacral area. The tumor deposits may appear as small nodules on the cord, conus medullaris, or nerve roots or present as diffuse, smooth, or nodular coating of the surface of the spinal cord ("sugar coating" or "zuckerguss"). Large, intrathecal masses in the subarachnoid space and nerve

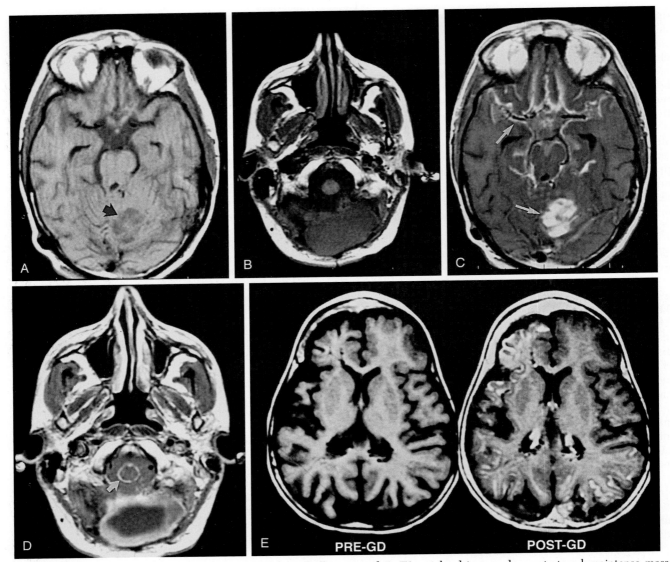

FIGURE 46–3 Recurrent grade III astrocytoma of the cerebellum. *A* and *B*, T1-weighted images demonstrate a hypointense mass in the vermis but no other specific abnormality *(arrow). C–E,* Gadolinium-enhanced images demonstrate both enhancement of the recurrent cerebellar tumor and diffuse enhancement of the leptomeningeal surfaces of the spinal cord, basilar cisterns, sulci, and cranial nerves at the base of the brain produced by extensive leptomeningeal tumor *(arrows in C and D).*

root sleeve filling defects are also seen. Myelography (which is reviewed elsewhere in this book) carries its own risks and is invasive, often requiring sedation for pediatric patients. In view of the poor visualization of noncontrast MRI for intracranial leptomeningeal metastasis, it is not surprising that early experience with MRI for the diagnosis of spinal leptomeningeal disease demonstrated poor results compared with myelography. The tumor deposits on the surface of the cord, roots, and thecal sac may be too small to distinguish against adjacent structures without the use of contrast material.[92, 93, 97] The small tumor nodules often have long T2 relaxation times, making them difficult to distinguish from adjacent hyperintense CSF on T2-weighted images. Larger tumor masses can usually be seen on MRI images of the spine without gadolinium enhancement. MRI including postgadolinium sequences is at least equal, or superior, to CT myelography in the

detection of intradural spinal metastases, allowing detection of tumor nodules as small as 1 to 2 mm.[98] The use of gadolinium enhancement also allows the differentiation of syringomyelia, which does not demonstrate any evidence of parenchymal or nodular enhancement, from tumor-related cysts, associated with enhancing masses or nodularity.[99–101] A comparison study of CT myelography and gadolinium MRI in children[102] found that MRI was positive in 65%, CT myelography in 47%, and CSF cytology (one sample) in only 29%. MRI with gadolinium was also superior at visualizing spinal cord nodules and sugar coating. CT myelography was more sensitive for nerve root sheath filling defects, but no cases of a positive CT myelogram without evidence of subarachnoid tumor with gadolinium-enhanced MRI were found. In some instances the MRI-detected disease was not seen on the CT myelogram. In a more recent prospective study of children and young adults with primary brain tumors,[103] the authors found that although equal numbers of patients had positive MRI examinations and CT myelograms, MRI detected more metastases overall and CT myelography did not detect any lesions not found by MRI. CSF cytology (one sample from lumbar puncture) was positive in 57% of patients with positive imaging studies but was also positive in 30% of patients with negative imaging studies. A myelogram may exacerbate a patient's symptoms if a subarachnoid block is present.[104] In sum, the study of choice for the evaluation of leptomeningeal metastatic disease is cranial and spinal gadolinium-enhanced MRI. Positive studies in the appropriate clinical setting are sufficient to diagnose spread of the tumor through the CSF, but a negative MRI study does not exclude the presence of tumor within the CSF.

MRI technique for imaging the spine for leptomeningeal disease typically includes T1-weighted sequences, 3 mm thick in the sagittal plane and 5 mm thick in the axial plane, both before and after the use of gadolinium contrast material. Fat-suppression techniques are useful in the lumbar spine to distinguish enhancing tumor from epidural fat.[105] False-positive spinal MRI findings may be seen if children are imaged in the immediate postoperative period.[106] In the subarachnoid space one may see areas of T1 signal (high signal intensity) due to hemorrhage during surgery and possible leakage of contrast material from areas of blood-brain barrier breakdown related to surgery. If evaluation for subarachnoid spread of tumor is to be performed, the postgadolinium MRI should ideally be obtained preoperatively, or 2 or more weeks after surgery.

Standard follow-up imaging for children with brain tumors at risk for subarachnoid spread, including PNET, medulloblastoma, ependymoma, germ cell tumors, and pineoblastomas, has included frequent myelography (at 6, 18, and 36 months after surgery in one commonly followed protocol[107]). With current technology it would be expected that the frequent myelography recommended in this protocol would be replaced with MRI. More recent evidence, in patients with medulloblastoma, suggests that surveillance scanning is of little clinical value.[108] No patients survived recurrent tumor, and most patients had clinical signs and symptoms of recurrence before or at the time of radiologic diagnosis. Only 17% of recurrences were detected radiographically in asymptomatic patients, and although this group appeared to survive longer after diagnosis, the survival difference may have represented lead-time bias from early detection. The authors believe that follow-up imaging in children with medulloblastoma should be done to assess the response to therapy and when clinical symptoms warrant further evaluation.

Evaluating the Effects of Radiation and Chemotherapy

After radiation or chemotherapy, changes in the brain from radionecrosis or chemonecrosis may develop. With increasing survival of children with brain tumors, recognition of these changes is important. Radiation changes may be divided clinically into acute injury, early delayed injury,

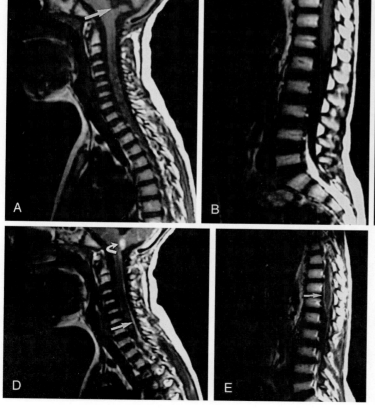

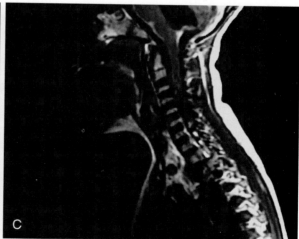

FIGURE 46–4 A 6-year-old child with leptomeningeal metastases from medulloblastoma. Sagittal T1-weighted images of the cervicomedullary junction (*A*) and lumbar spine (*B*) demonstrate postoperative changes to the cerebellum (*arrow*) but no intrathecal masses. Flow-related artifact overlies the thoracic cord. *C–E,* Gadolinium-enhanced images demonstrate diffuse enhancement of the operative site and of the surfaces of the pons, medulla, thoracic spinal cord, and conus medullaris (*straight arrows* in *D* and *E*) consistent with metastatic disease. Also note a nodular recurrence of tumor at the tonsils (*curved arrow* in *D*).

and late radiation injury.[109] Acute injury appears during radiation therapy as a transient worsening of pre-existing symptoms; however, patients imaged during therapy do not appear to have accompanying MRI changes attributable to the radiation.[110] Early delayed radiation changes may be seen from a few weeks up to 3 months after radiation therapy. The symptoms typically resolve within 6 weeks. CT shows nonspecific low-density changes in the basal ganglia, cerebral peduncles, and deep white matter that resolve. As these findings are also seen with late radiation injury, the diagnosis is one of exclusion made on the basis of resolution of the patient's symptoms and imaging findings. Pathologic evaluation has shown disseminated demyelination in a few extreme, fatal cases.[109]

Delayed radiation injury presents from a few months to 10 years or more after radiation therapy and is irreversible, progressive, and a major limiting factor of the dose used in radiation therapy. Focal and diffuse changes are seen and have been noted with CT in 26% of patients treated with cranial irradiation.[111] Focal radiation necrosis presents as an enhancing mass with focal neurologic symptoms and increased intracranial pressure (Fig. 46–5). Focal radiation necrosis typically affects the white matter, and areas of white matter adjacent to tumors appear more susceptible to this injury, possibly related to the presence of vasogenic edema. Focal radiation necrosis can have an identical appearance on CT and MRI to recurrent or residual tumor masses.[112] Radiologic distinction of tumor from radiation necrosis can be aided with nuclear medicine techniques discussed later.

Diffuse white matter changes vary considerably, from small foci of increased T2-weighted MRI signal at the angles of the ventricles to confluent periventricular and centrum semiovale signal extending to the corticomedullary junction (Fig. 46–6). White matter lesions may appear more frequently in younger (less than 3 years old)

children than in older children and may reflect increased sensitivity of the younger children's white matter to radiation during myelination. Comparison of MRI and CT has demonstrated the superiority of MRI in the detection of white matter radiation changes, and MRI can show abnormalities when CT is normal.[113] Typically, the brain stem, cerebellum, internal capsule, basal ganglia,[114] and corpus callosum[113] are relatively spared. More white matter changes are seen with whole-brain versus local radiation therapy, and in adults, the changes may mimic the normal white matter changes of aging.[115] The incidence of white matter abnormalities found with MRI after radiation therapy varies but has been found in all patients in a study of children treated with cranial irradiation who had neurologic symptoms at the time of imaging, although patients with intellectual damage but without focal neurologic deficits typically have either cortical atrophy or no pathologic abnormalities at autopsy.[116] Other studies, although also reporting radiation-related white matter abnormalities with MRI in all patients, found severe changes in only 20% of children. The prevalence of severe abnormalities seems to increase with age, the volume of brain irradiated, the radiation dose, and the interval between therapy and imaging,[115] although some studies have not found any correlation with age, radiation dose, or the use of steroids or concurrent chemotherapy.[117] Pathologic examination reveals fibrinoid necrosis of small arteries and arterioles, and focal or diffuse demyelination, in both diffuse white matter change and masslike radiation necrosis.[118] MRI, although superior to CT, likely underestimates the extent of radiation injury in the white matter.[119]

Ventricular shunt placement is performed on children with obstructive hydrocephalus produced by tumors of the posterior fossa, tectal region, and foramina of Monro. Increased white matter T2 signal intensity along the course of uncomplicated shunts appears to be common.[116]

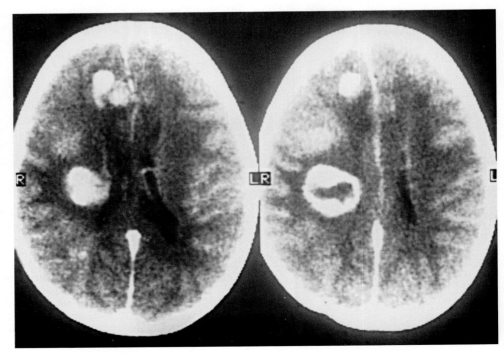

FIGURE 46–5 An 8-year-old boy with radiation necrosis, biopsy proven. The patient underwent whole brain irradiation for medulloblastoma 5 years previously. Contrast-enhanced computed tomography (CECT) demonstrates multiple, bilateral, ring- and solidly enhancing masses, predominantly in the white matter. The appearance is similar to that of other white matter lesions (malignancy, demyelination) but would represent an unusual presentation of either metastatic medulloblastoma or demyelinating disease in a child.

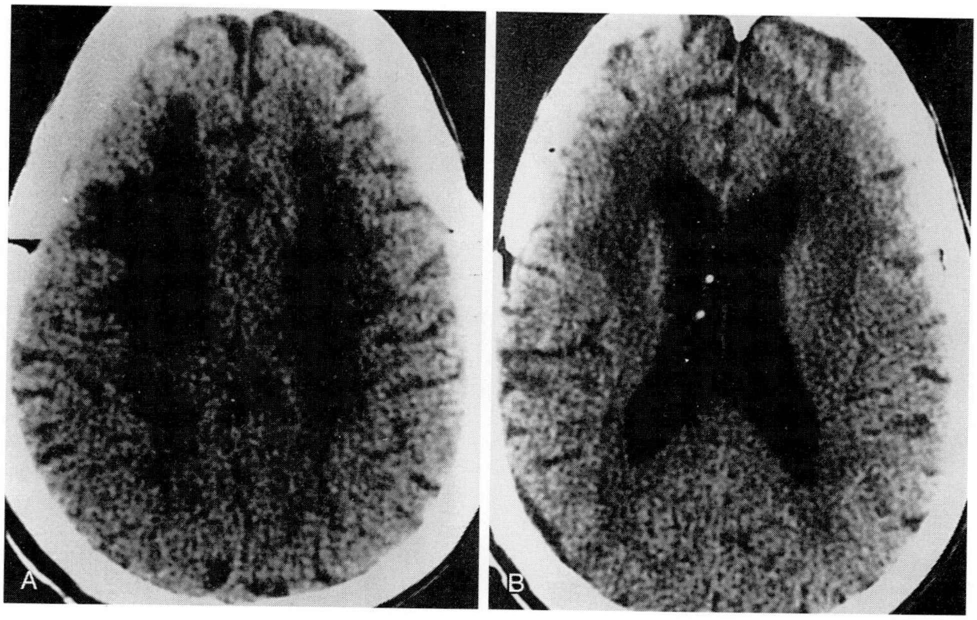

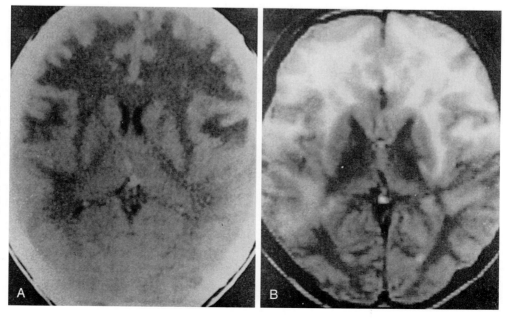

FIGURE 46–6 Postradiation white matter changes in a patient treated for anaplastic astrocytoma. *A* and *B*, Axial computed tomography (CT) scans show ventricular enlargement and diffuse low density in the white matter. (*A* and *B*, From Valk PE, Dillon WP. Radiation injury of the brain. AJNR 1991;12:46–62.)

Necrotizing leukoencephalopathy is seen after chemotherapy, with or without associated radiation therapy. It was first described in children treated with intrathecal methotrexate for leukemia.[120] The latency for this type of injury is shorter than that of radiation damage; the condition presents a few weeks after therapy, with rapid clinical progression. Children may have learning and speech difficulties and associated neuroendocrine dysfunction.[121] Pathologically there is axonal swelling, multifocal demyelination, coagulation necrosis, and gliosis, similar to radiation necrosis, but without the arterial hyalinization and fibrinoid necrosis typical of radiation damage. Periventricular and centrum semiovale regions are both affected,[122] with increased white matter signal intensity on T2-weighted images involving the periventricular regions,

which may extend into the more peripheral white matter (Fig. 46–7).

Mineralizing microangiopathy with dystrophic calcification is common in children treated for cancer and may be seen in up to 30% of children treated with intrathecal methotrexate and cranial radiation[123] and has also been noted in 28% of children treated with radiation therapy alone.[111] The calcification, best seen on CT, is found in the basal ganglia, particularly the putamen, and in the border zone between basal ganglia and cortical perforating vessels. Cortical calcification may also be present along with white matter hypointensity and cortical atrophy (Fig. 46–8). MRI may demonstrate areas of high signal intensity on T1-weighted images.[124] The T1 shortening has been attributed to the surface relaxation mecha-

FIGURE 46–7 Necrotizing leukoencephalopathy after radiation. *A*, CT scan shows diffuse low density in the anterior white matter. *B*, Axial T2-weighted MRI study shows high signal intensity of edema in a corresponding distribution. (*A* and *B*, From Valk PE, Dillon WP. Radiation injury of the brain. AJNR 1991;12:46–62.)

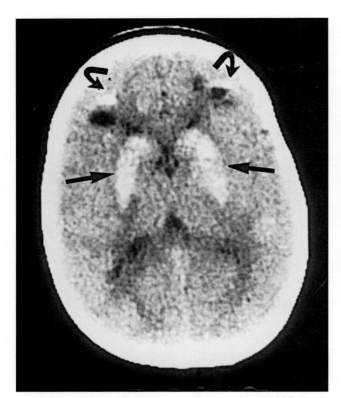

FIGURE 46–8 Mineralizing angiopathy in a 6-year-old boy who underwent irradiation therapy for optic nerve glioma several years previously. Noncontrast computed tomography (NCCT) demonstrates calcifications in the basal ganglia *(straight arrows)*. Subcortical calcifications *(curved arrows)* are also present, accompanied by apparently cystic regions that may represent radiation necrosis.

nism of deposited calcium.[125] The correlation with patient symptoms is unclear, as many patients do not appear to be adversely affected.[126]

Atrophy is a frequent late finding after cerebral radiation therapy, possibly related to diffuse white matter disease from injury to deep perforating arteries; it is important to include steroid therapy and inanition as potential causes of this finding.

Arterial damage to large cerebral arteries may occasionally be seen after radiation therapy. Rather than the fibrinoid necrosis seen in small and medium-sized arteries, the pathologic changes are those of atherosclerosis. Radiation can only be causally implicated in children (compared with adults), who are unlikely to have such vascular disease.[127] Large vessel disease produced by radiation is in general rare. Patients present with relatively acute neurologic changes, months to 20 years or more after radiation therapy, and may be diagnosed angiographically as intracranial carotid and proximal branch occlusions, with or without a moyamoya pattern, or as an angiographic appearance similar to that of cerebral vasculitis.[128] A moyamoya-like pattern has been noted in young patients treated for craniopharyngioma with irradiation to the sellar and suprasellar regions; MRI demonstrates occlusion of the supraclinoid carotid artery and watershed infarctions (Fig. 46–9).[129]

Large, symptomatic hemorrhage in the brain and spinal cord has occurred years after aggressive multimodal therapy for childhood primary malignant tumors.[130] The hematomas were not associated with tumor recurrence but were located in irradiated regions, and abnormal microscopic vessels were noted histologically.

Radiation-induced telangiectasias, appearing as punctate foci of hemosiderin deposition, have been noted in otherwise normal appearing white matter in children and young adults after cranial irradiation therapy.[131] They are best seen as small areas of signal loss near the corticomedullary junction, with "blooming" of their borders on gradient-echo images (Fig. 46–10). Without a history of irradiation therapy these may be difficult to distinguish from small cavernous angiomas. Most patients are asymptomatic, although these lesions have been associated with symptomatic hemorrhages. Pathologic examination reveals clusters of dilated, thickened, small-caliber vessels with hemosiderin in or around the walls resembling ectatic venules and capillaries. The development of these lesions may be related to radiation-induced veno-occlusive disease.[131]

Childhood leukemia is the most common form of childhood cancer. Primary central nervous system manifestations of leukemia include leptomeningeal infiltration, brain parenchymal involvement, and cerebrovascular infiltration. Effects related to therapy include white matter disease and arterial damage related to chemotherapy and radiation as discussed previously. In addition, treatment with asparaginase can lead to depletion of plasma proteins involved in both coagulation and fibrinolysis, producing infarcts, intracerebral hemorrhage, and dural sinus thrombosis.[132, 133]

Survivors of childhood leukemia may have an increased incidence of secondary malignancies, including brain tumors, with an overall annual incidence of 62.3 secondary malignancies per 100,000 patients per year.[134] The most common of the brain tumors are gliomas after therapy for acute lymphoblastic leukemia. Cranial irradiation as well as immunosuppressive drugs has been implicated in the development of these tumors.[135] In some cases, the early development of the secondary brain tumor, in as few as 3 to 5 years after therapy, suggests a genetic predisposition to the development of the malignancy.[136]

Applications of Nuclear Medicine and Magnetic Resonance Spectroscopy in the Imaging of Pediatric Brain Neoplasms

A limited amount of experience in the utilization of nuclear medicine techniques for the evaluation of pediatric brain neoplasms exists. The small number of studies specifically of children may reflect the need for sedation during the acquisition of tomographic images and a desire to keep the radiation exposure in this age group to a minimum. Ethical concerns restrict the imaging of normal controls as well. The use of nuclear medicine techniques for imaging of pediatric brain tumors is briefly reviewed here.

Positron emission tomography (PET) using fluorine-18–fluorodeoxyglucose (FDG) has been shown to be use-

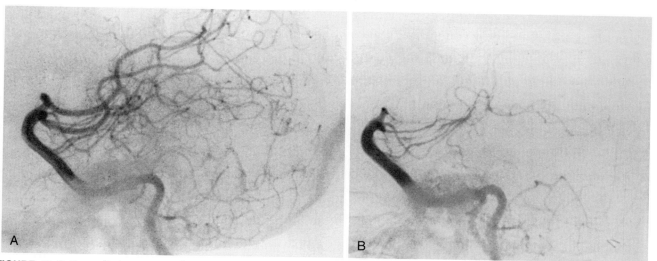

FIGURE 46–9 Postradiation angiopathy. Lateral views of left vertebral arteriogram in a patient treated with 65 Gy (6500 rads) for ependymoma show the normal appearance before treatment *(A)* and severe narrowing of both posterior cerebral arteries 4 months after radiation *(B)*. *(A and B,* From Brant-Zawadski M, Anderson M, DeArmond SJ, et al. Radiation-induced large intracranial vessel occlusive vasculopathy. AJR 1980;134:51–55.)

ful in the differentiation of residual or recurrent brain tumors from posttreatment (radiation or chemotherapy) changes, but most experience is with adult neoplasms. FDG is taken up by cells using the same active transport mechanism as glucose but once phosphorylated is trapped and cannot be transported out through cell membranes or further metabolized along the glycolytic pathway. FDG distribution is felt to correlate with metabolic activity, which is directly linked to blood flow in most instances; ischemia with luxury perfusion is a notable exception. Early studies demonstrated very high sensitivity and specificity for the detection of recurrent tumor,[137–139] although more recent experience has not produced such strong

results, with a sensitivity and specificity of only 81% and 40%, respectively, in a more recent study.[140] Regions of necrosis have reduced glucose utilization relative to normal adjacent or contralateral brain compared with residual or recurrent tumor (ratio of activity of abnormal area compared with normal brain of 0.34 to 0.54 for radio- or chemonecrosis versus 2.5 to 2.8 for residual or recurrent tumor[139]). False-positive PET scans may be seen in cases of seizure during administration of the radiopharmaceutical, whereas false-negative studies may be seen with necrotic tumors, low-grade tumors, or a discrepancy in glucose uptake versus the proliferative potential of a tumor. High-dose corticosteroid therapy has been noted to de-

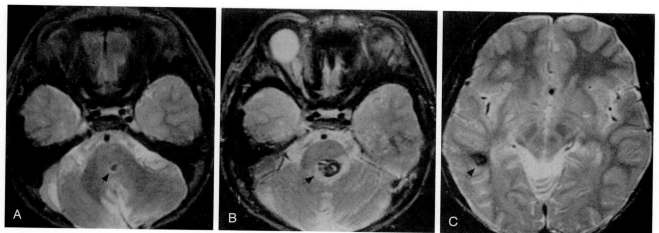

FIGURE 46–10 Telangiectasia in a 10-year-old boy after radiation. The patient had a medulloblastoma resected at 4 years of age and subsequently had whole brain radiation and posterior fossa boost radiation. *A,* Axial T2-weighted image 39 months after treatment showed a very small focus of hemosiderin deposition within the pons *(arrow)*. *B,* When the patient was 10 years old, evaluation of the pons showed a larger, more acute area of hemorrhage *(arrow)*. *C,* T2-weighted image at a higher level shows another region of hemosiderin deposition as low signal intensity *(arrow)*, with a central focus of higher signal intensity probably due to more recent hemorrhage. Pontine telangiectasia was pathologically confirmed by surgical resection. *(A–C,* From Gaensler EH, Dillon WP, Edwards MS, et al. Radiation-induced telangiectasia in the brain simulates cryptic vascular malformations at MR imaging. Radiology 1994;193:629–636.)

crease the apparent volume of some gliomas,[141–143] but FDG uptake is not affected by steroid therapy, or during imaging in the postoperative period.[144, 145] In adults, FDG-PET has also been shown to demonstrate hypermetabolism in low-grade gliomas that have degenerated into grade III or IV astrocytomas, anaplastic astrocytomas, or glioblastomas.[146] The tumors demonstrated quantitative glucose utilization similar to that of de novo high-grade tumors and visible areas of hypermetabolism relative to contralateral brain (Fig. 46–11).

FDG-PET has been useful in the differentiation of low-grade from high-grade gliomas.[147–149] High-grade tumors typically have FDG uptake greater than normal cortex, whereas low-grade tumors have uptake less than that of white matter (Fig. 46–12). Lesions falling between these two groups may be separated by uptake ratios, with a tumor to white matter ratio of 1.5 or higher indicating a high-grade tumor (sensitivity and specificity of 94% and 77%, respectively, in a recent study[150]). It should be noted that in some authors' experience, quantitative values of FDG uptake—a measurement of metabolic activity requiring sampling of arterial or arterialized venous blood—overlap more than visual interpretations, so the visual analysis of the images is still likely to be important.[151] Avoiding invasive blood monitoring by using visual analysis or activity ratios would be desirable in the pediatric population. Preoperative grading of tumors can potentially alter therapy if the lesion is in eloquent brain and may guide biopsy toward the most atypical, high-grade region of a tumor. Information about the accuracy of grading of pediatric gliomas with PET, and the clinical usefulness of such information as demonstrated by an outcome study, has not been obtained. A study of FDG-PET in pediatric posterior fossa tumors has been reported.[152] This qualitative study (which avoids the need for invasive blood sampling) found that in general the degree of uptake was higher with more malignant tumors.

Medulloblastomas typically had the highest uptake, followed by juvenile pilocytic astrocytomas and brain stem gliomas. Appearance was not predictive of histologic type, and variable, heterogeneous uptake was seen after therapy.

FDG-PET has shown applicability in the determination of the prognosis of patients with brain tumors, but most experience to date has been in adults.[153, 154] When the metabolic activity of the tumor (FDG uptake) is compared with that of the contralateral normal brain, shorter survival is associated with greater FDG uptake; in one study a ratio less than 1.4 was associated with a median survival of 19 months, whereas high metabolic activity and a ratio greater than 1.4 was associated with a median survival of 5 months. These features were superior to histologic grade in predicting the prognosis.[155] Although grade III or IV gliomas tended to have a worse prognosis, glucose utilization was a better predictor of survival, with all of the highly metabolic tumors having a poor prognosis regardless of whether the tumor was grade III or IV. Only a few of the tumors were nonenhancing on CECT, but the lack of enhancement was not a useful prognostic factor in patients with grade III or IV tumors.[156]

Brain tumors, especially gliomas, may be histologically heterogeneous, and biopsy specimens may be inadequate to demonstrate the true grade of the tumor or may fail to produce a diagnosis.[157] Even with experience, stereotactic biopsy may produce inaccurate diagnosis or grading and fail to provide a diagnosis of brain neoplasm in 5% of patients.[158, 159] In one study, FDG-PET was used to help guide stereotactic biopsy of adult brain tumors.[160] Targets with FDG uptake higher than normal surrounding brain were mostly high-grade gliomas, whereas hypometabolic lesions were low-grade tumors. Nondiagnostic biopsies were found only in patients with no evidence of hypermetabolic tumor regions. PET may be useful when plan-

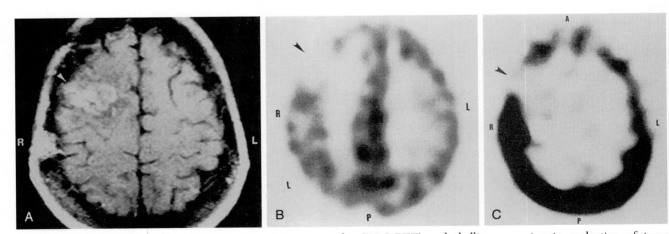

FIGURE 46–11 Fluorodeoxyglucose positron-emission tomography (FDG-PET) and thallium scanning in evaluation of tumor recurrence versus radiation necrosis. *A,* Axial gadolinium-enhanced T1-weighted MRI study in a woman treated with surgery and radiation for anaplastic astrocytoma 11 months previously shows an enhancing mass in the region of the surgical bed *(arrowhead). B,* Axial FDG-PET image shows very low, nearly absent activity in the corresponding location *(arrowhead). C,* Axial image from thallium-201 single-photon emission computed tomography (SPECT) scan shows a similar low level of activity *(arrowhead).* The hot rim around the brain is scalp activity. Very low activity on both scans is consistent with radiation necrosis. *(A–C,* From Kahn D, Follett KA, Bushnell DL, et al. Diagnosis of recurrent brain tumor: Value of [201]Th SPECT vs ^{18}F-Fluorodeoxyglucose PET. AJR 1994;163:1459–1465.)

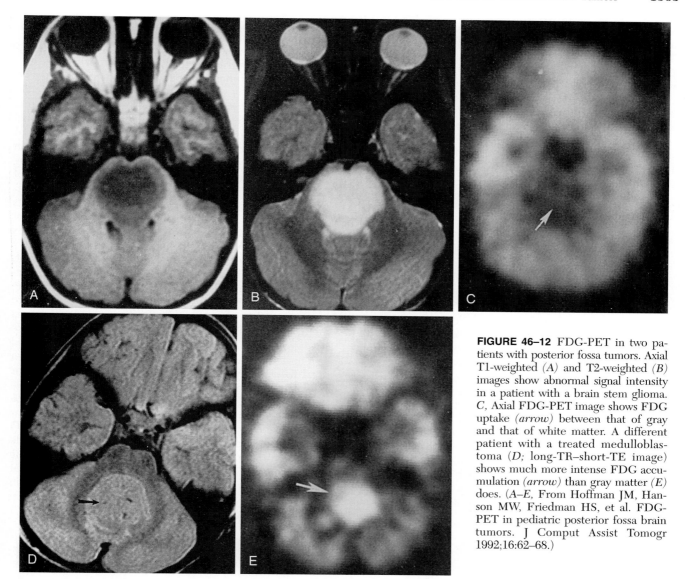

FIGURE 46–12 FDG-PET in two patients with posterior fossa tumors. Axial T1-weighted *(A)* and T2-weighted *(B)* images show abnormal signal intensity in a patient with a brain stem glioma. *C,* Axial FDG-PET image shows FDG uptake *(arrow)* between that of gray and that of white matter. A different patient with a treated medulloblastoma *(D;* long-TR–short-TE image) shows much more intense FDG accumulation *(arrow)* than gray matter *(E)* does. (A–E, From Hoffman JM, Hanson MW, Friedman HS, et al. FDG-PET in pediatric posterior fossa brain tumors. J Comput Assist Tomogr 1992;16:62–68.)

ning stereotactic biopsy of a heterogeneous lesion in order to maximize the yield and grade of the specimens and would also be expected to be useful when enhancement is present in nonneoplastic lesions such as radionecrosis.

An additional PET imaging agent, carbon-11–L-methionine, has been studied in children with brain tumors.[161] Increased uptake of the tracer was seen with a variety of neoplasms including ependymomas, medulloblastomas, and astrocytomas but was less intense in low-grade tumors. Uptake of the L-methionine was competitively reduced by L-phenylalanine in about 70% of patients, but not in areas of radiation injury, suggesting that a two-phase study (two doses, one after the oral administration of L-phenylalanine) with this agent may be useful for distinguishing radiation injury from recurrent tumor in children.

In sum, PET imaging has applications in the evaluation of patients with brain tumors, especially after therapy and in cases of histologically heterogeneous tumors. There are few large-scale studies of and little experience with pediatric brain tumor patients, whose tumors are histologically diverse and can demonstrate different clinical behavior than adult neoplasms. There is also a need for outcome-based studies of clinical PET imaging, as it has limited availability and is expensive; a recent report found that in only 2 of 39 patients evaluated for brain tumors with FDG-PET did the results of the study alter therapy.[162] Further experience in the pediatric population is required.

Thallium-201 (^{201}Tl) is a well-recognized tumor-imaging agent in adults. It is thought that thallium behaves biologically like potassium, although the exact mechanism of its localization is unknown. Potential mechanisms include variable blood flow, tumor viability, sodium-potassium–ATPase system activity, calcium ion channel exchange, vascular immaturity with leakage, and increased cell membrane permeability.[163] Preferential uptake into tumor cells has been demonstrated with high-grade astrocytomas.[164] In general, thallium uptake is minimal or negative in radionecrosis and resolving hematomas and is not affected by corticosteroid therapy. Low or absent uptake may also be seen in low-grade neoplasms.[163] The greatest advantage of thallium in the imaging of pediatric brain tumors is the larger volume of experience with this agent as well as its greater availability and lower cost than FDG-PET. Cerebral thallium studies are often combined with a brain perfusion study using technetium-99m-hexamethylpropyleneamine oxime (^{99m}Tc-HMPAO). This lipophilic agent crosses the blood-brain barrier with rapid first-pass uptake and has no significant late redistribution. Its uptake is proportional to regional cerebral blood flow. Imaging of both agents is readily accomplished with single-photon emission computed tomography (SPECT) equipment (Fig. 46–13).

A study of combined thallium-HMPAO cerebral imaging in children with treated brain tumors found an overall sensitivity and specificity of 77% and 93%, respectively, in the detection of recurrent or residual tumor.[165] These values are somewhat lower than those reported in adults, mostly with astrocytomas, in whom thallium brain tumor imaging is well established.[166, 167] Uptake was seen in a variety of tumors including medulloblastoma, astrocytoma, and ependymoma. Uptake of thallium is normally seen in the choroid plexus. The ratio of tumor to normal brain uptake was 2.5, similar to adult values.[168] Perfusion, as measured with HMPAO, was extremely variable, and this is different from the usual decrease in perfusion seen in adults. In this study, HMPAO did not improve the reliability of tumor detection and did not correlate with tumor activity. In some cases, the tumor status was correctly identified with SPECT but not with MRI. However, some tumors were missed, and the reliability of a normal thallium scan appears to be less than that of a positive study. The authors regard thallium as the imaging agent of choice for the evaluation of tumor activity as its tumor avidity is comparable to that of PET agents, but it is more widely available and less expensive.

The technetium-based imaging agent hexakis(2-methoxyisobutylisonitrile) technetium (I) (MIBI) shares similar properties to thallium in that it is a myocardial perfusion agent and is almost totally excluded by the intact blood-brain barrier. It is easily made on site at any time from a commercial kit and the eluate from the usual technetium generators used in nuclear medicine. MIBI has also been noted to be concentrated in other human tumors. A study of thallium versus MIBI SPECT imaging in childhood brain tumors found similar distribution of the two agents, with the exception that MIBI demonstrates more avid choroid plexus uptake.[169] Both agents demonstrated a sensitivity of 67% but a specificity of 100% with MIBI and 91% with thallium. Tumor edges are better seen with MIBI, likely due to the favorable γ energy and higher photon flux of this technetium agent. Thallium shows some advantage with deep or periventricular lesions because of the avid uptake of MIBI by the choroid plexus.[170] MIBI uptake by tumors also appears to be greater than that of thallium or of the PET agents methionine and FDG. Tumor to normal brain uptake ratios were 7.88 for thallium and 27.1 for MIBI.

The combination of thallium and HMPAO has been used in adults with high-grade gliomas to evaluate for recurrent glioma after treatment. Ratios of tumor to normal scalp thallium uptake greater than 3.5 had a 92% positive predictive value for tumor recurrence.[171] In patients with low or moderate thallium uptake, an HMPAO tumor to cerebellum ratio of 0.5 or less helped to exclude recurrent tumor. HMPAO uptake alone was nonspecific for the evaluation of tumor recurrence, similar to that described previously in children, and has been noted in other studies as well.[172] The reduced HMPAO activity in

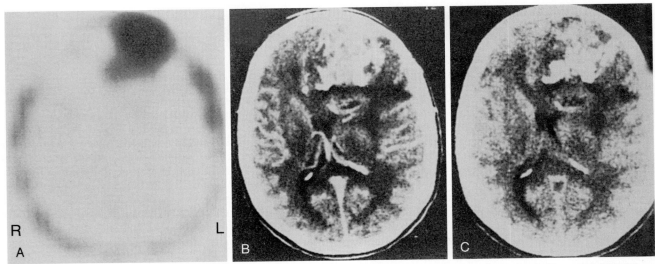

FIGURE 46–13 SPECT thallium scan localizes malignant components of tumor. *A,* Axial image from the thallium-201 SPECT scan shows a region of increased uptake in the left frontal lobe with two components, a very intense region near the frontal pole and a less-intense portion posterior to that. CT scans after *(B)* and prior to *(C)* contrast administration show a heavily calcified mass *(B)* with enhancement. CT does not distinguish the two portions of the tumor. The more posterior portion, corresponding to the lower activity on the thallium scan, was a low-grade oligodendroglioma, and the more anterior portion, corresponding to the intense uptake, was a high-grade mixed glioblastoma and anaplastic oligodendroglioma. (*A–C,* From Black KL, Hawkins RA, Kim KT, et al. Use of thallium-201 SPECT to quantitate malignancy grade of gliomas. J Neurosurg 1989;71:342–346.)

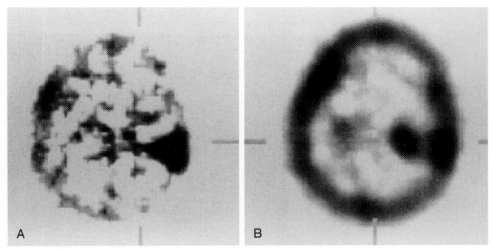

FIGURE 46–14 SPECT hexakis(2-methoxyisobutylisonitrile) technetium (I) (MIBI) of recurrent anaplastic ependymoma. Thallium-201 (*A*) and MIBI (*B*) SPECT scans show increased uptake in the left parietal lobe. Recurrence after surgery, chemotherapy, and radiation was confirmed pathologically. (*A* and *B*, Reprinted by permission of the Society of Nuclear Medicine from: O'Tuama LA, et al. Thallium-201 versus technetium-99m-MIBI SPECT in evaluation of childhood brain tumors: A within-subject comparison. Journal of Nuclear Medicine 1993;34:1046–1051.)

areas of posttherapy reactive changes is probably due to endothelial proliferation and thickening of the arterial walls with thrombosis and reduced blood flow.[171] High-grade tumors tend to have increased metabolic rates and possess abnormal vasculature, favoring the delivery and uptake of HMPAO. It appears that the usefulness of thallium and MIBI imaging in the evaluation of pediatric brain tumors is to identify recurrent disease when MRI and CT findings are equivocal and to evaluate suspected cases of posttherapy necrosis (Fig. 46–14).

FDG-PET is useful in the evaluation of possible radionecrosis, as discussed previously. SPECT imaging is less expensive and more widely available and would be a desirable alternative. In adults and children with high-grade astrocytomas a study utilizing thallium and HMPAO with visual assessment of tracer uptake has been performed to evaluate radiation necrosis versus recurrent tumor.[173] Patients with high uptake of thallium relative to the contralateral scalp (greater than 2.0) had recurrent tumor, and HMPAO perfusion equal to or greater than normal contralateral brain was also observed. Those with intermediate thallium uptake ratios (1.0 to 2.0) could be better differentiated by reviewing HMPAO perfusion; those with decreased perfusion usually had only reactive changes at biopsy, whereas those with HMPAO activity equal to or greater than normal brain tended to have recurrent tumor. Patients with low thallium and low HMPAO uptake had only reactive changes. An intermediate level of thallium uptake alone does not seem to be helpful for diagnosis as such uptake may be seen in areas of blood-brain barrier breakdown associated with radiation damage as well as hematomas, infarctions, and abscesses. The addition of perfusion information from HMPAO studies can improve the diagnostic specificity of thallium SPECT brain tumor imaging.

In a manner similar to that of using FDG uptake ratios, quantitative thallium has been used to determine the grade of gliomas in adults.[168] A ratio of tumor thallium uptake to contralateral normal brain uptake of 1.5 or higher predicted a high-grade tumor with 89% accuracy. Low-grade gliomas, by histologic type, with an uptake ratio greater than 1.5 behaved more like high-grade lesions, with some patients experiencing rapid tumor progression. The technique may also be useful in localizing dedifferentiated, high-grade portions of histologically heterogeneous tumor. Thallium uptake has also been shown to correlate with the grade of adult gliomas, the proliferative potential (as measured by bromodeoxyuridine incorporation after preoperative administration of this thymidine analogue, which is incorporated into the DNA synthetic phase [S phase] of the cell cycle), and clinical prognosis.[174]

Comparison among HMPAO, thallium, and FDG-PET imaging has been made. A small study of children with brain tumors imaged with all three modalities demonstrated the best performance overall with thallium SPECT.[175] A more recent study of adults imaged with thallium SPECT and FDG-PET found no significant differences in the sensitivity and specificity of thallium SPECT versus FDG-PET for the detection of recurrent tumor or radiation necrosis, although FDG-PET was more sensitive for small lesions and low-grade tumors.[140] With further experience, nuclear medicine techniques may become commonplace in the evaluation of children after therapy for brain tumors.

Magnetic resonance spectroscopy (MRS) can provide a noninvasive analysis of cellular chemistry. Initial attempts to characterize metabolism of tumors were made with phosphorus-31, but as the basic energy metabolism of different cell types does not vary greatly, the diagnostic specificity of ^{31}P-MRS to identify different types of tumors is low.[176–178] The technique works best in large tumors that can provide sufficient tumor volume for good-quality spectra.

The normal ^{31}P spectrum of human brain demonstrates seven prominent peaks: phosphomonoester/sugar phos-

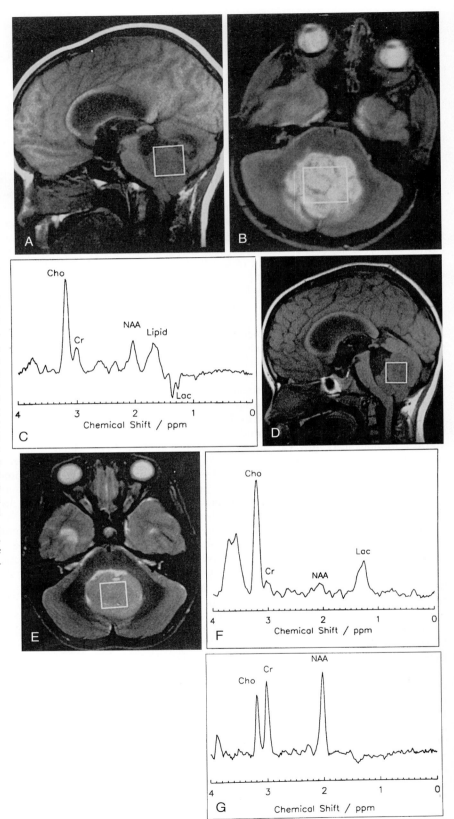

FIGURE 46–15 Differences between tumor types seen with magnetic resonance spectroscopy. Two morphologically similar tumors demonstrate abnormal but different spectra. A cerebellar astrocytoma shows low signal intensity on a T1-weighted image (A) and increased signal intensity on a T2-weighted axial image (B). C, Spectrum obtained using a spin-echo sequence shows a low ratio of creatine (Cr) to choline (Cho) and a low ratio of N-acetyl-L-aspartate (NAA) to choline. Lac, lactate. Cerebellar PNET in a different patient has a similar appearance on a T1-weighted image (D) and mildly increased signal intensity relative to brain on a T2-weighted sequence (E), but the NAA to Cho ratio (F; spectrum with stimulated echo acquisition mode [STEAM] sequence) is even lower than in the astrocytoma. G, Normal spectrum from cerebellar tissue is shown for comparison. (A–C, From Wang Z, Sutton LN, Cnaan A, et al. Proton MR spectroscopy of pediatric cerebellar tumors. AJNR 1995;16:1821–1833.)

phate, inorganic phosphate, phosphodiester, phosphocreatine, and the γ, α, and β peaks of adenosine triphosphate (ATP). The β-ATP peak is used as the reference for quantitation of ATP and to normalize other peaks in the form of ratios. Phosphomonoester and phosphodiester levels can be increased in tumor tissue[179] but are also increased in immature brain undergoing myelination.[180] The relative amounts of phosphocreatine, ATP, and inorganic phosphate reflect the bioenergetic state of the tissue sampled, and a decrease in the phosphocreatine to inorganic phosphate ratio is felt to indicate tissue ischemia.[181] A study of ^{31}P-MRS in large pediatric brain tumors has been performed.[182] Benign tumors had spectra essentially indistinguishable from those of normal brain. Malignant tumors had decreased phosphocreatine peaks and lower phosphocreatine to inorganic phosphate ratios (0.85 in malignant tumors versus 2.0 in benign masses). Phosphomonoester to β-ATP levels and pH were not different between malignant and benign tumors. It appears that there is not a specific metabolic appearance of childhood brain tumors, but some malignant tumors show evidence of ischemia.

Proton (hydrogen) MRS can identify a variety of chemical compounds in the brain. For tumor imaging the most important peaks are produced by choline, lactate, lipid, and creatine. *N*-Acetyl-L-aspartate (NAA), which appears to be found only in cells of neuronal origin, is also readily identifiable.[183] Studies of adult and pediatric brain tumors with proton MRS typically show a marked loss of the NAA peak and a decreased NAA to choline ratio that decreases with increasing tumor grade; however, the different grades cannot be separated by NAA to choline ratios alone.[184] Lactate and lipid peaks, the latter due to necrotic degradation products, are variable. Choline appears to be increased in all tumors because of increased membrane turnover and cell proliferation.[185] Anaplastic gliomas have widely different spectra, consistent with their morphologic and histologic heterogeneity.

Proton MRS appears to provide some contribution to brain tumor imaging by providing information about histologic grade. In a study of adults and children with brain tumors, low-grade gliomas could be separated from high-grade tumors reliably.[186] Low-grade tumors typically showed increased choline peaks and decreased NAA and lactate peaks, but no lipid peaks, whereas high-grade tumors often had undetectable or markedly reduced NAA and creatine peaks and often had elevated lipid and lactate peaks. In vivo[187] and in vitro[188] proton MRS studies specifically of pediatric brain tumors demonstrate elevated choline to NAA ratios in both benign and malignant tumors, with higher ratios found in the malignant tumors such as PNET. These ratios have been used to accurately separate posterior fossa astrocytomas from ependymomas and PNETs, with about 85% of the tumors accurately classified (Figs. 46–15 and 46–16).[189] The future role of proton MRS in the imaging of pediatric brain tumors includes improving the accuracy of diagnosis of atypical-appearing tumors on conventional MRI and CT and may help in the choice of optimal treatment of these tumors in the future. Additional uses of nuclear medicine techniques and MRS in neuroimaging are reviewed elsewhere in this book.

CLASSIFICATION OF CENTRAL NERVOUS SYSTEM TUMORS

"That practical, everyday tumor classification is not yet an exact science is a consequence of the incomplete understanding of histologic and clinical features, as well as an even more incomplete grasp of the ultimate detail of molecular anatomy."[190]

Most classification schemes of central nervous system tumors are based on the Bailey and Cushing system, in which tumors were related to a specific cell lineage, with tumors identified as primitive (-*blastic*), or differentiated (-*cytic*).[191] Lesions classified as fibrillary, diffuse astrocytic tumors (astrocytoma, anaplastic astrocytoma, glioblastoma) were classed as astrocytoma, astroblastoma, and spongioblastoma multiforme, respectively. Embryonal tumors (small, blue cell tumors with various degrees of differentiation) were categorized as medulloepithelioma,

FIGURE 46–16 Scattergram of creatine to choline and *N*-acetyl-L-aspartate to choline ratios in astrocytoma, ependymoma, PNET, and normal cerebellar tissue. (From Wang Z, Sutton LN, Cnaan A, et al. Proton MR spectroscopy of pediatric cerebellar tumors. AJNR 1995;16:1821–1833.)

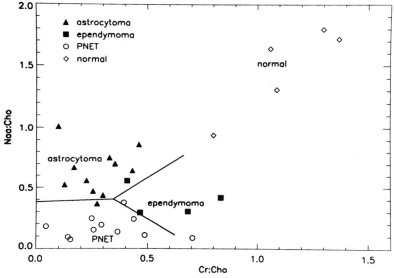

TABLE 46–1 Histologic Classification of Tumors of the Central Nervous System

Tumors of Neuroglia and Choroid Plexus Epithelium	Embryonal Tumors
Astrocytic neoplasms	Primitive neuroectodermal tumor
Fibrillary or diffuse astrocytic tumors	Medulloepithelioma
Astrocytoma	Neuroblastoma and ganglioneuroblastoma
Anaplastic astrocytoma	Ependymoblastoma
Glioblastoma multiforme	Medulloblastoma
Gliosarcoma	Medullomyoblastoma and melanotic medulloblastoma
Protoplasmic astrocytoma	**Tumors of the Pineal Gland**
Gliomatosis cerebri	Pineocytoma
Other astrocytic tumors	Pineoblastoma
Pilocytic astrocytoma	Pineal cyst
Pleomorphic xanthoastrocytoma	Gliomas
Subependymal giant cell astrocytoma	**Germ Cell Tumors**
Infantile desmoplastic astrocytoma	**Craniopharyngiomas**
Gliofibroma	Adamantinomatous craniopharyngioma
Oligodendroglial neoplasms	Papillary craniopharyngioma
Oligodendroglioma and anaplastic oligodendroglioma	**Benign Cystic Lesions**
Ependymal neoplasms	Colloid cyst of the third ventricle
Ependymoma and anaplastic ependymoma	Rathke's cleft cyst
Subependymoma	Choroid plexus cysts
Choroid plexus neoplasms	Arachnoid cysts
Choroid plexus papilloma	Pineal cysts
Choroid plexus carcinoma	**Tumor-Like Lesions of Maldevelopmental Origin**
Neuronal and Glioneuronal Tumors	Hypothalamic hamartoma
Gangliocytoma and ganglioglioma	
Desmoplastic infantile ganglioglioma	
Central neurocytoma	
Dysembryoplastic neuroepithelial tumor	

Modified from Burger PC, Scheithaner BW. Tumors of the Central Nervous System, Fasc. 10, Ser. 4. Atlas of Tumor Pathology. Washington, DC, Armed Forces Institute of Pathology, 1994.

neuroepithelioma, and various blastomas, the most common being the familiar medulloblastoma.

Kernohan and Sayre modified the Cushing and Bailey system of glial tumor classification. They considered the glial tumors to represent a spectrum of differentiation, and the astrocytoma, astroblastoma, and spongioblastoma become the more familiar astrocytomas, grades 1 to 4.[192] This approach dealt with the tendency of gliomas to transform to higher-grade tumors as well as the histologic heterogeneity seen in these tumors.

Russell and Rubenstein recognized the uniqueness of the pilocytic astrocytoma and the complexity of the embryonal cell tumors and added two new entities, ependymoblastoma and primitive polar spongioblastoma, to the work of Bailey and Cushing and Kernohan and Sayre. More recent editions of their classic text Pathology of Tumors of the Nervous System have included pleomorphic xanthoastrocytoma, central neurocytoma, and infantile desmoplastic ganglioglioma,[193] all of which are distinct tumors of children or young adults.

The World Health Organization (WHO), as part of its attempt to standardize nomenclature for all human neoplasms, established a consensus classification of brain tumors.[194] In this first attempt, the glioblastoma and medulloblastoma were combined under poorly differentiated and embryonal tumors, in response to a lack of consensus regarding the origins of these tumors, especially the medulloblastoma. The first WHO classification did refine a grading system for gliomas, based on histologic factors:

grade I tumors are the benign astrocytomas, subependymal giant cell astrocytomas, and pilocytic astrocytomas. Diffuse or fibrillary astrocytic tumors are grouped into three additional grades: grade II (astrocytoma), grade III (anaplastic astrocytomas), and grade IV (glioblastoma). This classification does suffer from a lack of precision in assigning grades, and from sometimes subtle differences between grade II (low-grade) and grade III or higher (high-grade) neoplasms, which may influence the decision to administer postoperative chemotherapy or radiation therapy.

The second WHO classification scheme is similar to the first but recognizes that glioblastoma is a high-grade diffuse astrocytoma, different from medulloblastoma. The new WHO scheme also recognizes central neurocytoma, dysembryoplastic neuroepithelial tumor, infantile desmoplastic ganglioglioma, pleomorphic astrocytoma, and papillary craniopharyngioma. Grading of astrocytomas was refined and made more rigid. Genetic alterations in astrocytomas were also acknowledged.[195] This classification is relatively straightforward and can be used as a framework to organize the various brain neoplasms encountered by neuroradiologists (Table 46–1). The WHO grading system reflects the likely biologic potential of tumors. Embryonal tumors continue to be a controversial topic among neuropathologists. Some classify most embryonal cell tumors as PNET, whereas others believe this to be an oversimplification. This chapter largely follows the second WHO classification scheme of restricting the term *PNET* as a generic term for both cerebellar medulloblastoma and neoplasms morphologically similar to the medulloblastoma but located at other sites in the central nervous system.

Tumors of the Posterior Fossa

In the pediatric population, posterior fossa neoplasms represent about 48% of brain tumors overall.[196] Medulloblastoma, cerebellar astrocytoma, ependymoma, and brain stem gliomas account for 95% of the tumors found in this compartment.[197]

Medulloblastoma

Medulloblastoma is the most common neoplasm of the posterior fossa in children, representing about one-third of neoplasms in this location.[198] The peak incidence is in the first decade, and there is a male to female predominance of from 2 to 1[199] to as high as 4 to 1.[200] The term *medulloblastoma* is best reserved for small cell neuroectodermal tumors of the cerebellum. Histogenesis of these tumors is controversial, but the external granular layer or cells in the posterior medullary velum have been implicated. It appears that these tumors arise from undifferen-

tiated cells of the medullary velum that migrate superiorly and laterally to form the external granular layer of the cerebellar hemispheres. This may explain the hemispheric location of medulloblastomas in older children and adults and the typical midline location in younger patients. It is likely that the term *medulloblastoma* encompasses more than one true tumor type. Almost half show some histologic evidence of differentiation, with neuronal, glial, mixed, and undifferentiated (classic) forms found.[190] These aggressive tumors frequently exit the intra-axial cerebellum, coating the subarachnoid space with neoplastic cells.

The typical appearance of medulloblastoma with CT is a midline, vermian, solid, hyperdense mass with some homogeneous diffuse enhancement.[201] "Atypical" features are in fact quite common and include cyst formation, (seen in up to 59%), calcification (in 21%), and combinations of cysts, calcification, and large cystic cavities.[199] The typical appearance was seen in only 30% of cases. A majority of tumors (70% to 90%) show homogeneous enhancement on CECT,[202] whereas the remainder have heterogeneous enhancement or do not enhance at all (Fig. 46–17).[200] Other atypical features include presentation as a cerebellopontine angle mass from exophytic

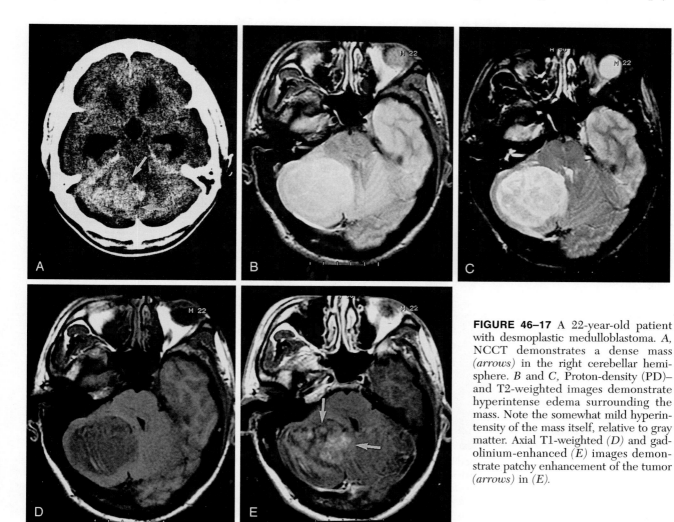

FIGURE 46–17 A 22-year-old patient with desmoplastic medulloblastoma. *A,* NCCT demonstrates a dense mass *(arrows)* in the right cerebellar hemisphere. *B* and *C,* Proton-density (PD)– and T2-weighted images demonstrate hyperintense edema surrounding the mass. Note the somewhat mild hyperintensity of the mass itself, relative to gray matter. Axial T1-weighted *(D)* and gadolinium-enhanced *(E)* images demonstrate patchy enhancement of the tumor *(arrows)* in *(E).*

growth and extension through fourth ventricle foramina (of Luschka and Magendie).[203] Hemorrhagic tumors have been reported. Hemorrhage may occur into intact tumor or into areas of tumor necrosis.[204] Multifocal tumors have been occasionally reported, and although these may represent early CSF dissemination, simultaneous tumor cannot be excluded.[205]

MRI features of medulloblastoma include hypointensity, isointensity, or a mixed appearance, relative to gray matter, on T1-weighted images, with intermediate to moderately high signal intensity with T2 weighting.[198] The density seen with CT, and the frequent occurrence of isointense or nearly isointense T2 signal, have been attributed to the marked cellularity and high nuclear to cytoplasmic ratio of medulloblastomas.[206] Signal heterogeneity on T2-weighted images is common and can represent areas of cyst, necrosis, calcifications, or small blood vessels. The cysts are seen even more frequently with MRI than with CT (in up to 77%), and their contents are usually isointense or slightly hyperintense, relative to CSF,

on both T1- and T2-weighted images;[203] the cysts likely contain proteinaceous fluid (Figs. 46–18 and 46–19).

CSF dissemination of medulloblastoma is common, present in up to half of patients at autopsy,[207] and the evaluation of such disease was described previously. Medulloblastoma is the third most common central nervous system tumor to exhibit systemic metastases, after glioblastoma and meningioma; the latter two tumors are distinctly less common in the pediatric population. The most common site of medulloblastoma metastasis is bone,[208] where the lesions are typically osteoblastic. MRI of skeletal medulloblastoma metastases to the spine shows focal areas of increased T2 signal intensity and decreased T1 signal intensity with gadolinium enhancement. The MRI signal abnormalities in the vertebral bodies have been observed with normal bone scintigraphy and can precede the development of sclerotic lesions on radiographs.[207]

Medulloblastoma may be seen in older children and adults, although it represents only 1% of brain tumors in

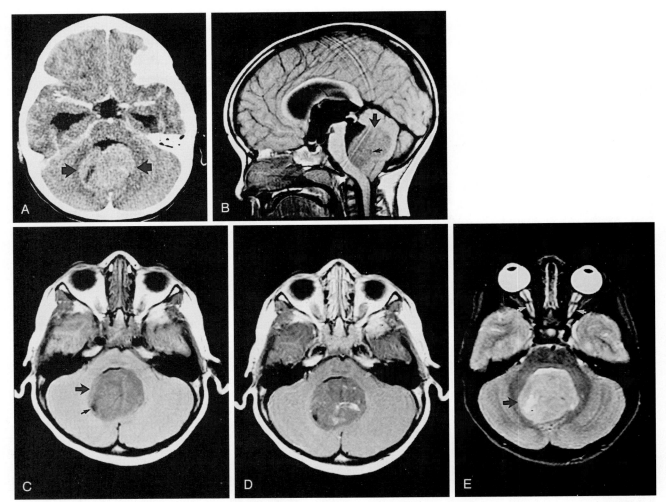

FIGURE 46–18 A 3-year-old child with medulloblastoma. *A*, CECT demonstrates an enhancing vermian mass *(arrows)* and dilatation of the temporal horns of the lateral ventricles from hydrocephalus. Sagittal *(B)* and axial *(C)* T1-weighted images demonstrate the vermian location of the hypointense mass *(large arrows)* and focal areas of low signal intensity likely representing cysts or necrosis *(small arrows)*, as calcification was not present on the CT scans. *D*, Mild patchy enhancement with gadolinium is present. *E*, T2-weighted image demonstrates only mild hyperintensity of the tumor *(black arrow)*. Fluid is present along the optic nerve sheaths *(white arrows)* from hydrocephalus.

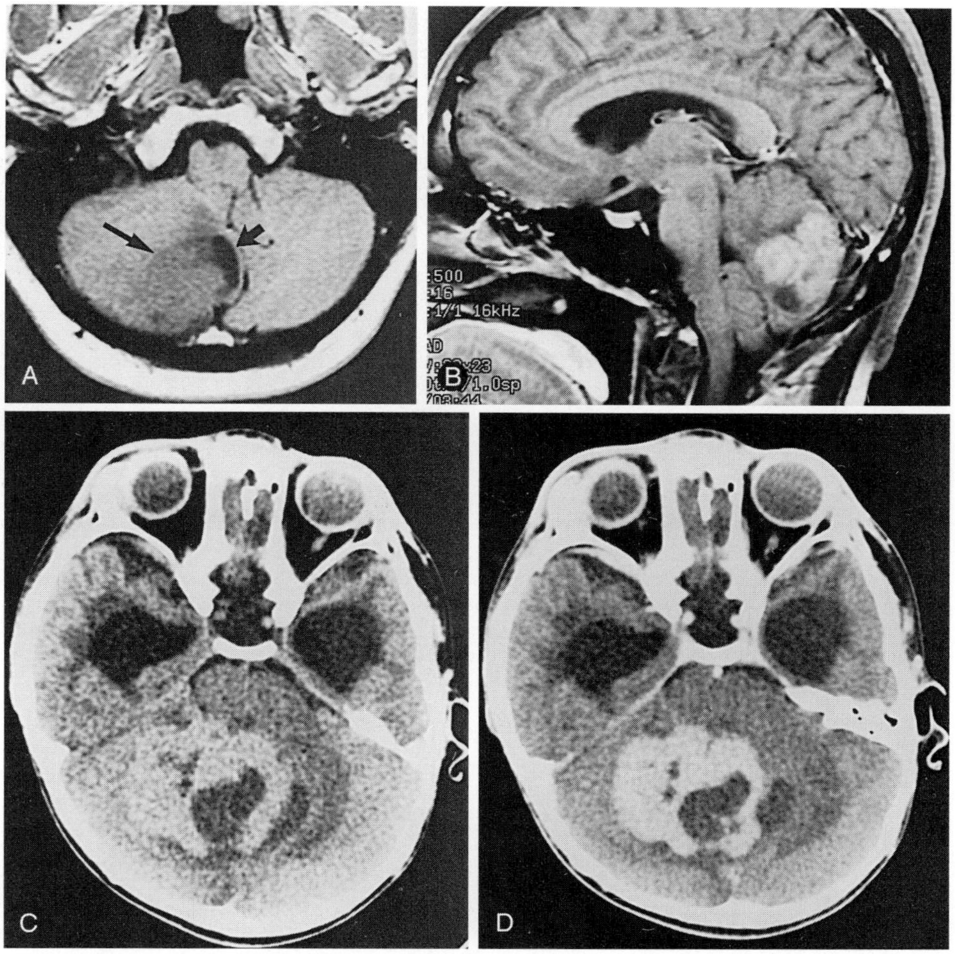

FIGURE 46–19 Medulloblastoma (two patients). *A*, T1-weighted axial image demonstrates a heterogeneous mass originating near the vermis *(long arrow)*, with apparently cystic areas *(short arrow)*. *B*, Gadolinium-enhanced T1-weighted sagittal image demonstrates avid, heterogeneous enhancement. *C*, NCCT of a different patient demonstrates a cystic and solid mass, hyperdense relative to brain. *D*, Enhancement of the solid portions of the tumor are seen with CECT.

the latter.[209] In these older patients, medulloblastomas are more likely to be located in the lateral aspect of the cerebellum and are even more likely to demonstrate hyperdensity on CT images; there may also be a tendency toward reduced T2 signal intensity due to the greater incidence of the desmoplastic variant seen in this age group.[210] It has been speculated that in children, medulloblastomas arise from undifferentiated cells of the floor of the fourth ventricle (posterior medullary velum) and are thus found in the midline, whereas adult tumors arise from the external granular layer of the cerebellar cortex, which forms from precursor cells that have migrated laterally from pluripotential cells of the posterior medullary velum. This may explain the difference in location between adults and children. The origin from the external granular layer also explains the more peripheral location of these tumors in the cerebellum in adults. The contiguity with brain surface and the cellularity of these tumors may mimic meningioma in the adult.[211]

Astrocytomas of the Cerebellum

Cerebellar astrocytomas account for 30% to 40% of posterior fossa tumors in childhood.[212] Both benign and anaplastic lesions are encountered, with the benign tumors (diffuse fibrillary astrocytoma and juvenile pilocytic astrocytoma) the most frequently encountered. The juvenile

pilocytic astrocytoma (JPA) constitutes 75% to 85% of all cerebellar astrocytomas, has a peak incidence in the first decade of life, and is associated with a nearly 90% 25-year survival rate.[213] The diffuse fibrillary type is more common in adolescents and young adults, represents up to 15% of pediatric posterior fossa astrocytomas, and is associated with a lower survival rate, 40% at 25 years. The diffuse type is more invasive and less easily resected than the sharply marginated JPA.[213] No gender predominance is observed with cerebellar astrocytomas.

The classic "biphasic" JPA is composed of loose stellate astrocytes with microcystic regions and compact tissue consisting of elongated fibrillated cells. Eosinophilic granular bodies and Rosenthal's fibers may be present. Although considered benign, pilocytic astrocytomas are noted to break through the pia and fill the adjacent subarachnoid space; this feature does not indicate aggressive behavior or leptomeningeal seeding.[190] The growth rate of such subarachnoid tumor can be very slow, with prolonged survival.[214] JPAs are typically large (>5 cm) at presentation, reflecting their indolent growth. Rare late malignant recurrence of pilocytic astrocytomas has been reported.[215] Radiation therapy–induced transformation as well as malignant transformation of a benign tumor have been implicated.

The typical appearance of a posterior fossa JPA is a

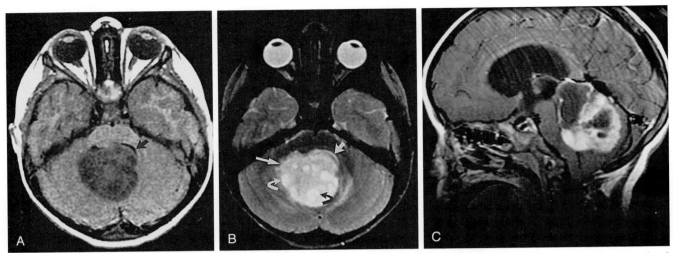

FIGURE 46–20 A 2-year-old child with juvenile pilocytic astrocytomas (JPAs) of the cerebellum. T1-weighted *(A)* and T2-weighted *(B)* images demonstrate a large, well-defined mass centered in the vermis. Note the anteriorly displaced fourth ventricle *(short arrow)* and heterogeneous signal intensity of the mass. Solid components are isointense on T1-weighted and hyperintense (relative to gray matter) on T2-weighted images *(long arrow)*, whereas areas isointense to cerebrospinal fluid (CSF) are likely cystic *(curved arrows)*. *C*, Sagittal T1-weighted image with gadolinium demonstrates intense enhancement of the solid portions of the tumor and dilated ventricles consistent with hydrocephalus.

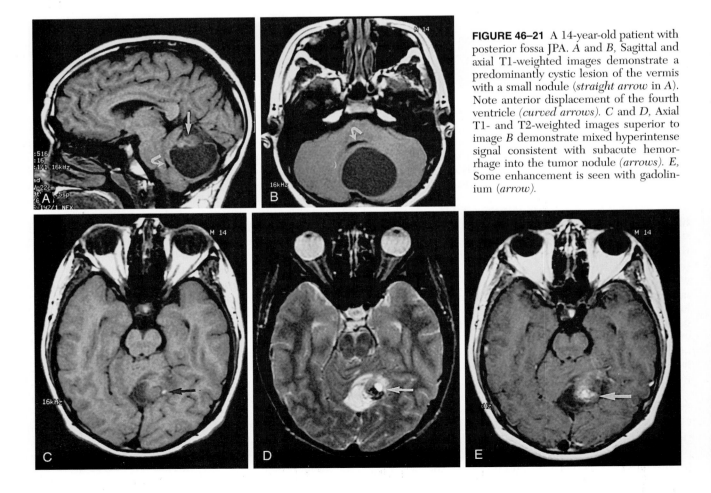

FIGURE 46–21 A 14-year-old patient with posterior fossa JPA. *A* and *B*, Sagittal and axial T1-weighted images demonstrate a predominantly cystic lesion of the vermis with a small nodule *(straight arrow* in *A)*. Note anterior displacement of the fourth ventricle *(curved arrows)*. *C* and *D*, Axial T1- and T2-weighted images superior to image *B* demonstrate mixed hyperintense signal consistent with subacute hemorrhage into the tumor nodule *(arrows)*. *E*, Some enhancement is seen with gadolinium *(arrow)*.

mass arising from the midline (85%) or cerebellar hemisphere (15%) that is cystic with a well-defined rounded or plaquelike mural nodule. With CECT, only the nodule is seen to enhance. This pattern is seen in about 50% of posterior fossa JPAs. The remainder usually have some evidence of cyst formation, including multiple cysts, with only 10% of lesions purely solid.[216] It is important to distinguish the large cyst with mural nodule variety from the partially solid lesion with intratumoral cysts; in the former, resection of the mural nodule and drainage of the cyst is curative, whereas in the later the entire mass needs to be resected.[213] The partially solid lesions tend to have multiple, multiloculated cysts in distinction to the solitary cyst of the typical JPA. Solid portions of these tumors, either the mural nodule or the tumor matrix in heterogeneous lesions, are hypo- or isodense with brain on noncontrast computed tomography (NCCT) and avidly enhance on CECT. Lesions are sharply demarcated, and edema is typically minimal or absent.[217] If present, calcifications are flecklike and seen in 10% to 20% of patients.

MRI features of posterior fossa JPA parallel those seen with CT. Cysts are seen in 80% of tumors; the cyst fluid is usually proteinaceous and tends to be slightly hyperintense on T1-weighted images and hyperintense on T2-weighted images, relative to CSF.[218] Solid components of the tumor, both mural nodules and the tumoral component of solid lesions, enhance avidly and tend to be hyperintense compared with gray matter on T2-weighted images, a useful differentiating feature from medulloblastoma.[219] Hemorrhage is rare in pediatric cerebellar astrocytomas (Figs. 46–20 through 46–22).[219]

The diffuse fibrillary low-grade astrocytomas of the cerebellum cannot always be differentiated radiographically from the pilocytic neoplasms. Poorly defined borders, hypodensity on NCCT, and lack of enhancement suggest a diffuse astrocytoma with poorer prognosis.[49]

Ependymoma

Ependymomas constitute 9% to 16% of all primary central nervous system tumors in children. They may be found in both the supratentorial and infratentorial compartments, but the majority are found in the posterior fossa.[213] Two age peaks are seen with posterior fossa tumors, the majority being found in children 5 years old and younger, with a smaller peak in adults aged 30 to 40 years.[220] These tumors are felt to arise from the ependymal lining of the fourth ventricle itself, typically from the floor more commonly than the roof, or from ependymal rests elsewhere in the neuroaxis. These rests may be found at sites where the ventricles are sharply angled, posterior to the occipital horns, at the ventral spur of the cerebral aqueduct, adjacent to the foramen of Luschka, near the ventricular outlets, along the tela choroidea, in the central canal of the spinal cord, and in the filum terminale.[221] The location of these rests is reflected by the various locations of ependymoma in the brain and spine. Posterior fossa tumors are largely intraventricular, but supratentorial tumors may have an extensive parenchymal component.

The classic ependymoma is characterized by a cellular pattern and the formation of perivascular pseudorosettes; some ependymomas express epithelial features with true

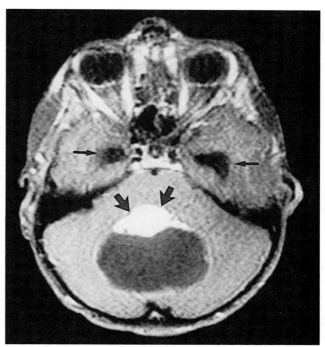

FIGURE 46–22 A 5-year-old boy with posterior fossa JPA. A gadolinium-enhanced T1-weighted image demonstrates a midline cerebellar mass, predominantly cystic with an intensely enhancing mural nodule *(large arrows)*. The fourth ventricle is not seen at this level and is displaced by the tumor, but dilated temporal horns consistent with hydrocephalus are present *(small arrows)*.

perivascular rosettes with central lumina.[190] The rarer papillary ependymomas exhibit extensive epithelial features. Myxopapillary ependymomas typically involve the filum terminale with only rare cases of tumors near the sacrum (probably arising from ectopic ependymal rests) and in intracranial locations.[222] The tanycytic variant of ependymoma is significant in its composition of elongated cells with fibrillar processes that may resemble a pilocytic astrocytoma. These tumors are well differentiated with few mitoses. There is no consensus on the grading of ependymomas or on the prognostic value of specific histologic features, but anaplastic tumors, highly cellular lesions with high mitotic activity, often in association with vascular proliferation, are more likely to recur and to do so more quickly.[223] Highly anaplastic malignant ependymomas are characterized by necrosis and pseudopalisading as seen in other central nervous system malignancies. Factors associated with improved survival are age greater than 6 years, gross total tumor resection at surgery, noninvasive tumors, and absent clinical signs of parenchymal invasion or lower cranial nerve involvement.[224] The majority of posterior fossa ependymomas are histologically benign, although malignant and embryonic subtypes exist.[225] The embryonic tumors (ependymoblastoma) are best considered as a small cell embryonal neoplasm with ependymoblastic rosettes, different from both conventional ependymoma and malignant ependymoma.[226] Recurrence is usually at the primary intracranial site, and symptomatic spinal (subarachnoid) spread does not occur frequently[227] despite the typical projection of these tumors into the ventricles. The malignant or anaplastic ependymoma does have a greater tendency to spread through the CSF. Ependymomas can infiltrate through the ependymal surface into adjacent brain, making complete surgical resection difficult, despite their typical intraventricular location.

NCCT features of a typical posterior fossa ependymoma are an isodense (80%) or heterogeneous mass with ill-defined borders filling and expanding the fourth ventricle. Calcification, usually nodular, is seen in about 50%.[221] Contrast enhancement is homogeneous in 40% and heterogeneous in 40% and may be absent in 10% to 20%. Small cysts may be seen but may be more common in supratentorial tumors. Intratumoral hemorrhage is uncommon, seen in about 10% of cases.[213] A well-known variant, the "plastic ependymoma,"[228] with extension out of the foramina of Luschka into the cerebellopontine angle and out of the foramen of Magendie with extension behind the brain stem, along with minimal expansion of the fourth ventricle, is seen in only a minority of cases. These tumors may demonstrate spread around the cervical cord.

MRI of ependymomas is also characterized by heterogeneous signal intensity. The solid tumor is typically isointense or hypointense compared with gray matter on T1-weighted images, with heterogeneous hyperintense signal on T2-weighted images. The heterogeneous signal intensity is due to the presence of calcification, small cystic areas, vascularity, hemorrhage, or a combination of these characteristics.[229] Gradient-echo MRI studies are more likely to detect the small nodular calcifications that are best seen with CT. Cystic areas are usually hyperintense on T2-weighted images, likely due to the increased protein content of the cyst fluid. Heterogeneous gadolinium enhancement is present in most ependymomas (Figs. 46–23 through 46–26).[216]

Brain Stem Gliomas

Brain stem gliomas represent 10% to 15% of infratentorial neoplasms in children, with 75% presenting before the age of 10 years and a mean age at presentation of 6 years.[230] Some authors have noted a male predominance with a male to female ratio of 2.5 to 1,[231] whereas others find an equal gender distribution of patients.[232] Histologic examination of 55% to 80% of brain stem gliomas in children reveals low-grade astrocytoma, usually a diffuse fibrillary astrocytoma.[233] Typical juvenile pilocytic astrocytomas may also be found in the brain stem but are distinctly less common. Anaplastic transformation, hemorrhage, and a histologic appearance consistent with high-grade glioma are found at the time of death in 60% to 80% of patients, and in 50% findings consistent with glioblastoma multiforme are present at autopsy.[231] It is unclear if this high incidence represents dedifferentiation of existing tumor or sampling error, as a heterogeneous histologic appearance is commonly present in these tumors, and extensive surgical resection is usually not ac-

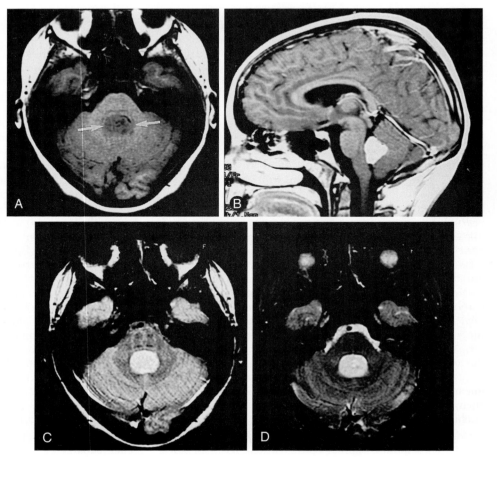

FIGURE 46–23 A 12-year-old patient with ependymoma. *A,* T1-weighted image demonstrates a sharply defined, slightly hypointense mass within the fourth ventricle with a few small cystic areas *(arrows). B,* Gadolinium-enhanced sagittal image better defines the intraventricular location of the mass. *C* and *D,* The mass is hyperintense on PD- and T2-weighted images.

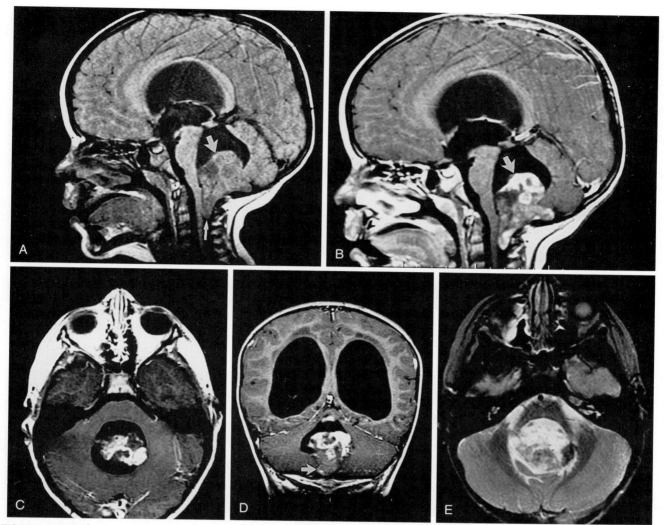

FIGURE 46–24 Plastic ependymoma in a young child. Sagittal T1-weighted *(A)* and gadolinium-enhanced T1-weighted *(B)* images demonstrate a heterogeneous, enhancing mass in the fourth ventricle *(large arrows)* with inferior extension through the foramen of Magendie *(small arrow* in *A)*. Tumor is seen extending beneath the cerebellar vermis and behind the upper cervical spinal cord. Axial *(C)* and coronal *(D)* gadolinium-enhanced images demonstrate marked hydrocephalus, the intraventricular location of the tumor, and extension of tumor through the foramen of Magendie *(arrow* in *D)*. *E,* Heterogeneous hyperintense signal is present on a T2-weighted image. The mass is within spaces normally filled by CSF and does not appear to invade adjacent brain to a great extent.

complished with brain stem gliomas except when the tumors are focal or exophytic. The presence of calcifications (microsopic), microcysts, and Rosenthal fibers suggests a less aggressive tumor, whereas a large number of mitoses, pleomorphism, and hyperchromatism suggest a worse prognosis.

The majority (54%) of brain stem gliomas are centered in the pons, with 32% found in the medulla and the remainder in the mesencephalon.[230] The tumors frequently infiltrate into the diencephalon or spinal cord, or through the peduncles into the cerebellum.[219]

Overall, these tumors have a poor prognosis with a mean survival of 4 to 15 months; in some series the 5-year survival rate is from 30%[234] to as low as 5%.[235] The inclusion of more benign brain stem gliomas significantly varies the survival rates in studies with up to a 50% 5-year survival when diencephalic or cervicomedullary

tumors are included in significant numbers. Series limited to tumors that infiltrate or enlarge the brain stem usually have survival rates under 20% at 3 years.[231] With current MRI techniques, the tumor location of brain stem gliomas may be determined accurately, correlated with survival, and used to guide treatment.

Because of their location within the brain stem, clinical presentation of brain stem tumors is different from that of lesions elsewhere in the posterior fossa. The classic presentation is a rapid onset of bilateral brain stem dysfunction, including multiple cranial nerve palsies and long-tract and cerebellar signs.[236] Cranial nerve palsies are present in up to 90% of patients at presentation,[237] with sixth and seventh cranial nerves the most frequently affected. Presentation with focal neurologic deficits, symptoms and signs referrable to the cerebellopontine angle, psychiatric symptoms, and failure to thrive (in

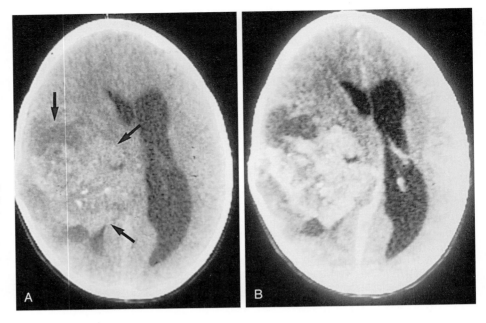

FIGURE 46–25 An 8-year-old girl with supratentorial papillary ependymoma. *A*, NCCT demonstrates a large hemispheric mass with small calcifications, significant effacement and shift of the right lateral ventricle, and surrounding vasogenic edema *(arrows)*. *B*, CECT reveals intense, heterogeneous enhancement.

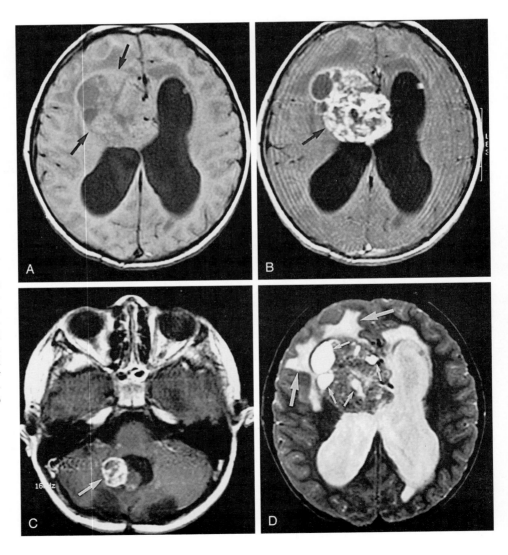

FIGURE 46–26 A 7-year-old child with recurrent ependymoma. Primary tumor was initially confined to the fourth ventricle. *A*, T1-weighted image demonstrates a large, cystic, invasive mass in the anterior horn of the right lateral ventricle *(arrows)*. *B* and *C*, Gadolinium-enhanced images demonstrate heterogeneous enhancement of the large mass as well as enhancing tumor nodules in the left lateral ventricle and the fourth ventricle *(arrows)*. *D*, T2-weighted image shows marked heterogeneity of the tumor with small cysts *(small arrows)* and edema *(large arrows)*, which may be related to invasion of the adjacent brain. Hydrocephalus is also present.

infants) is also reported.[238] Hydrocephalus is unusual, found in about 10% to 15% of patients[239] when exophytic growth into the fourth ventricle is present.

Brain stem gliomas may be classified as diffuse tumors, focal medullary tumors with or without exophytic growth into the fourth ventricle, and cervicomedullary lesions.[240] Diffuse tumors are almost always anaplastic astrocytomas with extension into contiguous regions and invasion into the cervical cord, cerebellum, or thalamus. Focal tumors of the medulla, when low grade, tend to be either limited and well defined, or exophytic with growth posteriorly into the fourth ventricle; growth superiorly is limited by transverse fibers of the pontomedullary barrier and caudally by fibers of the cervicomedullary junction. Cervicomedullary tumors resemble intramedullary spinal cord neoplasms caudally, with rostral growth limited at the cervicomedullary junction by decussating fibers in a manner similar to that of the focal tumors of the medulla. Most of these focal brain stem tumors are low-grade astrocytomas, with a smaller number of anaplastic tumors and gangliogliomas.[240] These anatomically focal tumors have a better prognosis than diffuse brain stem gliomas and may be identified radiologically.

The typical NCCT appearance of a brain stem glioma is a hypo- or isodense mass that expands the affected portion of the brain stem. Narrowing of the prepontine space and posterior displacement of the fourth ventricle are useful radiologic features.[216] Some authors have correlated hypodensity on NCCT with a worse prognosis, compared with isodensity.[241] Other CT signs of poor prognosis include extension into the cerebellopontine angle and large cystic tumors with enhancement of the cyst wall itself.[242] Hypodense nonenhancing tumors had an 18.3% 2-year survival versus a 60% rate for isodense lesions; an MRI signal equivalent has not been reported. The CECT appearance is variable, with enhancement reported as being unusual, or heterogeneous and present in up to 50% of cases (Fig. 46–27).[233] The presence of enhancement does not appear to correlate with survival in some authors' experience,[241] whereas others have noted that isodense tumors that enhance avidly on CECT have a better prognosis.[242] The tumors may be exophytic anterior to the pons and engulf the basilar artery. Calcification is uncommon in brain stem tumors,[243] but hemorrhage and cysts may be present. At presentation, 26% of brain stem gliomas show radiographic evidence of necrosis.[244] Over time, virtually all patients develop evidence of necrosis, and the time between the initial diagnosis of brain stem tumor and the development of necrosis correlates with survival. Although radiation therapy is commonly used to treat brain stem gliomas, the development of necrosis does not correlate with the radiotherapy technique used (conventional versus hyperfractionated) and was described in pontine tumors before the development of radiation therapy.[244, 245] Necrosis is probably part of the natural history of these tumors.

CT is limited by beam-hardening artifact in the posterior fossa, so it is not surprising that MRI is superior for delineation of the extent of brain stem neoplasms.[246–248] The typical appearance is an expansile mass with hypointensity on T1-weighted images and hyperintensity on T2-weighted images, relative to gray matter.[249] Images in the

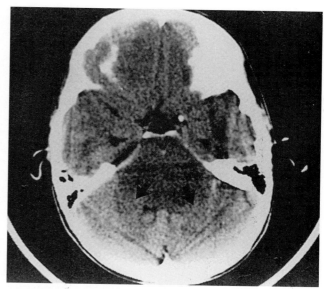

FIGURE 46–27 Diffuse pontine astrocytoma in a 5-year-old girl. Axial nonenhanced CT shows a low-density mass (*arrows*) within the pons expanding the brain stem. (From Kane AG, Robles HA, Smirniotopoulos JG, et al. Radiologic-pathologic correlation. Diffuse pontine astrocytoma. AJNR 1993;14:941–945.)

sagittal plane are particularly useful, and the T2-weighted images can demonstrate more extensive abnormalities than T1-weighted images (Fig. 46–28).[250] Brain stem gliomas typically do not have large amounts of surrounding edema, and the use of T2-weighted images to determine the extent of aggressive or diffuse brain stem gliomas is important. However, postradiation changes, ischemia, or extensive edema from high-grade lesions may produce T2-signal abnormalities that extend beyond the true extent of tumor. Edema surrounding low-grade astrocytomas is usually insignificant,[251] but as noted previously, there is an increased incidence of the development of a high-grade malignancy over time in brain stem glioma patients. The reported incidence of contrast enhancement of brain stem tumors varies considerably in the literature, from 25%[202] to as high as 80%;[49] typically the enhancement is heterogeneous. Overall, cystic areas are seen with MRI in about 25%.[230]

As noted previously, brain stem gliomas may be focal lesions (Fig. 46–29). Dorsally exophytic brain stem gliomas may penetrate the ependyma and extend into the fourth ventricle, occasionally with spread into the cisterna magna. These represent about 22% of brain stem gliomas. Despite the apparent invasiveness of these tumors, with transependymal spread, their prognosis is good.[252] These exophytic tumors are typically low-grade astrocytomas, present with more indolent symptoms than diffuse tumors, are isodense or slightly hypodense on NCCT, may have cysts, and enhance avidly. MRI of the dorsally exophytic gliomas demonstrates sharply defined lesions with low signal intensity on T1-weighted images, hyperintensity relative to gray matter on T2-weighted images, and avid enhancement of noncystic areas.[253] Unlike the diffuse brain stem gliomas, primary treatment for these tumors

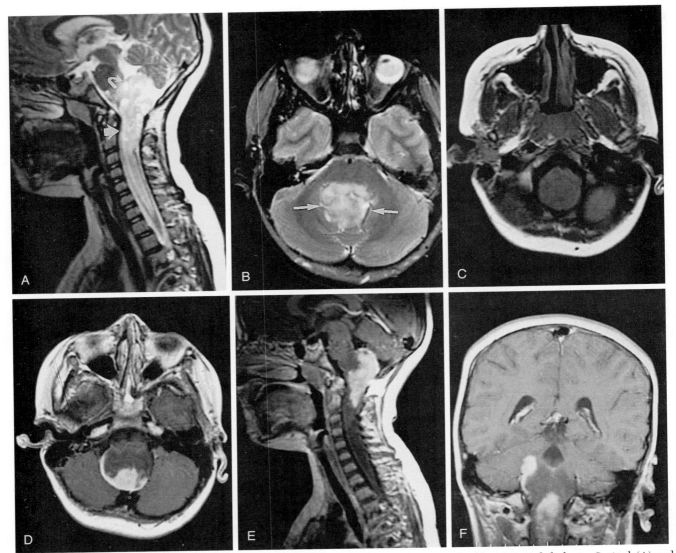

FIGURE 46–28 An 8-year-old child with cervicomedullary glioma. The patient presented with ataxia and diplopia. Sagittal (A) and axial (B) T2-weighted images demonstrate extensive expansion of the medulla and spinal cord by a hyperintense mass (straight arrows). The lesion's extent is poorly defined but appears to extend interiorly as far as the T1 level. An exophytic component is also present extending into the fourth ventricle (curved arrow in A). The tumor is hypointense on T1-weighted images (C) and demonstrates variable enhancement of some but not all of the tumor on gadolinium-enhanced images (D–F).

is frequently surgical, with radiation therapy for recurrent tumor. In an analogous manner, focal tumors of the cervicomedullary junction also have a better prognosis compared with diffuse tumors, are usually (88%) low-grade tumors with a longer duration of symptoms, and seem to respond favorably to surgery.[254]

It is important to recognize that there is a differential diagnosis for focal brain stem lesions in children, including hemorrhages, cavernous angiomas, and other vascular malformations.[233] Imaging characteristics of these three lesions may be seen with MRI and are described elsewhere in this book. Other diagnostic possibilities include tuberculoma, lymphoma, brain stem encephalitis, and acute disseminated encephalomyelitis.[216] The clinical course and evolution of these entities are important in evaluating a focal mass lesion of the brain stem.

Diffuse brain stem gliomas present a challenge in management, with treatment consisting primarily of radiation therapy. With current MRI techniques, the identification of a diffuse, expansile lesion of the brain stem in a child is sufficiently diagnostic of an infiltrative glioma that biopsy is probably unnecessary; biopsy is associated with its own morbidity, and the results of obtaining tissue seldom alter therapy.[255]

Difficulty may be encountered when evaluating a diffuse brain stem glioma after therapy. New enhancement may be present and due to radiation therapy rather than tumor recurrence,[50] but the presence of an enlarging mass with or without cyst formation usually represents tumor recurrence rather than radionecrosis.[251] Hemorrhage or cyst development alone may not signal tumor recurrence but may produce worsening of clinical symptoms.

Although experience is limited, FDG-PET may be

useful in the detection of recurrent brain stem glioma when MRI images are unchanged but the patient demonstrates clinical decline, or when transient radiographic or clinical deterioration occurs after radiation therapy.[256]

Pineal Region Neoplasms

The pineal region is anatomically diverse. The normal pineal gland is attached to the posterior border of the third ventricle, in the midline within the CSF of the quadrigeminal plate cistern. Adjacent structures include the cistern of the velum interpositum; tectum and tegmentum; thalami; splenium of the corpus callosum; internal cerebral veins; and vein of Galen. Overall, pineal region neoplasms are rare, representing only 1% to 3% of all intracranial neoplasms[257] and 3% to 8% of intracranial

tumors in children.[258] The incidence is higher in Asia. The median age of presentation is 13 years. The unique location of masses in this region produces some specific symptoms—precocious puberty, hypogonadism, and diabetes insipidus, as well as hydrocephalus from aqueductal compression. Precocious puberty may arise from interference with the normal antigonadotropic effect of the pineal gland, invasion into the diencephalon with destruction of the sexual inhibitory function of the median eminence, or ectopic production of gondadotropins.[257] Diabetes insipidus may occur if the mass invades or seeds, through CSF dissemination, the anterior and inferior recesses of the third ventricle or the hypothalamus itself.

A classic presentation of pineal region tumors is Parinaud's syndrome, with paralysis of conjugate upward gaze and occasional loss of ocular convergence. This syndrome

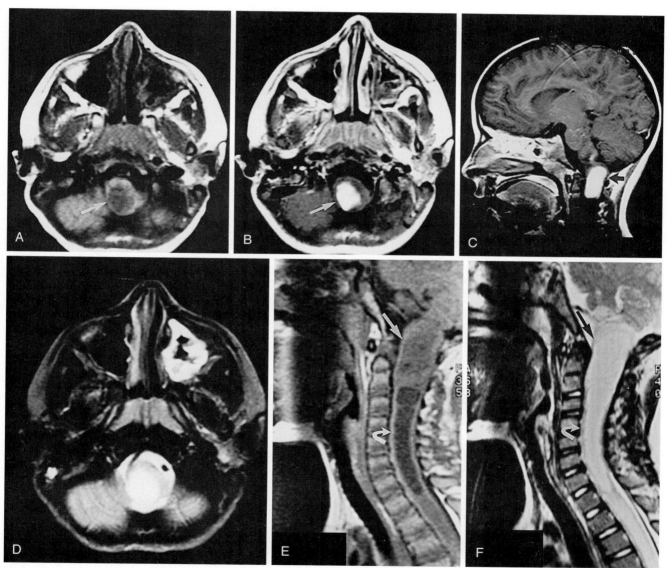

FIGURE 46–29 A 7-year-old with JPA of the brain stem. Pre- *(A)* and postgadolinium *(B and C)* images demonstrate hypointense expansion of the cervicomedullary junction *(arrows)*. The mass avidly enhances with gadolinium. *D,* T2-weighted image demonstrates hyperintensity of the mass. Sagittal T1-weighted *(E)* and T2-weighted *(F)* images demonstrate both the intramedullary mass *(straight arrows in E and F)*, which is isointense on T1-weighted and hyperintense on T2-weighted sequences, and a more interiorly located syrinx *(curved arrows)*, which is isointense to fluid.

TABLE 46–2 Pineal Region Masses

Germ Cell Tumors

Embryonic differentiation
  Germinoma
  Teratomas
Extraembryonic differentiation
  Choriocarcinoma
  Endodermal sinus tumor

Pineal Parenchymal Neoplasms

Pineocytoma
Pineoblastoma
Astrocytoma

Tumors of Supporting Elements or Adjacent Tissues

Astrocytoma
Ependymoma
Meningioma
Lymphoma

Nonneoplastic Masses

Pineal cyst
Lipoma
Arachnoid cyst
Dermoid and epidermoid
Vascular malformations

Metastatic Neoplasms

Modified from Smirniotopoulos JG, Rushing EJ, Mena HM. Pineal region masses: Differential diagnosis. Radiographics 1992;12:577–596.

results from compression on the reflex nuclei of the tectum.

A variety of pineal region tumors have been reported in children (Table 46–2); however, germinoma and astrocytoma account for the majority of tumors in this area.[258] With the availability of MRI, tumors in this region frequently (but not always) can be localized to the pineal gland itself, the tectum, or the tegmentum, and their location can be used to help narrow the differential of a pineal mass.

The normal pineal gland measures about 4 mm wide.[257] With MRI, the normal pineal gland may be visualized as a nodule, crescent, or ringlike structure, with cysts (5 mm or larger) noted in 0.6% of children and 2.6% of adults.[259] Histologic evidence of cysts is seen in 25% to 40% of pineal glands at autopsy.[260] The fluid within the cysts appears slightly hyperintense to CSF on both T1- and T2-weighted MRI images, likely due to its protein content and lack of cardiac-produced pulsation within the fluid of the cyst itself.[261, 262] The large majority of pineal cysts are asymptomatic, but symptomatic, nonneoplastic pineal cysts have been reported to produce neurologic symptoms and hydrocephalus.[263] The cysts have a distinct laminated wall whose inner-layer histologic appearance resembles that of a pilocytic astrocytoma. Correlation with MRI findings is helpful in making the correct diagnosis. Only about one-half of the cysts demonstrated enhancement;[263] this peripheral enhancement represents enhancement of surrounding normal pineal tissue, which does not have an intact blood-brain barrier (Fig. 46–30).

Calcifications are commonly seen in the pineal gland with NCCT but are not noted in children younger than 5 years and only in 11% of children up to the age of 14 years.[264] The presence of such calcification in young children, or abnormal displacement of the calcifications in a normal gland, are CT features of pineal tumors.

Ninety-five percent of the cells of the normal pineal gland are neuronal with dendritic processes (pinealocytes), and the remainder are neuroglial cells resembling astrocytes. However, about two-thirds of masses of the pineal region itself are multipotential embryonic germ cell derivatives that are identical to gonadal tumors.[257] These tumors, benign or malignant, arise from germ cells that originate in the yolk sac wall and normally migrate to the genital ridges but become misguided and embedded in the pineal gland. The pineal gland forms around 5 to 8 gestational weeks, during which time normal germ cell migration is occurring.

Pineal Germinoma

Germinomas represent two-thirds of the pineal germ cell tumors and are the most common tumor of the pineal overall. Eighty percent of germinomas are found in the pineal with the remainder in the suprasellar region.[257]

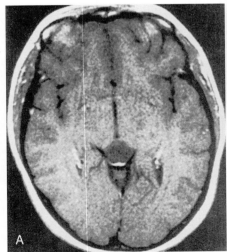 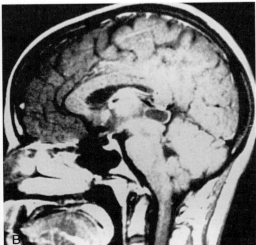

FIGURE 46–30 Pineal cyst. Axial (*A*) and sagittal (*B*) contrast-enhanced T1-weighted images show an oval fluid collection in the pineal region with signal intensity slightly greater than that of CSF and a crescent of enhancement in the residual pineal tissue. (*A* and *B* From Smirniotopoulos JG, Rushing EJ, Mena H. Pineal region masses. Differential diagnosis. Radiographics 1992;12:577–596.)

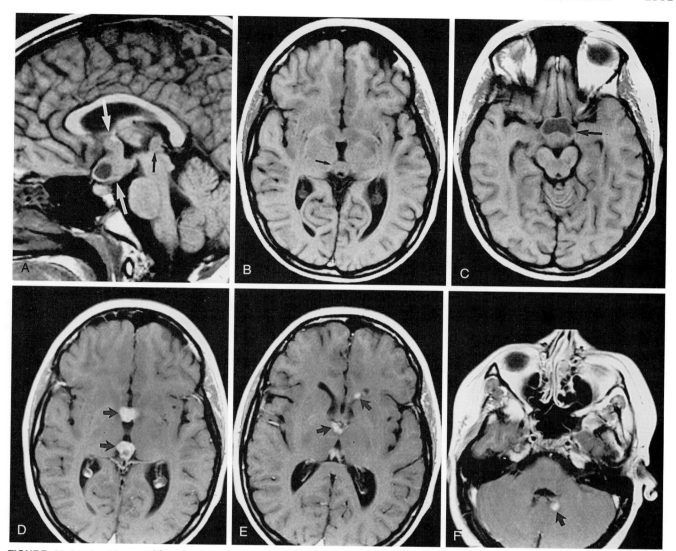

FIGURE 46–31 An 18-year-old with germinoma. *A–C,* T1-weighted images demonstrate an isointense mass of the pineal tissue *(small arrows)* as well as a larger sellar and suprasellar mass *(large arrows)* containing a central cyst or focus of necrosis. *D–F,* Gadolinium-enhanced images demonstrate enhancing tumor in the pineal region, third ventricle, fourth ventricle, and anterior horn of the lateral ventricle *(arrows).* The primary tumor may have arisen from either the pineal or the sellar region.

There is a strong gender predominance ranging from 2 to 17 times the incidence in males versus females. Children younger than 10 years may present with precocious puberty. The tumors are unencapsulated and histologically identical to testicular seminoma; these may disseminate through the CSF. The peak age of presentation is the second decade of life, with few patients older than 30 years. The tumors are responsive to radiation, and the 5-year survival rate with radiation alone is 75%.[257]

With NCCT, germinomas are noted to be slightly denser than normal brain, with calcifications of the tumor itself seen in 50%.[265] Calcifications within the normal pineal gland are almost always present, even in young patients not expected normally to have calcified pineal glands,[266, 267] and the tumor tends to abut or engulf the normal, calcified pineal gland. Moderate to marked enhancement is seen with CECT. MRI of germinomas typically demonstrates near isointensity to adjacent normal

brain on both T1- and T2-weighted sequences,[268] with some authors noting slight hyperintensity on T2-weighted images[269] and intense enhancement with gadolinium. Although germinomas are capable of invading adjacent structures, peritumoral edema surrounding germinomas is uncommon,[268] and the tumors are usually well-defined masses. MRI can occasionally demonstrate small, apparently cystic areas[270] that may be due to collections of proteinaceous fluid or necrosis (Figs. 46–31 and 46–32).[271]

Placental alkaline phosphatase levels are sometimes dramatically elevated in patients with pineal germinomas and can be a useful (but not diagnostic) tumor marker for germinoma.[272]

Pineal Teratoma

Teratomas are the second most common pineal tumor, accounting for 15% of pineal tumors. A strong male predominance is also noted for these tumors, with two to

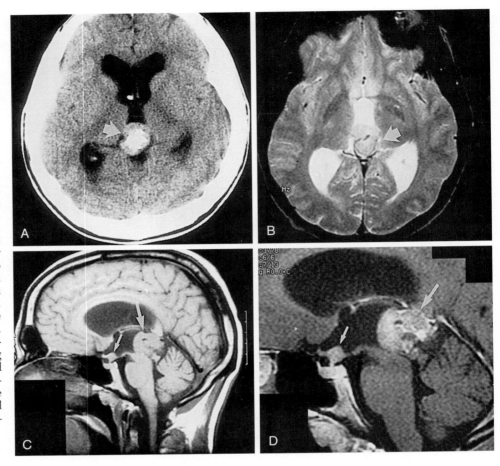

FIGURE 46–32 A 19-year-old man with pineal and suprasellar germinoma. *A,* NCCT demonstrates a large, calcified pineal region mass *(arrow).* The density at the septum pellucidum is the tip of a ventriculostomy catheter placed for hydrocephalus. *B,* T2-weighted image demonstrates enlarged ventricles and a mildly hyperintense pineal mass *(arrow).* T1-weighted unenhanced *(C)* and gadolinium-enhanced *(D)* images demonstrate a mass, centered at the pineal region, with focal hypointense regions that may represent small cysts or calcifications *(large arrows).* Also note the small suprasellar region mass *(small arrows),* probably in the floor of the third ventricle. Both of the masses demonstrate enhancement with gadolinium. Although both masses were present on the patient's first imaging study, the large pineal mass and smaller suprasellar mass that appears to lie in the floor of the third ventricle suggest a pineal origin of this patient's germinoma.

eight times the incidence seen in females.[257] Teratomas may be divided into mature and immature types.[190] They contain tissues from two or three of the three embryonic germ cell layers. Mature tumors contain fully differentiated tissues, whereas the more common immature tumors are composed of fetal-appearing tissue such as developing neuroectodermal structures; islands of cartilage; bands of striated muscles, skin, and adnexa; and endodermal derivatives such as intestinal epithelium. Teratomas may be associated with malignant germ cell components such as embryonal cell carcinoma or malignant tissues of conventional tissue types such as adenocarcinoma or rhabdomyosarcoma; descriptive terms are preferred over the broad category of *teratocarcinoma.*[190]

The histologic heterogeneity of teratomas is reflected in their imaging characteristics, with CT density and MRI signal intensity typical for soft tissues, fluid, fat, and calcification. NCCT may clearly demonstrate areas of lipid (fat) and calcified structures such as teeth.[267] Teratomas are typically sharply demarcated, and enhancement is not seen with CECT.[265] With MRI, heterogeneity is again seen, with fatty areas appearing hyperintense on T1-weighted images. Ringlike enhancement with gadolinium has been reported.[270] In rare instances, teratomas may rupture and spill their contents through the CSF.[273] Teratomas with malignant tissues (teratocarcinomas) have been noted to be invasive[274] and to have leptomeningeal

spread of the malignant component at presentation,[275] in addition to the heterogeneous appearance of their benign components (Figs. 46–33 and 46–34).

Choriocarcinoma

Choriocarcinomas represent less than 5% of pineal masses; a male predominance is seen with these tumors as well. The pure choriocarcinomas represent development of pluripotential cells into extraembryonic tissues and have a characteristic bilaminar histologic appearance[190] similar to that of normal placenta. Imaging findings are nonspecific; however, these tumors are hypervascular. MRI signal intensity consistent with subacute hemorrhage and the presence of neovascularity with small areas of aneurysmal dilatation on catheter angiography have been noted.[274] The ability of choriocarcinoma to produce elevated serum and CSF human chorionic gonadotropin levels is more useful for differential diagnosis than the imaging appearance is.[276]

Endodermal Sinus (Yolk Sac) Tumors

Endodermal sinus (yolk sac) tumors are uncommon and arise from differentiation of pleuripotential cells into cells resembling yolk sac endoderm and mesoblasts. No specific radiologic features have been noted, but invasive tumors isointense to adjacent brain on T1-weighted images and heterogeneous on T2-weighted images have been noted with MRI[274] as have cystic areas and calcifications with NCCT (Fig. 46–35).[267] Pure endodermal sinus tumors are rare; frequently portions of mixed germ cell tumors are noted to contain areas of this tumor. The presence of elevated α-fetoprotein levels in patients with endodermal sinus tumors is the most useful differential feature.[276]

Embryonal Cell Carcinoma

Pure embryonal cell carcinomas are rare, but they are more commonly seen as a component of mixed germ cell tumors. They are composed of large, undifferentiated epithelial cells, are malignant, and may disseminate through the CSF.[257] Hemorrhage and necrosis may be present. NCCT has demonstrated hyperdense masses with intense enhancement on CECT,[265] and tumor calcifications have been noted.[265]

Pineal Parenchymal Tumors

Parenchymal tumors of the pineal gland represent less than 15% of pineal region masses.[277] These tumors are felt to arise from the pineocytes, which are pineal parenchymal cells that represent specially modified neurons related to retinal photoreceptors. The tumors exist in a spectrum from well-differentiated pineocytomas to poorly differentiated pineoblastomas; mixed and intermediate forms are recognized as well.[190]

Pineocytomas are the most well differentiated of the pineal parenchymal tumors. Their histologic appearance is characterized by an unencapsulated, moderately cellular tumor with pineocytomatous rosettes.[278] The presence of these distinctive rosettes is felt to represent neuronal differentiation, and tumors with this feature have a better prognosis and lower recurrence rate than undifferentiated pineocytomas whose clinical behavior is characterized by

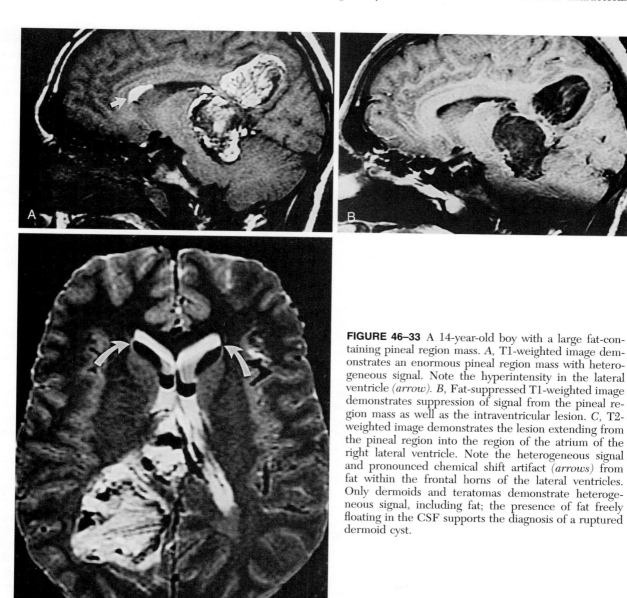

FIGURE 46–33 A 14-year-old boy with a large fat-containing pineal region mass. *A*, T1-weighted image demonstrates an enormous pineal region mass with heterogeneous signal. Note the hyperintensity in the lateral ventricle *(arrow)*. *B*, Fat-suppressed T1-weighted image demonstrates suppression of signal from the pineal region mass as well as the intraventricular lesion. *C*, T2-weighted image demonstrates the lesion extending from the pineal region into the region of the atrium of the right lateral ventricle. Note the heterogeneous signal and pronounced chemical shift artifact *(arrows)* from fat within the frontal horns of the lateral ventricles. Only dermoids and teratomas demonstrate heterogeneous signal, including fat; the presence of fat freely floating in the CSF supports the diagnosis of a ruptured dermoid cyst.

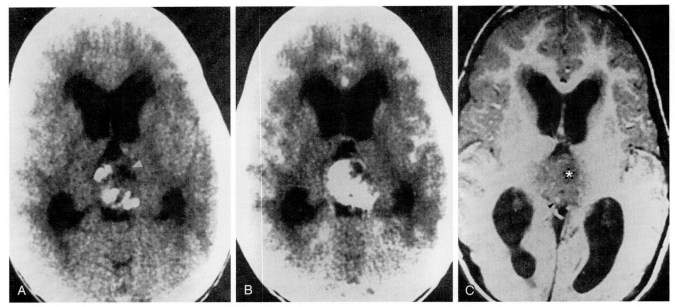

FIGURE 46–34 Pineal teratoma in a 4-year-old boy. *A,* CT shows a mixed-density mass in the pineal region, with low attenuation in a cystic region *(arrowhead)* and chunky calcifications. *B,* After contrast administration, there is enhancement of the noncystic portions of the mass. *C,* Axial T1-weighted MRI study shows a heterogeneous mass, with high signal intensity of lipid *(arrowhead)* and increased signal of fluid in the cyst *(asterisk)* relative to CSF, presumably due to proteinaceous fluid. *(A–C,* From Smirniotopoulos JG, Rushing EG, Mena H. Pineal region masses: Differential diagnosis. Radiographics 1992;12:577–596.)

recurrence and dissemination similar to that of pineoblastoma. Pineocytomas are found over a wide age range, from 8 to 63 years in one large study, with most patients less than 39 years old,[277] whereas others report a uniform distribution throughout life, with the incidence peaking slightly during the sixth decade.[279] They represent about 11% of pineal tumors in children.[280] No gender predominance is noted in most studies.[281, 282] The typical NCCT appearance of a pineocytoma is a well-defined, isodense or hypodense mass, associated with calcifications. In about half, the calcifications are peripheral and represent the normal, calcified pineal gland, whereas while in the remainder the calcifications are central, either within an undisturbed pineal gland or in the tumor itself. Occasional hyperdense pineocytomas are noted.[277] CECT demonstrates heterogeneous enhancement in most cases. MRI is nonspecific, with hypointensity or isointensity on T1-weighted images and hyperintensity on T2-weighted images; heterogeneous enhancement is usually present. In adult populations, pineocytomas are usually indolent,[281] but others have noted a higher incidence of aggressive behavior with up to 50% of patients developing recurrent tumor or leptomeningeal dissemination of pineocytoma (Fig. 46–36).[280]

Pineoblastomas are distinctly different from the more benign pineocytomas. These are highly cellular, aggressive neoplasms that resemble other PNETs and are seen in young children. Some pineoblastomas form Flexner-Wintersteiner rosettes, which are typical of photoreceptor differentiation and are also noted to be present in pineal retinoblastomas.[190] Some studies have noted a male gender predominance for pineoblastoma.[281] The clinical behavior of these tumors is also similar to that of PNET

elsewhere in the CNS, with early CSF dissemination. NCCT typically demonstrates a large, hyperdense tumor without calcification; CECT shows intense homogeneous enhancement. MRI demonstrates a lobulated tumor with hypointensity or isointensity on T1-weighted images and usually hypointensity or isointensity on T2-weighted images,[277] similar to that of medulloblastoma in the posterior fossa. Intense heterogeneous enhancement is typical (Fig. 46–37).

Other Pineal Tumors

Lipomas may be found associated with the pineal gland. Like other midline intracranial lipomas, these are congenital developmental lesions arising from the meninx primitiva[283] and are discussed elsewhere in this book. Unlike the more anteriorly located callosal lipomas, only about one-third of the pineal region lipomas are associated with other developmental defects.[284] Astrocytomas are found in the pineal region. Many of these tumors likely arise from adjacent structures including the tectum, but astrocytomas arising from the pineal gland itself have been reported. These tumors appear to be very rare, and most reported cases are in adults.[285, 286] Meningiomas may be found in the pineal region, usually arising from the junction of the falx and tentorium, the free edge of the tentorium, or meningiothelial cells in the velum interpositum.[287] Most patients are adults, with only a few pediatric cases reported. The MRI appearance is typical of meningiomas elsewhere in the central nervous system.[288] Isolated reports of pineal tuberculomas and hemangiopericytomas exist, but there are no specific imaging findings of these unusual pineal region lesions.[289]

Pineoblastoma with bilateral retinoblastoma *(trilateral*

retinoblastoma) radiographically appears as a mass of the pineal region. It develops in 3% to 10% of patients with bilateral retinoblastoma, and about 65% of patients with trilateral retinoblastoma have a family history of retinoblastoma as well.[290, 291] The pineal lesion typically develops about 3 years after the ocular lesions are discovered, and other midline tumors may occasionally be found in the suprasellar region.[292] The pineal region masses are typically isointense on T1-weighted images, avidly enhance with gadolinium, and display isointensity on T2-weighted images typical of other densely cellular primitive neuroectodermal tumors. Imaging of ocular retinoblastoma is reviewed elsewhere in this book.

Focal Midbrain Tumors

Neoplasms arising in the midbrain, although technically brain stem tumors, have distinct clinical and imaging features that separate them from the other brain stem tumors. The location of the tectum and tegmentum near the pineal gland allows their discussion among pineal region tumors.

Tumors of the tectum are characteristically indolent and nonprogressive neoplasms.[293] The majority of these tumors, when biopsied, are pilocytic or low-grade astrocytomas, although anaplastic astrocytomas have also been reported in this location.[294] Before the development of MRI, many of these tumors were misdiagnosed, at least initially, as benign aqueductal stenosis.[295] MRI is far superior to CT for the detection of tectal tumors and has been recommended to evaluate patients over the age of 6 months presenting with aqueductal stenosis.[296] Patients with lesions confined to the tectum present with hydrocephalus and increased intracranial pressure; some have

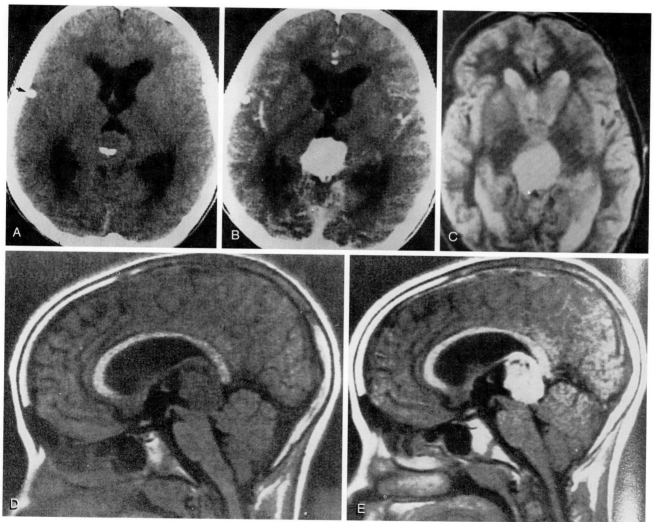

FIGURE 46–35 Pineal yolk sac tumor in a 9-year-old boy. *A,* Axial CT scan shows a round pineal region mass with central pineal calcifications. (*Arrow* points to an incidental dural calcification.) *B,* After contrast enhancement, there is homogeneous enhancement of the mass. *C,* Axial T2-weighted image shows increased signal intensity of the mass relative to gray matter. Sagittal T1-weighted MRI studies show intermediate signal intensity of the mass before contrast administration (*D*) and intense, slightly heterogeneous enhancement (*E*) after gadolinium administration. (*A–E,* From Smirniotopoulos JG, Rushing EJ, Mena H. Pineal region masses: Differential diagnosis. Radiographics 1992;12:577–596.)

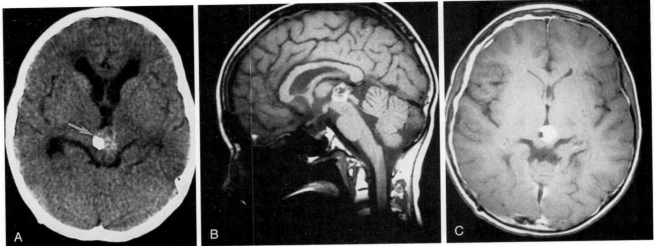

FIGURE 46–36 A 13-year-old girl with pineocytoma. *A,* NCCT demonstrates a calcified pineal mass *(arrow).* Mildly dilated frontal horns of the lateral ventricles are present, consistent with hydrocephalus. *B,* T1-weighted sagittal image demonstrates mixed signal intensity of the lesion. The hyperintensity may be due to soft tissue calcification or prior hemorrhage. *C,* Gadolinium-enhanced T1-weighted image demonstrates a more homogeneous appearance of the lesion, suggesting some enhancement, as well as dural enhancement owing to previous ventriculostomy catheter placement.

visual disturbances as well. The mean age of presentation is around 9 years[297] to 19 years.[298] No strong gender predominances have been noted.

CT may be normal in up to one-third of patients with tectal gliomas. Tectal distortion, calcifications, and cysts may also be seen with NCCT, and some enhancement has been noted with CECT in up to one-half of cases.[299] Others have noted transient CECT enhancement in a minority of cases, which became less prominent over time as the lesions calcified.[300] The typical appearance with MRI is a distorted, expanded tectal plate that is hypointense relative to adjacent brain on T1-weighted images and hyperintense on T2-weighted images. Extension into the thalamus can be present, and enhancement with gadolinium is minimal or absent.[301] Tectal gliomas are usually solid.[302] Gadolinium enhancement of tectal tumors, although usually felt to be an unusual finding, has been reported in from 10% of patients at presentation[297] in one study to 100% in another series.[302] Some authors have noted that patients with gadolinium enhancement of tectal neoplasms at presentation were more likely to demonstrate rapid tumor progression, whereas focal, nonenhancing tumors remained stable. Patients who did demonstrate tumor progression sometimes developed new enhancement in their tectal tumors.[297] The presence of enhancement, cysts, calcification, and exophytic growth into the CSF spaces surrounding the pineal gland does not correlate well with tumor grade, although exophytic growth can potentially mimic a primary tumor of the pineal gland itself (Figs. 46–38 through 46–40).[299] Tectal tumors typically have very indolent clinical courses, and treatment usually consists of ventricular shunting with follow-up MRI imaging; surgery can be deferred unless clinical or radiographic progression is seen.[296] Other authors believe that histologic diagnosis is important, although surgery of the tectum is not without significant morbidity.[298] Tumors that have progressed with growth into adjacent structures

have been biopsied and found to be benign astrocytomas and low-grade astrocytomas as well as mixed and anaplastic gliomas. Long-term survival after radiation therapy for progressive disease can be seen.[296]

Other reported neoplasms of the tectum include lymphoma and ependymomas. Exophytic astrocytomas (resembling primary pineal neoplasms) and cavernous angiomas may also be found in this region and present with hydrocephalus.[301]

Primary tumors of the tegmentum present with symptoms other than aqueductal compression. These tumors of the superior midbrain present with motor deficits, cranial neuropathies, and ocular symptoms and are typically low-grade astrocytomas as well.[302] The MRI appearance is a hypointense mass of the tegmentum on T1-weighted images, hyperintensity on T2-weighted images, and variable amounts of enhancement with gadolinium. These lesions may be larger at presentation than tectal tumors, and surgical decompression may be indicated in patients with brain stem signs (Fig. 46–41).[303]

In summary, a variety of neoplasms may be found in the pineal region. Although MRI allows improved localization of these tumors to the pineal gland itself, the tectum, or the tegmentum, the imaging appearance of these tumors is frequently nonspecific. Large neoplasms may defy anatomic localization. Correlation with tumor markers (α-fetoprotein, human chorionic gonadotropin placental alkaline phosphatase) can be helpful. Early experience with surgical resection of pineal region masses had high morbidity and mortality, but current operative techniques, advances in neuroanesthesia, and the use of stereotactic biopsy allow histologic confirmation of pineal tumors with acceptable complication rates.[258] Overall, 36% to 50% of pineal tumors are either benign or radioresistant.[304] With current surgical techniques and the lack of specificity of imaging findings, histologic confirmation of these tumors is usually made to guide appropriate therapy.[272]

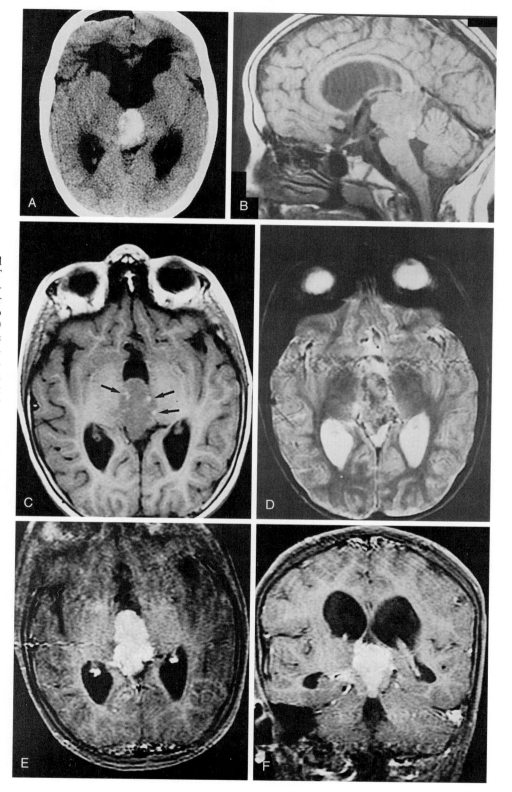

FIGURE 46–37 An 8-year-old girl with pineoblastoma. *A,* NCCT demonstrates a large, calcified pineal region mass. Intraventricular and extra-axial air is related to prior ventriculostomy. Sagittal *(B)* and axial *(C)* T1-weighted images demonstrate a large mass centered in the pineal region, predominantly isointense but with some small hyperintense foci that may be related to calcification or hemorrhage *(arrows in C). D,* T2-weighted image demonstrates a heterogeneously hypointense mass. *E* and *F,* Avid enhancement with gadolinium is present. The T2-weighted hypointensity may be related to either diffuse calcification or dense cellularity analogous to that seen with medulloblastoma.

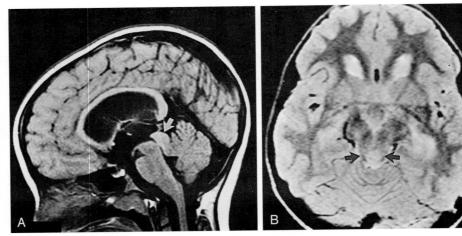

FIGURE 46–38 A 7-year-old child with tectal glioma. The patient had a long history of macrocrania before imaging. *A,* Sagittal T1-weighted image demonstrates expansion and loss of the normal contours of the tectal plate *(arrow).* There was no enhancement with gadolinium (not shown). *B,* Axial T2-weighted image shows subtle increased signal surrounding the aqueduct and extending into the tectum *(arrows).*

Sellar Region Tumors in Children

Sellar region tumors constitute 15% to 20% of all intracranial tumors in children.[305] The location of these tumors produces a wide variety of symptoms including visual disturbances, increased intracranial pressure and hydrocephalus, endocrinopathies, and the diencephalic syndrome (emaciation, pallor, alertness, and hyperactivity). The most commonly encountered childhood masses in this region include craniopharyngioma, gliomas of the visual pathways, germinomas and teratomas, and nonneoplastic tumors such as suprasellar arachnoid cysts, Rathke's cleft cysts, and hypothalamic hamartomas. The characteristic imaging findings of these neoplasms is dis-

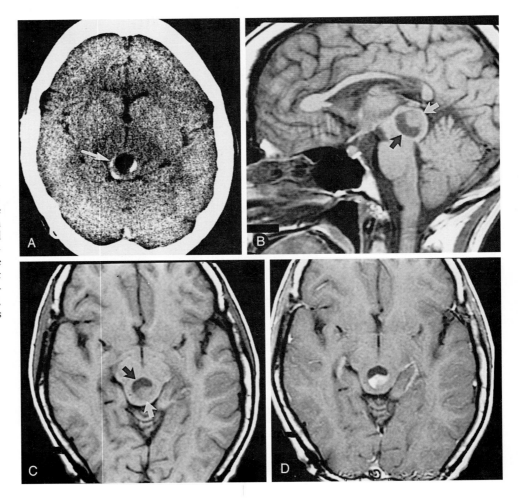

FIGURE 46–39 JPA of the tectum, pathologically proven. *A,* NCCT demonstrates a cystic mass expanding the tectum *(arrow)* with some peripheral calcifications. *B* and *C,* T1-weighted images show a cystic mass of the tectum *(black arrows)* with a peripherally located nodule *(white arrows). D,* The nodule intensely enhances with gadolinium.

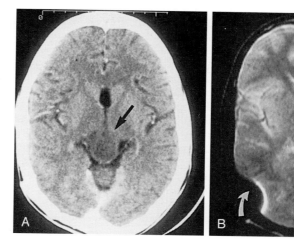

FIGURE 46–40 A 13-year-old boy with presumed tectal glioma. *A,* CECT demonstrates expansion of the tectum by a hypodense, nonenhancing mass *(arrow)* consistent with a low-grade glioma. *B,* T2-weighted MRI study demonstrates hyperintensity in the same region *(straight arrow).* Metallic artifact produced by a ventriculostomy is present over the right parietal lobe *(curved arrow).*

cussed here; skull base lesions and tumors of the pituitary itself are reviewed elsewhere in this book.

Craniopharyngioma

Craniopharyngiomas are the most common nonglial pediatric brain tumor, representing 6% to 9% of pediatric tumors and about half of all pediatric sellar region tumors.[306] The peak childhood incidence is seen at 5 to 10 years of age. A second peak of incidence is noted during the fourth to sixth decades of life. Some studies have noted a male preponderance, but it is more likely that there is no gender predominance.[306]

Craniopharyngiomas are epithelial neoplasms with two major histologic variants, the classic adamantinomatous variety and the papillary craniopharyngioma.[190] The adamantinomatous variant closely resembles the adamantinoma of the jaw, is most commonly seen in the pediatric population, in which it presents as a sellar region mass, and is frequently calcified. These tumors are almost always cystic, the cysts being filled with dark brown "ma-

chine oil" fluid containing cholesterol crystals. Nodules of necrobiotic squames with dystrophic calcification are also typical as is peripheral palisading of epithelial cells.[190]

Papillary craniopharyngiomas are usually encountered in adults as a solid, noncalcified mass, often within the third ventricle. The typical appearance is an isodense mass with NCCT and homogeneous enhancement with CECT. MRI reveals an intraventricular lesion that is isointense on T1-weighted images, is hyperintense compared with adjacent brain structures on T2-weighted images, and enhances homogeneously with gadolinium.[307, 308]

Craniopharyngiomas arise along the path of the craniopharyngeal canal, the path taken by Rathke's pouch from the oropharynx to the floor of the third ventricle.[309] The tumors can arise anywhere along this canal, and overall about 70% of tumors are both intra- and suprasellar, 20% are purely suprasellar, and about 10% are purely intrasellar.[309] Rare infrasellar lesions in the sphenoid sinus have been reported.[309, 310]

Craniopharyngiomas are slow-growing tumors that

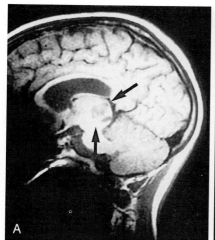
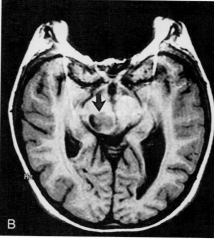
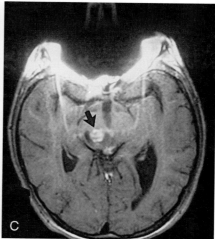

FIGURE 46–41 A 12-year-old girl with midbrain glioma. *A,* Sagittal T1-weighted image demonstrates expansion of the midbrain by a heterogeneous, apparently cystic and solid mass *(arrows).* *B,* T1-weighted axial image confirms the location of the tumor in the midbrain adjacent to the right cerebral peduncle *(arrow).* Note the cystic and hypointense solid portions. *C,* Gadolinium-enhanced image demonstrates nodular enhancement of some of the solid tumor *(arrow).* Metallic artifact from dental braces distorts the anterior portions of the images.

produce symptoms by compression of adjacent structures. When large they can obstruct CSF pathways and present with hydrocephalus and increased intracranial pressure. Young children may be unaffected by severe visual symptoms, but presentation with visual deficits may be seen in older children and adults. Craniopharyngiomas are not active hormonally but may present with anterior pituitary dysfunction by direct compression of the pituitary itself or interruption of the hypothalamic-pituitary portal system, producing growth failure.[216] Short stature, hypothyroidism, and diabetes insipidus are the three most common endocrinologic abnormalities produced by craniopharyngiomas.[306] Interference with the neurohypophysis can produce diabetes insipidus, whereas a mass effect on the optic chiasm and third ventricle/foramen of Monro can produce visual disturbance and hydrocephalus, respectively. Craniopharyngiomas are frequently cystic tumors, and spill of cyst contents, either spontaneously or during surgery, can produce a chemical meningitis.[311] The tumors induce an intense glial reaction of adjacent brain and can be adherent to the hypothalamus and other adjacent structures. Brain invasion is more frequently seen in children and in the adamantinomatous variant of tumor. The most significant factor associated with tumor recurrence is the extent of initial surgical resection; brain invasion in totally resected tumors does not predict a higher rate of recurrence.[312, 313] Recurrence is seen in 71% of children with subtotal resection, usually within 5 to 10 years, but in only 25% with total gross resection.[306] Tumor recurrence may be asymptomatic, detected only with neuroimaging studies, and can occur even after what is felt to be a total tumor resection.[314] Difficulty in separating the tumor from the hypothalamus may lead to postsurgical endocrine dysfunction. Therapy typically consists of surgery combined with radiation, and overall survival of children with craniopharyngioma is good, with 91% survival at 10 years.[315]

On neuroimaging studies, childhood craniopharyngioma demonstrates a typical heterogeneous appearance. With NCCT, a cystic or complex mass is seen, with the childhood tumors almost always demonstrating calcification.[316] The calcification may be seen as rimlike calcification surrounding cystic areas or as nodules of calcified tumor. By detecting the presence of fluid within tumor cysts and calcifications, CT may be more specific for the diagnosis of craniopharyngioma, but MRI better delineates the extent of the tumor and involvement of adjacent neural structures.[317] CT and MRI are best considered complementary in the diagnosis of craniopharyngioma. Contrast enhancement of the solid portions of the tumor is usually seen with CECT.[316] Compared with adult tumors, pediatric tumors are more likely to demonstrate calcification, cystic areas, and contrast enhancement,[316] with calcification and enhancement present in 90% of cases.[216] Cystic areas may occasionally demonstrate increased density with NCCT, beyond what is expected for collections of fluid, corresponding with collections of proteinaceous fluid.

MRI allows better definition of the tumor's relation to the sella, chiasm, hypothalamus, and temporal lobes. The appearance on MRI is remarkable for its heterogeneity, even within a single tumor. Cystic areas may demonstrate

T1-weighted signal intensity ranging from isointensity compared with CSF to isointensity compared with adjacent brain, to marked hyperintensity.[318] Analysis of the fluid within the cysts has been performed.[319] Hyperintensity on T1-weighted images corresponds with a high protein content, methemoglobin from prior hemorrhage, or both, rather than the presence of cholesterol crystals or triglycerides. This hyperintensity correlates with the "machine oil" fluid encountered surgically.[320] Cysts lacking blood degradation products or high protein content are isointense with CSF or brain on T1-weighted images. Cystic regions are typically hyperintense on T2-weighted images, whereas solid portions of the tumors are hypo- to isointense on T1-weighted images, and iso- to hyperintense, compared with adjacent brain, on T2-weighted images.[320] Craniopharyngiomas with enormous cysts extending into the frontal fossa, into the posterior fossa third ventricle, laterally into the middle cranial fossa, and into the sphenoid sinus and nasopharynx have been described.[321] Calcifications, if visible on MRI, appear as regions of low signal intensity on all sequences. Increased T2 signal within the optic chiasm and tracts has been described with craniopharyngiomas,[322] probably due to edema or reactive gliosis rather than extension of tumor.

With gadolinium, solid portions of the tumor show moderate enhancement, which may be heterogeneous, especially in areas of calcification. Cyst wall enhancement may also be present.[305] T1-weighted images overall best delineate the extent of tumor, whereas gadolinium improves the visualization of tumor margins and can demonstrate cavernous sinus invasion in some cases (Figs. 46–42 through 46–44).[323]

Rathke's Cleft Cysts

Rathke's cleft cysts are typically described as benign epithelial-lined sellar region cysts containing mucoid material. Most commonly, the cysts are an incidental finding at autopsy, found in 2% to 26% of cases. A female predominance (2 to 1) has been noted with symptomatic cysts, with an age range at presentation of 4 to 73 years.[324] Both symptomatic and asymptomatic cysts may be found in childhood.[325] The classic Rathke's cleft cyst is an intra- or suprasellar cyst lined by cuboidal or columnar epithelium with ciliated and goblet cells. Squamous metaplasia may be present as well.[190]

During fetal development of the pituitary, a cleft remains between the anterior and posterior lobes in the region of the pars intermedia. This cleft (*Rathke's cleft*) is commonly seen at autopsy in normal glands, is an ectodermal derivative, and has been considered to be the origin of both craniopharyngiomas and Rathke's cleft cysts.[326] Overlap lesions with histologic features of both craniopharyngioma and Rathke's cleft cyst have been noted and may be reflected on neuroimaging studies as well.[326]

Symptomatic Rathke's cleft cysts most commonly present with pituitary dysfunction, usually hypopituitarism with multiple endocrinopathies. In a large review of symptomatic cysts, 69% of patients under 18 years of age, and all patients less than 10 years old, had evidence of pituitary dwarfism.[324] Hyperprolactinemia may be secondary to the cyst, interfering with the secretion or transport

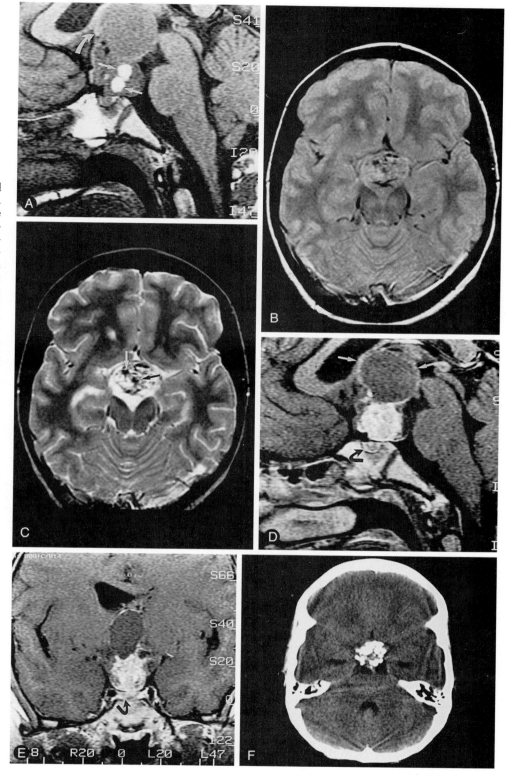

FIGURE 46–42 A 13-year-old child with craniopharyngioma. *A,* Sagittal T1-weighted image of the sellar region demonstrates a heterogeneous well-defined suprasellar mass. Portions of the mass are both isointense and hyperintense compared with adjacent brain; the hyperintense areas *(straight arrows)* likely correspond to proteinaceous fluid. A large cystic component extends up into the third ventricle, displacing the optic chiasm superiorly *(curved arrow).* PD-weighted *(B)* and T2-weighted *(C)* images demonstrate marked heterogeneity, and hypointense foci within the tumor *(arrows in C),* which correspond to large calcifications. *D* and *E,* Gadolinium-enhanced T1-weighted images demonstrate enhancement of both the solid components of the tumor and of the cyst walls *(straight arrows in D).* The adenohypophysis *(curved arrows)* appears separate from the mass. *F,* NCCT demonstrates prominent calcifications in the periphery of the tumor.

of prolactin-inhibiting factor.[327] Visual disturbance and headache may also be present.

The typical appearance of a Rathke's cleft cyst with NCCT is a cystic low-density noncalcified lesion; intrasellar, suprasellar, or combined intra- and suprasellar cysts are seen.[328] The MRI appearance is variable. Intrasellar

components of the cyst are usually in the anterior sella between the pars distalis and the pars nervosa.[320] Hypointensity on T1-weighted images and hyperintensity on T2-weighted images, similar to CSF signal, correlates with CSF-like fluid at surgery, whereas hyperintensity on T1-weighted images, similar to fat, with isointensity to brain

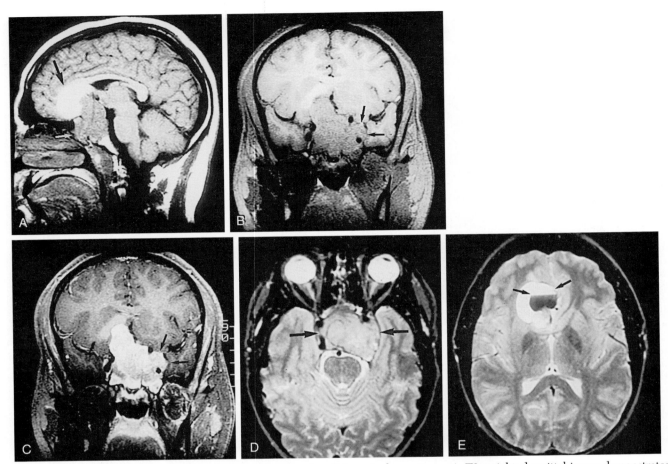

FIGURE 46–43 A 16-year-old boy with a large, predominantly solid craniopharyngioma. *A*, T1-weighted sagittal image demonstrates a large, heterogeneous sellar and suprasellar mass. Note the extension into the sphenoid sinus *(white arrow)* and a superiorly located, hyperintense portion *(black arrow)*, likely representing a cystic component containing proteinaceous fluid. *B* and *C*, Pre- and postgadolinium coronal T1-weighted images demonstrate intense enhancement of the solid component and prominent invasion of the left cavernous sinus *(arrows)*. *D* and *E*, Axial T2-weighted images demonstrate an isointense, heterogeneous suprasellar mass *(large arrows in D)*. More superiorly, a tumor cyst with a fluid level, likely calcific debris or hemorrhage, is present *(small arrows in E)*.

on T2-weighted images correlates with mucoid material or proteinaceous fluid containing mucopolysaccharides.[329–331] Hyperintensity on both T1- and T2-weighted images can be explained by hemorrhage,[329, 332] with hemorrhage from thin-walled blood vessels in granulation tissue found in the lining of some cysts. The signal intensity of the cyst contents is generally homogeneous, with heterogeneous signal intensity seen in cysts containing milky fluid and waxy mural nodules.[333] Heterogeneous signal with MRI and increasing density on NCCT, approaching that of normal adjacent brain, seems to correlate with transitional forms of Rathke's cleft cysts, with features of both cyst and craniopharyngioma.[328, 334] The cysts have been noted to range in size from small, 3-mm to 4-cm incidental lesions.[324] Ringlike peripheral enhancement on CECT has been noted in up to half of Rathke's cleft cysts;[324] however, the improved anatomic distinction of the cyst from the adjacent normal pituitary gland with postgadolinium MRI demonstrates that the enhancement is usually produced by displaced, normal pituitary tissue.[333, 335] The normal gland is usually located anterior

and inferior to the Rathke's cleft cyst but can be superior, posterior, or surrounding the entire cyst. True, faint ring-like enhancement of the cyst wall has been reported. This enhancement may correlate with the presence of inflammatory changes that result from degeneration of the cyst wall, followed by metaplasia of the cyst lining into squamous epithelium and consequent enhancement on CECT and postgadolinium MRI. However, enhancement does not always correlate with the histologic presence of squamous metaplasia or chronic inflammation.[336, 337] Rarely, calcification of Rathke's cleft cysts is present with NCCT (Fig. 46–45).[324]

The main differential of a Rathke's cleft cyst is craniopharyngioma and pituitary adenoma. When the typical appearance of a nonenhancing, uncalcified, homogeneous cystic mass is present, with normal-appearing pituitary gland within the sella, the diagnosis is not difficult. Delayed enhancement relative to the normal gland on dynamic enhancement MRI sequences (reviewed in the section on pituitary imaging), intrasellar or intra- and suprasellar location, and a lack of calcification and cyst

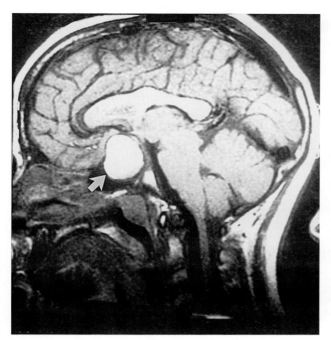

FIGURE 46–44 A 16-year-old girl with a predominantly cystic craniopharyngioma. An unenhanced T1-weighted image demonstrates a sellar and suprasellar mass predominantly consisting of a large cyst filled with proteinaceous fluid, producing T1-weighted hyperintensity (*arrow*).

formation suggest the diagnosis of a pituitary adenoma, a rare tumor in children. However, the presence of atypical features (calcification, enhancement) in a Rathke's cleft cyst may produce identical imaging findings to a craniopharyngioma and not allow presurgical diagnosis.[338] Therapy of Rathke cleft cysts consists of cyst drainage and biopsy of the wall,[339] and recurrence is rare.

Suprasellar Arachnoid Cysts

Arachnoid cysts are of developmental origin and may be found in a variety of intracranial locations. Suprasellar arachnoid cysts are rare, but the majority of patients with symptomatic suprasellar arachnoid cysts are children.[340] Typical clinical symptoms include hydrocephalus, impaired visual acuity, endocrinopathy (including precocious puberty, depressed growth hormone and corticotropin levels, and hypopituitarism), and the bobble-head doll syndrome. This syndrome is characterized by a to-and-fro bobbing and nodding of the head and trunk that was first described in children with suprasellar arachnoid cysts.[341] A male predominance has been noted.[342] Suprasellar arachnoid cysts represent about 9% of all arachnoid cysts diagnosed during childhood.[320]

Most arachnoid cysts are primary congenital lesions that develop within a splitting or duplication of leptomeningeal tissue.[343] The mechanism of growth of arachnoid cysts has been debated. Proposed mechanisms include osmotically induced filtration and unidirectional CSF flow (*ball-valve trapping*).[344] The ultrastructure of the cysts demonstrates that they are intra-arachnoid lesions whose walls consist of sheets of arachnoid cells that join with normal arachnoid at the cyst margins, and that the cells lining the cyst are capable of secretory activity. It is felt that most arachnoid cysts are thus nonneoplastic congenital lesions that grow by the secretion of fluid.[345] Other alternatives proposed for the origin of arachnoid cysts in children include the sequelae of trauma or infective processes and adhesive arachnoiditis, but evidence for such origins appears scant.[346] These cysts should be differentiated from the true posttraumatic leptomeningeal cyst (*growing skull fracture of childhood*) as well as loculations of CSF surrounded by arachnoidal scarring from prior trauma or inflammation.

A unique origin for suprasellar arachnoid cysts has

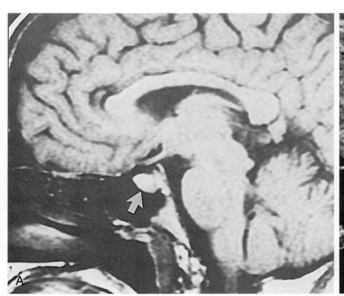 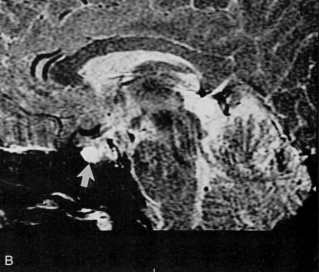

FIGURE 46–45 Rathke's cleft cyst. The lesion is likely an incidental finding in an MRI study obtained for headaches; the patient had no endocrine or visual symptoms. *A,* T1-weighted sagittal image demonstrates a well-defined intrasellar mass that is hyperintense (*arrow*). *B,* The cyst (*arrow*) remains hyperintense on the T2-weighted image. No abnormal enhancement was seen on postgadolinium images (not shown).

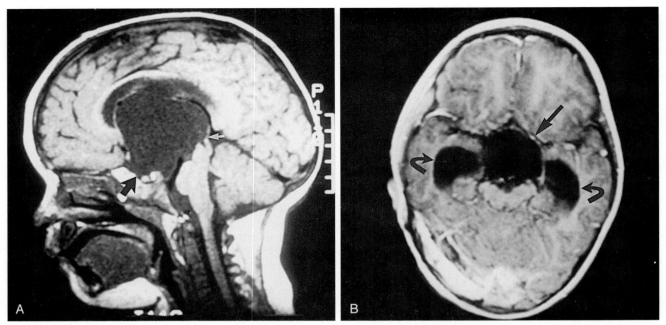

FIGURE 46–46 A 2-year-old child with a suprasellar arachnoid cyst. Sagittal *(A)* and axial *(B)* T1-weighted images demonstrate a large suprasellar lesion that is isointense to CSF. Note the dilatation of the suprasellar and interpeduncular cisterns *(straight black arrows)*. Superior extension of the cyst has obstructed the outflow of the third ventricle, producing dilatation of the posterior recesses of the third ventricle and proximal aqueduct *(white arrow)*. Dilated temporal horns *(curved arrows)* consistent with hydrocephalus are also present.

been proposed. These cysts may arise from an upward and forward diverticulum of the arachnoid membrane of Liliequist, a thin arachnoid veil between the dorsum sellae and apex of the interpeduncular fossa.[347] It is postulated that perforations in this membrane are occluded by infection, inflammation, maldevelopment, or subarachnoid hemorrhage.[50]

Suprasellar arachnoid cysts have characteristic CT and MRI appearances that allow them to be distinguished from the other cystic masses of the sellar region. With NCCT, the cysts appear as rounded well-demarcated thin-walled homogeneous masses isodense with CSF. Calcification is not seen, and the cyst wall does not enhance with CECT.[348] Dilatation of the basilar cisterns below the displaced membrane of Liliequist or an arachnoid web may be seen, with prominence of the suprasellar, interpeduncular, and pontine cisterns. The cyst may extend superiorly through the hypothalamus into the third ventricle, but the ventricle itself is not dilated and its posterior recesses are not enlarged unless hydrocephalus is present.[348] CT cisternography, performed with intrathecal injection of 3 ml of a nonionic radiocontrast material containing 180 mg of iodine per milliliter, demonstrates the cyst's smooth, sharply defined borders.[50]

MRI of suprasellar arachnoid cysts demonstrates the lesions as sharply defined thin-walled masses isointense to CSF on most pulse sequences.[349] The optic chiasm is frequently elevated and displaced anteriorly.[320] The lack of enhancement, calcifications, and significant soft tissue components, and isointensity and isodensity of the cyst contents relative to CSF, usually allow these lesions to be distinguished from the other sellar masses in children. Potential mimics include cysticercosis cysts, which may

have an appearance identical to that of suprasellar arachnoid cysts. Serum immunologic titers and the clinical setting as well as identification of a scolex along the cyst wall are useful for identifying cysticercosis. Epidermoid cysts may potentially mimic arachnoid cysts but tend to present in adulthood, are somewhat hyperintense relative to CSF on intermediate-weighted (PD-weighted) MRI images, have characteristic fronds that fill with contrast material on cisternography, and tend to encase adjacent arteries and cranial nerves whereas arachnoid cysts displace them.[350] Diffusion-weighted MRI techniques also allow solid epidermoids to be distinguished from arachnoid cysts (Fig. 46–46).

Hypothalamic Hamartoma

Hypothalamic hamartomas (hamartomas of the tuber cinereum), although pathologically not neoplastic, may be encountered while imaging children with endocrinopathy and should be distinguished from true neoplasms. Hypothalamic hamartomas classically present with isosexual central precocious puberty or gelastic ("laughing") seizures[351] and are the most common known (identifiable) cause of true precocious puberty.[352] Precocious puberty occurs in 74% of patients with histologically proven hypothalamic hamartomas, and in patients with precocious puberty 19% to 33% have such hamartomas.[353] Patients tend to present with early onset of puberty, usually younger than 3 years. Gelastic seizures and precocious puberty may be present together in the same patient.[354] A male gender predominance has been noted.[50]

Hypothalamic hamartomas characteristically are composed of well-differentiated neuroglial tissue that mimics the structure of the normal hypothalamus. Neurons that stain for luteinizing hormone–releasing hormone as well as growth hormone, corticotropin, and thyroid-stimulating hormone have been demonstrated.[190] These lesions are felt to arise from abnormal migration of neurons, including neurons that secrete luteinizing hormone–releasing hormone, from the medial olfactory placode of the developing nose. Normally these neurons come to rest in the septal-preoptic area and hypothalamus, but they are felt to migrate beyond these regions to the tuber cinereum and region of the mammillary bodies where they function as an uninhibited source of luteinizing hormone–releasing hormone.[352] The origin of seizures in hypothalamic hamartomas is uncertain. Neuronal connections from the hamartoma itself to the limbic system have been proposed and may explain the reduced number of seizures after surgical resection of the hamartoma.[355] Other congenital intracranial abnormalities have been associated with hypothalamic hamartomas including callosal agenesis, optic malformation, and hemispheric dysgenesis including heterotopia and microgyria.[356] These abnormalities may also play a role in the genesis of seizures in these patients.

Hypothalamic hamartomas may rarely be an incidental asymptomatic finding in adults and as such have been associated with polysyndactyly, possibly transmitted in an autosomal dominant manner.[357–359] A syndrome of hypothalamic hamartoma, imperforate anus, polydactyly, and hypopituitarism, with both autosomal recessive and autosomal dominant transmission, has been reported.[360, 361]

Imaging findings of hypothalamic hamartomas are specific. With NCCT, a mass adjacent to the tuber cinereum is seen; it is isodense to adjacent brain and does not demonstrate enhancement on CECT.[362] Calcifications, fat, and small cysts have been rarely reported within the masses, which range in size from 4 mm to 4 cm.[362] The lesions are noninvasive and do not change in size over time.

MRI is advantageous in determining the location of the hamartoma relative to the other midline structures. The lesions may be sessile or pedunculated but typically are connected to the tuber cinereum or a mammillary body directly or by a small stalk that may be seen with MRI.[355] Unattached hamartomas and lesions with multiple connections to the hypothalamus have also been reported.[355] On T1-weighted images, the lesions are isointense relative to adjacent brain and do not enhance, whereas T2-weighted images usually demonstrate hyperintensity relative to brain, similar to CSF,[363, 364] although isointensity on T2-weighted images has been reported in infants.[365] Intermediate-weighted (PD-weighted) images demonstrate variable signal, with slight to marked hyperintensity or isointensity relative to adjacent brain (Fig. 46–47).[366] Some studies have noted that the shape of

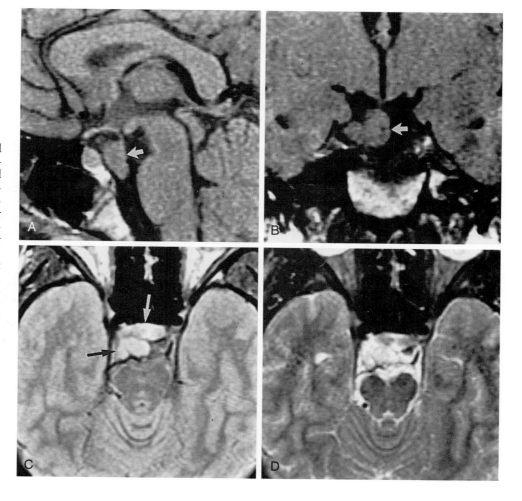

FIGURE 46–47 A 13-year-old child with hamartoma of the tuber cinereum. Sagittal *(A)* and coronal *(B)* T1-weighted images demonstrate a pedunculated mass attached to the tuber cinereum. The mass extends interiorly into the interpeduncular and prepontine cisterns *(arrows)*. No enhancement was present with gadolinium (not shown). PD-weighted *(C)* and T2-weighted *(D)* images show hyperintensity of the mass *(arrows in C)*, especially on the PD (first-echo) image.

the tumor correlates with symptoms, with pedunculated lesions associated with precocious puberty. Sessile lesions, especially lesions larger than 1.5 cm,[356] have been associated with seizures, perhaps due to a mass effect, although the associated cortical malformations, discussed previously, may play a role in the pathogenesis of the seizures.[352] Therapy for patients with precocious puberty and hypothalamic hamartomas is controversial, with both medical (luteinizing hormone–releasing hormone agonists) and surgical approaches used.[367] Some patients with seizures have shown improvement of the symptoms but not cures of their seizure disorder after resection.[368]

Sellar Region Germ Cell Tumors

Germinomas are the second most common sellar region mass in children,[49] with about 37% of all germ cell tumors arising in the sellar region. The sellar region is the second most common location for intracranial germ cell tumors after the pineal region.[276] Germinomas are the most common histologic variant of germ cell tumor in the sellar region, and for all intracranial germinomas, if multifocal tumors are included, 57% involve the sellar region. Nongerminomatous germ cell tumors predominate in the pineal region, with 68% of these tumors found near the pineal gland.[369] Synchronous germ cell tumors, the majority of which are germinomas, are present in the sellar and pineal regions in 6% to 12.8% of patients.[369, 370] Most patients with synchronous tumors are males, although the male predominance is not as strong as it is for isolated germ cell tumors of the pineal region. It is uncertain if these synchronous tumors represent dissemination through the CSF or true, multicentric tumors.[370] When the tumor involves both the sellar and the pineal region, the presenting symptoms are typically due to the sellar lesion rather than the pineal mass.[370] Germ cell tumors with involvement limited to the sellar region have been noted to have a slight female predominance, unlike the pineal tumors. Like patients with pineal lesions, patients affected with suprasellar germ cell tumors appear to present most commonly in Asia.[369, 370] The histologic appearance of the sellar region germ cell tumors is identical to that of the pineal and gonadal germ cell tumors.[371] Most of the sellar germ cell tumors are germinomas, with teratomas[372] and occasional choriocarcinomas and embryonal cell carcinomas reported in this region.[370]

In children, a classic triad of symptoms (diabetes insipidus, visual deficit, and hypopituitarism) may be seen with sellar region germ cell tumors,[373] whereas larger tumors, extending superiorly to the region of the foramen of Monro, may present with increased intracranial pressure and hydrocephalus. A mass effect on the optic chiasm may produce visual disturbances. Diabetes insipidus has been noted to be the initial and most prominent symptom in most germinomas, whereas teratomas have been noted to present most commonly with visual symptoms.[372] Sellar germ cell tumors most commonly present at the end of the first or during the second decade of life.[374] Many of these tumors arise in or near the diencephalic centers for the regulation of gonadotropic activity, and puberty with its increase in gonadotropins may be responsible for the age peak in adolescence.[369] Sellar region germinomas are radiosensitive. Previous experience suggested that sellar

germinomas were more malignant than pineal germinomas, with a less effective response to radiation and a lower survival rate.[375] More recent experience reports a very favorable prognosis for sellar germinomas, with 10-year survival as high as 90%.[376] Nongerminomatous germ cell tumors have a worse prognosis, with 5-year survival rates less than 25%.[376] Like pineal tumors, germ cell tumors of the sellar region, with the exception of benign teratomas, may disseminate through the CSF, with the frequency of metastatic disease reported between 10% and 57%.[376] Although prognosis of germ cell tumors does not appear to depend on the site of origin (pineal versus sellar region), involvement of the hypothalamus and third ventricle is associated with a worse prognosis.[369]

Sellar region germ cell tumors do not have specific imaging characteristics, and the typical therapeutic approach consists of surgical resection with radiation or chemotherapy, as indicated by the histologic appearance of the tumor.

Sellar region germinomas may be located within the sella itself,[377] in both intra- and suprasellar positions, or in the region of the floor of the third ventricle. The tumors are also frequently noted to arise from the region of the posterior lobe of the pituitary, or the infundibulum,[378] with small tumors appearing as enhancement and thickening of the infundibulum and floor of the third ventricle. NCCT demonstrates an isodense or slightly hyperdense sellar region mass; calcifications, hemorrhage, cysts, and necrosis are not common.[374] The masses are well circumscribed, and if present the hyperdensity is useful in distinguishing these tumors from opticochiasmatic-hypothalamic gliomas.[216] With CECT, diffuse enhancement is seen. Calcification within the native pineal gland is known to be more common with pineal germ cell tumors, but it is uncertain if a similar process occurs with the sellar region tumors, with some, but not all, studies finding an increase in pineal gland calcifications.[276, 266] MRI demonstrates lesions that are round or nodular, isointense or slightly hypointense relative to adjacent brain on T1-weighted images; slight hyperintensity relative to brain on PD- and T2-weighted images; and enhancement of both the primary tumor and any tumor disseminated through the CSF (Fig. 46–48).[49] Heterogeneous signal may be produced by microcysts.[305] Sellar germinomas may invade adjacent structures and can extend to the third ventricle, to the interpeduncular cistern, and into the optic chiasm, extending along the optic nerves.[305]

Differential diagnosis of a sellar region germinoma includes opticochiasmatic-hypothalamic gliomas, which may be distinguished by their hypodensity on NCCT and by the clinical course. Diabetes insipidus is far more common with sellar region germinoma, whereas visual disturbances and an association with neurofibromatosis type 1 (NF-1) are noted with the gliomas. The sellar germinomas usually displace the optic chiasm, whereas gliomas of this structure expand it. Calcifications are common with childhood craniopharyngioma as are cysts with differing signal intensity, findings unusual in germinoma. A small, entirely intrasellar germinoma may mimic a rare pituitary tumor. Diabetes insipidus is rare in patients with pituitary adenoma, and its presence is an important

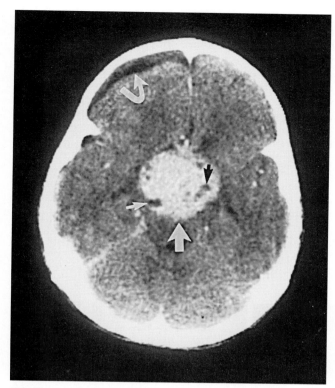

FIGURE 46–48 An 8-year-old girl with suprasellar germinoma. CECT demonstrates a large, enhancing suprasellar mass *(large arrow)* with small cystic areas *(small arrows)*. The subdural fluid collection *(curved arrow)* is a chronic subdural hematoma from previous ventriculostomy catheter placement.

clinical feature. Loss of the posterior pituitary "bright spot" has been reported in patients with diabetes insipidus[379–381] and is present in cases of intrasellar germinoma as well.[378]

Langerhans cell histiocytosis may clinically and radiographically mimic a small germinoma of the sellar region. The most common imaging appearance in the central nervous system is a thickened, enhancing infundibulum and, with MRI, loss of the posterior pituitary bright spot, often in the presence of clinical or subclinical diabetes insipidus.[382–384] Isolated disease of the central nervous system in Langerhans cell histiocytosis is rare.[385] Radiographic evaluation of other potential locations of histiocytosis (pulmonary, skeletal system, temporal bones) can be helpful in difficult cases.

Teratoma

Sellar region teratomas have a strong male predominance, with most of these tumors found in males in the first 3 decades of life.[386] With NCCT, a typical heterogeneous appearance is seen with areas of calcification and hypodense areas of cyst formation or fat. CECT demonstrates minimal enhancement; the presence of striking soft tissue enhancement suggests the presence of a mixed tumor with malignant germ cell tumor elements.[386] The presence of well-defined osseous structures or teeth in a sellar region mass is a rare but diagnostic imaging finding in teratoma.[387–389]

MRI of sellar region teratomas demonstrates heterogeneity in keeping with the histologic variability found in these lesions. A heterogeneous appearance with areas of hyper- and isointensity on T1-weighted images corresponding to fat and soft tissue components, and variable T2-weighted intensity from fat and cystic areas as well as solid components and larger portions of calcification, is typically seen.[390, 305] Some heterogeneous enhancement may be present. Teratomas isointense with brain on all pulse sequences have been noted[391] and may consist only of soft tissue components with few areas of fat to produce T1 hyperintensity.

Visual Pathway Glioma

This section discusses gliomas of the optic chiasm and tracts; optic nerve gliomas confined to the orbits are described in the orbital imaging sections.

Overall, visual pathway gliomas (VPGs) constitute 3% to 5% of all primary pediatric brain tumors. From 60% to 80% of the tumors involve the optic nerves, chiasm, and tracts, whereas 20% to 36% involve only the prechiasmatic portions of the visual pathway.[392] A strong association with NF-1 is noted with VPGs, with NF-1 present in 15% to 35% of patients with VPG, whereas 5% to 21% of NF-1 patients have VPG.[392, 393] Most patients present younger than 10 years,[376] and it has been suggested that patients with chiasmatic VPG are younger in those with NF-1. VPG are also the most common central nervous system tumor in children with NF-1[394] and are found with equal frequency in both sexes.[395]

Surgical therapy is frequently deferred for chiasmatic VPG, but when biopsied, most tumors are found to be pilocytic astrocytomas (WHO grade I) in keeping with their indolent clinical course.[393] Oligodendroglial elements are sometimes present in chiasmatic VPG.[396]

Overall, gliomas of the optic pathways (all types, including tumors confined entirely to the orbits) are indolent, with 10-year survival rates of 60% to 100%; lesions confined to the optic nerve alone may be resected completely and have 10-year survival rates of 85% to 100%.[397] Tumors involving the chiasm, or extending posteriorly, present greater difficulty in management, as total surgical resection is usually not possible, and the central location of the tumor would subject a significant portion of normal brain to radiation, limiting the dose used. Relapse-free rates for these tumors are thus lower, in the range of 56% to 90%.[397] VPGs are more likely to be multicentric in patients with NF-1,[398] and these patients appear to be at risk for the development of chiasmatic VPG after resection for tumors confined to the optic nerve.[396] The effect of NF-1 on the prognosis of tumors confined to the chiasm is uncertain, with some authors reporting an improved prognosis,[392] some an unchanged prognosis.[396] Children younger than 2 years have a worse prognosis, with more rapid and aggressive tumor growth despite a benign histologic appearance.[396] Determining the clinical course and ideal therapy of VPG is complicated by the long clinical course of these tumors. About half of purely intraorbital tumors will not progress and will stabilize without treatment over time; most of these patients have NF-1.[397] Posteriorly located VPG, involving the chiasm, have also been noted to stabilize or even regress,[399] but up to 20% of childhood chiasmatic tumors behave aggressively and are fatal.[400]

VPGs may be divided into three broad categories for imaging purposes.[395] Prechiasmatic lesions are confined to the optic nerves themselves. Diffuse chiasmatic lesions appear as enlargement and thickening of the optic chiasm and may extend into the optic nerves and tracts. With MRI, these tumors can be diagnosed radiographically, especially in the presence of NF-1. Exophytic chiasmatic-hypothalamic tumors present as large, bulky masses in the suprasellar region. Delineation of the optic nerves and chiasm, as well as the point of origin of these tumors, may be difficult to determine radiographically. Tumors confined to the optic chiasm are likely to present with visual disturbances, but the large exophytic lesions may present in younger children with failure to thrive, diencephalic syndrome, macrocephaly, or endocrinopathy. Large tumors may compress or extend into the third ventricle and produce hydrocephalus.

There is no consensus on the ideal therapy for VPG. Prechiasmatic tumors can be cured by total resection, but tumors with few symptoms, often found during screening MRI examinations of NF-1 patients, may be followed by serial MRI examinations. Diffuse chiasmatic tumors rarely are amenable to surgery; radiation has been traditionally used for progressive tumor or worsening symptoms, and careful serial MRI can play a part in the management of these lesions. The exophytic tumors show some palliation from surgical resection.[395]

Optic gliomas are uncommonly found in adults. These rare tumors are not associated with NF-1 and are either anaplastic astrocytomas or glioblastomas. The tumors may mimic optic neuritis clinically, have a poor prognosis, and are rapidly fatal.[401]

The typical NCCT appearance of a chiasmatic VPG is an isodense mass consisting of thickening of the optic chiasm, and, if involved by tumor, the optic nerves and tracts as well. Globular suprasellar masses consistent with

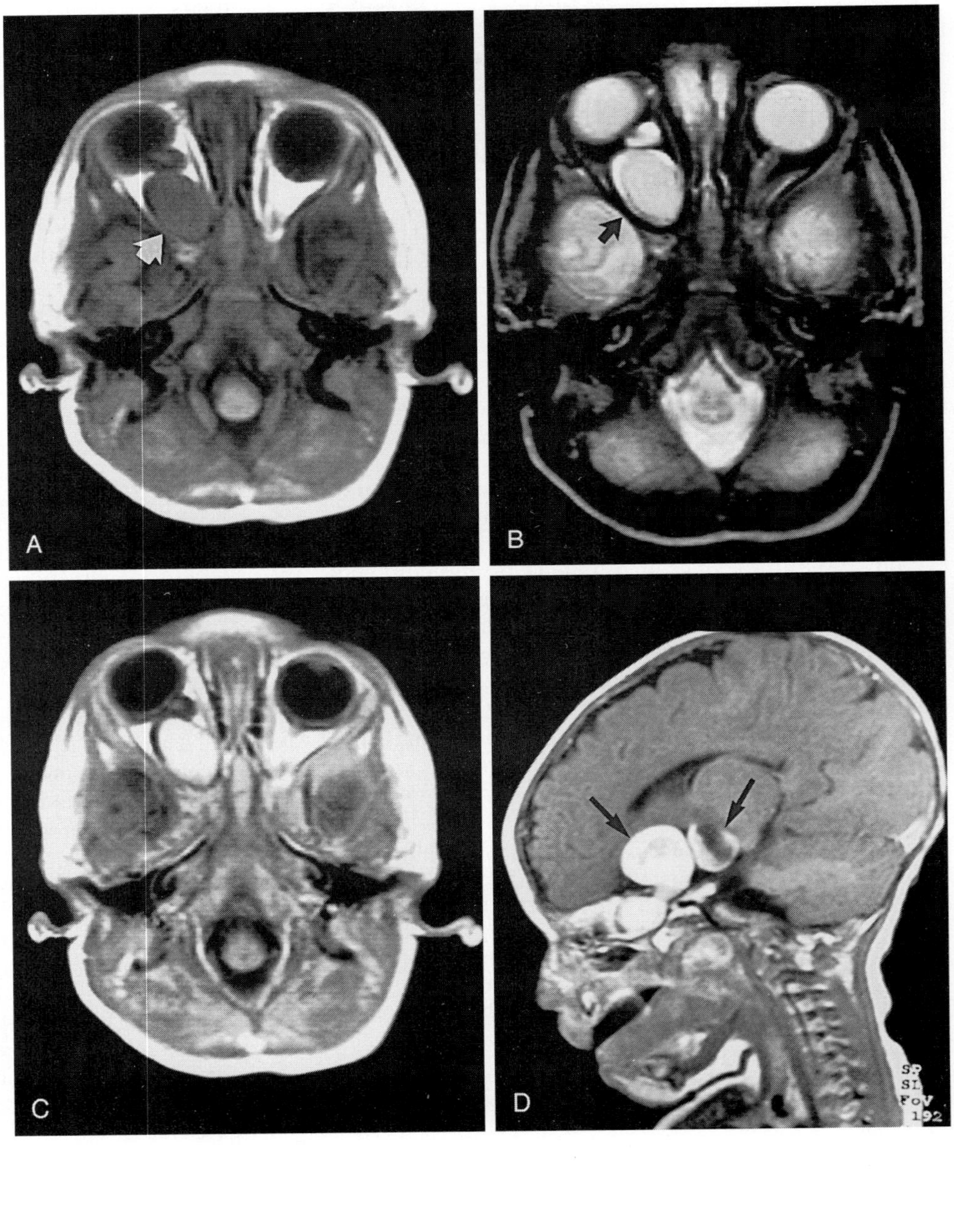

FIGURE 46–49 A 4-year-old child with opticochiasmatic visual pathway glioma. Axial T1-weighted (*A*) and T2-weighted (*B*) images demonstrate a well-defined intraconal mass isointense to brain on both sequences (*arrows*). *C* and *D*, Gadolinium-enhanced images demonstrate intense enhancement of the mass and extension of the lesion through the optic canal into the chiasm. A large suprasellar component is present extending into the third ventricle and hypothalamus (*arrows* in *D*).

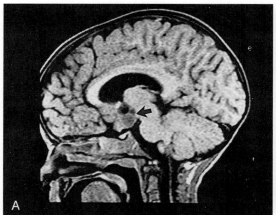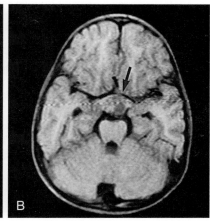

FIGURE 46–50 A 2-year-old child with hypothalamic region glioma. Sagittal (*A*) and axial (*B*) T1-weighted images demonstrate a well-defined cystic and solid mass centered in the hypothalamus (*arrows*). The optic chiasm cannot be delineated from the tumor, whose exact anatomic origin is difficult to determine.

exophytic gliomas are also noted. Calcification is rare but may be seen in the optic tracts, when they are involved, and in lesions after radiation therapy. Giant tumors with multiple lobulations or cysts suggest the presence of anaplastic gliomas, but the overall correlation of tumor size, or change in size, with the patient's vision is poor.[402, 403] With CECT, enhancement is usually present and may be marked, but nonenhancing VPGs are sometimes observed. Enhancement produced by tumor spread through the optic tracts to the lateral geniculate bodies and optic radiation can be present.[404]

MRI better defines the extent of tumor spread, as well as its relation to adjacent structures,[405] which is particularly important with large lesions whose point of origin may be within the hypothalamus, or with exophytic lesions that may be surgically treated. With large and invasive lesions that involve the optic chiasm, tracts, and hypothalamus, it may be difficult to determine the site of origin even with MRI. Images demonstrate thickening of the optic chiasm and nerves with hypo- to isointensity on T1-weighted images, and mild to marked hyperintensity on T2-weighted images (Figs. 46–49 and 46–50).[406] Spread of tumor, or edema, along the optic tracts and into the geniculate bodies and radiations may be seen with T2-weighted images as areas of hyperintensity. The involved optic radiations may have little mass effect despite the presence of invasive neoplasm.[407, 408] Signal abnormality in the posterior pathways may also represent demyelination, gliosis, or wallerian degeneration.[216] Gadolinium enhancement of VPG is variable. With lesions confined to the optic chiasm and nerves, enhancement can be mild or absent, whereas tumors with extension into the posterior pathways usually demonstrate marked enhancement,[409] which is heterogeneous and can involve the lateral geniculate bodies and proximal optic radiations. Microcysts, and rarely macrocysts, may be present.[216] In a few cases, the T2 hyperintensity, gadolinium enhancement, and thickening of presumed chiasmatic gliomas have been noted to regress spontaneously; similar changes were also noted in the lateral geniculate bodies and optic radiations and reflect the potentially indolent course of these tumors.[410]

Astrocytomas of the Cerebral Hemispheres and Thalami

Hemispheric supratentorial astrocytomas represent about 20% to 52% of reported supratentorial tumors in children,

whereas thalamic tumors represent about 10% of all pediatric brain tumors.[411–413] The hemispheric tumors peak around the age of 7 to 8 years, demonstrate a slight male predominance, and frequently have a benign course.[411] Most hemispheric tumors (56%) are pilocytic astrocytomas, with about 30% fibrillary or protoplasmic astrocytomas, 10% mixed tumors (frequently oligoastrocytomas), and occasional gemistocytic astrocytomas.[411] Hemispheric astrocytomas typically present with signs and symptoms related to the adjacent cerebral cortex including seizures and hemiparesis. Headache and vomiting as well as increased intracranial pressure are seen later. The tumors are most commonly located in the frontal and temporal lobes, but any portion of the supratentorial brain can be involved. With low-grade tumors, the prognosis is excellent after surgical resection alone, up to 93% at 10 years,[414] with the best prognosis seen with pilocytic astrocytomas. An older age at presentation, compared with cerebellar and diencephalic pilocytic astrocytomas, has been noted with the supratentorial variety, which may present into adulthood.[415] The later age at presentation may be due to better tolerance of a mass effect from supratentorial tumors.

Hemispheric pilocytic astrocytomas have a gross and histologic appearance identical to that found in the cerebellum, and the radiologic appearance of these tumors reflects these similarities. The typical NCCT appearance is a large cyst with a solid or slightly hypodense (relative to adjacent brain) mural nodule, mural plaque, or multiple mural masses packed together. The medial aspect of the cyst typically is contiguous with the wall of the lateral ventricle but is separated from it by ependyma. Solid pilocytic astrocytes are also found in the hemispheres. With CECT, enhancement of the solid portions of the tumor is always seen.[416] The tumors are smooth and well demarcated and usually do not demonstrate peritumoral edema even with MRI. The lack of edema and typical cystic appearance with focal enhancement, although not pathognomonic of pilocytic astrocytoma, are useful features distinguishing these tumors from malignant or infiltrative gliomas.[415] Calcification may be seen in any cell type of astrocytoma, but in childhood astrocytomas calcification appears unusual, and its presence should suggest another tumor type including oligodendroglioma, ganglioglioma, or supratentorial PNET.[417] The MRI appearance of a pilocytic astrocytoma in the hemispheres is a well-

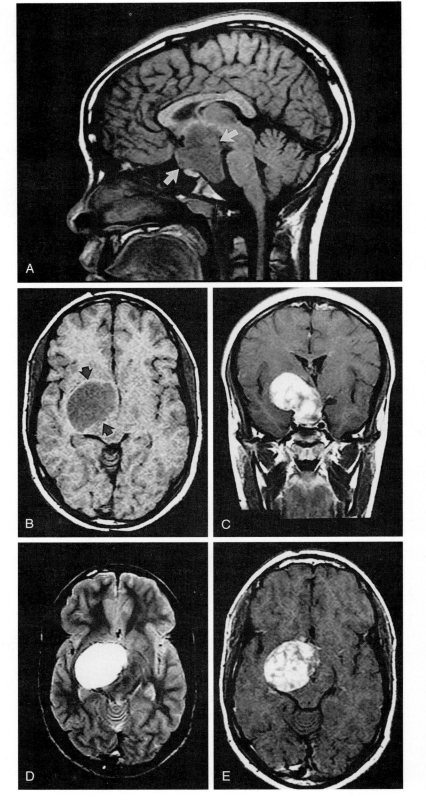

FIGURE 46–51 A 12-year-old child with hypothalamic–parasellar region JPA. *A* and *B*, T1-weighted images demonstrate a large hypointense mass in the suprasellar and prepontine spaces *(arrows)*. *C*, Coronal T1-weighted image with gadolinium demonstrates involvement of the hypothalamus and extension into the adjacent cerebrum. The mass enhances intensely. T2-weighted *(D)* and gadolinium-enhanced T1-weighted *(E)* axial images demonstrate diffuse enhancement of the mass and marked T2-weighted hyperintensity, but no prominent cystic-appearing areas.

defined tumor with sharp margins, with the solid portion demonstrating low signal intensity on T1-weighted images, increased T2 signal intensity, and dense enhancement (Figs. 46–51 and 46–52). Poorly defined margins and the absence of enhancement suggest a fibrillary astrocytoma, and the presence of necrosis, hemorrhage, and marked edema can be found in anaplastic astrocytomas or the rare pediatric glioblastoma.[49, 216, 414]

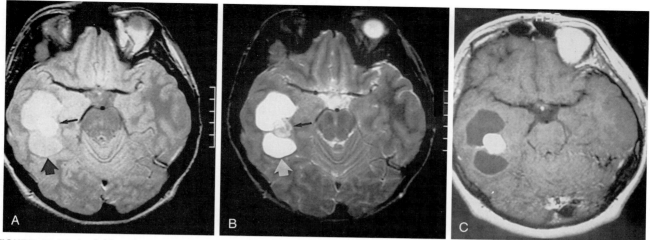

FIGURE 46–52 A child with temporal lobe JPA. The patient presented with temporal lobe epilepsy. PD-weighted *(A)* and T2-weighted *(B)* images demonstrate a temporal lobe lesion containing proteinaceous fluid that is hyperintense on the PD-weighted image, relative to CSF, and isointense on T2-weighted images *(large arrows)*. A solid nodule *(small arrows)* is present and is hyperintense relative to brain on both pulse sequences. *C,* The nodule intensely enhances with gadolinium.

Low-grade hemispheric fibrillary astrocytomas are infiltrative tumors of the white matter. Enhancement, calcification, and cyst formation are less common than in the pilocytic tumors, and hemorrhage is rare. CT demonstrates a hypodense mass that usually does not enhance, whereas MRI demonstrates a homogeneous mass that is hypointense on T1-weighted images and hyperintense on T2-weighted images. Occasional irregular enhancement may be present.[418]

Malignant glioma of the hemispheres, although a common primary brain tumor in adults, is rare in children; only 3% of glioblastoma multiforme (GBM) cases are found in children, representing about 7% to 11% of primary brain tumors in children overall.[419] The age at presentation is older than with the benign astrocytomas (13 years median age at diagnosis), and prognosis is poor, with a 10-year survival of 32% for malignant (grade III) astrocytoma, and 0% at 10 years for GBM.[420] Tumor dissemination through the CSF is common, seen in up to 30%, and tumoral hemorrhage may be found in 18%.

The outlook for pediatric patients with malignant glioma, although poor, is more favorable than in adult patients, especially in younger (than 12 years) children.[419] A significant number of these tumors represent second malignant neoplasms, arising at the site of previous radiation therapy, in patients with genetic predisposition to develop brain tumors (including NF-1), and in children with leukemia and prophylactic whole brain irradiation.[419] It has been suggested that up to 20% of these tumors may reflect malignant transformation of a benign lesion in patients with evolution of symptoms lasting 6 months or more.[421] The appearance and location of GBM in children and adults are similar, with the tumors found most often in the frontal and temporal lobes.[422] Presentation with signs and symptoms of increased intracranial pressure or seizures is typical of both adults and children with GBM. CT typically demonstrates a heterogeneous lesion, with a patchy appearance, irregular borders, marked perilesional edema, and ring enhancement. The lesions may be solid, cystic, or hyperdense (Fig. 46–53).[422, 423]

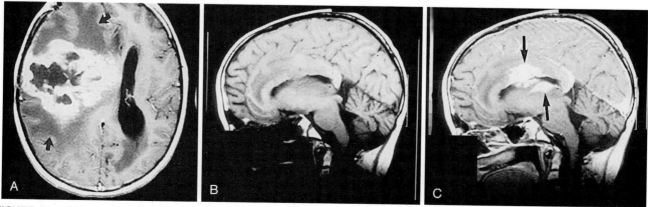

FIGURE 46–53 An 11-year-old boy with glioblastoma multiforme. *A,* T1-weighted gadolinium-enhanced image demonstrates a huge, enhancing, necrotic mass of the right cerebral hemisphere with a marked mass effect and shift of the right lateral ventricle. Note the extensive surrounding edema *(arrows)*. Sagittal T1-weighted image *(B)* and a gadolinium-enhanced T1-weighted image *(C)* demonstrate enhancing tumor invading the thalamus and crossing and expanding the corpus callosum *(arrows)*. The appearance is identical to that of a high-grade glioma in an adult.

Primary thalamic gliomas typically present with increased intracranial pressure or focal neurologic deficits. About half of all thalamic tumors are low-grade tumors, mostly pilocytic astrocytomas, oligodendrogliomas, or giant cell astrocytomas, with the remainder malignant astrocytomas or GBM.[424] CT has typically demonstrated solid masses with less than 20% of tumors demonstrating cystic components. Enhancement is seen in about one-half of thalamic tumors, and its presence does not correlate with the histologic grade (Fig. 46–54). Overall prognosis is poor.[412] Rare glial tumors in the septal area, including astrocytomas, oligodendrogliomas, and ependymomas, are found in children presenting with hydrocephalus. The few pediatric cases reported involved the septum pellucidum as well as the medial part of the floor of one or both frontal horns and may have arisen from multipotential cells in the septal area.[425]

Gliomatosis cerebri is a term used to describe a diffuse proliferation of glial elements infiltrating normal nervous tissue with destruction of myelin sheaths but little damage to neurons or axons. Cells typical of astrocytoma and oligodendroglioma may be found.[426] The disease may represent multicentric transformation, a dedifferentiation of astrocytes, or the extreme end of a spectrum of diffuse, infiltrating, and typically low-grade glioma. The age at presentation is from birth to 80 years, with a mean age of 42; clinical signs may be quite mild in the presence of marked MRI abnormality and include headache, seizure, and mental status changes. Intractable epilepsy, corticospinal tract deficits, and developmental delay may be seen in children.[427–429] CT can be normal but typically demonstrates diffuse hypointensity of the white matter, expansion of the cerebral structures, and no enhancement, whereas MRI, which demonstrates the extent of disease better than CT, shows diffuse white matter hypointensity or isointensity on T1-weighted images, and dif-

fusely increased, poorly defined PD and T2 signal. Infrequent focal parenchymal or leptomeningeal enhancement may be seen, and loss of a distinct gray-white junction may be present.[430–432] Involvement of two or more lobes of the brain, lack of a grossly distinct mass, no tissue necrosis, and little destruction of involved brain tissue are typical. Involvement of the optic chiasm, thalamus, hypothalamus, pons, basal ganglia, and cerebellum may be present.[433] It is important to recognize that in the pediatric patient, gliomatosis cerebri may mimic multiple sclerosis with confluent extensive lesions, viral encephalitides, adrenoleukodystrophy, metachromatic leukodystrophy, and subacute sclerosing panencephalitis.[428] The prognosis is poor, as the lesion is too diffuse to benefit from surgical therapy and typically does not respond well to radiation, as most lesions are low-grade gliomas.[434]

Germinomas of the Basal Ganglia and Thalamus

The basal ganglia and thalamus represent a rare location for germinomas, accounting for 5% to 16% of intracranial germinomas. The incidence of basal ganglia and thalamic germinomas is higher in Japan than in the United States.[435, 436] Patients are virtually all male, usually in the second decade of life, who present with focal neurologic symptoms including paresis and hemihypesthesia as well as dystonic movement, seizures, and precocious puberty. Ipsilateral hemicerebral atrophy is common at presentation as well.[437]

CT of basal ganglia and thalamic germinomas demonstrates a distinctly different appearance from pineal or sellar region germinomas. Slightly hyperdense masses with irregular borders are seen with little mass effect although the tumors can frequently be several centimeters at presentation. Calcification and cysts of various sizes

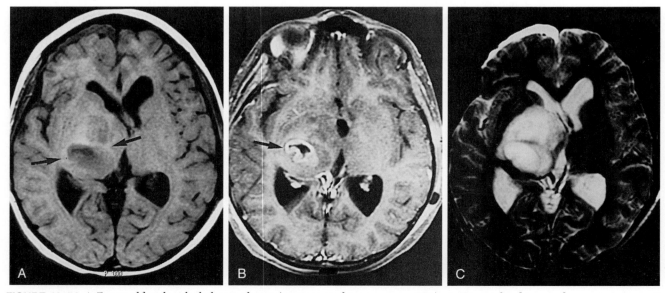

FIGURE 46–54 A 7-year-old girl with thalamic glioma (stereotactic biopsy-proven JPA). *A*, T1-weighted image demonstrates a cystic and solid mass in the right thalamus *(arrows)*. *B*, Gadolinium-enhanced image demonstrates ring enhancement in part of the lesion *(arrow)*. *C*, T2-weighted image demonstrates hyperintensity, consistent with tumor or edema, or both, throughout the right thalamus and basal ganglia. Subdural fluid is likely related to a decrease in hydrocephalus after ventriculostomy.

are common, and CECT demonstrates mild to moderate heterogeneous enhancement.[438, 435] The tumors are located in the lentiform nuclei and thalamus, and bilateral basal ganglia and thalamic tumors have been reported; they may be due to spread of the tumor through connecting white matter tracts. Like the sellar and pineal region tumors, these germinomas likely arise from migration of totipotential cells that are deviated off the midline by the developing third ventricle.[439, 440]

MRI of these germinomas demonstrates solid, cystic, or mixed-appearing masses. The solid portions are isointense or slightly hypointense relative to gray matter on T1-weighted images, are hyperintense on T2-weighted images, and enhance heterogeneously in all cases; both solid and rimlike enhancement may be seen. Peritumoral edema is seen in only one-third of cases, despite the frequently large size of the tumors. The calcifications usually are not seen on MRI but may occasionally appear as areas of hyperintensity on T1-weighted images. Areas of hyperintensity on T1- and T2-weighted images consistent with blood degradation products may be seen. The evidence of hemorrhage is seen less easily with NCCT.[435, 438] The cerebral atrophy, as well as atrophy of the ipsilateral cerebral peduncle, is likely due to involvement of adjacent white matter tracts by the tumor and is more common when the tumors have irregular margins involving the internal capsule.[441] Like germinomas elsewhere, basal ganglia and thalamic germinomas are radiosensitive. Mixed germ cell tumors may be found in the basal ganglia and thalamus and are less radiosensitive than pure tumors. Tumor markers are useful in their identification.

The combination of areas of cyst formation and hemorrhage, enhancement on MRI, and hyperdensity with frequent calcifications on NCCT is helpful in making the preoperative diagnosis of basal ganglia and thalamic germinoma. Gliomas are the most common tumor of the basal ganglia and thalamus in children but are usually isoor hypodense on NCCT. Lymphoma may have a similar appearance and location but is very uncommon in children, whereas cerebral PNET, although also a densely cellular and hyperdense tumor, is more often hemispheric and superficial (Fig. 46–55).

Ganglion Cell Tumors

Ganglioglioma and Gangliocytoma

Gangliogliomas are defined by the presence of both a neoplastic glial element and a component composed of abnormal neurons. The less common gangliocytoma consists of only abnormal neurons. These two terms are not distinct as a spectrum of pathologic lesions exists, and the term *ganglion cell tumor* is used to encompass these neoplasms. The glial elements are usually astrocytic and low grade, and foci of oligodendroglial elements may be found in these tumors as well.[190, 442]

Gangliogliomas constitute about 1.2% to 7.6% of all pediatric brain tumors and have a mean presentation age of 12.5 years. Series of both adults and children with gangliogliomas have found presentations well into adulthood, but the mean age is still young, around 25 years. No significant gender predominance is seen. Patients most commonly present with seizures, with behavioral disturbances and learning disabilities less common. Focal neurologic signs and increased intracranial pressure are distinctly unusual. These are indolent tumors, and the duration of symptoms is long, with a history of seizures present up to 45 years before diagnosis.[443–445] Patients presenting with seizures usually have complex partial seizures that are progressive or resistant to medication. MRI of patients with complex partial seizures in general demonstrates tumors in a little over 20% of cases, with ganglion cell tumors the most common cell type found, especially in patients younger than 12 years.[446, 447]

Gangliogliomas may be found anywhere in the CNS, with the cerebral hemispheres, especially the temporal lobes, the most common location. Other less common locations include the region of the third ventricle, cerebellum, brain stem, thalamus, and spinal cord. Hemispheric tumors have good prognosis, with most patients having a significant decrease in seizure frequency after surgical resection alone. The prognosis seems to be most dependent on the completeness of surgical resection.[448, 449] Posterior fossa tumors are seen more commonly in children than in adults. Midline tumors in the hypothalamus and cervicomedullary junction may present with focal neurologic defects such as blindness and paraparesis, present at a younger age, and have a shorter duration of symptoms. Prognosis is worse for these tumors as surgical therapy is difficult, and multiple operations, chemotherapy, and radiation therapy may be required for control of these tumors.[450] Malignant gangliogliomas are rare; usually it is the glial component that degenerates[451] from 5 to more than 20 years after the initial diagnosis,[452] although anaplastic gangliogliomas exist.[190]

Gangliogliomas are frequently calcified, a useful radiographic feature that can be present on conventional radiographs in one-third of cases,[453] as can focal thinning of the calvarium from the long-standing presence of the tumor. With NCCT, calcifications have been reported in up to 41% of cases.[445] The calcifications may appear as small flecks or large calcified masses, and in some instances calcification may be the only NCCT finding in smaller tumors.[454–456]

The typical NCCT appearance of a ganglioglioma is a low-density lesion in the cerebral hemisphere, most often the temporal lobe. The lesions are hypodense in up to 59% of patients. However, solid lesions that are slightly hypodense or isodense are common, and occasional hyperdense masses may be seen. Although about two-thirds of gangliogliomas appear cystic or have areas of low CT density, many of these lesions are found to be composed of solid but gelatinous tumors at surgery. The tumors may be any size, from small cortical lesions seen only on MRI to large masses occupying much of a lobe, but edema and a significant mass effect on adjacent brain is distinctly mild with these tumors, reflecting their slow, indolent growth. With CECT, some enhancement of the solid portions of the tumor, including ringlike enhancement and enhancing mural nodules in apparently cystic tumors, is seen in up to 50% of patients. When present the enhancement is typically reported as mild.[444, 457–460]

MRI demonstrates a wide range of signal intensities in gangliogliomas. Areas of decreased signal intensity on T1-

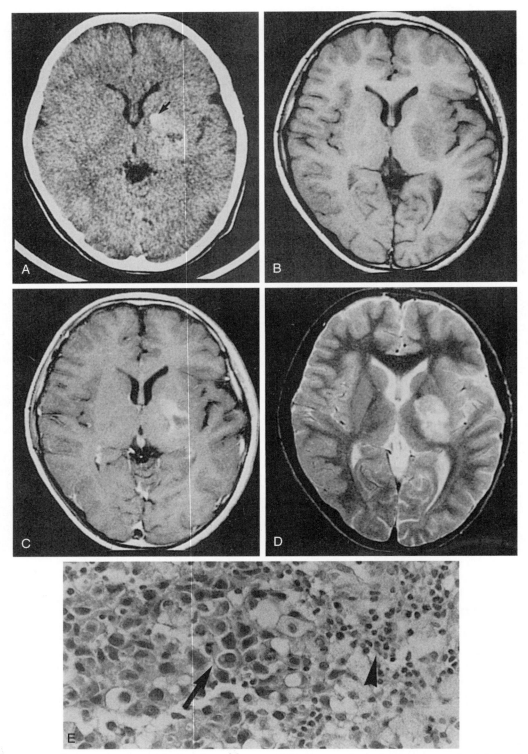

FIGURE 46–55 Germ cell tumor arising in the basal ganglia. *A,* NECT shows a hyperdense mass in the left basal ganglia with a central lower-density region and peripheral calcification *(arrow).* The mass shows low signal intensity on a T1-weighted image *(B)* and partial enhancement after gadolinium administration *(C). D,* Heterogeneous signal intensity is present on a T2-weighted image. *E,* Photomicrograph of tumor tissue shows a mixture of lymphocytes *(arrowhead)* and larger polygonal and spherical cells *(arrow).* (*A–E,* From Higano S, Takahashi S, Ishii, K, et al. Germinoma originating in the basal ganglia and thalamus: MR and CT evaluation. AJNR 1994;15:1435–1441.)

weighted images and increased PD and T2 signals, relative to gray matter, are commonly seen, and, although the tumors may appear cystic, solid tumor is frequently found at surgery. Solid tumors typically are isointense or slightly hypointense or even hyperintense, relative to gray matter, and frequently enhance with gadolinium. About one-half of the tumors have a mixed cystic and solid appearance on MRI, with most others appearing entirely solid. Occasionally, tumors with MRI appearances typical of a cystic lesion with no solid elements are found. Some studies have noted that in lesions with hyperintensity on PD- and T2-weighted images, relative to gray matter, the PD hyperintensity is more pronounced than that of the T2-weighted images and correlates with solid tumor rather than fluid. As expected, calcifications are less frequently identified with MRI than with CT. In young infants, the tumors may appear more hyperintense on T1-weighted images and hypointense on T2-weighted images than expected, probably due to the differing signal characteristics of the unmyelinated brain in this age group.[445, 456, 461–463] Perilesional edema is typically minimal or absent with gangliogliomas. Pathologic findings consistent with mesial temporal (hippocampal) sclerosis have been identified in excised temporal lobes from patients with temporal lobe gangliogliomas and may be produced by repetitive seizure activity (Figs. 46–56 and 46–57).[464]

Local involvement of the adjacent subarachnoid space may be produced by gangliogliomas and is not uncom-

mon.[465] Widespread dissemination is rare and usually produced by the glial element of the tumor. The few reported cases with radiographic findings have included diffuse leptomeningeal enhancement with gadolinium or the presence of multiple hyperintense cystlike lesions in the subarachnoid space.[466, 467]

Cerebellomedullary gangliogliomas have been noted to be hypodense or isodense relative to adjacent brain with NCCT. Most demonstrate enhancement, and calcifications are occasionally seen. MRI demonstrates isointensity relative to adjacent brain on T1-weighted images and hyperintensity on T2-weighted images. Both CECT and postgadolinium MRI demonstrate enhancement. The appearance is not specific and does not allow the distinction from brain stem glioma, but the clinical course may be more indolent with ganglioglioma, especially with exophytic lesions.[468, 469]

Pure gangliocytomas are very rare, overall representing only 0.1% of central nervous system tumors, and few reports of their radiographic appearance exist. NCCT demonstrates slight hyperdensity with little or no enhancement with CECT. The absence of a mass effect, cysts, or calcifications has been noted. A serpiginous appearance as well as a normal-appearing CT scan have been noted. With MRI, the lesions are found in the cortex of the hemispheres and may be difficult to identify on T1-weighted images, on which they appear isointense or slightly hyperintense. PD-weighted images demon-

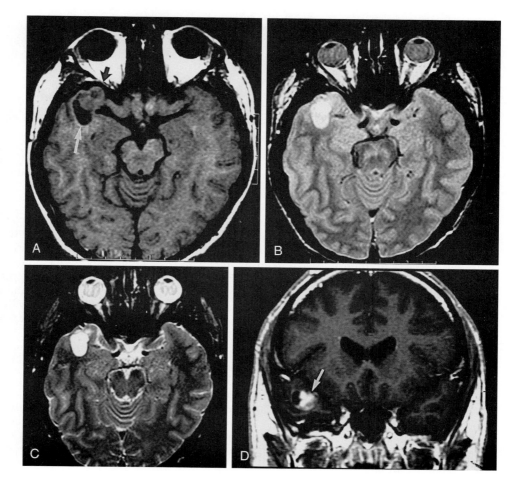

FIGURE 46–56 An 18-year-old with ganglioglioma. The patient presented with seizures. *A*, T1-weighted image demonstrates a temporal lobe lesion with a small cyst *(white arrow)* and solid cortical portions *(black arrow)*. The cystic component demonstrates progressive hyperintensity on PD-weighted *(B)* and T2-weighted *(C)* images whereas the solid portion is only mildly hyperintense. No edema is present. *D*, Avid gadolinium enhancement of the solid portion is seen *(arrow)*.

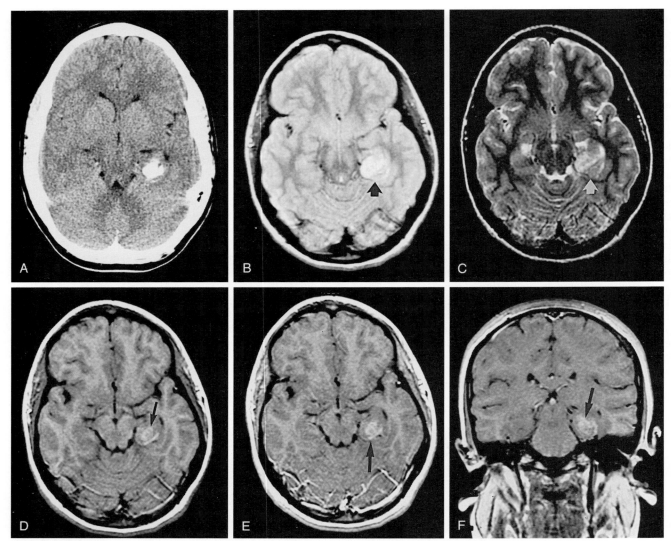

FIGURE 46–57 A 15-year-old girl with a mild seizure disorder. *A*, NCCT demonstrates a densely calcified mass in the left medial temporal lobe. The mass is hyperintense on PD-weighted *(B)* and T2-weighted *(C)* images *(arrows)*. *D*, T1-weighted image demonstrates mild focal central hyperintensity *(arrow)* possibly due to calcification. *E* and *F*, Faint enhancement *(arrows)* is seen with gadolinium. The appearance and location of the tumor are consistent with either oligodendroglioma or ganglion cell tumor.

strate intermediate to high signal, whereas on T2-weighted images the lesions are intermediate or hypointense relative to gray matter.[470, 471] Little or no mass effect is present. The lack of dramatic signal intensity seen with these lesions correlates with their pathologic resemblance to hamartomas (Fig. 46–58).

Oligodendroglioma

Oligodendrogliomas are uncommon infiltrating gliomas that account for only 4% to 5% of all primary brain tumors, with only 6% diagnosed in children, in which they represent only 1% to 2% of primary brain tumors.[472] The median age of incidence is 40 to 50 years, and a slight male predominance has been noted in some studies.[473] Most oligodendrogliomas are located in the cerebral hemispheres, most frequently in the frontal lobes (in up to one-half of cases) followed by the temporal and parietal

lobes. The tumors are typically cortical or subcortical with rare involvement of the deep gray structures as well as the posterior fossa reported.[473] Most patients with hemispheric tumors, including children,[474] present with seizures, whereas the rare posterior fossa tumors, which appear to be more common in children than in adults, present with obstructive hydrocephalus from a mass effect, or with intratumoral hemorrhage producing brain stem symptoms.[475]

Oligodendrogliomas are infiltrative neoplasms composed of oligodendrocytes but may appear well defined both on imaging studies and at gross inspection. Oligodendrogliomas have a significant tendency to calcify and to demonstrate intratumoral hemorrhage relative to other CNS tumors, and these findings on neuroimaging studies can be useful in suggesting the correct diagnosis.[190] Younger patients in general are more likely to have frontal lobe lesions, low-grade tumors, and a slightly improved prognosis relative to older patients.[476-478] Histologically pure oligodendrogliomas and the presence of calcification (histologic and radiographic) have been correlated with improved survival.[479] Surgical resection is the primary therapy; a detailed study of the optimal treatment, role of radiation and chemotherapy, and prognosis in children is difficult with this infrequently encountered tumor.

The typical NCCT appearance of an oligodendroglioma is a hypodense (57%), isodense (23%), heterogeneous, or occasionally hyperdense mass. In some series, low density with CT has been noted to be present in at least a portion of all tumors.[480] Tumor margins have been reported as both irregular and sharp but seem to appear even better defined with MRI. Hyperdensity on NCCT can be due to hemorrhage. With CECT, some enhancement is seen in 46% to 60%; the enhancement is usually faint. Although some tumors fail to enhance at all, a tendency for mixed tumors (oligoastroctyoma) and higher-grade, anaplastic tumors to enhance more frequently than pure tumors is seen. Tumors containing well-defined foci of both oligodendrocytic and astrocytic neoplastic cells are common.[190] High-grade tumors or mixed tumors can pathologically and radiographically resemble glioblastoma multiforme.[481] Calcification by CT has been noted in around 40% of pediatric and adolescent tumors and appears less common than the reported incidence of calcification in adult tumors, which ranges from 10% to as high as 91% (Fig. 46-59).[482]

MRI findings of oligodendrogliomas typically include hypointensity or occasional mixed hypo- and hyperintensity, relative to white matter on T1-weighted images. T2-weighted images usually demonstrate hyperintensity relative to white matter. Cystic-appearing regions are not frequently seen (0% to 20% of cases) and perilesional edema is rare (Fig. 46-60; also see Fig. 46-59). Tumor margins often appear well defined on MRI despite the infiltrative nature of the tumor, and a mass effect is often minimal, noted in less than one-half of patients. Enhancement with gadolinium is common, seen in up to 80% of cases, but seems less common with younger patients.[481, 482] The lower incidence of calcification and enhancement in younger patients, compared with adults, may reflect the greater proportion of pure oligodendrogliomas in younger patients. Posterior fossa oligodendrogliomas have presented as hypo- to hyperdense masses in the cerebellar vermis, fourth ventricle, or cerebral peduncles, or attached to the brain stem, with heterogeneous enhancement on CECT. The posterior fossa tumors may have a greater tendency for early leptomeningeal dissemination compared with the hemispheric tumors.[475]

The differential diagnosis includes ganglioglioma and low-grade astrocytoma. Both of these tumors are more

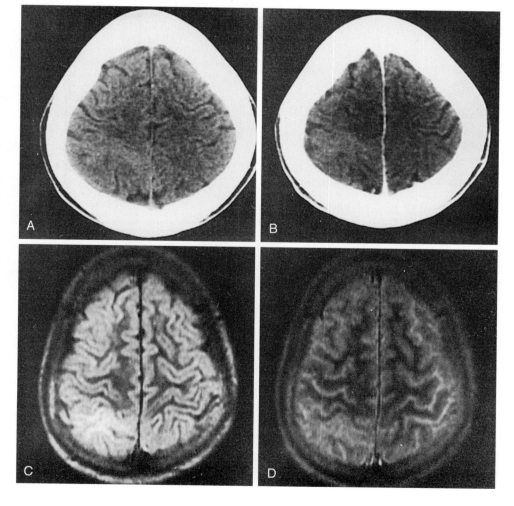

FIGURE 46-58 Gangliocytoma. *A,* Unenhanced CT scan of a 15-year-old boy with intractable seizures shows increased attenuation in the right posterior lobe. *B,* After contrast administration, there is no enhancement. Axial long-TR–short-TE *(C)* and T2-weighted *(D)* images from MRI studies show increased signal intensity in a corresponding location. (*A–D,* From Altman NR. MR and CT characteristics of gangliocytoma: A rare cause of epilepsy in children. AJNR 1988;9:917–921.)

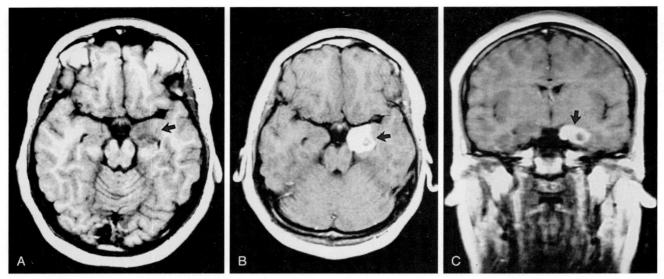

FIGURE 46–59 An 11-year-old with oligodendroglioma of the temporal lobe. The patient had a long history of partial complex seizures. *A,* T1-weighted image demonstrates hypointensity and expansion of the left uncus by the tumor *(arrow). B* and *C,* Gadolinium-enhanced images demonstrate an intensely enhancing mass with a focal area of hypointensity *(arrows)* consistent with a small cyst.

FIGURE 46–60 Oligodendroglioma. A 20-year-old patient presented with seizures. *A,* NCCT demonstrates a mildly hypodense mass *(large arrows)* with focal calcification in the right frontal lobe *(small arrow). B,* T2-weighted image demonstrates a well-defined hyperintensity involving the cortex and white matter with a mild mass effect. T1-weighted *(C)* and gadolinium-enhanced T1-weighted *(D)* images demonstrate the lesion as subtle hypointensity *(arrows* in *C),* similar in signal to normal gray matter, with no enhancement.

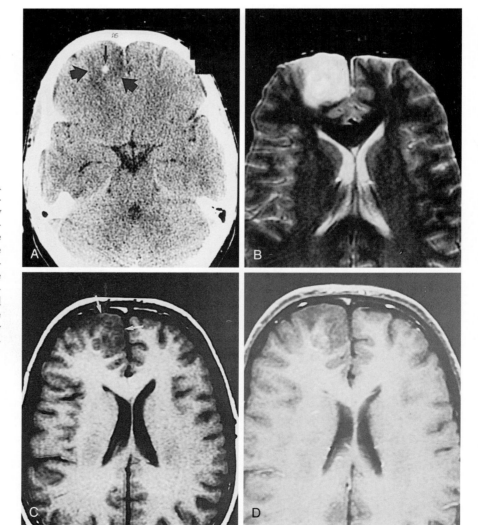

common than oligodendrogliomas in the pediatric population. Gangliogliomas are most frequently found in the temporal lobe but may otherwise have an identical appearance to oligodendrogliomas, and radiographic evidence of white matter tract infiltration by astrocytomas may be noted.

Pleomorphic Xanthoastrocytoma

Pleomorphic xanthoastrocytoma (PXA) is a superficially located astrocytic neoplasm with a distinct, pleomorphic histologic appearance and frequent xanthomatous change. Patients are typically older children or young adults presenting with a history of seizures (in 78%), sometimes with a long-standing history of a seizure disorder. The age range at presentation is from 2.5 years to the mid-30s, with a mean age of 14 years.[483, 484] The tumors most commonly involve the temporal lobe, alone or in combination with the adjacent lobes. Frontal and occipital tumors are less common. Involvement of the leptomeninges is very common and characteristic of this tumor, and, although the lesions appear grossly well demarcated, invasion of the cerebral cortex is often found at surgery.[484] Imaging findings frequently reveal a cystic-appearing area, but, unlike the findings in gangliogliomas, gross inspection of these tumors often reveals a fluid-filled cyst.[190]

The histologic appearance of PXA is characterized by cellular pleomorphism and variable accumulation of lipid droplets. Bizarre giant cells and occasional mitotic figures are seen, and these tumors have been confused pathologically with mesenchymal tumors such as malignant fibrous histiocytoma and fibrous xanthomas as well as anaplastic astrocytomas and glioblastomas. Necrosis is characteristically absent, and cells stain positively for glial fibrillary acidic protein (GFAP), as do other astrocytic tumors. Electron microscopy supports the subpial astrocyte as the cell of origin.[190, 485]

PXA characteristically has a good prognosis, with most patients experiencing long-term survival and improvement in their seizure frequency after surgical resection. Some patients, however, demonstrate good outcomes initially but may have late recurrences of malignant gliomas, sometimes years after their initial surgery. In these cases the development of malignant glioma likely represents malignant transformation of the tumor. In a few instances, early postoperative recurrence with rapid progression of the tumor has been noted, and the misdiagnosis of a malignant glioma with lipidized foamy cells as a PXA may account for some of these cases. Prediction of tumor prognosis based on the histologic appearance remains difficult, and the role of therapy beyond primary surgical resection and follow-up imaging is not well defined.[486-488]

On imaging studies PXA often may have a characteristic appearance that allows the diagnosis to be suggested in patients with prolonged histories of seizures. NCCT typically demonstrates a low-density or cystic lesion (with cysts present in about one-half of cases) involving the surface of the brain. Calcification is not usually seen, and solid portions of the tumor enhance on CECT. Solid enhancing lesions and serpiginous enhancement have also been noted.[489, 490] The cyst wall, if present, does not

enhance and is not neoplastic but is composed of reactive glial cells. The cyst itself is filled with proteinaceous fluid.[491] The superficial location of these tumors is characteristic. In some cases of avidly enhancing solid tumors, the radiographic appearance, including external carotid arterial supply with dense tumor blush and apparent extra-axial location, has been noted to be similar to a meningioma or other dural mesenchymal tumor.[492] Cases of skull and dural invasion have also been noted.[491]

MRI allows better definition of large cystic areas relative to the adjacent cortex and is useful for presurgical planning. Characteristic features seen with MRI include a superficial location and involvement of the cortex and gray-white junction. Extension to the leptomeningeal surface of the brain is seen in over 70%.[493] Nodular or solid areas are usually slightly hypo- to isointense with gray matter on T1-weighted images and are hyperintense on T2-weighted images. The solid portions of the tumors always enhance. Like the mass effect of other indolent tumors, the mass effect from PXA is often mild, and edema may be mild or absent; some studies have suggested that edema correlates with a more aggressive tumor.[494] Tumor margins are well defined, and dural enhancement has been occasionally noted. The cyst contents have an MRI signal similar to that of CSF, and irregularly marginated cysts typical of necrotic tumors are not seen (Figs. 46–61 through 46–63).[493, 495-497]

The differential diagnosis of PXA is extensive, with solid tumors mimicking meningiomas or malignant fibrous histiocytomas, both rare tumors in children. The appearance and temporal lobe location can be identical to those of ganglioglioma or hemispheric pilocytic astrocytoma, whereas the histologic pleomorphism and lipid content of the tumor cells can mimic a malignant glioma including glioblastoma multiforme. Fortunately, gangliogliomas and pilocytic astrocytomas are both indolent tumors as well, whereas glioblastoma is unusual in children. Calcification in PXA has not been frequently reported but is common with both gangliogliomas and oligodendrogliomas. Correlation of the radiographic findings with the histologic appearance can be helpful in suggesting the correct diagnosis.

Choroid Plexus Tumors

Choroid Plexus Papilloma and Choroid Plexus Carcinoma

Choroid plexus tumors (CPTs) are rare tumors of the central nervous system, overall representing only 0.5% of central nervous system neoplasms in all ages, but about 3% to 5% of brain tumors in children.[498] These are tumors primarily of young children and infants, with the median age at presentation as low as 10 months and an age range of 6 days to 16 years of age. Sixty-five percent of patients are 1 month to 2 years old, and 86% of patients present in the first 5 years of life.[499] A slight male predominance (3 to 2, male to female) has been noted.[500] About 10% to 20% of CPTs are malignant (choroid plexus carcinomas [CPCs]),[501] and virtually all of these carcinomas are found in children.

When all ages are considered, the location of choroid plexus papilloma (CPP) follows that of the normal choroid

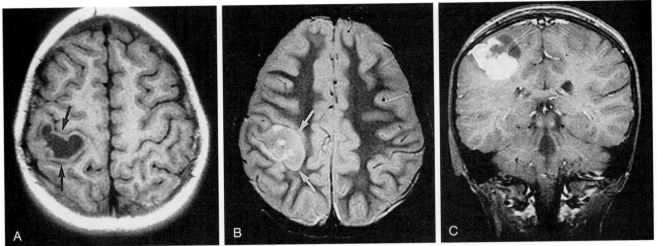

FIGURE 46–61 A 5-year-old boy with pleomorphic xanthoastrocytoma. The patient presented with focal motor seizures. *A,* T1-weighted image demonstrates a well-defined, peripheral, hemispherical, cystic mass *(arrows)*. *B,* PD-weighted image obtained slightly inferior to image *A* demonstrates the solid component of the tumor *(arrows)*, which is isointense to gray matter. *C,* Gadolinium-enhanced coronal image demonstrates intense enhancement of the solid component of the tumor. The appearance is identical to that of other low-grade astrocytomas, including JPA.

plexus, with 43% of tumors in the lateral ventricles, 39% in the fourth ventricle, 10% in the third ventricle, and 9% in the cerebellopontine angle.[498] Multiple tumors occur in 3.7% of patients, and it is important to note that both benign tumors (CPPs) and malignant tumors (CPCs) may disseminate through the CSF.[502, 503] A slight preference for the left lateral ventricle has been noted.[498] Fourth ventricular tumors are more common in adults. The distribution of CPTs in children favors the supratentorial location, with 80.2% in the lateral ventricles, 15.7% in the fourth ventricle, and 4.1% in the third ventricle. A slight tendency for the right lateral ventricle has been reported in children. CPTs of the cerebellopontine angle are extremely uncommon in children.[504] When present, these tumors are connected via the foramen of Luschka

with tumor in the fourth ventricle, whereas adult cerebellopontine angle tumors can be isolated masses.[500]

Children with CPC have a similar age distribution to those with CPP, from the neonatal period to 12 years, with most patients presenting between 2 and 4 years of age, and a mean age at presentation of 28 to 32 months.[505] A slight male predominance is also noted for CPCs, and the location of these malignant tumors is similar to that of CPPs, with 80% to 83% in the lateral ventricles, 10% to 20% in the fourth ventricle, and 4.3% in the third ventricle.[505]

Most patients with CPP present with signs and symptoms of increased intracranial pressure, which correlates with the common finding of hydrocephalus on imaging studies. Children with CPC seem to have a lower inci-

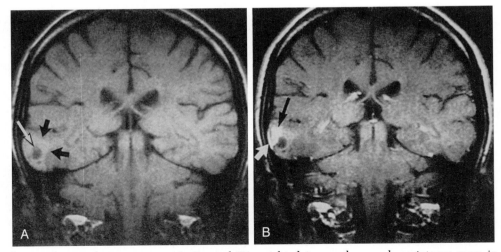

FIGURE 46–62 Pleomorphic xanthoastrocytoma. *A,* Coronal T1-weighted image shows a hyperintense mass in the right lateral temporal lobe *(short arrows)* with a low-signal-intensity cystic component *(long arrow)*. *B,* After gadolinium administration, there is intense contrast enhancement *(black arrow)* and adjacent leptomeningeal enhancement *(white arrow)*. (A and B, From Tien RD, Cardenas CA, Rajagopalan S. Premorphic xanthoastrocytoma of the brain: MR findings in six patients. AJR 1992;159:1287–1290.)

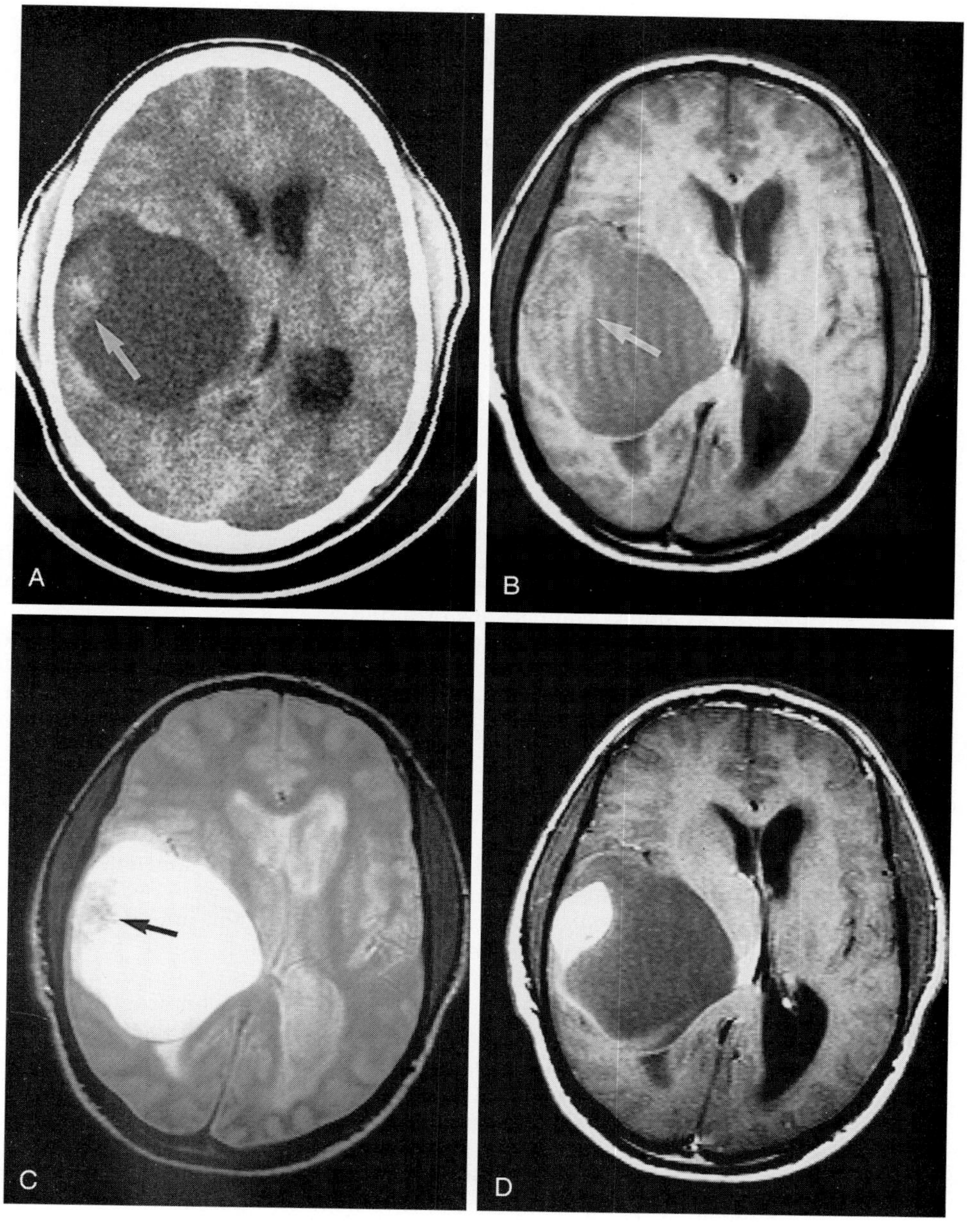

FIGURE 46–63 Pleomorphic xanthoastrocytoma. *A*, NCCT demonstrates a large cystic lesion in the right hemisphere with a considerable mass effect. An isodense peripherally located nodule (*arrow*) is present. T1-weighted (*B*) and T2-weighted (*C*) images demonstrate that the nodule (*arrows*) is nearly isointense to gray matter, whereas the cystic component is slightly more intense than CSF on the T1-weighted image. *D*, The nodule enhances intensely with gadolinium.

dence of clinically evident increased intracranial pressure, and their invasive tumors instead produce focal neurologic signs and symptoms.

A strong association of hydrocephalus with CPT, more commonly with CPP than CPC, is known. The origin of the hydrocephalus has been the subject of debate for many years. Proposed causes include overproduction of CSF by the papilloma itself, which is supported by clinical and ultrastructural studies; direct physical obstruction of the ventricles themselves, especially with third-ventricular tumors that may have mobile attachments to the normal choroid; and obstruction at the level of the arachnoid granulations from tumor-produced hemorrhage, secretion of proteinaceous material, or desquamation of tumor cells and debris, which may explain the persistent hydrocephalus seen after total surgical resection of some tumors.[506–509] CPP of the third ventricle can present with acute me-

chanical obstructive hydrocephalus and sudden death from obstruction at the foramen of Monro similar to that produced by a colloid cyst of the anterior third ventricle.[510]

CPPs appear as well-circumscribed, lobular, cauliflower-like intraventricular masses that may extend into the brain parenchyma along a broad, compressive indenting front, rather than by true invasion.[190] CPCs are distinguished at inspection by their invasiveness and the presence of necrosis and a mass effect on the involved brain. Microscopically, CPTs span a spectrum from well-differentiated papillomas to highly anaplastic malignant tumors with little obvious epithelial differentiation. Focal glial and ependymal differentiation is sometimes noted. Cytologic atypia may be present and does not equate with malignancy;[190] high cellularity, architectural disarray, poorly formed papillae, and nuclear evidence of malignancy with a high mitotic index are required for the histologic diagnosis of malignancy. The rare papillary ependymoma may have a histologic appearance similar to that of a CPT but can be distinguished by its widely positive staining for glial fibrillary acidic protein and negative staining for cytokeratin, whereas CPTs stain positive for cytokeratin, reflecting their epithelial nature. Foci of glial differentiation that stain positive for GFAP may be present and do not correlate with the prognosis.[190]

Rare cases of malignant transformation of benign-appearing CPPs to CPTs after incomplete resection have been noted,[190] as has metastatic spread of CPC to the lungs and bone, and through ventriculoperitoneal shunts with subsequent malignant ascites.[505] The overall prognosis with CPP is very favorable, with survival of 88% reported; currently it is probably even better with modern surgical and anesthetic techniques.[500, 511] Therapy is primarily surgical for both CPP and CPC, with a goal of total resection. Chemotherapy has been utilized for incomplete resection of tumors, especially invasive CPC, but with the small number of patients with CPC diagnosed each year (about 20 in the United States) comparisons of different therapeutic approaches are difficult. Radiation therapy is often avoided in patients with CPTs because of their young age and risk for intellectual and endocrinologic sequelae.[511–513] Survival with CPC is only around 45% to 50%.

The imaging of CPP reflects its origin from normal choroid plexus. NCCT typically demonstrates a well-defined, slightly lobulated mass associated with the normal choroid. When tumor is in the lateral ventricle, the atrium is the most common location. The tumors are often large at presentation, typically 3 to 6 cm in diameter. The masses are often slightly hyperdense or of mixed density on NCCT, relative to adjacent brain. The hyperdense areas, seen in two-thirds of patients, may be due to the vascularity of these tumors, the presence of microscopic calcification, or edema, which is sometimes noted to be present in the brain adjacent to CPPs (21% of patients) and CPCs (43% of patients). One-third of tumors appear isodense on NCCT. Small flecks of calcification are seen in 20% to 50% of patients, and calcification and intratumoral hemorrhage appear to be more common in adult cases of CPP. Adult tumors are more likely to

demonstrate cystic degeneration and a heterogeneous CT appearance. Hydrocephalus is a frequent finding, and asymmetric enlargement of the ventricles is sometime noted, with the side containing the tumor more prominent than the contralateral ventricle. This asymmetry has been attributed to local obstructive interference with CSF flow by the tumor. Cystic-appearing areas are frequent on CT and present in up to 50% of tumors. With CECT, avid homogeneous enhancement is virtually always seen.[499, 514–517]

CPPs arise from the choroid plexus and tend to engulf rather than displace the glomus of the choroid plexus. This is a useful feature for distinguishing large CPPs from other more aggressive neoplasms. The tumors can have a stalklike attachment to the normal choroid and tend to be found adjacent to the inferior portion of the trigone of the lateral ventricle, roof of the third ventricle, or posterior medullary vellum in the fourth ventricle.[501] When angiography is performed, intense tumor blush is present with arterial supply to the tumor from the anterior, medial posterior, or lateral posterior choroid arteries.[514]

MRI of CPPs demonstrates their intraventricular appearance well. The tumors are typically isointense on T1-weighted images and only mildly hyperintense on T2-weighted images, relative to gray matter. In some instances the tumors are nearly isointense compared with the adjacent brain, and this feature is useful for suggesting the diagnosis of CPP. PD-weighted images usually demonstrate intermediate signal intensity. A heterogeneous appearance is common and has been attributed to the presence of small cystic areas in the tumor, with signal intensity similar to that of CSF, and calcifications and arterial flow voids presenting as small focal areas of absent signal. Enhancement with gadolinium is intense but heterogeneous.[216, 501] When present, extension through the foramen of Monro by third or lateral ventricular CPP is a helpful diagnostic finding.[518] Increased periventricular PD and T2 signal intensity, best seen on the PD-weighted images, may be seen when hydrocephalus is present (Figs. 46–64 through 46–66).

MRI findings of CPC are variable and nonspecific. Findings that suggest the diagnosis of an invasive malignancy include marked edema, especially when focal; mid-

FIGURE 46–64 A 3-month-old child with choroid plexus papilloma in the trigone of the lateral ventricle. *A,* NCCT demonstrates a well-defined lobulated mass in the right trigone, with small cystlike areas *(straight arrows).* Hydrocephalus is present, as is edema where the tumor contacts the ependymal surface of the ventricle *(curved arrows). B,* CECT shows intense enhancement of the mass.

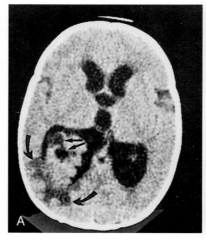
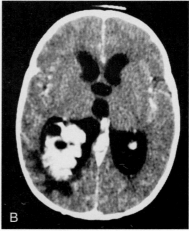

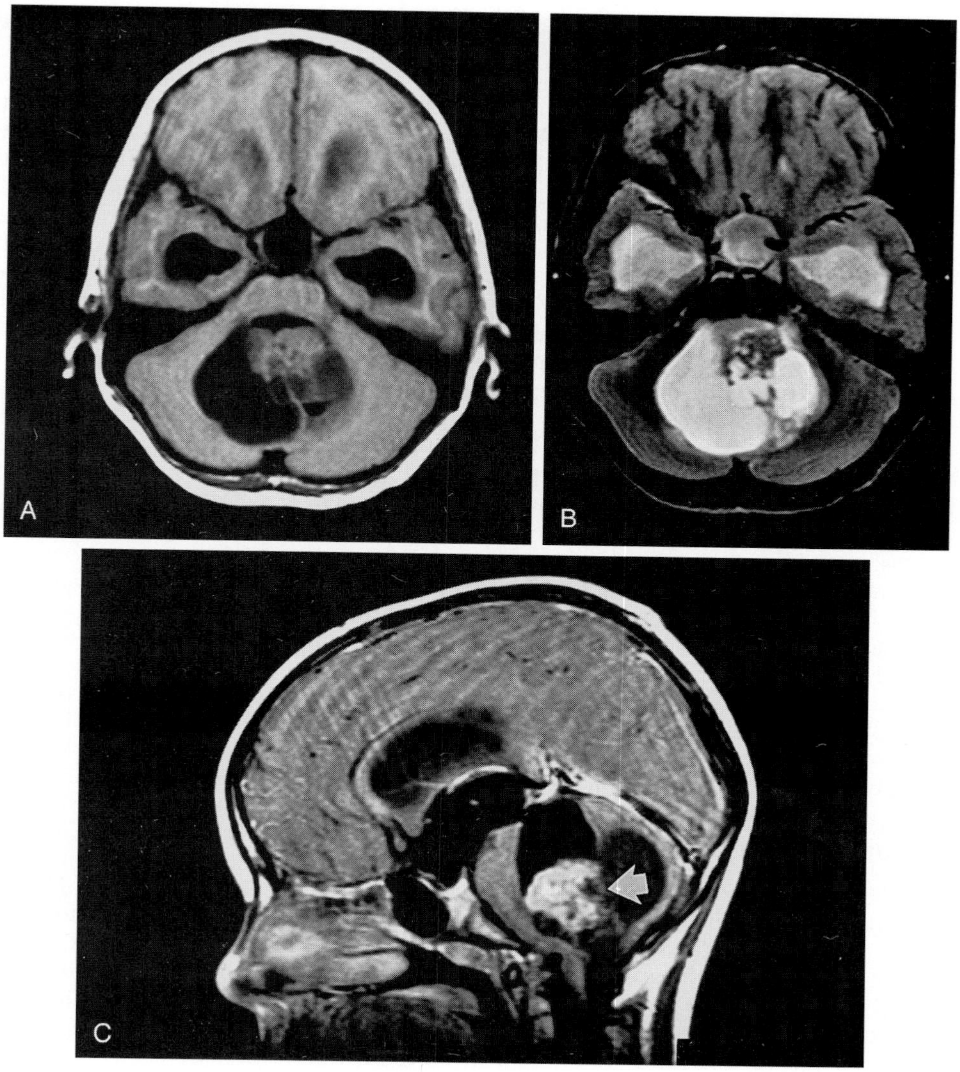

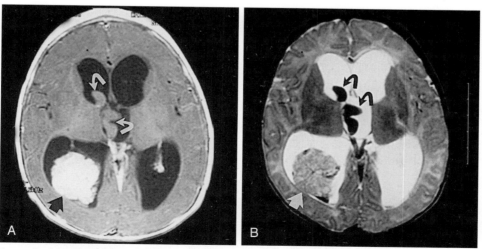

FIGURE 46–65 A 7-year-old with choroid plexus papilloma of the fourth ventricle. *A,* T1-weighted image demonstrates hydrocephalus and an intraventricular mass in an expanded fourth ventricle. *B,* T2-weighted image shows the mass to be well defined but with heterogeneous signal with apparent cystic areas. *C,* Gadolinium-enhanced image shows intense enhancement of the mass *(arrow).*

FIGURE 46–66 A 5-month-old boy with choroid plexus papilloma. *A,* T1-weighted image with gadolinium enhancement demonstrates an intensely enhancing intraventricular mass in the right ventricular atrium *(black arrow).* Note the serpentine mass in the right frontal horn and third ventricle *(curved arrows).* *B,* T2-weighted image demonstrates the mass as a hypointense lesion with small signal voids that may represent calcifications or vessels *(straight arrow).* The serpentine intraventricular lesion is markedly hypointense *(curved arrows)* and likely represents an intraventricular clot from tumor hemorrhage, containing deoxyhemoglobin. Also note the markedly hydrocephalic ventricles.

line shift; gross invasion of adjacent brain; and focal areas of decreased T1 and increased T2 signal with irregular borders representing necrosis. Tumor margins are indistinct or irregular. CT density is often more heterogeneous in CPP, and calcifications can be present. Blood degradation products from hemorrhage may be seen. Leptomeningeal disease as an isolated finding with an otherwise benign-appearing CPT is not helpful since both benign and malignant CPTs can disseminate through the CSF (Fig. 46–67).[501, 511, 519]

The differential diagnosis of a CPP includes other intraventricular masses in children such as central neurocytomas, colloid cysts, and unusual gliomas with exophytic growth into the ventricles or arising from the septum pellucidum. Metastatic disease may involve the choroid plexus but is usually seen in adults. Colloid cysts are very rare in children and show minimal peripheral enhancement and a smooth rim. Central neurocytomas are seen closer to adulthood and may be densely calcified. Choroid plexus xanthogranulomas are benign lesions that present with hydrocephalus but are almost exclusively seen in adults.[520] In a child, the aggressive appearance of a CPC cannot be distinguished from a supratentorial PNET or ependymoma, cerebral neuroblastoma, ependymoblastoma, or aggressive astrocytoma. Large subependymal giant cell astrocytomas may appear similar, but clinical and radiographic evidence of tuberous sclerosis is useful in identifying these tumors.

Subependymal Giant Cell Astrocytoma

Subependymal giant cell astrocytomas (SGCAs) are well-demarcated predominantly intraventricular tumors found in the region of the foramen of Monro. The tumors are strongly associated with tuberous sclerosis complex (TS), and SGCA is seen in 2% to 26% (average about 17%) of patients with TS. The peak age at presentation is 8 to 18 years, but the tumors have been found in newborns, in whom they are presumably congenital, and in patients as old as 40 years.[521–523] The tumors are characterized by slow indolent growth and if symptomatic can produce hydrocephalus by obstruction at the foramen of Monro. Increasingly, as TS patients are routinely imaged, the tumors may be identified by sequential radiographic studies. Presentation of SGCA with suddenly increased intracranial pressure and death from obstructive hydrocephalus has occurred.[524] The tumors are characteristically noninvasive, and focal neurologic signs are not commonly seen at presentation. Although most SGCAs are found in patients with a known diagnosis of TS, patients may initially present with symptoms of increased intracranial pressure or chronic headaches, be diagnosed with SGCA, and then be noted to have the clinical and radiographic findings of TS.[525] Up to one-third of patients with SGCA who are found to have TS have the diagnosis of TS determined for the first time after the initial CT.[526]

TS is characterized by the presence of giant cells that have features of both astrocytic and neuronal differentiation, and the giant cell appears to be a product of a dysgenetic event early in development. The radiographic features of TS, described elsewhere in this book, also reflect a disorder of migration of neuroblasts from the germinal matrix of the ventricular zone to the cortical plate. Although it has been hypothesized that SGCAs arise from cells of the germinal matrix that have failed to migrate, the tumors more likely arise from the subependymal nodules (SENs) commonly found in TS. Thus the SENs and the SGCAs that develop from them represent an arrest of migration of dysgenetic cells, the giant cells, in patients with TS.[521, 527] Sequential studies of patients with TS have shown the development of SGCAs from SENs located at the foramen of Monro, whereas the nodules located elsewhere along the ependymal surface of the ventricles remained stable.[527]

Grossly, the tumors are smooth, firm masses that frequently contain calcification found along the ventricular

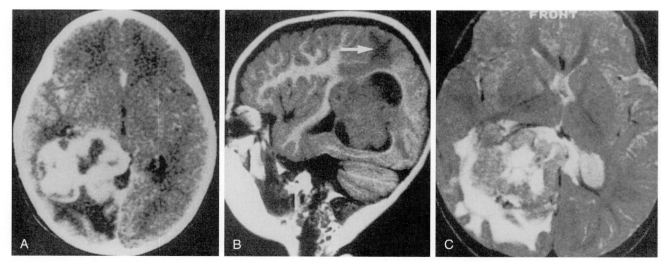

FIGURE 46–67 Choroid plexus carcinoma in a 15-month-old child. *A*, CECT scan shows a large mass with intense enhancement, central necrosis, and surrounding low-density edema. *B*, Sagittal T1-weighted MRI study shows the mass in the atrium of the lateral ventricle. Low-signal-intensity edema *(arrow)* extends above the tumor. *C*, The mass appears heterogeneous on an axial T2-weighted image, with central areas of necrosis and adjacent vasogenic edema of high signal intensity. (*A–C*, From Coates TL, Hinshaw DB Jr, Peckman N, et al. Pediatric choroid plexus neoplasms: MR, CT, and pathologic correlation. Radiology 1989;173:81–88.)

surface at the foramen of Monro. They can be densely adherent to adjacent brain and very vascular, but evidence of gross or microscopic invasion into adjacent brain is not seen. A thin covering of ependyma along the ventricular aspect of the tumor is seen.[190, 528] The histologic appearance of SGCA is characterized by microscopic variation and giant cells with morphologic and immunohistochemical qualities of both neuronal and glial development; confusion with other more aggressive neoplasms is possible but made less likely when the clinical history of TS and typical radiographic findings of TS and SGCA are made. Features of high-grade tumors such as focal necrosis and a high mitotic index have been noted in some cases but do not correlate with aggressive behavior clinically.[529] True malignant transformation into an aggressive glioma is rare.[530]

It is clear that SGCAs develop from SENs, and patients have been followed for several years with the development of tumors and hydrocephalus. These indolent tumors are not radiosensitive, and therapy is essentially surgical. Some authors recommend surgery only when the tumors are symptomatic, whereas others recommend earlier surgery when the growth of the lesion is first detected in order to avoid sudden death from a rapid onset of increased intracranial pressure and to make surgical management of these deeply located lesions easier.[527, 531–534]

The SENs of both TS and SGCA have characteristic imaging findings that have been well described. SENs are found most commonly along the thalamostriate groove but can be anywhere along the lateral margins of the lateral ventricles. Their deep portions may appear embedded in the caudate nucleus or thalamus and they project into the ventricles. The number of SENs does not appear to correlate with the overall clinical severity of symptoms in patients with TS, unlike the various cortical abnormalities seen in this condition.[535, 536]

NCCT typically demonstrates the SENs as isointense masses; the nodules are found in almost all (96%) patients with TS. Calcification is extremely common and characteristic and seen in 88% of nodules.[537] Patients may have up to one dozen or more nodules. Typically, they measure 1 to 12 mm in diameter and do not produce hydrocephalus.[521] With CECT, nonneoplastic SENs are not reported to enhance.[538] MRI of the SENs demonstrates isointensity compared with white matter and slight hyperintensity or isointensity compared with gray matter on T1-weighted images, and hyperintensity on PD- and T2-weighted images. Central calcification, if prominent, may produce a focal hypointensity in the center of the nodule on T2-weighted images. The nodules are best seen with T1-weighted images or inversion recovery images designed to suppress CSF (fluid attenuated inversion recovery [FLAIR]) and may be difficult to detect against the adjacent CSF signal on T2-weighted images. With gadolinium, up to 80% of SENs show some enhancement, and the presence of enhancement alone does not equate with the diagnosis of a SGCA.[539–541] The increased rate of enhancement with MRI compared with CECT is probably due to the increased sensitivity to blood-brain barrier alterations by MRI, the higher tissue contrast seen with MRI, or the histologic similarity of SENs to SGCAs, as

the nodules can be indistinguishable from the giant cell astrocytomas.[542]

Giant cell astrocytomas typically are larger than the SENs seen in TS, measuring 21 to 47 mm in diameter. They are almost always found at the foramen of Monro and often have associated hydrocephalus.[521] CT demonstrates masses that are isodense or mildly hyperdense and on CECT enhance intensely and homogeneously.[543, 544] MRI demonstrates SGCA as heterogeneous and, compared with brain, somewhat hypointense or isointense lesions on T1-weighted images and hyperintense on the PD- and T2-weighted images. Small areas of decreased T2 signal corresponding to calcifications or arterial flow voids may be observed.[521] SGCA may appear somewhat more nodular than SEN but otherwise have a very similar appearance to SEN. The similarity is made even greater by the observation that almost all SENs at the foramen of Monro enhance, and this is the most common location of SGCAs as well (Figs. 46–68 and 46–69).

The diagnosis of an SGCA versus a stable SEN of TS is made on MRI by the presence of a moderate or large mass at the foramen of Monro, with serial growth on imaging studies; a degree of enhancement that is more pronounced than that of the SEN; a more heterogeneous signal; and the presence of serpentine flow voids.[521, 541] SGCAs grow slowly when followed on sequential studies, are noninvasive, and typically do not have perilesional edema. Overall, the appearance of SENs and SGCAs can overlap to a significant degree.

Unusual imaging characteristics of SGCA include intratumoral and intraventricular hemorrhage, and an unusual appearance of these tumors in the rare neonatal cases. Newborn infants with SGCA demonstrate a hyperdense mass on NCCT, hyperintensity on T1-weighted MRI images, and hypointensity on T2-weighted MRI images, relative to brain parenchyma. This reversal of the typical density and signal characteristics of SGCA seen in adults likely reflects the immature myelination and relatively increased water content of the brain in infants.[545]

Intraventricular Neurocytoma

Intraventricular neurocytoma is a relatively recently described brain tumor of older children and young adults.[546] Patients present with a predominantly intraventricular mass involving the lateral ventricles and third ventricle, producing hydrocephalus and increased intracranial pressure. Visual symptoms have also been reported. Symptoms are usually present for 2 to 6 months, but presentation with sudden onset of coma has also been reported.[547] Occasionally patients may present with seizures, and the lesion has been found incidentally in patients imaged for head injury. Patients have a reported age range of 17 to 53 years, with a mean of 31 years.[548]

Grossly, the masses are well-circumscribed masses found near the septum pellucidum; frequently the mass is attached to the septum as well as the walls of the lateral ventricles. Microscopic examination reveals a cellular tumor that closely resembles oligodendroglioma, ependymoma, or neuroblastoma.[190] Ependymoma can usually be identified by its involvement with brain tissue adjacent to the ventricles and the presence of some GFAP staining in specimens. Difficulties arise in distinguishing the neurocytoma from an oligodendroglioma. The histologic appearance of these two tumors as well as radiographic features may be identical, and tumors diagnosed as intraventricular oligodendrogliomas have been found to be neurocytomas on review. The most important pathologic feature of intraventricular neurocytoma is immunostaining for synaptophysin, a glycoprotein of presynaptic vesicles seen in neuroendocrine-derived tumors, which is found in neurocytomas but not in oligodendrogliomas.[190] Staining for neuron-specific enolase (NSE) is usually positive in neurocytomas as well. Electron microscopy is also essential, revealing ultrastructural details similar to those seen in mature neurons. Both immunohistochemical and electron microscopic studies should be obtained when the radiographic findings suggest neurocytoma.[549]

The radiographic appearance of central neurocytoma is characterized by a large mass predominantly involving the lateral ventricles or third ventricle with associated hydrocephalus. The masses demonstrate calcifications in more than 50% of cases; they can be fine or very coarse and conglomerate. Uncalcified portions of the tumor are isodense with brain parenchyma and demonstrate moderate enhancement with CECT. MRI of this tumor is significant for a very heterogeneous appearance produced by the prominent calcifications, which appear as hypointensities, especially on T2-weighted images. Noncalcified areas are typically isointense or slightly hyperintense compared with gray matter on T1-weighted images and slightly hyperintense or isointense to gray matter on T2-weighted images. Moderate contrast enhancement is seen with gadolinium, and heterogeneity from the calcifications as well as flow voids may be present. Intratumoral intraventricular hemorrhage has been observed, but edema of the adjacent brain is not commonly seen.[550, 551] Areas compatible with cysts, with fluid density on CT and near isointensity to CSF on T1- and T2-weighted MRI images, are very common, seen in 60% of cases (Figs. 46–70 and 46–71).

Extension of the neurocytoma through the foramen of Monro into the third ventricle and through the aqueduct into the fourth ventricle and extraventricular extension

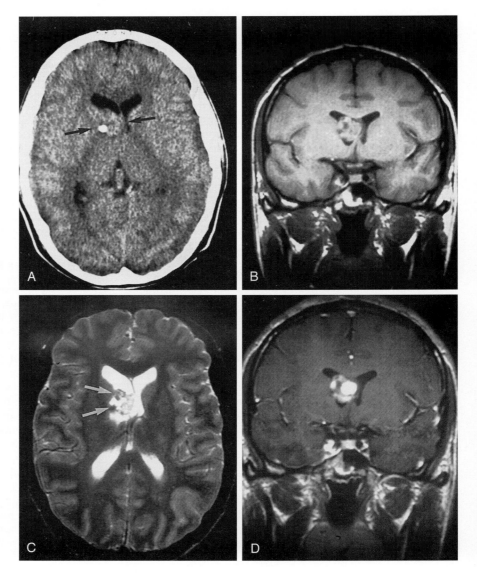

FIGURE 46–68 A 13-year-old boy with subependymal giant cell astrocytoma. *A,* NCCT demonstrates a calcified mass at the foramen of Monro *(arrows)*. The mass appears heterogeneous on the coronal T1-weighted image *(B)*, with focal hypointensities probably representing calcifications or intratumoral cysts, seen as hyperintensities *(arrows)* on the T2-weighted image *(C)*. *D,* Avid enhancement is present with gadolinium. Interestingly, the images did not demonstrate any other findings to suggest tuberous sclerosis.

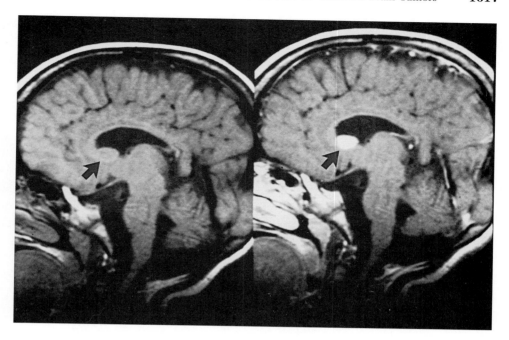

FIGURE 46–69 Giant cell astrocytoma. Sagittal T1-weighted images before *(left)* and after *(right)* gadolinium administration show a mass *(arrows)* near the foramen of Monro.

into adjacent brain have been noted and correlated with the anaplastic histologic appearance.[552]

Attachment of the tumor to the septum pellucidum has been a frequent finding, and it has been proposed that the septum is the site of origin of intraventricular neurocytoma.[547] Other authors have noted frequent broad attachment to the superolateral wall of the body of the lateral ventricle, suggesting that the tumor originates from the subependymal layer covering the medial aspect of the caudate nucleus, possibly from a neuroectodermal precursor cell found in this location.[552, 553]

Intraventricular neurocytoma behaves in a benign manner and carries a good prognosis without evidence of early recurrence. Complete surgical removal is the goal of therapy, and even patients with subtotal resections do well. Correct identification of the tumor's histologic type is essential to avoid misdiagnosis of the lesion as a more aggressive tumor.[554] Radiation therapy is usually not used except for the few cases demonstrating invasive or malignant behavior.

The differential diagnosis of central neurocytoma compared with other intraventricular masses includes intraventricular oligodendroglioma and unusual cases of astrocytoma, meningioma, ependymoma, subependymoma, colloid cyst, germ cell tumor, craniopharyngioma, and CPP. Oligodendrogliomas may have an identical appearance[555] without electron microscopic and immunohistochemical studies. Before such studies were available, neurocytomas were often likely to have been classified as intraventricular oligodendrogliomas. Meningiomas and colloid cysts are both rare in children. The colloid cyst has few calcifications and a different enhancement pattern, and meningiomas are usually found in the trigone. Astrocytomas are common in children but are less likely to calcify, usually originate in the brain substance itself, and are more likely to have associated edema. Pilocytic tumors may present as cystic lesions with enhancing mural nodules. Subependymal giant cell astrocytomas are

centered at the striatothalamic groove and associated with other MRI findings in TS. CPPs, as described previously, enhance intensely and do not have large calcifications as a prominent feature. Extension through the foramen of Monro to involve the third and portions of the lateral ventricles may be seen with CPP. They tend to be hyperdense but not heavily calcified on NCCT and are somewhat hypointense on T2-weighted images. They are usually found in younger patients than neurocytomas are. CPCs are invasive, aggressive-appearing tumors. Ependymomas are usually found at a younger age than intraventricular neurocytomas, arise within the brain parenchyma, and can be invasive. Craniopharyngiomas occasionally involve the third ventricle in an isolated manner. Third ventricular craniopharyngiomas, as described previously, are predominantly solid tumors. The various signal intensities of the cysts in craniopharyngiomas arising from the sellar region into the third ventricle are also useful diagnostic findings. Rare germ cell tumors may be isolated to the third ventricle.

Colloid Cyst

Colloid cysts are rare cysts located in the anterior third ventricles that usually produce symptoms in adults related to increased intracranial pressure from obstruction at the foramen of Monro. The reported age range at presentation is from 2 months to 79 years of age, but the lesions are extremely rare in children.[556] Children can present with headaches, seizures, nausea, and signs of increased intracranial pressure. Most patients have symptoms for days to months, but acute obstructive hydrocephalus and sudden death have been reported.[557] Patients have also died from an unsuspected, asymptomatic cyst after lumbar puncture.[558] The origin of these nonneoplastic cysts has been the subject of debate, but immunohistochemical and ultrastructural analysis supports an origin from endo-

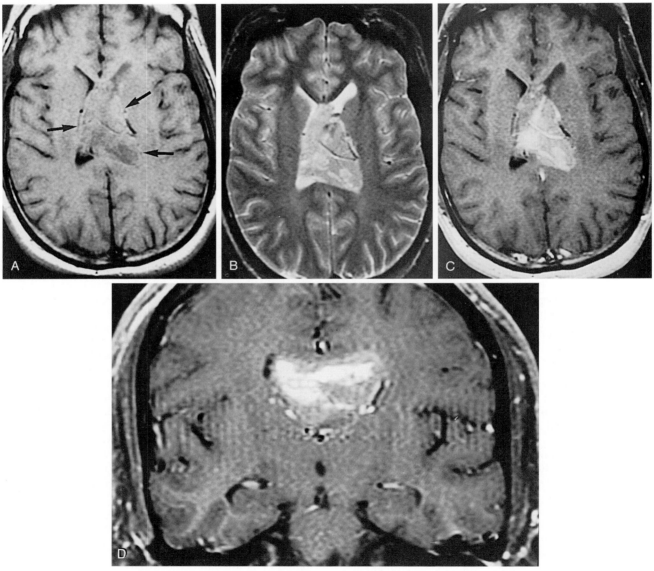

FIGURE 46–70 A 25-year-old patient with central neurocytoma. *A,* T1-weighted image demonstrates an intraventricular mass *(arrows),* isointense to gray matter. *B,* T2-weighted image demonstrates mild hyperintensity, heterogeneous signal, and no significant edema in the adjacent cerebrum. *C* and *D,* Gadolinium-enhanced images demonstrate intense but heterogeneous enhancement of the mass. Note that the septum pellucidum cannot be identified separately from the mass, and the tumor appears adherent to portions of the ependymal surface of the lateral ventricular wall.

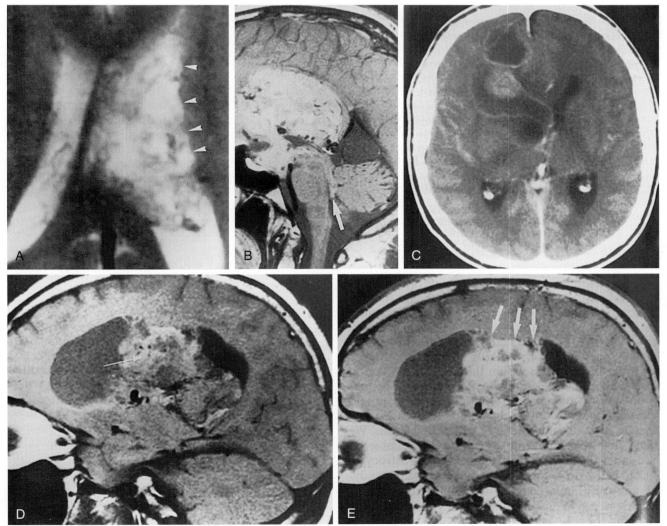

FIGURE 46–71 Central neurocytoma, four different patients. *A,* Axial T2-weighted MRI study shows a heterogeneous mass within the body of the left lateral ventricle. There is ipsilateral hydrocephalus. Calcifications are hypointense. There is a broad attachment to the lateral ventricular wall *(arrowheads)*. *B,* Sagittal T1-weighted image after gadolinium administration demonstrates inhomogeneous enhancement of a large mass within the lateral ventricle with extension through the third ventricle into the fourth ventricle *(arrow)*. *C,* Axial CECT shows a mass within the right frontal horn extending into the right frontal lobe, with large eccentric cysts. This was an anaplastic central neurocytoma. Parasagittal T1-weighted images before *(D)* and after *(E)* gadolinium administration show a large, heterogeneous mass in the body of the lateral ventricle with low-signal-intensity calcification and higher-signal-intensity solid portions *(arrow in D)*. There is inhomogeneous enhancement and broad attachment to the superolateral wall of the ventricle *(arrows in E)*. *(A–E,* From Wichmann W, Schubiger O, von Deimling A, et al. Neuroradiology of central neurocytoma. Neuroradiology 1991;33:143–148).

dermal epithelium, most likely the respiratory endothelium, rather than neuroepithelium.[559, 560]

The imaging characteristics of colloid cysts have been well described in adults and are discussed elsewhere in this book. The pediatric patients do not appear to differ in imaging characteristics from adults, typically demonstrating well-defined, smooth masses at the foramen of Monro, with iso- or hypodensity compared with brain parenchyma on NCCT, and distinctly variable appearance with MRI, the most common combination of signal intensities being hyperintense compared with gray matter on T1-weighted images and hypointense on T2-weighted images.[561, 562] The childhood cases have been reported to have cyst diameters of 1 to 2 cm, similar to adult cases.[558] Calcification and hemorrhage are not common, and enhancement, if present, is mild and confined to the wall of the cysts. The minimal mass effect, absence of invasion into adjacent structures, absence of calcification and significant enhancement, and distinct location at the foramen of Monro allow colloid cysts to be distinguished from neoplasms involving this location in children, such as neurocytomas, oligodendrogliomas, and subependymal giant cell astrocytomas.

Desmoplastic Supratentorial Neuroepithelial Tumors

Desmoplastic Infantile Ganglioglioma and Desmoplastic Cerebral Astrocytoma

These two tumors, whose radiographic appearance and clinical characteristics are similar, present as typically large, supratentorial, peripheral lesions of young children with a conspicuous cystic component. Desmoplastic infantile gangliogliomas (DIGs) are mixed glioneuronal neoplasms containing both ganglion cells and astrocytic cells resembling those of fibrillary astrocytomas. Desmoplastic cerebral astrocytomas (DCAs) are histologically identical to DIGs except for the absence of ganglion cells.[190] Both tumors are characterized histologically by collagenous tissue that, despite its mesenchymal appearance, is of neuroepithelial origin and is immunoreactive for GFAP. Ganglion cells may be scattered among the glial cells or

desmoplastic tissue and can be identified with NSE and synaptophysin stains.[190]

Clinical characteristics of the tumors are nearly identical, with both tumors presenting between the ages of 1.5 to 18 months with increased intracranial pressure, macrocephaly, seizures, or headaches. Focal neurologic signs are not commonly present. The lesions are most commonly located in the frontal and parietal lobes, involve the dura, and are grossly cystic. A slight male predominance is present in the reported cases of DIG.[563, 564] It is possible that the two tumors represent different degrees of differentiation of a single lesion, as variability in the amount and type of cell differentiation is observed.[564]

The radiographic appearance of these tumors is fairly distinct. The masses are often huge, 10 cm or more in diameter, with an obvious cystic component on NCCT. The cystic area can be part of the tumor itself, or can represent a reaction to the tumor and be composed of gliotic brain parenchyma. The solid component is iso- or hyperdense compared with brain parenchyma and is not calcified. CECT demonstrates intense enhancement of the solid component of the tumor, with the enhancing solid component characteristically extending to the meninges. The enhancing area corresponds with neural and glial elements as well as the desmoplastic element. MRI demonstrates that the cystic components, which may be multilocular, are isointense to CSF, whereas the solid component resembles gray matter on T1- and T2-weighted images but enhances strongly with gadolinium.[563, 565–567] Despite the large size, the mass effect and peritumoral edema are mild (Fig. 46–72).

Although usually reported in infants and young children, DIG has been reported in adolescence and in a 25-year-old adult. The MRI appearance of both cases was similar to that of younger patients.[568]

An extremely rare tumor, the gliofibroma, has been described in adults and children in both the supratentorial brain and the posterior fossa and spinal cord. The rarity of this lesion makes determination of its imaging characteristics difficult, and it has been suggested that gliofibromas and DCAs may in fact represent the same basic

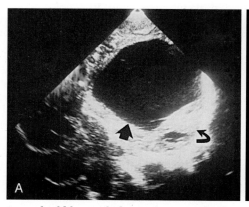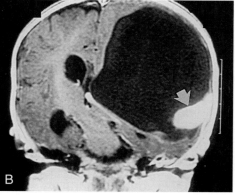

FIGURE 46–72 A 4-month-old boy with desmoplastic cerebral astrocytoma. *A,* Ultrasonographic image obtained in the coronal plane through the anterior fontanelle demonstrates a huge cystic mass that distorts the intracranial anatomy *(straight arrow).* An echoic mural nodule is present *(curved arrow). B,* T1-weighted image with gadolinium enhancement demonstrates the huge cystic mass with an intensely enhancing peripheral mural nodule, abutting the surface of the cerebral hemisphere *(arrow).*

tumor, whereas the DIG differs from these two tumors by demonstrating neuronal differentiation.[569]

Recognition of DCA and DIG is important, as prognosis is very favorable, with most patients having long-term survival after surgery alone. The diagnosis should be suggested when the typical imaging findings are present in a very young child or infant, and appropriate ultrastructural and immunohistochemical studies should be obtained.[570, 571] The differential diagnosis in a young child with this lesion includes PNET, ependymoma, astrocytoma, and pleomorphic astrocytoma. Supratentorial PNET and ependymomas are usually more deeply located tumors with frequent calcifications and heterogeneous appearance and enhancement on MRI, and astrocytomas of the hemispheres are not common in infants. PXAs may have an appearance similar to that of DIG, including leptomeningeal involvement, but are typically seen in the temporal lobe in older patients.

Dysembryoplastic Neuroepithelial Tumor

The dysembryoplastic neuroepithelial tumor (DNT) is a relatively recently described supratentorial lesion presenting in children and young adults with complex partial seizures. Patients present with their onset of seizures from 1 week to 30 years of age with a mean age of 9.5 years and frequently have a prolonged history of epilepsy before surgery (age 7 months to 37 years, with a mean age at surgery of 17 years).[572] Almost all patients have symptoms confined to seizures, with focal neurologic symptoms and evidence of increased intracranial pressure distinctly infrequent. The lesions are most commonly located in the frontal and temporal lobes. Although rare, representing only 0.4% to 1.3% of all primary brain tumors, the lesion is more common in epilepsy surgery series, where it may constitute up to 13% of resected tumors.[573]

The lesions are characterized pathologically by an intracortical location, a heterogeneous cellular composition including astrocytes, oligodendrocytes, and neurons, and a multinodular architecture. There is frequent association with nonneoplastic cortical dysplasia consisting of disturbed lamination, architectural disarray, and abnormal neurons. The presence of a "specific glioneuronal element" consisting of bundles of axons, oligodendrocytes, and neurons that seem to float in interstitial fluid is also helpful in making the diagnosis. Small biopsy samples of DNT can be identical to oligodendroglioma or a ganglion cell tumor, and the architectural pattern seen in larger samples, and sometimes in MRI, is important in making the correct diagnosis.[190, 574-576]

DNT is a very indolent tumor, with therapy usually limited to surgical resection. Even partially resected tumors do not appear to recur in most instances. It has been suggested that these tumors, with multiple lines of differentiation, arise from the subpial granular layer, a secondary germinal center. However, the association with cortical dysplasia and the benign course of these tumors has led to the suggestion that they are hamartomatous in nature.[577]

The neuroimaging characteristics of DNT are nonspecific. The tumors are found in the temporal or frontal lobes in most instances. NCCT demonstrates a well-demarcated moderately or markedly low-density lesion, with no associated edema or mass effect. Tumoral hemorrhage is not common. Calvarial thinning adjacent to the lesion from long-standing tumors has been noted in up to 60%. Calcifications are occasionally seen (about 23%). Enhancement with CECT is also uncommon, seen in about 18% of cases, and is usually focal, punctate, or marginal. It has been suggested that peripheral enhancement may be due to blood-brain barrier breakdown from frequent seizures rather than from the tumor itself.[578, 579] In a few cases, slow growth of the tumors has been observed by serial CT scans (a finding not expected in a hamartoma), but no evidence of malignant tumor was found at surgery.[573] CT images may be normal with small lesions or in areas of the brain obscured by beam-hardening artifact.

MRI allows a more detailed view of this lesion and can reveal some features useful in differentiating the DNT from other low-grade supratentorial tumors. Cortical involvement by the tumor is always present, and a thickened gyrus or a nodular appearance is evident. The most characteristic MRI feature is the presence of multiple nodules that appear isointense with CSF on T1- and T2-weighted images. PD-weighted images of these nodular regions demonstrate mildly decreased or increased signal or isointensity compared with CSF, suggesting that they are not truly cystic in nature. Pathologically, tumor cysts are not typical of the DNT, and these nodular areas correspond with the nodular architecture seen histologically. The nodules have a significant myxoid interstitial component and low cellularity compared with other areas of the tumor, accounting for the MRI signal, which is similar but not identical to that of CSF. These nodular areas are usually multiple, measure between 1 and 3 cm, appear to be present in many although not all DNTs, and may be the only MRI evidence of the tumor. The solid components of the tumor are typically isointense with gray matter on T1-weighted images, moderately hyperintense compared with gray matter on PD-weighted images, and mildly to markedly hyperintense on T2-weighted images. The solid portions may be located eccentrically to or intermixed within the nodular cystic-appearing components. Enhancement is seen in about one-half of the solid components and is usually focal or punctate or occasionally ringlike. Tumor margins on MRI are often well demarcated (in 50% to 80% of cases), and peritumoral edema is distinctly uncommon, as is a large amount of mass effect (Figs. 46-73 and 46-74).[573, 579, 580, 581] A single case suggestive of bilateral tumors in the temporal lobes has been noted, but histologic proof was not obtained.[572] DNT studied with thallium SPECT demonstrated no radiopharmaceutical uptake and very low HMPAO and iodine-123 iodoamphetamine (IMP) uptake, all of which are less than is typically seen even with low-grade gliomas, in keeping with the hamartomatous-like nature of this lesion.[582]

The differential diagnosis of DNT includes oligodendroglioma, astrocytoma, ganglion cell tumors, and glioneuronal malformations. Astrocytomas usually infiltrate the white matter and do not involve the cortex itself. Pleomorphic xanthoastrocytomas can show cortical and

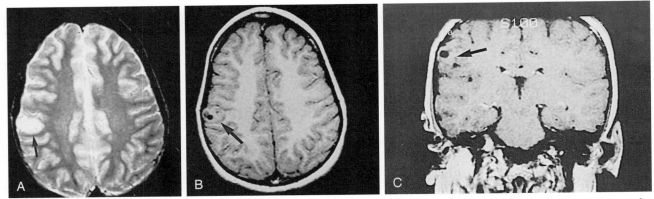

FIGURE 46–73 11-year-old boy with dysembryoplastic neuroepithelial tumor. The patient presented with seizures. *A,* PD-weighted image demonstrates subtle cortical and white matter hyperintensity *(arrow)*. *B,* T1-weighted image demonstrates the nodular, cortical, and cystic appearance of the tumor *(arrow)*. *C,* Gadolinium-enhanced image demonstrates no evidence of enhancement *(arrow)*.

meningeal involvement and almost always enhance on postgadolinium MRI studies. Oligodendrogliomas have a frontal lobe predominance and are seen in older patients, and calcification and enhancement are both more commonly seen than with DNT.

Ganglion cell tumors have radiologic and pathologic appearances similar to those of DNT. Gangliogliomas demonstrate enhancement more frequently (up to 80% of cases) and are more likely to calcify (up to 50% of cases). The multicystic appearance seen with DNT is not commonly seen with gangliogliomas, and 43% of gangliogliomas are entirely solid.[445] Glioneuronal malformations are typically solid and noncalcified and do not enhance.[573] Overall, the most important imaging findings seen in DNT that allow this tumor to be preoperatively diagnosed are an intracortical location, a thickened nodular or gyral configuration, and a multicystic appearance produced by multiple nodules containing a myxoid interstitial component. Low-power microscopic inspection demonstrating the cortical location and nodular architecture, along with the presence of multiple cell lines and the specific glioneuronal element, remains necessary for the diagnosis.

Primary Malignant Rhabdoid Tumor

Malignant rhabdoid tumor (MRT) is a rare childhood neoplasm typically arising in the kidney and was originally thought to represent a sarcomatous variant of Wilms' tumor. Extrarenal MRT has been found in the paravertebral region, chest wall, heart, liver, pelvis, and reproductive tract.[583] MRT of the central nervous system is usually found in young children, often younger than 2 years, who present with lethargy, signs and symptoms of increased intracranial pressure, or visual disturbances. Dissemination through the CSF is common, and the prognosis is poor, with most patients dying within 12 months of diagnosis.[584] Both supratentorial and posterior fossa tumors have been reported, with a cerebellar location the most frequent.[585]

The origin of this tumor is unknown. Conventional histologic examination demonstrates a "rhabdoid" appear-

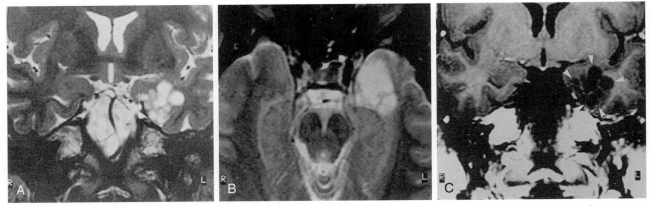

FIGURE 46–74 Dysembryoplastic neuroepithelial tumor in a 28-year-old patient with onset of seizures at 12 years of age. Coronal *(A)* and axial *(B)* T2-weighted images show a mass in the left medial temporal lobe with multiple cystic-appearing components. *C,* Coronal gadolinium-enhanced T1-weighted image shows low signal intensity in the cystic-appearing areas *(arrowheads)* with no enhancement. The tumor causes a minimal mass effect. (*A–C,* From Ostertun B, Wolf HK, Campos MG, et al. Dysembryoplastic neuroepithelial tumors MR and CT evaluation. AJNR 1996;17:419–430).

ance of the tumor, but no histochemical or ultrastructural evidence of myogenous differentiation is seen,[586] indicating that the tumor is unrelated to either Wilms' tumor or rhabdomyosarcoma. Evidence of differentiation along neuroglial and epithelial lines is noted in MRT found in the CNS but is not usually seen in the renal variant of rhabdoid tumor. Both a neuroectodermal origin, with the CNS tumor representing a variant of PNET, and origin from a meningiothelial precursor cell, equivalent to the serosal mesothelial precursor cells surrounding the kidneys, have been postulated.[585, 587] Associations of CNS medulloblastoma, pineoblastoma, PNET, medulloepithelioma (all primitive, embryonal tumors), and malignant SGCA with a history of renal malignant rhabdoid tumor have also been noted.[585]

The neuroimaging characteristics of MRT can only be based on the few cases reported. NCCT demonstrates an isodense or hyperdense mass, sometimes with small flecks of calcification. Large calcifications are not reported. The tumors, which are often several centimeters in diameter when supratentorial, may be found in the cerebellum, in the cerebral hemispheres, and in an intraventricular location associated with the lateral ventricles. The masses are lobulated and have been associated with extensive peritumoral edema when located within the brain parenchyma. Intense enhancement with CECT has been reported. MRI demonstrates a heterogeneous mass that is often nearly isointense with gray matter on both T1- and T2-weighted images. Small cysts and necrosis are present, and patchy enhancement after gadolinium administration is seen. Subarachnoid dissemination is often present at diagnosis or on follow-up imaging (Fig. 46–75).[583, 588–590] Cases presenting as large masses of the inferior frontal region with marginal cysts, resembling olfactory neuroblastoma, and as a large cystic congenital tumor resembling hydranencephaly have been reported.[591, 592]

The differential diagnosis includes the various supratentorial primitive neuroectodermal tumors (described later), medulloblastoma (in the posterior fossa), and supratentorial ependymoma and teratoma, both found in infants and young children.

Supratentorial Ependymoma

The supratentorial compartment is a less frequent location of ependymomas than the posterior fossa is, with 20% to 49% of the tumors (30% of childhood ependymomas) found in this location.[219, 593] A slight male predominance has been noted, and patients typically present with a variety of symptoms, including focal neurologic findings, seizures, and increased intracranial pressure.[594] The peak age of incidence of childhood supratentorial ependymomas is 1 to 6 years, but the tumors are found over a fairly broad age range (1.5 to 43 years with a mean of 18.4 years) in some series, and congenital tumors have also been reported.[219, 595, 596] Hydrocephalus is a less common finding with the supratentorial tumors compared with the posterior fossa neoplasms.

Ependymomas are commonly thought to be associated with the ependymal lining of the brain, but the supratentorial tumors are frequently (up to 85%[219]) located off the midline, within the frontal or parietal lobes. The tumor

grade increases, and prognosis worsens, for lesions located off the midline, compared with tumors in the ventricles. About two-thirds of supratentorial ependymomas in children are malignant (grade 3) tumors. Supratentorial ependymomas located adjacent to the ventricular surface are often found at the ends and flexures of the lateral ventricles and the ventricular outlets, where ependymal cell rests are frequently found. The purely extraventricular hemispheric tumors probably arise from nests of ependymal cells incorporated into the brain parenchyma during embryogenesis.[595] Third ventricular ependymomas are rare (less than 8% of all specifically localized tumors) and found in adult patients.[597]

Therapy of supratentorial ependymomas is primarily surgical, with radiation reserved for histologically malignant tumors, recurrent tumors, and subtotal resections of tumors near eloquent brain. Dissemination of tumor through the CSF is not common, and prophylactic spinal irradiation may not be indicated. When the outcome of therapy for supratentorial versus infratentorial ependymomas is compared, patients with supratentorial tumors do better, with up to two-thirds of patients alive at 10 years. Invasion into critical structures by the infratentorial tumors, making surgical resection difficult, may account for some of this difference in prognosis.[593, 598]

Supratentorial ependymomas have a nonspecific but heterogeneous appearance on neuroimaging studies. The tumors are well demarcated and often large, greater than 4 cm in diameter. They may be entirely parenchymal, located at the ventricular border, or intraventricular. NCCT demonstrates a heterogeneous mass with hypodense solid components, although slightly hyperdense solid components, possibly related to diffuse fine calcification, and isodense tumors may also be seen. Calcification, appearing as flecks, large masses, or even as rimlike peripheral calcification, is common and seen in 38% to 80% of cases. Cyst formation is also very common and seen in 70% of cases. CECT usually demonstrates enhancement of the solid portions of the tumors. Peritumoral edema is also seen in more than one-half of cases.[219, 596, 599, 600] Hemorrhage into ependymomas is unusual and seen in less than 15% of supratentorial tumors.[601] Up to 40% of ependymomas may contain clusters of cells that resemble oligodendrogliomas, but these tumors have not been noted to have imaging characteristics different from those of pure tumors.[600]

MRI also demonstrates a heterogeneous appearance of supratentorial ependymomas. Solid components are iso- or hypointense relative to white matter on T1-weighted images and hyperintense on T2-weighted images. Areas of hyperintensity on T1-weighted images may be seen, due to the presence of calcification or blood degradation products. The solid components always show enhancement with gadolinium. Heterogeneity of the tumors is produced by the presence of cystic areas, which are isointense with CSF on T1-weighted images and iso- or hyperintense with CSF on T2-weighted images. The hyperintensity of the cyst fluid noted on T2-weighted images may be due to its protein content or restricted flow, with shielding from motion within the CSF (see Fig. 46–25). Tumors within the lateral ventricle may ex-

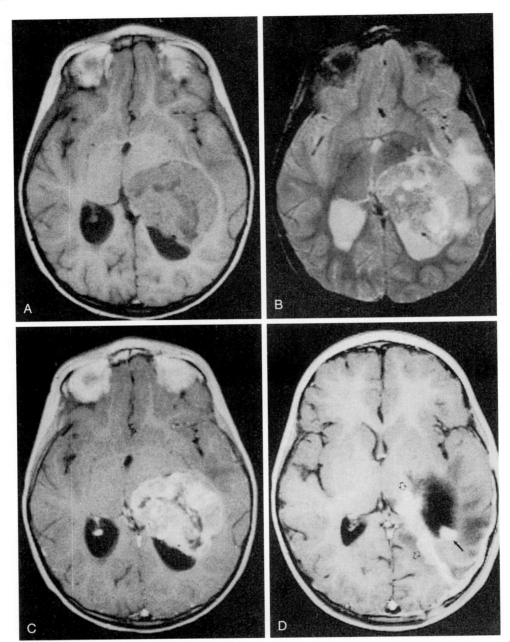

FIGURE 46–75 Primary malignant rhabdoid tumor in a 5-year-old girl. *A*, Axial T1-weighted image shows a large, somewhat heterogeneous mass in the atrium of the left lateral ventricle. *B*, T2-weighted image at the same level shows nearby vasogenic edema. *C*, Patchy enhancement is present after gadolinium administration. *D*, On a later scan after resection, a gadolinium-enhanced T1-weighted image shows tumor recurrence in the surgical bed *(arrows)*. (*A–D*, From Hanna SL, Langston JW, Parnham DM, Douglass EC. Primary malignant rhabdoid tumor of the brain: Clinical, imaging, and pathologic findings. AJNR 1993;14:107–115.)

tend through the foramen of Monro into the third ventricle.[600, 602]

The differential diagnosis includes both benign and malignant CPTs and PNET, all of which may have an appearance identical to that of ependymoma in the supratentorial brain. Low-grade astrocytomas typically are not calcified and do not demonstrate extensive enhancement, other than the pilocytic types, but are more common than ependymomas in the supratentorial compartment and should also be considered as a diagnostic possibility. Sub-

ependymal giant cell astrocytomas typically do not have peritumoral edema and are primarily found at the foramen of Monro. Calcification is also common in SGCA, but the presence of radiographic findings associated with TS is helpful in its identification.

Subependymoma

Subependymomas are rare tumors in adults and even less common in children. Only about 37% of subependymomas become symptomatic, usually producing obstructive hydrocephalus. About half of such tumors are located in the supratentorial compartment, unlike the asymptomatic tumors found at autopsy or as incidental imaging findings, which more commonly show a fourth ventricular location.[603, 604] Adults with symptomatic supratentorial tumors present with heterogeneous, cystic-appearing masses on MRI and CT involving the lateral ventricle and septum pellucidum. These tumors can be distinguished from ependymomas and intraventricular neurocytomas by a lack of calcification and perilesional edema, and only mild or no contrast enhancement. Posterior fossa subependymomas almost always extend into the ventricle, whereas supratentorial ependymomas are more frequently parenchymal or at the border of the ventricle.[605, 606]

The few cases of symptomatic subependymomas in children have been patients with fourth ventricular masses and hydrocephalus. Histologically, these tumors were mixed tumors consisting of cellular ependymoma and subependymoma. Unlike the excellent prognosis of adult pure subependymoma, these mixed tumors have been associated with poor outcomes, possibly due to the invasive nature of the ependymomatous component.[607] Fourth ventricular subependymomas may demonstrate significant calcification and enhancement, making distinction from ependymoma difficult, especially in a child.[605]

Supratentorial Primitive Neuroectodermal Tumors

The concept of PNET was introduced to describe malignant, predominantly undifferentiated tumors of the cerebrum in children. The tumors were believed to share a common neuroepithelial origin and could have areas of differentiation along neuronal or glial cell lines. The term initially was limited to largely undifferentiated tumors, with at least 90% of the tumor consisting of undifferentiated small blue cells and the remaining portions demonstrating differentiation along variable cell lines.[608] The concept of the PNET was subsequently expanded to include all primitive tumors that could share common neuroepithelial precursors, including tumors in the cerebellum, brain stem, spinal cord, and locations outside the neuroaxis itself (esthesioneuroblastoma or olfactory neuroblastoma of the olfactory bulbs, retinoblastoma, and melanotic progonoma of the maxilla). This expanded utilization of the term *PNET* has generated considerable controversy. Some neuropathologists prefer to apply the term *PNET* to all these tumors, along with qualification of the degree and type of differentiation.[609] With this approach a *primary cerebral neuroblastoma* is a PNET with neuronal differentiation, and *ependymoblastoma* is a PNET with ependymal differentiation. Problems with this approach include differences in the clinical behavior of the various subtypes of PNET and difficulty in determining the origin of these tumors, which potentially could arise from a truly undifferentiated multipotent precursor cell, from a cell committed to a particular line of differentiation, or from differentiated cells that have undergone malignant transformation into a more primitive type.[609] Overall, supratentorial PNETs are rare tumors, constituting 1% to 5% of all pediatric brain tumors.[216, 418]

The prognosis of supratentorial PNET is poor, with frequent leptomeningeal dissemination and occasional metastatic disease beyond the central nervous system. The overall 3-year survival is only 57%, with more than one-half of patients demonstrating tumor progression during the first 3 years after surgery, and up to one-third with evidence of dissemination of tumor through the CSF or distant metastatic disease at presentation.[610]

Childhood PNETs are most frequently found in the cerebral hemispheres, and dividing the cytogenesis of the forebrain into discrete stages can be used as an approach to understand the origin of these tumors. Malignant transformation at one of these stages can give rise to PNET with different lines of differentiation.[611]

The embryonic neural tube contains multipotential cells that produce all neuroectodermal elements of the central nervous system. These cells are found in the germinal matrix lining the ventricles up to the 30th week of gestation, after which the layer thins, with residual cells found only at the caudothalamic groove at birth. The residual germinal matrix has usually disappeared by 1 year of age, but nests of matrix cells may persist in the frontal lobe periventricular white matter, reflecting the frontal lobe location of some PNETs.

The cytogenesis of the forebrain may be divided into three stages, with malignant transformation at each stage producing a characteristic subtype of PNET. Stage I is characterized by constantly dividing neuroepithelial cells without differentiation. Transformation at this stage corresponds to the medulloepithelioma, the most undifferentiated tumor. These tumors are very rare (1% of all brain tumors in children) and are seen early in life, usually before the age of 5 years with a mean age of 2 years. Patients present with a rapidly expanding mass, increased intracranial pressure, seizures, and focal neurologic signs. The histologic appearance and immunohistochemistry are characterized by the formation of glandlike structures with epithelial surfaces, resembling the embryonic neural tube, and multiple lines of glial, neuronal, and mesenchymal differentiation. The tumors are found in both supra- and infratentorial locations. The prognosis is very poor, with frequent dissemination through the CSF, and survival less than 1 year.[190, 612] These cerebral tumors should be distinguished from the ocular medulloepithelioma, which has a similar histologic appearance and arises from the ciliary body, but, unlike the cerebral tumor, frequently has benign behavior and a good outcome after enucleation of the affected orbit.

Stage II of forebrain cytogenesis is characterized by the differentiation of some matrix cells into neuroblasts, which migrate outward toward the cortex. The corresponding tumor at this stage is the primary cerebral neuroblastoma. These tumors typically (80%) present during the first decade of life, without a gender predominance, although adult cases have been reported. They represent only 2% of all neuroblastomas in children.[613] Most patients present with increased intracranial pressure and a short duration of symptoms lasting less than 6 months. The tumors are found anywhere in the cerebrum with a slight preference for the frontal or frontoparietal regions.[611, 614] The histologic appearance of cerebral neuroblastoma is characterized by neuronal differentiation,

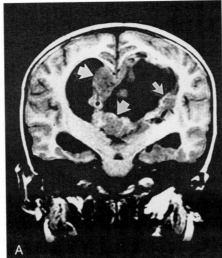
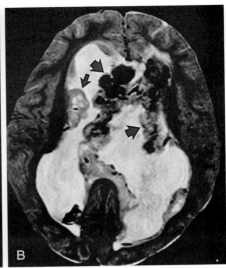

FIGURE 46–76 An infant with intraventricular cerebral PNET. T1-weighted (*A*) and T2-weighted (*B*) images demonstrate enlarged ventricles and multiple masses lining the ventricles (*arrows*). Note the marked heterogeneity of signal intensities present, with some focal areas markedly hypointense on T2-weighted images; this may represent calcification.

including fibrillary areas of neuronal processes, reactivity for NSE and synaptophysin, and the presence of ganglion cells. Homer-Wright rosettes are typically observed, and desmoplastic variants containing connective tissue are also seen. Electron microscopy can demonstrate neurosecretory granules. Rare partial differentiation into mature neuronal cells is sometimes seen, analogous to the maturation of peripheral neuroblastomas arising from the autonomic ganglia. The prognosis does not appear to be related to the degree of differentiation but is said to be better than that of other subtypes of PNET, with overall survival of 60% at 3 years.[615] Therapy consists of surgical resection and local radiotherapy. The efficacy of chemotherapy and spinal radiation therapy is uncertain, with the former utilized for residual tumor after subtotal resection and the latter when there is evidence of spinal leptomeningeal dissemination.[614] Primary cerebral neuroblastoma (and all other PNET subtypes) can disseminate through the CSF, leading to the use of prophylactic radiation of the entire neuroaxis in some institutions. Distant metastatic disease from primary cerebral neuroblastoma has been found in the lung, liver, bone marrow, pericardium, cervical lymph nodes, and skin and may be accelerated in the presence of dural sinus invasion.[616]

Stage III of forebrain cytogenesis is characterized by the differentiation of matrix cells into primitive glial cells (glioblasts or spongioblasts) that give rise to astrocytes and oligodendrocytes. Differentiation of matrix cells in the subependymal region into ependymal cells also occurs during stage III. Stage III PNETs therefore are typified by the ependymoblastoma and spongioblastoma.

The spongioblastoma (primitive polar spongioblastoma) is a tumor composed of elongated bipolar cells arranged in palisades. There has been debate about the very existence of this tumor as well as its exact origin, whether this lesion is a distinct entity or a nonspecific tissue pattern found in a variety of neuroectodermal tumors. Current WHO classification places the spongioblastoma among tumors of uncertain origin.[190]

These very rare tumors are found in the periventricular region or in the cerebellum of young children. The histologic appearance is characterized by bipolar cells in pali-

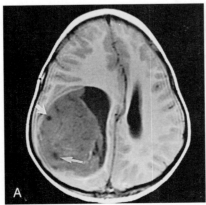
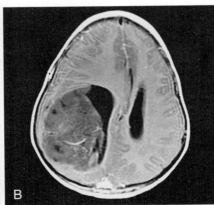
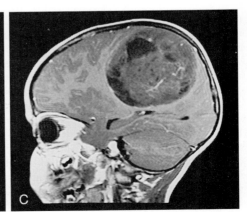

FIGURE 46–77 A 2-year-old with cerebral PNET (primary cerebral neuroblastoma). *A*, T1-weighted image demonstrates a large hemispheric and intraventricular mass. Note the heterogeneity of the mass with focal areas of hypointensity that may represent cysts, necrosis, or calcifications (*arrows*). *B* and *C*, Gadolinium-enhanced images demonstrate mild and heterogeneous enhancement. Note the lack of edema in the surrounding brain despite the large size of the mass.

sades, with immunohistochemical features of both neuronal and glial differentiation. The tissue pattern of polar spongioblastoma may be found in more ordinary tumors including oligodendroglioma and pilocytic astrocytoma. The characteristic pattern has also been observed in ependymomas and cerebral neuroblastomas, and some authors doubt its separate existence from the other subtypes of PNET. The clinical behavior of this tumor is also not well characterized.[617, 618]

The ependymoblastoma is a small cell neoplasm characterized histologically by the presence of ependymoblastic rosettes, consisting of multilayered rosettes with small lumina formed of mitotically active cells. The tumor should not be confused with malignant or anaplastic ependymoma. Like the other PNETs, ependymoblastoma presents at young age (mean of 2 years, with a reported range of birth to 36 years of age) and carries a poor prognosis, with common CSF dissemination and median survival after surgery of 12 months. Patients typically present with large hemispheric masses.[619, 620]

It should be noted that mixed embryonal tumors with characteristics of more than one subtype of PNET may be demonstrated histologically. A rare childhood tumor of the vermis, the medullomyoblastoma, has been de-

scribed and resembles a posterior fossa medulloblastoma with areas of muscle differentiation. This unusual tumor may represent myogenic and neuronal differentiation of neuroepithelial cells; radiographic findings have not been described.[621]

The variable approach to the classification and nosology of supratentorial PNET extends to the imaging literature. Reports of the imaging appearance of primary cerebral neuroblastoma as a distinct entity exist, as do descriptions of the appearance of supratentorial PNET, but in many cases the subtypes of the tumors described are not included. Fortunately, no radiologic differences between the various subtypes of PNET have been described, and they probably can be considered as a group with regard to their neuroimaging appearance (Figs. 46–76 through 46–79).[49]

The reported appearance of primary cerebral neuroblastoma is a large hemispheric mass with calcification and cyst formation. The masses frequently abut the lateral ventricular surface and contain intratumoral hemorrhage. Spontaneous intraventricular hemorrhage may occasionally be seen. The tumor density on NCCT is usually mixed, and heterogeneous enhancement on CECT is always present to some degree. Calcification is very com-

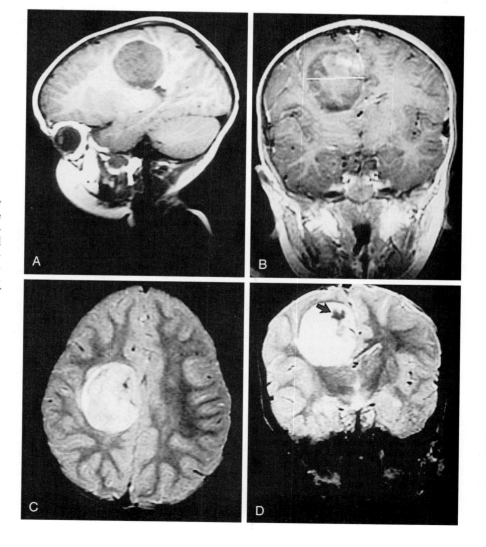

FIGURE 46–78 A 21-month-old boy with PNET. *A,* T1-weighted image demonstrates a well-defined, heterogeneous mass. *B,* Gadolinium-enhanced image demonstrates mild heterogeneous enhancement. *C* and *D,* T2-weighted images demonstrate hyperintensity of the lesion. Note the lack of significant surrounding edema and the focal area of hypointensity *(arrow in D)* representing a large calcification.

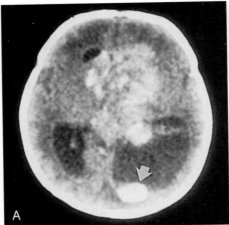 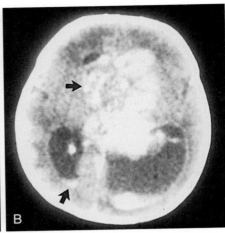

FIGURE 46–79 A 16-day-old infant with PNET (ependymoblastoma). *A,* NCCT demonstrates a large calcified mass and hydrocephalus. *B,* CECT demonstrates heterogeneous enhancement. Note the apparently calcified tumor nodule in the left ventricle occipital horn (*arrow* in *A*) and enhancing tumor abutting the occipital and frontal horns of the right lateral ventricle (*arrows* in *B*).

mon in primary cerebral neuroblastoma, reported in 50% to 80% of cases. MRI demonstrates heterogeneous signal, with hypointense areas corresponding to hemosiderin or calcification; hyperintense regions on T1-weighted images may also be seen and correspond with subacute hemorrhage. In general, the tumors are very well defined, and tumor definition is improved on postgadolinium images. Solid portions of the tumors are isointense on T1-weighted images and hyperintense on T2-weighted images. Enhancement with gadolinium is always present, usually heterogeneous, and variable in intensity. Peritumoral edema is distinctly minimal or absent, despite the large size of these tumors. Dural sinus invasion by cerebral neuroblastoma may be seen with MRI and by allowing the tumor access to distant sites may predispose the patient to metastatic disease beyond the central nervous system.[616, 622–624]

The reported appearance of supratentorial PNET with NCCT is a large hemispheric mass, usually greater than 6 cm and up to 15 cm in diameter at presentation, with some preference for the frontal and temporal regions. The masses are well defined, with minimal or no edema, and have a heterogeneous appearance. Cystic or necrotic areas are common, seen in up to 65% of cases. Calcifications are also very common and reported in 50% to 71% of cases. Solid portions of the tumor are iso- to hyperdense, and intense but heterogeneous enhancement on CECT is nearly always present. Enhancement may be solid, nodular, or ringlike, surrounding cystic or necrotic cavities. Intratumoral or intracystic hemorrhage is common as well. The reported CT appearances of supratentorial PNET versus cerebral neuroblastoma overlap, but it has been suggested that PNETs are denser than cerebral neuroblastomas. Differences in neuropathologic nomenclature make comparisons somewhat difficult. Dissemination through the CSF intracranially with studding of the ventricular surfaces or masses in the subarachnoid space is common even at presentation and may be seen as enhancing tumor with CECT in up to 70% of patients.[625–628]

The MRI appearance of primary cerebral neuroblastoma is characterized by markedly heterogeneous signal, with areas of hyper- and hypointensity on both T1- and T2-weighted images produced by the combination

of solid tumor, cysts, necrosis, calcifications, and blood degradation products of various ages. Evidence of intratumoral hemorrhage is seen in about one-half of cases evaluated with MRI. Enhancement of the solid portions is present, and dilated arteries supplying the tumor may be visualized as flow voids.[49, 216, 629]

The MRI appearance of ependymoblastoma has been described as a well-circumscribed hemispheric mass with no significant surrounding edema, hypointense on T1-weighted images and hyperintense with heterogeneous signal on T2-weighted images, with mild enhancement on postgadolinium images.[620] Similar findings with medulloepithelioma have been reported.[612] In both cases, the MRI appearance is not distinct from that of the other supratentorial PNETs. In a young child with a hemispheric mass demonstrating marked heterogeneity, calcification, cystic or necrotic areas, and hemorrhage, the diagnosis of PNET should be considered. The absence of significant peritumoral edema is a helpful imaging finding. The differential diagnosis of supratentorial PNET includes ependymoma, choroid plexus tumors, and astrocytomas.

Brain Tumors During the First 2 Years of Life

Brain tumors presenting in the first 2 years of life differ from those of older children in their location, tumor type, and presenting symptoms. As a group, tumors presenting during the first 2 years of life represent 7% to 18% of pediatric brain tumors, and those presenting during the first year of life account for 1.9% to 8.5% of pediatric brain tumors.[630–632]

Compared with older children, younger children have a distinct increase in the incidence of supratentorial tumors, with 59% of tumors found in the supratentorial compartment. Others have noted an equal supra- and infratentorial location during the first year of life, with supratentorial tumors dominating during the second year.[630, 631] During the first 2 years of life, the most common tumor reported is astrocytoma, most often a low-grade (I or II) tumor, followed by medulloblastoma and ependymoma. The sellar region and the region adjacent to the lateral ventricles are the most common supraten-

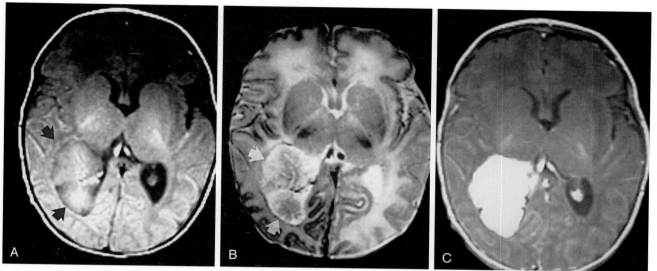

FIGURE 46–80 A 21-day-old infant with congenital choroid plexus papilloma. T1-weighted (A) and T2-weighted (B) images demonstrate a lobulated mass within the atrium of the right lateral ventricle (arrows). C, Avid enhancement is seen with gadolinium. Note that the lesion appears to be separate from the ependyma of the ventricle (best appreciated on the T1-weighted image), suggesting a nonaggressive tumor.

torial locations, whereas the inferior cerebellar vermis and fourth ventricle are the most common infratentorial locations.[633] Many of the astrocytomas present as large hemispheric masses, but visual pathway gliomas and hypothalamic gliomas account for some of the astrocytomas seen in this age group.[634] The tumors, although often large, do not present with focal neurologic symptoms. Most commonly, increased intracranial pressure or seizures are seen. In infants whose sutures and fontanelles are open, progressive macrocrania is a common presentation. Intracranial pressure may be normal in these patients as the calvarium expands to contain the growing tumor. Diencephalic region tumors, including visual pathway gliomas, may present in infants as failure to thrive.

Tumors presenting with symptoms during the first 2 months of life are often considered congenital lesions, representing about 0.5% to 1.9% of all pediatric brain tumors. About two-thirds of these tumors are supratentor-ial, and more than one-half of the patients in this young age group have either PNET (including typical posterior fossa medulloblastoma) or teratoma, with teratoma the single most common brain tumor encountered in infants. Other common congenital tumors include astrocytomas (both benign and high grade, including glioblastoma), CPPs, ependymomas, germinomas, meningiomas, and gangliogliomas.[635] Other series note a somewhat different distribution of tumor types during the first 2 years of life, with 36% represented by teratomas and 50% from neuroepithelial origin including 11.5% medulloblastomas, 9.5% astrocytomas, 7.5% CPPs, and 7% ependymomas. An increased incidence of congenital abnormalities, involving either the CNS or other parts of the body, is noted with brain tumors presenting during the first 2 months of life and supports a congenital origin of these tumors.[636]

Prognosis of these young children with brain tumors is

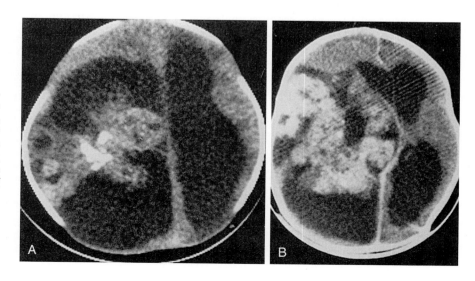

FIGURE 46–81 Supratentorial teratoma. A, Axial CT scan shows chunky calcification within a heterogeneous mass, with associated hydrocephalus. B, After contrast administration, there is heterogeneous enhancement. (A and B, From Buetow PC, Smirniotopoulos JG, Done S. Congenital brain tumors: A review of 45 cases. AJNR 1990;11:793–799).

FIGURE 46–82 Fetus-in-fetu. *A,* Nonenhanced CT scan of a 2-month-old child at the level of the frontal and occipital horns shows hydrocephalus and a mass near the pineal region with mixed soft tissue, calcium, and fat attenuation *(arrow). B,* Axial image at a higher level shows a portion of an extremity, with fat surrounding a central bony structure, probably a femur *(arrow).* (*A* and *B,* From Yang ST, Leow SW. Intracranial fetus-in-fetu. CT diagnosis. AJNR 1992;13:1326–1329.

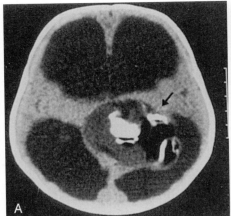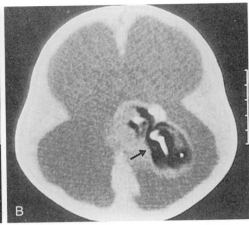

in general poor, with 5-year survival rates of 20% to 30% for the tumors presenting in the first year of life and of 74% during the second year of life.[630, 637] Patients with congenital teratomas have a mean survival as short as 21 days,[635] but rare cases of intracranial teratomas located superficially or predominantly involving the neck with only minor intracranial portions have long survival.[638, 639] CPPs are amenable to complete surgical resection and have 5-year survivals as high as 100%.[632]

The neuroimaging appearance of the various tumors encountered in young children has been described previously in this chapter. Congenital medulloblastoma has been reported as a predominantly hyperdense posterior fossa mass by NCCT in a newborn.[640] Gliomatosis cerebri has mimicked agyria by CT.[641] Congenital CPP can present as intraventricular masses, similar to those seen in older children, and as homogeneous echogenic masses within the ventricles on transcranial ultrasonography, which may be the first diagnostic test used in these infants (Fig. 46–80).[642]

Three forms of congenital teratomas have been described: massive intracranial teratoma replacing the intracranial contents of a neonate, smaller intracranial masses producing hydrocephalus, and intracranial masses with extension into the neck or orbit. The exact site of origin of these tumors, especially the massive ones, is difficult to determine, but they may arise from the pineal region, quadrigeminal plate, or walls of the third ventricle.[643]

When detected with NCCT, congenital teratomas are heterogeneous masses with areas of large, dense calcifications, and cystic- and solid-appearing portions. The solid areas are typically isodense to soft tissue and demonstrate some patchy enhancement on CECT. The calcifications are more prominent and massive than those typically seen in PNET in this age group. Fat, if present, allows the diagnosis to be made confidently.[635, 644–646] MRI, as expected, reflects this heterogeneity with variable signal intensity, including hyperintense T1 signal from fat, cystic-appearing areas, and areas of signal void compatible with calcification.[647] Teratomas, as congenital lesions, may be diagnosed with obstetric ultrasonography, during which they appear as very heterogeneous masses with solid and cystic portions and areas of shadow-producing calcifications. The tumors reported are usually of the

massive type, replacing most of the intracranial contents, with only a thin surrounding rim of native brain. The maternal history may include polyhydramnios or a uterine size greater than expected for gestational age.[648, 649] Maternal MRI can be used to demonstrate the large, very heterogeneous mass as well.[650] Intracranial teratoma should be distinguished from the extremely rare intracranial fetus-in-fetu, a variant of incomplete twinning of monozygotic twins whose CT appearance may mimic teratoma but is distinguished by the presence of well-formed limbs or vertebrae (Figs. 46–81 and 46–82).[651]

REFERENCES

1. Pollack IF. Brain tumors in children. N Engl J Med 1994; 331:1500–1507.
2. Zimmerman RA. Posterior fossa pediatric tumors. In Categorical Course on Neoplasms of the Central Nervous System, pp. 33–35. American Society of Neuroradiology, 1990.
3. Enzmann DR, Norman D, Levin V, et al. Computed tomography in the follow-up of medulloblastomas and ependymomas. Radiology 1978;128:57–63.
4. Devkota J, El Gammal T, Brooks BS, et al. Role of computed tomography in cases of cranial metastatic neuroblastoma. J Comput Assist Tomogr 1981;5:654–659.
5. Pedersen H, McConnell J, Harwood-Nash DC, et al. Computed tomography in intracranial, supratentorial metastases in children. Neuroradiology 1989;31:19–23.
6. Cordier S, Iglesias M-J, Le Goaster C, et al. Incidence and risk factors for childhood brain tumors in the Ile de France. Int J Cancer 1994;59:776–782.
7. Mueller BA, Gurney JG. Epidemiology of pediatric brain tumors. Neurosurg Clin N Am 1992;3:715–721.
8. Kuijten RR, Bunin GR. Risk factors for childhood brain tumors. Cancer Epidemiol Biomarkers Prev 1993;2:277–288.
9. Young JL Jr, Miller RW. Incidence of malignant tumors in U.S. children. J Pediatr 1975;86:254–258.
10. Lannering B, Marky I, Nordberg C. Brain tumors in childhood and adolescence in west Sweden 1970–1984: Epidemiology and survival. Cancer 1990;66:604–609.
11. Devesa SS, Blot WJ, Stone BJ, et al. Recent cancer trends in the United States. J Natl Cancer Inst 1995;87:175–182.
12. Duffner PK, Cohen ME, Myers MH, et al. Survival of children with brain tumors: SEER program, 1973–1980. Neurology 1986;36:597–601.
13. Stiller CA, Nectoux J. International incidence of childhood brain and spinal tumors. Int J Epidemiol 1994;23:458–464.
14. Radhakrishnan K, Bohen NI, Kurland LT. Epidemiology of brain tumors. In Morantz RA, Walsh JW (eds): Brain Tumors: A Comprehensive Text, pp. 1–18. New York, Marcel Dekker, 1993.
15. Radhakrishnan K, Mokri B, Parisi JE, et al. The trends in incidence

of primary brain tumors in the population of Rochester, Minnesota. Ann Neurol 1995;37:67–73.

16. Thorne RN, Pearson ADJ, Nicoll JAR, et al. Decline in incidence of medulloblastoma in children. Cancer 1994;74:3240–3244.

17. Gold EB, Leviton A, Lopez R, et al. The role of family history in risk of childhood brain tumors. Cancer 1994;73:1302–1311.

18. Choi NW, Schuman LM, Gullen WH. Epidemiology of primary central nervous system neoplasms. II. Case-control study. Am J Epidemiol 1970;91:467.

19. Modan B, Mart H, Baidatz D, et al. Radiation-induced head and neck tumors. Lancet 1974;1:277–279.

20. Zaridze DG, Li N, Men T, et al. Childhood cancer incidence in relation to distance from the former nuclear testing site in Semipalatinsk, Kazakhstan. Int J Cancer 1994;59:471–475.

21. McCredie M, Maisonneuve P, Boyle P. Antenatal risk factors for malignant brain tumors in New South Wales children. Int J Cancer 1994;56:6–10.

22. Gold EB, Leviton A, Lopez R, et al. Parental smoking and risk of childhood brain tumors. Am J Epidemiol 1993;137:620–628.

23. Preston-Martin S, Yu MC, Benton B, et al. N-Nitroso compounds and childhood brain tumors: A case-control study. Cancer Res 1982;42:5240–5245.

24. John EM, Savitz DA, Sandler DP. Prenatal exposure to parents' smoking and childhood cancer. Am J Epidemiol 1991;133:123–132.

25. Wertheimer N, Leeper E. Electrical wiring configurations and childhood cancer. Am J Epidemiol 1979;109:273–284.

26. Moulder JE, Foster KR. Biological effects of power-frequency fields as they relate to carcinogenesis. Proc Soc Exp Biol Med 1995;209:309–324.

27. Savitz DA, John EM, Kleckner RC. Magnetic field exposure from electrical appliances and childhood cancer. Am J Epidemiol 1990;131:763–773.

28. Wilkins JR 3rd, Hundley VD. Paternal occupational exposure to electromagnetic fields and neuroblastoma in offspring. Am J Epidemiol 1990;131:995–1008.

29. Nasca PC, Baptiste MS, MacCubbin PA, et al. An epidemiologic case-control study of central nervous system tumors in children and parental occupational exposures. Am J Epidemiol 1988;128:1256–1265.

30. Tomenius L. 50-Hz electromagnetic environment and the incidence of childhood tumors in Stockholm County. Bioelectromagnetics 1986;7:191–207.

31. Savitz DA, Wachtel H, Barnes FA, et al. Case-control study of childhood cancer and exposure to 60-Hz magnetic fields. Am J Epidemiol 1988;128:21–38.

32. Feychting M, Ahlbom A. Magnetic fields and cancer in children residing near Swedish high-voltage power lines. Am J Epidemiol 1993;138:467–481.

33. Macklis RM. Magnetic healing, quackery, and the debate about the health effects of electromagnetic fields. Ann Intern Med 1993;118:376–383.

34. Wilson R, Shlyakhter A. Re: "Magnetic fields and cancer in children residing near Swedish high-voltage power lines." Am J Epidemiol 1995;141:378–379.

35. Kraut A, Tate R, Tran N. Residential electric consumption and childhood cancer in Canada (1971–1986). Arch Environ Health 1994;49:156–159.

36. Hughes JT. Electromagnetic fields and brain tumors: A commentary. Teratog Carcinogen Mutagen 1994;14:213–217.

37. Shao T. EMF-cancer link: The ferritin hypothesis. Med Hypotheses 1993;41:28–30.

38. Goodman EM, Greenebaum B, Marron MT. Effects of electromagnetic fields on molecules and cells. Int Rev Cytol 1995;158:279–338.

39. Fairbairn DW, O'Neill KL. The effect of electromagnetic field exposure on the formation of DNA single strand breaks in human cells. Cell Mol Biol (Noisy-le-grand) 1994;40:561–567.

40. Berger MS, Keles GE, Geyer JR. Cerebral hemispheric tumors of childhood. Neurosurg Clin N Am 1992;3:839–852.

41. Mercuri S, Russo A, Palma L. Hemispheric supratentorial astrocytomas in children. Long-term results in 29 cases. J Neurosurg 1989;71:316–326.

42. Vezina L-G, Packer RJ. Infratentorial brain tumors of childhood. Neuroimaging Clin N Am 1994;4:423–436.

43. Bille B. Migraine in school children. Acta Pediatr 1962;51 (Suppl 136):1–151.

44. Sillanapaa M. Changes in the prevalence of migraine and other headaches during the first seven school years. Headache 1983;23:15–19.

45. Dooley JM, Campfield PR, O'Neill M, et al. The value of CT scans for children with headaches. Can J Neurol Sci 1990;17:309–310.

46. Chu ML, Shinnar S. Headaches in children younger than 7 years of age. Arch Neurol 1992;49:79–82.

47. Maytal J, Bienkowski RS, Patel M, et al. The value of brain imaging in children with headaches. Pediatrics 1995;96:413–416.

48. Honig PJ, Charney EB. Children with brain tumor headaches. Am J Dis Child 1982;136:121–124.

49. Fitz C. Magnetic resonance imaging of pediatric brain tumors. Top Magn Reson Imaging 1993;5:174–189.

50. Barkovich AJ. Pediatric Neuroimaging, 2nd ed. Philadelphia, Lippincott-Raven, 1995.

51. Tice HM, Jones KM, Mulkern RV, et al. Fast spin-echo imaging of intracranial neoplasms. J Comput Assist Tomogr 1993;17:425–431.

52. Kjos BO, Umansky R, Barkovich AJ. MR of the brain in children with developmental retardation of unknown cause. AJNR 1990;11:1035–1040.

53. Ge HL, Hirsch WL, Wolf GL, et al. Diagnostic role of gadolinium-DTPA in pediatric neuroradiology: A retrospective review of 655 cases. Neuroradiology 1992;34:122–125.

54. Brasch RC (ed). MRI Contrast Enhancement in the Central Nervous System: A Case Study Approach. Philadelphia, Lippincott-Raven, 1993.

55. Kilgore DP, Breger RK, Daniels DL, et al. Cranial tissues: Normal MR appearance after intravenous injection of Gd-DTPA. Radiology 1986;160:757–761.

56. Berry I, Brant-Zawadzki M, Osaki L, et al. Gd-DTPA in clinical MR of the brain. 2. Extraaxial lesions and normal structures. AJNR 1986;7:789–793.

57. Gadian DG, Payne JA, Bryant DJ, et al. Gadolinium-DTPA as a contrast agent in MR imaging: Theoretical projections and practical observations. J Comput Assist Tomogr 1985;9:242–251.

58. Byrd SE, Darling CF, Allen E. Contrast agents in neuroimaging. Neuroimaging Clin N Am 1994;4:9–26.

59. Ball WS, Parker JR, Davis PC, et al. Efficacy of gadoteridol for contrast-enhanced magnetic resonance imaging in children. Invest Radiol 1992;27:545–552.

60. Bird CR, Drayer BP, Medina M, et al. Gd-DTPA-enhanced MRI imaging in pediatric patients after brain tumor resection. Radiology 1988;169:123–126.

61. Elster AD, Rieser GD. Gd-DTPA-enhanced cranial MR imaging in children: Initial clinical experience and recommendations for its use. AJNR 1989;10:1027–1030.

62. Ball WS Jr, Nadel SN, Zimmerman RA, et al. Phase III multicenter clinical investigation to determine the safety and efficacy of gadoteridol in children suspected of having neurologic disease. Radiology 1993;186:769–774.

63. Shellock FG, Kanal E. Magnetic Resonance. Bioeffects, Safety, and Patient Management. Philadelphia, Lippincott-Raven, 1994.

64. Wolff SD, Balaban RS. Magnetization transfer contrast (MTC) and tissue water proton relaxation in vivo. Magn Reson Med 1989;10:135–144.

65. Wolff SD, Balaba RS. Magnetization transfer contrast: Method for improving contrast in gradient-recalled-echo images. Radiology 1991;179:133–137.

66. Kurki T, Niemi P, Valtonen S. MR of intracranial tumors: Combined use of gadolinium and magnetization transfer. AJNR 1994;15:1727–1736.

67. Kurki TJI, Niemi PT, Lundbom N. Gadolinium-enhanced magnetization transfer contrast imaging of intracranial tumors. J Magn Reson Imaging 1992;2:401–406.

68. Dickman CA, Rekate HL, Bird CR, et al. Unenhanced and gadolinium-DTPA-enhanced MR imaging in postoperative evaluation in pediatric brain tumors. J Neurosurg 1989;71:49–53.

69. Elster AD, DiPersio DA. Cranial postoperative site: Assessment with contrast-enhanced MR imaging. Radiology 1990;174:93–98.

70. Lanzieri CF, Som PM, Sacher M, et al. The postcraniectomy site: CT appearance. Radiology 1986;159:165–170.

71. Laster DW, Moody DM, Ball MR. Resolving intracerebral hematoma: Alteration of the ring sign with steroids. AJR 1978;130:935–939.

72. Meyding-Lamadé U, Forsting M, Albert F, et al. Accelerated

methaemoglobin formation: Potential pitfall in early postoperative MRI. Neuroradiology 1993;35:178–180.

73. Hudgins PA, Davis PC, Hoffman JC. Gadopentetate dimeglumine–enhanced MR imaging in children following surgery for brain tumor: Spectrum of meningeal findings. AJNR 1991;12:301–307.

74. Kun LE. The brain and spinal cord. In Moss WT, Cox JD (eds). Radiation Oncology. Rationale, Technique, Results, p. 597. St. Louis, Mosby, 1989.

75. Eisenberg HM, Barlow CF, Lorenzo AV. Effect of dexamethasone on altered brain vascular permeability. Arch Neurol 1970;23:18–22.

76. Sze G, Soletsky S, Bronen R, et al. MR imaging of the cranial meninges with emphasis on contrast enhancement and meningeal carcinomatosis. AJNR 1989;10:965–975.

77. Mathews VP, Kuharik MA, Edwards MK, et al. Gd-DTPA-enhanced MR imaging of experimental bacterial meningitis: Evaluation and comparison with CT. AJNR 1988;9:1045–1050.

78. Packer RJ, Siegel KR, Sutton LN, et al. Leptomeningeal dissemination of primary central nervous system tumors of childhood. Ann Neurol 1985;18:217–221.

79. Stanley P, Senac MO Jr, Segall HD. Intraspinal seeding from intracranial tumors in children. AJNR 1984;5:805–809.

80. Kandt RS, Shinnar S, D'Souza BJ, et al. Cerebrospinal metastases in malignant childhood astrocytomas. J Neurooncol 1984;2:123–128.

81. Grabb PA, Albright AL, Pang D. Dissemination of supratentorial malignant gliomas via the cerebrospinal fluid in children. Neurosurgery 1992;30:64–71.

82. Chamberlain MC. A review of leptomeningeal metastases in pediatrics. J Child Neurol 1995;10:191–199.

83. Olson M, Chernik N, Posner J. Infiltration of the leptomeninges by systemic cancer. A clinical and pathologic study. Arch Neurol 1974;30:122–137.

84. Little J, Dale A, Okazaki H. Meningeal carcinomatosis: Clinical manifestations. Arch Neurol 1974;30:138–143.

85. Theodore WH, Gendelman S. Meningeal carcinomatosis. Arch Neurol 1981;38:696–699.

86. Glass J, Melamed M, Chernik N, et al. Malignant cells in cerebrospinal fluid (CSF): The meaning of a positive CSF cytology. Neurology 1979;29:1369–1375.

87. Wasserstrom WH, Glass J, Posner J. Diagnosis and treatment of leptomeningeal metastases from solid tumors: Experience with 90 patients. Cancer 1982;49:759–772.

88. Kaplan J, DeSouza T, Farkash A, et al. Leptomeningeal metastases: Comparison of clinical features and laboratory data of solid tumors, lymphomas, and leukemias. J Neurooncol 1990;92:225–229.

89. Lee Y, Glass JP, Geoffrey A, et al. Cranial-computed tomographic abnormalities in leptomeningeal metastasis. AJR 1984;143:1035–1039.

90. Jaeckle KA, Krol G, Posner JB. Evolution of computed tomographic abnormalities in leptomeningeal metastasis. Ann Neurol 1985;17:85–89.

91. Ascherl GF, Hilal SK, Brisman R. Computed tomography of disseminated meningeal and ependymal malignant neoplasms. Neurology 1981;31:567–574.

92. Barloon TJ, Uyuh WT, Yang CJ. Spinal subarachnoid tumor seeding from intracranial metastasis: MR findings. J Comput Assist Tomogr 1987;11:242–244.

93. Davis PC, Freedman NC, Fry SM. Leptomeningeal metastasis: MR imaging. Radiology 1987;163:449–454.

94. Sze G, Soletsky S, Bronen R, et al. MR imaging of the cranial meninges with emphasis on contrast enhancement and meningeal carcinomatosis. AJNR 1989;10:965–975.

95. Chamberlain MC, Sandy AD, Press GA. Leptomeningeal metastasis: A comparison of gadolinium-enhanced MR and contrast-enhanced CT of the brain. Neurology 1990;40:435–438.

96. Krol G, Sze G, Malkin M, et al. MR of cranial and spinal meningeal carcinomatosis: Comparison with CT and myelography. AJNR 1988;9:709–714.

97. Davis PC, Hoffman JC Jr, Ball TL, et al. Spinal abnormalities in pediatric patients: MR imaging findings compared with clinical, myelographic, and surgical findings. Radiology 1988;166:679–685.

98. Blews DE, Wang H, Kumar AJ, et al. Intradural spinal metastases in pediatric patients with primary intracranial neoplasms: Gd-DTPA enhanced MR vs CT myelography. J Comput Assist Tomogr 1990;14:730–735.

99. Sze G, Krol G, Zimmerman RD, et al. Intramedullary disease of the spine: Diagnosis using gadolinium-DTPA enhanced MR imaging. AJR 1988;151:1193–1204.

100. Dillon WP, Norman D, Newton TH, et al. Intradural spinal cord lesions: Gd-DTPA enhanced MR imaging. Radiology 1989;170:229–237.

101. Slasky BS, Bydder GM, Niendorf HP, et al. MR imaging with gadolinium-DTPA in the differentiation of tumor, syrinx and cyst of the spinal cord. J Comput Assist Tomogr 1987;11:845–850.

102. Kramer ED, Rafto S, Packer RJ, et al. Comparison of myelography with CT follow-up versus gadolinium MRI for subarachnoid metastatic disease in children. Neurology 1991;41:46–50.

103. Heinz R, Wiener D, Friedman H, et al. Detection of cerebrospinal fluid metastasis: CT myelography or MR? AJNR 1995;16:1147–1151.

104. Kochi M, Mihara Y, Takada A, et al. MRI of subarachnoid dissemination of medulloblastoma. Neuroradiology 1991;33:264–268.

105. Barkovich AJ. Neuroimaging of pediatric brain tumors. Neurosurg Clin N Am 1992;3:739–769.

106. Wiener MD, Boyko OB, Friedman HS, et al. False-positive spinal MR findings for subarachnoid spread of primary CNS tumor in postoperative pediatric patients. AJNR 1990;11:1100–1103.

107. Kun LE, D'Souza B, Tefft M. The value of surveillance testing in childhood brain tumors. Cancer 1985;56:1818–1823.

108. Torres CF, Rebsamen S, Silber JH, et al. Surveillance scanning of children with medulloblastoma. N Engl J Med 1994;330:892–895.

109. Valk PE, Dillon WP. Radiation injury of the brain. AJNR 1991;12:45–62.

110. Jena A, Rath GK, Ravichandran R, et al. Effects of radiation therapy on the human normal brain (white matter) visualized by MR imaging. Magn Reson Imaging 1991;9:959–961.

111. Davis PC, Hoffman JC, Pearl GS, et al. CT evaluation of effects of cranial radiation therapy in children. AJR 1986;147:587–592.

112. Dooms GC, Hecht S, Brant-Zawadzki M, et al. Brain radiation lesions: MR imaging. Radiology 1986;155:149–155.

113. Curnes JT, Laster DW, Ball MR, et al. MRI of radiation injury to the brain. AJR 1986;147:119–124.

114. Tsuruda JS, Kortman KE, Bradley WG, et al. Radiation effects on cerebral white matter: MR evaluation. AJR 1987;149:165–171.

115. Constine LS, Konski A, Ekholm S, et al. Adverse effects of brain irradiation correlated with MR and CT imaging. Int J Radiat Oncol Biol Phys 1988;15:319–330.

116. Packer RJ, Zimmerman RA, Bilaniuk LT. Magnetic resonance imaging in the evaluation of treatment-related central nervous system damage. Cancer 1986;58:635–640.

117. Curran WJ, Hecht-Leavitt C, Schut L, et al. Magnetic resonance imaging of cranial radiation lesions. Int J Radiat Oncol Biol Phys 1987;13:1093–1098.

118. DeReuck J, VanderEecken H. The anatomy of the late radiation encephalopathy. Eur Neurol 1975;13:481–494.

119. Oppenheimer JH, Levy ML, Sinha U, et al. Radionecrosis secondary to interstitial brachytherapy: Correlation of magnetic resonance imaging and histopathology. Neurosurgery 1992;31:336–343.

120. Kay HEM, Knapton PJ, O'Sullivan JP, et al. Encephalopathy in acute leukemia associated with methotrexate therapy. Arch Dis Child 1972;47:344–354.

121. Packer RJ, Meadows AT, Rorke LB, et al. Long-term sequelae of cancer treatment on the central nervous system in childhood. Med Pediatr Oncol 1987;15:241–253.

122. Rubinstein LJ, Herman MM, Long TF, et al. Disseminated necrotizing leukoencephalopathy: A complication of treated central nervous system leukemia and lymphoma. Cancer 1975;35:306–318.

123. Bleyer WA, Griffin TW. White matter necrosis, mineralizing microangiopathy, and intellectual abilities in survivors of childhood leukemia. In Gilbert HA, Kagan AR (eds). Radiation Damage to the Central Nervous System: A Delayed Therapeutic Hazard, pp. 155–174. Philadelphia, Lippincott-Raven, 1980.

124. Chen C-Y, Zimmerman RA, Faro S, et al. Childhood leukemia: Central nervous system abnormalities during and after treatment. AJNR 1996;17:295–310.

125. Henkelman RM, Watts JF, Kucharczyk W. High signal intensity in MR imaging of calcified brain tissue. Radiology 1991;179:199–206.

126. Price RA, Birdwell DA. The central nervous system in childhood leukemia. III. Mineralizing microangiopathy and dystrophic calcification. Cancer 1978;42:717–728.

127. Painter MJ, Chutorian AM, Hilal SK. Cerebrovasculopathy following irradiation in children. Neurology 1975;25:189–194.

128. Brant-Zawadzki M, Anderson M, DeArmond SJ, et al. Radiation-induced large intracranial vessel occlusive vasculopathy. AJR 1980;134:51–55.

129. Wilms G, Marchal G, VanFraeyenhoven L, et al. Unilateral moyamoya disease: MRI findings. Neuroradiology 1989;31:442.

130. Allen JC, Miller DC, Budzilovich GN, et al. Brain and spinal cord hemorrhage in long-term survivors of malignant pediatric brain tumors: A possible late effect of therapy. Neurology 1991;41:148–150.

131. Gaensler EHL, Dillon WP, Edwards MSB, et al. Radiation-induced telangiectasia in the brain simulates cryptic vascular malformations at MR imaging. Radiology 1994;193:629–636.

132. Priest JR, Ramsay NKC, Steinherz PG, et al. A syndrome of thrombosis and hemorrhage complicating L-asparaginase therapy for childhood acute lymphoblastic leukemia. Pediatrics 1982; 100:984–989.

133. Ramsay NKC, Coccia PF, Krivit W, et al. The effect of L-asparaginase on plasma coagulation factors in acute lymphoblastic leukemia. Cancer 1977;4:1398–1401.

134. Miké V, Meadows AT, D'Angio GJ. Incidence of second malignant neoplasms in children: Results of an international study. Lancet 1982;2:1326–1331.

135. Zarrabi MH, Rosner F, Grünwald HW. Second neoplasms in acute lymphoblastic leukemia. Cancer 1983;52:1712–1719.

136. Malone M, Lumley H, Erdohazi M. Astrocytoma as a second malignancy in patients with acute lymphoblastic leukemia. Cancer 1986;57:1979–1985.

137. Valk PE, Budinger TF, Levin VA, et al. PET of malignant cerebral tumors after interstitial brachytherapy: Demonstration of metabolic activity and correlation with clinical outcome. J Neurosurg 1988;69:830–838.

138. Patronas NJ, DiChiro G, Brooks RA, et al. Work in progress: [18F] Fluorodeoxyglucose and positron emission tomography in the evaluation of radiation necrosis of the brain. Radiology 1982;144:885–889.

139. Kim EE, Chung SK, Haynie TP, et al. Differentiation of residual or recurrent tumors from post-treatment changes with F-18 FDG PET. Radiographics 1992;12:269–279.

140. Kahn D, Follett KA, Bushnell DL, et al. Diagnosis of recurrent brain tumor: Value of 201Tl SPECT vs F-fluorodeoxyglucose PET. AJR 1994;163:1459–1465.

141. Cairncross JG, Macdonald DR, Pexman JHW, et al. Steroid-induced CT changes in patients with recurrent malignant glioma. Neurology 1988;38:724–726.

142. Hatam A, Bergstrom M, Yu Z-Y, et al. Effect of dexamethasone treatment on volume and contrast enhancement of intracranial neoplasms. J Comput Assist Tomogr 1983;7:295–300.

143. Gerber AM, Savolaine ER. Modification of tumor enhancement and brain edema in computerized tomography by corticosteroid: Case report. Neurosurgery 1980;6:282–284.

144. Hanson MW, Hoffman JM, Glantz MJ, et al. FDG PET in the early postoperative evaluation of patients with brain tumor. [Abstract] J Nucl Med 1990;31:799.

145. Glantz MJ, Hoffman JM, Coleman RE, et al. Identification of early recurrence of primary central nervous system tumors by [18F]fluorodeoxyglucose positron emission tomography. Ann Neurol 1991;29:347–355.

146. Francavilla TL, Miletich RS, DiChiro G, et al. Positron emission tomography in the detection of malignant degeneration of low-grade gliomas. Neurosurgery 1989;24:1–5.

147. DiChiro G, DeLaPaz RL, Brooks RA, et al. Glucose utilization of cerebral gliomas measured by [18F]fluorodeoxyglucose and positron emission tomography. Neurology 1982;32:1323–1329.

148. Patronas NJ, Brooks RA, DeLaPaz RL, et al. Glycolytic rate (PET) and contrast enhancement (CT) in human cerebral gliomas. AJNR 1983;4:533–535.

149. Kim CK, Alavi JB, Alavi A, et al. New grading system of cerebral gliomas using positron emission tomography with F-18 fluorodeoxyglucose. J Neurooncol 1991;10:85–91.

150. Delbeke D, Meyerowitz C, Lapidus RL, et al. Optimal cutoff levels of F-18 fluorodeoxyglucose uptake in the differentiation of low-grade from high-grade brain tumors with PET. Radiology 1995;195:47–52.

151. DiChiro G, Brooks RA. PET quantitation: Blessing and curse. J Nucl Med 1988;29:1603–1604.

152. Hoffman JM, Hanson MW, Friedman HS, et al. FDG-PET in pediatric posterior fossa brain tumors. J Comput Assist Tomogr 1992;16:62–68.

153. DiChiro G. Positron emission tomography using [18F]fluorodeoxyglucose in brain tumors: A powerful diagnostic and prognostic tool. Invest Radiol 1986;22:360–371.

154. Alavi JB, Alavi A, Chawluk J, et al. Positron emission tomography in patients with glioma: A predictor of prognosis. Cancer 1988;62:1074–1078.

155. Coleman RE, Hoffman JM, Hanson MW, et al. Clinical application of PET for the evaluation of brain tumors. J Nucl Med 1991;32:616–622.

156. Patronas NJ, DiChiro G, Kufta C, et al. Prediction of survival in glioma patients by means of positron emission tomography. J Neurosurg 1985;62:816–822.

157. Brucher JM. Neuropathological diagnosis with stereotactic biopsies. Possibilities, difficulties, and requirements. Acta Neurochir 1993;124:37–39.

158. Feiden W, Steude U, Bise K, et al. Accuracy of stereotactic brain tumor biopsy: Comparison of the histologic findings in biopsy cylinders and resected tumor tissue. Neurosurg Rev 1991;14:51–56.

159. Black PM. Brain tumors (first of two parts). N Engl J Med 1991;324:1471–1476.

160. Levivier M, Goldman S, Pirotte B, et al. Diagnostic yield of stereotactic biopsy guided by positron emission tomography with [18F]fluorodeoxyglucose. J Neurosurg 1995;82:445–452.

161. O'Tuama LA, Phillips PC, Strauss LC, et al. Two-phase [11C]L-methionine PET in childhood brain tumors. Pediatr Neurol 1990;6:163–170.

162. Olivero WC, Dulebohn SC, Lister JR. The use of PET in evaluating patients with primary brain tumours: Is it useful? J Neurol Neurosurg Psychiatry 1995;58:250–252.

163. Nadel HR. Thallium-201 for oncological imaging in children. Semin Nucl Med 1993;23:243–254.

164. Mountz JM, Raymond PA, McKeever PE, et al. Specific localization of thallium 201 in human high-grade astrocytoma by microautoradiography. Cancer Res 1989;49:4053–4056.

165. O'Tuama LA, Janicek MJ, Barnes PD, et al. 201Tl/99mTc-HMPAO SPECT imaging of treated childhood brain tumors. Pediatric Neurol 1991;7:249–257.

166. Lindegdard MW, Skretting A, Hager B, et al. Cerebral and cerebellar uptake of 99mTc-(d,l)-hexamethyl-propyleneamine oxime (HM-PAO) in patients with brain tumor studied by single photon emission tomography. Eur J Nucl Med 1986;12:417–420.

167. Langen KJ, Roosen N, Herzog H, et al. Investigations of brain tumours with 99mTc HMPAO SPECT. Nucl Med Commun 1989; 10:325–334.

168. Black KL, Hawkins RA, Kim KT, et al. Use of thallium-201 SPECT to quantify malignancy grade of gliomas. J Neurosurg 1989; 71:342–346.

169. O'Tuama LA, Treves ST, Larar JN, et al. Thallium-201 versus technetium-99m-MIBI SPECT in evaluation of childhood brain tumors: A within-subject comparison. J Nucl Med 1993;34:1045–1051.

170. O'Tuama LA, Larar JM, Kwan A, et al. Tc-99m MIBI/Tl-201 SPECT in childhood brain tumors. [Abstract] J Nucl Med 1992;33:844.

171. Carvalho PA, Schwartz RB, Alexander E, et al. Detection of recurrent gliomas with quantitative thallium-201/technetium-99m HMPAO single-photon emission computerized tomography. J Neurosurg 1992;77:565–570.

172. Holman BL, Tumeh SS. Single-photon emission computed tomography (SPECT): Applications and potential. JAMA 1990;263:561–564.

173. Schwartz RB, Carvalho PA, Alexander E, et al. Radiation necrosis vs high-grade recurrent glioma: Differentiation by using dual-isotope SPECT with 210Tl and 99mTc-HMPAO. AJNR 1991; 12:1187–1192.

174. Oriuchi N, Tamura M, Shibazaki T, et al. Clinical evaluation of thallium-201 SPECT in supratentorial gliomas: Relationship to histologic grade, prognosis, and proliferative activities. J Nucl Med 1993;34:2085–2089.

175. Maria BL, Drane WE. Single-photon emission computed tomography of pediatric brain tumors: A comparative study of thallium-201 chloride, ^{18}F fluorodeoxyglucose, and ^{99}Tc hexamethylpropyleneamineoxime. [Abstract] Ann Neurol 1994;36:505.

176. Glickson JD. Clinical NMR spectroscopy of tumors: Current status and future directions. Invest Radiol 1989;24:1011–1016.

177. Hubesch B, Sappey-Marinier D, Roth K, et al. P-31 MR spectroscopy of normal human brain and brain tumors. Radiology 1990;174:401–409.

178. Heindel W, Bunke J, Glathe S, et al. Combined [1]H-MR imaging and localized ^{31}P-spectroscopy of intracranial tumors in 43 patients. J Comput Assist Tomogr 1988;12:907–916.

179. Maris JM, Evans AE, McLaughlin AC, et al. [31]P nuclear magnetic resonance spectroscopic investigation of human neuroblastoma in situ. N Engl J Med 1985;312:1500–1505.

180. Younkin DP, Delivoria-Papadopoulos M, Leonard JC, et al. Unique aspects of human newborn cerebral metabolism evaluated with phosphorus. Nucl Magn Reson Spectrosc 1984;16:581–586.

181. Hilberman M, Subramanian VH, Haselgrove J, et al. In vivo time resolved brain phosphorus nuclear magnetic resonance. J Cereb Blood Flow Metab 1984;4:334–342.

182. Sutton LN, Lenkinski RE, Cohen BH, et al. Localized ^{31}P magnetic resonance spectroscopy of large pediatric brain tumors. J Neurosurg 1990;72:65–70.

183. Gill SS, Small RK, Thomas DGT, et al. Brain metabolites as ^{1}H NMR markers of neuronal and glial disorders. NMR Biomed 1989;2:196–200.

184. Ott D, Henning J, Ernst T. Human brain tumors: Assessment with in vivo proton MR spectroscopy. Radiology 1993;186:745–752.

185. Bruhn H, Frahm J, Gyngell ML, et al. Noninvasive differentiation of tumor with the use of localized H-1 MR spectroscopy in vivo: Initial experience in patients with cerebral tumors. Radiology 1989;172:541–548.

186. Poptani H, Gupta RK, Roy R, et al. Characterization of intracranial mass lesions with in vivo proton MR spectroscopy. AJNR 1995;16:1593–1603.

187. Sutton LN, Wang Z, Gusnard D, et al. Proton magnetic resonance spectroscopy of pediatric brain tumors. Neurosurgery 1992;31:19.

188. Sutton LN, Wehrli SL, Gennarelli L, et al. High-resolution [1]H-magnetic resonance spectroscopy of pediatric posterior fossa tumors in vitro. J Neurosurg 1994;81:443–448.

189. Wang Z, Sutton LN, Cnaan A, et al. Proton MR spectroscopy of pediatric cerebellar tumors. AJNR 1995;16:1821–1833.

190. Burger PC, Scheithauer BW. Tumors of the Central Nervous System. Fascicle 10, Third Series. Atlas of Tumor Pathology. Washington, D.C., Armed Forces Institute of Pathology, 1994.

191. Bailey P, Cushing H. A classification of tumors of the glioma group. Philadelphia, JB Lippincott, 1926.

192. Kernohan JW, Sayre GP. Tumors of the Central Nervous System, Section X, Fascicles 35 and 37. Atlas of Tumor Pathology. Washington, D.C., Armed Forces Institute of Pathology, 1952.

193. Russell DS, Rubinstein LJ. Pathology of Tumors of the Nervous System, 5th ed. Baltimore, Williams & Wilkins, 1989.

194. Zülch KJ. Histological Typing of Tumours of the Central Nervous System. Geneva, World Health Organization, 1979.

195. Kleihues P, Burger PC, Scheithauer BW. The new WHO classification of brain tumours. Brain Pathol 1993;3:255–268.

196. Harwood-Nash DC. Primary neoplasms of the central nervous system in children. Cancer 1991;67:1223–1228.

197. Albright L. Posterior fossa tumors. Neurosurg Clin N Am 1992; 3:881–891.

198. Meyers SP, Kemp SS, Tarr RW. MR imaging features of medulloblastomas. AJR 1992;158:859–865.

199. Nelson M, Diebler C, Forbes WS. Paediatric medulloblastoma: Atypical CT features at presentation in the SIOP II trial. Neuroradiology 1991;33:140–142.

200. Sandhu A, Kendall B. Computed tomography in management of medulloblastomas. Neuroradiology 1987;29:444–452.

201. Zimmerman RA, Bilaniuk LT, Pahlajani H. Spectrum of medulloblastomas demonstrated by computed tomography. Radiology 1978;126:137–141.

202. Vézina L-G, Packer, RJ. Infratentorial brain tumors of childhood. Neuroimaging Clin N Am 1994;4:423–436.

203. Mueller DP, Moore SA, Sato Y, et al. MRI spectrum of medulloblastoma. Clin Imaging 1992;16:250–255.

204. Weinstein ZR, Downey EF Jr. Spontaneous hemorrhage in medulloblastomas. AJNR 1983;4:986–988.

205. Shen W-C, Yang C-F. Multifocal cerebellar medulloblastoma: CT findings. J Comput Assist Tomogr 1988;12:894.

206. Atlas SW. Intraaxial brain tumors. In Atlas SW (ed). Magnetic Resonance Imaging of the Brain and Spine, Philadelphia, Lippincott-Raven, 1990. p. 149–203.

207. Algra PR, Postma T, VanGroeningen CJ, et al. MR imaging of skeletal metastases from medulloblastoma. Skeletal Radiol 1992; 21:425–430.

208. Vieco PT, Azouz EM, Hoeffel JC. Metastases to bone in medulloblastoma. A report of five cases. Skeletal Radiol 1989;18:445–449.

209. Maleci A, Cervoni L, Delfini R. Medulloblastoma in children and in adults: A comparative study. Acta Neurochir (Wein) 1992; 119:62–67.

210. Bourgouin PM, Tampieri D, Grahovac SZ, et al. CT and MR imaging findings in adults with cerebellar medulloblastoma: Comparison with findings in children. AJR 1992;159:609–612.

211. Koci TM, Chiang F, Mehringer CM, et al. Adult cerebellar medulloblastoma: Imaging features with emphasis on MR findings. AJNR 1993;14:929–939.

212. Schneider JH, Raffel C, McComb G. Benign cerebellar astrocytomas of childhood. Neurosurgery 1992;30:58–63.

213. Gusnard DA. Cerebellar neoplasms in children. Semin Roentgenol 1990;25:263–278.

214. Mishima K, Nakamura M, Nakamura H, et al. Leptomeningeal dissemination of cerebellar pilocytic astrocytoma. J Neurosurg 1992;77:788–791.

215. Ushio Y, Arita N, Yoshimine T, et al. Malignant recurrence of childhood cerebellar astrocytoma: Case report. Neurosurgery 1987;21:251–255.

216. Maroldo TV, Barkovich AJ. Pediatric brain tumors. Semin Ultrasound CT MR 1992;13:412–448.

217. Lee Y-Y, VanTassel P, Bruner JM, et al. Juvenile pilocytic astrocytomas: CT and MR characteristics. AJNR 1989;10:363–370.

218. Zimmerman RA, Bilaniuk LT, Rebsamen S. Magnetic resonance imaging of pediatric posterior fossa tumors. Pediatr Neurosurg 1992;18:58–64.

219. Naidich TP, Zimmerman RA. Primary brain tumors in children. Semin Roentgenol 1984;19:100–114.

220. Zee C, Segal HD, Ahmadi J, et al. Computed tomography of intracranial ependymomas in childhood. Surg Neurol 1983;20:221–226.

221. Swartz JD, Zimmerman RA, Bilaniuk LT. Computed tomography of intracranial ependymomas. Radiology 1982;143:97–101.

222. Marujama R, Koga K, Nakahara T, et al. Cerebral myxopapillary ependymoma. Hum Pathol 1992;23:960–962.

223. Schiffer D, Chiò A, Cravioto H, et al. Ependymoma: Internal correlations among pathological signs: The anaplastic variant. Neurosurgery 1991;29:206–210.

224. Nazar GB, Hoffman HJ, Becker LE, et al. Infratentorial ependymomas in childhood: Prognostic factors and treatment. J Neurosurg 1990;72:408–417.

225. Rorke LB. Relationship of morphology of ependymoma in children to prognosis. Prog Exp Tumor Res 1987;30:170–174.

226. Mørk SJ, Rubinstein LJ. Ependymoblastoma. A reappraisal of a rare embryonal tumor. Cancer 1985;55:1536–1542.

227. Lyons MK, Kelly PJ. Posterior fossa ependymomas: Report of 30 cases and review of the literature. Neurosurgery 1991;28:659–665.

228. Courville CB, Broussalian SL. Plastic ependymomas of the lateral recess. Report of eight verified cases. J Neurosurg 1961;18:792–799.

229. Spoto GP, Press GA, Hesselink JR, et al. Intracranial ependymoma and subependymoma: MR manifestations. AJNR 1990;11:83–91.

230. Kane AG, Robles HA, Smirniotopoulos JG, et al. Radiologic-pathologic correlation. Diffuse pontine astrocytoma. AJNR 1993;14:941–945.

231. Zee CS, Segall HD, Nelson M, et al. Infratentorial tumors in children. Neuroimag Clin N Am 1993;3:705–714.

232. Packer RJ, Nicholson HS, Vezina LG, et al. Brainstem gliomas. Neurosurg Clin N Am 1992;3:863–879.

233. Smith RR. Brain stem tumors. Semin Roentgenol 1990;25:249–262.

234. Petronio JA, Edwards MSB. Management of brainstem tumors in children. Contemp Neurosurg 1989;11:1–6.

235. Fulton DS, Levin VA, Wara WM, et al. Chemotherapy of pediatric brain-stem tumors. J Neurosurg 1981;54:721–725.
236. Edwards MSB, Wara WM, Ciricillo SF, et al. Focal brain-stem astrocytomas causing symptoms of involvement of the facial nerve nucleus: Long-term survival in six pediatric cases. J Neurosurg 1994;80:20–25.
237. Albright AL, Price RA, Guthkelch AN. Brain stem gliomas of children. A clinicopathologic study. Cancer 1983;52:2313–2319.
238. Maria BL, Rehder K, Eskin TA, et al. Brainstem glioma. I. Pathology, clinical features, and therapy. J Child Neurol 1993;8:112–128.
239. Mariz BL, D'Souza BJ. Brain stem glioma. Contemp Neurosurg 1984;6:1–16.
240. Epstein FJ, Farmer J-P. Brain-stem glioma growth patterns. J Neurosurg 1993;78:408–412.
241. Albright AL, Guthkelch AN, Packer RJ, et al. Prognostic factors in pediatric brain stem gliomas. J Neurosurg 1986;65:751–755.
242. Stroink AR, Hoffman HJ, Hendrick EB, et al. Diagnosis and management of pediatric brain-stem gliomas. J Neurosurg 1986;65:745–750.
243. Bilaniuk LT, Zimmerman RA, Littman P, et al. Computed tomography of brain stem gliomas in children. Radiology 1980;134:89–95.
244. Nelson MD, Soni D, Baram TZ. Necrosis in pontine gliomas: Radiation induced or natural history? Radiology 1994;191:279–282.
245. Buckley RC. Pontine gliomas: A pathologic study and classification of twenty-five cases. Arch Pathol 1930;9:779–819.
246. Lee BCP, Kneeland JB, Walker RW, et al. MR imaging of brain-stem tumors. AJNR 1985;6:159–163.
247. Packer RJ, Zimmerman RA, Bilanuik LT, et al. Magnetic resonance imaging of lesions of the posterior fossa and upper cervical cord in childhood. Pediatrics 1985;76:84–90.
248. Hueftle MG, Han JS, Kaufman B, et al. MR imaging of brain stem gliomas. J Comput Assist Tomogr 1985;9:263–267.
249. Byrne JV, Kendall BE, Kingsley DPE, et al. Lesions of the brain stem: Assessment by magnetic resonance imaging. Neuroradiology 1989;31:129–133.
250. Barkovich AJ, Krischer J, Kun LE, et al. Brain stem gliomas: A classification system based on magnetic resonance imaging. Pediatr Neurosurg 1990–1991;16:73–83.
251. Smith RR, Zimmerman RA, Packer RJ, et al. Pediatric brainstem glioma. Post-radiation clinical and MR follow-up. Neuroradiology 1990;32:265–271.
252. Stroink AR, Hoffman HJ, Hendrick EB, et al. Transependymal benign dorsally exophytic brain stem gliomas in childhood: Diagnosis and treatment recommendations. Neurosurgery 1987;20:439–444.
253. Khatib ZA, Heideman RL, Kovnar EH, et al. Predominance of pilocytic histology in dorsally exophytic brain stem tumors. Pediatr Neurosurg 1994;20:2–10.
254. Robertson PL, Allen JC, Abbott IR, et al. Cervicomedullary tumors in children: A distinct subset of brainstem gliomas. Neurology 1994;44:1798–1803.
255. Albright AL, Packer RJ, Zimmerman R, et al. Magnetic resonance scans should replace biopsies for the diagnosis of diffuse brain stem gliomas: A report from the children's cancer group. Neurosurgery 1993;33:1026–1030.
256. Bruggers CS, Friedman HS, Fuller GN, et al. Comparison of serial PET and MRI scans in a pediatric patient with a brainstem glioma. Med Pediatr Oncol 1993;21:301–306.
257. Smirniotopoulos JG, Rushing EJ, Mena HM. Pineal region masses: Differential diagnosis. Radiographics 1992;12:577–596.
258. Edwards MSB, Hudgins RJ, Wilson CB, et al. Pineal region tumors in children. J Neurosurg 1988;68:689–697.
259. Sener RN. The pineal gland: A comparative MR imaging study in children and adults with respect to normal anatomical variations and pineal cysts. Pediatr Radiol 1995;25:245–248.
260. Golzarian J, Balériaux D, Bank WO, et al. Pineal cyst: Normal or pathological? Neuroradiology 1993;35:251–253.
261. Lee DH, Norman D, Newton TH. MR imaging of pineal cysts. J Comput Assist Tomogr 1987;4:586–590.
262. Mamourian AC, Towfighi J. Pineal cysts: MR imaging. AJNR 1986;7:1081–1086.
263. Fain JS, Tomlinson FH, Scheithauer BW, et al. Symptomatic glial cysts of the pineal gland. J Neurosurg 1994;80:454–460.
264. Zimmerman RA, Bilaniuk LT. Age-related incidence of pineal calcification detected by computed tomography. Radiology 1982;142:659–662.
265. Ganti SR, Hilal SK, Stein BM, et al. CT of pineal region tumors. AJNR 1986;7:97–104.
266. Chang CG, Kageyama T, Yoshida J, et al. Pineal tumors: Clinical diagnosis, with special emphasis on the significance of pineal calcification. Neurosurgery 1981;8:656–668.
267. Zimmerman RA, Bilaniuk LT, Wood JH, et al. Computed tomography of pineal, parapineal, and histologically related tumors. Radiology 1980;137:669–677.
268. Kilgore DP, Strother CM, Starshak RJ, et al. Pineal germinoma: MR imaging. Radiology 1986;158:435–438.
269. Müller-Forell W, Schroth G, Egan PJ. MR imaging in tumors of the pineal region. Neuroradiology 1988;30:224–231.
270. Zee C-S, Segall H, Apuzzo M, et al. MR imaging of pineal region neoplasms. J Comput Assist Tomogr 1991;15:56–63.
271. Koide O, Watanabe Y, Sato K. A pathological survey of intracranial germinoma and pinealoma in Japan. Cancer 1980;45:2119–2130.
272. Baumgartner JE, Edwards MSB. Pineal tumors. Neurosurg Clin N Am 1992;3:853–862.
273. Ghoshhajra K, Baghai-Naiini P, Hahn HS, et al. Spontaneous rupture of pineal teratoma. Neuroradiology 1979;17:215–217.
274. Tien RD, Barkovich AJ, Edwards MSB. MR imaging of pineal tumors. AJNR 1990;11:557–565.
275. Raaijmakers C, Wilms G, Demaerel P. Pineal teratocarcinoma with drop metastases: MR features. Neuroradiology 1992;34:227–229.
276. Chang T, Teng MMH, Guo W-Y, et al. CT of pineal tumor and intracranial germ-cell tumors. AJNR 1989;10:1039–1044.
277. Chiechi MV, Smirniotopoulos JG, Mena H. Pineal parenchymal tumors: CT and MR features. J Comput Assist Tomogr 1995;19:509–517.
278. Borit A, Blackwood W, Mair WGP. The separation of pineocytoma from pineoblastoma. Cancer 1980;45:1408–1418.
279. Vaquero J, Ramiro J, Martinez R, et al. Clinicopathological experience with pineocytomas: Report of five surgically treated cases. Neurosurgery 1990;27:612–619.
280. D'Andrea AD, Packer RJ, Rorke LB, et al. Pineocytomas of childhood. A reappraisal of natural history and response to therapy. Cancer 1987;59:1353–1357.
281. Herrick MK, Rubinstein LJ. The cytological differentiating potential of pineal parenchymal neoplasms (true pinealomas). Brain 1979;102:289–320.
282. Disclafani A, Hudgins RJ, Edwards MSB, et al. Pineocytomas. Cancer 1989;63:302–304.
283. Truwit CL, Barkovich AJ. Pathogenesis of intracranial lipoma: An MR study in 42 patients. AJNR 1990;11:665–674.
284. Tart RP, Quisling RG. Curvilinear and tubulonodular varieties of lipoma of the corpus callosum: An MR and CT study. J Comput Assist Tomogr 1991;15:805–810.
285. Benjamin JC, Furneaux CE, Scholtz CL. Pineal astrocytoma. Surg Neurol 1985;23:139–142.
286. Barnett DW, Olson JJ, Thomas WG, et al. Low-grade astrocytomas arising from the pineal gland. Surg Neurol 1995;43:70–76.
287. Piatt JH, Campbell GA. Pineal region meningioma: Report of two cases and literature review. Neurosurgery 1983;12:369–375.
288. İplikçioglu AC, Bayar MA, Fökes F, et al. Pineal meningioma: MRI. Neuroradiology 1993;35:539–540.
289. Gouliamos AD, Kalovidouris AE, Kotoulas GK, et al. CT and MR of pineal region tumors. Magn Reson Imaging 1994;12:17–24.
290. Blach LE, McCormick B, Abramson DH, et al. Trilateral retinoblastoma—incidence and outcome: A decade of experience. Int J Radiat Oncol Biol Phys 1994;29:729–733.
291. Provenzale JM, Weber AL, Klintworth GK, et al. Radiologic-pathologic correlation. Bilateral retinoblastoma with coexistent pineoblastoma (trilateral retinoblastoma). AJNR 1995;16:157–165.
292. Smirniotopoulos JG, Bargallo N, Mafee MF. Differential diagnosis of leukokoria: Radiologic-pathologic correlation. Radiographics 1994;14:1059–1079.
293. Boydston WR, Sanford RA, Muhlbauer MS, et al. Gliomas of the tectum and periaqueductal region of the mesencephalon. Pediatr Neurosurg 1991;17:234–238.
294. Raffel C, Hudgins R, Edwards MSB. Symptomatic hydrocephalus: Initial findings in brainstem gliomas not detected on computed tomographic scans. Pediatrics 1988;82:733–737.
295. Pendl G, Vorkapic P, Koniyama M. Microsurgery of midbrain lesions. Neurosurgery 1990;26:641–648.
296. Pollack IF, Pang D, Albright AL. The long-term outcome in

children with late-onset aqueductal stenosis resulting from benign intrinsic tectal tumors. J Neurosurg 1994;80:681–688.

297. Squires LA, Allen JC, Abbott R, et al. Focal tectal tumors: Management and prognosis. Neurology 1994;44:953–956.

298. Lapras CL, Bognar L, Turjman T, et al. Tectal plate gliomas. Part I. Microsurgery of the tectal plate gliomas. Acta Neurochir (Wien) 1994;126:76–83.

299. Bognar L, Turjman F, Villanyi E, et al. Tectal plate gliomas. Part II. CT scans and MR imaging of tectal gliomas. Acta Neurochir (Wien) 1994;127:48–54.

300. May PL, Blaser SI, Hoffman HJ, et al. Benign intrinsic tectal "tumors" in children. J Neurosurg 1991;74:867–871.

301. Friedman DP. Extrapineal abnormalities of the tectal region: MR imaging findings. AJR 1992;159:859–866.

302. Vandertop WP, Hoffman HJ, Drake JM, et al. Focal midbrain tumors in children. Neurosurgery 1992;31:186–194.

303. Robertson PL, Muraszko KM, Brunberg JA, et al. Pediatric midbrain tumors: A benign subgroup of brainstem gliomas. Pediatr Neurosurg 1995;22:65–73.

304. Hoffman HJ, Yoshida M, Becker LE, et al. Pineal region tumors in childhood. Experience at the Hospital for Sick Children. In Humphreys RP (ed). Concepts in Pedatric Neurosurgery 4. Basel, S. Karger, 1983.

305. Kollias SS, Barkovich AJ, Edwards MSB. Magnetic resonance analysis of suprasellar tumors of childhood. Pediatr Neurosurg 1991–1992;17:284–303.

306. Sanford RA, Muhlbauer MS. Craniopharyngioma in children. Neurol Clin 1991;9:453–465.

307. Ikezaki K, Fujii K, Kishikawa T. Magnetic resonance imaging of an intraventricular craniopharyngioma. Neuroradiology 1990;32:247–249.

308. Matthews FD. Intraventricular craniopharyngioma. AJNR 1983;4:984–985.

309. Hillman TH, Peyster RG, Hoover ED, et al. Infrasellar craniopharyngioma: CT and MR studies. J Comput Assist Tomogr 1988;12:702–704.

310. Akimura T, Kameda H, Abiko S, et al. Infrasellar craniopharyngioma. Neuroradiology 1989;31:180–183.

311. Patrick CK, DeGirolami U, Earle KM. Craniopharyngiomas: A clinical and pathological review. Cancer 1976;37:1944–1952.

312. Weiner HL, Wisoff JH, Rosenberg ME, et al. Craniopharyngiomas: A clinicopathological analysis of factors predictive of recurrence and functional outcome. Neurosurgery 1994;35:1001–1011.

313. Miller DC. Pathology of craniopharyngiomas: Clinical import of pathological findings. Pediatr Neurosurg 1994;21(Suppl 1):11–17.

314. Hoffman HJ, DeSilva M, Humphreys RP, et al. Aggressive surgical management of craniopharyngiomas in children. J Neurosurg 1992;76:47–52.

315. Hetelekidis S, Barnes PD, Tao ML, et al. 20-year experience in childhood craniopharyngioma. Int J Radiat Oncol Biol Phys 1993;27:189–195.

316. Fitz CR, Wortzman G, Harwood-Nash DC, et al. Computed tomography in craniopharyngiomas. Radiology 1978;127:687–691.

317. Freeman MP, Kessler RM, Allen JH, et al. Craniopharyngioma: CT and MR imaging in nine cases. J Comput Assist Tomogr 1987;11:810–814.

318. Pusey E, Kortman KE, Flannigan BD, et al. MR of craniopharyngiomas: Tumor delineation and characterization. AJNR 1987;8:439–444.

319. Ahmadi J, Destian S, Apuzzo MLJ, et al. Cystic fluid in craniopharyngiomas: MR imaging and quantitative analysis. Radiology 1992;182:783–785.

320. Hershey BL. Suprasellar masses: Diagnosis and differential diagnosis. Semin Ultrasound CT MR 1993;14:215–231.

321. Young SC, Zimmerman RA, Nowell MA, et al. Giant cystic craniopharyngiomas. Neuroradiology 1987;29:468–473.

322. Youl BD, Plant GT, Stevens JM, et al. Three cases of craniopharyngioma showing optic tract hypersignal on MRI. Neurology 1990;40:1416–1419.

323. Hald JK, Eldevik OP, Brunberg JA, et al. Craniopharyngiomas—the utility of contrast medium enhancement for MR imaging at 1.5T. Acta Radiol 1994;35:520–525.

324. Voelker JL, Campbell RL, Muller J. Clinical, radiographic, and pathological features of symptomatic Rathke's cleft cysts. J Neurosurg 1991;74:535–544.

325. Ito H, Shoin K, Hwang W-Z, et al. Preoperative diagnosis of Rathke's cleft cyst. Childs Nerv Syst 1987;3:225–227.

326. Harrison MJ, Morgello S, Post KD. Epithelial cystic lesions of the sellar and parasellar region: A continuum of ectodermal derivatives? J Neurosurg 1994;80:1018–1025.

327. Woodruff WW Jr, Heinz ER, Djang WT, et al. Hyperporlactinemia: An unusual manifestation of suprasellar cystic lesions. AJNR 1987;8:113–116.

328. Kucharczyk W, Peck WW, Kelly WM, et al. Rathke cleft cysts: CT, MR imaging, and pathologic features. Radiology 1987;165:491–495.

329. Asari S, Ito T, Tsuchida S, et al. MR appearance and cyst content of Rathke cleft cysts. J Comput Assist Tomogr 1990;14:532–535.

330. Mize W, Ball WS, Towbin BK, et al. Atypical CT and MR appearance of a Rathke cleft cyst. AJNR 1989;10(Suppl):S83–S84.

331. Nemoto Y, Inoue Y, Fukuda T, et al. MR appearance of Rathke's cleft cysts. Neuroradiology 1988;30:155–159.

332. Oka H, Kawano N, Suwa T, et al. Radiological study of symptomatic Rathke's cleft cysts. Neurosurgery 1994;35:632–637.

333. Sumida M, Uozumi T, Mukada K, et al. Rathke cleft cysts: Correlation of enhanced MR and surgical findings. AJNR 1994;15:525–532.

334. Whyte AM, Sage MR, Brophy BP. Imaging of large Rathke's cleft cysts by CT and MRI: Report of two cases. Neuroradiology 1993;35:258–260.

335. Hua F, Asato R, Miki Y, et al. Differentiation of suprasellar nonneoplastic cysts from cystic neoplasms by Gd-DTPA MRI. J Comput Assist Tomogr 1992;16:744–749.

336. Okamoto S, Handa H, Yamashita J, et al. Computed tomography in intra- and suprasellar epithelial cysts (symptomatic Rathke cleft cysts). AJNR 1985;6:515–519.

337. Naylor MF, Scheithauer BW, Forbes GS, et al. Rathke cleft cysts: CT, MR, and pathology of 23 cases. J Comput Assist Tomogr 1995;19:853–859.

338. Christophe C, Flamant-Durand J, Hanquinet S, et al. MRI in seven cases of Rathke's cleft cyst in infants and children. Pediatr Radiol 1993;23:79–82.

339. Ross DA, Norman D, Wilson CB. Radiologic characteristics and results of surgical management of Rathke's cysts in 43 patients. Neurosurgery 1992;30:173–179.

340. Hoffman HJ, Hendrick EB, Humphreys RP, et al. Investigation and management of suprasellar arachnoid cysts. J Neurosurg 1982;57:597–602.

341. Benton JW, Nellhaus G, Huttenlocher PR, et al. The bobble-head doll syndrome. Report of a unique truncal tremor associated with third ventricular cyst and hydrocephalus in children. Neurology 1966;16:725–729.

342. Pierre-Kahn A, Capelle L, Brauner R, et al. Presentation and management of suprasellar arachnoid cysts. J Neurosurg 1990;73:355–359.

343. McCullough DC, Harbert JC, Manz HJ, et al. Large arachnoid cysts at the cranial base. Neurosurgery 1980;6:76–81.

344. Harsh GR, Edwards MSB, Wilson CB. Intracranial arachnoid cysts in children. J Neurosurg 1986;64:835–842.

345. Go KG, Houthoff HJ, Blaauw EH, et al. Arachnoid cysts of the sylvian fissure. Evidence of fluid secretion. J Neurosurg 1984;60:803–810.

346. DiRocco C, Caldarelli M, DiTrapani G. Infratentorial arachnoid cysts in children. Childs Brain 1981;8:119–133.

347. Fox JL, Al-Mefty O. Suprasellar arachnoid cysts: An extension of the membrane of Liliequist. Neurosurgery 1980;7:615–618.

348. Gentry LR, Smoker WRK, Turski PA, et al. Suprasellar arachnoid cysts. 1. CT recognition. AJNR 1986;7:79–86.

349. Weiner SN, Pearlstein AE, Eiber A. MR imaging of intracranial arachnoid cysts. J Comput Assist Tomogr 1987;11:236–241.

350. Quint DJ. Retroclival arachnoid cysts. AJNR 1992;13:1503–1504.

351. Berkovic SF, Andermann F, Melanson D, et al. Hypothalamic hamartomas and ictal laughter: Evolution of a characteristic epileptic syndrome and diagnostic value of magnetic resonance imaging. Ann Neurol 1988;23:429–439.

352. Mahachoklertwattana P, Kaplan SL, Grumbach MM. The luteinizing hormone–releasing hormone-secreting hypothalamic hamartoma is a congenital malformation: Natural history. J Clin Endocrinol Metab 1993;77:118–124.

353. Robben SGF, Oostdijk W, Drop SLS, et al. Idiopathic isosexual

central precocious puberty: Magnetic resonance findings in 30 patients. Br J Radiol 1995;68:34–38.

354. Marliani AF, Tampieri D, Melancon D, et al. Magnetic resonance imaging of hypothalamic hamartomas causing gelastic epilepsy. Can Assoc Radiol J 1991;42:335–339.

355. Nishio S, Fujiwara S, Aiko Y, et al. Hypothalamic hamartoma. Report of two cases. J Neurosurg 1989;70:640–649.

356. Diebler C, Ponsot G. Hamartomas of the tuber cinereum. Neuroradiology 1983;25:93–101.

357. Cheng K, Sawamura Y, Yamauchi T, et al. Asymptomatic large hypothalamic hamartoma associated with polydactyly in an adult. Neurosurgery 1993;32:458–460.

358. Löw M, Moringlane JR, Reif J, et al. Polysyndactyly and asymptomatic hypothalamic hamartoma in mother and son: A variant of Pallister-Hall syndrome. Clin Genet 1995;48:209–212.

359. Grebe TA, Clericuzio C. Autosomal dominant inheritance of hypothalamic hamartoma associated with polysyndactyly: Heterogeneity or variable expressivity? Am J Med Genet 1996;66:129–137.

360. Hall JG, Pallister PD, Clarren SK, et al. Congenital hypothalamic hamartoblastoma, hypopituitarism, imperforate anus, and postaxial polydactyly—a new syndrome? Part I. Clinical, casual and pathogenetic considerations. Am J Med Genet 1980;7:47–74.

361. Topf KF, Kletter GB, Kelch RP, et al. Autosomal dominant transmission of the Pallister-Hall syndrome. J Pediatr 1993;123:943–946.

362. Burton EM, Ball WS, Crone K, et al. Hamartoma of the tuber cinereum: A comparison of MR and CT findings in four cases. AJNR 1989;10:497–501.

363. Barral V, Brunelle F, Brauner R, et al. MRI of hypothalamic hamartomas in children. Pediatr Radiol 1988;18:449–452.

364. Hahn FJ, Leibrock LG, Huseman CA, et al. The MR appearance of hypothalamic hamartoma. Neuroradiology 1988;30:65–68.

365. Hubbard AM, Egelhoff JC. MR imaging of large hypothalamic hamartomas in two infants. AJNR 1989;10(Suppl):1277.

366. Boyko OB, Curnes JT, Oakes WJ, et al. Hamartomas of the tuber cinereum: CT, MR, and pathologic findings. AJNR 1991;12:309–314.

367. Albright AL, Lee PA. Neurosurgical treatment of hypothalamic hamartomas causing precocious puberty. J Neurosurg 1993;78:77–82.

368. Sato M, Ushio Y, Arita N, et al. Hypothalamic hamartoma: Report of two cases. Neurosurgery 1995;16:198–206.

369. Jennings MT, Gelman R, Hochberg F. Intracranial germ-cell tumors: Natural history and pathogenesis. J Neurosurg 1985;63:155–167.

370. Sugiyama K, Uozumi T, Kiya K, et al. Intracranial germ-cell tumor with synchronous lesions in the pineal and suprasellar regions: Report of six cases and review of the literature. Surg Neurol 1992;38:114–120.

371. Shokry A, Janzer RC, VonHochstetter AR, et al. Primary intracranial germ-cell tumors. J Neurosurg 1985;62:826–830.

372. Nishio S, Inamura T, Takeshita I, et al. Germ cell tumor in the hypothalamo-neurohypophysial region: Clinical features and treatment. Neurosurg Rev 1993;16:221–227.

373. Hoffman HJ, Otsubo H, Hendrick EB, et al. Intracranial germ-cell tumors in children. J Neurosurg 1991;74:545–551.

374. Zimmerman RA. Imaging of intrasellar, suprasellar, and parasellar tumors. Semin Roentgenol 1990;25:174–197.

375. Legido A, Packer RJ, Sutton LN, et al. Suprasellar germinomas in childhood. Cancer 1989;63:340–344.

376. Rutka JT, Hoffman HJ, Drake JM, et al. Suprasellar and sellar tumors in childhood and adolescence. Neurosurg Clin N Am 1992;3:803–820.

377. Frank G, Galassi E, Fabrizi AP, et al. Primary intrasellar germinoma: Case report. Neurosurgery 1992;30:786–788.

378. Fujisawa I, Asato R, Okumura R, et al. Magnetic resonance imaging of neurohypophyseal germinomas. Cancer 1991;68:1009–1014.

379. Fujisawa I, Nishimura K, Asato R, et al. Posterior lobe of the pituitary in diabetes insipidus. J Comput Assist Tomogr 1987;11:221–225.

380. Fujisawa I, Asato R, Kawata M, et al. Hyperintense signal of the posterior pituitary on T1-weighted MR images: An experimental study. J Comput Assist Tomogr 1990;13:371–377.

381. Mark LP, Haughton VM, Hendrix J, et al. High-intensity signals within the posterior pituitary fossa: A study with fat-suppression MR techniques. AJNR 1991;12:929–932.

382. Manelfe C, Louvet J-P. Computed tomography in diabetes insipidus. J Comput Assist Tomogr 1979;3:309–316.

383. Tien RD, Newton TH, McDermott MW, et al. Thickened pituitary stalk on MR images in patients with diabetes insipidus and Langerhans cell histiocytosis. AJNR 1990;11:703–708.

384. Maghnie M, Arico M, Villa A, et al. MR of the hypothalamic-pituitary axis in Langherhans cell histiocytosis. AJNR 1992;13:1365–1371.

385. Nishio S, Mizuno J, Barro DL, et al. Isolated histiocytosis-X, the pituitary gland: Case report. Neurosurgery 1987;21:718–721.

386. Chambers AA, Lukin RR, Tomsick TA. Suprasellar masses. Semin Roentgenol 1984;19:84–90.

387. Jallu A, Rahm B, Kanaan I, et al. Pituitary tooth: Case report of a suprasellar teratoma. Childs Nerv Syst 1990;6:368–369.

388. Konovalov AN, Lichterman BL, Korshunov AG. Endo-suprasellar teratoma with teeth formation. Case report. Acta Neurochir (Wien) 1992;118:181–184.

389. Kobayashi N. Suprasellar teratoma. [Letter] Childs Nerv Syst 1991;7:117–119.

390. Karnaze MG, Sartor K, Winthrop JD, et al. Suprasellar lesions: Evaluation with MR imaging. Radiology 1986;161:77–82.

391. Lee BCP, Deck MDF. Sellar and juxtasellar lesion detection with MR. Radiology 1985;157:143–147.

392. Cohen ME, Duffner PK. Optic pathway tumors. Neurol Clin 1991;9:467–477.

393. Kuenzle Ch, Weissert M, Roulet E, et al. Follow-up of optic pathway gliomas in children with neurofibromatosis type 1. Neuropediatrics 1994;25:295–300.

394. Riccardi VM. Neurofibromatosis: Past, present, and future. N Engl J Med 1991;324:1283–1285.

395. Wisoff JH. Management of optic pathway tumors of childhood. Neurosurg Clin Am 1992;3:791–802.

396. Alvord EC, Lofton S. Gliomas of the optic nerve or chiasm. J Neurosurg 1988;68:85–98.

397. Jenkin D, Angyalfi S, Becker L, et al. Optic gliomas in children: Surveillance, resection, or irradiation. Int J Radiat Oncol Biol Phys 1993;25:215–225.

398. Stern J, DiGiacinto GV, Housepian EM. Neurofibromatosis and optic glioma: Clinical and morphological correlations. Neurosurgery 1979;4:524–528.

399. Venes JL, Latack J, Kandt RS. Postoperative regression of opticochiasmatic astrocytoma: A case for expectant therapy. Neurosurgery 1984;15:421–423.

400. Imes RK, Hoyt WY. Childhood chiasmal gliomas: Update of the facts of patients in the 1969 San Francisco study. Br J Ophthalmol 1986;70:179–182.

401. Millar WS, Tartaglino LM, Sergott RC, et al. MR of malignant optic glioma of adulthood. AJNR 1995;16:1673–1676.

402. Fletcher WA, Imes RK, Hoyt WF. Chiasmal gliomas: Appearance and long-term changes demonstrated by computerized tomography. J Neurosurg 1986;65:154–159.

403. Savoiardo M, Harwood-Nash DC, Tadmor R, et al. Gliomas of the intracranial anterior optic pathways in children. Radiology 1981;138:601–610.

404. Lourie GL, Osborne DR, Kirks DR. Involvement of posterior visual pathways by optic nerve gliomas. Pediatr Radiol 1986;16:271–274.

405. Brown EW, Riccardi VM, Mawad M, et al. MR imaging of optic pathways in patients with neurofibromatosis. AJNR 1987;8:1031–1036.

406. Aoki S, Barkovich AJ, Nishimura K, et al. Neurofibromatosis types 1 and 2: Cranial MR findings. Radiology 1989;172:527–534.

407. Imes RK, Hoyt WF. MR imaging signs of optic nerve gliomas in neurofibromatosis 1. Am J Ophthalmol 1991;111:729–734.

408. Bognanno JR, Edwards MK, Lee TA, et al. Cranial MR imaging in neurofibromatosis. AJR 1988;151:381–388.

409. Menor F, Martí-Bonmatí L, Mulas F, et al. Imaging considerations of central nervous system manifestations in pediatric patients with neurofibromatosis type 1. Pediatr Radiol 1991;21:389–394.

410. Parazzini C, Triulzi F, Bianchini E, et al. Spontaneous involution of optic pathway lesions in neurofibromatosis type 1: Serial contrast MR evaluation. AJNR 1995;16:1711–1718.

411. Mercuri S, Russo A, Palma L. Hemispheric supratentorial astrocytomas in children. J Neurosurg 1981;55:170–173.

412. Krouwer HGJ, Prados MD. Infiltrative astrocytomas of the thalamus. J Neurosurg 1995;82:548–557.

413. Balestrini MR, Zanette M, Micheli R, et al. Hemispheric cerebral tumors in children. Childs Nerv Syst 1990;6:143–147.

414. Pollack IF, Claassen D, Al-Shboul Q, et al. Low-grade gliomas of the cerebral hemispheres in children: An analysis of 71 cases. J Neurosurg 1995;82:536–547.

415. Katsetos CD, Krishna L. Lobar pilocytic astrocytomas of the cerebral hemispheres. I. Diagnosis and nosology. Clin Neuropathol 1994;13:295–305.

416. Palma L, Guidetti B. Cystic pilocytic astrocytomas of the cerebral hemispheres. J Neurosurg 1985;62:811–815.

417. Finizio FS. CT and MRI aspects of supratentorial hemispheric tumors of childhood and adolescence. Childs Nerv Syst 1995;11:559–567.

418. Pfleger MJ, Gerson LP. Supratentorial tumors in children. Neuroimaging Clin N Am 1993;3:671–687.

419. Dropcho EJ, Wisoff JH, Walker RW, et al. Supratentorial malignant gliomas in childhood: A review of fifty cases. Ann Neurol 1987;22:355–364.

420. Marchese MJ, Chang CH. Malignant astrocytic gliomas in children. Cancer 1990;65:2771–2778.

421. Hoppe-Hirsch E, Hirsch JF, Lellouch-Tubianna A, et al. Malignant hemispheric tumors in childhood. Childs Nerv Syst 1993;9:131–135.

422. Artico M, Cervoni L, Celli P, et al. Supratentorial glioblastoma in children: A series of 27 surgically treated cases. Childs Nerv System 1993;9:7–9.

423. Pedersen H, Cjerris F, Klinken L. Malignancy criteria in computed tomography of primary supratentorial tumors in infancy and childhood. Neuroradiology 1989;31:24–28.

424. Bernstein M, Hoffman HJ, Halliday WC. Thalamic tumors in children. J Neurosurg 1984;61:649–656.

425. Page LK, Clark R. Gliomas of the septal area in children. Neurosurgery 1981;8:651–655.

426. Artigas J, Cervos-Navarro J, Iglesias JR, et al. Gliomatosis cerebri: Clinical and histologic findings. Clin Neuropathol 1985;4:135–148.

427. Felsberg GJ, Silver SA, Brown MT, et al. Radiologic-pathologic correlation. Gliomatosis cerebri. AJNR 1994;15:1745–1753.

428. del Carpio-O'Donovan R, Korah I, Salazar A, et al. Gliomatosis cerebri. Radiology 1996;198:831–835.

429. Jennings MT, Frenchman M, Shehab T, et al. Gliomatosis cerebri presenting as intractable epilepsy during early childhood. J Child Neurol 1995;10:37–45.

430. Shin YM, Chang KH, Han MH, et al. Gliomatosis cerebri: Comparison of MR and CT features. AJR 1993;161:859–862.

431. Geremia GK, Wollman R, Foust R. Computed tomography of gliomatosis cerebri. J Comput Assist Tomogr 1988;12:698–701.

432. Dexter MA, Parker GD, Besser M, et al. MR and positron emission tomography with fludeoxyglucose F 18 in gliomatosis cerebri. AJNR 1995;16:1507–1510.

433. Spagnoli MV, Grossman RI, Packer RJ, et al. Magnetic resonance imaging determination of gliomatosis cerebri. Neuroradiology 1987;29:15–18.

434. Ross IB, Robitaille Y, Villemure JG, et al. Diagnosis and management of gliomatosis cerebri: Recent trends. Surg Neurol 1991;36:431–440.

435. Higano S, Takahashi S, Ishii K, et al. Germinoma originating in the basal ganglia and thalamus: MR and CT evaluation. AJNR 1994;15:1435–1441.

436. Ho DM, Liu H-C. Primary intracranial germ cell tumor. Pathologic study of 51 patients. Cancer 1992;70:1577–1584.

437. Soejima T, Takeshita I, Yamamoto H, et al. Computed tomography of germinomas in basal ganglia and thalamus. Neuroradiology 1987;29:366–370.

438. Moon WK, Chang KH, Kim I-O. Germinomas of the basal ganglia and thalamus: MR findings and a comparison between MR and CT. AJR 1984;162:1413–1417.

439. Kobayashi T, Yoshida J, Kida Y. Bilateral germ cell tumors involving the basal ganglia and thalamus. Neurosurgery 1989;24:579–583.

440. Komatsu Y, Narushima K, Kobayashi E, et al. CT and MR of germinoma in the basal ganglia. AJNR 1989;10:S9–S11.

441. Mutoh K, Okuno T, Ito M, et al. Ipsilateral atrophy in children with hemispheric tumors: CT findings. J Comput Assist Tomogr 1988;12:740–743.

442. Smith NM, Carli MM, Hanieh A, et al. Gangliogliomas in childhood. Childs Nerv Syst 1992;8:258–262.

443. Demierre B, Stichnoth FA, Hori A, et al. Intracerebral ganglioglioma. J Neurosurg 1986;65:177–182.

444. Sutton LN, Packer RJ, Zimmerman RA, et al. Cerebral gangliogliomas of childhood. Prog Exp Tumor Res 1987;30:239–246.

445. Zentner J, Wolf HK, Ostertun B, et al. Gangliogliomas: Clinical, radiological, and histopathological findings in 51 patients. J Neurol Neurosurg Psychiatry 1994;57:1497–1502.

446. Kuznieck R, Murro A, King D, et al. Magnetic resonance imaging in childhood intractable partial epilepsies: Pathologic correlations. Neurology 1993;43:681–687.

447. Brooks BS, King DW, Gammal TE, et al. MR imaging in patients with intractable complex partial epileptic seizures. AJNR 1990;11:93–99.

448. Khajavi K, Comair YG, Prayson RA, et al. Childhood ganglioglioma and medically intractable epilepsy. A clinicopathological study of 15 patients and a review of the literature. Pediatr Neurosurg 1995;22:181–188.

449. Johannsson JH, Rekate HL, Roessmann U. Gangliogliomas: Pathological and clinical correlation. J Neurosurg 1981;54:58–63.

450. Mickle JP. Ganglioglioma in children. A review of 32 cases at the University of Florida. Pediatr Neurosurg 1992;18:310–314.

451. Russell DS, Rubinstein LJ. Ganglioglioma: A case with long history and malignant evolution. J Neuropathol Exp Neurol 1962;21:185–193.

452. Silver JM, Rawlings CE, Rossitch E, et al. Ganglioglioma: A clinical study with long-term follow-up. Surg Neurol 1991;35:261–266.

453. Garrido E, Becker LF, Hoffman HJ, et al. Gangliogliomas in children. A clinicopathological study. Childs Brain 1978;4:339–346.

454. Rommel T, Hamer J. Development of ganglioglioma in computed tomography. Neuroradiology 1983;24:237–239.

455. Diepholder HM, Schwechheimer K, Mohadjer M, et al. A clinicopathologic and immunomorphologic study of 13 cases of ganglioglioma. Cancer 1991;68:2192–2201.

456. Tampieri D, Moumdjian R, Melanson D, et al. Intracerebral gangliogliomas in patients with partial complex seizures: CT and MR imaging findings. AJNR 1991;12:749–755.

457. Nass R, Whelan MA. Gangliogliomas. Neuroradiology 1981;22:67–71.

458. Sutton LN, Packer RJ, Rorke LB, et al. Cerebral gangliogliomas during childhood. Neurosurgery 1983;13:124–128.

459. Haddad SF, Moore SA, Menezes AH, et al. Ganglioglioma: 13 years of experience. Neurosurgery 1992;31:171–178.

460. Dorne HL, O'Gorman AM, Melanson D. Computed tomography of intracranial gangliogliomas. AJNR 1986;7:281–285.

461. Castillo M, Davis PC, Takei Y, et al. Intracranial ganglioglioma: MR, CT, and clinical findings in 18 patients. AJNR 1990;11:109–114.

462. Benitez WI, Glasier CM, Husain M, et al. MR findings in childhood gangliogliomas. J Comput Assist Tomogr 1990;14:712–716.

463. Hashimoto M, Fujimoto K, Shinoda S, et al. Magnetic resonance imaging of ganglion cell tumors. Neuroradiology 1993;35:181–184.

464. Otsubo H, Hoffman HJ, Humphreys RP, et al. Detection and management of gangliogliomas in children. Surg Neurol 1992;38:371–378.

465. Wacker MR, Cogen PH, Etzell JE, et al. Diffuse leptomeningeal involvement by a ganglioglioma in a child. J Neurosurg 1992;77:302–306.

466. Tien RD, Tuori SL, Pulkingham N, et al. Ganglioglioma with leptomeningeal and subarachnoid spread: Results of CT, MR and PET imaging. AJR 1992;159:391–393.

467. Harle TS, Carrol CL, Leeds NE, et al. Image interpretation session: 1994. Radiographics 1995;15:211–233.

468. Blatt GL, Ahuja A, Miller LL, et al. Cerebellomedullary ganglioglioma: CT and MR findings. AJNR 1995;16:790–792.

469. Martin LD, Kaplan AM, Hernried LS, et al. Brainstem gangliogliomas. Pediatr Neurol 1986;2:178–182.

470. Duchowny MS, Resnick TJ, Alvarez L. Dysplastic gangliocytoma and intractable partial seizures in childhood. Neurology 1989;39:602–604.

471. Altman NR. MR and CT characteristics of gangliocytoma: A rare cause of epilepsy in children. AJNR 1988;9:917–921.

472. Dohrmann J, Farwell JR, Flannery JT. Oligodendrogliomas in children. Surg Neurol 1978;10:21–25.

473. Peterson K, Cairncross JG. Oligodendrogliomas. Neurol Clin 1995;13:861–873.

474. Favier J, Pizzolato GP, Berney J. Oligodendroglial tumors in childhood. Childs Nerv Syst 1985;1:33–38.

475. Packer RJ, Sutton LN, Rorke LB, et al. Oligodendrogliomas of the posterior fossa in childhood. Cancer 1985;56:195–199.

476. Ludwig CL, Smith MT, Godfrey AD, et al. A clinicopathological study of 323 patients with oligodendrogliomas. Ann Neurol 1986;19:15–21.

477. Nijjar TS, Simpson WJ, Gadalla T, et al. Oligodendroglioma. The Princess Margaret Hospital experience (1958–1984). Cancer 1993;71:4002–4006.

478. Kros JM, Pieterman H, vanEden CG, et al. Oligodendroglioma: The Rotterdam-Dijkzigt experience. Neurosurgery 1994;34:959–966.

479. Shimizu KT, Tran LM, Mark RJ, et al. Management of oligodendrogliomas. Radiology 1993;186:569–572.

480. Vonofakos D, Marcu H, Hacker H. Oligodendrogliomas: CT patterns with emphasis on features indicating malignancy. J Comput Assist Tomogr 1979;3:783–788.

481. Lee YY, Tassel PV. Intracranial oligodendrogliomas: Imaging findings in 35 untreated cases. AJNR 1989;10:119–127.

482. Tice H, Barnes PD, Goumnerova L, et al. Pediatric and adolescent oligodendrogliomas. AJNR 1993;14:1293–1300.

483. Davies KG, Maxwell RE, Seljeskog E, et al. Pleomorphic xanthoastrocytoma—report of four cases, with MRI scan appearances and literature review. Br J Neurosurg 1994;8:681–689.

484. Thomas C, Golden B. Pleomorphic xanthoastrocytoma: Report of two cases and brief review of the literature. Clin Neuropathol 1993;12:97–101.

485. Kepes JJ, Rubinstein LJ, Eng LF. Pleomorphic xanthoastrocytoma: A distinctive meningocerebral glioma of young subjects with relatively favorable prognosis. Cancer 1979;44:1839–1852.

486. Weldon-Linne CM, Victor TA, Groothuis DR, et al. Pleomorphic xanthoastrocytoma. Ultrastructural and immunohistochemical study of a case with a rapidly fatal outcome following surgery. Cancer 1983;52:2055–2063.

487. Whittle IR, Gordon A, Misra BK, et al. Pleomorphic xanthoastrocytoma. Report of four cases. J Neurosurg 1989;70:463–468.

488. Macaulay RJ, Jay V, Hoffman HJ, et al. Increased mitotic activity as a negative prognostic indicator in pleomorphic xanthoastrocytoma. Case report. J Neurosurg 1993;79:761–768.

489. Blom RJ. Pleomorphic xanthoastrocytoma: CT appearance. J Comput Assist Tomogr 1988;12:351–352.

490. Yoshino MRT, Lucio R. Pleomorphic xanthoastrocytoma. AJNR 1992;13:1330–1332.

491. Petropoulou K, Whiteman MLH, Altman NR, et al. CT and MRI of pleomorphic xanthoastrocytoma: Unusual biologic behavior. J Comput Assist Tomogr 1995;19:860–865.

492. Brown JH, Chew FS. Pleomorphic xanthoastrocytoma. AJR 1993;160:1272.

493. Lipper MH, Eberhard DA, Phillips CD, et al. Pleomorphic xanthoastrocytoma, a distinctive astroglial tumor: Neuroradiologic and pathologic features. AJNR 1993;14:1397–1404.

494. Bicik I, Raman R, Knightly JJ, et al. PET-FDG of pleomorphic xanthoastrocytoma. J Nucl Med 1995;36:97–99.

495. Mascalchi M, Muscas GC, Galli C, et al. MRI of pleomorphic xanthoastrocytoma: Case report. Neuroradiology 1994;36:446–447.

496. Tien RD, Cardenas CA, Rajagopalan S. Pleomorphic xanthoastrocytoma of the brain: MR findings in six patients. AJR 1992;159:1287–1290.

497. Rippe DJ, Boyko OB, Radi M, et al. MRI of temporal lobe pleomorphic xanthoastrocytoma. J Comput Assist Tomogr 1992;16:856–859.

498. Rovit RL, Schechter MM, Chodroff P. Choroid plexus papillomas. Observations on radiographic diagnosis. AJR 1970;110:608–617.

499. Shoemaker EI, Romano AJ, Gado M. Neuroradiology case of the day 2: Choroid plexus papilloma, third ventricle. AJR 1989;152:133–135.

500. Ellenbogen RG, Winston KR, Kupsky WJ. Tumors of the choroid plexus in children. Neurosurgery 1989;25:327–335.

501. Coates TL, Hinshaw DB, Peckman N, et al. Pediatric choroid plexus neoplasms: MR, CT, and pathologic correlation. Radiology 1989;173:81–88.

502. Spallone A, Pastore FS, Giuffre R, et al. Choroid plexus papillomas in infancy and childhood. Childs Nerv Syst 1990;6:71–74.

503. Cila A, Ozturk C, Senaati S. Bilateral choroid plexus carcinoma of the lateral ventricles. Pediatr Radiol 1992;22:136–137.

504. Pascual-Castroviejo I, Villarejo F, Perez-Higueras A, et al. Childhood choroid plexus neoplasms. A study of 14 cases less than 2 years old. Eur J Pediatr 1983;140:51–56.

505. Pierga JY, Kalifa C, Terrier-Lacombe MJ, et al. Carcinoma of the choroid plexus: A pediatric experience. Med Pediatr Oncol 1993;21:480–487.

506. Kahn EA, Luros JT. Hydrocephalus from overproduction of cerebrospinal fluid (and other experiences with papillomas of the choroid plexus). J Neurosurg 1952;9:59–67.

507. Eisenberg HM, McComb JG, Lorenzo AV. Cerebrospinal fluid overproduction and hydrocephalus associated with choroid plexus papilloma. J Neurosurg 1974;40:381–385.

508. Milhorat TH, Davis DA, Hammock MK. Choroid plexus papilloma. II. Ultrastructure and ultracytochemical localization of Na-K-ATPase. Childs Brain 1976;2:290–303.

509. McDonald JV. Persistent hydrocephalus following removal of papillomas of the choroid plexus of the lateral ventricles. J Neurosurg 1969;30:736–740.

510. Schijman E, Monges J, Raimondi AJ, Tomita T. Choroid plexus papillomas of the III ventricle in childhood. Childs Nerv Syst 1990;6:331–334.

511. Packer RJ, Perilongo G, Johnson D, et al. Choroid plexus carcinoma of childhood. Cancer 1992;69:580–585.

512. Sharma R, Rout D, Gupta AK, et al. Choroid plexus papillomas. Br J Neurosurg 1994;8:169–177.

513. St. Clair SK, Humphreys RP, Pillay PK, et al. Current management of choroid plexus carcinoma in children. Pediatr Neurosurg 1991–1992;17:225–233.

514. Kendall B, Reider-Grosswasser I, Valentine A. Diagnosis of masses presenting within the ventricles on computed tomography. Neuroradiology 1983;25:11–22.

515. Ken JG, Sobel DF, Copeland B, et al. Choroid plexus papillomas of the foramen of Luschka: MR appearance. AJNR 1991;12:1201–1203.

516. Jelinek J, Smirniotopoulos JG, Parisi JE. Lateral ventricular neoplasms of the brain: Differential diagnosis based on clinical, CT, and MR findings. AJNR 1990;11:567–574.

517. Matsushima T, Kitamura K, Fukui M, et al. Choroid plexus papillomas. Prog Exp Tumor Res 1987;30:181–193.

518. Hopper KD, Foley LC, Nieves NL, et al. The intraventricular extension of choroid plexus papillomas. AJNR 1987;8:469–472.

519. Tien RD. Intraventricular mass lesions of the brain: CT and MR findings. AJR 1991;157:1283–1290.

520. Gaskill SJJ, Saldivar V, Rutman J, et al. Giant bilateral xanthogranulomas in a child: Case report. Neurosurgery 1992;31:114–117.

521. Braffman BH, Bilaniuk LT, Naidich TP, et al. MR imaging of tuberous sclerosis: Pathogenesis of this phakomatosis, use of gadopentetate dimeglumine, and literature review. Radiology 1992;183:227–238.

522. Tien RD, Hesselink JR, Duberg A. Rare subependymal giant-cell astrocytoma in a neonate with tuberous sclerosis. AJNR 1990;11:1251–1252.

523. Holanda FJCS, Holanda GMP. Tuberous sclerosis: Neurosurgical indications in intraventricular tumors. Neurosurg Rev 1980;3:139–150.

524. Prahlow JA, Teot LA, Lantz PE, et al. Sudden death in epilepsy due to an isolated subependymal giant cell astrocytoma of the septum pellucidum. Am J Forensic Med Pathol 1995;16:30–37.

525. Rieger E, Binder B, Starz I, et al. Tuberous sclerosis complex: Oligosymptomatic variant associated with subependymal giant-cell astrocytoma. Pediatr Radiol 1991;21:432.

526. Kingsley DPE, Kendall BE, Fitz CR. Tuberous sclerosis: A clinicoradiological evaluation of 110 cases with particular reference to atypical presentation. Neuroradiology 1986;28:38–46.

527. Morimoto K, Mogami H. Sequential CT study of subependymal giant-cell astrocytoma associated with tuberous sclerosis. Case report. J Neurosurg 1986;65:874–877.

528. Whittle IR. Anterior lateral ventricular subependymal giant cell astrocytomas. Microsurgical aspects of two cases. Acta Neurochir (Wien) 1992;118:176–180.

529. Chow CW, Klug GL, Lewis EA. Subependymal giant-cell astrocytoma in children. An unusual discrepancy between histological and clinical features. J Neurosurg 1988;68:880–883.

530. Fitz CR, Harwood-Nash DCF, Thompson JR. Neuroradiology of tuberous sclerosis in children. Radiology 1974;110:635–642.

531. Roszkowski M, Drabik K, Barszcz S, et al. Surgical treatment of intraventricular tumors associated with tuberous sclerosis. Childs Nerv Syst 1995;11:335–339.

532. Fujiwara S, Takaki T, Hikita T, et al. Subependymal giant-cell astrocytoma associated with tuberous sclerosis. Do subependymal nodules grow? Childs Nerv Syst 1989;5:43–44.

533. Boesel CP, Paulson GW, Kosnik EJ, et al. Brain hamartomas and tumors associated with tuberous sclerosis. Neurosurgery 1979;4:410–417.

534. Eisenberg HM. Supratentorial astrocytoma. In American Association of Neurological Surgeons (eds). Pediatric Neurosurgery. Surgery of the Developing Nervous System, pp. 429–432. New York, Grune & Stratton, 1982.

535. Shepherd CW, Houser OW, Gomez MR. MR findings in tuberous sclerosis complex and correlation with seizure development and mental impairment. AJNR 1995;16:149–155.

536. Martin N, Debussche C, DeBroucker T, et al. Gadolinium-DTPA enhanced imaging in tuberous sclerosis. Neuroradiology 1990;31:492–497.

537. Altman NR, Purser RK, Post MJD. Tuberous sclerosis: Characteristics at CT and MR imaging. Radiology 1988;167:527–532.

538. Lee BCP, Gawler J. Tuberous sclerosis: Comparison of computed tomography and conventional neuroradiology. Radiology 1978;127:403–407.

539. McMurdo SK, Moore SG, Brant-Zawadzki M, et al. MR imaging of intracranial tuberous sclerosis. AJNR 1987;8:77–82.

540. Nixon JR, Houser OW, Gomez MR, et al. Cerebral tuberous sclerosis: MR imaging. Radiology 1989;170:869–873.

541. Menor F, Marti-Bonmati L, Mulas F, et al. Neuroimaging in tuberous sclerosis: A clinicoradiological evaluation in pediatric patients. Pediatr Radiol 1992;22:485–489.

542. Wippold FJ, Baber WW, Gado M, et al. Pre- and postcontrast MR studies in tuberous sclerosis. J Comput Assist Tomgr 1992;16:69–72.

543. Moran V, O'Keeffe F. Giant cell astrocytoma in tuberous sclerosis: Computed tomographic findings. Clin Radiol 1986;37:543–545.

544. Winter J. Computed tomography in diagnosis of intracranial tumors versus tubers in tuberous sclerosis. Acta Radiol 1982;23:337–343.

545. Hahn JS, Bejar R, Gladson CL. Neonatal subependymal giant cell astrocytoma associated with tuberous sclerosis: MRI, CT, and ultrasound correlation. Neurology 1991;41:124–128.

546. Hassoun J, Gambarelli D, Grisoli F, et al. Central neurocytoma. An electron microscopic study of two cases. Acta Neuropathol (Berl) 1982;56:151–156.

547. Barbosa MD, Balsitis M, Jaspan T, et al. Intraventricular neurocytoma: A clinical and pathological study of three cases and review of the literature. Neurosurgery 1990;26:1045–1054.

548. Goergen SK, Gonzales MF, McLean CA. Intraventricular neurocytoma: Radiologic features and review of the literature. Radiology 1992;182:787–792.

549. Yuen ST, Fung CF, Ng THK, et al. Central neurocytoma: Its differentiation from intraventricular oligodendroglioma. Childs Nerv Syst 1992;8:383–388.

550. Bolen JW, Lipper MH, Caccamo D. Case report. Intraventricular central neurocytoma: CT and MR findings. J Comput Assist Tomogr 1989;13:495–497.

551. Chang KH, Han MH, Kim DG, et al. MR appearance of central neurocytoma. Acta Radiol 1993;34:520–526.

552. Wichmann W, Schubiger O, Deimling AV, et al. Neuroradiology of central neurocytoma. Neuroradiology 1991;33:143–148.

553. Nishio S, Fujiwara S, Tashima T, et al. Tumors of the lateral ventricular wall, especially the septum pellucidum: Clinical presentation and variations in pathological features. Neurosurgery 1990;27:224–230.

554. Maiuri F, Spaziante R, DeCaro ML, et al. Central neurocytoma: Clinico-pathological study of 5 cases and review of the literature. Clin Neurol Neurosurg 1995;97:219–228.

555. Dolinskas CA, Simeone FA. CT characteristics of intraventricular oligodendrogliomas. AJNR 1987;8:1077–1082.

556. Read EJ. Colloid cyst of the third ventricle. Ann Emerg Med 1990;19:1060–1062.

557. Byard RW, Moore L. Sudden and unexpected death in childhood due to a colloid cyst of the third ventricle. Forensic Sci 1993;38:210–213.

558. Macdonald RL, Humphreys RP, Rutka JT, et al. Colloid cysts in children. Pediatr Neurosurg 1994;20:169–177.

559. Lach B, Scheithauer BW, Gregor A, et al. Colloid cyst of the third ventricle. A comparative immunohistochemical study of neuraxis cysts and choroid plexus epithelium. J Neurosurg 1993;78:101–111.

560. Ho KL, Garcia JH. Colloid cyst of the third ventricle: Ultrastructural features are compatible with endodermal derivation. Acta Neuropathol (Berl) 1992;83:605–612.

561. Maeder PP, Holtas SL, Basibuyuk LN, et al. Colloid cysts of the third ventricle: Correlation of MR and CT findings with histology and chemical analysis. AJNR 1990;11:575–581.

562. Wilms G, Marchal G, VanHecke P, et al. Colloid cysts of the third ventricle: MR findings. J Comput Assist Tomogr 1990;14:527–531.

563. Taratuto AL, Monges J, Lylyk P, et al. Superficial cerebral astrocytomas attached to dura. Report of six cases in infants. Cancer 1984;54:2505–2512.

564. Paulus W, Schlote W, Perentes E, et al. Desmoplastic supratentorial neuroepithelial tumours of infancy. Histopathology 1992;21:43–49.

565. Martin DS, Levy B, Awwad EE, et al. Desmoplastic infantile ganglioglioma: CT and MR features. AJNR 1991;12:1195–1197.

566. Tenreiro-Picon OR, Kamath SV, Knorr JR, et al. Desmoplastic infantile ganglioglioma: CT and MRI features. Pediatr Radiol 1995;25:540–543.

567. Serra A, Strain J, Ruyle S. Desmoplastic cerebral astrocytoma of infancy: Report and review of the imaging characteristics. AJR 1996;166:1459–1461.

568. Kuchelmeister K, Bergmann M, vonVild K, et al. Desmoplastic ganglioglioma: Report of two non-infantile cases. Acta Neuropathol 1993;85:199–204.

569. Rushing EJ, Rorke LB, Sutton L. Problems in the nosology of desmoplastic tumors of childhood. Pediatr Neurosurg 1993;19:57–62.

570. VandenBerg SR, May EE, Rubinstein LJ, et al. Desmoplastic supratentorial neuroepithelial tumors of infancy with divergent differentiation potential ("desmoplastic infantile gangliogliomas"). Report on 11 cases of a distinctive embryonal tumor with favorable prognosis. J Neurosurg 1987;66:58–71.

571. Duffner PK, Burger PC, Cohen ME, et al. Desmoplastic infantile gangliogliomas: An approach to therapy. Neurosurgery 1994;34:583–589.

572. Raymond AA, Halpin SFS, Alsanjari N, et al. Dysembryoplastic neuroepithelial tumour. Features in 16 patients. Brain 1994;117:461–475.

573. Ostertun B, Wolf HK, Campos MG, et al. Dysembryoplastic neuroepithelial tumors: MR and CT evaluation. AJNR 1996;17:419–430.

574. Daumas-Duport C, Scheithauer BW, Chodkiewicz JP, et al. Dysembryoplastic neuroepithelial tumor: A surgically curable tumor of young patients with intractable partial seizures. Neurosurgery 1988;23:545–556.

575. Taratuto AL, Pomata H, Sevlever G, et al. Dysembryoplastic neuroepithelial tumor: Morphological, immunocytochemical, and deoxyribonucleic acid analyses in a pediatric series. Neurosurgery 1995;36:474–481.

576. Daumas-Duport C. Dysembryoplastic neuroepithelial tumours. Brain Pathol 1993;3:283–295.

577. Prayson RA, Estes ML. Dysembryoplastic neuroepithelial tumor. Am J Clin Pathol 1992;97:398–401.

578. Vali AM, Clarke MA, Kelsey A. Dysembryoplastic neuroepithelial tumour as a potentially treatable cause of intractable epilepsy in children. Clin Radiol 1993;47:255–258.

579. Kuroiwa T, Bergey GK, Rothman MI, et al. Radiologic appearance of the dysembryoplastic neuroepithelial tumor. Radiology 1995;197:233–238.

580. Kuroiwa T, Kishikawa T, Kato A, et al. Dysembryoplastic neuroepithelial tumors: MR findings. J Comput Assist Tomogr 1994;18:352–356.

581. Koeller KK, Dillon WP. Dysembryoplastic neuroepithelial tumors: MR appearance. AJNR 1992;13:1319–1325.

582. Abe M, Tabuchi K, Tsuji T, et al. Dysembryoplastic neuroepithelial tumor: Report of three cases. Surg Neurol 1995;43:240–245.

583. Hanna SL, Langston JW, Parham DM, et al. Primary malignant

rhabdoid tumor of the brain: Clinical, imaging, and pathologic findings. AJNR 1993;14:107–115.

584. Satoh H, Goishi J, Sogabe T, et al. Primary malignant rhabdoid tumor of the central nervous system: Case report and review of the literature. Surg Neurol 1993;40:429–434.

585. Chou SM, Anderson JS. Primary CNS malignant rhabdoid tumor (MRT): Report of two cases and review of the literature. Clin Neuropathol 1991;10(1):1–10.

586. Biggs PJ, Garren PD, Powers JM, et al. Malignant rhabdoid tumor of the central nervous system. Hum Pathol 1987;18:332–337.

587. Weeks DA, Malott RL, Zuppan CW, et al. Primitive cerebral tumor with rhabdoid features: A case of phenotypic rhabdoid tumor of the central nervous system. Ultrastruct Pathol 1994;18:23–28.

588. Ho PSP, Lee WH, Chen CY, et al. Primary malignant rhabdoid tumor of the brain: CT characteristics. J Comput Assist Tomogr 1990;14:461–463.

589. Agranovich AL, Ang LC, Griebel RW, et al. Malignant rhabdoid tumor of the central nervous system with subarachnoid dissemination. Surg Neurol 1992;37:410–414.

590. Youssef Booz MMKA, Koelma I, Unnikrishnan M. Case report: Primary malignant rhabdoid tumour of the brain. Clin Radiol 1996;51:65–66.

591. Munoz A, Carrasco A, Munoz MJ, et al. Cranial rhabdoid tumor with marginal tumor cystic component and extraaxial extension. AJNR 1995;16:1727–1728.

592. Velasco ME, Brown JA, Kini J, Ruppert ES. Primary congenital rhabdoid tumor of the brain with neoplastic hydranencephaly. Childs Nerv Syst 1993;9:185–190.

593. Palma L, Celli P, Cantore G. Supratentorial ependymomas of the first two decades of life. Long-term follow-up of 20 cases (including two subependymomas). Neurosurgery 1993;32:169–175.

594. Marsh WR, Laws ER. Intracranial ependymomas. Prog Exp Tumor Res 1987;30:175–180.

595. Ernestus RI, Wilcke O, Schroder R. Supratentorial ependymomas in childhood: Clinicopathological findings and prognosis. Acta Neurochir (Wien) 1991;111:96–102.

596. Centeno RS, Lee AA, Winter J, et al. Supratentorial ependymomas. Neuroimaging and clinicopathological correlation. J Neurosurg 1986;64:209–215.

597. Oppenheim JS, Strauss RC, Mormino J, et al. Ependymomas of the third ventricle. Neurosurgery 1994;34:350–353.

598. Rawlings CE, Giangaspero F, Burger PC, et al. Ependymomas: A clinicopathologic study. Surg Neurol 1988;29:271–281.

599. Armington WG, Osborn AG, Cubberley DA, et al. Supratentorial ependymomas: CT appearance. Radiology 1985;157:367–372.

600. Furie DM, Provenzale JM. Supratentorial ependymomas and subependymomas: CT and MR appearance. J Comput Assist Tomogr 1995;19:518–526.

601. Mork SJ, Loken AC. Ependymoma. A follow-up study of 101 cases. Cancer 1977;40:907–915.

602. Spoto GP, Press GA, Hesselink JR. Intracranial ependymoma and subependymoma: MR manifestations. AJNR 1990;11:83–91.

603. Scheithauer BW. Symptomatic subependymoma. J Neurosurg 1978;49:689–696.

604. Lobato RD, Sarabia M, Castro S, et al. Symptomatic subependymoma: Report of four new cases studied with computed tomography and review of the literature. Neurosurgery 1986;19:594–598.

605. Chiechi MV, Smirniotopoulos JG, Jones RV. Intracranial subependymomas: CT and MR imaging features in 24 cases. AJR 1995;165:1245–1250.

606. Hoeffel C, Boukobza M, Polivka M, et al. MR manifestations of subependymomas. AJNR 1995;16:2121–2129.

607. Rea GL, Akerson RD, Rockswold GL, et al. Subependymoma in a 2 1/2-year-old boy. J Neurosurg 1983;59:1088–1091.

608. Hart MN, Earle KN. Primitive neuroectodermal tumors of the brain in children. Cancer 1973;32:890–896.

609. Rorke LB, Gilles FH, Davis RL, et al. Revision of the World Health Organization classification of brain tumors for childhood brain tumors. Cancer 1985;56:1869–1886.

610. Cohen BH, Zeltzer PM, Boyett JM, et al. Prognostic factors and treatment results for supratentorial primitive neuroectodermal tumors in children using radiation and chemotherapy: A Childrens Cancer Group randomized trial. J Clin Oncol 1995;13:1687–1696.

611. Robles HA, Smirniotopoulos JG, Figueroa RE. Understanding the

radiology of intracranial primitive neuroectodermal tumors from a pathological perspective: A review. Semin Ultrasound CT MR 1992;13:170–181.

612. Molloy PT, Yachnis AT, Rorke LB, et al. Central nervous system medulloepithelioma: A series of eight cases including two arising in the pons. J Neurosurg 1996;84:430–436.

613. David R, Lamki N, Fan S, et al. The many faces of neuroblastoma. Radiographics 1989;9:859–882.

614. Berger MS, Edwards MSB, Wara WM, et al. Primary cerebral neuroblastoma. Long-term follow-up review and therapeutic guidelines. J Neurosurg 1983;59:418–423.

615. Bennett JP, Rubinstein LJ. The biological behavior of primary cerebral neuroblastoma: A reappraisal of the clinical course in a series of 70 cases. Ann Neurol 1984;16:21–27.

616. Wiegel B, Harris TM, Edwards MK, et al. MR of intracranial neuroblastoma with dural sinus invasion and distant metastases. AJNR 1991;12:1198–1200.

617. Ng HK, Tang NLS, Poon WS. Polar spongioblastoma with cerebrospinal fluid metastases. Surg Neurol 1994;41:137–142.

618. Schiffer D, Cravioto H, Giordana MT, et al. Is polar spongioblastoma a tumor entity? J Neurosurg 1993;78:587–591.

619. Mork SJ, Rubinstein LJ. Ependymoblastoma. A reappraisal of a rare embryonal tumor. Cancer 1985;55:1536–1542.

620. Dorsay TA, Rovira MJ, Ho VB, et al. Ependymoblastoma: MR presentation. A case report and review of the literature. Pediatr Radiol 1995;25:433–435.

621. Schiffer D, Giordana MT, Pezzotta S, et al. Medullomyoblastoma: Report of two cases. Childs Nerv Syst 1992;8:268–272.

622. Zimmerman RA, Bilaniuk LT. CT of primary and secondary craniocerebral neuroblastoma. AJR 1980;135:1239–1242.

623. Chambers EF, Turski PA, Sobel D, et al. Radiologic characteristics of primary cerebral neuroblastomas. Radiology 1981;139:101–104.

624. Davis PC, Wichman RD, Takei Y. Primary cerebral neuroblastoma: CT and MR findings in 12 cases. AJNR 1990;11:115–120.

625. Ganti SR, Silver AJ, Diefenbach P, et al. Computed tomography of primitive neuroectodermal tumors. AJNR 1983;4:819–821.

626. Kingsley DPE, Harwood-Nash DCF. Radiological features of the neuroectodermal tumours of childhood. Neuroradiology 1984; 26:463–467.

627. Altman N, Fitz CR, Chuang S, et al. Radiologic characteristics of primitive neuroectodermal tumors in children. AJNR 1985;6:15–18.

628. Hinshaw DB, Ashwal S, Thompson JR, et al. Neuroradiology of primitive neuroectodermal tumors. Neuroradiology 1983;25:87–92.

629. Figueroa RE, El Gammal T, Brooks BS. MR findings on primitive neuroectodermal tumors. J Comput Assist Tomogr 1989;13:773–778.

630. Murshid WR, Siquiera E, Rahm B, et al. Brain tumors in the first 2 years of life in Saudi Arabia. Childs Nerv Syst 1994;10:430–432.

631. Balestrini MR, Micheli R, Giordano L, et al. Brain tumors with symptomatic onset in the first two years of life. Childs Nerv Syst 1994;10:104–110.

632. Haddad SF, Menezes AH, Bell WE, et al. Brain tumors occurring before 1 year of age: A retrospective review of 22 cases in an 11-year period (1977–1987). Neurosurgery 1991;29:8–13.

633. DiRocco C, Ceddia A, Iannelli A. Intracranial tumors in the first year of life. A report on 51 cases. Acta Neurochir (Wein) 1993;123:14–24.

634. Tadmor R, Harwood-Nash DCF, Savoiardo M, et al. Brain tumors in the first two years of life: CT diagnosis. AJNR 1980;1:411–417.

635. Buetow PC, Smirniotopoulos JG, Done S. Congenital brain tumors: A review of 45 cases. AJNR 1990;11:793–799.

636. Wakai S, Arai T, Nagai M. Congenital brain tumors. Surg Neurol 1984;21:587–609.

637. Tomita T, McLone DG. Brain tumors during the first twenty-four months of life. Neurosurgery 1985;17:913–919.

638. Hunt SJ, Johnson PC, Coons SW, et al. Neonatal intracranial teratomas. Surg Neurol 1990;34:336–342.

639. Ulreich S, Hanieh A, Furness ME. Positive outcome of fetal intracranial teratoma. J Ultrasound Med 1993;3:163–165.

640. Kayama T, Yoshimoto T, Shimizu H, et al. Neonatal medulloblastoma. Neurooncol 1993;15:157–163.

641. Barth PG, Stam FC, Hack W, et al. Gliomatosis cerebri in a newborn. Neuropediatrics 1988;19:197–200.

642. Schellhas KP, Siebert RC, Heithoff KB, et al. Congenital choroid

portant to determine which of the structures are predominantly affected: the thalamus, the globus pallidus, or the corpus striatum (the caudate and putamen). When the thalamus is affected, there is usually more diffuse involvement of all the deep gray matter, and ischemic, hypoglycemic, and toxic lesions predominate. When the globus pallidus is primarily involved and appears typically bright on T2-weighted sequences, carbon monoxide, kernicterus, methylmalonic acidemia, or propionic acidemia should be considered. When the globus pallidus appears dark on T2-weighted sequences, the cause in children is almost always iron secondary to Hallervorden-Spatz disease, although chronic hemochromatosis has a similar appearance. Dense calcifications may also appear as dark lesions on T2-weighted sequences but should be easily recognized by the clinical history, such as calcifying microangiopathy secondary to radiation, or from the appearance on CT scanning. Involvement of the striatum suggests mitochondrial disorders, including Leigh's disease, mitochondrial encephalomyopathy with lactic acidosis and strokelike events (MELAS), glutaric aciduria, Wilson's disease, and Huntington's disease.

3. Disorders of cortical gray matter, or poliodystrophies: These include ceroid-lipofuscinoses, trichopoliodystrophy, and Menkes' disease. These uncommon disorders may be best recognized by the presence of cortical atrophy, manifested by widening of the sulci. Fluid attenuated inversion recovery (FLAIR) imaging demonstrates the abnormal bright signal in the cortex more than do routine T2-weighted sequences.

4. Disorders with both gray and white matter involvement: Many diseases that predominantly affect only the gray or only the white matter may also be included in this category because of the occasional presentation with diffuse involvement of both the gray and the white matter. Several disorders virtually always involve both the gray and the white matter. When there is evidence of cortical dysplasia or migrational disorder in addition to white and gray matter lesions, peroxisomal disorders, including Zellweger's syndrome, are the usual cause. Other diseases apparently unrelated to the inherited disorders of metabolism may have similar MRI findings. Fukuyama's muscular dystrophy and Walker-Warburg syndrome, probably related disorders, appear similar to Zellweger's syndrome. Tuberous sclerosis may also have lesions in both the gray and the white matter but is more easily differentiated by the presence of subependymal nodules.

5. Mucopolysaccharidoses: These diseases, involving cortical gray matter early, but also commonly showing lesions in the white matter, are considered separately because of the more widespread involvement of the skeleton and viscera that usually makes the diagnosis secure clinically before imaging studies are considered.

DISORDERS OF WHITE MATTER

Of all the metabolic disorders, diseases involving white matter are the most common. These may involve the periventricular white matter or the subcortical white matter predominantly. When the subcortical white matter is predominantly affected, it is important to note whether or not the subcortical U-fibers are also involved. The arcuate U-fibers, a thin white matter band immediately below the cortex, assumes a characteristic "u" configuration as it curves around the cortex at the depths of the sulci. The clinical condition of the patient should also be determined. The age of onset of the disease, the sex of the patient, the presence of nystagmus, a history of other affected family members, and the size of the patient's head are all important clinical factors. Another common method of categorizing white matter diseases is to divide them into demyelinating diseases, those in which normal myelin is later destroyed, and dysmyelinating diseases, in which myelin is abnormally formed. Multiple sclerosis is the most common demyelinating disease; inborn errors of metabolism are common examples of dysmyelinating diseases.

Peripheral White Matter

Late in the course of most inherited metabolic diseases, the appearance on MRI is similar to that of diffuse white matter abnormality, atrophy, and frequently, gray matter abnormalities as well. For that reason, it is helpful to determine which portion of the brain is affected early in the course of the disease and to establish a list of differential diagnoses based on the early MRI appearance of the disease. There are several difficulties with this approach, especially the similarity of the appearance of many of these diseases, but also the variations in presentation and involvement with different portions of the white matter. Acknowledging these difficulties, the pattern approach to these diseases still appears to be the most promising way of narrowing the diagnostic considerations. Canavan's disease and Alexander's disease should be considered in patients with macrocephaly and predominant involvement of the peripheral white matter.

Canavan's Disease

Canavan's disease, formerly known as *spongiform leukodystrophy,* is a rare inherited neurologic disorder of children. Similar to Tay-Sachs and Niemann-Pick disease, Canavan's disease is most commonly found in Ashkenazi Jews. There is an autosomal recessive pattern of inheritance. The biochemical basis for the disease has been discovered to be a deficiency in the enzyme aspartoacylase, resulting in *N*-acetylaspartic aciduria.[3, 4]

There are three forms of Canavan's disease, based on the time of onset:[5] (1) The congenital form presents at birth or in the first few days of life with hypotonia, lethargy, and feeding difficulties. These children die within a few weeks. (2) The infantile form is the most common. These children are normal at birth but become hypotonic within the first 6 months. Macrocephaly and seizures are common presenting features. Spasticity, deteriorating mental capacity, and blindness develop during the next 2 years.[3, 5] Most patients die before 4 years of age. (3) The juvenile form is uncommon, with children presenting after 5 years of age and death usually by late adolescence. The juvenile form differs from other forms of Canavan's disease in that it is inherited by sporadic mutations and does not have macrocephaly.

Brain biopsy reveals characteristic replacement of the white matter by a network of fine glial stranding separating small fluid-containing cysts, accounting for the name of *spongy degeneration.*[6] This network is most prominent in the subcortical regions. The internal capsule is rarely involved.

On imaging studies, diffuse symmetric lesions of the entire cerebral white matter are demonstrated, with relative sparing of only the internal capsule and only when scanned early (Fig. 47–1).[5] Late in the disease, diffuse atrophy may be seen. Proton spectroscopy demonstrates enlargement of the *N*-acetyl aspartate peak. This enlargement is believed to be specific for Canavan's disease.[7]

Alexander's Disease

In patients with inherited leukodystrophy and macrocephaly, the second major consideration is Alexander's disease, also known as *fibrinoid leukodystrophy.* Children with Alexander's disease present during the first year of life with developmental delay and macrocephaly. There is progressive neurologic deterioration with psychomotor retardation and death by early childhood.[3, 8] An autosomal recessive pattern of inheritance is seen. Alexander's disease remains one of the leukodystrophies without a clear enzymatic defect or genetic mutation.[6] The diagnosis is made by the characteristic clinical course and imaging findings. CT and MRI studies demonstrate white matter abnormality in the frontal region, which progresses posteriorly to involve the entire white matter (Fig. 47–2). The internal and external capsule regions are involved later. Late in the disease, there may be cystic degeneration.[3]

Cockayne's Syndrome

Cockayne's syndrome, an autosomal recessive disease, is one of the less well defined of the sudanophilic leukodys-

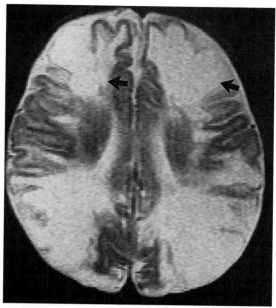

FIGURE 47–2 Alexander's disease. T2-weighted images show extensive areas of abnormal bright signal in the white matter of both the frontal lobes and the parieto-occipital regions. Areas of cystic encephalomalacia are present *(arrows).*

trophies, which are diseases with sudanophilic droplets composed of cholesterol and triglycerides. Other sudanophilic leukodystrophies are Pelizaeus-Merzbacher disease and the Jervis type of sudanophilic leukodystrophy. The clinical presentation of Cockayne's syndrome is unusual and characteristic, with the appearance of the face resembling old age.[6] The wrinkled facies is due to lack of subcutaneous fat and cutaneous photosensitivity. Patients suffer from psychomotor retardation in late infancy, with progressive growth and developmental delays. Other common findings are severe kyphoscoliosis, dwarfism, retinal degeneration, deafness, gait abnormalities, and microcephaly.[2, 6]

Imaging of Cockayne's syndrome reveals progressive atrophy and severe white matter abnormalities. Calcifications of the basal ganglia and dentate nuclei of the cerebellum are seen on CT scans and gradient-echo MRI images (Fig. 47–3).

Galactosemia

Galactosemia, inherited by autosomal recessive transmission, is caused by galactose-1-phosphate-uridyl transferase deficiency. Patients usually present in early infancy with signs of increased intracranial pressure, such as vomiting. Marked neurologic deterioration, seizures, choreoathetosis, and liver failure develop in the untreated child.[3, 9] Dietary restriction of galactose delays the onset of the disease and prevents the most severe complications, but some clinical and MRI evidence of neurologic deterioration is almost always found, even in compliant patients. CT and MRI show abnormalities in the peripheral, subcortical white matter with progressive atrophy of both the cerebral and the cerebellar hemispheres (Fig. 47–4).[10]

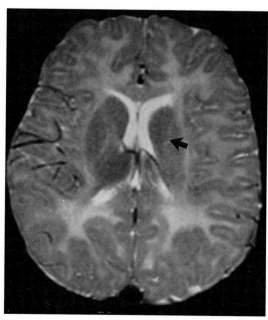

FIGURE 47–1 Canavan's disease. T2-weighted images show an abnormal bright signal throughout the white matter, with relative sparing of only the internal capsule *(arrow).*

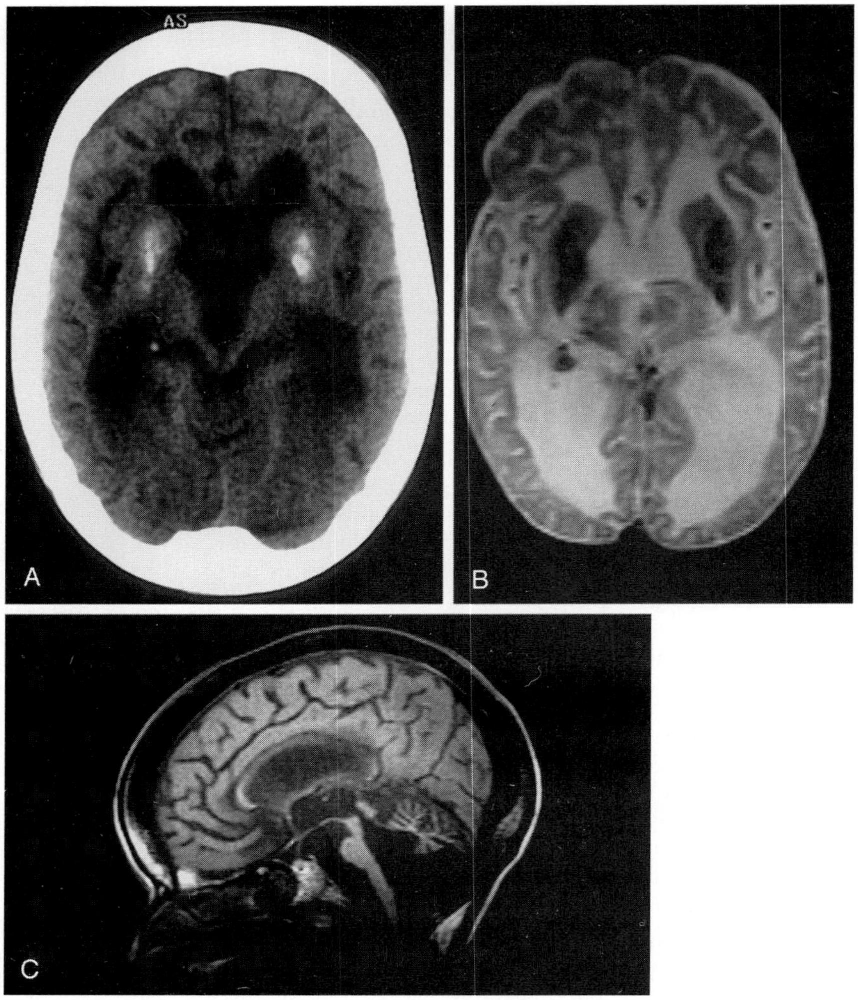

FIGURE 47–3 Cockayne's syndrome. *A,* Precontrast axial computed tomography (CT) scan shows bilateral basal ganglia calcifications. *B,* Axial T2-weighted image shows marked T2 shortening due to the calcification and abnormal bright signal in the periventricular white matter. *C,* Sagittal T1-weighted image shows advanced cerebellar atrophy.

Central White Matter

The following diseases typically present with involvement of the periventricular white matter early in the course of the disease.

Metachromatic Leukodystrophy

Metachromatic leukodystrophy includes several disorders that have in common a deficiency in the activity of arylsulfatase A. The function of arylsulfatase A is to break down myelin for reuse in the central and peripheral nervous system. When there is a disorder in the function of this enzyme, there is an abnormality in myelination and accumulation of sulfatides in macrophages and Schwann cells resulting in metachromatic staining of lipid-rich granules in the cells. Severe demyelination of the white matter leads to focal cavitation.

Of the several forms of metachromatic leukodystrophy, the most common is the late infantile form, presenting in the second or third year of life with marked motor delay. Frequent falls result from weakness and ataxia.[3] There is rapid progression within 3 to 6 months with deterioration of speech, psychomotor retardation, spasticity, and optic atrophy. Seizures and decerebrate or decorticate posturing are usually present before death at 6 to 7 years of age.[11]

The juvenile forms of metachromatic leukodystrophy are less common, presenting with either early onset, at 4 to 6 years, or late onset, after age 6 years. Both juvenile forms are similar to the infantile form with gait disturbances, psychomotor retardation, and extrapyramidal signs, but neurologic deterioration progresses more slowly. The adult form is even more uncommon.[11, 12]

Metachromatic leukodystrophy is one of the most difficult dysmyelinating diseases to diagnose by imaging studies. The white matter is abnormal in the periventricular region in a symmetric pattern with areas of normal myelination preserved. Although the MRI appearance may mimic other diseases of periventricular white matter, such as periventricular leukodystrophy, acute disseminated encephalomyelitis, or multiple sclerosis, the clinical presentation of normal development and later progressive deterioration should help establish the diagnosis of metachromatic leukoencephalopathy. Peripheral white matter involvement and atrophy are seen late in the disease (Fig. 47–5).[11, 12]

Krabbe's Disease

Krabbe's disease, also known as *globoid cell leukodystrophy,* is the result of β-galactocerebrosidase deficiency,

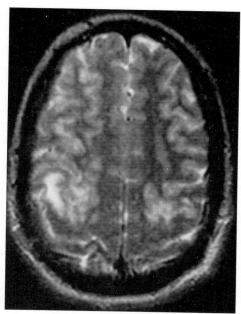

FIGURE 47–4 Galactosemia. Axial T2-weighted image shows peripheral, subcortical white matter lesions with associated focal atrophy.

which causes a destruction of oligodendrocytes and an accumulation of psychosine within the cells. Transmission is autosomal recessive. The diagnosis may be made prenatally, and it is possible to detect healthy carriers of this disease.

The disease is detected when the infant is usually between 3 and 6 months of age, and neonatal diagnoses may even be made. The initial presentation is extreme

irritability, with hypersensitivity to sensory stimuli, especially sound.[13] Infants with Krabbe's disease develop feeding problems, intermittent fever, and developmental regression.[13] Seizures may be the problem that first brings the child to the neurologist. The disease progresses quickly, with progressive motor deterioration and abnormal posturing, hypertonic extremities, extended legs, flexed arms, and thrown-back head.[13, 14] Blindness and flaccidity follow. Death comes early, and few children live beyond 2 years. The diagnosis is made from an assay of β-galactosidase in leukocytes or skin cells.

Imaging findings may help direct the neuroradiologist to consider Krabbe's disease in the early stages. Early in the disease, there are areas of increased density on CT scan in the thalamus, caudate nuclei, and corona radiata.[13] Atrophy develops quickly. On MRI, initial studies may demonstrate a paramagnetic effect with short T2 and T1 lesions (Fig. 47–6).[13] Later, abnormal bright signal on T2-weighted sequences is seen in the deep gray matter structures and deep white matter, in the cerebellum as well as the cerebrum.[13, 14] The pattern is quite symmetric and is usually most severe in the parietal regions.[14] Contrast enhancement is rarely seen (Fig. 47–7).

Adrenoleukodystrophy

Adrenoleukodystrophy is the most common of the peroxisomal disorders, a group of diseases with a single enzyme defect preventing the oxidation of very-long-chain fatty acids (>26 carbon atoms) and resulting in the accumulation of these fatty acids within the cells. The peroxisomes are small intracellular organelles with a single membrane that function to oxidize very-long-chain fatty acids for reuse within the cells.[3] The name *peroxisomes* comes from the hydrogen peroxide within the organelle used to oxidize the fatty acids. When the very-long-chain fatty

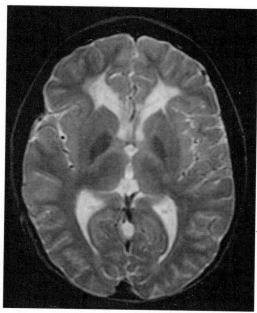

FIGURE 47–5 Metachromatic leukodystrophy. Axial T2-weighted image shows an abnormal bright signal surrounding both frontal horns of the lateral ventricles.

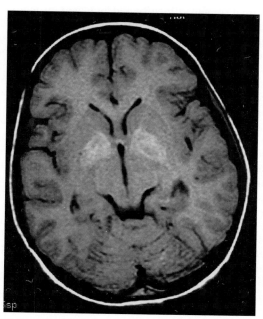

FIGURE 47–6 Krabbe's disease. Early involvement with the disease is manifest on the axial T1-weighted image as a bright signal in the deep gray matter.

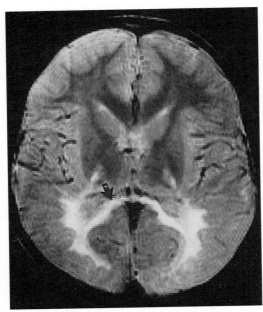

FIGURE 47–7 Late involvement with Krabbe's disease on the axial T2-weighted image shows an abnormal bright signal symmetrically surrounding the atria, extending through the posterior corpus callosum (*arrow*).

acids cannot be broken down, they are used to help form myelin, which is then unstable. Because this defect exists in all cells, the diagnosis can be made by assays of very-long-chain fatty acids in plasma and fibroblasts, and prenatal diagnosis is possible.

Classic adrenoleukodystrophy is an X-linked disorder, presenting between 5 and 10 years of age with a typical clinical picture of gradual motor and intellectual deterioration in a previously healthy boy.[15, 16] The first symptoms are frequently gait difficulty and behavior problems. Abnormal skin pigmentation and other signs of adrenal insufficiency are variable findings, occasionally preceding the neurologic signs but more often seen late or not at all.[16] The disease progresses rapidly to loss of hearing and visual acuity, hypotonia, seizures, and ataxia. A less common form of the disease presents in adolescence and adulthood and is called *adrenomyeloneuropathy*.[16, 17]

The imaging of adrenoleukodystrophy is rewarding because of the typical pattern on CT and MRI, which makes the diagnosis fairly secure in most patients. On both CT and MRI, there is a symmetric zone of demyelination beginning in the periventricular white matter, spanning the corpus callosum, which then progresses to involve greater and greater amounts of the surrounding white matter.[2, 3, 18] The leading edge of this process frequently shows enhancement on CT and MRI.[18] On CT, the zone of demyelination is of decreased density; on MRI, the zone is bright on T2-weighted images and dark on T1-weighted images. The cerebellar white matter and cortical spinal tracts in the brain stem are frequently involved. The peripheral white matter becomes abnormal in the later stages of the disease. The progression of the disease from central to peripheral has been categorized on pathologic examination as Schaumburg's zones.[2] Schaumburg's

zone 3, located most centrally, represents the oldest area of involvement, with widespread demyelination on pathologic examination and bright signal on MR imaging. Zones 1 and 2, representing the most acute and most peripheral areas of involvement, show inflammatory reaction and enhancement on imaging studies (Fig. 47–8). Although two-thirds of patients present with this typical pattern, other patterns are also common, with frontal involvement preceding the occipital involvement in several patients (Fig. 47–9). Unilateral disease has also been seen (Fig. 47–10).

Adrenomyeloneuropathy involves the cerebellum and brain stem more commonly than does adrenoleukodystrophy (Fig. 47–11).[16, 17] Proton spectroscopy demonstrates decreased *N*-acetyl-aspartate; increased choline, glutamine, and glutamate; decreased *myo*-inositol; and increased aliphatic hydrocarbon peaks.[19] These abnormalities on magnetic resonance spectroscopy (MRS) may precede the abnormalities on MRI.[19]

Other Peroxisomal Disorders

Other peroxisomal disorders fall into two categories: (1) those similar to classic X-linked adrenoleukodystrophy with the peroxisomal disorder confined primarily to the nervous system and (2) those similar to Zellweger's (cerebrohepatorenal) syndrome with a generalized disorder of the peroxisomes.[3] Refsum's disease and rhizomelic chondrodysplasia calcificans punctata are two disorders similar to classic adrenoleukodystrophy, with bright lesions on T2-weighted images involving the white matter of the brain and brain stem (Fig. 47–12).[20] Zellweger's syndrome, neonatal adrenoleukodystrophy, and hyperpipecolic acidemia are generalized peroxisomal disorders. These diseases present shortly after birth with severe abnormalities of most organ systems. They share the features of severe hypotonia, developmental delay, retardation, seizures, abnormal facies, and abnormal liver function. Zellweger's syndrome is the most severe of the peroxisomal disorders, with ocular and cardiac anomalies as well.[15, 21] The diagnosis may be made from electron microscopic examination of liver tissue. Most children die within the first year of life. Because siblings are commonly affected, the mode of inheritance is presumed to be autosomal recessive.

On MRI, there is virtually complete loss of white matter throughout both hemispheres, causing a small head size and atrophic corpus callosum (Fig. 47–13). Cortical dysplasia, characterized by polymicrogyria, and gray matter heterotopia may be seen.

Pelizaeus-Merzbacher Disease

Pelizaeus-Merzbacher disease is the best understood of the sudanophilic leukodystrophies, which are diseases with the accumulation of sudan-staining droplets composed of cholesterol and triglycerides. Cockayne's syndrome is also one of the sudanophilic leukodystrophies.

Pelizaeus-Merzbacher disease is a rare X-linked recessive disorder with severe abnormalities of white matter, usually presenting in the infantile period with severe neurologic dysfunction and nystagmus.[22] The first signs of the disease are most often seen in the first months of life. These include wandering eye movements, truncal

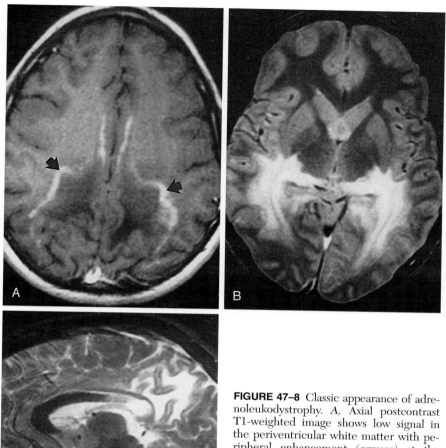

FIGURE 47–8 Classic appearance of adrenoleukodystrophy. *A,* Axial postcontrast T1-weighted image shows low signal in the periventricular white matter with peripheral enhancement *(arrows)* at the leading edge. *B,* Occipital white matter. There is sparing of the subcortical U fibers. *C,* Sagittal T2-weighted image shows involvement of the splenium of the corpus callosum.

hypotonia, limb spasticity, and microcephaly. Discoveries have been made concerning the genetic mutation responsible for Pelizaeus-Merzbacher disease. In this disease, there is a defect in the production of the proteolipid protein, one of the components of myelin. This defect has been localized to the Q arm of the X chromosome. Several different defects in this chromosome (duplications, deletions, abnormal sequence) at different locations can result in a similar appearance on MRI but have different severity in clinical presentation.[22] With increasing understanding of the genetic basis of this disease, more patients with less severe clinical presentations are being included. In classic Pelizaeus-Merzbacher disease, the disease presents in the first months of life and progresses to death by adolescence or early adulthood.

The MRI appearance of Pelizaeus-Merzbacher disease is a complete lack of myelination, without significant atrophy or destruction of white matter. There is an unusually complete distribution of bright signal throughout all visualized white matter, even including the corpus callosum, internal capsule, external capsule, white matter bands of the pons, and cerebellum (Fig. 47–14).[3, 12] A tigroid pattern of preserved myelination is an unusual MRI pattern, although it has been described commonly in histopathologic examinations (Fig. 47–15). Late in the disease, the cortical sulci may show slowly progressive enlargement.

Maple Syrup Urine Disease

Maple syrup urine disease is a rare autosomal recessive disorder in which the biochemical defect causes an accumulation of aromatic branched-chain amino acids in the urine, with the characteristic aroma from which the disease is named. Normal oxidative decarboxylation is interrupted, and the branched-chain amino acids (leucine, isoleucine, and valine) cannot be broken down and reused in normal cell metabolism.[23, 24] If the disease is not recognized early, affected infants become quite ill, progressing from poor feeding to dystonia, seizures, coma, and death

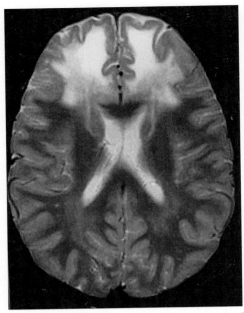

FIGURE 47–9 Atypical frontal lobe involvement with adrenoleu-kodystrophy. Axial T2-weighted image shows an abnormal bright signal within the frontal periventricular white matter.

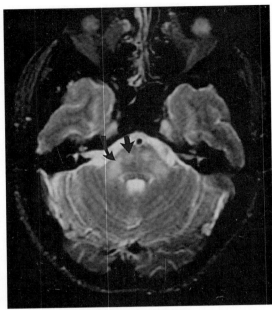

FIGURE 47–11 Adrenomyeloneuropathy. Axial T2-weighted image in the posterior fossa shows an abnormal bright signal in the cortical spinal tracts (*straight arrow*) and brachium pontis (*curved arrow*).

within weeks of birth. Treatment may prevent the most severe effects of the disease.[23, 24]

By the time infants become symptomatic, imaging studies demonstrate profound white matter edema in areas of active myelination. These include the deep white matter, dorsum of the brain stem, cerebral peduncles,

posterior limb of the internal capsule, and globus pallidus (Fig. 47–16).[23, 24] These areas appear quite bright on T2-weighted images. FLAIR imaging sequences demonstrate subtle lesions more clearly than standard T2-weighted abnormalities. If the child is suffering from increased intracranial pressure, there may be more generalized edema superimposed on focal areas of abnormality. In infants who are treated, there is a variable degree of

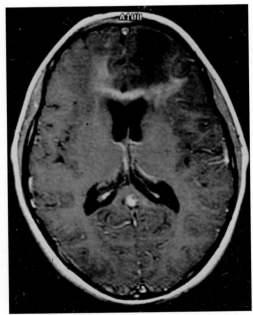

FIGURE 47–10 Atypical asymmetric involvement in adrenoleu-kodystrophy. Contrast-enhanced axial T1-weighted images show an abnormal dark signal in the left frontal white matter with a leading edge of enhancement. On the right, there is no low signal; only the acute enhancing leading edge is seen.

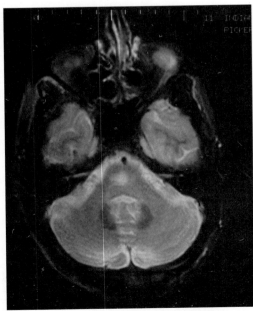

FIGURE 47–12 Refsum's disease. Axial T2-weighted image in the posterior fossa shows an abnormal bright signal in the pons, similar to central pontine myelinolysis.

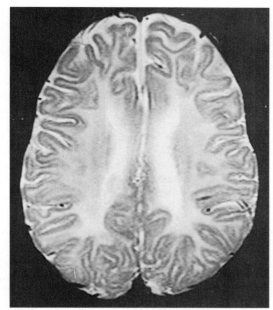

FIGURE 47–13 Zellweger's syndrome. Complete loss of normal white matter is demonstrated on the axial T2-weighted image.

white matter injury, reflecting the severity of the disease at the time treatment was begun.[3, 23, 24]

Trichothiodystrophy

Trichothiodystrophy is a rare autosomal recessive disease resulting from abnormal synthesis of high-sulfur–containing proteins.[25] Another name for trichothiodystrophy is *sulfur-deficient brittle hair disease*. The clinical presentation of the disease varies in severity. All patients

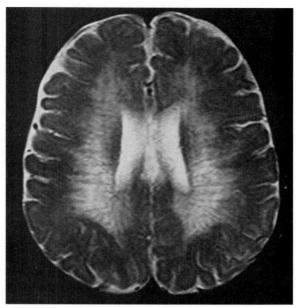

FIGURE 47–15 Pelizeaus-Merzbacher disease with tigroid appearance. Axial T2-weighted image shows an abnormal bright signal of the periventricular white matter with a striated appearance.

have a hair defect, and for some this is the only abnormality. The remaining patients may have all or some of the following findings: psychomotor retardation; short stature; decreased fertility; immunodeficiency; cataracts; and a variety of cutaneous abnormalities, including ichthyosis, photosensitivity, and nail dystrophy.[25] Although the clinical presentation is varied, the imaging pattern is similar, with diffuse lack of myelination of the white matter simi-

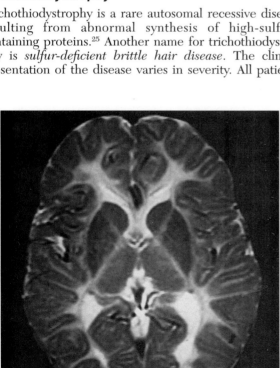

FIGURE 47–14 Classic Pelizeaus-Merzbacher disease. Axial T2-weighted image shows an abnormal bright signal replacing the entire white matter. No atrophy is seen.

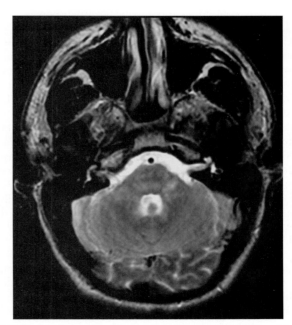

FIGURE 47–16 Maple syrup urine disease. Axial T2-weighted image of the posterior fossa shows an abnormal bright signal within the dorsum brain stem and cerebral peduncles.

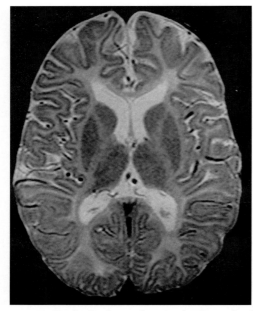

FIGURE 47–17 Trichothiodystrophy. Axial T2-weighted image shows a diffuse abnormal bright signal throughout all visualized white matter tracts.

lar to that of Pelizaeus-Merzbacher disease (Fig. 47–17).[3, 25]

Phenylketonuria

Phenylketonuria, also known as *hyperphenylalanemia,* is an autosomal recessive disorder, similar to the majority of metabolic diseases of the brain. This disease usually results from a deficiency of phenylalanine hydroxylase, which has the effect of blocking the transformation of phenylalanine to tyrosine.[23] An overproduction of toxic compounds containing the phenyl group (phenylpyruvic acid, phenylacetic acid, and phenylacetylglutamine) results. Most patients can be well controlled with treatment. Rigorous dietary restriction of all compounds containing phenylalanine is the mainstay of treatment, although occasionally dietary supplements are used.[23] This diet can be difficult to maintain because phenylalanine is present in most diet sodas and many common foods. Patients who are untreated or who are not cooperative with the dietary restrictions manifest global developmental delay; short stature; eczema; hypopigmentation; and a characteristic odor of the urine, skin, and hair. In some patients with phenylketonuria, there is a more complicated biochemical defect, with a cofactor deficiency in the enzyme dihydropteridine reductase, which is a prerequisite in the conversion of tyrosine to L-dopa and tryptophan to 5-hydroxytryptamine. This cofactor deficiency therefore not only creates an accumulation of phenylalanine but also impairs the biosynthesis of vital neurotransmitters, causing severe neurologic abnormalities.[2] In these patients with the severe cofactor deficiency, dietary restriction of phenylalanine is supplemented by replacement of cofactor and neurotransmitter precursors.

The imaging appearances of both forms of phenylketonuria are similar, varying in severity depending on the extent to which serum levels of phenylalanine can be controlled. In infants and children, MRI and CT scans may be normal or subtle, showing only abnormal signal corresponding to delayed myelination (Fig. 47–18).[26] These findings are most prominent initially in the periventricular white matter with sparing of the subcortical regions.[26] In older patients or those with advanced disease, cerebral and cerebellar atrophy may be seen, appearing as enlargement of the ventricles and widening of the cortical sulci. Confluent white matter abnormalities may be demonstrated (Fig. 47–19). In some patients who are newly diagnosed and in whom therapy has been started after MRI findings are present, there may be significant improvement in the clinical and imaging findings after dietary restriction has been started.[26]

Lowe's Syndrome

Lowe's syndrome, also known as *oculocerebrorenal syndrome,* is an X-linked recessive disorder characterized by several findings in all affected children and several more variable clinical findings. Consistent findings in all affected patients include dense cataracts, growth failure, and severe mental retardation.[3, 27] Renal tubular dysfunction may be absent at birth but increases in severity with age.[27] Other frequent findings are glaucoma, frequently with buphthalmos, corneal scarring, hypotonia, diminished deep tendon reflexes, metabolic acidosis, hyperaminoaciduria, and tubular proteinuria.[27] Cryptorchidism is frequently found. Rickets is a late manifestation, the result of the severe renal disease. There is a characteristic facial appearance, the result of blindness, mental retardation, and hypotonia. These children have a characteristic high-pitched scream. Death in childhood usually results from infection or dehydration and electrolyte imbalance.[2, 27] Children rarely live beyond adolescence. The imaging

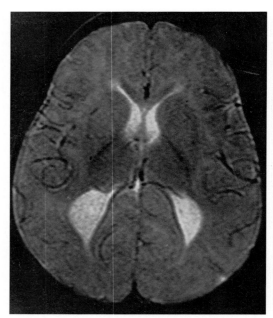

FIGURE 47–18 Early phenylketonuria. Axial T2-weighted image shows only delayed myelination. No abnormal signal lesions are present.

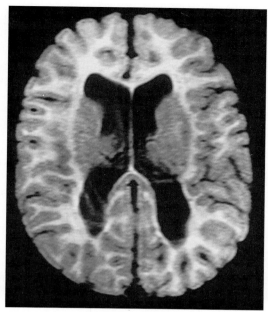

FIGURE 47–19 Late phenylketonuria. Axial fluid attenuated inversion recovery (FLAIR) sequence demonstrates severe atrophy and diffuse delay in myelination.

pattern is nonspecific, with scattered bright signal areas on T2-weighted images, which are dark on T1-weighted images (Fig. 47–20).[27] Later, confluent areas of bright signal that initially spare the subcortical regions can be seen.[27]

Central Pontine Myelinolysis

Central pontine myelinolysis is a demyelinating disorder commonly associated with rapid correction of hypona-

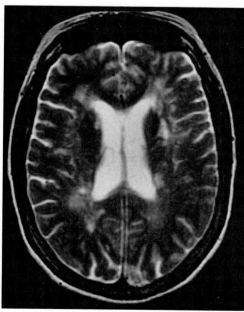

FIGURE 47–20 Lowe's syndrome. Axial T2-weighted image shows nonspecific scattered abnormal white matter lesions in an asymmetric distribution.

tremia. Although this disorder is most frequently seen in adults, children with electrolyte disturbances may also develop central pontine myelinolysis. The symptoms are quadriparesis, pseudobulbar palsy, and changing levels of consciousness. Many patients progress to death after a state of pseudocoma (locked-in syndrome). With improved awareness of the syndrome, many more patients have survived with varying degrees of residual neurologic deficits.[28] The MRI findings are bright signal within the pons on T2-weighted sequences, with extrapontine sites of myelinolysis commonly seen cephalad to the pons (Fig. 47–21).[28]

Diseases with Nonspecific Involvement of Peripheral and Deep White Matter

Diseases with nonspecific involvement may involve deep or superficial white matter and may even have gray matter involvement on occasion.

Toxic Effects of Radiation and Chemotherapy

In children, as in adults, arteritis and secondary ischemic lesions of brain may be caused by radiation or chemotherapy.[29–31] Determining whether the child's symptoms are due to an exacerbation of the neoplasm or to the effects of therapy can be a confusing clinical question. Symptoms of intracranial masses are similar to those of therapy-induced arteritis: seizures, headaches, confusion, and focal neurologic deficits. MRI is frequently used to help differentiate primary from secondary neurologic dysfunction.

Radiation-induced injury follows a predictable pattern, depending on the dose and time after the radiation. Acute reactions occur 1 to 6 weeks after treatment. These are usually transient, asymptomatic areas of mild localized edema seen as focal areas of brightness in the white matter on T2-weighted sequences (Fig. 47–22). No mass effect or contrast enhancement is present in the lesions. Early delayed reactions occur 3 weeks to several months after treatment and appear similar to acute reactions (Fig. 47–23). Late delayed reactions present several months to years after treatment, with marked changes in the brain and devastating clinical sequelae. Late delayed reaction results from injury to the endothelium of small arterioles and capillaries, leading to blood-brain barrier breakdown and exudation of fibrin from the blood vessels. The endothelium then becomes hyalinized, and proliferation of the hyaline compromises the lumen of the vessel and decreases local blood flow, with resultant white matter infarction.[30, 31] On histologic examination, there are areas of necrosis, with thinning and fragmentation of myelin and cellular disruption.[30, 31] Widespread leukomalacia, calcifying microangiopathy, and atrophy are frequently present.[30, 31] Patients may develop localized neurologic deficits or obtundation. Focal atrophy of any portion of the central nervous system can occur, including the optic nerves, resulting in optic atrophy; the pituitary gland, resulting in panhypopituitarism; and even the amygdaloid nuclei, resulting in Klüver-Bucy syndrome.[29]

In children, the younger the patient at the time of radiation therapy, the more devastating the clinical result.

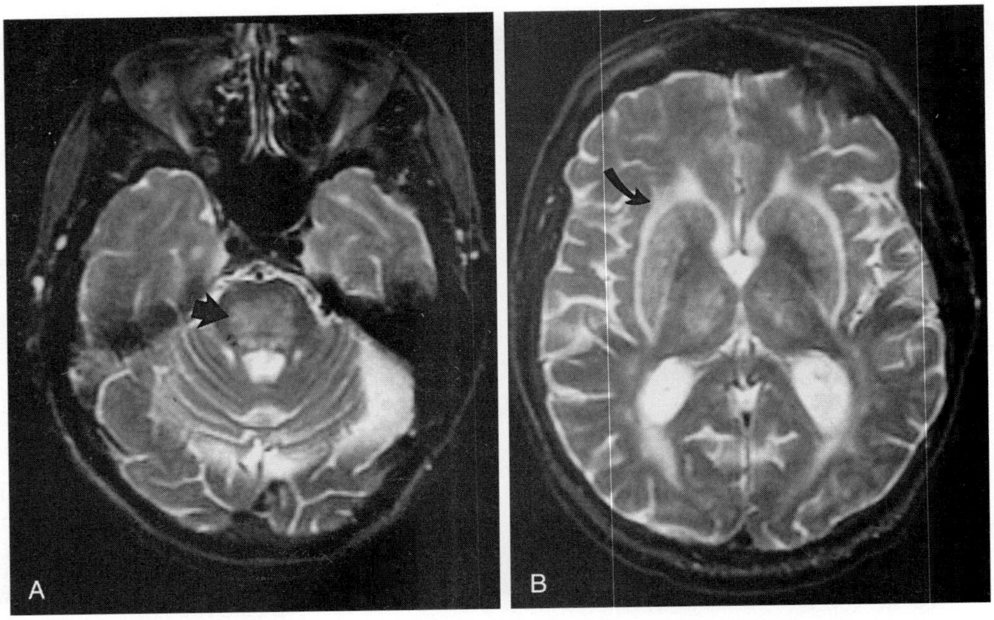

FIGURE 47–21 Central pontine myelinolysis. Axial T2-weighted images of the pons (*A*) and at the level of the basal ganglia (*B*) show pontine (*arrow* in *A*) and extrapontine (*arrow* in *B*) lesions of abnormal bright signal.

Radiation therapy to the brain is virtually never given to children younger than 2 years of age and only rarely given to children between 2 and 3 years. Even in children older than age 3, the late effects of radiation include severe psychomotor retardation. In combination with chemotherapy, the effects of radiation may be even more severe. Subacute leukoencephalopathy is seen as a consequence of the combination of intrathecal methotrexate and irradiation of the central nervous system.

Areas of radiation necrosis can be focal or disseminated within the white matter. Radiation necrosis appears acutely as an area of abnormal signal brightness of T2-weighted sequences, with variable contrast enhancement. Mass ef-

fect and edema are common findings in radiation necrosis (Fig. 47–24). Later in the course of the disease, ventricular enlargement and atrophy predominate. When diffuse, the changes of radiation therapy appear as extensive, confluent white matter lesions, scalloped laterally, adjacent to the cortical gray matter, reflecting involvement of the arcuate, U-fiber damage. The corpus callosum is usually spared. Petechial hemorrhage may be present, appearing as multifocal areas of bright signal on T1-weighted sequences and dark signal on T2-weighted sequences.[32] It is helpful to know the location of the radiation ports when assessing possible radiation therapy injury.[32]

Chemotherapeutic agents are commonly associated with white matter injury. The drugs currently recognized as causing leukoencephalopathy are cyclosporine, methotrexate, cisplatin, arabinosyl cytosine, carmustine, and thiotepa.[33–36] Most white matter abnormalities caused by chemotherapy are transient and disappear after cessation of therapy. Not all children with obvious chemotherapy-induced white matter lesions on MRI are symptomatic (Fig. 47–25). The pattern of white matter injury tends to be symmetric, widespread, and often diffuse. There is often sparing of the corpus callosum, and in contrast to the injury of radiation therapy, there is sparing of the subcortical U-fibers. Contrast enhancement is uncommon and is not cavitary. L-Asparaginase, an enzyme used in treating acute leukemia, has been associated with intracranial sinus thrombosis in 1% to 2% of children. Hemorrhagic infarcts, the result of sinus thrombosis, present as seizures, obtundation, headache, or hemiparesis. MRI has been of great value in the early detection of sinus thrombosis in children treated with L-asparaginase and in documenting subcortical white matter changes.[6]

Any exposure to unusual substances may be suspected to be the cause of acute neurologic symptoms and abnormalities on MRI scans. A herpes-type encephalopathy with temporal lobe lesions on MRI has been found after aluminum exposure, caused by treatment of a petrous bone defect with aluminum-containing cement.[37]

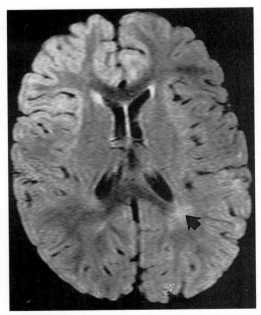

FIGURE 47–22 Acute radiation injury. Axial FLAIR sequence shows an abnormal bright signal (*arrow*).

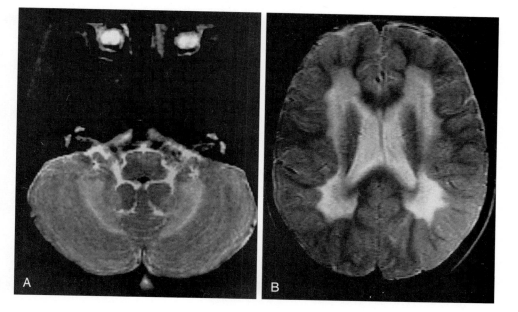

FIGURE 47–23 Delayed radiation injury. *A,* Early delayed injury on axial T2-weighted image of the posterior fossa with an abnormal bright signal in the brachium pontis. *B,* Late delayed injury on axial T2-weighted with a widespread abnormal bright signal in the centrum semiovale.

Late effects of high-dose chemotherapy for cancer and bone marrow transplantation have been observed 1 to 2 months after cytotoxic therapy (Fig. 47–26). Patients developed neurologic symptoms of seizures, confusion, and lethargy and were found to have multifocal, asymmetric, and predominantly white matter lesions that were reversible.[28]

Nonketotic Hyperglycinemia

Nonketotic hyperglycinemia, an autosomal recessive inherited disease, is a disorder of amino acid metabolism caused by a disturbance in the breakdown of glycine.[3] This disturbance results in a large accumulation of glycine in plasma, urine, and cerebrospinal fluid. Patients present in infancy with seizures, dystonia, and severe psychomotor retardation.

Imaging studies demonstrate cerebral and cerebellar atrophy with a nonspecific pattern of bright signal in the white matter and thinning of the corpus callosum (Fig. 47–27).[38] An abnormal glycine peak at 3.56 ppm is seen on proton spectroscopy.[39] This finding is present in affected children with normal MRI studies and has the potential of becoming the preferred method of monitoring the disease in children with nonketotic hyperglycinemia.[39]

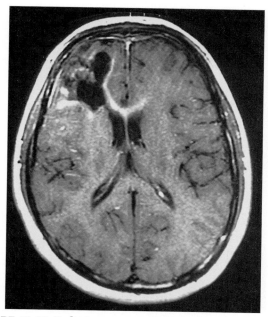

FIGURE 47–24 Radiation necrosis. Enhanced axial T1-weighted image shows an abnormal bright signal caused by enhancement surrounding an area of cavitation.

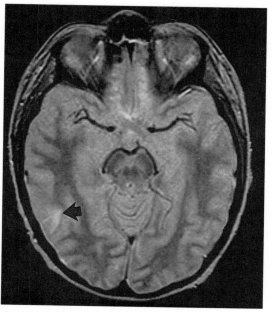

FIGURE 47–25 Chemotherapy toxicity from cyclosporine. Axial T2-weighted image shows a small focus of abnormal bright signal in the posterior right temporal lobe *(arrow).*

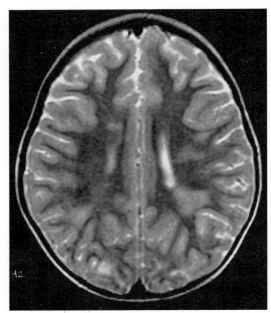

FIGURE 47–26 Late effects of chemotherapy. Two months after administration of multiagent chemotherapy, axial T2-weighted image shows an abnormal bright signal in the right occipital lobe.

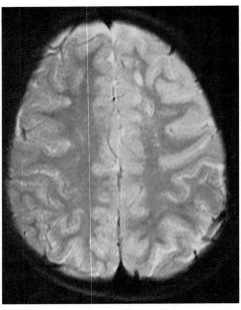

FIGURE 47–28 Carbamyl transferase deficiency. Focal asymmetric white matter lesions are present in the frontal white matter on the axial T2-weighted image.

Urea Cycle Disorders

Several disorders result in the accumulation of ammonia, owing to the inability to eliminate nitrogen waste products. Some of these disorders are ornithine carbamyl transferase deficiency, carbamyl phosphate synthetase deficiency, argininosuccinic aciduria, citrullinemia, and hyperargininemia. Increased ingestion of protein or in-

creased breakdown of protein, such as occurs in illness, can exacerbate these diseases. During periods of increased ammonemia, patients experience neurologic dysfunction manifested by movement disorders, seizures, ataxia, or confusion.[3]

There is a nonspecific imaging pattern in these diseases. Initially, there may be a pattern of diffuse edema. Later, MRI may demonstrate focal or diffuse areas of asymmetric increased signal intensity on T2-weighted se-

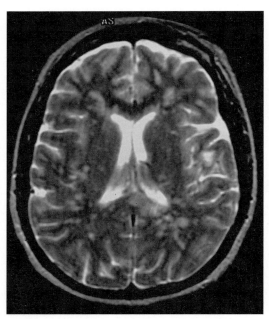

FIGURE 47–27 Nonketotic hyperglycemia. Atrophy and nonspecific white matter bright signal lesions are seen on the axial T2-weighted image.

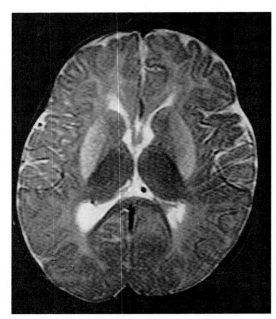

FIGURE 47–29 Hepatic encephalopathy. Bilaterally symmetric lesions of the basal ganglia are present on the axial T2-weighted image.

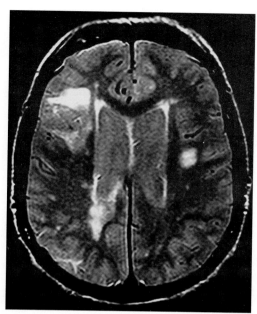

FIGURE 47–30 Multiple sclerosis in 14-year-old girl. Scattered bright lesions are present in the periventricular and subcortical white matter on the axial T2-weighted image.

quences (Fig. 47–28). Gray matter and subcortical U-fiber involvement may be present in the acute phase.[3]

Hepatic Encephalopathy

In neonates, hyperbilirubinemia (also known as *kernicterus*) is a well-recognized cause of brain damage. In neonates, the most common cause of hyperbilirubinemia is the hemolysis of red cells, typically resulting from blood group incompatibility, such as AB-O or Rh factor incompatibilities. Intrinsic defects of red blood cell membranes or the breakdown of blood products in hematomas can also release large amounts of bilirubin. Deposits of

manganese in the brain in patients with chronic liver failure have been implicated in hepatic encephalopathy.[40] Polycythemia and inherited defects in bilirubin metabolism are less common causes of hyperbilirubinemia. Cirrhosis of the liver, from any cause, produces hyperbilirubinemia and similar findings on MRI.[41] The initial neurologic picture in children with hyperbilirubinemia includes lethargy and poor tone. Seizures may occur but are uncommon. Increased tone and spasticity occur later. Permanent deficits result from persistently high levels of bilirubin, and developmental delay may be severe. MRI shows lesions in the basal ganglia on T2-weighted sequences (Fig. 47–29).[42] Marked improvement in the MRI pattern has been seen after liver transplantation.[43]

Autoimmune and Infectious Disorders

Multiple sclerosis, typically considered a disease of adults, commonly presents initially in childhood or adolescence. The onset is rare before the age of 7 years, but there have been occasional reports of children affected before the age of 3 years.[44] Up to 2% of cases of multiple sclerosis present in childhood.[45, 46] The clinical presentation is similar to that in adults, with optic neuritis, nystagmus, cerebellar syndrome, brain stem and spinal cord dysfunction, hemiplegia, dysesthesia, sphincter problems, paraplegia, and meningeal signs commonly seen.[46] In contrast to adults, fever is frequent in children. There is elevation of the cerebrospinal fluid protein and cells in half of cases.[44–46] Oligoclonal bands and decreased T cells are frequent findings in the cerebrospinal fluid in active multiple sclerosis. The imaging findings are similar to those in adults, with scattered white matter lesions appearing as bright areas on T2-weighted sequences, frequently oriented as a radial pattern surrounding the lateral ventricles (Fig. 47–30).[46] In contrast to adults, tumefactive plaques are somewhat more common, with marked edema and contrast enhancement in the acute phase (Fig. 47–31).[47] MRS shows a decrease in *N*-acetyl-

FIGURE 47–31 Tumefactive multiple sclerosis. *A*, Contrast-enhanced T1-weighted axial image shows an acute zone of active demyelination as bright enhancement surrounding areas of dark cystic necrosis. *B*, Axial T2-weighted image shows fulminant edema throughout the white matter. Marked mass effect mimics tumor.

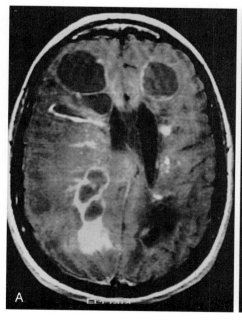
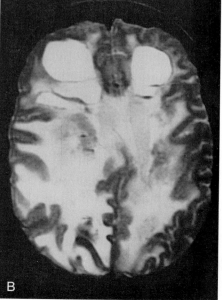

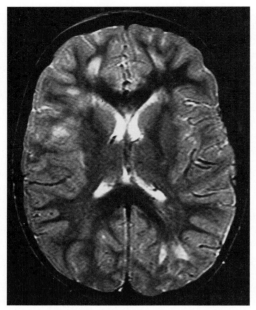

FIGURE 47–32 Typical white matter involvement with acute disseminated encephalomyelitis (ADEM). Axial T2-weighted image shows a scattered abnormal bright signal, predominantly in the subcortical white matter.

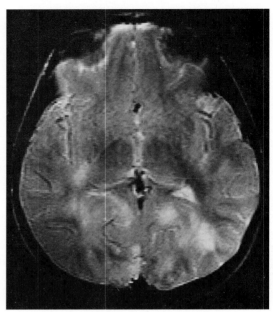

FIGURE 47–33 Gray matter involvement in ADEM. Axial T2-weighted image shows an abnormal bright signal in both the white and the gray matter.

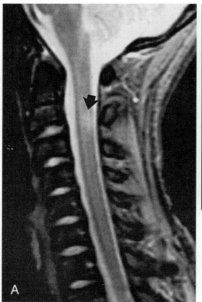

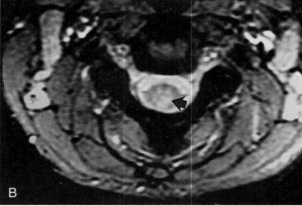

FIGURE 47–34 Brain stem involvement in ADEM. Sagittal *(A)* and axial *(B)* T2-weighted images of the cervical spinal cord show abnormal bright signal at C2 *(arrows)*.

aspartate and creatines and an increase in cholines and myo-inositol peaks. There may be reduced N-acetyl-aspartate in cortical gray matter.[3]

Acute disseminated encephalomyelitis or postinfectious encephalomyelitis is a monophasic acute inflammatory demyelinating disease, somewhat more common in children than adults.[48] It most commonly follows a viral illness but may also occur after immunization, bacterial infection, or serum administration.[48, 49] The most common presentation is the abrupt onset of fever and altered mental status, often associated with seizures and multifocal neurologic signs. Mild mononuclear pleocytosis and protein elevation is usually present in the cerebrospinal fluid. Less fulminant cases may present with headache, fever, irritability, drowsiness, or vomiting. Most patients recover completely over a period of a few weeks, although 10% to 20% have some permanent residual neurologic deficits.[49, 50] Histologic examination reveals perivenular inflammation and demyelination predominantly in the white matter. Cortical and deep gray matter structures are more commonly involved than in multiple sclerosis. It has been postulated that acute disseminated encephalomyelitis is an autoimmune disease, although cell-mediated immunity has not been well studied.

During the acute phase, edema is seen, and this edema is likely the cause of permanent disability in acute disseminated encephalomyelitis. The most common locations for permanent deficits are the optic nerves and spinal cord—confined areas where swelling might cause enough compression to result in ischemia. MRI of acute disseminated encephalomyelitis demonstrates a dynamic, asymmetric pattern of demyelination predominantly in the subcortical white matter (Fig. 47–32).[49, 50]

Gray matter involvement, both cortical and deep, is somewhat more common than with multiple sclerosis (Fig. 47–33). The brain stem, spinal cord, and cerebellar white matter are also frequently affected (Fig. 47–34). The pattern changes rapidly, with areas of enhancement appearing and then clearing and migrating areas of involvement during the acute phase of the disease. The disease responds quickly to steroid administration but may recur as steroids are tapered. Acute hemorrhagic encephalomyelitis is a more fulminant variant of acute disseminated encephalomyelitis, with rapid development of hemorrhagic necrosis within the brain (Fig. 47–35).[3] Most children die within the first week of the illness, but aggressive steroid administration may be beneficial.

Progressive multifocal leukoencephalitis is an acute demyelinating disease caused by a papovavirus in immunosuppressed patients. Asymmetric areas of bright signal are seen on T2-weighted sequences within the subcortical white matter (Fig. 47–36).[3] Mass effect and contrast enhancement are rarely present because of the inability of the immunosuppressed host to mount an inflammatory response to the illness. The disease is relentlessly progressive, with death occurring within months after the onset of the illness.

The collagen vascular disorders are immune-mediated diseases in which antigen-antibody response occurring in many parts of the body results in multiorgan dysfunction. In children, the most common collagen vascular disease is systemic lupus erythematosus.

METABOLIC DISEASES PRIMARILY OF GRAY MATTER

Several metabolic diseases have a predilection for gray matter involvement. Most of these result in abnormal bright signal within the basal ganglia on T2-weighted images. The areas of involvement commonly calcify. In the later stages of many of these diseases, white matter involvement is present in addition to the deep gray matter disease.

Ceroid-Lipofuscinosis

Ceroid-lipofuscinosis is an uncommon progressive encephalopathy inherited by autosomal recessive transmis-

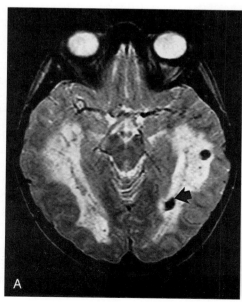
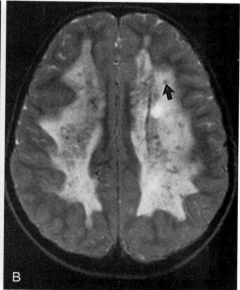

FIGURE 47–35 Acute hemorrhagic leukoencephalopathy variant of ADEM. Axial T2-weighted images at the level of the atria of the lateral ventricles (A) and the centrum semiovale (B) show abnormal bright signal diffusely throughout the white matter, with punctate foci of dark signal caused by hemorrhage (arrows).

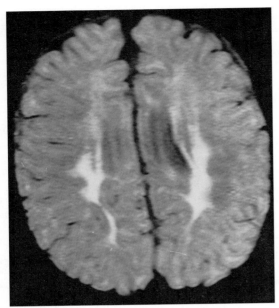

FIGURE 47–36 Progressive multifocal leukoencephalopathy. Axial FLAIR image shows an abnormal bright signal predominantly in the subcortical regions.

sion that causes gray matter degeneration within the cerebral cortex.[51–53] The pattern on MRI is that of cortical atrophy with relative sparing of the underlying white matter (Fig. 47–37).[54] Cortical gray matter is markedly hypointense on T2-weighted images.[55]

Hallervorden-Spatz Disease

Hallervorden-Spatz disease is an unusual metabolic disease in that an abnormality of iron metabolism causes

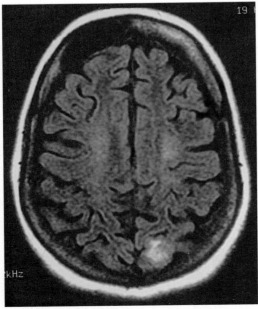

FIGURE 47–37 Ceroid lipofuscinosis. Axial FLAIR image shows an abnormal bright signal in the left occipital cortex.

iron deposition in the basal ganglia, resulting in a markedly dark signal on T2-weighted images.[56, 57] This pattern is unique and highly recognizable on MRI.

Patients with Hallervorden-Spatz disease usually present in the second decade of life with progressive gait problems that gradually result in rigidity of all extremities, movement disorders, dysarthria, and deteriorating higher cortical functions.[15, 21]

Initially, MRI is highly characteristic with an abnormally dark signal in the globus pallidus (Fig. 47–38).[56] This signal may become more complex as the disease progresses, with the development of foci of bright signal within the large areas of dark signal in the basal ganglia. The foci of bright signal are believed to represent cellular injury, death, and glial scarring.[57]

Juvenile Huntington's Disease

When Huntington's disease presents in childhood, the typical clinical presentation is quite different than that in adults. Patients with juvenile Huntington's disease present with rigidity rather than the choreoathetoid movements characteristic of adult Huntington's disease. Children also develop accelerated mental deterioration and seizures. Huntington's disease has an autosomal dominant form of transmission.

The imaging characteristics of juvenile Huntington's disease are similar to those in adults except for the early onset.[58] As in adults, affected children have abnormal bright signal in the caudate heads on T2-weighted sequences, which progresses to atrophy, first of the caudate, then of the putamen (Fig. 47–39).[58] Cortical atrophy is a late finding.

METABOLIC DISEASES WITH BOTH GRAY AND WHITE MATTER ABNORMALITIES

Mucopolysaccharidoses

The diseases that make up the mucopolysaccharidoses are characterized by a disorder in the lysosomes, intracellular storage sacs that contain enzymes that help degrade mucopolysaccharides. Lysosomes are named for their appearance and function; they contain enzymes that break down substances (*lysis*), and they are small bodies (*soma*). In all of the lysosomal storage disorders, there is a deficiency in one of the enzymes that degrades a specific macromolecule. In the mucopolysaccharidoses, the deficiency is of a specific exoglycosidase, an enzyme that normally breaks down the mucopolysaccharides, which are long chains of repeating disaccharide units. As the mucopolysaccharides collect, they fill the lysosomes and interfere with the degradation of other macromolecules.[12] These macromolecules as well as mucopolysaccharides accumulate in tissues and are excreted in the urine.[12]

The large category of the mucopolysaccharidoses comprises a group of several different diseases. These different diseases have different target organs that are most affected by the accumulation of mucopolysaccharide within the lysosomes. Table 47–1 summarizes the different diseases and their most frequent manifestations.

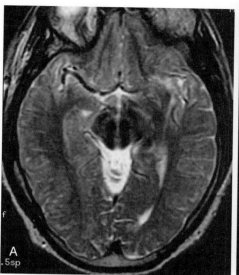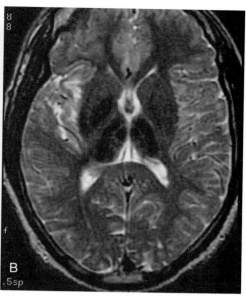

FIGURE 47–38 Hallevorden-Spatz disease. Axial T2-weighted images at the level of the midbrain *(A)* and basal ganglia *(B)* show characteristic abnormal dark signal lesions caused by iron deposition in the brain stem, basal ganglia, and thalamus.

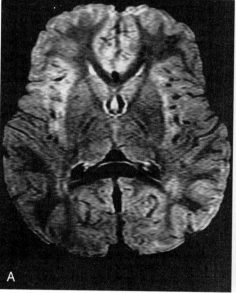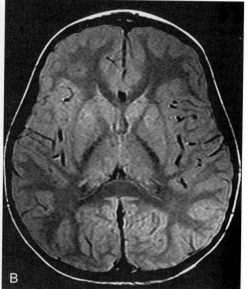

FIGURE 47–39 Juvenile Huntington's disease. Axial proton-density–weighted *(A)* and axial FLAIR *(B)* images show a subtle abnormal bright signal in the caudate nucleus.

TABLE 47–1 Mucopolysaccharidoses

Type	Disease Name	Target Organ System Involvement	Urinary Excretion
1H	Hurler's	Severe CNS, skeletal and visceral	Dermatan sulfate
1S(V)	Scheie's	No CNS, skeletal and visceral disease	Heparan sulfate
II	Hunter's	Mild-to-moderate CNS, skeletal and visceral	Dermatan or heparan sulfate
III	Sanfilippo's	Only CNS, mental deterioration	Heparan sulfate
IV	Morquio's	Severe skeletal, no CNS or visceral	Keratan sulfate
VI	Maroteaux-Lamy	Only skeletal, no CNS or visceral	Dermatan sulfate
VII	Sly's	Variable CNS, skeletal and visceral	Dermatan or heparan sulfate
VIII	Diferrante's	Only skeletal, no CNS or visceral	Dermatan or heparan sulfate

Abbreviation: CNS, central nervous system.

Neuropathologic examination of the brain in patients with central nervous system involvement reveals storage bodies in the neurons, astrocytes, and capillary pericytes. This involvement is especially severe in the white matter, where the periadventitial spaces are markedly dilated and filled with fluid, prompting the name *gargoyle cells*.[59, 60] The release of the viscous fluid from these cells into the subarachnoid space may cause scarring, resulting in arachnoid cysts (frequently in the sellar region) and communicating hydrocephalus.

The transmission of the mucopolysaccharidoses is by autosomal recessive inheritance except in Hunter's disease, which is sex-linked recessive. Mental retardation, hydrocephalus, and spinal cord compression, most commonly at C1, are the most common neurologic problems.[60] The spinal abnormalities are most common in mucopolysaccharidosis types IV and VI. Patients frequently are deaf, and extreme kyphosis, with a gibbous deformity in the lower thoracic spine, is common. There is a constellation of other skeletal and visceral manifestations of the mucopolysaccharidoses, including dwarfism with short limbs; abnormal facies with depression and widening of the nasal bridge; hypertrichosis; hepatosplenomegaly; and umbilical herniation.[60]

Imaging of patients with known mucopolysaccharidosis is usually reserved for evaluation of suspected hydrocephalus or spinal cord compression. The brain shows progressive atrophy, delayed myelination, white matter lesions, and variable hydrocephalus or arachnoid cysts.[61] The white matter lesions appear as focal areas of abnormally bright signal on T2-weighted images and dark on T1-weighted images.[61, 62] These appear as discrete areas isointense with cerebrospinal fluid and most likely represent mucopolysaccharide-filled spaces. Later in the disease, the abnormal white matter lesions may become more widespread and confluent, representing more diffuse infarction and demyelination (Fig. 47–40).

Wilson's Disease

Wilson's disease, an autosomal recessive disorder of copper metabolism, is characteristically seen with cirrhosis of the liver and brain degeneration that is predominantly of the basal ganglia.[63–65] The genetic defect in Wilson's disease is rare, and consanguinity is frequent. Large amounts of copper accumulate in the brain and liver. Elevated serum copper and ceruloplasmin levels and diminished fecal copper elimination can be demonstrated. When copper is deposited in the periphery of the cornea, a green Kayser-Fleischer ring may suggest the diagnosis. The disease may present with liver failure in children, nodular cirrhosis, jaundice, or portal hypertension.[65, 66] When neurologic symptoms are most prominent, the disease usually does not present until the teens.[66] Patients may present with signs of dysarthria, difficulty swallowing, tremor, dystonia, and psychiatric disorders. Schizophrenia or emotional disorders may be the only presenting signs in rare cases.

Pathologic examination of the brain reveals a marked red pigmentation and spongy degeneration in the putamen. Small cavities, decreased numbers of neurons, axonal degeneration, and large numbers of astrocytes are

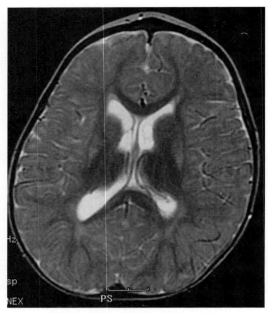

FIGURE 47–40 Mucopolysaccharidosis, although appearing frequently as normal on magnetic resonance imaging, this patient's axial T2-weighted image shows a very subtle bright signal in the white matter.

seen. Although the thalamus and putamen are the most commonly involved portions of the brain, abnormalities have also been demonstrated in the frontal lobe, brain stem, dentate nucleus, and substantia nigra.[67]

MRI of patients with Wilson's disease reveals increased signal in the thalamus, putamen, and caudate nuclei on T2-weighted sequences and dark signal on T1-weighted sequences.[67] Bright signal may also be seen in the globus pallidus and dorsal midbrain on T1-weighted images in patients with liver failure. This finding is typical of kernicterus and is not due primarily to copper deposition. Diffuse white matter abnormalities are frequently present, and cerebral cortical lesions, appearing bright on T2-weighted sequences, are generally bilaterally symmetric (Fig. 47–41).[68] Atrophy is present in the majority of patients. Improvement in the high-signal lesions and in neurologic function was demonstrated after copper-trapping therapy with chelating agents (D-penicillamine or zinc sulfate), but brain atrophy did not change.[67, 69, 70] A report of decreased signal intensities within the basal ganglia on T2-weighted imaging after therapy suggests that iron or calcium deposition in exchange for copper might occur.[71]

MITOCHONDRIAL ABNORMALITIES

The entities that constitute the mitochondrial disorders are a heterogeneous group with the common abnormalities of the function, number, and structure of the mitochondria.[72] Even though these disorders have been categorized into several different syndromes, there is considerable overlap among these, and different patients within the same family may resemble different syndromes. For this reason, it is suggested that the syn-

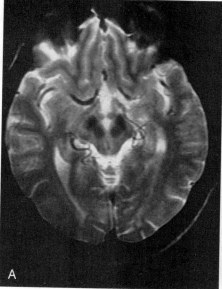
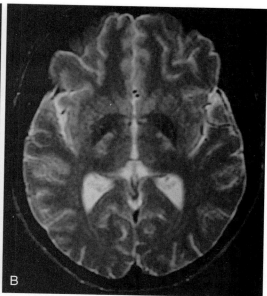

FIGURE 47–41 Wilson's disease. Mixed bright and dark lesions are present on axial T2-weighted images at the level of the midbrain (A) and basal ganglia (B).

dromes that constitute the mitochondrial disorders should be considered different manifestations of a spectrum of mitochondrial diseases rather than separate disease entities.[73, 74] Table 47–2 summarizes the mitochondrial disorders that have central nervous system findings. The diseases are arranged according to age at onset and are discussed in this order. These are not arranged in order of frequency, however, because mitochondrial encephalomyopathy with lactic acidosis and strokelike events (MELAS) syndrome and Leigh's disease are more common than the other disorders. Because myoclonic epilepsy with ragged-red fibers (MERRF) is an adult disease, it is not discussed here.[75]

TABLE 47–2 Mitochondrial Disorders

Disease	Usual Age at Presentation	Signs and Symptoms
Trichopolio- dystrophy	Infants	Hypotonia, failure to thrive, seizures, kinky hair, early death
Glutaric aciduria I and II	Infants	Hypotonia, acidosis, encephalopathy
Leigh's disease	0–2 yr	Variable CNS manifestations and progression
Alpers' disease	0–3 yr	Liver disease, epilepsy, severe progressive CNS deterioration
MELAS	10–20 yr	Acute episodes of cerebral infarction
Kearns-Sayre syndrome	10–20 yr	Progressive external ophthalmoplegia, weakness, short stature
MERRF	Adults	Bursts of myoclonus with weakness, short stature

Abbreviations: CNS, central nervous system; MELAS, mitochondrial encephalopathy with lactic acidosis and strokelike episodes; MERRF, myoclonic epilepsy with ragged-red fibers.

Trichopoliodystrophy or Menkes' Disease

Menkes' (kinky-hair) disease, also known as *trichopoliodystrophy,* is a rare (1:35,000 live births) X-linked recessive disease caused by abnormal copper metabolism.[76] Prenatal diagnosis is possible. Patients frequently present with low birth weight and prematurity. Hypotonia, unstable temperatures, seizures, drowsiness, and lack of spontaneous movements are typically seen in the infantile period. Kinky hair, the most commonly recalled feature of the disease, is not seen at birth. Infants are born with normal hair, which later becomes twisted, depigmented, and fragile, breaking off and leaving short stubble.[76] Progressive neurologic deterioration results in early death, usually between 4 and 6 months of age. The diagnosis can be made from low serum copper and ceruloplasmin levels and low urinary copper excretion. There is no known treatment. Pathologic examination reveals diffuse atrophy of both the gray and the white matter of the cerebrum and cerebellum. Multiple small fluid-filled spaces are present in the gray matter, with spongiform degeneration progressing to cavitation.

MRI and CT reveal rapidly progressive cerebral atrophy and large subdural spaces (Fig. 47–42).[77] When scanned early, abnormalities within the gray matter of the cerebral cortex can be seen as bright signal on T2-weighted images.[77–80] Menkes' disease is one of the differential considerations when presented with an imaging picture that may resemble shaken baby syndrome.[79, 80]

Glutaric Aciduria Types I and II

The two types of glutaric aciduria both result from mitochondrial defects.[81–83] Type I glutaric aciduria, with an autosomal recessive form of inheritance, is the result of a deficiency of glutaryl-coenzyme A dehydrogenase, an enzyme within the mitochondria.[81] The usual clinical presentation of glutaric aciduria type I is an infant who is normal during the first few months of life, who then

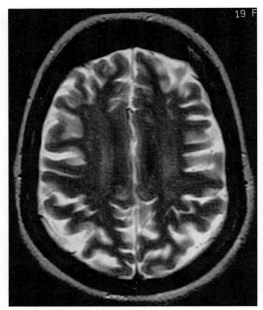

FIGURE 47–42 Menkes' kinky-hair disease. Axial T2-weighted image shows nonspecific atrophy.

develops acute encephalopathy. In some patients, a more slowly progressive neurologic deterioration occurs, with developmental delay, hypotonia, movement disorders, and eventually, tetraplegia. Seizures are common, and death occurs in childhood. Defective myelination and degeneration of the basal ganglia are found at autopsy. MRI demonstrates delay in myelination with abnormal basal ganglia, bright on T2-weighted and dark on T1-weighted images (Fig. 47–43). Atrophy is seen late in the course of the disease.

Glutaric aciduria type II is a rare disorder with the defect of the mitochondria located at the level of the electron transport chain at coenzyme Q.[82, 83] Most patients present in infancy with severe hypoglycemia, hypotonia, and acidosis, and death occurs within the first few weeks of life. A rare mild variant of this disease exists, with a few patients presenting in later infancy and even adulthood.

Leigh's Disease

Leigh's disease, an autosomal recessive disorder of pyruvate metabolism, is also known as *subacute necrotizing encephalomyelopathy.* There are several genetic and biochemical disorders of the mitochondria involving pyruvate metabolism with the clinical pattern of Leigh's disease.[84–86] For this reason, the term *Leigh's syndrome* has been used to describe the disorders that share similar clinical features, and the term *Leigh's disease* has been reserved for patients with classic pathologic findings.[87] The biochemical defects of patients with Leigh's syndrome include pyruvate dehydrogenase deficiency, pyruvate carboxylase deficiency, and cytochrome *c* oxidase deficiency.[84, 85, 87]

This syndrome typically presents in young children—two-thirds present younger than 2 years—but older children and even adults may be affected. In Leigh's disease as with most of the metabolic diseases, the older the onset, the more mild the course of the disease.[84, 85] The disease may be acute or slowly progressive. Even within the same family, there is great variability in the onset and course of the disease. The clinical course is characterized by seizures and neurologic deterioration, including spasticity, blindness, deafness, and dementia. There are multiple progressive neurologic problems, including ophthalmoplegia, apnea, ataxia, spasticity, paresis, extrapyramidal signs, feeding problems, and mental deterioration.[85]

Imaging findings are symmetric areas of bright signal on T2-weighted images and dark signal on T1-weighted images, most commonly of the basal ganglia (especially

FIGURE 47–43 Glutaric aciduria type I. *A,* Axial T2-weighted image at the level of the middle cranial fossa shows bilateral arachnoid cysts, found in 60% of patients with glutaric aciduria. *B,* Axial T2-weighted image at the level of the basal ganglia demonstrates an abnormal bright signal in the external capsule.

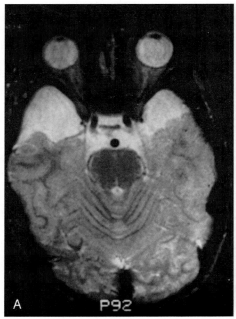

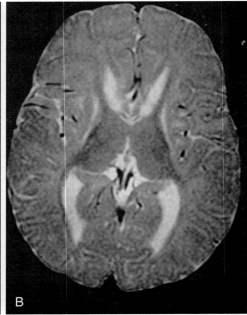

the putamen) but also within the midbrain in the periaqueductal region and cerebral peduncles.[83, 84] Involvement of the cortical gray matter, hypothalamus, dorsal pons, and white matter is also seen (Fig. 47–44). MRS has shown some promise in confirming the diagnosis of Leigh's disease, with elevation of the lactate peak and decreased N-acetyl-aspartate in areas most affected on MRI.[86]

Alpers' Disease

Progressive cerebral poliodystrophy, first described by Alpers, is an autosomal recessive disease with multisystem involvement of the brain, liver, heart, and muscles.[74] As with Leigh's syndrome, several different disease entities share the name *Alpers' disease,* all with the clinical findings of poliodystrophy and mitochondrial abnormalities.[74] Because Alpers' disease is only a collection of similar clinical and metabolic entities, there is a variable clinical presentation. Although a few infants are diagnosed with Alpers' disease, most patients present several years after normal early development. Liver disease may or may not precede neurologic symptoms, but abnormalities in liver chemistries can usually be detected.[89] Progressive mental retardation, epilepsy, dementia, movement disorders, vomiting, and failure to thrive are common symptoms. The epilepsy of Alpers' disease is particularly difficult to control, and several patients die from status epilepticus.

The disease is characterized histologically by atrophy with diffuse cystic deterioration of the cerebral cortex, particularly in the occipital lobes. Neuronal loss, gliosis, and microglial proliferation are seen. Involvement of the cerebellum, thalamus, basal ganglia, and brain stem is frequent.[74] In most patients, white matter atrophy is present.

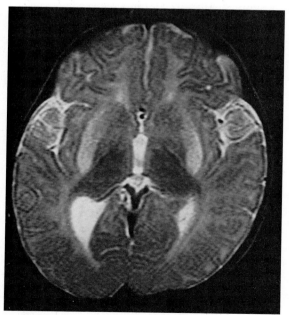

FIGURE 47–44 Leigh's disease. Axial T2-weighted image shows the characteristic, symmetric abnormal bright signal in the putamen.

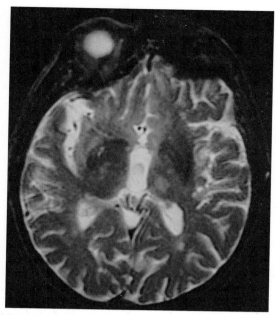

FIGURE 47–45 Alpers' disease. Atrophy with an abnormal bright signal in gray and white matter on the axial T2-weighted image.

The imaging characteristics of Alpers' disease are diffuse atrophy of both the white and the gray matter, with particular thinning of the corpus callosum.[11, 74] Focal lesions in both gray and white matter accompanied by atrophy and delayed myelination have been reported (Fig. 47–45).[90]

MELAS Disease

MELAS disease is a collection of disorders of mitochondrial function presenting with a characteristic clinical picture of acute episodes resembling cerebral infarction (hemiparesis, hemianesthesia, hemianopsia), which may be permanent or reversible.[89, 90] Other symptoms include episodic vomiting, tiredness, weakness, seizures, deafness, progressive mental retardation, and short stature. It has been suggested that the strokelike events are the result of mitochondrial dysfunction in the smooth muscles of the small arteries in the brain.[3] Although MELAS may present at any age, most patients are normal until their teens, when they present with progressive neurologic deterioration.[89]

Imaging studies are nonspecific, with abnormal areas of bright signal seen in any affected area of the brain.[89, 91] In patients with few or mild symptoms, the MRI scan is usually normal. It is common to see migrating areas of T2-weighted hyperintensities appear and resolve with exacerbation and improvement in the clinical symptoms.[88, 91] With time, however, and numerous strokelike episodes, most patients have permanent lesions.[91] Lesions appear as bright areas on T2-weighted images, dark areas on T1-weighted images, and lucent on CT scans (Fig. 47–46).[91, 93, 94] The distribution is variable, but temporal/parietal and occipital cortical and subcortical involvement is most frequent.[93, 94] Atrophy is a late finding.

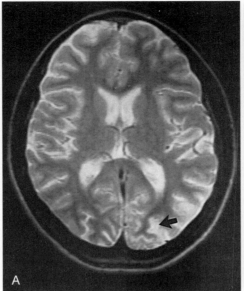
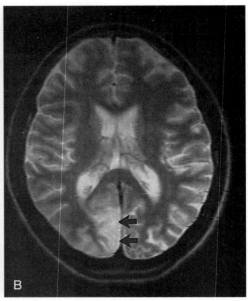

FIGURE 47–46 Mitochondrial encephalomyopathy with lactic acidosis and strokelike events (MELAS) syndrome. *A* and *B,* Axial T2-weighted images, obtained 3 months apart, show a changing pattern of abnormal areas of bright signal within the occipital cortex *(arrows).*

Kearns-Sayre Syndrome

Kearns-Sayre syndrome is a poorly characterized collection of disease entities with the clinical picture of chronic progressive external ophthalmoplegia, weakness, cardiac conduction defects, and retinitis pigmentosa.[2, 11, 95] Onset of symptoms is before age 20 years. Other neurologic signs include ataxia, sensorineural deafness, seizures, and dementia. Short stature, elevated cerebrospinal fluid protein, elevated serum and cerebrospinal fluid lactate, and endocrine abnormalities may be found. In some patients, renal abnormalities are present, with glycosuria, hyperphosphaturia, and aminoaciduria.

MRI reveals symmetric areas of abnormal bright signal within the basal ganglia and thalamus on T2-weighted images.[3] White matter lesions in a less symmetric distribution in the subcortical region are also common. Early involvement of the subcortical U-fibers is seen (Fig. 47–47).[3, 95]

ENDOCRINE LESIONS IN CHILDHOOD

Abnormalities of pituitary function may result from congenital or acquired lesions. Hypoplasia of the pituitary gland is an uncommon abnormality that is almost always associated with other congenital lesions. The most common of these lesions in the brain is septo-optic dysplasia, discussed with the other congenital brain lesions. Other associated anomalies include lesions or hypoplasia of the adrenal gland, thyroid, testes, ovaries, and penis. Patients with pituitary hypoplasia commonly present with short stature secondary to growth hormone deficiency. Older children may present with precocious puberty, and teenagers may be evaluated for delayed sexual development. Other symptoms of pituitary hormone dysfunction, such as thyroid or adrenal insufficiency, are rarely severe enough to cause the family to bring the child in for evaluation.

Imaging features of pituitary hypoplasia include a small sella and pituitary gland, hypoplasia of the infundibular stalk, and presence of a high-intensity posterior lobe of the pituitary gland in the region of the median eminence of the hypothalamus.[96] When seen in this region, the term *ectopic pituitary bright spot* is used to describe the aberrant location of the neurohypophysis (Fig. 47–48).[96] Although the neurohypophysis is aberrant in location, it functions normally, and these children have normal antidiuretic hormone function.[96, 97]

Pituitary dysfunction can result from compression from adjacent tumors (Fig. 47–49) as well as from damage

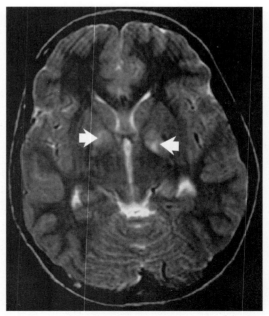

FIGURE 47–47 Kearns-Sayre syndrome. Axial T2-weighted image shows an abnormal bright signal in the deep gray matter *(arrows)* as well as scattered white matter lesions.

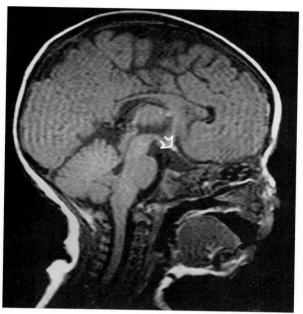

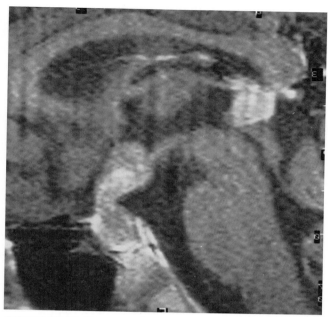

FIGURE 47–48 Ectopic posterior pituitary gland. Midsagittal T1-weighted, nonenhanced image demonstrates a small pituitary gland with hypoplastic infundibular stalk. The posterior pituitary bright spot is located at the upper extent of the infundibulum at the level of the median eminence of the hypothalamus *(arrow)*.

FIGURE 47–50 Pituitary adenoma causing symptoms of galactorrhea and amenorrhea in a 15-year-old girl. Midsagittal T2-weighted enhanced image shows a large mass extending cephalad through the diaphragma sella to the infundibular stalk.

owing to radiation or trauma. Intrinsic tumors of the pituitary gland are rare in preadolescent children (Fig. 47–50). Pituitary adenomas are occasionally found in adolescents and teenagers and appear identical to adenomas in adults.

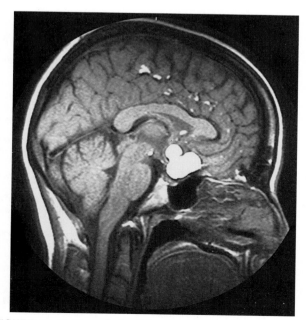

FIGURE 47–49 Hypoplasia of the pituitary gland associated with a suprasellar dermoid tumor. Midsagittal T1-weighted, nonenhanced image demonstrates a large mass with bright signal.

References

1. van der Knaap MS, Valk J, Barth PG, et al. Leukoencephalopathy with swelling in children and adolescents: MRI patterns and differential diagnosis. Neuroradiology 1995;37:679–686.
2. Diebler C, Dulac O. Pediatric Neurology and Neuroradiology. Berlin, Springer-Verlag, 1987.
3. Barkovich AJ. Toxic and metabolic brain disorders. In Barkovich AJ (ed). Pediatric Neuroimaging, pp. 55–105. New York, Raven, 1995.
4. Matalon R, Michals K, Sebesta D, et al. Aspartoacylase deficiency and N-acetylaspartic aciduria in patients with Canavan disease. Am J Med Genet 1988;29:463–471.
5. Brismar J, Brismar G, Gascon G, et al. Canavan disease: CT and MRI of the brain. AJNR 1990;11:805–810.
6. Valk J, van der Knaap MS. Magnetic Resonance of Myelin, Myelination, and Myelination Disorders. Berlin, Springer-Verlag, 1989.
7. Grodd W, Krageloh-Mann I, Petersen D, et al. In vivo assessment of N-acetylaspartate in brain in spongy degeneration (Canavan's disease) by proton spectroscopy. [Letter] Lancet 1990;2:437–438.
8. Farrell K, Chuang S, Becker LE. Computed tomography in Alexander's disease. Ann Neurol 1984;15:605–609.
9. Snodgrass SR. Abnormalities of carbohydrate metabolism. In Berg B (ed). Neurologic Aspects of Pediatrics, pp. 93–124. Boston, Butterworth-Heinemann, 1992.
10. Nelson MD Jr, Wolff JA, Cross CA, et al. Galactosemia: Evaluation with MRI. Radiology 1992;184:255–261.
11. Kendall BE. Disorders of lysosomes, peroxisomes, and mitochondria. AJNR 1992;13:621–653.
12. Becker LE. Lysosomes, peroxisomes and mitochondria: Function and disorder. AJNR 1992;13:609–620.
13. Bernardi B, Fonda C, Franzoni E, et al. MRI and CT in Krabbe's disease: Case report. Neuroradiology 1994;36:477–479.
14. Zafeiriou DI, Michelakaki EM, Anastasiou AL, et al. Serial MRI and neurophysiological studies in late-infantile Krabbe disease. Pediatr Neurol 1996;15:240–244.
15. Moser HW, Mihalik SJ, Watkins PA. Adrenoleukodystrophy and other peroxisomal disorders that affect the nervous system, including new observations on L-pipecolic acid oxidase in primates. Brain Dev 1989;11:80–90.
16. Moser H, Moser A, Naidu S, et al. Clinical aspects of adrenoleukodystrophy and adrenomyeloneuropathy. Dev Neurosci 1991;13:254–261.

17. Snyder RD, King JN, Keek GM, et al. MRI of the spinal cord in 23 subjects with ALD-AMN complex. AJNR 1991;12:1095–1098.

18. Kumar AJ, Rosenbaum AE, Naidu S, et al. Adrenoleukodystrophy: Correlating MRI with CT. Radiology 1987;165:497–504.

19. Tzkika A, Ball W Jr, Vigneron D, et al. Childhood adrenoleukodystrophy: Assessment with proton MRS. Radiology 1993;189:467–480.

20. Dubois J, Sebag G, Argyropoulou M, et al. MR findings in infantile Refsum disease: Case report of two family members. AJNR 1991;12:1159–1161.

21. Naidu S, Moser AE, Moser HW. Phenotypic and genotypic variability of generalized peroxisomal disorders. Pediatr Neurol 1988;4:5–12.

22. Wang PJ, Young C, Liu HM, et al. Neurophysiologic studies and MRI in Pelizaeus-Merzbacher disease: Comparison of classic and connatal forms. Pediatr Neurol 1995;33:47–53.

23. Sweetman L, Haas RH. Abnormalities of amino acid metabolism. In Berg BO (ed). Neurologic Aspects of Pediatrics, pp. 3–32. Boston, Butterworth-Heinemann, 1992.

24. Brismar J, Aqueel A, Brismar G, et al. Maple syrup urine disease. AJNR 1990;11:1219–1228.

25. Price VH. Trichothiodystrophy: Update. Pediatr Dermatol 1992;9:369–370.

26. Shaw DW, Maravilla KR, Weinberger E, et al. MRI of phenylketonuria. AJNR 1991;12:403–406.

27. Carroll WJ, Woodruff WW, Cadman TE. MR findings in oculocerebrorenal syndrome. AJNR 1993;14:449–451.

28. Tahsildar HI, Remler BF, Creger RJ, et al. Delayed, transient encephalopathy after marrow transplantation: Case reports and MRI findings in four patients. J Neurooncol 1996;27:241–250.

29. Thajeb P. Progressive late delayed postirradiation encephalopathy with Klüver-Bucy syndrome: Serial MRI and clinico-pathological studies. Clin Neurol Neurosurg 1995;97:264–268.

30. Valk PE, Dillon WP. Radiation injury of the brain. AJNR 1991;12:45–62.

31. Ball WS Jr, Prenger EC, Ballard ET. Neurotoxicity of radio/chemotherapy in children: Pathologic and MR correlation. AJNR 1992;13:761–776.

32. Young-Poussaint T, Barnes P, Burrows P, et al. Hemorrhagic radiation vasculopathy of the central nervous system in childhood: Diagnosis and follow-up. Radiology 1993;189:194.

33. Lien HH, Blomlie V, Saeter G, et al. Osteogenic sarcoma: MR signal abnormalities of the brain in asymptomatic patients treated with high dose methotrexate. Radiology 1991;179:547–550.

34. Ebner F, Ranner G, Slavc I, et al. MR findings in methotrexate-induced CNS abnormalities. AJNR 1989;10:959–964.

35. Wilson CA, Nitschke R, Bowman ME, et al. Transient white matter changes on MR images in children undergoing chemotherapy for acute lymphocytic leukemia: Correlation with neuropsychologic deficiencies. Radiology 1991;180:205–209.

36. Kay HEM, Knapton PJ, O'Sullivan JP, et al. Encephalopathy in acute leukemia associated with methotrexate therapy. Arch Dis Child 1972;47:344–354.

37. Leveque C, Soulie D, Sarrazin JL, et al. Toxic aluminum encephalopathy: Predominant involvement of the limbic system on MRI. J Neuroradiol 1996;23:168–172.

38. Press GA, Barshop BA, Haas RH, et al. Abnormalities of the brain in nonketotic hyperglycinemia: MR manifestations. AJNR 1989;10:315–321.

39. Heindel W, Kugel H, Roth B. Noninvasive detection of increased glycine content by proton MRS in the brains of two infants with nonketotic hyperglycinemia. AJNR 1993;14:629–635.

40. Barron TF, Devenyi AG, Mamourian AC. Symptomatic manganese neurotoxicity in a patient with chronic liver disease: Correlation of clinical symptoms with MRI findings. Pediatr Neurol 1994;10:145–148.

41. Weissenborn K, Ehrenheim C, Hori A, et al. Pallidal lesions in patients with liver cirrhosis: Clinical and MRI evaluation. Metab Brain Dis 1995;10:219–231.

42. Chamuleau RA, Vogels BA, Bosman DK, et al. In vivo brain magnetic resonance imaging (MRI) and magnetic resonance spectroscopy (MRS) in hepatic encephalopathy. Adv Exp Med Biol 1994;386:23–31.

43. Skehan S, Norris S, Hegarty J, et al. Brain MRI changes in chronic liver disease. Eur Radiol 1997;7:905–909.

44. Hanefeld F, Bauer HJ, Christen H-J, et al. Multiple sclerosis in childhood: Report of 15 cases. Brain Dev 1991;13:410–416.

45. Ebner F, Millner MM, Justich E, et al. Multiple sclerosis in children: Value of serial MR studies to monitor patients. AJNR 1990;11:1023–1027.

46. Osborn AG, Harnsberger HR, Smoker WR, et al. Multiple sclerosis in adolescents: CT and MR findings. AJNR 1990;11:489–494.

47. Dousset V, Gorssman RI, Ramer KN, et al. Experimental allergic encephalomyelitis and multiple sclerosis: Lewion characterization with magnetization transfer imaging. Radiology 1992;182:483–491.

48. Nasralla CAW, Pay N, Goodpasture HC, et al. Postinfectious encephalopathy in a child following *Campylobacter jejuni* enteritis. AJNR 1993;14:444–448.

49. Atlas SW, Grossman RI, Goldberg HI, et al. MR diagnosis of acute disseminated encephalomyelitis. J Comput Assist Tomogr 1986;10:798–801.

50. Caldmeyer KS, Harris TM, Smith RR, et al. Gadolinium enhancement in acute disseminated encephalomyelitis. J Comput Assist Tomogr 1991;15:673–675.

51. Autti T, Raininko R, Vanhanen SL, et al. MRI of neuronal ceroid lipofuscinosis: I. Cranial MRI of 30 patients with juvenile neuronal ceroid lipofuscinosis. Neuroradiology 1996;38:476–482.

52. Vanhanen SL, Liewendahl K, Raininko R, et al. Brain perfusion SPECT in infantile neuronal ceroid-lipofuscinosis (INCL): Comparison with clinical manifestations and MRI findings. Neuropediatrics 1996;27:76–83.

53. Wisniewski K, Kida E, Connell F, et al. New subform of the late infantile form of neuronal ceroid lipofuscinosis. Neuropediatrics 1993;24:155–163.

54. Vanhanen SL, Raininko R, Autti T, et al. MRI evaluation of the brain in infantile neuronal ceroid-lipofuscinosis: Part 2. MRI findings in 21 patients. J Child Neurol 1995;10:444–450.

55. Vanhanen SL, Raininko R, Santavuori P, et al. MRI evaluation of the brain in infantile neuronal ceroid-lipofuscinosis: Part 1. Postmortem MRI with histopathologic correlation. J Child Neurol 1995;10:438–443.

56. Farley TJ, Ketonen LM, Bodensteiner JB, et al. Serial MRI and CT findings in infantile Krabbe disease. Pediatr Neurol 1992;8:455–458.

57. Feliciani M, Curatolo P. Early clinical and imaging (high-field MRI) diagnosis of Hallervorden-Spatz disease. Neuroradiology 1994;36:247–248.

58. Harris GJ, Pearlson GD, Peyser CE, et al. Putamen volume reduction on magnetic resonance imaging exceeds caudate changes in mild Huntington's disease. Ann Neurol 1992;31:69–73.

59. McKusick VA, Neufeld EF. The mucopolysaccharide storage diseases. In Stanbury JB (ed). The Metabolic Basis of Inherited Disease, pp. 751–823. New York, McGraw-Hill, 1983.

60. Becker LE, Yates A. Inherited metabolic disease. In Davis R, Robertson D (eds). Textbook of Neuropathology, 2nd ed, pp. 331–427. Baltimore, Williams & Wilkins, 1990.

61. Lee C, Dineen TE, Brack M, et al. Mucopolysaccharidoses: Characterization by cranial MRI. AJNR 1993;14:1285–1292.

62. Murata R, Nakajima S, Tanaka A, et al. MRI of the brain in patients with mucopolysaccharidosis. AJNR 1989;10:1165–1170.

63. Mochizuki H, Kamakura K, Masaki T, et al. Atypical MRI features of Wilson's disease: High signal in globus pallidus on T1-weighted images. Neuroradiology 1997;39:171–174.

64. Aisen AM, Martel W, Gabrielsen TO, et al. CT of Wilson's disease. AJNR 1985;4:429–430.

65. Yoshii F, Takahashi W, Chinohara Y. A Wilson's disease patient with prominent cerebral white matter lesions: Five-year follow-up by MRI. Eur Neurol 1996;36:392–393.

66. Magalhaes AC, Caramelli P, Menizes JR, et al. Wilson's disease: MRI with clinical correlation. Neuroradiology 1994;36:97–100.

67. Roh JK, Lee TG, Wie BA, et al. Initial and follow-up brain MRI findings and correlation with the clinical course in Wilson's disease. Neurology 1994;10:1064–1068.

68. Prayer L, Wimberger D, Kramer J, et al. Cranial MRI in Wilson's disease. Neuroradiology 1990;32:211–212.

69. Huang CC, Chu NS. Wilson's disease: Resolution of MRI lesions following long-term oral zinc therapy. Acta Neurol Scand 1996;93:215–218.

70. Schlaug G, Hefter H, Engelbrecht V, et al. Neurological impairment and recovery in Wilson's disease: Evidence from PET and MRI. J Neurol Sci 1996;136:129–139.

71. Engelbrecht V, Schlaug G, Hefter H, et al. MRI of the brain in Wilson disease: T2 signal loss under therapy. J Comput Assist Tomogr 1995;19:635–638.

72. DiMauro S, Bonilla E, Lombes A, et al. Mitochondrial encephalo-myopathies. Neurol Clin 1990;8:483–506.

73. Wallace DC. Mitochondrial genetics: A paradigm for aging and degenerative diseases? Science 1992;256:628–632.

74. Tulinius MH, Holme E, Kristiansson B, et al. Mitochondrial encephalo-myopathies in childhood: II. Clinical manifestations and syndromes. J Pediatr 1991;119:251–259.

75. Rowland LP, Blake DM, Hirano M, et al. Clinical syndromes associated with ragged red fibers. Rev Neurol 1991;147:467–473.

76. Menkes JH. Genetic disorders of mitochondrial function. J Pediatr 1987;110:255–259.

77. Faerber EN, Grover WD, DeFilipp GJ, et al. Cerebral MR of Menkes kinky-hair disease. AJNR 1989;10:190–192.

78. Blaser SI, Berns DH, Ross JS, et al. Serial MR studies in Menkes disease. J Comput Assist Tomogr 1989;13:113–115.

79. Ichihashi K, Yano S, Kobayashi S, et al. Serial imaging of Menkes disease. Neuroradiology 1990;32:56–59.

80. Johnsen DE, Coleman L, Poe L. MR of progressive neurodegenerative change in treated Menkes' kinky hair disease. Neuroradiology 1991;33:181–182.

81. Altman NR, Rovira MJ, Bauer M. Glutaric aciduria type I: MR findings in two cases. AJNR 1991;12:966–968.

82. Goodman SI, Frerman FE, Loehr JP. Recent progress in understanding glutaric acidemias. Enzyme 1987;38:76–79.

83. Sugita K, Kakinuma H, Okajima Y, et al. Clinical and MRI findings in a case of D-2 hydroxyglutaric aciduria. Brain Dev 1995;17:139–141.

84. Koch TK, Yee M, Hutchinson H, et al. Magnetic resonance imaging in subacute necrotizing encephalomyelopathy (Leigh's disease). Ann Neurol 1986;19:605–607.

85. Paltiel HJ, O'Gorman PM, Meagher-Villemure K, et al. Subacute necrotizing encephalomyelopathy (Leigh disease): CT study. Radiology 1987;162:115–118.

86. Shevell MI, Matthews PM, Scriver CR, et al. Cerebral dysgenesis and lactic acidemia: An MRI/MRS phenotype associated with pyruvate dehydrogenase deficiency. Pediatr Neurol 1994;11:224–229.

87. Medina L, Chi TI, DeVivo DC, et al. MR findings in patients with subacute necrotizing encephalomyelopathy (Leigh syndrome): Correlation with biochemical defect. AJNR 1990;11:379–384.

88. Kimura S, Osaka H, Saitou K, et al. Improvement of lesions shown on MRI and CT scan by administration of dichloroacetate in patients with Leigh syndrome. J Neurol Sci 1995;134:103–107.

89. Rosen L, Phillips S, Enzmann D. Magnetic resonance imaging in MELAS syndrome. Neuroradiology 1990;32:168–171.

90. Harding BN. Progressive neuronal degeneration of childhood with liver disease (Alpers-Huttenlocher syndrome): A personal review. J Child Neurol 1990;5:273–287.

91. Abe K, Invi T, Hirono N, et al. Fluctuating MR images with mitochondrial encephalomyopathy, lactic acidosis, stroke-like syndrome (MELAS). Neuroradiology 1990;32:77.

92. Clark JM, Marks MP, Adalsteinsson E, et al. MELAS: Clinical and pathologic correlations with MRI, xenon/CT, and MRS. Neurology 1996;46:223–227.

93. Damian MS, Reichmann H, Seibel P, et al. MELAS syndrome: Clinical aspects, MRI, biochemistry and molecular genetics. Nervenarzt 1994;65:258–263.

94. Huang CC, Wai YY, Chu NS, et al. Mitochondrial encephalomyopathies: CT and MRI findings and correlations with clinical features. Eur Neurol 1995;35:199–205.

95. Demange P, Gia HP, Kalifa G, et al. MR of Kearns-Sayre syndrome. AJNR 1989;10:S91.

96. Kelly WM, Kucharczyk W, Kucharczyk J, et al. Posterior pituitary ectopia: An MR feature of pituitary dwarfism. AJNR 1988;9:453–460.

97. Abrahams JJ, Trefelner E, Boulware SD. Idiopathic growth hormone deficiency: MR findings in 35 patients. AJNR 1991;12:155–160.

C H A P T E R

48

Imaging of Congenital Abnormalities of the Face

MAURICIO CASTILLO, M.D.
SURESH K. MUKHERJI, M.D.

This chapter addresses the imaging features of congenital malformations of the face with emphasis on the central portion. Knowledge of the embryology of this complex region is essential for the understanding of the imaging findings. Because of its complexity, both computed tomography (CT) and magnetic resonance imaging (MRI) are required.

EMBRYOLOGY

The formation of the face is primarily determined by the migration of cranial neural crest cells.[1] Cells from the region of the fifth cranial nerve nuclei migrate initially in a wavelike fashion into the orbits and maxillary and mandibular regions. A second wave of migrating neural crest cells establishes the skeletal and connective tissues of the face. These neural crest cells will form the lower, mid and superior, and orbital (including the eye) regions of the face (Fig. 48–1). The lower facial component comprises the upper neck, mandible, and external ear structures, which are derived from the branchial apparatuses. The mandible forms from the first branchial arches. The first and second branchial arches give rise to the pinnae; tympanic membranes; malleuses; incuses; superstructures of the stapes; styloid processes; hyoid bone; trigeminal and facial nerves; and the muscles of mastication and facial expression.[2] The pinnae (auricles) and the external auditory canals are derived from the first branchial groove and the mesoderm of the first and second branchial arches. The pinnae continue to grow and are fully formed by the third week of life. By the eighth week, the primary external auditory meatuses are formed and will eventually become the cartilaginous portions of the external auditory canals. These deepen and contact the tubotympanic recesses, which derive from the first pharyngeal pouches.[3] Epidermal plugs will cover these openings and dissolve at about the 28th week, resulting in the tympanic membranes and patent external auditory canals. The formation of the mastoid bones, middle ear cavities, ossicles, and labyrinths is beyond the scope of this chapter.

The oral opening separates the lower face from the midface. This opening derives from the oral placode. It eventually divides into the proper mouth opening and the buccal cavity, which derives from the stomodeum.[3] The cephalic portion of the pharyngeal gut is separated from the stomodeum by the buccopharyngeal membrane. This membrane disappears by the fourth week of life, and a communication is established between the gut and the mouth. The embryologic remnant of the buccopharyngeal membrane is Waldeyer's ring. The midface is basically formed by the nasal cavities and the nose. The midface is continuous with the superior face, which is mainly formed by the forehead. The developments of the midface and superior face are intimately related, and it is better to consider them as a unit. Also, the formation of the nose and its cavities is intimately related to the formation of the orbits and lacrimal apparatuses. The nasal placode deepens to form the nasal pits, which separate

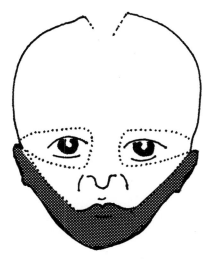

FIGURE 48–1 Facial segments. The lower aspect of the face (*shaded*) derives from the branchial apparatus. The orbits (*dotted lines*) arise from the specialized optic placodes. The midface derives from the frontal, nasal, and maxillary processes. (From Castillo M, Mukherji SK. Imaging of the Pediatric Head, Neck, and Spine. Philadelphia, Lippincott-Raven, 1996.)

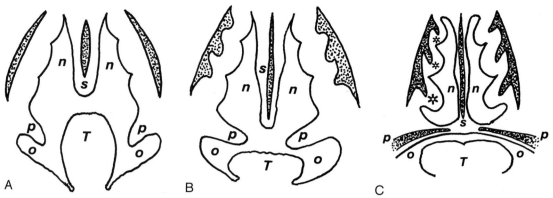

FIGURE 48–2 Formation of the nasal cavities. *A*, At 6 weeks of life, the nasal cavities (n) communicate with the oral cavity (o) and tongue (T). The nasal septum (s) and palatal shelves (p) are rudimentary. *Shaded areas* indicate cartilage. *B*, At 8 weeks, the septum (s) has elongated inferiorly and the palatal shelves (p) have a more midline position. The nasal cavities (n) still communicate with the oral cavity (o) and the tongue (T). *C*, At 10 weeks, the septum (s) and palate (p) have fused, separating the nasal cavities (n) from the oral cavity (o) and tongue (T). The rudimentary nasal conchae (asterisks) are present. (*A–C*, From Castillo M, Mukherji SK. Imaging of the Pediatric Head, Neck, and Spine. Philadelphia, Lippincott-Raven, 1996.)

the nasomedial and nasolateral processes.[4] The nasal pits will form the nostrils, and together with the nasal processes they will form the piriform (or anterior) nasal apertures. The primitive nasal cavities are present at 6 weeks and are separated from the buccal cavity by the rudimentary palatal shelves, which derive from fusion of the maxillary and frontal processes (Fig. 48–2A). The nasal cavities are separated in the midline by a cartilaginous septum. At 8 weeks, the palatal shelves begin to migrate medially and the nasal septum inferiorly (Fig. 48–2B). At 10 weeks, the palatal shelves fuse in the midline, and also with the inferior border of the nasal septum, and with the posterior margins of the primary palate, which is located in the anteriormost aspect of the buccal cavity (Fig. 48–2C). At this stage, the lateral walls of both nasal cavities contain excrescences that will form the nasal conchae. Posteriorly, the embryonic nasal cavities are separated from the buccal cavity by the bucconasal membrane. This membrane eventually dissolves, establishing a communication between both cavities and also possibly forming the soft palate. The posterior nasal cavities canalize and form the primary or temporary choanae. These openings become occluded by epithelial plugs that later resorb and finally establish the secondary or permanent posterior choanae. The naso-optic grooves extend from the inferior aspects of the nasal cavities to the medial orbits (Fig. 48–3). Superiorly, they give rise to the lacrimal canaliculi and sacs and, inferiorly, to the valves of Hasner, which are located under the inferior turbinates. Their midportion will form the nasolacrimal ducts.[5] The superior portion of the nasomedial process extends rostrally to fuse with the frontal prominence and produce the nasal bones; cartilaginous nasal capsule (which produces mainly the nasal septum and the ethmoid sinus complexes); the central portion of the upper lip and of the superior alveolus; central incisors; the anteriorly located primary palate; and the frontal bones. From the inferior portion of the nasomedial process, the maxillary processes merge and give origin to the columella and the philtrum. During the fourth to eighth weeks of life, the nasolateral

processes fuse with maxillary processes and give origin to the nasal alae. At this stage, the outer segment maxillary processes merge with the mandibular arches and establish the lateral margins of the mouth. The maxillary processes also fuse with the frontal process to form the lateral two-thirds of the upper lip and superior alveoli, and the palatal shelves. The formation of the paranasal sinuses is not addressed here.

The superior portion of the nose fuses with the frontal bones. At around 7 to 8 weeks of life, the nasofrontal region develops.[6] Both frontal and nasal components derive from intramembranous ossification centers. The posterior margin of the nasofrontal region is the cartilaginous nasal capsule and the anterior skull base. Between the primitive nasal bones and the cartilaginous capsule is the prenasal space (Fig. 48–4A). During its development, this space contains a dural cerebrospinal fluid–filled diverticulum. This diverticulum regresses into the cranial cavity,

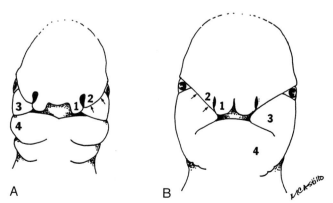

FIGURE 48–3 Formation of the midface. *A*, Face at 5 weeks of life. *B*, Face at 7 weeks. 1, nasal medial process; 2, nasolateral process; 3, maxillary process; 4, mandibular process. *Arrows* indicate the naso-optic grooves. (*A* and *B*, From Castillo M. Congenital abnormalities of the nose: CT and MR findings. AJR 1994;162:1211–1217.)

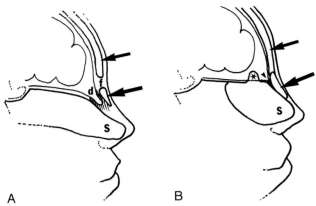

FIGURE 48–4 Development of the nasofrontal region. *A,* During fetal life, the prenasal space *(shaded area)* contains a dural diverticulum (d) that separates the nasal bones *(large arrow)* from the cartilaginous nasal capsule (S). The fonticulus frontalis (f) is located between the nasal and the frontal bones *(small arrow). B,* With growth, the prenasal space is obliterated and the nasal septum (S) and nasal bones *(large arrow)* fuse. The foramen cecum *(arrowhead)* is the remnant of the diverticulum and is located anterior to the crista galli *(asterisk).* The nasal and frontal bones *(small arrow)* fuse, closing the fonticulus frontalis.

leaving behind the foramen cecum, which lies anterior to the crista galli. Between the primitive nasal bones and the frontal bones is a tiny fontanelle known as the *fonticulus frontalis.* Fusion of the nasal and frontal bones obliterates this space, leaving behind the nasofrontal suture (Fig. 48–4B).

During the fourth week of life, the formation of the orbits begins. The optic sulci extend outward from the forebrain and later invaginate on themselves to produce the optic vesicles.[7] Progressive elongation of the optic vesicles leads to formation of the optic nerves. Invagination of the optic vesicles produces the optic cups. The ectoderm, which invaginates into the anterior aspects of the optic cups, is known as the *lenticular vesicles.* The lenticular vesicles become incorporated into the optic cups. The lenticular vesicles will form the lenses, anterior chambers, and corneas. The embryonic fissures fuse and finish the closing of the optic cups. The hyaloid arteries are trapped inside the cups by these fissures. These hyaloid arteries supply the vascular mesenchymes that will eventually form the vitreouses. Neuroectoderm will eventually form the optic nerves and the retinas. Detailed discussion of this region is beyond the scope of this presentation.

From this discussion it is obvious that the development of the face occurs mainly from the fourth to the eighth weeks of life. Although the face is formed by different components, their development is interrelated, and an anomaly in one component usually affects the development of others (Table 48–1). For example, an arrest in the midline fusion of neural crest cells in the face commonly leads to midfacial clefts and to incomplete closure of the optic embryonic fissure, resulting in colobomas; hypoplasia of branchial apparatus derivatives results in hemifacial microsomia and also in an ipsilateral small orbit with microphthalmos. In addition, the formation of

the midline facial structures is related to the formation of the midline intracranial structures such as the corpus callosum, pituitary-hypothalamic axis, and ventricles. Children with midline facial anomalies may have midline cerebral defects.

MALFORMATIONS OF THE LOWER AND LATERAL FACE

Malformations of the lower and lateral face result from anomalous development of the first to fourth branchial arches on either side. These malformations comprise mandibular hypoplasia and hypoplasia or aplasia of the ipsilateral auricle, external auditory canals, and middle ear cavity.[8] The ipsilateral malleus and incus are commonly involved.

Crouzon's syndrome is also known as *craniofacial dysostosis.*[9] It is commonly inherited as an autosomal

TABLE 48–1 Common Anomalies Resulting from Anomalous Development of Different Facial Regions

Facial Region Involved	Resulting Anomaly
Lower and lateral face	Crouzon's disease, Goldenhar's syndrome, maxillofacial dysostosis, Nager's anomaly, Treacher Collins syndrome, and other hemifacial hypoplasias
Mouth region	Transverse facial clefts and syndromes associated with macrostomia, common facial clefts
Midline face	Midline facial clefting syndromes, holoprosencephalies, Apert's syndrome, primary or secondary cleft palate and lip, agenesis of the nose, polyrhinia, common facial clefts
Off-midline facial regions	Hypoplasia of the nasal alae, nasolacrimal duct anomalies, lateral nasal clefting, proboscis lateralis, common facial clefts
Posterior nasal passages	Stenosis or atresia of posterior choanae, nasopharyngeal atresia, secondary cleft palate, bifid uvula
Anterior nasal passages	Piriform nasal aperture stenosis, distal nasolacrimal duct cysts, agenesis of the nose
Nasofrontal region Prenasal space	Dermoids, epidermoids, dermal sinuses, intranasal heterotopias,° nasoethmoid encephalocele
Fonticulus frontalis	Extranasal heterotopias,° frontonasal encephalocele

°Also referred to as *nasal gliomas.*

dominant trait but may also be sporadic. The maxilla is typically small. The external auditory canals are narrowed and are occasionally absent. The malleus and incus are deformed and may be fused to each other or fused to the tegmen tympani. The middle ear cavity is small. Proptosis and hypertelorism are present. Synostosis may involve any suture and result in brachycephaly, oxycephaly, dolichocephaly, or trigonocephaly. Hydrocephalus may be present.

Goldenhar's syndrome is also known as *oculoauriculovertebral dysplasia*. This syndrome does not have a known pattern of inheritance, and most cases are sporadic. The mandible and maxilla are small (Fig. 48–5). The auricles are malformed and preauricular skin tags may be seen. The external auditory canal may be narrowed or absent.[10] The malleus and incus may also be deformed or absent. The middle ear cavity is small. The labyrinth is abnormal. Ocular colobomas may be present. The cervical spine may harbor segmentation defects and block (fused) vertebrae.

Nager's anomaly or syndrome is also known as *acrofacial dysostosis*. Its pattern of inheritance is not known. The mandible and the zygomatic arches are small and the auricles are deformed (Fig. 48–6). Ocular colobomas may be present.

Treacher Collins syndrome is also known as *mandibulofacial dysostosis*. It is inherited as an autosomal dominant trait. The mandible and the zygomas are small (Fig. 48–7). The external auditory canals may be small or absent and there may be preauricular skin tags. The middle ear cavities and the mastoid air cells may be hypoplastic. The malleus and incus may be absent, deformed, or fused.[11] The hard palate may be absent, giving rise to a cleft. The orbits are slanted in an antimongoloid fashion. Ocular colobomas may be present.

In the hemifacial microsomia syndrome, the mandible

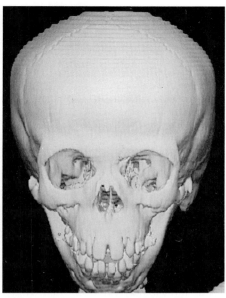

FIGURE 48–6 Nager's anomaly. Frontal three-dimensional re-formation of CT data shows a small mandible and shallow zygomatic arches.

and maxilla are small. The temporomandibular joints may be malformed. The ipsilateral auricle is often small. The external auditory canal is narrowed or absent. The malleus and incus may be deformed or fused. Ocular colobomas may be present.

These anomalies are well evaluated by CT using a spiral (helical) technique with 3-mm-thick sections at an equal distance of table travel (pitch of 1). The images are reconstructed with 3-mm-thick sections. This allows future three-dimensional re-formation of the data. If craniosynostosis is present, the skull also needs to be imaged. This may be done with the same data volume if the CT unit permits, and if not, a second spiral volume should be obtained with a similar technique. The images are processed using the high-resolution (edge enhancement) bone algorithm and soft tissue window settings. This should also be done for the images of the skull in order to evaluate the brain. Detailed evaluation of middle and inner ear malformations may not be possible with this technique. If these malformations are a consideration, it may be necessary to complement the initial study with direct coronal 1-mm-thick sections (nonspiral) through the temporal bones.

MALFORMATIONS OF THE MOUTH

Malformations of the mouth result from incomplete, late, or exaggerated and early fusion of the maxillary processes with the mandibular arches. There is great variability in the size of the mouth. A large mouth is also known as *macrostomia* and is probably a variation of bilateral transverse facial clefts.[12] However, transverse facial clefts may be unilateral. These should be distinguished from facial deformities produced by amniotic bands, which may have a similar clinical appearance. Macrostomia may be an isolated anomaly or be found in combination with

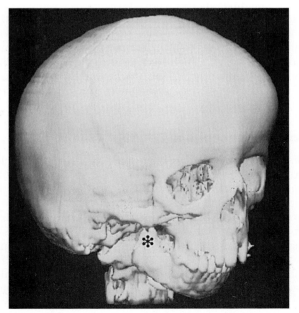

FIGURE 48–5 Goldenhar's syndrome. Oblique three-dimensional re-formation of computed tomography (CT) data shows a severely hypoplastic mandible (*asterisk*) with an absent condyle and coronoid process.

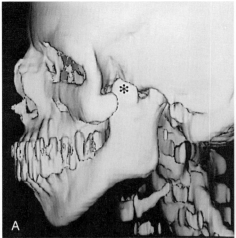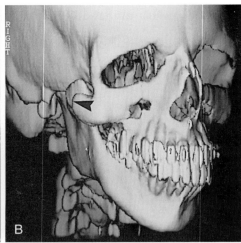

FIGURE 48–7 Treacher Collins syndrome. *A,* Lateral three-dimensional re-formation of CT data shows a somewhat small mandible with a small condyle and compensatory overgrowth of the coronoid process *(asterisk). B,* Oblique view shows a hypoplastic right zygomatic arch *(arrowhead)* and deformity of the mandible.

Treacher Collins and Goldenhar's syndromes.[9] On rare occasions, the mouth may be very small (microstomia). These anomalies generally do not require imaging.

MALFORMATIONS OF THE MIDLINE FACE

Malformations of the midline face can be classified into those that have facial clefts with hypertelorism (midline facial cleft syndromes), facial clefts with normal interocular distance (common facial clefts), and those with or without clefts and hypotelorism (holoprosencephalies and variants).

Midline Cleft Syndromes

The midline facial cleft syndromes are very rare and constitute less than 1% of all facial clefts.[13] They are inherited in a sporadic fashion, but a few familial cases are known to exist. These have been either autosomal dominant or recessive and may also occur in twins. The cleft may or may not be visible clinically; however, hypertelorism is always present (Fig. 48–8A; Table 48–2). For practical purposes, these clefting anomalies may be divided into high (group A) and low (group B) syndromes. Some patients have features of both groups. In the low syndrome, the cleft involves the upper lip, the hard and soft palates, and only rarely the nose. (Fig. 48–8B).[3] The cleft is mostly midline and in the nose may be covered by skin. Intracranially, midline lipomas and dysgenesis of the corpus callosum may be present. Basal cephaloceles may also occur. The arrest in midline facial fusion concurs with an arrest of closure of optic embryonic fissure that leads to dysplasias of the optic nerves such as colobomas, optic pits, and megalopapilla. (Fig. 48–8C). In the high group, the midline cleft involves the nose and the forehead but only rarely the upper lip and palate (Fig. 48–8D and E).[14] The cleft is commonly covered by skin and may be seen as a shallow depression in the bridge of the nose and forehead. The tip of the nose may be bifid. Hypertelorism is prominent. The anterior hairline is low with a "widow's peak" configuration. The cleft continues

from the forehead into the region of the bregma. A larger bone defect covered by skin (cranium bifidum occultum) is commonly present. Isolated cranium bifidum occultum is the mildest form of this syndrome. Intracranially, interhemispheric lipomas and dysgenesis of the corpus callosum may accompany this syndrome (Fig. 48–8F). There may be intraorbital or frontoethmoid (frontobasal) cephaloceles. The globes may be small (microphthalmos) or absent (anophthalmos). It is in this group of patients (high syndrome) that the syndrome may be familial. Other associated anomalies are hydrocephalus, sutural synostosis, preauricular skin tags, mental retardation, and scoliosis.

Imaging of patients with midline facial cleft syndromes requires both CT and MRI. CT is ideal for imaging of the face. Contiguous axial 3-mm-thick slices (preferably using spiral techniques) should be obtained from the lower mandible to the skull vertex. Three-dimensional data re-formations provide valuable information to the otolaryngologist and the plastic surgeon. CT images (also 3-mm-thick sections) may be continued through the brain and processed with high-resolution (edge enhancement) bone algorithms to evaluate bony defects and sutural synostosis. However, examination of the brain is better performed with MRI.

Holoprosencephalies

The holoprosencephalies are a group of disorders characterized by the lack of normal diverticulation and separation of the cerebral hemispheres as well as failure of midline cleavage of the face.[15] These anomalies are always accompanied by decreased interocular distance (hypotelorism) except in the less severe forms (Fig. 48–9A. See also Table 48–2). Alobar and semilobar types commonly have midfacial clefts (Fig. 48–9B). Patients with lobar holoprosencephaly and septo-optic dysplasia generally have no facial clefts, and the interocular distance tends to be normal. Holoprosencephaly occurs in approximately 1 in 16,000 live births and is associated with maternal diabetes, bleeding during early pregnancy, dizygotic twinning, radiation exposure, and several chromosomal anomalies.[15] The appearance of the face indicates the condition

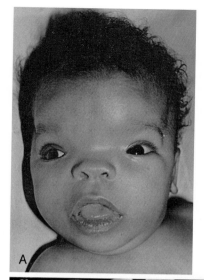

FIGURE 48–8 Median cleft syndrome. *A*, Child with hypertelorism and a flat nasal bridge (high median facial cleft syndrome). *B*, Axial CT scan in a child with low median facial cleft syndrome shows the cleft involving the upper lip and palate. *C*, Axial CT scan in the same patient shows bilateral colobomas *(arrows)* and microphthalmia. *D*, Three-dimensional re-formation of CT data in a different case of high median cleft syndrome shows the cleft *(arrowheads)* extending from the maxilla to a large cranium bifidum defect. *E*, Three-dimensional re-formation of CT data in a different patient shows an occult cranium bifidum defect and calcification *(arrow)* of the anterior falx cerebri. *Small arrow* indicates the nasal cleft. *F*, Axial CT scan in the same patient as in *E* shows agenesis of the corpus callosum and an interhemispheric lipoma (L). (*A–F*, From Castillo M, Mukherji SK. Imaging of the Pediatric Head, Neck, and Spine. Philadelphia, Lippincott-Raven, 1996.)

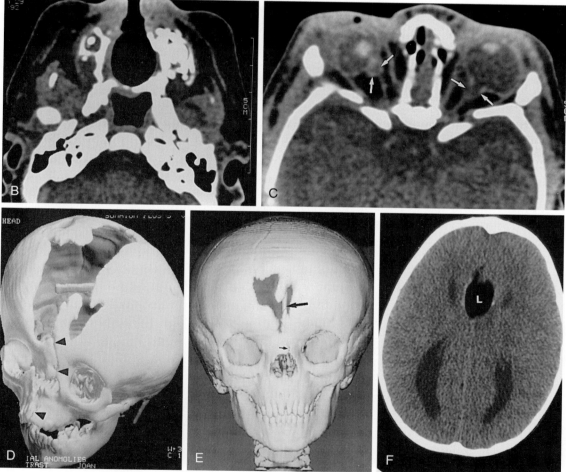

of the brain, but a "normal" face does not mean a "normal" brain. Severe facial deformities are always accompanied by severe cerebral anomalies. The most severe type of hypotelorism is fusion of both orbits resulting in a single midline eye (cyclopia). These children have a supraophthalmic tube of soft tissue (proboscis) protruding from their foreheads. They may also have two orbits

accompanied by a proboscis, two orbits with a rudimentary nose that has only one nostril, median cleft lip with hypotelorism, and isolated hypotelorism.[15] Generally, only children with the latter two facial expressions survive past infancy. Patients with severe facial anomalies tend to be stillborn. The bridge of the nose is flat in all patients with holoprosencephaly. Occasionally, a single midline upper

TABLE 48–2 Relationship of Facial Clefts to Interocular Distance

Facial Anomaly or Interocular Distance	Midline Facial Cleft Syndromes	Holoprosen- cephalies	Common Facial Clefts
Hypertelorism	+		
Hypotelorism		+	
Normal			+

central incisor is present and may be accompanied by cerebral anomalies and stenosis of the nasal piriform apertures. A lateral proboscis is not commonly associated with holoprosencephaly. Survivors commonly have spasticity, athetoid movements, and mental retardation. Holoprosencephaly has been classically divided into three categories according to order of severity: alobar, semilobar, and lobar. Septo-optic dysplasia may also be a part of lobar holoprosencephaly.[16] In reality, the classification of holoprosencephalies is artificial, as many patients have anomalies that are difficult to fit into a single type. It is better to consider the holoprosencephalies as a single disorder with different expressions of severity.

Patients with alobar holoprosencephaly are always microcephalic. The lateral ventricles are fused into a single horseshoe-shaped ventricle with no septum pellucidum (Fig. 48–9C). This ventricle may communicate with a dorsal interhemispheric cyst. The brain is flat and there is no interhemispheric fissure, no falx cerebri, and no corpus callosum. The third ventricle is absent and the thalami are fused. Venous and arterial anomalies are common.

The intermediate form of the spectrum is semilobar holoprosencephaly. Microcephaly is common. The mono-

ventricle shows rudimentary temporal horns. The septum pellucidum is absent.[17] The posterior aspect of the interhemispheric fissure and falx cerebri may be present. The splenium of the corpus callosum may also be present.

The least severe type is lobar holoprosencephaly. Patients are normocephalic. The lateral ventricles are almost normal in shape, but the septum pellucidum is absent. The third ventricle is present and the thalami are separated. The interhemispheric fissure and falx cerebri are near normal but may be dysgenetic anteriorly.

The septum pellucidum is also absent in patients with septo-optic dysplasia; therefore, this disorder may be considered as the mildest form of holoprosencephaly (Fig. 48–10A).[16] Approximately 50% of patients with septo-optic dysplasia present with seizures, and the other half present with hormonal anomalies. In the former group, a schizencephaly is present. In the latter group, the pituitary gland is absent and the posterior lobe is translocated to the hypothalamus (Fig. 48–10B and C). The optic nerves and the chiasm are hypoplastic in both groups. Optic nerve hypoplasia may be difficult to establish reliably on imaging studies, but funduscopy readily establishes the presence of small optic nerve disks.

It is not imperative to image the face in children with holoprosencephaly. The imaging of the brain is better done with MRI.

Common Facial Clefts

More than 95% of all facial clefts fall into the category of common facial clefts. In these patients, the interocular distance is normal, (see Table 48–2). Most of these clefts are isolated anomalies without central nervous system anomalies. Embryologically, the hard palate is formed by the posterior and shelflike secondary palates and the

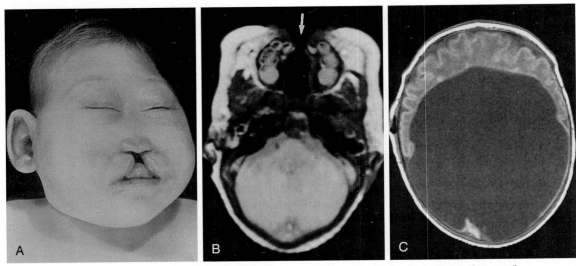

FIGURE 48–9 Holoprosencephalies. *A*, Stillborn child with alobar holoprosencephaly shows hypotelorism, flat nose, and midline facial cleft. *B*, Axial proton-density magnetic resonance imaging (MRI) study in a different case shows a midline cleft *(arrow)*. *C*, Axial T1-weighted MRI study in the same patient as in *B* shows a large monoventricle communicating with a dorsal cerebrospinal fluid cyst. There are no midline cerebral structures in this case of alobar holoprosencephaly. (*A–C*, From M Castillo, TW Bouldin, JH Scatliff, K Suzuki. Radiologic-pathologic correlation. Alobar holoprosencephaly. AJNR 14[5]:1151–1156, 1993, © by American Society of Neuroradiology.)

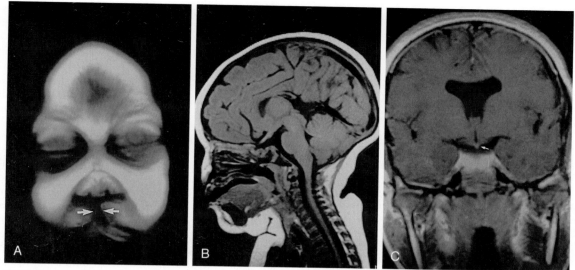

FIGURE 48–10 Septo-optic dysplasia. *A,* Frontal T1-weighted MRI study shows a midline cleft *(arrows)* involving the upper lip. *B,* Midsagittal T1-weighted MRI study in the same case shows an absent pituitary gland. *C,* Coronal T1-weighted MRI study in the same case shows a bright posterior pituitary lobe *(arrow)* translocated to the hypothalamus. *(A–C,* From Castillo M, Mukherji SK. Imaging of the Pediatric Head, Neck, and Spine. Philadelphia, Lippincott-Raven, 1996.)

anterior and triangular primary palate. Lack of fusion of one of the sides of the primary palate with its corresponding secondary palate results in an anterior and slightly off-center primary cleft. Lack of midline fusion of the secondary palates results in a posterior, midline, and secondary cleft. The most benign form of secondary cleft is a bifid uvula. These clefts are commonly unilateral, but occasionally they may be bilateral. All these clefts are eccentric in location. True midline clefts involving the upper lip are part of the midline facial cleft syndromes. Externally, primary common cleft palate may extend into the upper lip. The cleft lip may be separated from the ipsilateral nostril (incomplete type) and extend into it (complete type). In the latter type, the nasal ala is flat, the columella is short, and the ipsilateral maxilla is hypoplastic. The nasal septum is deformed. If bilateral, the intermaxillary segment may undergo disproportionate growth and present as a bony or soft tissue mass protruding anteriorly through the clefts.

Surgical correction of all common facial clefts is better accomplished between 8 and 10 years of age. Earlier intervention may preclude the normal growth of the face. Patients with common facial clefts have no associated brain anomalies and therefore do not require imaging studies.

Polyrhinia

Underdevelopment of the frontonasal process leads to separation of the medial nose into two lateral halves and induction of each nasal medial process.[18] As these grow, two noses are produced. This is an extremely rare malformation. Clinically, the eyes appear far apart when indeed there is no true hypertelorism. Atresia of the posterior choanae may be present. We have never seen this anomaly personally.

MALFORMATIONS OF THE OFF-MIDLINE FACIAL REGIONS

Hypoplasia of the Nasal Alae

Hypoplasia of the nasal alae is obvious at birth and does not require imaging. Surgical correction is done based on clinical findings. There are no intracranial anomalies.

Nasolacrimal Duct Cysts

Canalization of the nasolacrimal duct system begins during the last trimester of pregnancy and may not be completed until several months postpartum. Crying after birth probably contributes to canalization. Patency of the nasolacrimal duct system is present in 6% to 73% of newborns.[5] Obstruction of the system at any level leads to accumulation of secretions, and dilatation. These dilatations may be called *mucoceles* or *retention cysts.* Proximal obstructions result in masses in the medial canthi of the orbits.[19] These masses should be differentiated mainly from hemangiomas, encephaloceles, epidermoids, dermoids, and nasal heterotopias. Obstruction of the distal nasolacrimal ducts results in dilatation of the duct, and masses that project under the inferior turbinates and occlude the inferior nasal passages (Fig. 48–11). These cysts are commonly due to inflammatory obstruction of the valves of Hasner. Clinically, these patients present with respiratory obstructions, which are similar to those seen in patients with the more common posterior choanal stenosis or atresia. However, in patients with distal nasolacrimal duct cysts, a nasogastric tube can be advanced only briefly into the nose. Forceful advancement of the tube may result in perforation and possibly resolution of these cysts. However, if not totally resected, recurrences or infections, or both, may supervene. Distal nasolacrimal

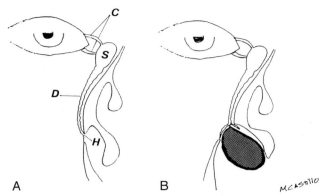

FIGURE 48–11 Normal nasolacrimal system and cysts. *A*, Normal anatomy. C, canaliculi; S, lacrimal sac; D, lacrimal duct; H, valve of Hasner. *B*, Location of an abnormal cyst *(shaded area)*. (*A* and *B*, From M Castillo, DF Merten, MC Weissler. Bilateral nasolacrimal duct mucocele, a rare cause of respiratory distress: CT findings in two newborns. AJNR 14[5]:1011–1013, 1993, © by American Society of Neuroradiology.)

duct cysts may be bilateral or unilateral (Fig. 48–12). When bilateral, they tend to be asymmetric in size. When unilateral, the nasal septum may be deviated toward the opposite side. The nasal septum may also be thin because of pressure erosion. The inferior turbinates may be thin and displaced superiorly. The remainder of the nasolacrimal ducts may also become dilated. Surgery is commonly performed immediately after their discovery and involves complete resection or marsupialization of the cysts.

CT is the diagnostic method of choice. We obtain 1- to 2-mm-thick sections through the region of interest. Data are processed with the high-resolution bone algorithm and soft tissue window settings. Axial images generally suffice, and we routinely do not obtain coronal views.

Lateral Nasal Clefting and Proboscis Lateralis

Anomalous fusion of the medial and lateral nasal processes results in lateral nasal clefts.[18] These clefts involve the alae and the lateral nasal walls. Clinically, these clefts may be subtle scarlike defects or triangular defects in which the soft tissues, cartilages, and bone are absent. Some patients have mild hypertelorism and are mentally retarded. These patients usually harbor brain anomalies. Surgery consists of local flaps and grafts of skin and cartilage harvested from the pinnae. In patients with isolated lateral clefts, normal interocular distance, and normal mentation, no imaging is needed.

The proboscis lateralis is a very unusual anomaly (1 in 100,000 births) in which failure of fusion of the medial and lateral nasal processes induces the ipsilateral maxillary process to fuse with the opposite nasal processes.[20] This results in a tubular soft tissue structure (proboscis) in the medial canthus of an orbit. The ipsilateral nasal cavity and paranasal sinuses may be absent or hypoplastic. The maxilla is hypoplastic in 38% of patients. The ipsilateral nasolacrimal apparatus is also absent. Intracranial anomalies include encephaloceles and holoprosencephaly in 19% of patients. Anomalies of the eye, mainly microphthalmia and colobomas, occur in 44% of patients.

MALFORMATIONS OF THE POSTERIOR NASAL PATHWAYS

Anomalous Posterior Choanae

Stenoses or atresia of the posterior nasal orifices, or both, occur in approximately 1 in 8000 live births and are more common in females.[21] The condition may be familial and is associated with multiple chromosomal anomalies and multiorgan syndromes. One-half of all patients with posterior choanal abnormalities have systemic abnormalities.[21] Most abnormalities are unilateral and tend to present late in childhood with chronic infections, sinusitis, and abundant secretions. In this age group, the main differential diagnosis is that of an intranasal foreign body. Therapy is aimed at controlling secretions, and surgical correction is commonly performed before the child begins school. Bilateral atresias and stenoses present in the immediate postpartum period. Moderate to severe stenoses behave clinically like atresias. The child is unable to nose breathe,

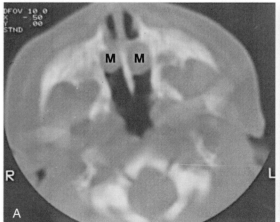
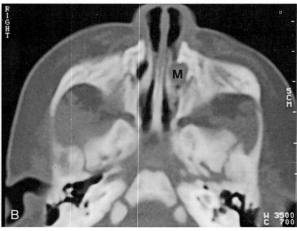

FIGURE 48–12 Distal nasolacrimal duct cysts. *A*, Axial CT scan shows bilateral cysts (M). *B*, Axial CT scan shows a unilateral left cyst (M).

and the dyspnea is commonly alleviated by crying. Symptoms are aggravated by feeding. A nasogastric tube can be advanced only 2 to 3 cm into the nasal cavities before meeting resistance. Since mouth breathing is not learned until 4 to 6 weeks of age, immediate establishment of an oral airway is imperative. Surgical correction is promptly performed after diagnosis via transnasal or, preferably, transpalatine approaches. CT is the imaging method of choice. Contiguous axial sections 1 to 1.5 mm thick are obtained with the gantry angled 5 degrees cephalad to the plane of the hard palate.[21] Both soft tissue window settings and high-resolution bone algorithms are needed. Parasagittal re-formations are helpful in illustrating the full extent of the abnormality. Using the CT unit's electronic calipers, one measures the region of maximal narrowing as well as the thickness of the posterior and inferior vomer. Pure membranous atresia is extremely rare (Fig. 48–13A). Membranes may be thin or thick and pluglike (Fig. 48–13B). Membranous atresia is commonly accompanied by some degree of stenosis. Stenosis is characterized by increased width of the vomer (Fig. 48–13C). Normally, the vomer measures less than 2.3 mm in newborns and should not exceed 5.5 mm.[13] The opening of the posterior choanae should not be less than 3.4 mm in diameter.[13]

Nasopharyngeal Atresia

Nasopharyngeal atresia is extremely rare. In this anomaly, the posterior border of the hard palate is fused with the ventral surface of the clivus (Fig. 48–14).[22] It is probably related to a lack of resorption of the bucconasal membrane. The posterior nasopharynx cavity and hard palate are absent. Clinically, the signs and symptoms are identical to those of posterior choanal atresia. Indeed, this anomaly may be considered a severe form of posterior choanal atresia. Because of the long-term management required, a tracheostomy tube is necessary in these children.

MALFORMATIONS OF THE ANTERIOR NASAL PASSAGES

Cysts of the distal nasolacrimal ducts and anterior cleft palate or lip have been discussed previously.

Piriform Aperture Stenosis

Piriform aperture stenosis is narrowing of the anterior nasal openings due to overgrowth of the medial processes of the maxilla (Fig. 48–15).[23] Clinically, it presents with respiratory difficulty after birth and an inability to pass a nasogastric tube into the nose. Stenosis of the piriform aperture may be an isolated anomaly or may be associated with holoprosencephaly (alobar or semilobar types). If the patient has a single, midline, upper megaincisor, the possibility of accompanying holoprosencephaly is high.[24] In the absence of a megaincisor, it is an isolated anomaly.

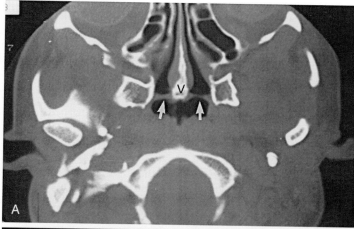
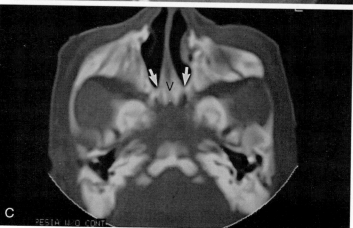
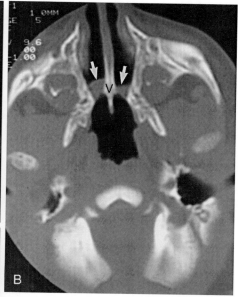

FIGURE 48–13 Posterior choanal anomalies. *A,* Axial CT scan shows pure membranous atresias *(arrows)* with a normal-size vomer (V). *B,* Axial CT scan in a different patient shows thick membranous atresias *(arrows)* with a normal-size vomer (V). *C,* Axial CT scan shows bilateral bony atresias *(arrows)* characterized by widening of the vomer (V). *(A–C,* From Castillo M. Congenital abnormalities of the nose: CT and MR findings. AJR 1994;162:1211–1217.)

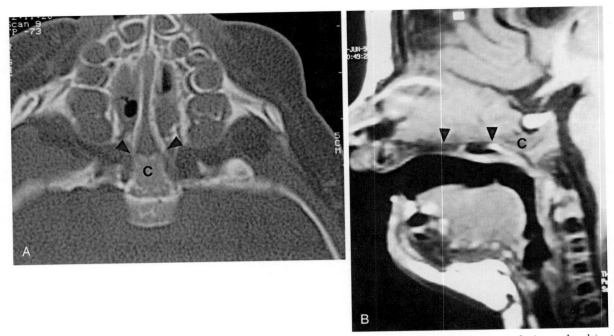

FIGURE 48–14 Nasopharyngeal atresia. *A*, Axial CT scan shows a widened vomer, which is fused posteriorly (*arrowheads*) with the clivus (C). *B*, Midsagittal T1-weighted MRI study in the same patient shows an absent nasopharynx and fusion of the palate (*arrowheads*) with the clivus (C). No soft palate is present. (*A* and *B*, From JK Smith, M Castillo, SK Mukherji, et al. Imaging of nasopharyngeal atresia. AJNR 16[9]:1936–1938, 1995, © by American Society of Neuroradiology.)

Other associated abnormalities include facial hemangiomas, clinodactyly, and endocrine dysfunctions. The latter may be due to anomalies of the hypothalamic-pituitary axis. Surgical correction is indicated and involves resection of the anteromedial maxilla and reconstruction of the anterior nasal openings. CT is the imaging method of choice, and the technique needed is similar to that described for the evaluation of posterior choanal abnormalities. There are no standard measurements for the diameter of the anterior nasal openings. However, less than 3 mm is definitively abnormal.

Agenesis of the Nose

Agenesis of the nose is an extremely rare anomaly in which the nasal bones, premaxilla, and anterior nasopharynx are absent (Fig. 48–16A).[18] The nostrils are also ab-

sent (Fig. 48–16B). Despite the severity of the abnormalities, these children have little respiratory distress at birth. Surgical correction is generally delayed until 5 years of age, when several upper incisors are extracted and a nasal cavity established. Narrowing of this neonasopharynx may occur with progressive growth. Prosthetic noses are used until full facial reconstruction is possible (this after facial growth has ceased).

MALFORMATIONS OF THE NASOFRONTAL REGION

Most malformations of the nasofrontal region manifest as symptomatic masses in the midline of the nose. At times, they may be associated with local infections or meningitis (particularly chronic and repetitive). They are found in

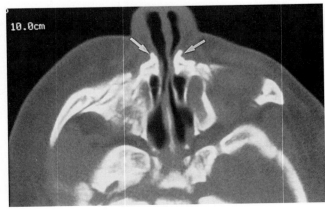

FIGURE 48–15 Piriform aperture stenosis. A CT scan shows overgrowth of the medial maxillary segments (*arrows*) with narrowing of the anterior nasal openings.

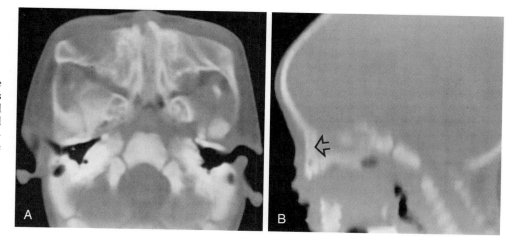

FIGURE 48–16 Agenesis of the nose. *A*, Axial CT scan shows complete absence of the nasal cavities, septum, turbinates, and nose. *B*, Midsagittal CT scan re-formation shows bone atretic plate *(arrow)*.

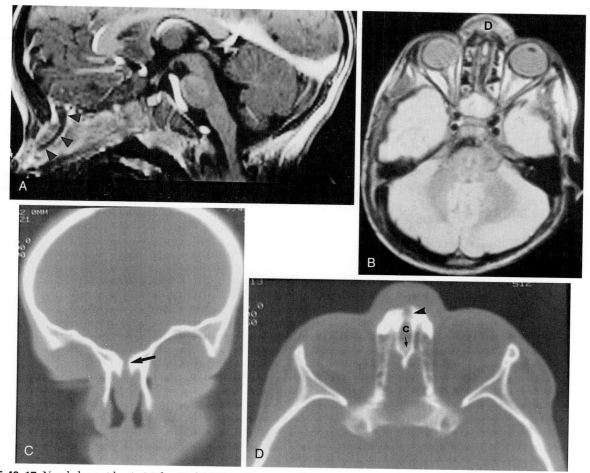

FIGURE 48–17 Nasal dermoids. *A*, Midsagittal MRI re-formation shows a nasal dermoid and tract *(arrowheads)* coursing through the prenasal region to the foramen cecum. *B*, Axial proton-density MRI study shows a dermoid (D) over the nasal bones. *C*, Coronal CT scan in the same patient as in *B* shows the tract *(arrow)*. *D*, Axial CT scan in the same patient as in *B* shows the tract through the nasal bones *(arrowhead)*, an enlarged foramen cecum (c), and a crista galli that is splayed anteriorly *(arrow)*. (*A–D*, From Castillo M, Mukherji SK. Imaging of the Pediatric Head, Neck, and Spine. Philadelphia, Lippincott-Raven, 1996.)

TABLE 48–3 Clinical Features of Nasofrontal Region Masses

	(Epi) Dermoid	Nasal Heterotopia	Encephalocele
Age at presentation	Children and adults	Children	Children
Clinical appearance	Solid, dimple, hairs	Reddish, solid	Bluish, soft, pulsatile
Meningitis	Rarely	Rarely	Yes
CSF leaks	Rarely	Rarely	Yes
Bone defects	None or very small	None or very small	Yes

Abbreviations: CSF, cerebrospinal fluid.

approximately 1 in 40,000 live births and have no gender predilection.[6] Up to one-half of these patients have intracranial abnormalities, including dysgenesis of the corpus callosum, interhemispheric lipomas, colloid cysts, and arachnoid cysts.

Malformations of the Prenasal Space

Dermal Sinuses, Epidermoids, and Dermoids

Dermal sinuses are skin-lined tracts extending from the surface of the nose to the region of the foramen cecum (Fig. 48–17A). The opening for these sinuses may be located in the glabella, dorsum, tip, or columella of the nose.[6] These patients may present with bilateral subfrontal intracranial abscesses. Epidermoids are relatively uncommon and present as eccentric masses. Approximately 50% have intracranial communication. They may also become infected.

Dermoids in this location account for 10% of all head and neck dermoids (Table 48–3). They are midline masses composed of ectoderm and mesoderm.[18] The presence of hair follicles, sweat glands, and sebaceous glands differentiates them from a simple epidermoid. They arise from sequestered tissues within a dermal sinus tract. They are

more common in the nasal dorsum, where they are often accompanied by a tiny external opening that usually contains extruding hair. Some dermoids are simple cysts that require only local resection, whereas others, which are associated with a dermal sinus, require resection of the tract for a complete cure. Resection is commonly performed between 2 and 5 years of age. If the foramen cecum is normal by CT, a subcribriform resection may be planned. However, if the foramen cecum is widened by CT, intracranial exploration should be considered. Both CT and MRI are helpful in imaging these patients. CT determines the appearance of the foramen cecum and the crista galli, which may be excavated or bifid when the abnormality has an intracranial component (Fig. 48–17B–D). MRI allows multiplanar imaging, further characterization of the mass, and evaluation of congenital abnormalities of infections of the brain. By MRI, epidermoids have signal-intensity characteristics similar to those of fluid on T1-weighted and T2-weighted images, whereas dermoids may be hyperintense on both imaging sequences. Unfortunately, the signal characteristics of both overlap, and thus differentiating them may not be possible. These masses do not enhance unless they have become infected. Internal septations are also rare in the absence of prior infection.

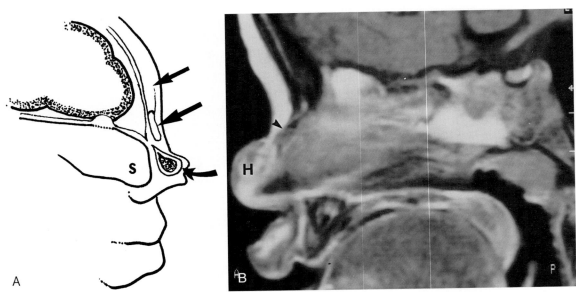

FIGURE 48–18 Intranasal heterotopia. *A,* Diagram shows brain heterotopia *(curved arrow)* sequestered inferior to the nasal bones *(straight arrows)* and superficial to the cartilaginous nasal capsule (S). *B,* Midsagittal T1-weighted MRI study shows heterotopia (H) inferior to the nasal bones *(arrowhead)* and superficial to the septum. (*A* and *B,* From Castillo M, Mukherji SK. Imaging of the Pediatric Head, Neck, and Spine. Philadelphia, Lippincott-Raven, 1996.)

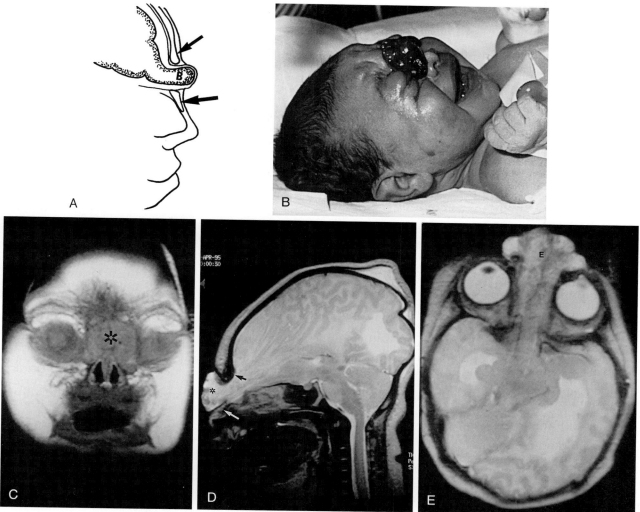

FIGURE 48–19 Frontonasal encephalocele. *A,* Diagram shows the brain (B) herniating between the frontal *(small arrow)* and the nasal *(large arrow)* bones. *B,* Frontonasal encephalocele in a newborn. *C,* Coronal T1-weighted MRI study in the same child as in *B* shows the encephalocele *(asterisk)* to be of the same signal intensity as gray matter. *D,* Midsagittal T1-weighted MRI scan in a different child shows the encephalocele *(asterisk)* between the frontal *(black arrow)* and the nasal *(white arrow)* bones. *E,* Axial T2-weighted MRI study shows the encephalocele (E) and hypertelorism. (*A,* From Castillo M, Mukherji SK. Imaging of the Pediatric Head, Neck, and Spine. Philadelphia, Lippincott-Raven, 1996.)

Nasoethmoid Encephaloceles

It is possible for brain to extend into the prenasal space.[6] These protrusions may contain brain (encephaloceles), meninges (meningoceles), or both (meningoencephaloceles). Encephaloceles are named according to the structures that form their roof and their floor. In these nasoethmoid encephaloceles, the roof is formed by the nasal bones and the floor by the ethmoid sinus complex. They constitute approximately 30% of sincipital cephaloceles.[25] By MRI, they have signal intensity similar to that of brain on T1-weighted images, but they may be hyperintense with respect to normal brain on T2-weighted images, probably secondary to trapped CSF spaces or gliosis, or both.

Intranasal Heterotopia

If the brain contained in the dural diverticulum of the prenasal space becomes separated from the brain, it becomes a heterotopia or nasal glioma[6] (Fig. 48–18; see also Table 48–3). Approximately 40% of all nasal gliomas are located in the prenasal space, and about 50% of them have a thin stalk joining them with brain (strictly, these may be categorized as encephaloceles).[13] This latter group will show some growth. These are commonly asymptomatic but may become infected. They have no malignant potential despite their nomenclature as *gliomas*. Although their signal intensity tends to parallel that of the normal brain in all sequences, they may be of increased signal intensity on T2-weighted MRI studies because of gliosis.

Malformations of the Fonticulus Frontalis

Frontonasal Encephaloceles

Frontonasal encephaloceles are secondary to herniation of frontal lobes via an enlarged fonticulus frontalis, which

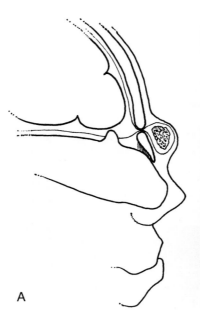
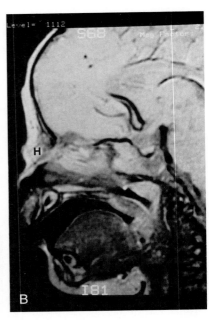

FIGURE 48–20 Extranasal heterotopia. *A,* Diagram shows heterotopic brain *(shaded area)* sequestered superficially to normal nasal and frontal bones. The fonticulus frontalis is closed. *B,* Midsagittal proton-density MRI study shows heterotopia (H) lying superficial to the intact nasofrontal region.

A

remains open (Fig. 48–19*A* and *B*; see also Table 48–3).[25] The roof of these encephaloceles is the frontal bones, and their floor is the nasal bones. They account for 40% to 60% of sincipital encephaloceles.[25] MRI readily establishes the diagnosis (Fig. 48–19*C–E*). Naso-orbital (lateral) encephaloceles are mentioned here for sake of completeness. These are rare, constituting less than 10% of encephaloceles in this region.[25] They occur when brain herniates between the frontal processes of the maxilla and the lacrimal bones and may be unilateral or bilateral.

Extranasal Heterotopias

Extranasal heterotopias occur when brain that has herniated through the fonticulus frontalis is separated from the frontal lobes secondary to closure of this fontanelle (Fig. 48–20*A*).[13] The sequestered brain is then located superficial to relatively intact nasal bones, nasofrontal suture, and frontal bones (Fig. 48–20*B*). They constitute over 60% of all nasal heterotopias. They are static masses that do not grow.[26]

References

1. Stool SE, Isaacson GC. Phylogenetic aspects and embryology. In Bluestone CD, Stool SE, Scheetz MD (eds). Pediatric Otolaryngology, 2nd ed., pp. 3–16. Philadelphia, WB Saunders, 1990.
2. Hiatt JL, Gartner LP. Head and Neck Anatomy, pp. 57–72. New York, Appleton-Century-Crofts, 1982.
3. Naidich TP, Osborn RE, Bauer BS, et al. Embryology and congenital lesions of the midface. In Som PM, Bergeron RT (eds). Head and Neck Imaging, 2nd ed., pp. 1–15. St Louis, CV Mosby, 1991.
4. Fairbanks DF. Embryology and anatomy. In Bluestone CD, Stool SE, Scheetz MD (eds). Pediatric Otolaryngology, 2nd ed., pp. 605–631. Philadelphia, WB Saunders, 1991.
5. Castillo M, Merten DF, Weissler MC. Bilateral nasolacrimal duct mucocele, a rare cause of respiratory distress: CT findings in two newborns. AJNR 1993;14:1011–1013.
6. Barkovich AJ, Vandermarck P, Edwards MSB, Cogen PH. Congenital nasal masses: CT and MR imaging features in 16 cases. AJNR 1991;12:105–116.
7. Moore KL. The eye and ear. In The Developing Human: Clinically Oriented Embryology, 4th ed., pp. 402–420. Philadelphia, WB Saunders, 1988.
8. Maniglia AJ. Embryology, teratology, and arrested developmental disorders in otolaryngology. Otolaryngol Clin North Am 1981;14:25–38.
9. Taybi H, Lachman RS. Radiology of Syndromes, Metabolic Disorders, and Skeletal Dysplasias, 3rd ed., pp. 460–461. Chicago, Year Book Medical, 1990.
10. Bergeron RT, Lo WWM, Swartz JD, et al. Temporal bone. In Som PM, Bergeron RT (eds). Head and Neck Imaging, 2nd ed., pp. 998–999. St Louis, CV Mosby, 1991.
11. Mafee MF, Selis JE, Yannias DA, et al. Congenital sensorineural hearing loss. Radiology 1984;150:427–434.
12. Parkin JL. Congenital malformations of the mouth and pharynx. In Bluestone CD, Stool SE, Scheetz MD (eds). Pediatric Otolaryngology, 2nd ed., pp. 850–859. Philadelphia, WB Saunders, 1990.
13. Castillo M. Congenital abnormalities of the nose: CT and MR findings. AJR 1994;162:1211–1217.
14. Thorne CH. Craniofacial clefts. Clin Plast Surg 1993;20:803–814.
15. Castillo M, Bouldin TW, Scatliff JH, Suzuki K. Alobar holoprosencephaly. AJNR 1993;14:1151–1156.
16. Barkovich AJ, Fram EK, Norman D. MR of septo-optic dysplasia. Radiology 1989;171:189–192.
17. Barkovich AJ, Norman D. Absence of the septum pellucidum: A useful sign in the diagnosis of congenital brain malformations. AJNR 1988;9:1107–1114.
18. Hengerer AS, Newburg JA. Congenital malformations of the nose and paranasal sinuses. In Bluestone CD, Stool SE, Scheetz MD (eds). Pediatric Otolaryngology, 2nd ed., pp. 718–728. Philadelphia, WB Saunders, 1990.
19. Rand PK, Ball WS, Lulwin DR. Congenital nasolacrimal mucoceles: CT evaluation. Radiology 1989;173:691–694.
20. Poe LB, Hochhauser L, Bryke C, et al. Proboscis lateralis with associated orbital cyst: Detailed MR and CT imaging and correlative embryopathy. AJNR 1992;13:1471–1476.
21. Chinwuba C, Wallman J, Strand R. Nasal airway obstruction: CT assessment. Radiology 1986;159:503–506.
22. Smith JK, Castillo M, Mukherji SK, Drake A. Nasopharyngeal atresia: CT and MR imaging. AJNR 1995;16:1936–1938.
23. Bignault A, Castillo M. Congenital nasal pyriform aperture stenosis. AJNR 1994;15:877–878.
24. Arlis H, Ward RF. Congenital nasal pyriform aperture stenosis. Arch Otolaryngol Head Neck Surg 1992;118:989–991.
25. Naidich TP, Altman NR, Braffman BH, et al. Cephaloceles and related malformations. AJNR 1992;13:655–690.
26. Castillo M, Mukherji SK. Imaging of the Pediatric Head, Neck, and Spine. Philadelphia, Lippincott-Raven, 1996.

49

Anoxic Ischemic Injury
in Children

ROSALIND B. DIETRICH, M.B.B.S.

Since Little first associated perinatal complications, premature birth, and spastic rigidity of the limbs in his classic paper of 1862, investigators have been trying to more fully understand the mechanisms leading to anoxic ischemic brain damage in children.[1] The topic remains of major significance to both neonatologists and pediatric neurologists, as perinatal asphyxia is a major cause of long-term neurologic sequelae in childhood and is the single most important perinatal cause of neurologic morbidity in the full-term as well as the low-birth-weight premature infant.[2, 3]

Anoxic ischemic injury affects between 0.5% and 1% of live term newborns, with as many as 10% of these suffering severe neurologic deficits or dying as a result of the insult.[2–4] An even higher number of premature newborns are affected.[5] It is reported that 5% to 15% of surviving infants with a birth weight of less than 1500 gm have major spastic motor deficits, and an additional 25% to 50% have milder developmental disabilities.[5, 6]

Current imaging techniques play an active role in both the early detection of injury and the demonstration of the resulting long-term sequelae. In addition, at the present time, experimental interventional strategies are actively under way to evaluate the neuronal protective effects of certain pharmaceutical agents. These experiments, currently using animal models, are evaluating the ability of specific agents to minimize the amount of brain damage occurring after an anoxic ischemic event.[2] If such agents also prove to be effective in infants, it will be vitally important to be able to recognize, soon after the insult, which infants have suffered early damage. Identified infants may then benefit from treatment in order to prevent additional damage from occurring. Along with other techniques, imaging will play a vital role in this regard, both to demonstrate the presence and location of such injury and to monitor the effects of the interventional agents once administered.

PATHOPHYSIOLOGY

The mechanisms underlying the development of brain damage from asphyxia are extremely complex (Fig. 49–1). Together, changes occurring in arterial oxygen content, carbon dioxide content, pH, and blood pressure due to the asphyxia ultimately lead to the development of ischemic brain injury.[7] Initially after the insult, compensatory responses come into operation to help protect the brain and temporarily lead to maintenance of cerebral blood flow by elevation of blood pressure and redistribution of blood flow to vital organs. As the insult continues, a concomitant increase in carbon dioxide levels and decrease in blood pressure lead to a subsequent loss of autoregulation, reducing cerebral blood flow and resulting in decreased brain perfusion.[2, 7] This results in the development of infarction. The decrease in oxygen concentration that also occurs leads to changes in capillary regulation and ultimately to capillary damage. When blood pressure is subsequently restored to normal values, resulting in reperfusion of previously injured tissue, hemorrhage may develop at the sites of previous capillary damage.[7]

Although the initial insult affects the whole brain, not all areas of the brain are equally injured, and different and distinct patterns of damage can be identified. The extent of injury seen correlates closely with the nature and duration of the insult and with the level of maturity of the immature brain at the time of injury.[8–11] For instance, the relative maturity of the brain at the time of

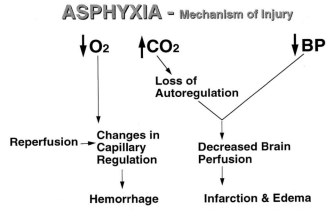

FIGURE 49–1 Mechanisms of injury after perinatal asphyxia. BP, blood pressure.

the insult influences where watershed infarction will occur, the site of resulting hemorrhage, and if gliosis will develop as a result of the insult.[11, 12] In order to understand why all areas of the brain are not equally affected, it is important to understand the concepts of *reversibility* and *selective vulnerability*. Reversibility explains why although large areas of the brain may initially appear to be injured by anoxia, damage in some or all of these areas may be reversible, resulting in recovery of structure and function. Selective vulnerability helps explain why certain areas of the brain are more vulnerable than others to damage at different stages of brain maturity.[13] At present three main theories help explain the selective vulnerability of different areas of the brain. They are the circulatory theory, the metabolic theory, and the excitotoxin theory.[2, 13]

Circulatory Theory

The blood supply of the developing brain changes as the brain matures. The premature infant's cortex and underlying white matter receive most of their blood supply from the ventriculopetal branches of blood vessels on the surface of the hemispheres. By contrast, the term infant's brain is supplied primarily by branches of the anterior, middle, and posterior cerebral arteries. Because of this, the effective watershed areas of the brain differ between the preterm and the term infant (Fig. 49–2). Before 36 weeks of gestation, effective watershed areas have been previously considered to be in the periventricular white matter, adjacent to the borders of the lateral ventricles (Fig. 49–2A).[14–17] This concept was based on classical anatomic studies of fetal brain blood supply and supported by clinical positron emission tomography perfusion studies.[18] More recently the accuracy of this early anatomic work has been refuted.[19, 20]

Later the watershed areas, like those of the adult, are at the borders between the major cerebral artery distributions, that is, between the anterior and middle cerebral and the middle and posterior cerebral circulations.[21, 22] Injury in these areas leads to the *parasagittal zones of injury*, as referred to by Volpe and colleagues (Fig. 49–2B and C).[22, 23]

Metabolic Theory

The areas of the brain that have high metabolic demands also change as the brain matures.[24] The metabolic theory states that the regions of the brain with the highest metabolic demands at the time the insult occurs will be the most vulnerable to injury.[25, 26] These areas will therefore be damaged first and to a greater degree during an anoxic insult than the rest of the brain. Alternatively, if the whole brain is initially affected but there is reversibility in some areas, the areas with the highest metabolic demands will be the most likely to sustain permanent damage. In the fetal and newborn brain, the areas of highest metabolic demand at a specific time are those that are actively myelinating. At term, these areas include the posterior brain stem, the lentiform nuclei and thalami, and the perirolandic areas of the cortex.[27–29] Earlier, during the third trimester, the areas actively myelinating are less extensive and confined to the thalami and posterior brain stem. There is strong correlation between these sites of early myelination, as seen by magnetic resonance imaging (MRI), and the high metabolic areas seen on positron emission tomography.[24]

Excitotoxin Theory

The excitotoxin theory is based on work describing the similarities of the location of anoxic damage in the infant brain (in the human fetus and in animal models) with the distribution of glutamate receptors.[30, 31] It is well known that during an anoxic event there is an excessive release of excitatory amino acids (or excitotoxins) from neuron end plates (Fig. 49–3). These substances are extremely important in the mediation of anoxic ischemic injury. The most significant of these, glutamate, spills into the synaptic cleft after release and is subsequently picked up by postsynaptic receptors. Three different types of postsyn-

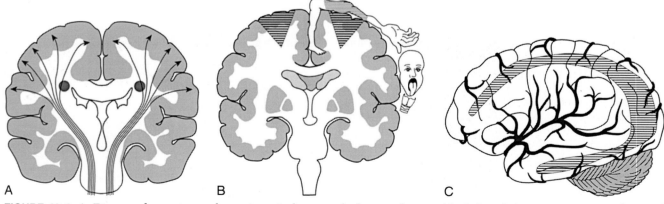

FIGURE 49–2 *A,* Diagram demonstrates the periventricular watershed zone of injury *(shaded circles)* seen in preterm infants and its relationship to the corticospinal tracts. *B,* Diagram demonstrates the parasagittal watershed zone of injury *(crosshatched wedges)* seen in term infants who suffer a prolonged period of hypoxia and its relationship to the homunculus of the cortical strip. *C,* Diagram demonstrates the parasagittal watershed zone of injury *(crosshatched area)* between the anterior and middle and the middle and posterior cerebral circulations.

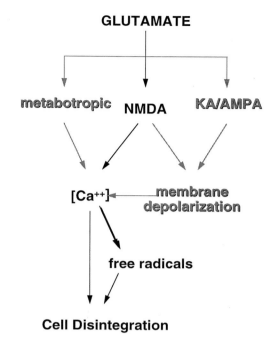

GLUTAMATE

metabotropic NMDA KA/AMPA

[Ca⁺⁺] ← membrane depolarization

free radicals

Cell Disintegration

FIGURE 49–3 Mechanisms of glutamate-induced brain injury. NMDA, N-methyl-D-aspartate; KA/AMPA, kainate/α-amino-3-hydroxy-5-methyl-4-isoxazole-propionic acid.

aptic receptors are recognized. One of particular interest is the N-methyl-D-aspartate receptor. When glutamate is picked up by this type of receptor, a chemical chain reaction is triggered that subsequently leads to the formation of free radicals and ultimately cell disintegration.[7] This glutamate-mediated cell death occurs in two phases, one with an immediate mechanism and one with a delayed mechanism. The immediate mechanism results in activation of receptors leading to depolarization of the cell membrane and intracellular influx of sodium and chloride, resulting in rapid osmotic cell lysis.[7] The delayed mechanism, which is thought to be the predominant one,

occurs within several hours of the insult. It involves intracellular influx of calcium through calcium ion channels and eventually causes formation of free radicals. It is this delayed mechanism that may be potentially blocked by certain pharmaceutical agents that function as excitatory amino acid antagonists, calcium channel blockers, or free radical scavengers.[2]

EARLY IMAGING FINDINGS

Term Brain

The earliest imaging findings in children who have suffered severe anoxic ischemic events may be very subtle but can be seen as early as the first day of life.[32] Although ultrasonography is often used as the screening modality for cerebral abnormality in neonates, it is less useful in the evaluation of the term brain that has suffered anoxic ischemic damage than it is in the premature brain, in which abnormalities are often centrally located and contain hemorrhage.[2] This is because in the term brain, abnormalities are more often peripherally, not centrally, located, and associated hemorrhage is less frequently present. The limited visualization of the subarachnoid space, cerebral cortex, and posterior fossa structures by ultrasonography and the subjective interpretation of diffuse altered echogenicity compound the problem.[2] Nonetheless, ultrasonography may detect abnormalities of generalized increased echogenicity in the brain parenchyma in the first few days after an insult suggesting diffuse neuronal injury.[33, 34] The presence of a more localized area of increased echogenicity suggests that a focal infarction may be present (Fig. 49–4). Occasionally increased echogenicity, localized to the basal ganglia, may also be identified,[35] but ultrasonography is less sensitive in its identification of abnormality in this area than MRI, and such abnormalities may be easily overlooked.[35, 36]

Some groups have extensive experience with computed tomography (CT) in the evaluation of anoxic ischemic injury.[36] Soon after an anoxic ischemic event, CT may

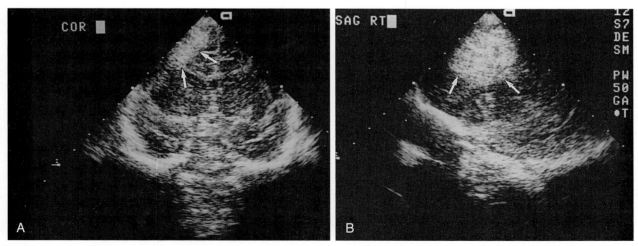

FIGURE 49–4 Focal infarction. *A,* Coronal ultrasound image demonstrates a focal area of increased echogenicity in the right parasagittal area *(arrows)* representing focal infarction. *B,* Right parasagittal ultrasound image more clearly defines the extent of infarction *(arrows).* (*A* and *B,* Courtesy of Valerie Hunter, M.D.)

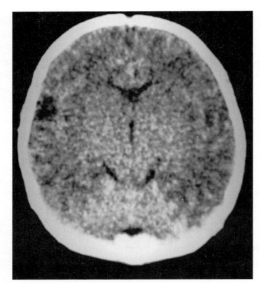

FIGURE 49–5 Diffuse edema on computed tomography (CT). An axial CT image shows loss of differentiation of gray and white matter and loss of definition of the basal ganglia and thalamus.

demonstrate a loss of gray-white matter differentiation and generalized decreased density in the supratentorial brain parenchyma, due to edema. The presence of this type of edema is a nonspecific finding, and involved parenchyma may or may not eventually evolve into damaged brain.[37] When the basal ganglia are also involved by this type of edema, the infant is reported to have a significantly worse prognosis than if these areas are spared (Fig. 49–5).[36]

MRI is more sensitive than the other modalities for the detection of anoxic ischemic injury in the first few days after the insult. At this time, abnormal findings include the presence of focal or diffuse edema (with or without infarction), basal ganglia T1-hyperintensity, and laminar necrosis.[32] Hemorrhage may also be identified within areas of infarction (Fig. 49–6).

Because of the inherent high signal intensity in the newborn brain, subtle increases of water content associated with areas of edema or infarction may be difficult to detect by the less experienced reader. Therefore, when anoxic ischemic damage is suspected clinically, the radiologic images should be reviewed carefully. When focal or diffuse edema is present, MRI studies may demonstrate findings related to a mass effect (as can be seen on CT) such as obscuration of sulci and gyri, and the presence of slitlike ventricles. The most sensitive sign, however, is loss of the gray-white matter differentiation pattern normally seen on T2-weighted images. In the newborn period, the signal intensity of the cortical ribbon is lower than that of the underlying high-signal-intensity white matter. When edema is present within the cortex, the inherent signal intensity of the gray matter becomes higher on T2-weighted images. This appearance occurs because of the increased water content present within the gray matter, which increases its inherent signal intensity to more closely approximate that of the underlying white matter. This obscures the differentiation between the two (see Fig. 49–15). The presence of edema within the brain parenchyma is much more easily appreciated using diffusion-weighted MRI sequences (Fig. 49–7).[38] In addition to being more sensitive to edema, such sequences also better demonstrate the full extent of the edema.

After episodes of hypoxia, peripherally located wedge-shaped areas of infarction may be identified in the parasagittal zones (see Figs. 49–4 and 49–6).[8, 23] On early images these areas appear echogenic on ultrasound images and hypodense on CT. The same lesions have low signal intensity on T1-weighted images and high signal intensity on T2-weighted images.

After severe insults, characteristic changes that evolve over time may be seen in the basal ganglia.[32, 39–43] The earliest finding, seen as early as day 1 after an anoxic ischemic event, is of diffuse high signal intensity in the basal ganglia on T1-weighted images (Fig. 49–8). This finding may be quite striking or more subtle. When images are evaluated for this finding, it is helpful, therefore, to remember that in normal infants the signal intensity of

FIGURE 49–6 Hemorrhagic parasagittal infarction. Axial spin-echo (SE) (600/20) *(A)* and SE (3500/120) *(B)* magnetic resonance imaging (MRI) studies show hemorrhagic parasagittal infarction *(arrows)* in the right frontal lobe. Diffuse edema is present with loss of gray-white matter differentiation on the T2-weighted image *(B)*.

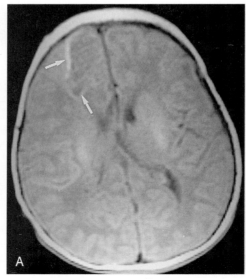
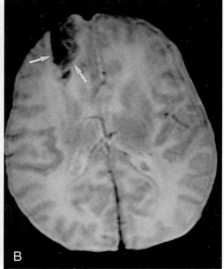

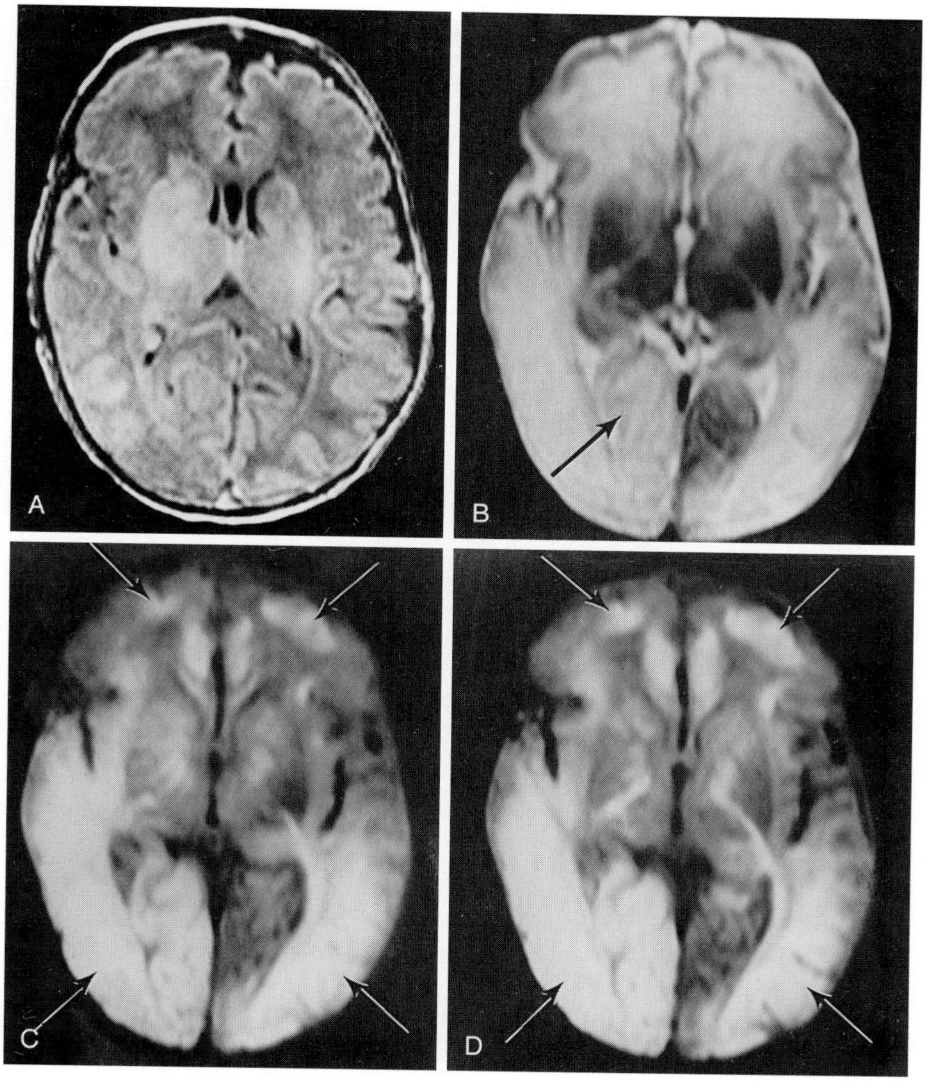

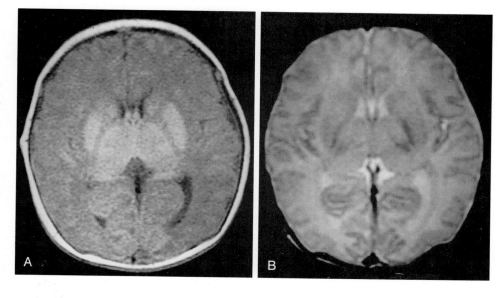

FIGURE 49–7 Diffusion-weighted MRI after anoxia. *A,* Axial SE (720/20) image shows areas of patchy high signal intensity in the basal ganglia and edema in the frontal white matter and the right occipital lobe. *B,* Axial SE (3000/120) shows edema in the white matter with loss of gray-white matter differentiation *(arrows)*. *C* and *D,* Diffusion-weighted imaging (SE pulse interval/200 msec). Left to right sensitization (b = 600 sec/mm²) *(C)* and through-plane sensitization (b = 600 sec/mm²) *(D)* show extensive areas of high signal intensity *(arrows)* demonstrating the full extent of tissue involved. (Courtesy of Graeme Bydder, M.B., Ch.B.)

FIGURE 49–8 Early basal ganglia findings after total anoxia. Axial SE (600/20) *(A)* and SE (3500/120) *(B)* in a 2-day-old infant. On T1-weighted images *(A)*, the lentiform, caudate nuclei, and thalami are swollen and demonstrate diffusely high signal intensity. In comparison, the T2-weighted image *(B)* appears relatively normal at this time.

the posterior limb of the internal capsule is always higher than that of the adjacent lentiform nucleus and thalamus on T1-weighted images. At this time, the same areas appear normal on T2-weighted images. It is not known for certain what the T1 hyperintensity represents; possibilities include hemorrhage, calcium, myelin breakdown products, free fatty acids, or free radicals.[8, 32] This early pattern of basal ganglia T1 hyperintensity may be seen for up to 7 to 10 days after the insult. This early basal ganglia appearance then transitions into an intermediate pattern in which focal or patchy increased T1 signal intensity and decreased T2 signal intensity are present (Fig. 49–9). This intermediate appearance may be due to the presence of calcium, as reported previously by Parisi and associates in a case with parallel CT findings and autopsy correlation.[44] After about day 17 a more chronic appearance may start to be seen, with areas of gliosis identified on T2-weighted images and T1-weighted images now demonstrating no abnormality, subtle hypointensity, or areas of cystic necrosis (see Fig. 49–26).[32, 35, 45–47] Similar areas of cystic necrosis may be seen on CT images, which are less sensitive for demonstrating these changes and may frequently be negative in such cases. Fig. 49–10 shows the time frame of these changes.

Cortical laminar necrosis may also be seen after an anoxic ischemic event. It may be first identified as gyriform or curvilinear high signal intensity on T1-weighted images in the inferior aspect of the cortex and is particularly prominent in the bases of the sulci (Fig. 49–11). On follow-up studies, low signal intensity may be seen in the same areas on T2-weighted sequences.[49–50] The distribution of injury is thought to occur because the cortex at the base of the sulcus is particularly vulnerable to anoxic ischemic injury because of its more precarious blood supply.[51]

Infants demonstrating this group of early findings are at risk for the development of long-term sequelae and should be closely followed. However, the demonstration of the presence of focal or diffuse edema after an insult does not necessarily correlate with a poor outcome. In some instances the edema seen on early images may be

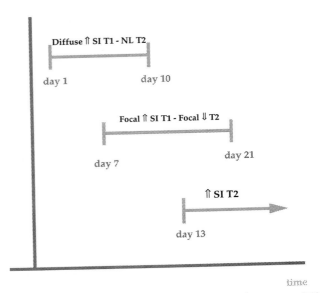

FIGURE 49–10 Time line of basal ganglia signal intensity (SI) after a period of total anoxia. NL, normal.

reversible, and infants demonstrating this finding may go on to develop into neurologically normal children.[37] This correlates with work by Vanucci and colleagues that suggests that although edema is frequently seen in association with anoxic ischemic events, its presence neither causes nor contributes to the ultimate brain damage that may develop.[37] A poor outcome is much more likely, however, in infants who develop the intermediate type of basal ganglia changes or show evidence of laminar necrosis on follow-up studies, or both.[32]

Preterm Brain

The early imaging findings seen in the preterm brain after an anoxic ischemic event include germinal matrix hemorrhage, periventricular venous infarction, and periventricular leukomalacia.[5] In the first week after an insult,

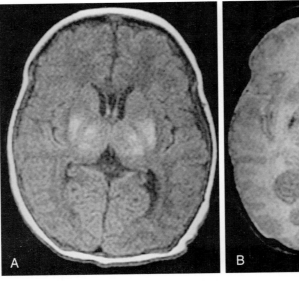
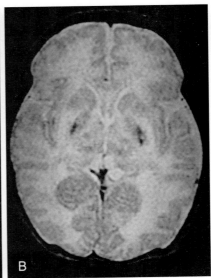

FIGURE 49–9 Intermediate basal ganglia findings after total anoxia. Axial SE (600/20) (A) and SE (3000/120) (B) images in a 16-day-old infant show a more patchy distribution of high signal intensity in the thalami and lentiform nuclei on the T1-weighted image (A). Areas of patchy low signal intensity are now apparent on the T2-weighted image (B).

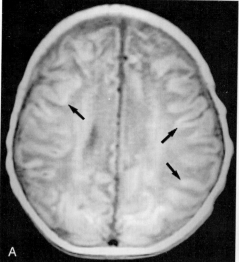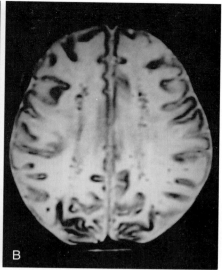

FIGURE 49–11 Laminar necrosis. Axial SE (600/20) *(A)* and SE (3500/120) *(B)* images show areas of T1 hyperintensity and T2 hypointensity in areas of the cortex, which are particularly prominent at the base of the sulci *(arrows in A).*

hemorrhage and edema may be identified. Because of the risks associated with moving premature infants out of the safe environment of the neonatal intensive care unit, ultrasonography is usually the initial imaging technique used to evaluate such infants. This modality is particularly useful in demonstrating and screening for hemorrhage adjacent to or within the ventricular system.[5]

Germinal matrix intraventricular hemorrhage is the most common type of hemorrhage found in the premature infant. By contrast, it is rarely seen in term infants. It is found in 35% to 55% of premature infants of less than 32 weeks of gestation and less than 1500 gm.[52]

The germinal matrix consists of a rich vascular stroma that is present in the subependymal region of the early fetal brain and is the origin of neuronal and glial development. Its blood supply is from the deep perforating branches of the anterior, middle, and posterior cerebral arteries. Although it originally surrounds the lateral ventricles, between 24 and 28 weeks of gestation it starts to regress and by 36 weeks is only present in the subependymal caudothalamic groove, adjacent to the frontal horns of the lateral ventricles, in the floor of the caudate nuclei. The causes of germinal matrix intraventricular hemorrhage are multifactorial and complex. However, it is known that the vessels of the germinal matrix, which are thin walled and lack connective tissue, are vulnerable to hemorrhage with fluctuations in arterial pressure. This type of hemorrhage may be seen in association with many varied conditions that occur in infancy including respiratory distress syndrome, pneumothorax, patent ductus arteriosus, noxious stimuli, and seizures.[53]

When hemorrhage occurs, it destroys the germinal matrix and may burst through the subependymal layer into the lateral ventricles. Blood products may then mix with cerebrospinal fluid and pass through the subarachnoid space. Noncommunicating or communicating hydrocephalus may develop if the presence of blood obstructs the flow of cerebrospinal fluid through the aqueduct or prevents its absorbtion by the arachnoid villi. The currently used four-point grading system for germinal matrix intraventricular hemorrhage was first described by

Burstein, Papile, and Burstein[54] and later adapted by Volpe.[5] It is described in (Table 49–1).

On ultrasonography, germinal matrix hemorrhage is initially identified as focal areas of increased echogenicity with mass effect (Fig. 49–12). After 1 to 2 weeks, the hemorrhage becomes less echogenic. Later it fades away, or undergoes liquefaction and eventually forms a cyst.[55] Germinal matrix hemorrhage is seen adjacent to the head of the caudate nucleus in the floor of the lateral ventricles on coronal images (Fig. 49–12). On sagittal images the echogenic area can be seen extending anterior to the caudothalamic groove, thereby differentiating it from the echogenic choroid plexus, which is positioned posteriorly. When hemorrhage is present within the ventricles (grades II and III), the echogenic blood clots fill all or part of the ventricle and may also distend it.[55] Screening for hemorrhage in premature infants is best performed at the end of the first week, as more than 90% of neonatal hemorrhage occurs before this time.[52] Serial ultrasound studies should be performed in infants with known germinal matrix intraventricular hemorrhage to detect the possible development of hydrocephalus.[56]

Grade IV hemorrhages are now known to occur by a different mechanism than grades I to III. Although previously thought to be extensions into the adjacent parenchyma of germinal matrix intraventricular hemorrhage, they are now known to represent periventricular hemorrhagic venous infarctions within the brain parenchyma.[5] They are thought to develop due to compression, by germinal matrix intraventricular hemorrhage on the ter-

TABLE 49–1 Grading of Germinal Matrix Intraventricular Hemorrhage

Grade I	Hemorrhage confined to the germinal matrix
Grade II	Intraventricular hemorrhage without ventricular dilatation
Grade III	Intraventricular hemorrhage with ventricular dilatation
Grade IV	Periventricular hemorrhagic venous infarction

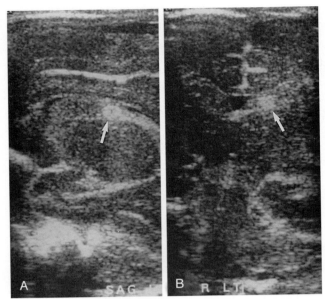

FIGURE 49–12 Germinal matrix hemorrhage, grade I. *A,* Sagittal ultrasound scan shows a discrete area of increased echogenicity located in the region of the caudothalamic groove *(arrow).* *B,* Coronal ultrasound scan shows the same focal area of echogenicity in the region of the left caudate nucleus causing compression of the adjacent frontal horn *(arrow).*

minal vein as it passes through the subependymal region of the caudate nucleus. The mass effect caused by the hemorrhage leads to the development of venous infarction.[5, 53]

On ultrasound studies these areas of hemorrhagic infarction are seen as poorly defined areas of mixed echogenicity and are frequently unilateral and almost always asymmetric (Fig. 49–13). This latter finding helps distinguish them from areas of hemorrhagic periventricular leukomalacia. Later the affected area becomes less echogenic, with liquefaction occurring peripherally first.[56] The entire hemorrhagic infarct becomes absorbed over several months. Infants with periventricular venous infarction have a much poorer prognosis, with 90% demonstrating major long-term neurologic sequelae compared with only 30% to 40% of infants with grade III hemorrhage.[56]

Hemorrhage may also be identified with CT or MRI.[54, 57–59] As in adults and older children, hemorrhage of less than a week is hyperdense compared with adjacent brain on CT, becoming isointense in the subacute phase. When MRI is used to image infants, hemorrhage in any location may be easily identified (Fig. 49–14). Extra-axial and peripherally located parenchymal hemorrhage, and that located in the posterior fossa, may be seen on MRI despite negative ultrasound and CT studies. The presence of hemorrhage within the ventricular system can be seen for a longer period of time using MRI, as hemosiderin may be seen staining the ependyma (Fig. 49–15). The age of the hemorrhage and its location and extent should be assessed using routine spin-echo T1- and T2-weighted images. In the newborn infant, the signal intensity of parenchymal hematomas follows similar sequential changes to those previously described in adult patients

despite the presence of fetal hemaglobin, which has a stronger oxygen affinity, in this age group. When there is a strong clinical suspicion that hemorrhage has occurred but none is identified on routine sequences, increased sensitivity may be obtained with gradient-echo T2°-weighted images (Fig. 49–16).[60]

Periventricular leukomalacia (PVL) is seen primarily in preterm fetuses and premature infants who are ventilator dependent and survive more than a few days. Although it is generally thought to be due to lack of cerebrovascular autoregulation in an acutely ill premature infant coupled with systemic hypotension,[61] its cause is not well understood. There is substantial work implicating an infectious cause in some cases.[62, 63] Adverse perinatal events that have been shown to correlate with the development of PVL include prenatal asphyxia, recurrent apnea, septicemia, hypocarbia, and prolonged mechanical ventilation.

The most common locations of PVL are the periventricular white matter at the trigone of the lateral ventricles and adjacent to the foramen of Monro.[64, 65] Lesions are characterized pathologically by areas of coagulation necrosis with subsequent macrophage activity, liquefaction, and cyst formation.[66, 67] By 3 to 4 weeks, cavities frequently have coalesced and communicated with the ventricles. Because of this, the white matter volume is greatly diminished and the ventricles become mildly enlarged. Hemorrhage has been reported to occur in areas of PVL in 25% of patients.[67]

Although ultrasound is the screening modality used to evaluate for the development of PVL, early PVL may be extremely difficult to diagnose using this modality. This is because the earliest imaging findings are subtle and due to the presence of edema within the periventricular white

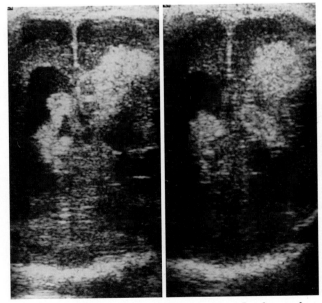

FIGURE 49–13 Germinal matrix intraventricular hemorrhage, grade IV *(left)* and grade III *(right).* Coronal ultrasound scan demonstrates echogenic blood clots bilaterally in the lateral ventricles, which are dilated. In addition, on the *left,* increased echogenicity is also seen in the adjacent parenchyma, representing periventricular hemorrhagic infarct.

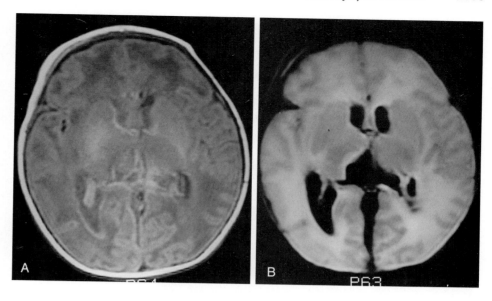

FIGURE 49–14 MRI studies of intraventricular acute hemorrhage in a 3-day-old infant. Axial SE (600/20) (A) and SE (3500/120) (B) images demonstrate hemorrhage completely filling the lateral ventricles. The hemorrhage is isointense to brain on T1-weighted images and markedly hypointense on T2-weighted images, consistent with deoxyhemoglobin. The ventricles are mildly dilated. In addition, there is loss of gray-white matter differentiation in multiple areas, consistent with the presence of diffuse edema.

matter. When seen, they consist of increased echogenicity in the periventricular white matter, which may have a coarse linear appearance, and mild ventricular compression (Fig. 49–17). Such findings may be easier to detect when asymmetric.[56] At this time it is not always possible to differentiate increased echogenicity due to early PVL from a normal halo of echogenicity that may be seen in the same area due to an anisotropic effect created as the sound beam hits axially traversing vessels.[68] Follow-up studies may have to be performed to distinguish the two. In the subacute stage (2 to 6 weeks) when cystic areas develop in the white matter adjacent to the trigone and the foramen of Monro, the diagnosis of PVL can be confirmed (Fig. 49–17). Later these peritrigonal cysts may

be no longer seen due to incorporation into the lateral ventricles.

Early PVL may also be seen with MRI.[69–71] Initially, areas of hemorrhage are seen in the periventricular white matter paralleling the borders of the lateral ventricles (Fig. 49–18). Later, as the hemorrhage resorbs, these areas become cystic. Serial studies may dramatically demonstrate incorporation of these lesions into the lateral ventricles, which subsequently enlarge and develop ragged borders (Fig. 49–18).

When preterm infants suffer catastrophic anoxic ischemic events either in the perinatal period or while in utero, they may also demonstrate basal ganglia changes similar to those previously described in term infants. The extent of basal ganglia involvement is usually less than that seen in the term infant, with the most severe damage occurring in the thalami and the posterior aspects of the midbrain and brain stem (Fig. 49–19).[72–76] The decreased area of involvement in this group is because the metabolically active areas of the brain and those areas that are actively myelinating are smaller in the preterm infant than at term. Because of this, the area of brain most vulnerable to anoxic ischemic damage is also less prevalent.

Older Child

When a severe anoxic ischemic insult occurs in older children, a different pattern of injury may be demonstrated. Clinically this is frequently seen in children who suffer a near-drowning episode. In this group of initially unstable patients, CT is usually the first imaging study performed. Early studies may show hypoattenuation of the basal ganglia and cortex.[77, 78] Later, diffuse cerebral edema may be seen with loss of gray–white differentiation (Fig. 49–20). Early MRI studies may show increased T2-signal intensity in the basal ganglia and cortex with sparing of the perirolandic cortex. Later studies may show diffuse atrophy, gliosis, and, occasionally, iron deposition (Fig. 49–21).[79]

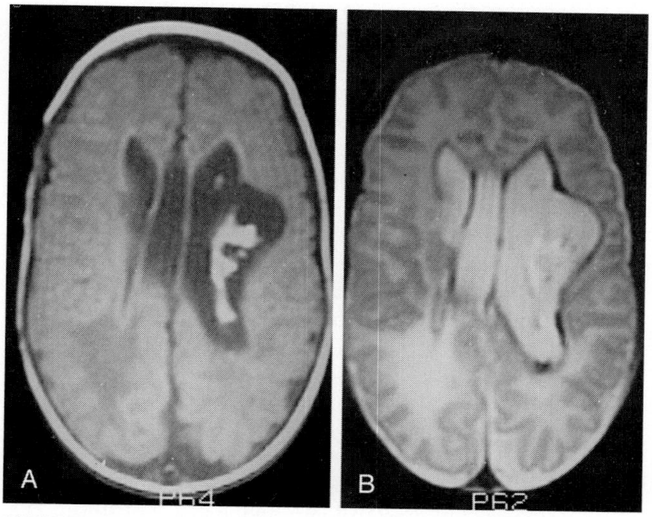

FIGURE 49–15 MRI studies of subacute intraventricular hemorrhage in a premature infant. Axial SE (600/20) (A) and axial SE (3500/120) (B) images demonstrate high-signal-intensity (on both T1- and T2-weighted images) subacute blood clots in the left lateral ventricle and an area of porencephaly. In addition, the T2-weighted image (B) shows low-signal-intensity hemosiderin staining along the ependyma bilaterally.

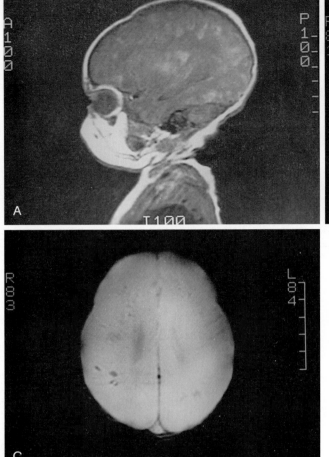

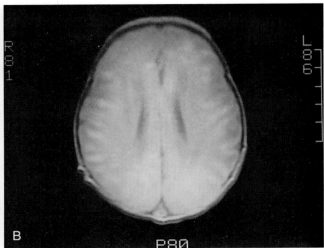

FIGURE 49–16 Visualization of hemorrhage using gradient-recalled echo sequences after anoxia. Sagittal SE (600/20) *(A)* and axial SE (3000/90) *(B)* images demonstrate diffuse edema with areas of laminar necrosis. *C*, Axial gradient-recalled echo (50/15/15°) shows several small areas of low-signal-intensity hemorrhage in the right posterior parietal region, not seen on other sequences.

IMAGING FINDINGS OF THE LATE SEQUELAE WITH CLINICAL CORRELATION

When children who have had previous anoxic ischemic damage are imaged, a variety of late sequelae may be identified. Table 49–2 summarizes the more common findings that may be seen both in children who were preterm and in those who were term infants at the time an anoxic ischemic event occurred. One of the major differences in the two subgroups is in their ability or inability to form gliosis as a result of the insult. Before 30 to 32 weeks of gestation the immature brain is incapa-

TABLE 49–2 Long-Term Sequelae of Anoxic Ischemic Injury

Premature	Term
Periventricular leukomalacia	Diffuse atrophy
Porencephaly	Ulegyria
	Gliosis
Cystic encephalomalacia	Cystic encephalomalacia
Delayed myelination	Delayed myelination

ble of forming gliosis as a response to an anoxic ischemic insult. Instead, affected areas necrose and subsequently develop cavitary areas of porencephaly.[10, 11, 80] After 32 weeks, in addition to the development of necrosis, areas of scarring or gliosis due to astrocystic proliferation may be seen. The presence or absence of gliosis in the brain of affected children has become a helpful aid in dating the timing of specific insults after the fact.[11]

In affected children, imaging may be required during the workup of a static neurologic deficit; in a previously diagnosed child imaging may be required if signs and symptoms appear to be evolving or for medicolegal reasons. MRI is now established as the imaging modality of choice for evaluation of the late sequelae of anoxic ischemic damage. Ultrasonography is no longer useful at this later time because closure of the fontanelles leads to loss of the imaging windows previously used.

Clinically, children who have suffered anoxic ischemic events develop static neurologic deficits that fit under the umbrella term of *cerebral palsy*.[81, 82] There are several different subtypes of cerebral palsy, and children with all subtypes may have associated seizures and intellectual impairment.

In the spastic subtypes of cerebral palsy, increased muscle tone may be seen predominantly involving the

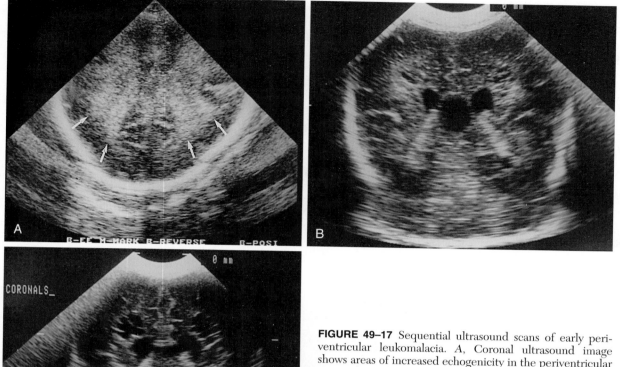

FIGURE 49–17 Sequential ultrasound scans of early peri-ventricular leukomalacia. *A*, Coronal ultrasound image shows areas of increased echogenicity in the periventricular region *(arrows)*. *B*, Follow-up study shows the early development of areas of cystic necrosis with areas of increased echogenicity. *C*, Later study shows more extensive cystic cavitation. *(A–C*, Courtesy of Valerie Hunter, M.D.)

FIGURE 49–18 MRI studies of incorporation of periventricular cysts into the lateral ventricles. *A*, Axial SE (800/20) image at 3 weeks. High-signal-intensity periventricular hemorrhage *(arrows)* is identified adjacent to the lateral ventricles. *B*, Axial SE (800/20) image at 8 weeks, after loss of white matter. The areas of hemorrhage are being incorporated into the lateral ventricles, and the latter are enlarging. *(A* and *B*, Courtesy of Craig McArdle, M.D.)

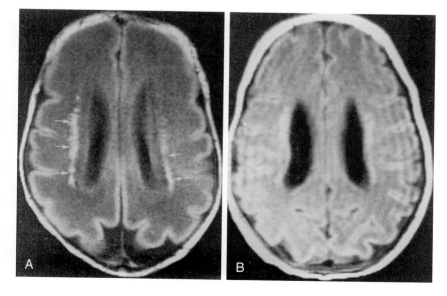

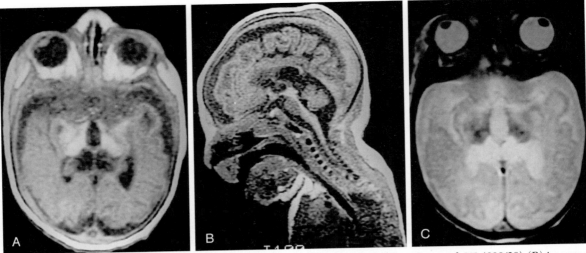

FIGURE 49–19 MRI findings of total anoxia to a preterm brain. Axial SE (600/20) (A) and sagittal SE (600/20) (B) images obtained on day 1 of life in an infant who suffered an anoxic event in the third trimester show areas of T1 hyperintensity predominantly involving the thalami and posterior brain stem. C, Axial SE (3500/120) image shows low signal intensity in the same areas.

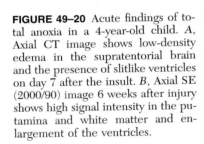

FIGURE 49–20 Acute findings of total anoxia in a 4-year-old child. A, Axial CT image shows low-density edema in the supratentorial brain and the presence of slitlike ventricles on day 7 after the insult. B, Axial SE (2000/90) image 6 weeks after injury shows high signal intensity in the putamina and white matter and enlargement of the ventricles.

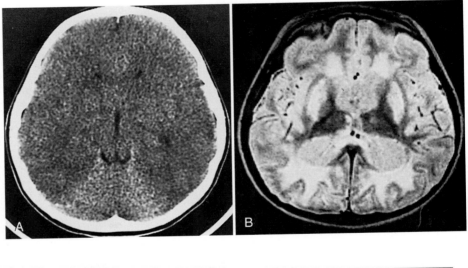

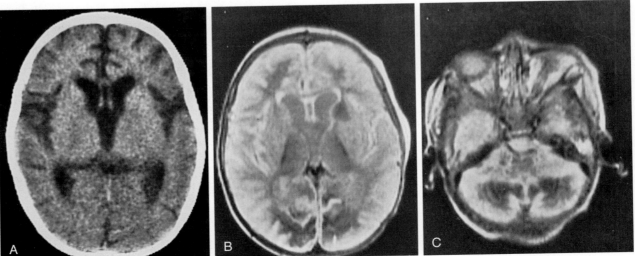

FIGURE 49–21 Chronic findings in total anoxia. A, Axial CT image shows diffuse atrophy. B and C, Axial SE (2000/84) MR images show enlarged ventricles and iron deposition in the occipital white matter and the dentate nuclei.

legs, the arms and trunk, or one side of the body. This subgroup includes spastic diplegia, spastic quadriplegia, and spastic hemiplegia. Infants with spastic diplegia demonstrate more severe involvement of the lower extremities than the upper. There is increased muscle tone in the legs, which are frequently maintained in extension (scissoring). In less severe forms, "toe-walking" and impaired coordination of fine and rapid finger movements may be present. In contrast, children with spastic hemiplegia (or infantile hemiplegia) have more severe involvement of one side of the body and of the upper extremities than of the lower. They frequently present with demonstration of hand dominance before its normal development at 2 to 4 years of age. Later, spasticity and flexion contractures are present in affected limbs, and "fisting" of the hand may be seen. Children with spastic quadriplegia demonstrate severe neurologic impairment with increased muscle tone and rigidity of all four limbs. Involvement is frequently more severe in the upper than lower limbs. Pseudobulbar signs when present lead to associated swallowing problems.

Children with extrapyramidal cerebral palsy do not show spasticity but instead manifest a variety of involuntary movements (hyperkinetic form) or postures (dystonic form), or both, due to defective regulation of muscle tone and coordination. It is important to realize that the manifestations of cerebral palsy are extremely varied, however, and a high percentage (13% to 21%) of children demonstrate mixed or atypical forms.[81]

Prolonged Hypoxia in the Preterm Infant

When the preterm brain suffers a single prolonged period or several intermittent periods of hypoxia, the most frequent abnormal finding seen is the development of PVL. The most common scenario of this type of event is of a ventilator-dependent premature infant with hyaline membrane disease.

Both CT and MRI are able to show the long-term sequelae in such patients. On both T1- and T2-weighted MRI studies, ventricles are enlarged with ragged borders due to white matter loss from infarction in the periventricular white matter regions (Fig. 49–22).[64, 83-85] As a result of the white matter loss, the sulci extend almost to

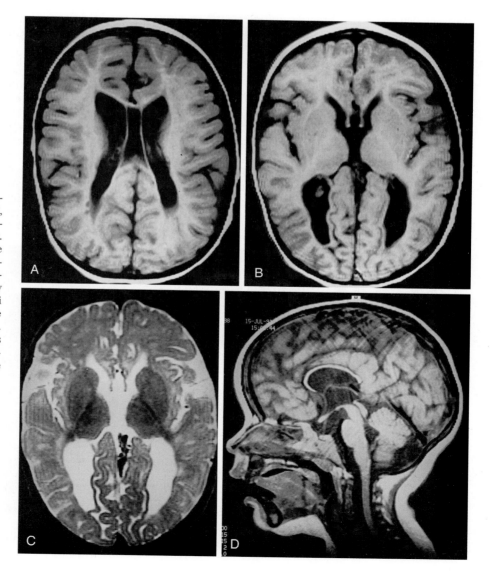

FIGURE 49–22 Late findings in periventricular leukomalacia. *A* and *B*, Axial (SE 600/20) images show enlarged ventricles with ragged borders. Small cysts are seen adjacent to the ventricles. *C*, Axial (SE 3000/90) image demonstrates the presence of gliosis in the white matter immediately next to the lateral ventricles. The sulci extend almost to the border of the ventricle in the region of the atria. *D*, Sagittal (SE 600/20) image shows marked thinning of the corpus callosum, especially in the region of the posterior body and the splenium.

the outer border of the ventricles (Fig. 49–22), especially in the region of the ventricular atria. Cystic areas may be present in the periventricular white matter adjacent to the ventricles and are more frequently seen in the region around the atria and the frontal horns. As a result of the loss of white matter, the corpus callosum does not undergo its normal postnatal development and appears abnormally thin on midline sagittal images, especially in the posterior portion of the body where the axons from the periatrial region are positioned (Fig. 49–22D). If the insult leading to the development of PVL occurs later than 30 to 32 weeks of gestation, then gliosis may also be seen in the periventricular region.[8] In addition, delayed myelination is often identified.

Clinically, children with PVL frequently develop spastic diplegia and may have additional visual problems.[83] As previously stated, the areas most severely involved in PVL are those adjacent to the lateral borders of the ventricles. Figure 49–22A demonstrates the relationship of these areas to the corticospinal tracts. The most medially located corticospinal tracts are those that pass directly to the lower extremities, thus explaining the predominant involvement of the lower extremity in infants with spastic diplegia. When more extensive injury occurs, a larger proportion of the corticospinal tracts are involved, and therefore the upper extremities and trunk may also be involved, leading to the development of spastic quadriplegia. Visual impairment is due to involvement of the geniculocalcarine tracts.

Prolonged Hypoxia in the Term Infant

Term infants may also undergo prolonged or intermittent periods of hypoxia, for example, an infant who develops lung disease after meconium aspiration. Follow-up images of these children demonstrate peripherally located, parasagittal infarctions,[13] the development of which is best explained by the circulatory theory. Imaging studies show wedge-shaped areas of encephalomalacia at the watershed junctions between the anterior and middle cerebral artery territories and the middle and posterior cerebral artery territories. When injury is more extensive, larger areas of the cerebral cortex and the underlying white matter may be involved, and affected gyri may have a characteristic mushroom shape.[8] This appearance, termed *ulegyria*, has been described at autopsies and is characteristic of hypoxic damage.[80] It is thought to occur because the blood supply to the base of the gyrus is more precarious than that to the tip. After the insult there is therefore more tissue destruction to the base of the gyrus, leading to the development of the characteristic mushroom shape.[8]

Children who have these types of injury characteristically develop infantile hemiplegia if the insult is predominantly unilateral, and spastic quadriplegia if the insult is bilateral. Those with infantile hemiplegia frequently demonstrate more severe involvement of the arm and trunk than the lower extremity. This is explained in Figure 49–2B by comparison of the location of the injury and siting on the motor strip of the homunculus of the various body parts.

Total Anoxia in Term and Preterm Infants

When a short but total period of anoxia occurs to either a preterm or a term child, the pattern of brain injury is predominantly to the brain stem, basal ganglia, thalamus, and perirolandic areas.[8] This type of injury usually occurs after catastrophic events such as placental abruption, nuchal cord, or severe placental hemorrhage.

The pattern of injury is best explained by the metabolic and excitotoxin theories. As a result of the predominant involvement of the basal ganglia and relative sparing of the cortical gray and the white matter, children who suffer this type of injury do not demonstrate spasticity but instead demonstrate extrapyramidal (choreoathetoid)

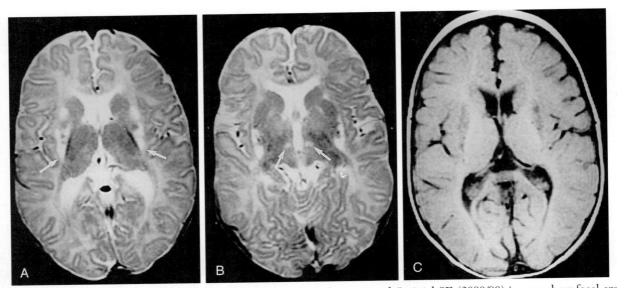

FIGURE 49–23 Late findings after a period of total anoxia to a term brain. *A* and *B*, Axial SE (3000/90) images show focal areas of high-signal-intensity gliosis in the posterior aspects of the lentiform nuclei and the ventrolateral thalami (*arrows*). *C*, On axial SE (600/20) image, the same areas demonstrate subtle decreased signal intensity.

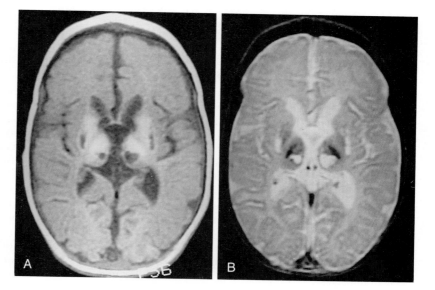

FIGURE 49–24 Cystic changes in the basal ganglia after a period of total anoxia (day 78). Axial SE (600/20) *(A)* and SE (3000/120) *(B)* images show areas of cystic necrosis in the lentiform nuclei and thalami bilaterally.

cerebral palsy.[45, 47] The basal ganglia injury incurred causes the development of choreoathetoid movements or posturing, or both.

MRI studies show late sequelae consisting of characteristic areas of gliosis or cavitation or both in the posterior aspects of the lentiform nuclei and ventrolateral aspects of the thalami bilaterally (Figs. 49–23 and 49–24).[35, 45–47] In addition, gliosis may be seen in the region of the centrum semiovale; and focal dilatation of the temporal horns of the lateral ventricles, when present, reflects hippocampal atrophy resulting from the episode of anoxia.

When the period of total anoxia is very prolonged, extensive damage occurs to the entire brain. All the theoretical mechanisms of injury (circulatory, metabolic, and excitotoxic) are probably involved when catastrophic injuries of this type occur. Large areas of the cortex and subcortical white matter are destroyed, and multicystic encephalomalacia results.[86] Children who demonstrate

these severe findings clinically usually have severe spastic quadriplegia.[81]

On T1- and T2-weighted MRI studies, the extensive areas of cystic necrosis with septations between them and associated gliosis that develop are easily seen (Fig. 49–25).[8, 46] The basal ganglia are generally not cystic, though, and demonstrate a relative lack of gliosis.

FOCAL INFARCTION

The causes of focal infarction in the pediatric age group are diverse. They include embolus, thrombosis, vasospasm (migraine), vascular malformations, tumors, and metabolic causes.[87]

Embolus may have several causes including cyanotic heart disease, cardiomyopathy, carotid dissection, and mitral valve prolapse. Thrombosis may form as a result of

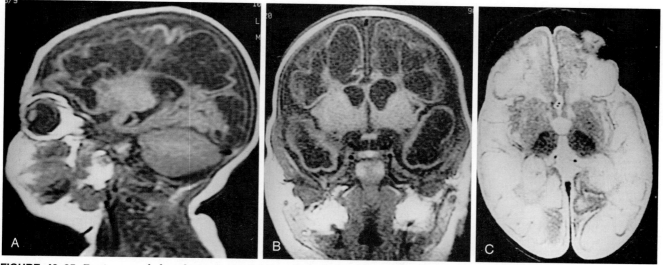

FIGURE 49–25 Cystic encephalomalacia. Sagittal *(A)* and axial (600/20) *(B)* images and axial SE (3000/120) *(C)* image show enlargement of the lateral ventricles and extensive cysts with septation between them replacing the cerebral hemispheres. There is relative sparing of the basal ganglia.

polycythemia, trauma leading to dissection, viral infection, meningitis, coagulopathies, maternal drug use (especially cocaine), and a host of vasculopathies. Metabolic causes of infarction are less frequently seen.

Focal infarction presents differently in newborns and infants than in older children and adults. In the term newborn, infarction may present with seizures or with nonspecific nonfocal findings, such as hypotonia. It may, therefore, be much more difficult to detect clinically at this age. The demonstration of hand preference in a child younger than 1 year may be the first indication of the presence of a unilateral hemiparesis due to a previous infarction. Older children, like adults, more frequently present with evidence of a focal neurologic deficit. Focal infarction is rare in premature infants but has been reported.[88] In this age group seizures usually do not occur as a result of the infarction.

The imaging findings of infarction may be subtle and more difficult to identify than in the adult. On ultrasound studies the infarcted area is seen as an ill-defined region of hyperechogenicity. If hemorrhage is present within the infarct, the area of hyperechogenicity may be more obvi-ous and well defined (Fig. 49–4). On CT studies infarction appears as an area of hypodensity compared with the adjacent normal brain. If it is peripherally located, it may appear wedge shaped (Fig. 49–2). When hemorrhage is present, increased density is seen in the involved paren-chyma in the acute period. After contrast administration, enhancement may be seen within the infarct from 5 days to approximately 1 month. Although MRI is very sensitive for demonstration of infarction, the findings may often be subtle, especially in the newborn infant, when the water content of the brain is still very high.

Areas of infarction may demonstrate a focal mass ef-fect, effacement of sulci and gyri, and loss of the distinct gray-white matter border, so well seen on T2-weighted images (Fig. 49–14). When hemorrhage is present, the signal intensity of the involved area changes depending on the age of the hemorrhage. When subacute, it demon-strates either high signal intensity on T1-weighted images and low signal intensity on T2-weighted images (intracel-lular methemoglobin) or high signal intensity on both T1- and T2-weighted images (extracellular methemoglobin). Recently, the use of diffusion MRI in the detection of

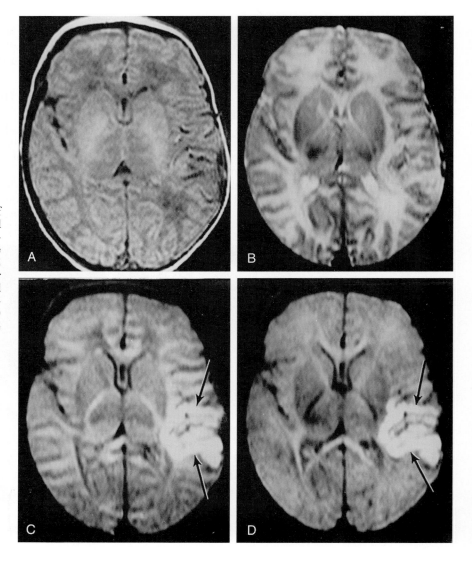

FIGURE 49–26 Diffusion MRI studies of acute stroke. Axial SE (720/20) *(A)* and SE (3000/120) *(B)* images show an ex-tremely subtle area of focal edema in the left parietal lobe. Diffusion-weighted SE (pulse interval/200 msec, anteroposterior sensitization, b = 600 sec/mm²) *(C)*, and SE (pulse interval/200 msec through-plane sensitization, b = 600 sec/mm²) *(D)* images demonstrate the full extent of the infarct *(arrows)*. (A–D, Courtesy of G. Bydder, M.B., Ch.B.)

FIGURE 49–27 MRI studies of early infarction after carotid dissection. *A,* Axial SE (650/15) image shows low signal intensity in the distribution of the left middle cerebral artery. The involved area demonstrates effacement of the overlying sulci and gyri and a mild mass effect on the frontal horn of the lateral ventricle. *B,* Axial SE (3000/90) image shows diffuse high signal intensity of the same region with total obliteration of the gray-white matter differentiation in this region.

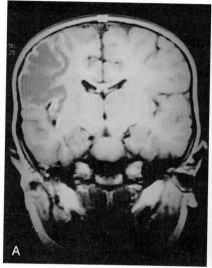 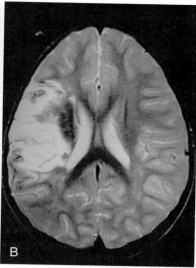

acute stroke in infants has been described. In the acute situation diffusion imaging demonstrates evidence of stroke that could not be or is difficult to identify on routine spin-echo images (Fig. 49–26).

In older children, as in adults, focal infarction is easier to identify and most frequently is seen as a wedge-shaped area of low signal intensity on T1-weighted images and high signal intensity on T2-weighted images in a vascular distribution (Fig. 49–27). Infarction involving the basal ganglia may show heterogeneous signal intensity of the deep gray matter and results from obstruction of the lenticulostriate and thalamoperforating vessels. Loss of signal void within intracranial vessels may be seen in the blood vessels supplying the affected area, and this sign should be actively sought in all cases of suspected infarction. Cerebral angiography or MR angiography[89, 90] may both be useful in identifying the cause of infarction in children.

References

1. Little WJ. On the influence of abnormal parturition, difficult labor, premature birth, and asphyxia neonatorum on the mental and physical conditions of the child, especially in relation to deformities. Trans Lond Obstet Soc 1862;3:293.
2. Hill A. Current concepts of hypoxic-ishemic injury in the term newborn. Pediatr Neurol 1991;7:317–325.
3. Volpe JJ. Hypoxic-ischemic encephalopathy. In Neurology of the Newborn, 2nd ed., pp. 159–280. Philadelphia, WB Saunders, 1987.
4. Roland E, Hill A. MR and CT evaluation of profound neonatal and infantile asphyxia. [Commentary] AJNR 1992;13:973–975.
5. Volpe JJ. Current concepts of brain injury in the premature infant. AJR 1989;153:243–251.
6. Volpe JJ. Brain injury in the premature infant: Current concepts of pathogenesis and prevention. Biol Neonate 1992;62:231–242.
7. Volpe JJ. Hypoxic-ischemic encephalopathy: Biochemical and physiological aspects. In Volpe JJ (ed). Neurology of the Newborn, 3rd ed., pp. 211–259. Philadelphia, WB Saunders, 1991.
8. Barkovich AJ. Destructive brain disorders of childhood. In Barkovich AJ (ed). Pediatric Neuroimaging, 2nd ed., pp. 107–175. Philadelphia, Lippincott-Raven, 1995.
9. Myers RE. Experimental models of perinatal brain damage: Relevance to human pathology. In Gluck L (ed). Intrauterine Asphyxia and the Developing Fetal Brain, pp. 37–97. Chicago, Year Book, 1977.
10. Raybaud C. Destructive lesions of the brain. Neuroradiology 1983;25:265–291.
11. Barkovich AJ, Truwit CL. MR of perinatal asphyxia: Correlation of gestational age with pattern of damage. AJNR 1990;11:1087–1096.
12. Gilles FH. Neuropathologic indicators of abnormal development. In Freeman JM (ed). Prenatal and Perinatal Factors Associated With Brain Disorders, pp. 53–107. Bethesda, NIH, 1985.
13. Volpe JJ. Neuropathology and pathogenesis. In Volpe JJ (ed). Neurology of the Newborn, 3rd ed., pp. 279–313. Philadelphia, WB Saunders, 1991.
14. DeReuck JL. Cerebral angioarchitecture and perinatal brain lesions in premature and full-term infants. Acta Neurol Scand 1984;70:391–395.
15. Van den Bergh R. Centrifugal elements in the vascular pattern of the deep intracerebral blood supply. Angiology 1969;20:88–94.
16. Takashima S, Tanaka K. Development of the cerebrovascular architecture and its relationship to periventricular leukomalacia. Arch Neurol 1978;35:11–16.
17. DeReuck J. The human periventricular arterial blood supply and the anatomy of cerebral infarctions. Eur Neurol 1971;5:321–334.
18. Volpe JJ, Herscovitch P, Perlman JM, Raichle ME. Positron emission tomography in the newborn: Extensive impairment of regional blood flow with intraventricular hemorrhage and hemorrhagic intracerebral involvement. Pediatrics 1983;72:589–595.
19. Kuban KCK, Gilles FH. Human telencephalic angiogenesis. Ann Neurol 1985;17:539–548.
20. Nelson MD Jr, Gonzalez-Gomez I, Gilles FH. The search for human telencephalic ventriculofugal arteries. AJNR 1991;12:215–222.
21. Meyer JE. Uber die lokalisation fruhkindlicher Hischaden in arteriellen Grenzgebieten. Arch Psychiatr Nervenchr 1953;190:328.
22. Volpe JJ, Herscovitch P, Perlman JM, et al. Positron emission tomography in the asphyxiated newborn: Parasagittal impairment of cerebral blood flow. Ann Neurol 1985;17:287–296.
23. Volpe JJ, Pasternak JF. Parasagittal cerebral injury in neonatal hypoxic-ischemic encephalopathy: Clinical and neuroradiological features. J Pediatr 1977;91:472–476.
24. Chugani HT, Phelps ME, Mazziotta JC. Positron emission tomography study of human brain functional development. Ann Neurol 1987;22:487–497.
25. Hasegawa M, Houdou S, Mito T, et al. Development of myelination in the human fetal and infant cerebellum: A myelin basic protein immunohistochemical study. Brain Dev 1992;14:1–6.
26. Dobbing J. Vunerable periods of brain development. In Dobbing J (ed). Lipids, Malnutrition and the Developing Brain, pp. 9–23. Amsterdam, Elsevier, 1972.
27. Johnson MA, Pennock JM, Bydder GM, et al. Clinical MR imaging of the brain in children: Normal and neurological disease. AJR 1983;141:1005–1018.
28. Dietrich RB, Bradley WG, Zagaroza EJ, et al. MR evaluation of early myelination patterns in normal and developmentally delayed infants. AJNR 1988;9:69–76.

29. Barkovich AJ, Kjos BO, Jackson DE Jr, et al. Normal maturation of the neonatal and infant brain: MR imaging at 1.5 T. Radiology 1988;166:173–180.

30. Greenamyre JT, Penney JB, Young AB, et al. Evidence for transient perinatal glutamatergic innervation of globus pallidum. J Neurosci 1987;7:1022–1030.

31. Barks JD, Silverstein FS, Sims K, et al. Glutamate recognition sites in human fetal brain. Neurosci Lett 1988;84:131–136.

32. Cohn MJ, Dietrich RB, Roth GM. Anoxic-ischemic events in infants: Early MR findings. 33rd Annual Meeting of American Society of Neuroradiology, Book of Abstracts, p. 81. 1995.

33. Siegel MJ, Shackelford GD, Perlman JM, Fulling KH. Hypoxic-ischemic encephalopathy in term infants: Diagnosis and prognosis evaluated by ultrasound. Radiology 1984;152:395–399.

34. Martin DJ, Hill A, Fritz CR, et al. Hypoxic-ischemic cerebral injury in the neonatal brain: A report of sonographic features with computed tomographic correlation. J Pediatr Radiol 1983;13:307–316.

35. Rutherford MA, Pennock JM, Murdoch-Eaton DM, et al. Athetoid cerebral palsy with cysts in the putamen after hypoxic-ischemic encephalopathy. Arch Dis Child 1992;67:846–850.

36. Phillips R, Brandberg G, Hill A, et al. Prevalence and prognostic value of abnormal CT findings in 100 term asphyxiated newborns. Radiology 1993;189P:287.

37. Vannucci RC, Christensen MA, Yager JY. Nature, time course, and extent of cerebral edema in perinatal hypoxic-ischemic brain damage. Pediatr Neurol 1993;9:29–34.

38. Cowan FM, Pennock JM, Hanrahan JD, et al. Early detection of cerebral infarction and hypoxic-ischemic encephalopathy in neonates using diffusion-weighted magnetic resonance imaging. Neuropediatrics 1994;25:172–175.

39. Barkovich AJ, Westmark KD, Partridge JC, et al. Perinatal asphyxia: MR findings in the first 10 days. AJNR 1995;16:427–438.

40. Westmark KD, Barkovich AJ, Sola A, et al. Patterns and implications of MR contrast enhancement in perinatal asphyxia: A preliminary report. Am J Neuroradiol 1995;16:685–692.

41. Baenziger O, Martin E, Steinlin M, et al. Early pattern recognition in severe perinatal asphyxia: A prospective MRI study. Neuroradiology 1993;35:437–442.

42. Christophe C, Clerex A, Blum D, et al. Early MR detection of cortical and subcortical hypoxic-ischemic encephalopathy in full-term-unfants. Pediatr Radiol 1994;24:581–584.

43. Rutherford MA, Pennock JM, Schwieso JE, et al. Hypoxic ischaemic encephalopathy: Early magnetic resonance imaging findings and their evolution. Neuropediatrics 1995;26:183–191.

44. Parisi JE, Collins GH, Kim RC, Crosley CJ. Prenatal symmetrical thalamic degeneration with flexion spasticity at birth. Ann Neurol 1983;13:94–97.

45. Dietrich RB, Kerrigan J, Chugani H, Gabriel R. Cerebral palsy: Correlation of MR imaging, history and clinical findings. 33rd Annual Meeting of the Society of Pediatric Radiology. Book of Abstracts, p. 46. 1990.

46. Barkovich AJ: MR and CT evaluation of profound neonatal and infantile asphyxia. AJNR 1992;13:959–972.

47. Menkes J, Curran JG. Clinical and magnetic resonance imaging correlates in children with extrapyramidal cerebral palsy. Am J Neuroradiol 1994;15:451–457.

48. Castillo M, Smith JK, Mukherji SK. MR appearance of cerebral cortex in children with and without a history of perinatal anoxia: Preliminary observations. AJR 1995;164:1481–1484.

49. Sawada H, Udaka F, Seriu N, et al. MRI demonstration of cortical laminar necrosis and delayed white matter injury in anoxic encephalopathy. Neuroradiology 1990;32:319–321.

50. Takahashi S, Higano S, Ishii K, et al. Hypoxic brain damage: Cortical laminar necrosis and delayed changes in white matter at sequential MR imaging. Radiology 1993;189:449–456.

51. Takashima S, Tanaka K. Subcortical leukomalacia, relationship to development of the central sulcus, and its vascular supply. Arch Neurol 1978;35:470–476.

52. Harlow C, Hay TC, Rumack CM. The pediatric brain. In Rumack CM (ed). Pediatric Sonography, pp 1009–1044. St. Louis, Mosby–Year Book, 1991.

53. Volpe JJ. Intracranial hemorrhage: Germinal matrix-intraventricular hemorrhage of the premature infant. In Volpe JJ (ed). Neurology

of the Newborn, 3rd ed., pp. 403–466. Philadelphia, WB Saunders, 1991.

54. Burstein J, Papile L, Burstein R. Intraventricular hemorrhage and hydrocephalus in premature newborns: A prospective study with CT. AJR 1979;132:631–635.

55. Hayden CK, Swischuk LE. The head and spine. In Hayden CK, Swischuk LE (eds). Pediatric Ultrasonography, pp. 3–77. Baltimore, Williams & Wilkins, 1987.

56. Babcock DS, Allison JW, Dietrich RB. Hypoxic-Ischemic Injury in the Preterm and Term Infant. RSNA Learning Center Program 1996. RSP 543.

57. McArdle CB, Richardson CJ, Hayden CK, et al. Abnormalities of the neonatal brain: MR imaging. I. Intracranial hemorrhage. Radiology 1987;163:387–394.

58. Keeney SE, Adcock EW, McArdle CB. Prospective observations of 100 high-risk neonates by high-field (1.5 Tesla) magnetic resonance imaging of the central nervous system. I. Intraventricular and extracerebral lesions. Pediatrics 1991;87:421–430.

59. Zuerrer M, Martin E, Boltshauser E. MR imaging of intracranial hemorrhage in neonates and infants at 2.35 Tesla. Neuroradiology 1991;33:223–229.

60. Kannegieter LS, Mann CI, Dietrich RB. Role of T2-weighted GRE in the evaluation of intracranial hemorrhage in infants. Annual Meeting of the Society for Magnetic Resonance Imaging, Book of Abstracts, p. 70. 1992.

61. Greisen G. Ischemia of the preterm brain. Biol Neonate 1992;62:243–247.

62. Leviton A, Gilles FH. Acquired perinatal leukoencephalopathy. Ann Neurol 1984;16:1.

63. Gilles FH, Averill DR, Kerr CS. Neonatal endotoxin encephalopathy. Ann Neurol 1977;2:49.

64. Flodmark O, Roland EH, Hill A, et al. Periventricular leukomalacia: Radiologic diagnosis. Radiology 1987;162:119–124.

65. DeReuck J, Chatta AS, Richardson EP Jr. Pathogenesis and evolution of periventricular leukomalacia in infancy. Arch Neurol 1972;27:229–236.

66. Banker BQ, Larroche JC. Periventricular leukomalacia in infancy. Arch Neurol 1962;7:386–410.

67. Armstrong D, Norman MG. Periventricular leukomalacia in neonates: Complications and sequelae. Arch Dis Child 1974;49:367–375.

68. Grant EG, Schellinger D, Richardson JD, et al. Echogenic periventricular halo: Normal sonographic finding or neonatal cerebral hemorrhage? Am J Neuroradiol 1983;4:43–46.

69. McArdle CB, Richardson CJ, Hayden CK, et al. Abnormalities of the neonatal brain: MR imaging. II. Hypoxic-ischemic brain injury. Radiology 1987;163:395–403.

70. Keeney SE, Adcock EW, McArdle CB. Prospective observations of 100 high-risk neonates by high-field (1.5 Tesla) magnetic resonance imaging of the central nervous system. II. Lesions associated with hypoxic-ischemic encephalopathy. Pediatrics 1991;87:431–438.

71. Schouman-Clays E, Henry-Fuegeas M-C, Roset F, et al. Periventricular leukomalacia: Correlation between MR imaging and autopsy findings during the first 2 months of life. Radiology 1993;189:59–64.

72. Roland EH, Hill A, Norman MG, et al. Selective brainstem injury in an asphyxiated newborn. Ann Neurol 1988;23:89–92.

73. Leech RW, Alvord EC Jr. Anoxic ischemic encephalopathy in the human neonatal period: The significance of brain stem involvement. Arch Neurol 1977;34:109–113.

74. Schneider H, Ballowitz L, Schachinger H, et al. Anoxic encephalopathy with predominant involvement of basal ganglia, brainstem and spinal cord in the perinatal period. Acta Neuropath (Berl) 1975;32:287–298.

75. Pasternak JE, Predey TA, Mikhael MA. Neonatal asphyxia: Vulnerability of basal ganglia, thalamus, and brainstem. Pediatr Neurol 1991;7:147–149.

76. Barkovich AJ, Sargent SK. Profound asphyxia in the premature infant: Imaging findings. AJNR 16:1837–1846.

77. Fitch SJ, Gerald B, Magill HL, Tonkin ILD. Central nervous system hypoxia in children due to near drowning. Radiology 1985;56:647–650.

78. Kjos BO, Brant-Zawadzki M, Young RG. Early CT findings of global central nervous system hypoperfusion. AJR 1983;141:1227–1232.

79. Dietrich RB, Bradley WG. Iron accumulation in the basal ganglia

following severe ischemic-anoxic insults in children. Radiology 1988;168:203–206.

80. Friede RL. Developmental Neuropathology, 2nd ed. Berlin, Springer-Verlag, 1989.
81. Menkes JH. Perinatal asphyxia and trauma. In Menkes JH (ed). Textbook of Child Neurology, 4th ed., pp. 284–326. Philadelphia, Lea & Febiger, 1990.
82. Volpe JJ. Hypoxic-ischemic encephalopathy: Clinical aspects. In Volpe JJ (ed). Neurology of the Newborn, 3rd ed., pp. 314–372. Philadelphia, WB Saunders, 1991.
83. Flodmark O, Lupton B, Li D, et al. MR imaging of periventricular leukomalacia in childhood. AJNR 1989;10:111–118.
84. Wilson DA, Steiner RE. Periventricular leukomalacia: Evaluation with MR imaging. Radiology 1986;160:507–511.
85. Baker LL, Stevenson DK, Enzmann DR. End stage periventricular leukomalacia: MR imaging evaluation. Radiology 1988;168:809–815.
86. Naidich T, Chakera MH. Cystic encephalomalacia: CT appearance and pathological correlation. J Comput Assist Tomogr 1984;8;631–636.
87. Menkes JH. Cerebrovascular disorders. In Menkes JH (ed): Textbook of Child Neurology, 4th ed., pp. 583–601. Philadelphia, Lea & Febiger, 1990.
88. DeVries LS, Regev R, Connell JA, et al. Localised cerebral infarction in the premature infant: A ultrasound diagnosis correlated with computed tomography and magnetic resonance imaging. Pediatrics 1988;81:36–40.
89. Mann CL, Dietrich RB, Schrader MT, et al. Posttraumatic carotid artery dissection in children: Evaluation with MR angiography. AJR 1993;160:134–136.
90. Maas KP, Barkovich AJ, Dong L, et al. Selected indications for and applications of magnetic resonance angiography in children. Pediatr Neurosurg 1994;20:113–125.

50

Hydrocephalus and Cerebrospinal Fluid Flow

WILLIAM G. BRADLEY, Jr., M.D., Ph.D.
WILLIAM W. ORRISON, Jr., M.D.

CEREBROSPINAL FLUID DYNAMICS

Cerebrospinal fluid (CSF) is produced as an altered filtrate of plasma by the choroid plexus within the ventricles of the brain at a rate of approximately 500 ml/day. There is 120 to 150 ml of CSF present within the body at all times with the cerebral ventricles containing about 40 ml. CSF normally flows inferiorly through the foramen of Monro, the aqueduct of Sylvius, and out the foramina of Luschka and Magendie in the fourth ventricle. Some of the CSF flows down around the spinal cord; most of it, however, flows up through the basal cisterns and over the cerebral convexities eventually to be absorbed by the arachnoidal villi (arachnoid granulations) on either side of the superior sagittal sinus.[1] There is also some CSF absorption through the ependymal lining of the ventricular system and along the spinal cord and meninges.[2, 3] Superimposed on this slow, steady egress of CSF from the ventricular system is a much more prominent to-and-fro motion secondary to cardiac pulsations, which is due to the systolic expansion and diastolic contraction of the brain. The high velocity associated with this motion produces relative signal loss of the CSF in the aqueduct and third and fourth ventricles known as the *CSF flow void* (Fig. 50–1).

HYDROCEPHALUS

A relative obstruction to the normal flow of CSF resulting in an increase in the size of the ventricular system is generally termed *hydrocephalus*. Hydrocephalus results from a mechanical imbalance between CSF production and absorption whereby production exceeds absorption in a manner sufficient for subsequent ventricular enlargement. Hydrocephalus is not secondary to either abnormal brain development or a loss of cerebral tissue.[2, 4] Therefore, all hydrocephalus is obstructive, and it is the goal of the neuroimaging evaluation to determine the exact level of this obstruction. It is possible for the obstruction to occur at any level in the normal pathway of CSF flow (Fig. 50–2). This pathway includes and occurs (1) within the lateral ventricles, (2) at the level of the foramen of Monro, (3) within the third ventricle, (4) at the level of the cerebral aqueduct, (5) within the fourth ventricle, (6) at the outlets of the fourth ventricle (foramina of Magendie and Luschka), (7) at the tentorial incisura, (8) over the cerebral convexities, and (9) at the level of the arachnoidal granulations. Common causes of obstructive hydrocephalus include subarachnoid hemorrhage, infection, intracranial masses, and congenital anomalies.[2, 4]

Although often thought of by the novice as a simple problem on neuroimaging studies, hydrocephalus is frequently missed, miscommunicated, or incompletely diagnosed. The goal of any imaging study performed for the exclusion or definition of hydrocephalus is to determine whether or not the condition is present and, if so, the exact nature of the obstruction. A number of types of hydrocephalus have been described in the literature. Hydrocephalus has classically been defined as either *communicating* or *noncommunicating*. Such a designation is not adequate to describe the findings on the advanced neuroimaging methods readily available today in most modern medical facilities. This nomenclature is still in use by many clinicians, however, and therefore it is imperative that the neuroimager understand what is meant by these terms. *Communicating hydrocephalus* in general refers to a form of hydrocephalus in which there is *communication* or free flow of CSF between the ventricular system and the subarachnoid spaces. This form of hydrocephalus is now commonly referred to as *extraventricular obstructive hydrocephalus* (EVOH).

Noncommunicating hydrocephalus implies that there is a block either at some level within the ventricular system or at the level of the outlets of the fourth ventricle. This obstruction prevents the free flow or communication between the ventricular system and the subarachnoid spaces, thus the designation of *noncommunicating* hydrocephalus. This type of hydrocephalus is now commonly referred to as *intraventricular obstructive hydrocephalus* (IVOH). In addition to EVOH (communicating) and IVOH (noncommunicating), the terms *hydrocephalus ex vacuo, external hydrocephalus, overproduction hydro-*

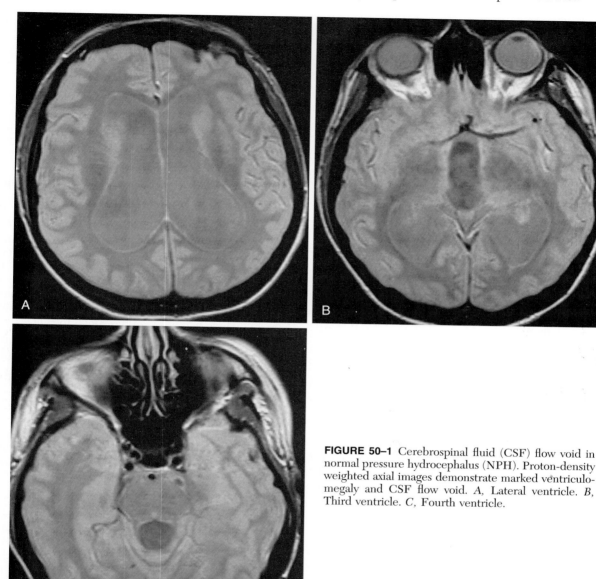

FIGURE 50–1 Cerebrospinal fluid (CSF) flow void in normal pressure hydrocephalus (NPH). Proton-density weighted axial images demonstrate marked ventriculomegaly and CSF flow void. *A*, Lateral ventricle. *B*, Third ventricle. *C*, Fourth ventricle.

cephalus, and *normal pressure hydrocephalus* (NPH) have been or are currently in use. This confusing array of terms can be more appropriately classified for modern neuroimaging.

The term *hydrocephalus ex vacuo* is a misnomer and should be abandoned.[2, 4, 5] *Hydrocephalus ex vacuo* simply refers to atrophy and therefore should be stated as such. It is recommended that the designation of atrophy as a form of hydrocephalus be abandoned to avoid the confusion caused by using the term *hydrocephalus* in the absence of obstruction. It is also important to prevent any clinical misunderstanding. For example, the term *hydrocephalus ex vacuo* might be construed by the uninitiated to imply that some type of invasive treatment should be considered. Therefore, *hydrocephalus ex vacuo* is considered obsolete terminology.

Benign external hydrocephalus is a form of EVOH in children generally younger than 9 months whose fontanelles are still open. The condition is self-limited and believed to result from immature arachnoid granulations that are not quite able to absorb adequate quantities of CSF. As a result, there is backup of CSF within the ventricles as well as in the subarachnoid space over the convexities, owing to the ability of the sutures to expand at this early age. Cortical vessels are seen to float freely in the enlarged subarachnoid spaces rather than to be compressed against the gyri as they would be by subdural collections. These patients should not be shunted.

The term *external hydrocephalus* has also been used inappropriately to describe extra-axial fluid collections of CSF density on computed tomography (CT), sometimes known by the outmoded term *subdural hygromas.* It is

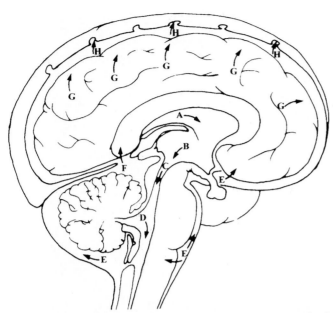

FIGURE 50–2 Normal flow pattern. A, lateral ventricles; B, third ventricle; C, cerebral aqueduct; D, fourth ventricle; E, basal cisterns; F, incisura; G, cerebral hemispheres; H, arachnoid granulations.

now clearly understood by magnetic resonance imaging (MRI) that the term *subdural hygromas* has been used to mean both chronic subdural hematomas and arachnoid rents leading to subdural accumulations of CSF. On MRI, the higher protein content (and higher signal intensity) of the chronic subdural hematoma clearly allows these two entities to be distinguished. For this reason, it is recommended that the term *subdural hygroma* be dropped in favor of the terms *chronic subdural hematoma* and *arachnoid rents leading to CSF accumulation in the subdural space*. The designation of *hydrocephalus* can continue to be appropriately reserved for obstructive conditions that are accompanied by ventricular enlargement.[2, 4]

Special consideration is often given to two forms of EVOH: (1) overproduction hydrocephalus and (2) NPH. Obstruction can occur at any level beyond the outflow of the fourth ventricle in EVOH, but when it occurs as a result of insufficient absorption or flow of CSF, it is generally considered more specifically. One of these conditions is confined almost exclusively to the very young and the other to the very old. The first of these forms of EVOH is the uncommon *overproduction hydrocephalus* that is seen most often in early childhood, typically in patients with choroid plexus neoplasms. An increase in the size of the ventricles can often be identified in these patients, and this is presumably due to increased production of CSF by the tumor. This overproduction of CSF results in the inability to absorb CSF sufficiently at a comparable rate. The relative obstruction then occurs at a level outside of the ventricular system. It also possible, however, for IVOH to occur in patients with a choroid plexus neoplasm as a result of mass effect from the neoplasm (Fig. 50–3).[2, 5–7] The second form of EVOH that is frequently given a separate designation is NPH.

This disorder appears to be a condition confined to the older population. Although sometimes difficult to diagnose, NPH is far from a rare disorder.

NORMAL PRESSURE HYDROCEPHALUS

Classically, NPH patients present with a clinical triad of gait apraxia, dementia, and incontinence.[8–10] Although the mean intraventricular pressure is normal in these patients, the pulse pressure (i.e., the change in CSF pressure over the cardiac cycle) is much greater than normal. A *waterhammer* pulse has been described in such patients when intraventricular pressure is monitored.[11, 12] Until now, the diagnosis of NPH has typically been based on three criteria: (1) the clinical presentation, (2) the radiographic pattern of ventricles enlarged out of proportion to cortical sulcal enlargement (to distinguish NPH from atrophy), and (3) radionuclide cisternography.

Before the advent of MRI, the radiographic picture and the appropriate clinical triad alone were not sufficient to predict which patients would respond to ventriculoperitoneal shunting, which is the primary treatment for NPH. When the local CSF velocity is sufficiently high (e.g., through the narrow aqueduct of Sylvius), a *CSF flow void*[13, 14] is normally produced on MRI that is similar to that seen with rapidly flowing blood.[15] When there is obstruction to CSF flow, as in aqueductal stenosis, this MRI flow void is not observed.[14] The magnitude of the aqueductal CSF flow void (see Fig. 50–1) has been used to predict which patients with clinical NPH would respond to shunting.[16] The CSF flow void is a normal

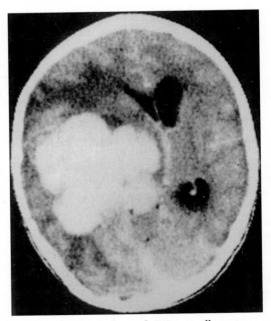

FIGURE 50–3 Contrast-enhanced CT scan illustrates mass effect and contralateral dilatation of the lateral ventricle secondary to obstruction at the level of the foramen of Monro. Enlargement of the ventricles may have started in this case as a result of *overproduction* of cerebrospinal fluid from the choroid plexus papilloma.

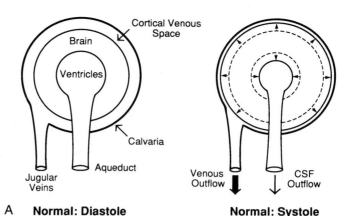

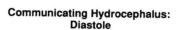

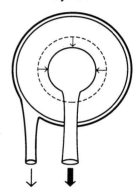

FIGURE 50–4 Schematic representation of cerebrospinal fluid (CSF) flow mechanism: Cause of hyperdynamic CSF flow state in communicating hydrocephalus. *A,* In normal patients, systolic expansion of cerebral hemispheres occurs outwardly, compressing cortical veins and, to a lesser extent, inwardly compressing the lateral ventricles. *B,* In communicating hydrocephalus, the brain has already expanded against the inner table of the calvaria. Because outward expansion of the brain is no longer possible, the entire increase in volume as a result of systolic expansion is directed inward, toward the lateral ventricles. The combination of this greater inward displacement and the mild aqueductal enlargement that accompanies communicating hydrocephalus leads to hyperdynamic CSF flow.

phenomenon, resulting from the pulsatile motion of CSF back and forth through the ventricular system during the cardiac cycle.[17] In the normal patient, there is space over the cerebral convexities occupied by the cortical veins and the CSF in the subarachnoid space (Fig. 50–4). When the brain expands during systole, it expands outwardly, compressing the cortical veins (leading to subsequent venous outflow), and it expands inwardly, compressing the lateral ventricles (leading to outflow of CSF through the aqueduct, which produces the normal flow void).[16] In EVOH, the brain has already expanded against the inner table of the calvaria, so that further outward expansion is not possible. Thus, during systole, all cerebral expansion is directed inward, compressing the lateral and third ventricles, leading to increased outflow of CSF through the aqueduct. This situation is the cause for the increased CSF flow void[10] in patients with EVOH and normal cerebral blood flow (Fig. 50–4). When the blood supply to the brain decreases because of atrophy, the main force behind the CSF pump decreases, and the CSF flow void is consequently also reduced.

In one study, there was a significant correlation between an increased CSF flow void (i.e., one extending from the third ventricle through the obex of the fourth

ventricle) and a successful response to ventriculoperitoneal shunting.[10] Patients with clinical NPH who did *not* have a hyperdynamic flow void failed to respond to shunting. This association was significant at the $P < .003$ level.[16] Thus, in the setting of an appropriate clinical triad for NPH and ventricular enlargement out of proportion to cortical sulcal dilatation, the presence of an increased aqueductal CSF flow void on MRI should prompt the neurosurgeon to perform a ventriculoperitoneal shunt. Younger patients with EVOH and normal cerebral blood flow may also have hyperdynamic CSF flow. Thus, the sign is not specific for NPH.

Because NPH is a disease of elderly patients, it appears that symptoms result from a *combined* insult related both to the ventricular enlargement (and *barotrauma* of the waterhammer pulse) and to the decreased perfusion of the periventricular region (i.e., the same process that leads to deep white matter ischemia and infarction).[18] It was originally postulated by Hakim that tangential shearing forces involving the periventricular (corona radiata) fibers led initially to the gait disturbance. Later, with continued ventricular enlargement, it was hypothesized that radial shearing forces involving the cortical gray matter led to the dementia. More recently, it has been postulated that the symptoms identified clinically in NPH may be secondary to impingement of the corpus callosum by the falx cerebri rather than resulting from ventricular dilatation.[7, 19]

COMPUTED TOMOGRAPHY AND MAGNETIC RESONANCE IMAGING

The CT and MRI findings in cases of hydrocephalus depend on the type of disorder (i.e., IVOH or EVOH), the length of time that the hydrocephalus has been present, and the age of the patient. In most cases of IVOH, the ventricular system is symmetrically dilated above the level of the obstruction and of normal size below the obstruction. The location of the obstruction in IVOH may be at any point within the lateral ventricles down to and including the foramina of Magendie and Luschka of the fourth ventricle. In general, MRI is superior to CT for localizing the exact level of obstruction and for identifying small obstructing pathology.

In acute EVOH, there is typically an initial enlargement of the temporal horns and the third ventricle followed by the lateral ventricles. There may be a marked delay before the fourth ventricle is seen to increase in size. It has been postulated that the early increase in size of the temporal horns and third ventricle is because of the smaller amount of white matter confining these structures compared with the remainder of the ventricular system. As the lateral ventricles increase in size, there is a corresponding decrease in the size of the cortical sulci, and in some instances, the basal cisterns may also become compressed. Subsequently, there is an increase in transependymal flow of CSF corresponding to increased intraventricular pressure in most cases. This transependymal flow of CSF is seen as a thick, irregular periventricular rim of decreased density on CT and as decreased signal on T1-weighted MRI in acute hydrocephalus. This periventricular rim of signal change is much easier to detect on proton-density and T2-weighted sequences and is best seen on fluid attenuated inversion recovery (FLAIR) imaging (Fig. 50–5). A thin rim may be seen in pediatric cases of IVOH or EVOH, but a thin rim of periventricular signal can normally be seen in older adult patients. A thick, irregular rim of signal is often indicative of acute hydrocephalus in adults, whereas a thinner rim may reflect a more chronic condition, such as NPH.[7, 20, 21]

MAGNETIC RESONANCE IMAGING TECHNIQUES USED TO MEASURE CEREBROSPINAL FLUID FLOW

A number of MRI observations and techniques have been employed to take advantage of signal changes associated with CSF flow. The aqueductal CSF flow void (see Fig. 50–1) noted on routine MRI images was the first indication of CSF motion.[13, 14] Subsequently, the CSF flow void was shown to be related to the cardiac cycle.[22] Although a CSF flow void may be appreciated on routine spin-echo and gradient-echo MRI images, the degree of signal loss is not consistent, and it does not change in a linear fashion with velocity.[1] Thus, by using the CSF flow void sign

alone, it may be difficult to appreciate when CSF flow is mildly abnormal. CSF flow void may not be visualized at all in areas where it is normally expected (e.g., the aqueduct); however, inferences can be made concerning obstruction.[14] Axial, single-slice, gradient-echo techniques that maximize flow-related enhancement[15] (entry phenomenon) have also been used[23] to evaluate aqueductal patency. The best observations of CSF flow, however, have been obtained using dedicated techniques, gated to the cardiac cycle.

In 1985, Feinberg and colleagues[24, 25] used MRI *velocity density imaging* to measure the velocity of CSF through the aqueduct as a function of the cardiac cycle. Subsequently, Edelman and associates[26] used saturation pulses and bolus tracking techniques , whereas Axel and Dougherty[22] used spatial modulation of magnetization (SPAMM) to measure CSF velocity. Today, most investigators use the phase contrast techniques.[27–29]

The phase contrast CSF velocity imaging techniques[27, 29] can be divided on the basis of the form of cardiac gating used (i.e., prospective or retrospective)[30] and on the basis of background phase determination.[31] Most investigators[27, 28] determine the background phase from an additional acquisition. This approach necessitates obtaining two interleaved acquisitions and then subtracting them. Others make the assumption of zero net flow[29] over the cardiac cycle and calculate the background phase (which entails a single acquisition in half the time).

The relationship between the phase shift θ and velocity v is given by the equation

$$\theta = \gamma \int_0^t G\,(t)vt\,dt$$

where θ is the phase shift, γ is the gyromagnetic ratio, $G(t)$ is the gradient strength as a function of time t, v is velocity, and t is the elapsed time.[32] Thus, for an appropriate gradient pulse of strength G and duration t, a linear relationship should exist between the phase shift (from 0 to ±180 degrees, depending on the direction of flow) and the CSF velocity. A new parameter, the V_{enc}, is the aliasing or *encoding* velocity, which leads to a 180-degree phase shift for flow in either direction.

There are two ways to do cardiac gating—prospectively and retrospectively. Prospective cardiac gating is most commonly used and is also called *electrocardiogram (ECG) triggering* (although this method also includes triggering from a finger plethysmograph). With prospective cardiac gating, acquisition starts as a predetermined time interval after the R wave and continues at approximately 50- to 75-msec intervals to within about 200 msec of the next R wave (to allow for respiratory variation).[27] The R wave can be determined electrically (from the ECG) or mechanically (from the finger plethysmograph). Because there is no sampling of CSF motion during the final 100 or 200 msec of the R-R interval (when flow is in a rostral or retrograde direction), there appears to be a large net flow of CSF in the systolic direction (i.e., craniocaudal) over this partially sampled cardiac cycle.[29]

With retrospective cardiac gating (Siemens) or *cine–phase contrast (PC)* (GE),[30] the computer keeps track of the R wave (defined electrically or mechanically), and data are acquired throughout the cardiac cycle, then ret-

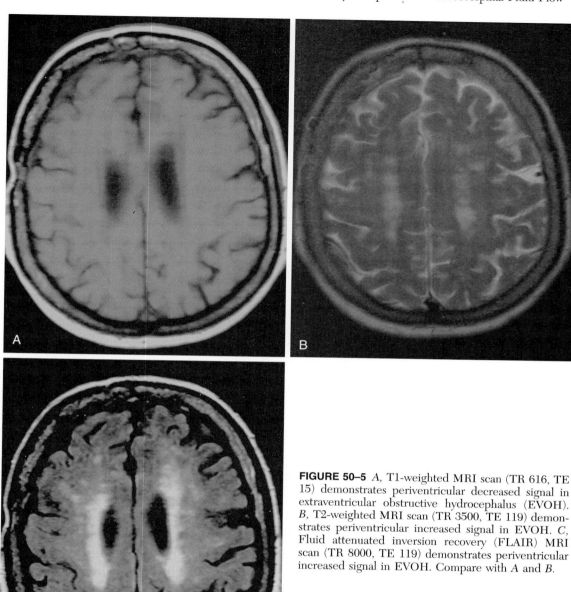

FIGURE 50–5 *A,* T1-weighted MRI scan (TR 616, TE 15) demonstrates periventricular decreased signal in extraventricular obstructive hydrocephalus (EVOH). *B,* T2-weighted MRI scan (TR 3500, TE 119) demonstrates periventricular increased signal in EVOH. *C,* Fluid attenuated inversion recovery (FLAIR) MRI scan (TR 8000, TE 119) demonstrates periventricular increased signal in EVOH. Compare with *A* and *B.*

rospectively *binned* into a predetermined number of cine frames.[30] The entire cardiac cycle is sampled; therefore, there is no time for eddy currents to build up, as they do during the 200-msec dead time when prospective cardiac gating is used.[29]

Two retrospective cardiac gating techniques are routinely used:[29] (1) a *routine resolution* sagittal acquisition in the midline (Fig. 50–6) and (2) a *high-resolution* angled axial acquisition through the aqueduct (Fig. 50–7). In the sagittal technique, a 4-mm slice is acquired in the midsagittal plane (Fig. 50–6) with velocity sensitization

along the readout axis, which is also the craniocaudal axis of the patient. It is better to perform cardiac gating with ECG leads rather than using finger plethysmography because the systolic motion of the brain may actually precede the systolic pulse in the finger.[29] The basic MRI technique is a flow-compensated, two-dimensional fast imaging with steady-state precision (FISP) (on Siemens) or a two-dimensional gradient-recalled acquisition in the steady state (GRASS)—with cine-PC (on GE) with a TR of 70 msec, a TE of 13 msec, and a 15-degree flip angle (Fig. 50–6). A 192 × 256 matrix is acquired over a 25-

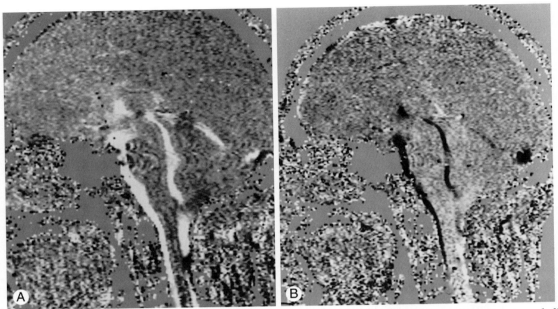

FIGURE 50–6 Sagittal phase contrast technique. *A,* During systole, cerebrospinal fluid (CSF) flow is down (craniocaudad), indicated by shades of *white. B,* During diastole, CSF flow is up (caudocraniad), indicated by shades of *black.* By placing a cursor over any point in the image, the velocity can be obtained as a function of the cardiac cycle.

cm field-of-view, providing in-plane spatial resolution of approximately 1 mm. The aliasing velocity is set to 100 mm/sec. Such images are routinely used in the head to document midsagittal CSF flow. Using a single excitation and taking 32 acquisitions before advancing the phase, this technique takes about 7 minutes. When a computer cursor is placed over any point on the phase contrast velocity image on the monitor, craniocaudal CSF velocities can be measured and plotted versus the phase of the cardiac cycle. This allows comparison of phase relationships of CSF motion at different points in the midline ventricular system, basal cisterns, and cervical subarachnoid space (Fig. 50–6).[29]

The measured velocity through the aqueduct on this sagittal acquisition also includes the stationary tissue in the midbrain on either side of the aqueduct in a 4-mm-thick slice. Therefore, the measured velocity is artifactually reduced because of partial volume effects.[29] To circumvent these effects, a high-resolution axial technique was developed.[29] In this technique, an angled axial slice is positioned perpendicular to the aqueduct so that it is viewed en face, without inclusion of adjacent stationary tissue (see Fig. 50–7). Velocity sensitization is provided by the slice-select gradient (i.e., for through-plane flow). A 512 × 512 matrix (half Fourier with 16 lines of oversampling) is used over a 16-cm field-of-view, provid-

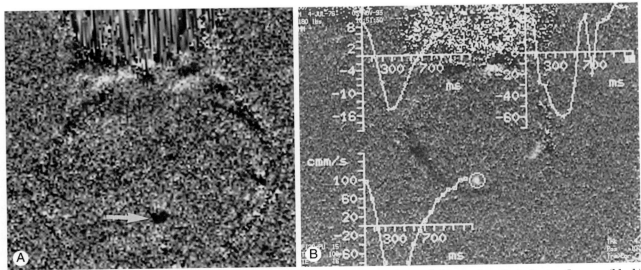

FIGURE 50–7 Axial phase contrast technique. *A,* High-resolution axial image obtained during diastole indicates flow up *(black)* in the aqueduct *(arrow). B,* During systole, flow is down *(white)* inside region of interest. The mean velocity *(left upper),* peak velocity *(right upper),* and volumetric flow rates *(left lower)* through the aqueduct are shown as a function of the cardiac cycle.

ing 0.3-mm pixels. Thirty such pixels can be placed in an average 2-mm diameter aqueduct. Similar to the sagittal technique, this is a modified two-dimensional FISP/GRASS technique with a 15-degree flip angle, a TR of 100 msec, and a TE of 16 msec. With a single excitation and 32 acquisitions per phase step, the process takes about 14 minutes.[29] An aliasing velocity of 200 mm/sec is routinely used. Integrating the volumetric flow rate over either the systolic or the diastolic phase of the cardiac cycle, an aqueductal CSF *stroke volume* can be calculated.[29] Using a pulsatile flow phantom, velocity and volumetric flow measurements have been validated.[33]

NORMAL CEREBROSPINAL FLUID FLOW IN THE BRAIN

In normals, the maximal downward wave of CSF movement through the aqueduct occurs 175 to 200 msec after the R wave; however, it is usually preceded by CSF flow out of the fourth ventricle through the foramen of Magendie.[28] Mixing occurs in the mid-fourth ventricle, resulting in turbulence.[29] Midway through the cardiac cycle, a diastolic cephalad (retrograde) wave of CSF can be seen rising through the aqueduct.[28] Variable degrees of CSF flow within the posterior third ventricle are observed; occasionally, flow at the level of the foramen of Monro is also seen in normals. Flow is less often observed in the lateral ventricles, however, because of the larger diameters involved. As a result of volume changes in the brain over the cardiac cycle, CSF also flows to-and-fro in the basal cisterns.[29]

Flow out of the inferior portion of the fourth ventricle through the foramen of Magendie is not simply a continuation of the flow coming down from the aqueduct. Such asynchrony may result from pulsations of the choroid plexus of the fourth ventricle.[28] In fact, the caudally directed CSF pulse wave is observed to start first in the fourth ventricle, followed approximately 100 msec later by caudal flow in the aqueduct.[28] Cranial flow of CSF back through the aqueduct may still be occurring when the first downward motion through the foramen of Ma-

gendie is seen. Clearly, therefore, this cephalad aqueductal CSF flow is not simply the result of retrograde flow from the basal cisterns into the fourth ventricle and upward.[28] The probable reasons for these normal variations are multiple but relate most likely to the size of the nearby vascular structures, the compliance of surrounding brain and spinal cord, the anatomy of the CSF spaces, the volume and vascularity of the choroid plexus, and the resulting systematic hydrodynamics.[28]

ABNORMAL CEREBROSPINAL FLUID FLOW IN THE BRAIN

Using phase contrast CSF velocity imaging, the hyperdynamic CSF flow of NPH (Fig. 50–8) can be distinguished from normal flow or from the decreased flow of atrophy. The high-resolution axial technique provides a reliable, quantitative measurement of the aqueductal CSF stroke volume. In a study of 18 patients with clinically suspected NPH, 12 were found to have hyperdynamic CSF flow (i.e., stroke volumes > 42 μl), whereas 6 were found to have hypodynamic flow.[34] All 12 of the patients with hyperdynamic flow responded favorably to ventriculoperitoneal shunting. Thus, in this series, this technique had a positive predictive value of 100%. Of the 6 patients who had stroke volumes less than or equal to 42 μl, 3 responded to shunting and 3 did not, probably reflecting the presence of concomitant atrophy in these patients. Of the 12 patients with hyperdynamic flow (as determined by the measured stroke volume), only 6 (50%) had hyperdynamic CSF flow voids on their routine MRI images. This finding most likely reflects the current widespread use of first-order flow compensation on the proton-density–weighted images, which was not available when the earlier study was performed.[16] Thus, quantitative CSF velocity imaging is an even better technique than routine MRI to determine the presence of *shunt-responsive* NPH.

CSF velocity imaging is also useful in the evaluation of potential shunt malfunction.[35] In patients who have been shunted for communicating hydrocephalus, the nor-

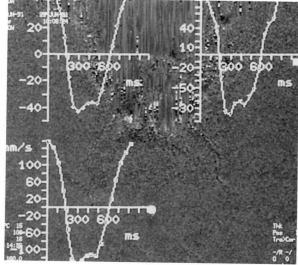

FIGURE 50–8 NPH. In this 78-year-old man with clinical NPH, hyperdynamic flow is demonstrated through the aqueduct.

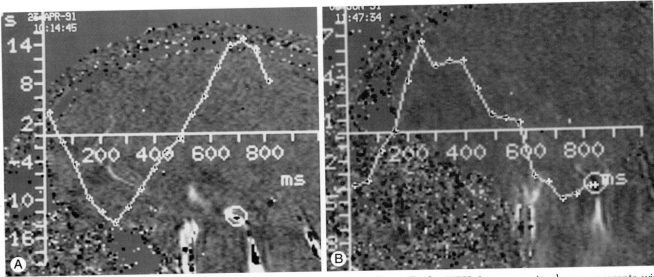

FIGURE 50–9 Shunt malfunction in NPH. *A,* A 73-year-old-man shunted initially for NPH 1 year previously now presents with recurrent symptoms and *normal* flow pattern through the aqueduct. *B,* Two months later, when the shunt has been revised and the patient is again asymptomatic, the cerebrospinal fluid flow pattern through the aqueduct is reversed (as expected with normal shunt function).

mal pattern of CSF flow through the aqueduct is exactly 180 degrees out of phase with what is normal with respect to the cardiac cycle (i.e., CSF flows caudocraniad during systole and craniocaudad during diastole) (Fig. 50–9). This finding probably reflects the fact that the shunt tube is the lowest resistance pathway to outflow of CSF after systolic expansion of both the cerebrum and the cerebellum. (The phase relationship between CSF flow and the cardiac cycle depends on how the R wave is acquired. Because the R wave reaches the finger approximately 400 msec after electrical systole, the use of finger plethysmography may give the false appearance of expected flow reversal through the aqueduct when the shunt is, in fact, nonfunctional.)

In patients with either IVOH or EVOH hydrocephalus, the high-resolution axial technique can also be used to assess flow through the shunt tube itself (Fig. 50–10). In cases of normal shunt function, CSF motion tends to be intermittent and unidirectional, rather than sinusoidal (as is normally seen through the aqueduct), reflecting the presence of the one-way valve.

Because the plane and position of both CSF velocity imaging techniques can be modified, they can also be used to distinguish cysts from enlarged CSF spaces. Within the cyst, the motion of CSF appears to rebound against the flowing CSF around it. This *cyst rebound sign*[36] is the finding of decreased CSF velocity (within the cyst) 90 degrees phase-advanced relative to the motion of the surrounding CSF (Fig. 50–11).

SLIT VENTRICLE SYNDROME

The *slit ventricle syndrome* (SVS) is a potential complication from extracranial ventricular shunt placement for hydrocephalus. SVS has been noted to be accompanied by a clinical triad of (1) chronic intermittent headache,

(2) slowly refilling shunt reservoir, and (3) markedly decreased ventricular size, the so-called slit ventricles.[37–40] The symptom complex associated with SVS is believed to result from a combination of intracranial hypotension and hypertension that is related to the ventricular shunt system.

SVS is theorized to result from a series of ventricular shunt–related dynamics that begins with excessive siphoning of CSF through the shunt system, resulting in an initial episode of intracranial hypotension. This episode allows the walls of the ventricles to collapse around the proximal end of the shunt system, causing shunt obstruction. The result of the obstructed shunt is an increase in intracranial pressure. Such intermittent ventricular shunt malfunction creates the development of an abnormally elastic brain. This condition is particularly sensitive to the intermittent intracranial pressure spikes that accompany SVS, so that the patients become increasingly symptomatic.[37, 38, 41–44]

It is important to recognize SVS on neuroimaging procedures because the treatment is often different for patients with SVS than those with other shunt-related disorders (Fig. 50–12).[37, 38, 42, 45–49] The management of SVS is frequently difficult and often requires removal of the shunt system.[37, 38, 41, 42, 46, 48] The neuroimaging study plays an essential role in establishing the diagnosis of SVS.

CONCLUSIONS

Overall, MRI is superior to CT in the evaluation of hydrocephalus. Not only can MRI assist in locating the anatomic position of a possible obstructing lesion in cases of IVOH, but also in many cases it may be able to evaluate CSF flow dynamics. The addition of newer MRI techniques to measure CSF flow can now assist in determining the diagnosis of conditions such as NPH and

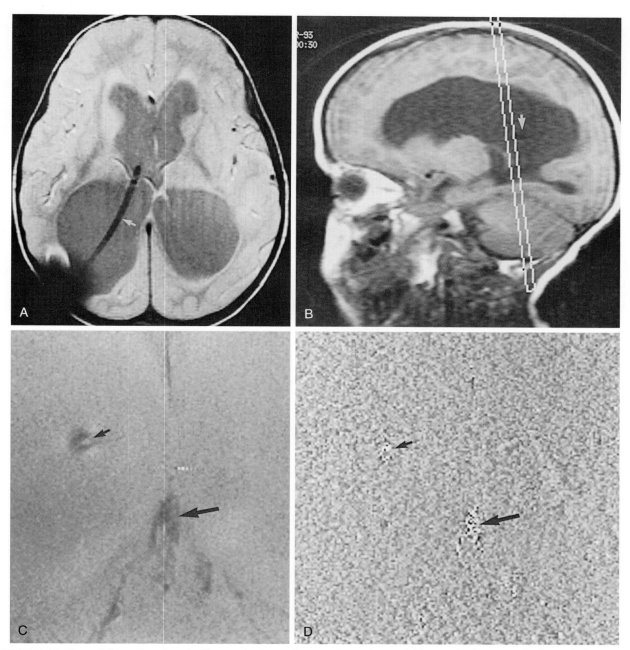

FIGURE 50–10 Normal shunt function. *A,* Shunt tube *(arrow)* is noted in a 2-year-old boy with obstructive hydrocephalus. *B,* Right parasagittal section demonstrates position of high-resolution acquisition plane perpendicular to dark shunt tube *(arrow)*. *C, Magnitude* image from high-resolution coronal acquisition, angled perpendicular to shunt tube *(small arrow)*, also demonstrates quadrigeminal plate cistern *(large arrow)*. *D,* Phase contrast image again demonstrates quadrigeminal plate cistern *(large arrow)* and high signal intensity *(small arrow)* in shunt, corresponding to forward flow.

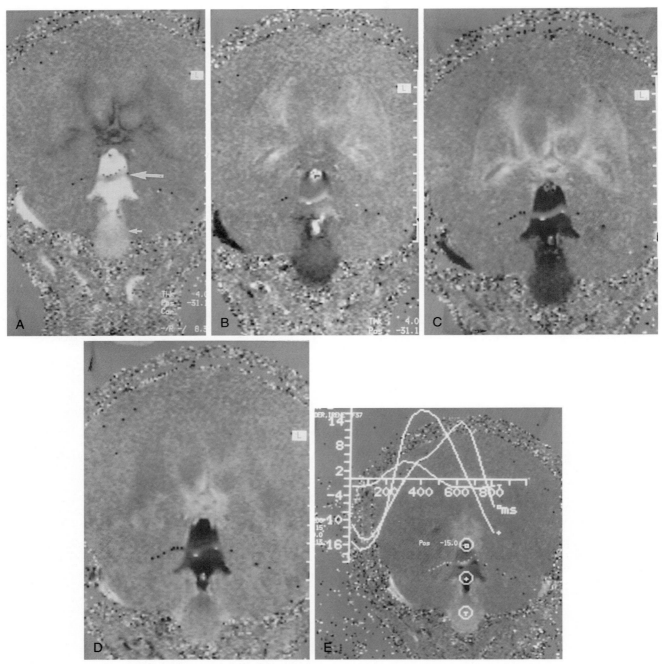

FIGURE 50–11 *Rebound sign* in arachnoid cyst. *A,* The qualitative (sagittal) technique has been rotated into the coronal plane with velocity encoding along the craniocaudal readout axis. White is flow down, and black is flow up. (No flow is gray.) During systole, flow in the fourth ventricle *(large arrow)* is down, whereas flow in the arachnoid cyst *(small arrow)* has stopped because of maximal deformation by the surrounding cerebrospinal fluid. *B,* 200 msec later, flow in the fourth ventricle has stopped (turning gray), whereas flow in the cyst has already started heading up (turning black). *C,* 200 msec later, flow in both the cyst and the fourth ventricle are up. *D,* 100 msec later, the cyst has become maximally deformed and has stopped flowing (turning gray), whereas flow continues in the caudocraniad direction in the fourth ventricle. *E,* By placing cursors on the fourth ventricle and the cyst, motion in the cyst is seen to be of lower amplitude and 90 degrees phase-advanced relative to flow within the fourth ventricle.

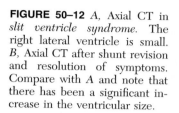
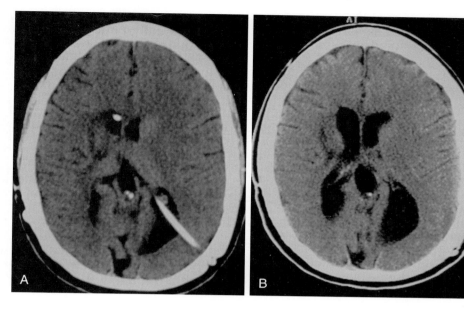

FIGURE 50–12 *A*, Axial CT in *slit ventricle syndrome*. The right lateral ventricle is small. *B*, Axial CT after shunt revision and resolution of symptoms. Compare with *A* and note that there has been a significant increase in the ventricular size.

may provide important information regarding the probable response to shunting procedures. In the neuroimaging of hydrocephalus, it is important to remember that the goal of the procedure is to determine the exact nature of the obstruction and to help determine the most appropriate mode of therapeutic intervention.

References

1. Bradley WG, Quencer RM. Hydrocephalus and CSF flow. In Stark DD, Bradley WG (eds). Magnetic Resonance Imaging, 3rd ed. St. Louis, Mosby–Year Book, 1999.
2. Orrison WW Jr. Introduction to Neuroimaging. Boston, Little, Brown, 1989.
3. Mettler FA, Guiberteau MJ. Essentials of Nuclear Medicine Imaging, 2nd ed. Orlando, FL, Grune & Stratton, 1986.
4. Harwood-Nash DC, Fitz CR. Neuroradiology in Infants and Children. St. Louis, CV Mosby, 1976.
5. Osborn AG. Diagnostic Neuroradiology. St. Louis, Mosby–Year Book, 1994.
6. Escourolle R, Poirier J, Bruinstein LJ. Manual of Basic Neuropathology. Philadelphia, WB Saunders, 1971.
7. Slager UT. Basic Neuropathology. Baltimore, Williams & Wilkins, 1970.
8. Hakim S. Some observations on CSF pressure: Hydrocephalic syndrome in adults with "normal" CSF pressure. Thesis No 957. Bogota, Colombia, Javerian University, School of Medicine, 1964.
9. Adams RD, Fisher CM, Hakim S, et al. Symptomatic occult hydrocephalus with "normal" cerebrospinal fluid pressure: A treatable syndrome. N Engl J Med 1965;273:117–126.
10. Hakim S, Venegas JG, Burton JD. The physics of the cranial cavity hydrocephalus and normal pressure hydrocephalus: Mechanical interpretation and mathematical role. Surg Neurol 1970;5:187–209.
11. Ekstedt J, Friden H. CSF hydrodynamics of the study of the adult hydrocephalus syndrome. In Shapiro K, Marmarou A, Portnoy H (eds). Hydrocephalus. New York, Raven, 1984.
12. Foltz EL. Hydrocephalus and CSF pulsatility: Clinical and laboratory studies. In Shapiro K, Marmarou A, Portnoy H (eds). Hydrocephalus. New York, Raven, 1984.
13. Bradley WG, Kortman KE, Burgoyne B. Flowing cerebrospinal fluid in normal and hydrocephalic states: Appearance on MRI images. Radiology 1986;159:611–616.
14. Sherman JL, Citrin CM. Magnetic resonance demonstration of normal CSF flow. AJNR 1986;7:3–6.
15. Bradley WG, Waluch V. Blood flow: Magnetic resonance imaging. Radiology 1985;154:443–450.
16. Bradley WG, Whittemore AR, Kortman KE, et al. Marked cerebrospinal fluid void: Indicator of successful shunt in patients with suspected normal pressure hydrocephalus. Radiology 1991;178:459–466.
17. DuBoulay GH. Pulsatile movements in the CSF pathways. Br J Radiol 1966;39:255–262.
18. Bradley WG, Whittemore AR, Watanabe AS, et al. Association of deep white matter infarction with chronic communicating hydrocephalus: Implications regarding the possible origin of normal pressure hydrocephalus. AJNR 1991;12:31–39.
19. Xiong G, Rauch RA, Hagino N, Jinkins JR. An animal model of corpus callosum impingement as seen in patients with normal pressure hydrocephalus. Invest Radiol 1993;28:46–50.
20. Cronqvist S. Hydrocephalus and atrophy. Riv di Neuroradiol 1990;3(suppl 2):25–28.
21. Gean AD. Imaging of Head Trauma. New York, Raven, 1994.
22. Axel L, Dougherty L. MR imaging of motion with spatial modulation of magnetization. Radiology 1989;171:841.
23. Atlas SW, Mark AS, Fram EK. Aqueductal stenosis: Evaluation with gradient-echo rapid MR imaging. Radiology 1988;169:449–456.
24. Feinberg DA, Crooks LE, Sheldon P, et al. Magnetic resonance imaging in the velocity vector components of fluid flow. Magn Reson Med 1985;2:555–556.
25. Feinberg DA, Mark AS. Human brain motion and cerebrospinal fluid circulation demonstrated with MRI velocity imaging. Radiology 1985;154:443–450.
26. Edelman RR, Mattle HP, Kleefield J, Silver MS. Quantification of blood flow with dynamic MRI imaging and presaturation bolus tracking. Radiology 1989;171:551–556.
27. Quencer RM, Donovan Post MJ, Hinks RS. Cine MRI in the evaluation of normal and abnormal CSF flow: Intracranial and intraspinal studies. Neuroradiology 1990;32:371–391.
28. Enzmann DR, Pelc NJ. Normal flow patterns of intracranial and spinal cerebrospinal fluid defined by phase-contrast cine MR imaging. Radiology 1991;178:467–747.
29. Nitz WR, Bradley WG Jr, Watanabe AS, et al. Flow dynamics of CSF: Assessment with phase contrast velocity MRI imaging performed with retrospective cardiac gating. Radiology 1992;8:676–681.
30. Spraggins TA. "Wireless retrospective gating" application to cine cardiac imaging. Magn Reson Med 1990;8:676–681.
31. Firmin DN, Nayler GL, Kilner PJ, Longmore DB. The application of phase shifts in NMR for flow measurement. Magn Reson Med 1990;14:230–241.
32. Moran PR. A flow velocity zeugmatographic interface for NMR imaging of humans. Magn Reson Imaging 1982;1:197–203.
33. Mullin WJ, Atkinson D, Hashemi R, et al. Cerebrospinal fluid flow quantitation: Pulsatile flow phantom comparison of three measurement methods. J Magn Reson Imaging 1993;3:55.
34. Bradley WG, Scalzo D, Queralt J, et al. Normal pressure hydrocephalus: Evaluation with cerebrospinal fluid flow measurements at MR imaging. Radiology 1996;198:523–529.

35. Bradley WG, Atkinson D, Chen D-Y, et al. Evaluation of ventriculoperitoneal shunt status with cerebrospinal fluid velocity imaging. Radiology 1993;189:223.
36. Herbst MD, Bradley WG, Nitz WR, et al. Reproduction of the arachnoid cyst rebound sign in a cerebrospinal fluid flow phantom. Radiology 1991;181:287.
37. Baskin JJ, Manwaring KH, Rekate HL. Ventricular shunt removal: The ultimate treatment of the slit ventricle syndrome. J Neurosurg 1998;88:478–484.
38. Holness RO, Hoffman HJ, Hendrick EB. Subtemporal decompression for the slit-ventricle syndrome after shunting in hydrocephalic children. Child Brain 1979;5:137–144.
39. Hyde-Rowan MD, Rekate HL, Nulsen FE. Re-expansion of previously collapsed ventricles: The slit ventricle syndrome. J Neurosurg 1982;56:536–539.
40. Rekate HL. Classification of slit-ventricle syndromes using intracranial pressure monitoring. Pediatr Neurosurg 1993;19:15–20.
41. Becker DP, Nulsen FE. Control of hydrocephalus by valve-regulated venous shunt: Avoidance of complications in prolonged shunt maintenance. J Neurosurg 1968;28:215–226.
42. Benzel EC, Reeves JD, Kesterson L, et al. Slit ventricle syndrome in children: Clinical presentation and treatment. Acta Neurochir 1992;117:7–14.
43. Walker ML, Fried A, Petronio J. Diagnosis and treatment of the slit ventricle syndrome. Neurosurg Clin North Am 1993;4:707–714.
44. Wisoff JH, Epstein FJ. Diagnosis and treatment of the slit ventricle syndrome. In Scott RM (ed). Hydrocephalus Concepts in Neurosurgery, Vol. 3, pp. 79–85. Baltimore, Williams & Wilkins, 1990.
45. Abbott R, Epstein FJ, Wisoff JH. Chronic headache associated with a functioning shunt: Usefulness of pressure monitoring. Neurosurgery 1991;28:72–77.
46. Baskin JJ, Manwaring KH. Endoscopic third ventriculostomy for obstructive hydrocephalus. In Rengachary SS, Wlkins RH (eds). Neurosurgical Operative Atlas, Vol. 1, 2nd ed., pp. 241–246. Park Ridge, IL, American Association of Neurological Surgeons, 1996.
47. Baskin JJ, Manwaring KH. Intraventricular endoscopy: Diagnostic ventriculoscopy, tissue biopsy, cyst fenestration, and shunting. In Rengachary SS, Wilkins RH (eds). Neurosurgical Operative Atlas, Vol. 1, 2nd ed., pp. 85–98. Park Ridge, IL, American Association of Neurological Surgeons, 1996.
48. Epstein F, Lapras C, Wisoff JH. Slit ventricle syndrome: Etiology and treatment. Pediatr Neurosci 1998;14:5–10.
49. Fouyas IP, Casey ATH, Thompson D, et al. Use of intracranial pressure monitoring in the management of childhood hydrocephalus and shunt-related problems. Neurosurgery 1996;38:726–732.

51

Neurocutaneous Syndromes

BLAINE L. HART, M.D.

MARK H. DEPPER, M.D.

CAROL L. CLERICUZIO, M.D.

Neurocutaneous syndromes are a diverse group of diseases that involve both skin and nervous systems. Other organs, especially the eyes but also the visceral organs, are also often involved. Despite being grouped together by tradition and for convenience in discussion, most of these diseases are unrelated to one another in cause or major clinical manifestations. Considerable progress has been made regarding the genetic basis of the most common of these conditions, and greater understanding of these diseases can be expected with further investigation. Several syndromes are of special interest because of autosomal dominant inheritance, a high rate of spontaneous mutation, and diverse clinical manifestations.

The term *phakomatoses* has often been applied to these syndromes. The term was first used by Van der Hoeve[1, 2] for tuberous sclerosis (TS) and neurofibromatosis (NF). He later included von Hippel–Lindau disease and Sturge-Weber syndrome in this classification.[3, 4] *Phakoma* is derived from Greek *phakos*, for lens or eye, although other suggested derivations have referred to *freckle* or *spot*. Although the word has been used as a general term for hamartomas and skin lesions found in the phakomatoses, it is also used specifically to refer to the retinal hamartoma that occurs commonly in TS.[5] Retinal lesions superficially similar to the phakoma of TS but consisting of myelinated patches of retinal nerve fibers occur in NF-1.

The most common neurocutaneous syndromes are NF-1 and TS. NF-2, von Hippel–Lindau disease, and Sturge-Weber syndrome are much less common but are also among the generally recognized neurocutaneous syndromes. All but Sturge-Weber syndrome are of autosomal dominant inheritance. In addition to these five conditions, several other rare conditions are notable for both cutaneous and central nervous system (CNS) manifestations. Many of these are autosomal recessive genetic conditions. These also may conveniently be considered neurocutaneous syndromes.

NEUROFIBROMATOSIS

The description of cutaneous tumors of NF dates to at least 1793, when Tilesius used the term *molluscum fibrosum*.[6, 7] Although common features, such as café au lait macules and neurofibromas, are easily recognized, the clinical expression of NF is highly variable. Because of the great variability in clinical manifestations, the existence of two distinct subtypes of NF was difficult to recognize. In fact, the genetic basis and natural history of each subtype is quite different. A National Institutes of Health (NIH) consensus development conference in 1987[8] established diagnostic criteria and terminology for these two conditions. Additional review of these criteria in 1997 resulted in no changes for criteria for NF-1 but minor modifications for NF-2.[9] Variants of neurofibromatosis were also reviewed in this collaborative effort by the National Neurofibromatosis Foundation Clinical Care Advisory Board.

Neurofibromatosis Type 1

Von Recklinghausen[10] in 1882 described the syndrome that subsequently received his name. *Von Recklinghausen's neurofibromatosis* is now known as NF-1. It is among the more common of the well-defined human genetic syndromes and also has a high incidence of spontaneous mutation. Particularly common features are cutaneous café au lait spots; neurofibromas, including plexiform neurofibromas; hamartomas of the iris (Lisch nodules); and abnormalities of the CNS, including white matter and deep gray matter signal abnormality on magnetic resonance imaging (MRI), optic pathway gliomas, and astrocytomas. A wide range of other clinical features can occur and are highly variable in expression.[11]

Genetics

The NF-1 gene on chromosome 17q was cloned in 1990 (band 11.2)[12, 13] and its protein product termed *neurofibromin*. The prevalence in the population is about 1 in 4000. The inheritance is autosomal dominant with high penetrance and variable expression. There is a high incidence of spontaneous mutation, about 50%;[14] that is, about half of NF-1 cases are thought to be due to spontaneous mutations.

NF-1 involves both neoplastic and dysplastic conditions. The nervous system, both CNS and neural crest origin peripheral system, displays dysplastic as well as neoplastic manifestations. Tissues of mesodermal origin, however, have dysplastic but not neoplastic features in NF-1.

Diagnostic Criteria

Diagnostic criteria were established at the NIH Consensus Development Conference and are listed in Table 51–1.[8] No changes were recommended in the 1997 review of NF-1 and NF-2.[9] The criteria are entirely clinical and depend on family history and physical findings. Molecular diagnostic evaluation of NF-1 is not widely available, owing to the high number of identified mutations of the large NF-1 gene. The various CNS abnormalities that are demonstrable by imaging techniques are not included in these formal criteria, although they lend additional support to a suspected diagnosis of NF-1.

Clinical Findings and Natural History

Café au lait spots are light brown macules that begin to appear early, often in the first year of life. They are not specific to NF-1. One or two such macules are common, sporadic, normal findings in the general population. Café au lait spots can also occur in McCune-Albright syndrome. Multiple such spots often occur in NF-1, however. Six or more café au lait spots greater than 5 mm in diameter before puberty or 15 mm after puberty constitute one of the diagnostic criteria for NF-1. Intertriginous freckling occurs in many patients, most commonly in axillary and inguinal regions, but also in inframammary locations and other areas where there are apposing skin surfaces.[15–17]

Neurofibromas are tumors that consist of intermixed neurons, Schwann cells, fibroblasts, mast cells, and vascular elements. They generally become apparent around the time of puberty, but they may increase in number throughout life. They occur in the skin and deeper nerves.

Plexiform neurofibromas are unencapsulated, tortuous, often fusiform masses that consist of Schwann cells, neurons, and collagen with intercellular matrix. They are congenital in origin. They are often locally aggressive, extending along the nerve of origin and causing mass effect.[18] Plexiform neurofibromas constitute one of the

TABLE 51–1 Diagnostic Criteria for Neurofibromatosis Type 1 (Von Recklinghausen)

≥2 of the following are present:
  ≥6 café au lait macules with greatest diameter >5 mm in prepubertal patients and >15 mm in postpubertal patients
  ≥2 neurofibromas of any type or 1 plexiform neurofibroma
  Freckling in axillary or inguinal region
  Optic glioma
  ≥2 Lisch nodules (iris hamartomas)
  A distinctive osseous lesion, such as sphenoid dysplasia or thinning of long bone cortex, with or without pseudarthrosis
  A parent, sibling, or child with neurofibromatosis 1 according to criteria above

From Neurofibromatosis Conference Statement: National Institutes of Health Consensus Development Conference. Arch Neurol 1988;45:575–578.

identifying features of NF-1 (see Table 51–1) and occur in about one-third of patients.[16] Plexiform neurofibromas can cause significant problems from mass effect. They may be associated with focal gigantism when present in an extremity.[17] Plexiform neurofibromas around the head can extend into the intracranial spaces, especially the orbits. The findings are discussed subsequently.

The *Lisch nodule* is a hamartoma of the iris, best detected with slit-lamp examination. The nodules begin to appear in childhood. Although the NIH criteria specify two or more Lisch nodules as diagnostic, the Lisch nodule is strongly associated with NF-1. Nearly all adults with NF-1 have Lisch nodules.[15, 16, 19]

A variety of skeletal manifestations can accompany NF-1. Hypertrophy of a limb may occur, especially when a plexiform neurofibroma is present. Pseudarthrosis is present in 0.5% to 1% of patients with NF-1; these constitute about half of all cases of congenital pseudarthrosis.[17] The tibia is the most common site, followed by the radius. Kyphoscoliosis requiring surgery occurs in about 5% of patients.[16] Posterior scalloping of the vertebral bodies is occasionally observed.[20] Ribbon-like, overconstricted ribs may accompany the scoliosis. Skull lesions include sphenoid wing dysplasia and lambdoid suture defects and are discussed in greater detail later.

The natural history of NF-1 is highly variable. Clinical manifestations range from minimal to severe. Approximately 8% to 9% of NF-1 patients have been estimated to have severe clinical symptoms and another 15% to have treatable complications.[16] Typical CNS signs or symptoms can result from intracranial masses. Other possible clinical features of this syndrome include developmental delay or learning disabilities; headaches; seizures; and endocrine dysfunction, such as short stature or precocious puberty. Cutaneous conditions may include pruritus and numerous neurofibromas. Limb deformity or kyphoscoliosis can cause complications. Vascular dysplasias can result in stroke or hypertension. Neurofibrosarcomas are an uncommon complication and sometimes arise from plexiform neurofibromas.[9, 21–23] Neurofibrosarcomas may involve the skull or spine as well as other sites.[23]

Optic Gliomas

Gliomas of the optic pathways are well known in NF-1. The incidence of optic gliomas is difficult to assess because of different patient populations and methods of ascertainment. Symptomatic optic pathway gliomas were reported to occur in fewer than 2% of patients in a population-based study,[16] and up to 15% of patients in referral centers are reported to have radiographically identifiable gliomas.[24–27] These are usually low-grade (pilocytic) astrocytomas and occur in childhood. Although they may grow, they are nearly always histologically stable.[28, 29] More aggressive forms can also occur.[30, 31] Spontaneous regression of optic glioma in NF-1 has been reported.[32] Among patients who present with optic glioma, the number with NF-1 has been estimated to range from 25%[33] to 50% among children.[25]

The optic nerves are most commonly involved. Less commonly, the optic chiasm and optic tracts can also be sites of such gliomas.[34] Extension beyond the lateral geniculate bodies into the optic radiations is rare. The

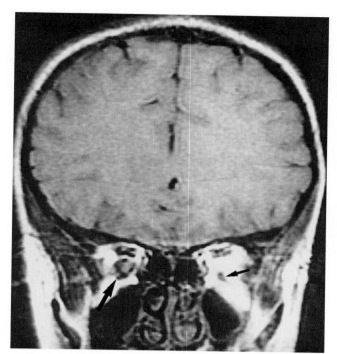

FIGURE 51–1 Optic glioma in a boy with neurofibromatosis type 1 (NF-1). Coronal T1-weighted magnetic resonance imaging (MRI) study demonstrates enlarged right optic nerve (*large arrow*). Compare with normal size of left optic nerve (*small arrow*). (From Hart BL, Benzel EC, Ford CC. Fundamentals of Neuroimaging. Philadelphia, WB Saunders, 1997.)

with optic nerve glioma to have NF-1.[37] Because of the less aggressive nature of most of these gliomas and lack of benefit of early treatment, neuroimaging is not recommended for asymptomatic patients with NF-1.[38] Serial ophthalmologic examination, however, is part of routine NF-1 evaluation; a screening protocol has been recommended by a task force.[38]

Fusiform enlargement of the optic nerves within the orbit can be recognized on computed tomography (CT) or MRI. Bone windows on CT may demonstrate an enlarged optic canal. MRI has the obvious advantage of avoiding exposure of the lens to ionizing radiation. Moreover, MRI is also superior to CT for evaluation of other intracranial abnormalities. Optic nerve gliomas usually appear nearly isointense to brain on short and long TR images (Fig. 51–1). Chiasmal and postchiasmal optic gliomas are more likely to demonstrate low signal intensity on T1-weighted images and higher signal intensity on T2-weighted images. Contrast enhancement is variable, ranging from absent or minimal to intense (Fig. 51–2).[29, 39–42]

A patulous optic nerve sheath is an uncommon manifestation of NF-1 that may be confused with optic glioma.[43] This condition may be indistinguishable from a glioma by CT, but MRI can separate dural ectasia of the nerve sheath from the presence of a solid tumor. Contrast enhancement indicates a solid mass, but not all masses enhance.

Other Glial Tumors

There is also an increased risk of primary brain tumors other than optic glioma in NF-1.[39, 44–50] Astrocytomas occur with increased frequency, especially in the tectum, brain stem, and hypothalamus. Most of these are pilocytic astrocytomas. Fibrillary and other infiltrative subtypes occur less commonly. Ependymoma, ganglioglioma, and

prognosis of gliomas that involve the chiasm is worse than those that involve only the optic nerves.[30, 35, 36] Because chiasmal involvement is less frequent, a patient who presents with chiasmal glioma is less likely than a patient

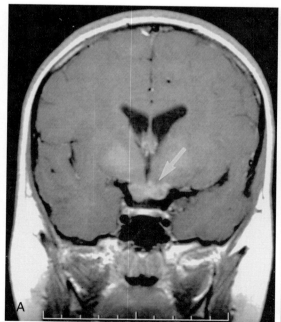
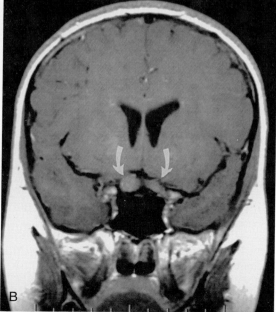

FIGURE 51–2 Chiasmal glioma. *A* and *B*, Coronal postgadolinium T1-weighted MRI studies show enhancing, thickened optic chiasm (*white arrow* in *A*) and prechiasmal optic nerves (*curved arrows* in *B*).

FIGURE 51–3 Astrocytoma in NF-1. *A,* Axial, noncontrasted computed tomography (CT) scan of a girl with NF-1 shows enlarged frontal and temporal horns, deviated third ventricle, and low density in the region of the right thalamus and midbrain (*arrows*). *B,* Axial T2-weighted MRI study demonstrates similar changes in the ventricles. Mixed signal intensity is present within the right thalamic mass. (*A* and *B,* From Hart BL, Benzel EC, Ford CC. Fundamentals of Neuroimaging. Philadelphia, WB Saunders, 1997.)

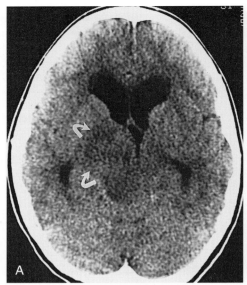
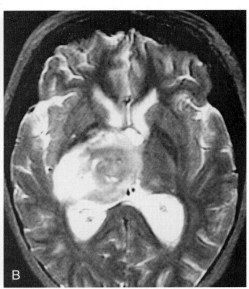

other tumors have been reported in association with NF-1 but are uncommon.[51, 52] Imaging findings of such brain tumors are described in detail elsewhere in this text. MRI is the best modality for detection and evaluation of such tumors (Fig. 51–3). Gadolinium-compound administration is often helpful, but both pilocytic astrocytomas (World Health Organization grade I, with low malignant potential) and high-grade infiltrative astrocytomas (with aggressive nature and poor prognosis) can demonstrate intense enhancement. Low-grade fibrillary astrocytomas often demonstrate little enhancement but have a worse prognosis than pilocytic astrocytomas. A common diagnostic challenge relates to the nonneoplastic areas of signal abnormality that are often detected on cranial MRI of NF-1 patients.

Magnetic Resonance Imaging Bright Areas

The most common MRI finding in the brain in NF-1 consists of multiple bright areas on intermediate-weighted and T2-weighted images.[47, 50, 53–57] These range from punctate to confluent regions greater than 2 cm in diameter. They are seen most often in the pons; cerebellum, especially the peduncles; midbrain; lentiform nucleus; and thalamus (Figs. 51–4 and 51–5). Other locations include the spinal cord, corpus callosum, and periventricular white matter. Usually there is no associated mass effect, edema, or contrast enhancement, and they are isointense to brain on T1-weighted images. Lesions in the globus pallidus behave somewhat differently; they may have mild mass effect and appear mildly hyperintense to brain on T1-weighted images as well as T2-weighted images (Fig. 51–6).[47, 53, 58] CT is less than one-third as sensitive for the detection of basal ganglia lesions in NF-1.[59]

These areas of signal abnormality are common in NF-1, occurring in 75% or more of patients.[50] They begin to appear in patients around the age of 3 years, increase in size and number until about 10 years of age, and then decrease.[60–61] They are seen less often in adulthood than in childhood. The criteria listed in Table 51–1 were defined by the NIH consensus group in 1987, before these

MRI findings were well appreciated. At this time, therefore, the signal abnormalities may, in fact, be highly suggestive of the diagnosis of NF-1 but are not included in the official list of diagnostic criteria.

The histologic correlates of these regions of signal abnormality are poorly understood. Hamartomas and atypical glial cells are known to occur in NF-1,[62–65] and these are possible causes for some of the areas of signal abnormality. The known tendency for regression of these MRI findings, however, argues against static lesions, such as hamartomas, as a single cause. Delayed or disordered myelination has also been suggested.[47, 50] Limited pathologic information has become available, and spongiotic changes and microcalcifications have been reported.[66] Postmortem examination of three patients with NF-1

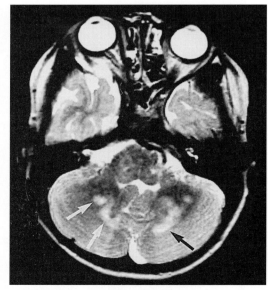

FIGURE 51–4 A 4-year-old with NF-1. T2-weighted MRI study demonstrates typical foci of hyperintensity in the deep white matter of the cerebellum (*arrows*) and pons.

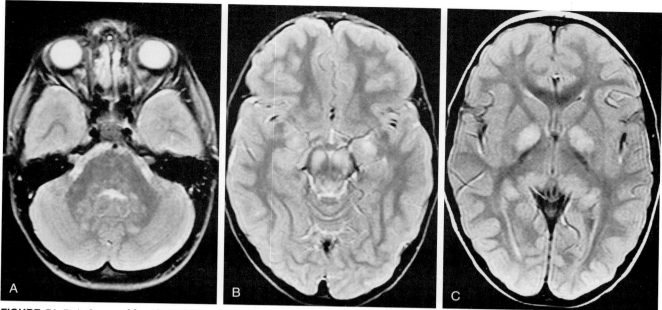

FIGURE 51–5 A 6-year-old with NF-1. *A–C,* T2-weighted MRI studies demonstrate typical hyperintense foci in the cerebellum, middle cerebellar peduncles, cerebral peduncles, and basal ganglia.

showed vacuolar changes in the myelin or spongiotic change, which is likely to explain the high signal intensity on T2-weighted images. Microcalcifications in the globus pallidus may be responsible for increased signal intensity on T1-weighted images.[66] The clinical significance of these nonneoplastic MRI abnormalities in NF-1 is also still unclear. A correlation with learning disabilities has been reported,[67] but other investigators have found no association.[68, 69]

Because of the potential for confusion with gliomas, a follow-up scan in 6 to 12 months after detection of these signal abnormalities has been recommended, especially if

an area of signal abnormality appears atypical.[50, 70] Because magnetic resonance spectroscopy of these nonneoplastic areas appears similar to normal brain and different from gliomas, there may be a role for spectroscopy in some cases.[68] In most cases, however, the low grade of astrocytomas in NF-1 safely permits follow-up MRI scans. Contrast administration for baseline brain MRI studies can increase confidence in the diagnosis of benign-appearing areas of signal abnormality probably representing vacuolar change and improve characterization of suspected tumors.[71] The typical location and appearance of nonneoplastic areas of MRI signal abnormality, however,

FIGURE 51–6 An 11-year-old with NF-1. *A,* T2-weighted MRI study demonstrates bilateral hyperintensities in the globus pallidus (*arrows*). *B,* T1-weighted MRI study shows the mild hyperintensity of these lesions (*arrows*), seen with lesions in this location but less commonly elsewhere in the brain.

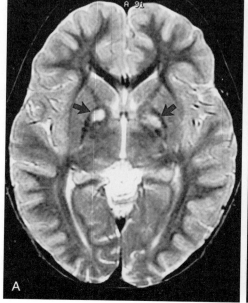
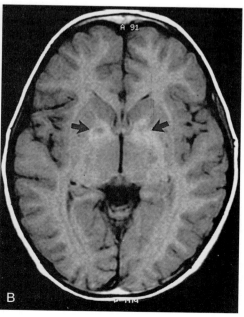

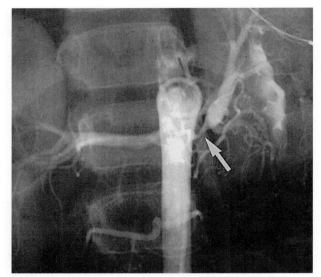

FIGURE 51–7 Renal artery stenosis in NF-1. Anteroposterior view from an abdominal aortogram of a teenage boy with hypertension shows a tight stenosis near the origin of the left renal artery (*arrow*). There is poststenotic dilatation.

are often readily recognized even without or before intravenous gadolinium administration and differ from the appearance of aggressive astrocytomas.

Other Central Nervous System Findings

Vascular dysplasias occur uncommonly in NF-1. Intimal proliferation is common and may result in narrowing or occlusion of the carotid or proximal middle or anterior cerebral arteries.[56, 72–74] Stenosis of the internal carotid artery may occur secondary either to this mesenchymal

dysplasia or to previous radiation for a tumor.[50] The result may be numerous enlarged collateral vessels, seen on imaging as a moyamoya pattern. Angiography shows occlusion or stenosis of the involved arteries. The *puff of smoke* pattern of multiple vessels in the basal ganglia occurs in some cases. Similar findings may be seen with magnetic resonance angiography. MRI demonstrates numerous enlarged arteries in the basal ganglia.

There is an increased risk of cerebral aneurysms in NF-1.[75–77] These may be saccular or fusiform. Ectasia and arteriovenous malformations or fistulas have also been reported.[78]

Intracranial vascular dysplasias are rare in NF-1 but can be significant when they do occur. In addition to primary vascular dysplasia, neurologic symptoms or signs may result from radiation arteritis in patients for tumor or from hypertension in patients with renal artery stenosis.[79] Extracranial arterial stenoses are more common in NF-1 than intracranial vascular dysplasias (Fig. 51–7). Pheochromocytoma is another condition of rare but relatively increased incidence in NF-1 compared to the general population that can cause hypertension and vascular disease.

Aqueductal stenosis can be caused by tectal glioma in NF-1 or may be due to nonneoplastic causes.[47, 55, 56] CT shows hydrocephalus, but MRI is best for demonstrating the findings of aqueductal stenosis and for evaluating for possible brain stem glioma.

Meningioangiomatosis is a rare hamartomatous lesion of the cerebral cortex, characterized by meningovascular fibroblastic proliferation. Approximately half of these patients have been reported to have NF.[80, 81] Leptomeningial calcification is frequently present. The cortex appears thickened, signal intensity on T2-weighted images is heterogeneous, and enhancement is variable (Fig. 51–8).

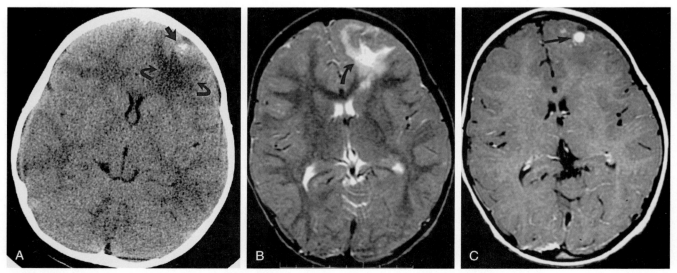

FIGURE 51–8 Meningioangiomatosis. *A*, Non–contrast-enhanced CT scan of a 3-year-old girl with seizures shows calcification (*straight arrow*) in the left frontal cortex and adjacent low attenuation (*curved arrows*). *B*, T2-weighted axial MRI study shows only slight hypointensity relative to gray matter in the region of the calcification. There is distortion of the cortex and surrounding high signal intensity extending into the nearby white matter (*arrow*). *C*, After gadolinium administration, there is a rounded area of intense enhancement (*arrow*). Nonenhanced T1-weighted MRI study (not shown) demonstrated no high signal intensity before gadolinium administration.

Skull Findings

Characteristic lesions of the skull are among the diagnostic criteria for NF-1 (see Table 51–1).[28, 33, 50, 82–85, 92] These are additional examples of mesodermal dysplasia. Deficiency of the sphenoid bone, most often the greater wing, results in an *empty orbit* appearance (Fig. 51–9). The adjacent temporal lobe can herniate into the posterior orbit, causing a pulsatile exophthalmos. A plexiform neurofibroma of the orbit is sometimes associated. Midline sphenoid body dysplasia is rare.[82] Deficiency of the greater sphenoid wing results in a characteristic empty orbit or harlequin appearance on plain film. CT or MRI can also demonstrate absence of the sphenoid bone.

Other skull abnormalities include macrocrania, deficiencies of the skull, and sequelae of dural ectasia. The most common location for cranial defects is in the region of the sphenoid wings, more often the greater wing.[82] Mastoid pneumatization is often deficient in these cases. Uncommon locations for defects are lambdoid suture, facial bones, petrous temporal bone, skull base, and dental structures. Dural ectasia in the internal auditory canal can result in enlargement of the canal, sometimes with clinical signs as well.[48, 86, 87] Although the internal auditory canals may be enlarged in both NF-1 and NF-2, enlargement in NF-1 is due to dural ectasia and an enlarged cerebrospinal fluid space, whereas enlargement in NF-2 is due to schwannoma.

Other Orbital Abnormalities

The orbit is a common location for plexiform neurofibromas, and mass effect in the confined space of the orbit can cause symptoms of exophthalmos and can impair motility.[17, 88–90] They usually arise from small nerves and tend to extend toward the brain.[50] The superior orbital fissure and cavernous sinus are frequently involved. On CT, these nonencapsulated neurofibromas appear poorly delineated and are usually of low attenuation (Fig. 51–10). Signal intensity on MRI is often heterogeneous. They are generally isointense to hypointense to brain on T1-weighted images and hyperintense on T2-weighted images. Contrast enhancement is variable, but some of the neurofibroma usually enhances. Low signal intensity regions on T2-weighted images may represent fibrous and myxoid elements (Figs. 51–11 through 51–13).

Congenital glaucoma can result from neurofibromatous involvement of ocular structures or abnormal development of anterior chamber angle, causing obstruction to outflow of the aqueous humor.[88] Buphthalmos, a congeni-

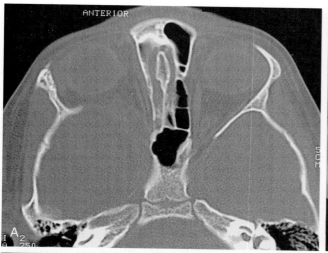
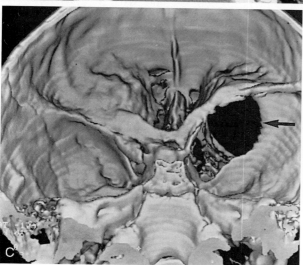
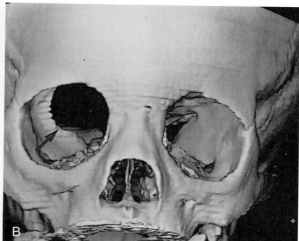

FIGURE 51–9 A 4-year-old with NF-1. *A,* Axial CT scan demonstrates hypoplasia of the sphenoid, predominantly the greater wing, producing an *empty orbit. B* and *C,* Three-dimensional re-formatted non–contrast-enhanced CT images (from front [*B*] and from behind [*C*]) further illustrate the appearance resulting from sphenoid dysplasia *(arrows).*

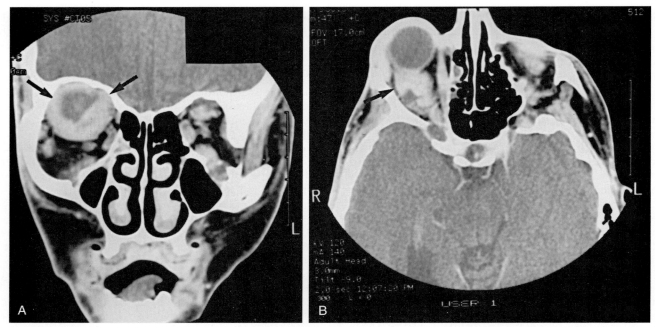

FIGURE 51–10 Plexiform neurofibroma. *A* and *B,* Contrast-enhanced CT images demonstrate a heterogeneously enhancing mass (*arrows*) in the superior portion of the right orbit, accompanied by proptosis and chronic remodeling and expansion of the walls of the orbit. Note that the lesion is separate from the optic nerve. The appearance is compatible with a plexiform neurofibroma in the distribution of the first division of the trigeminal nerve.

tally enlarged globe that results from glaucoma, has been reported in approximately half of cases with sphenoid dysplasia.[91]

Spine Findings

Abnormalities of the spine are common in NF-1. These include both neoplasms and mesenchymal dysplasias that cause bony and dural anomalies.

Neoplasms

Nerve sheath tumors are common but not unique to NF-1. Isolated nerve sheath tumors are not uncommon as sporadic occurrences in the general population. They are often multiple in NF-1, however. Schwannomas originate from the Schwann cells that surround the nerve. The tumors are eccentric to the nerve itself. Neurofibromas generally encompass and infiltrate the nerve, meaning that nerve cannot be readily separated from the tumor. The cell of origin is thought to be the fibroblast. Spinal nerve sheath tumors in NF-1 are most often neurofibromas, and these are relatively characteristic of NF-1.[18, 84, 92–95]

These tumors commonly occur along the exiting spinal nerves, most often along the dorsal roots. They are usually intradural extramedullary lesions but often also have a mixed extradural component. A dumbbell appearance is common, with both an intradural extramedullary component and extension through the neural foramen (Figs. 51–14 and 51–15). Spinal neurofibromas are often multiple in NF-1 but are usually fewer in number (several) compared to spinal masses in NF-2 (often ≥10). Contrast-enhanced spinal MRI of 28 patients with NF-1 revealed 16 with bony abnormalities (see following section),

6 with spinal tumors, 1 with an intramedullary tumor (astrocytoma), 3 with dural ectasia, and 11 normal patients.[93]

Plain film radiographs of the spine often show an enlarged neural foramen at the level of a nerve sheath tumor. The pedicles are thinned but without evidence of erosion. On CT, nerve sheath tumors usually demonstrate lower attenuation than muscle. MRI displays the tumors well. Signal intensity is usually greater than that of muscle on T1-weighted and T2-weighted images. Heterogeneity of signal intensity is not uncommon. The central portion, in particular, often demonstrates lower signal intensity on T2-weighted images, probably as a result of high collagen content.[18, 50, 92, 94] The tumors demonstrate contrast enhancement on both CT and MRI. Myelography or postmyelography CT can show the relationship of the tumor to the spinal cord. MRI can give the same information noninvasively.

Intramedullary neoplasms are uncommon in NF-1, but astrocytomas have been reported. Nonneoplastic areas of MRI signal abnormality similar to those in the brain can also be detected in the spinal cord.

Skeletal and Dural Abnormalities

Kyphoscoliosis occurs in at least 2% of patients with NF-1.[17, 82–84] Thoracic and lumbar locations are frequent (Fig. 51–16; see also Fig. 51–15). Cervical kyphosis is a finding strongly suggestive of NF-1 and is often also associated with vertebral scalloping and wedging. Most cases of scoliosis in NF-1 are thought to be due to a primary mesenchymal dysplasia, but in a smaller percentage of cases, nerve sheath tumors can be associated with scoliosis.[17] In addition to the usual idiopathic spinal curve, NF-

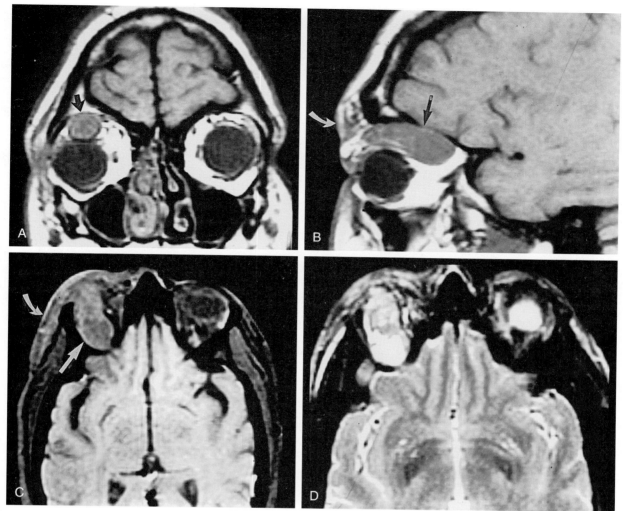

FIGURE 51–11 A 22-year-old with NF-1 and orbital plexiform neurofibroma. *A–C,* T1-weighted MRI studies demonstrate a well-defined extraconal mass in the right orbit, with heterogeneous signal (*straight arrows*). Note extension into adjacent subcutaneous soft tissues (*curved arrows*). *D,* T2-weighted MRI study demonstrates mixed hyperintensity of the mass.

1 patients also may have an uncommon but characteristic short segment kyphoscoliosis with sharp angulation.[96]

Dural ectasia in NF-1 can result in meningoceles in NF-1.[23, 28, 82–84, 93, 97–100] The thoracic spine is the most common location. Multiple thoracic lateral meningoceles may occur. Pedicle thinning may be seen on radiographs in such cases, but CT and MRI clearly show that the mass is isodense or isointense with cerebrospinal fluid (see Fig. 51–15). The meningoceles are generally attributed to a mesenchymal dysplasia affecting the dura. Similar dural dysplasia may be responsible for posterior scalloping of the vertebral bodies that is often observed in NF-1.

Pheochromocytoma

There appears to be an increased incidence of pheochromocytoma in NF-1 compared to the general population. In a population-based study, pheochromocytoma occurred in 1% of patients. The tumors occur in adults and are histologically identical to sporadically occurring pheochromocytomas.[17, 101]

Neurofibromatosis Type 2

NF-2 is about one-tenth as common as NF-1, with an incidence of about 1 in 30,000 to 40,000 births.[102] Skin manifestations are less prominent than in NF-1. The hallmarks are multiple cranial nerve schwannomas, especially bilateral vestibular schwannomas, and multiple meningiomas.[47, 48, 103, 104] Ependymomas of the spinal cord and nerve sheath tumors (schwannomas) are also common. Most intracranial manifestations are thus tumors of the tissues along surfaces of the brain and cranial nerves, as opposed to the prominent intra-axial features of NF-1.[47]

Genetics

The NF-2 gene on chromosome 22q was cloned in 1993 and its protein product termed *merlin* or *schannomin.*[105, 106] Similar to NF-1, the pattern of inheritance is autosomal dominant. There is evidence for abnormalities of chromosome 22 in patients with familial meningiomas but not NF-2. Multiple meningiomatosis without

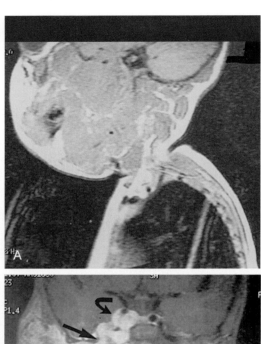
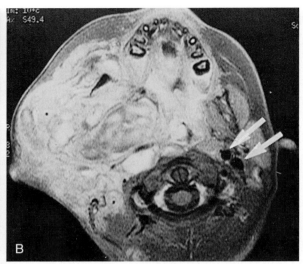
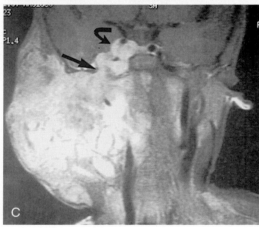

FIGURE 51–12 A 2-year-old girl with NF-1 and giant plexiform neurofibroma. T1-weighted sagittal (*A*) and axial (*B*) gadolinium-enhanced MRI studies demonstrate an enormous mass involving multiple soft tissue compartments of the neck, with heterogeneous enhancement and distortion of normal anatomy. Normal internal carotid and jugular signal voids are present on the left (*arrows in B*) but cannot be identified on the right side of the neck. *C,* Coronal gadolinium-enhanced MRI study demonstrates involvement of the skull base, with enhancing tumor extending through an expanded foramen ovale (*straight arrow*) and into the cavernous sinus (*curved arrow*).

other features of NF-2 is a separate syndrome from NF-2 and is linked to a different site on chromosome 22.[107] Loss of heterozygosity for markers on the long arm of chromosome 22 has also been reported in sporadically occurring spinal schwannomas from non-NF-2 patients, suggesting that there is a common locus involved in Schwann cell tumorigenesis.[108] As would be expected with an autosomal dominant disorder, there is no convincing evidence of a male/female difference in severity of disease.[48]

Diagnostic Criteria

Diagnostic criteria for NF-2 established at the NIH Consensus Development Conference were revised in 1997 and are listed in Table 51–2.[9] Recognizing that the rigidity of these criteria may be too exclusive, a category of *presumptive or probable NF-2* was created (Table 51–2). As in NF-1, the diagnosis of NF-2 remains a strictly clinical one. The limitations of diagnostic molecular testing are similar for NF-1 and NF-2, and such testing is not widely practical. The central role of eighth nerve schwannomas in this disease is underlined by the NIH criteria. NF-2 is established by these criteria if there are either bilateral vestibular schwannomas or a positive family history plus one vestibular schwannoma or two of

other specific abnormalities, including schwannomas and meningiomas.[8]

Clinical Findings and Natural History

The pleomorphic nature of von Recklinghausen's disease (now NF-1) meant that for many years the features of NF-2 were easily confused with NF-1, despite the completely different genetic causes. Many older reports on clinical features of NF combined the two conditions. Because of this situation, the relatively recent clinical definition of NF-2 as a separate syndrome, and the much lower incidence of NF-2 compared to NF-1, the full spectrum of clinical manifestations and natural history of NF-2 is still being fully defined. The name *neurofibromatosis* is perhaps inappropriate for this condition because neurofibromas are not characteristic of NF-2. Smirniotopoulos and Murphy[28] have suggested the term *MISME syndrome* as a concise summary of the features: *m*ultiple *i*nherited *s*chwannomas, *m*eningiomas, and *e*pendymomas.

Onset of symptoms in NF-2 is often later than that in NF-1 because the NF-2 tumors are generally not apparent until after puberty. Clinical symptoms from vestibular schwannomas may begin in the teens, and the peak age for detection of these tumors is in the 20s.[101, 109] Mean age of presentation of sporadic vestibular schwannomas

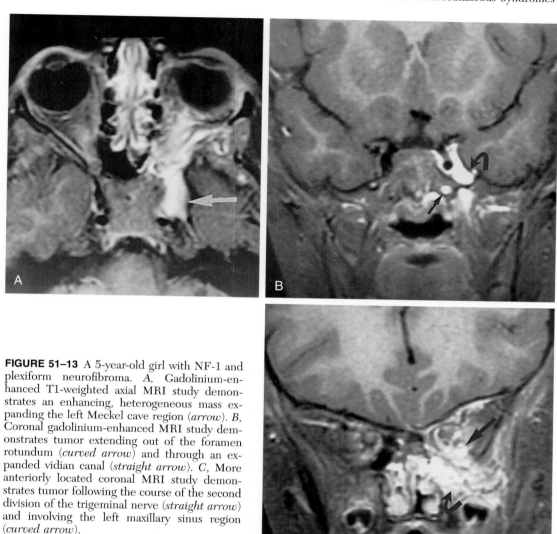

FIGURE 51–13 A 5-year-old girl with NF-1 and plexiform neurofibroma. *A*, Gadolinium-enhanced T1-weighted axial MRI study demonstrates an enhancing, heterogeneous mass expanding the left Meckel cave region (*arrow*). *B*, Coronal gadolinium-enhanced MRI study demonstrates tumor extending out of the foramen rotundum (*curved arrow*) and through an expanded vidian canal (*straight arrow*). *C*, More anteriorly located coronal MRI study demonstrates tumor following the course of the second division of the trigeminal nerve (*straight arrow*) and involving the left maxillary sinus region (*curved arrow*).

is later, in the 40s. Cranial nerve symptoms from other schwannomas may occur, especially the trigeminal nerve. Meningiomas can cause mass effect. The age of presentation of meningiomas in NF-2 is also often earlier than for patients with sporadic meningiomas.[101] Approximately one-fourth of children with meningiomas have other stigmata of NF-2.[110] Schwannomas and meningiomas are discussed in greater detail in subsequent sections. Cognitive impairment and learning disabilities, seen in up 30% of patients with NF-1, are not features of NF-2.[16, 48, 104]

Café au lait spots are generally sparse or not observed in NF-2, in contrast to NF-1. Among the 61 patients examined by Mulvihill and colleagues,[48] 52% had no café au lait macules, 46% had one to four, and only 1 patient had more than six.[48] Axillary and inguinal freckling is not a feature of NF-2.[48]

Tumors of the skin are common in NF-2, more so than has sometimes been suggested in the past.[48, 103] Approximately two-thirds of NF-2 patients have skin tumors,

although they may require careful examination to detect in some cases. The tumors appear either as soft, raised areas, often hyperpigmented and hypertrichotic, or as spherical subcutaneous masses along peripheral nerves. The frequent existence of skin tumors may contribute to the clinical confusion between NF-1 and NF-2. In contrast to NF-1, however, in which the tumors are neurofibromas, the skin tumors in NF-2 appear to be schwannomas.[103] Given the skin, intracranial, and spinal findings, NF-2 is more accurately a *schwannomatosis* than *neurofibromatosis*. A small number of NF-2 patients have peripheral neuropathy that appears not to be related to tumors of the skin or CNS.[103, 111–113] The cause is not known.

Several ocular abnormalities can occur in NF-2. Multiple Lisch nodules are not a feature of NF-2. As mentioned earlier, they are probably pathognomonic for NF-1. Presenile posterior subcapsular opacities of the lens do occur in NF-2 as well as cortical opacities.[114–118] Cataracts eventually occur in up to 80% of NF-2 patients. Although

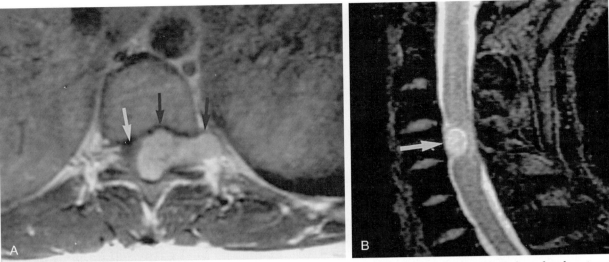

FIGURE 51–14 Cervical spine neurofibroma. *A,* Axial gadolinum-enhanced MRI study shows dumbbell-shaped enhancing tumor (*black arrows*) in the spinal canal and left neural foramen. The spinal cord is severely displaced to the right (*white arrow*). *B,* Sagittal T2-weighted MRI study shows the neurofibroma (*arrow*) displacing the spinal cord posteriorly. (*A* and *B,* From Hart BL, Benzel EC, Ford CC. Fundamentals of Neuroimaging. Philadelphia, WB Saunders, 1997.)

optic nerve gliomas do not occur with increased frequency in NF-2, meningiomas of the optic nerve sheath are another possible cause of decreased vision, in addition to cataracts. Moreover, retinal and choroidal hamartomas and epiretinal membranes occur in approximately 10% to 20% of patients.[48] Macular involvement by these hamartomas can lead to strabismus and is a third possible cause of visual loss in NF-2.[119–123] These combined hamartomas differ from the astrocytic retinal *mulberry-like* hamartomas (phakomas) of TS. When visual loss or diplopia is the cause of initial symptoms in NF-2 patients, it often presents in patients younger than 10 years old.[48]

TABLE 51–2 Diagnostic Criteria for Neurofibromatosis Type 2 (NF-2)

Individuals with the following clinical features have confirmed (definite) NF-2
  One of the following is present:
    Bilateral vestibular schwannomas seen on CT or MRI
    A parent, sibling, or child with NF-2 and either unilateral vestibular schwannoma (detected before age 30 yr) or any two of the following: meningioma, glioma, schwannoma, or juvenile posterior subcapsular lenticular opacity
Individuals with the following clinical features should be evaluated for NF-2 (presumptive or probable NF-2)
  Unilateral vestibular schwannoma (detected before age 30 yr) plus at least one of the following: meningioma, glioma, schwannoma, juvenile posterior subcapsular lenticular opacities/juvenile cortical cataract
  Multiple meningiomas (≥2) plus unilateral vestibular schwannoma (detected before age 30 yr) or one of the following: glioma, schwannoma, juvenile posterior subcapsular lenticular opacities/juvenile cortical cataract

From Gutmann DH, Aylsworth A, Carey JC, et al. The diagnostic evaluation and multidisciplinary management of neurofibromatosis 1 and neurofibromatosis 2. JAMA 1997;278:51–57.

In a group of 58 symptomatic patients with NF-2, mean age of initial symptoms was 20.3 years.[48] The most common cause of symptoms was vestibular schwannomas (48%), followed by other schwannomas and meningiomas (24%), with skin tumors and ocular symptoms responsible for the remainder (14% each). Five additional asymptomatic patients had been identified through screening. Among these 63 patients, all but 1 had vestibular schwannomas; bilateral vestibular schwannomas were present in 58 (92%). Nearly half of the patients had meningiomas, usually multiple, and nearly one-fourth had schwannomas other than those of the eighth nerve. More than two-thirds of those who had MRI of the spine had spine tumors.

Several subtypes of NF-2 have been proposed. Statistical analysis provides evidence for two types. A mild (Gardner) form presents later in life and has fewer meningiomas and spinal tumors than the more severe (Wishart) type.[9, 48, 103]

Cranial Nerve Schwannomas

Schwannomas arise from the Schwann cells surrounding the cranial nerves.[27, 124] The most common cranial nerve schwannomas in NF-2 are those of the eighth cranial nerve; most arise from the vestibular division.[125] Following the eighth cranial nerve in frequency are the fifth, ninth, and tenth.[27, 126, 127] Any of the third through twelfth cranial nerves may be involved, however, and detection of an unusual intracranial schwannoma or detection of multiple schwannomas should prompt consideration of the possibility of NF-2.

Vestibular schwannomas are common in NF-2 and in about 45% of patients are the cause of initial symptoms in NF-2.[47, 48, 128] Such symptoms include hearing loss, tinnitus, poor balance, and facial weakness, in decreasing order of frequency. Although most eighth nerve schwannomas originate in the vestibular divisions, as in

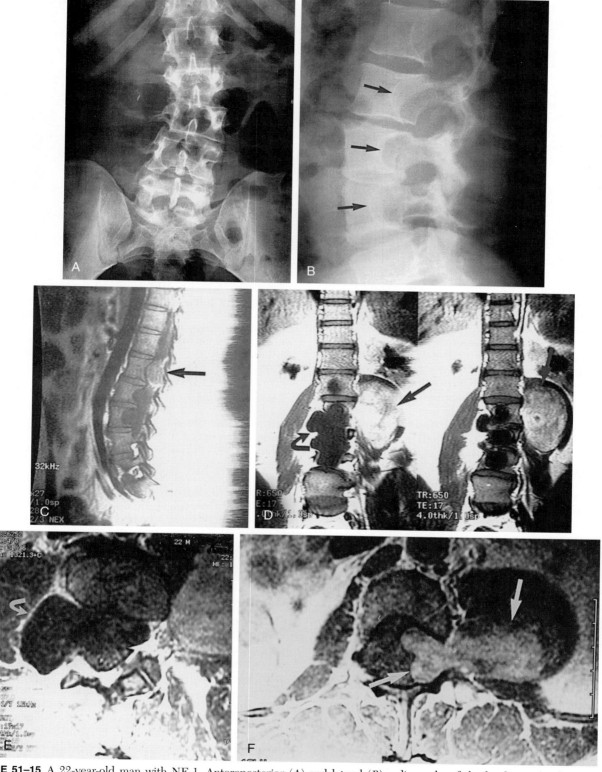

FIGURE 51–15 A 22-year-old man with NF-1. Anteroposterior (*A*) and lateral (*B*) radiographs of the lumbar spine demonstrate a levoconvex scoliosis and pronounced posterior vertebral body scalloping (*arrows* in *B*) as a result of dural ectasia. *C,* Gadolinium-enhanced T1-weighted sagittal MRI study of the lumbar spine also demonstrates posterior vertebral body scalloping, which spares the intervertebral disks, as well as an enhancing intrathecal mass (*arrow*), consistent with a nerve sheath tumor. *D,* Coronal gadolinium-enhanced T1-weighted image demonstrates the extraspinal component of the tumor (*straight arrow*) seen in *C.* A lateral meningocele is also present (*curved arrow*). *E,* Gadolinium-enhanced axial T1-weighted MRI study at the level of the meningocele demonstrates the pouch of dura, containing cerebrospinal fluid (*curved arrow*). *F,* Axial MRI study through the nerve sheath tumor demonstrates the typical *dumbbell* configuration and enhancement of a spinal nerve sheath tumor (*arrows*).

sporadic eighth nerve schwannomas, there is a much greater tendency in NF-2 for the facial and cochlear nerves to be encompassed or compressed. In contrast, sporadically occurring vestibular schwannomas typically are eccentric to the nerve and spare the other nerves within the internal auditory canal for a time, making nerve-sparing surgery more often possible.[128–130]

Vestibular schwannomas usually originate within the internal auditory canal.[131] Small, intracanalicular schwannomas may be difficult to detect. Contrast-enhanced MRI is the most sensitive imaging technique and shows the schwannomas as small, enhancing masses (Fig. 51–17).[47, 132, 133] Work has also demonstrated nearly equal sensitivity of high-resolution, nonenhanced, fast spin echo T2-weighted MRI for detection of intracanalicular schwannomas.[134–136] Routine CT is insensitive for small vestibular schwannomas, but gas cisternography CT can demonstrate intracanalicular tumors. In this technique, 1 or 2 cm³ of air is injected into the subarachnoid space in the lumbar spine, and the patient is positioned with the head up and turned to the side such that the air rises to the cerebellopontine angle. Air in the internal auditory canal then outlines the nerves and a small neoplasm, if present, on thin-section CT. The technique is less sensitive than MRI and more invasive. It is therefore reserved now for patients who cannot receive MRI.

The natural history of vestibular schwannomas is continued growth into the cerebellopontine angle. A mushroom-like or ice cream cone shape results. Larger masses are more rounded and typically deviate the adjacent brain stem and cerebellum. The signal intensity on MRI is usually similar to brain on T1-weighted images and mildly hyperintense on T2-weighted images. Heterogeneity on T2-weighted images in larger lesions is common. Intense contrast enhancement is usually present on T1-weighted images after intravenous gadolinium administration (Figs. 51–17 through 51–20). Necrotic regions without enhance-

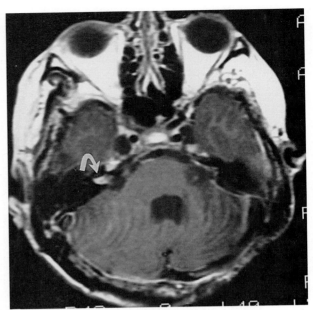

FIGURE 51–17 Intracanalicular vestibular schwannoma in neurofibromatosis type 2 (NF-2). Axial gadolinium-enhanced T2-weighted MRI study in a woman with NF-2 shows enhancing within the right internal auditory canal (*arrow*). There has been previous surgery on the patient's left internal auditory canal. (From Hart BL, Benzel EC, Ford CC. Fundamentals of Neuroimaging. Philadelphia, WB Saunders, 1997.)

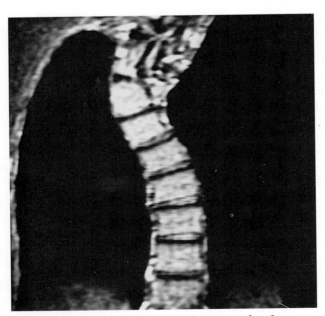

FIGURE 51–16 Coronal T1-weighted MRI study of a patient with NF-1 shows high thoracic scoliosis.

ment may be present. Cysts may occur but are not a common feature. CT, preferably using high-resolution technique and contrast enhancement, can show cerebellopontine angle masses, although with less detail than MRI. The schwannomas of NF-2 are individually not different from those occurring sporadically, although bilateral schwannomas are diagnostic criteria of NF-2.

Imaging findings of schwannomas of cranial nerves III through XII are similar to vestibular schwannomas except for location.[137] MRI is also better than CT for visualization of these. Intense contrast enhancement follows gadolinium administration (see Figs. 51–18 through 51–20).

Meningiomas

There is a high incidence of meningiomas in NF-2, and multiple meningiomas are common.[47, 138] Imaging characteristics are similar to those of sporadically occurring meningiomas: extra-axial, dural-based masses that demonstrate intense contrast enhancement. Attenuation on CT before contrast agent administration is often higher than that of brain. Calcification can contribute to this density, but a major factor in most cases is the high nuclear to cytoplasmic ratio of the cells. Cyst formation is rare. Signal intensity of meningiomas is variable on MRI but is often similar to that of brain on all pulse sequences.[47, 139] Angiography typically demonstrates an early, dense blush that persists well into the venous phase. Intraventricular meningiomas may also occur in NF-2. Contrast-enhanced MRI is the most sensitive technique for detection of meningiomas and can be especially helpful for detection of multiple lesions in NF-2 (see Figs. 51–18 and 51–20).[140, 141] Small, extra-axial lesions around the skull base

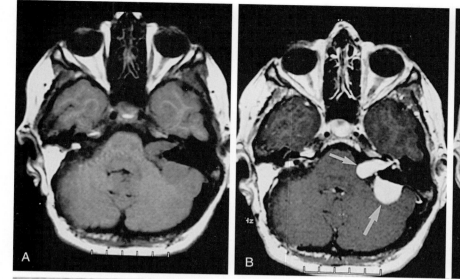
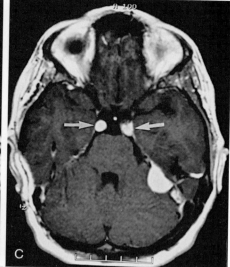

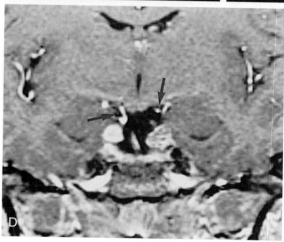

FIGURE 51–18 A 31-year-old man with NF-2. T1-weighted axial nonenhanced (*A*) and gadolinium-enhanced (*B*) MRI studies demonstrate homogeneously enhancing extra-axial masses at the left cerebellopontine angle. One mass (*small arrow* in *B*) expands and extends into the internal auditory canal, consistent with an acoustic schwannoma, whereas the other (*large arrow* in *B*) extends from the dura of the petrous ridge and is a meningioma. Postoperative changes and fat-packing are present in the right petrous temporal bone from prior resection of an additional acoustic schwannoma. More superiorly located gadolinium-enhanced axial (*C*) and coronal (*D*) MRI studies demonstrate small extra-axial tumors (*arrows*), likely other cranial nerve schwannomas.

in NF-2, which may be either schwannomas or meningiomas, may present a similar appearance to one another. Thin-slice thickness and multiple planes can be helpful in these cases to distinguish a schwannoma from meningioma based on location on a cranial nerve.

Spine Findings

Both schwannomas and meningiomas can occur along the spine, usually as intradural extramedullary masses.[23, 93, 142] The nerve sheath tumors of NF-2, in contrast to the neurofibromas of NF-1, are schwannomas.[94] These masses can also appear as dumbbell-shaped lesions extending through the neural foramen. Schwannomas in NF-2 can also appear as intramedullary masses. Spinal schwannomas in NF-2 are frequently multiple, with greater average number than spinal neurofibromas in NF-1. In a study of NF-1 and NF-2 patients, all nine of the NF-2 patients had extramedullary spinal masses, on average 12 tumors, whereas 39% of the NF-1 patients had no spine tumors.[93] Mulvihill and colleagues[48] found numerous spinal tumors in 30 of 40 patients who received imaging of the entire spine.

Contrast enhancement, especially with MRI, increases

sensitivity greatly. Multiple enhancing schwannomas are often seen along the spinal nerve roots (see Figs. 51–19 and 51–20). Coronal images can be helpful in demonstrating the location of multiple schwannomas along the nerve roots. Axial MRI better demonstrates the relationship of masses to the spinal cord. Myelography and postmyelography CT can also show these masses, although MRI has clear advantages for patients able to receive it.

There is also an increased frequency of intramedullary ependymomas in the spine in NF-2.[93, 142] Single ependymomas are usually in the conus or filum region. Multiple ependymomas can also occur throughout the spinal cord. MRI is clearly the best technique for detection of these intramedullary masses.

Other Features of Neurofibromatosis Type 2

Intracranial calcifications not associated with tumors have been reported in NF-2 in the choroid plexus, cerebellar cortex, and surface of the cerebral cortex.[63, 103, 143–145]

Other Forms of Neurofibromatosis

Many types of NF have been proposed. At present, only types 1 and 2, already discussed, have clearly defined

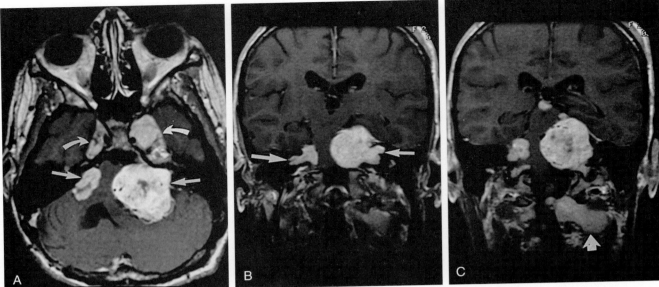

FIGURE 51–19 A 20-year-old woman with NF-2. *A* and *B,* Gadolinium-enhanced T1-weighted MRI studies demonstrate typical bilateral acoustic schwannomas (*straight arrows*). Marked expansion of both cavernous sinuses is also present (*curved arrows* in *A*) and is probably produced by schwannomas of other cranial nerves. *C,* Gadolinium-enhanced MRI study of the skull base also demonstrates a large, dumbbell-shaped tumor of the upper cervical spine (*arrow*).

genetic characteristics. As Gutmann and colleagues[9] have noted, ". . . Subclassifying variable clinical presentations of NF-1 or NF-2 as separate forms of neurofibromatosis is not warranted."[9] A segmental or mosaic form of NF-1 or NF-2 can present in which neural and cutaneous manifestations are limited to one region of the body.[9] Confusion regarding overlap syndromes has arisen in some cases because skin schwannomas can be confused with neurofibromas. This is most likely to occur in NF-2 with an unusual number of café au lait spots and skin tumors. The clinical criteria for NF-1 may thus be apparently met, but family history and other, characteristic features of NF-1 would be lacking.[48] Other conditions that may sometimes be confused with NF but that have different genetic origin include familial café au lait spots, schwannomatosis, and multiple meningiomas.

TUBEROUS SCLEROSIS COMPLEX

TS complex is an autosomal dominant condition characterized by multiple hamartomas of the brain, eye, skin, and kidneys. Hamartomas of the heart, lungs, and other organs can also occur. Neurologic manifestations include infantile spasms, seizures, and mental retardation. Subependymal giant cell astrocytomas are a significant cause of morbidity and mortality.

As with others of the neurocutaneous syndromes, eponyms are associated with this condition. Bourneville described the syndrome in 1880, and TS is also known as *Bourneville's disease.*[7] The classic triad of adenoma sebaceum, mental retardation, and seizures is also known as *Vogt's triad.* Adenoma sebaceum is sometimes referred to by the name of *Pringle's disease. Epiloia* and *cerebral sclerosis* are older terms that have also been applied to TS.

Genetics

TS complex has at least two genetic causes, TSC1 on chromosome 9q and TSC2 on chromosome 16p. The TSC1 gene was cloned in 1997 and the TSC2 gene in 1993. It is estimated that two-thirds of affected individuals are the result of sporadic new mutations. Each of the two identified mutations accounts for up to 50% of the familial cases.[146]

Diagnostic Criteria

The diagnosis of TS complex remains an entirely clinical one, with criteria set forth in 1992 and outlined in Table 51–3.[147] Definitive diagnosis of TS is straightforward when multiple, classic features are present. Some patients, however, have only a few findings. In the absence of a commercially available DNA diagnostic test, the criteria listed in Table 51–3 are used. The findings are classified as primary, secondary, and tertiary features, and combinations of these lead to a diagnosis of definite, probable, or suspected TS complex. Some of these criteria depend on histologic confirmation, but others can be determined on the basis of radiologic evidence alone (Table 51–3). Modifications in these criteria can be expected with further clinical and genetic research, but radiologic findings will continue to be important in identifying patients and evaluating complications.

Clinical Findings and Natural History

Mental retardation and seizures are the most common clinical neurologic manifestations of TS complex. Mental retardation is noted in approximately 60%, with a wide range of severity from borderline to profound.[148]

Seizures, including complex seizures, are common in

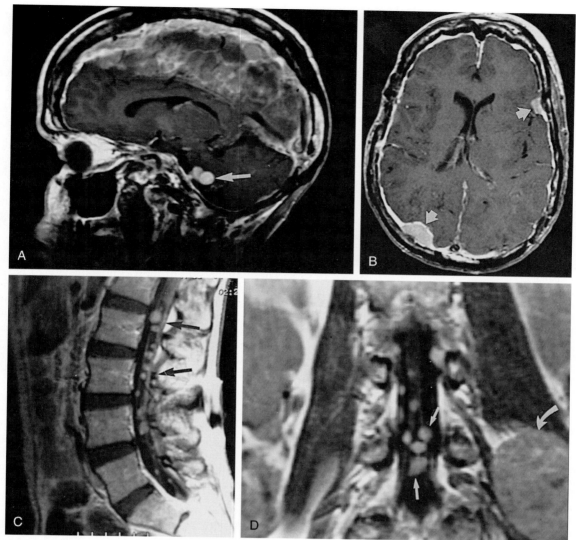

FIGURE 51–20 A 32-year-old man with NF-2. *A* and *B*, Gadolinium-enhanced T1-weighted MRI studies demonstrate multiple focal extra-axial masses (*arrows* in *B*) consistent with meningiomas and a small enhancing tumor (*arrow* in *A*) at the cerebellopontine angle consistent with schwannoma of the fifth cranial nerve. Diffuse dural enhancement is also present, probably resulting from multiple prior surgeries for tumor resections. *C* and *D*, Gadolinium-enhanced sagittal and coronal T1-weighted MRI studies of the lumbar spine demonstrate multiple small tumors of the cauda equina (*straight arrows*) as well as a larger paraspinal mass (*curved arrow*) consistent with multiple schwannomas.

older patients. Infantile spasms represent a common presentation of TS complex, and overall 80% to 90% of individuals with TS complex have some form of seizure disorder.[149] Early onset of seizures is associated with a greater risk of mental retardation.[150, 151] Approximately 20% of TS complex patients have seizures but are of normal intelligence.[152]

Skin manifestations of TS include ash-leaf macules, adenoma sebaceum, shagreen patches, and subungual fibromas. The earliest skin manifestations are usually hypopigmented, oval macules with irregular margins. These *ash-leaf* macules are sometimes best visualized with Wood's lamp.[153] The term *adenoma sebaceum* is a misnomer because the lesions are neither adenomas nor of sebaceous origin. Rather, the reddish, raised macules are angiofibromas, a type of dermal hamartoma. They appear

earliest in the nasolabial folds and spread to cover the infraorbital face and the nose. They usually appear between 2 and 6 years of age and are found in 90% of affected adults.[154] Angiofibromas can also be found elsewhere on the body, especially the trunk and periungual regions. Shagreen patches are leathery macules that are most common in the lumbar region. Ungual fibromas are also hamartomas. They are seen almost exclusively in TS (see Table 51–3). Café au lait macules have a similar incidence in TS complex patients as in the general population.[155]

Although the classic clinical triad of Vogt is well known, it, in fact, occurs in a minority of patients.[156] Patients with TS have decreased survival in comparison with the general population. In a review of 355 patients with TS complex, Shepherd and colleagues[157] found 40 of these

**TABLE 51–3 Diagnostic Criteria for Tuberous
Sclerosis**

Primary features
  Facial angiofibromas°
  Multiple ungual fibromas°
  Cortical tuber (histologically confirmed)
  Subependymal nodule or giant cell astrocytoma
    (histologically confirmed)
  Multiple calcified subependymal nodules protruding into the
    ventricle (radiographic evidence)
  Multiple retinal astrocytomas°
Secondary features
  Affected first-degree relative
  Cardiac rhabdomyoma (histologic or radiographic
    confirmation)
  Other retinal hamartoma or achromic patch°
  Cerebral tubers (radiographic confirmation)
  Noncalcified subependymal nodules (radiographic
    confirmation)
  Shagreen patch°
  Forehead plaque°
  Pulmonary lymphangiomyomatosis (histologic confirmation)
  Renal angiomyolipoma (radiographic or histologic
    confirmation)
  Renal cysts (histologic confirmation)
Tertiary features
  Hypomelanotic macules°
  Confetti skin lesions°
  Renal cysts (radiographic evidence)
  Randomly distributed enamel pits in deciduous or
    permanent teeth
  Hamartomatous rectal polyps (histologic confirmation)
  Bone cysts (radiographic evidence)
  Pulmonary lymphangiomyomatosis (radiographic evidence)
  Cerebral white matter *migration tracts* or heterotopias
    (radiographic evidence)
Gingival fibromas°
  Hamartoma of other organs (histologic confirmation)
  Infantile spasms
Definite TSC   1 primary feature, 2 secondary features, or 1
  secondary plus 2 tertiary features
Probable TSC   1 secondary plus 1 tertiary feature or 3
  tertiary features
Suspect TSC   1 secondary feature or 2 tertiary features

From Roach ES, Smith M, Huttenlocher P, et al. Report of the
Diagnostic Criteria Committee of the National Tuberous Sclerosis Asso-
ciation. *J Child Neurol* 1992;7:221–224. Reprinted with permission from
B.C. Decker, Inc.
  Abbreviation: TSC, tuberous sclerosis complex.
  °Histologic confirmation is not required *if* the lesion is clinically ob-
vious.

clinic patients who had died of complications of the disease. Nine additional patients had died of unrelated diseases. The commonest single cause of death, in 11 of 40,
was renal complications, including renal failure, bleeding
angiomyolipoma, and renal cell carcinoma. Brain abnormalities directly or indirectly led to almost half of the
deaths. Ten patients died from brain tumors (known or
presumed to be subependymal giant cell astrocytoma)
or complications of treatment for brain tumor. Thirteen
additional patients with severe mental retardation died
of status epilepticus or bronchopneumonia. Thus, brain
tumors or seizures pose significant risks to patients with

TS complex. Cardiac causes, including cardiac rhabdomyoma and ruptured thoracic aortic aneurysm, occurred in
infants or children, and lymphangiomyomatosis of the
lung caused death only in patients 40 years old or older.
The findings emphasize the potential value of detecting
and treating CNS complications in TS complex.

Central Nervous System Manifestations

The lesions of TS in the brain include cortical, white
matter, and subependymal hamartomas and subependymal giant cell ependymomas. MRI is the single most
sensitive imaging technique, but CT can also be helpful,
especially because of the high frequency of calcifications.
Histologically, these all consist of abnormal, large cells
with astrocytic and neuronal features.[158]
   Hamartomas occur commonly in the brain of TS patients in a subependymal location (up to 95% of patients).
These nodules occur most commonly along the ventricular surface of the caudate nucleus, especially along the
striothalamic groove just posterior to the foramen of
Monro. They also occur elsewhere in the ventricular system. Initially isodense to brain on CT, they often calcify
with increasing age (Figs. 51–21 and 51–22).[150] On both
CT and MRI, the nodules protrude into the ventricle. In
infants, the signal intensity of subependymal nodules is
higher than that of brain on T1-weighted images and
lower on T2-weighted images (Fig. 51–22). Signal intensity becomes closer to that of white matter as myelination
progresses. Signal intensity on T2-weighted images may
be heterogeneous. Densely calcified nodules demonstrate
low signal intensity on MRI, especially on gradient-recall
sequences (Fig. 51–23).[59, 83, 159–162] Multiple calcified
subependymal nodules on CT constitute one of the

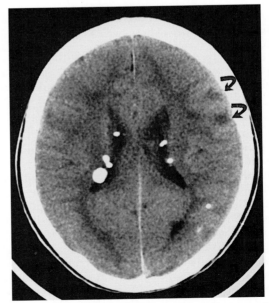

FIGURE 51–21 Calcified hamartomas in tuberous sclerosis.
Non–contrast-enhanced CT scan shows multiple periventricular
calcifications and left posterior peripheral calcifications in
hamartomas. Low-density cortical tubers (*arrows*) are present
in the left frontal lobe.

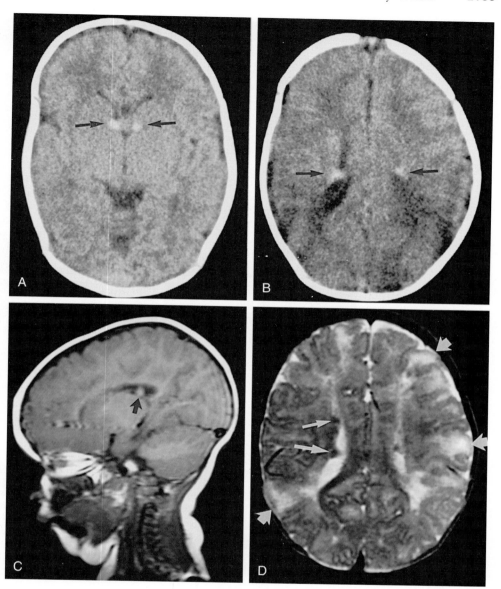

FIGURE 51–22 Tuberous sclerosis. *A* and *B,* Non–contrast-enhanced CT images of an infant demonstrate foci of increased density at the foramina of Monro and along the ependyma of the lateral ventricles consistent with subependymal nodules *(arrows)*. *C,* T1-weighted MRI study of the same patient obtained at age 1.5 years demonstrates the nodules are isointense with brain *(arrow)*. *D,* T2-weighted MRI study demonstrates multiple, nearly isointense nodules *(long arrows)* as well as several gyri that are expanded by hyperintense tubers *(short arrows)*.

primary diagnostic features of TS complex and lead to a definitive diagnosis. Enhancement is variable on MRI, ranging from none to mild, but occasionally intense (Fig. 51–23).[83, 163, 164]

Cortical hamartomas are smooth, firm, raised nodules found in nearly all patients with TS. The name *tuberous sclerosis* derives from these tubers. The tubers contain giant cells with abnormal, mixed astrocytic and neuronal components and lack of a normal six-layered cortex. They are usually multiple and can occur throughout the cerebral cortex. The frontal lobe is the most common location, followed by parietal, occipital, and temporal lobes. Calcification also occurs with increasing age, with about 50% of TS complex patients reported to have calcified tubers by age 10 (see Figs. 51–21 through 51–23).[150] Unusual gyriform calcification has been reported in TS, simulating that of Sturge-Weber syndrome.[165] The presence of other features, such as subependymal nodules, should differentiate the two conditions. Broadening of the involved gyrus

is often demonstrable on both CT and MRI. Low attenuation within a broadened gyrus is seen in infants, but the attenuation approaches that of brain in older children and adults.

As with subependymal nodules, cortical tubers appear hyperintense to white matter on T1-weighted images and hypointense on T2-weighted images early in life. The pattern reverses as the brain myelinates, with decreased central signal intensity on T1-weighted images and increased intensity on T2-weighted images.[83, 160, 161, 163] This altered signal intensity usually appears immediately below the cortex, which has been referred to as a *gyral core* (Figs. 51–24 and 51–25).[162] Fluid-attenuated inversion recovery (FLAIR) sequences are sensitive for detection of TS lesions and are especially helpful for detection of subcortical and gyral core lesions (Fig. 51–25).[166] A central depression or umbilication is sometimes visible on MRI.[83] This umbilication is more common with increasing age, presumably because of atrophy and degeneration

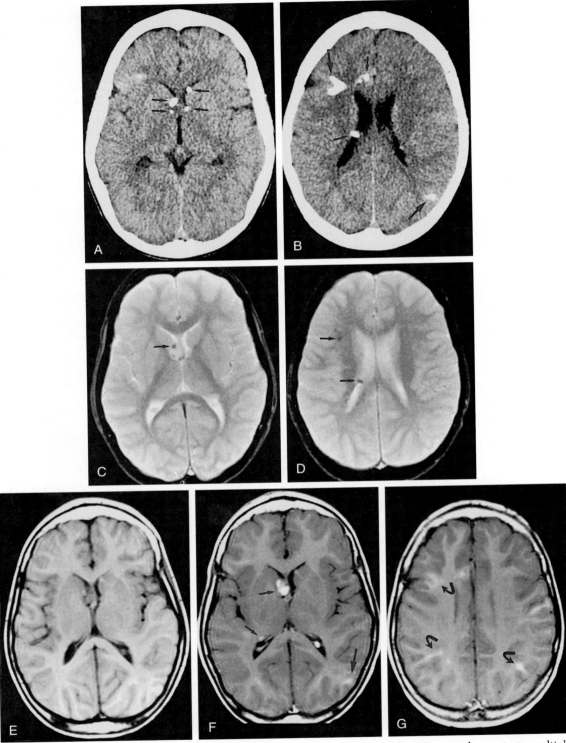

FIGURE 51–23 A 10-year-old with tuberous sclerosis. *A* and *B*, Non–contrast-enhanced CT images demonstrate multiple calcified subependymal nodules at the foramen of Monro and lining the ependymal surfaces of the lateral ventricles (*small arrows*) as well as some tubers with calcification (*large arrows* in *B*). *C* and *D*, T2-weighted MRI studies demonstrate some of the calcifications as focal hypointensities (*arrows*). *E*, T1-weighted MRI study demonstrates only the largest nodule as an isointense mass. *F* and *G*, Gadolinium-enhanced MRI studies demonstrate intense enhancement of the nodules (*small arrows* in *F*) as well as some enhancement of the tubers (*large arrows* in *F*). Enhancement of the tubers is an unusual finding, likely produced by degenerative changes, and when present is seen with calcification on CT. The enhancing nodule at the foramen of Monro (*small arrows* in *F*) could represent a subependymal giant cell astrocytoma, and follow-up MRI study is important. At a higher level, areas of white matter signal abnormality are visible (*curved arrows* in *G*).

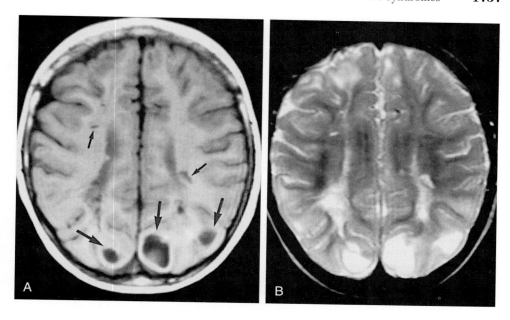

FIGURE 51–24 Cystic changes in tuberous sclerosis in a 4-year-old patient. T1-weighted (A) and T2-weighted (B) MRI studies demonstrate unusual, cystic-appearing cortical tubers with hypointense T1-weighted and hyperintense T2-weighted signal (*large arrows* in A). Small, cystlike regions are present in the white matter (*small arrows* in A). These small white matter cysts are relatively common; they may represent enlarged perivascular spaces or areas of degeneration.

within the tuber, and corresponds to the type 2 tubers described by Pellizzi.[7, 167] Tubers with a smooth surface are Pellizzi type 1. The distinction has no known clinical significance.

Calcification can lead to low signal intensity or a heterogeneous appearance. High signal intensity on T1-weighted images can also accompany calcification. A small proportion of tubers can appear cystic on MRI (see Fig. 51–24).[83] Enhancement can occur in degenerated cortical tubers (<5%).[83] When it occurs, enhancement is usually nodular, with gyral enhancement rarely observed.[83, 168] Cerebellar hamartomas occur in about 10% of patients and have a similar imaging appearance to cortical tubers.[83, 150] CT is more limited for the detection of cerebel-

lar lesions because of the usual artifacts that occur in the posterior fossa. Nuclear medicine studies with technetium 99m hexamethylpropyleneamineoxime single-photon emission computed tomography show less uptake in cortical tubers than in normal cortex,[169] and positron emission tomography (PET) studies have shown decreased metabolism of tubers.[170]

In addition to subependymal nodules and cortical tubers, similar regions containing disordered cells also occur in the white matter. When large enough, these regions can be identified on CT and MRI (see Figs. 51–23 and 51–25). They demonstrate low density on CT unless calcified. Signal characteristics are generally similar to those of cortical tubers. They can be linear, wedge-

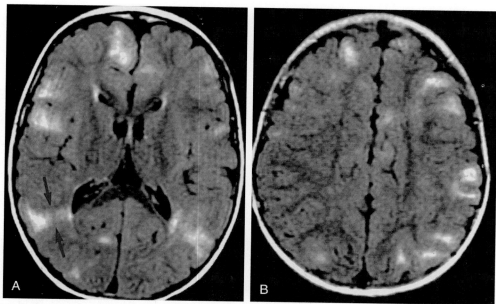

FIGURE 51–25 Fluid-attenuated inversion recovery (FLAIR) imaging of tuberous sclerosis. A and B, FLAIR sequence highlights the gyral core of the cortical tubers as bright areas. A white matter band is visible extending from the cortex to the periventricular region (*arrows* in B).

shaped, or more conglomerate. In older patients, they are most easily seen as high-signal-intensity lesions on T2-weighted sequences.[83, 160, 161, 163] White matter lesions can occur uncommonly in the cerebellum. A small percentage of white lesions can enhance. A radial pattern of linear or curvilinear signal abnormality is often seen extending from the cortex through the white matter to the periventricular region.[83, 171, 172] This pattern is likely to reflect the underlying abnormality of TS in the brain.

It has been hypothesized that dysplastic stem cells early in development in TS result in abnormal differentiation and myelination.[158, 173–175] This can result in abnormal cells along the pathway from the germinal matrix to the cortex, and a radial pattern is sometimes seen (see Fig. 51–25). The giant cells within TS lesions of the brain can have features of primitive neurons, astrocytes, or a spectrum of intermediate or undecided forms. The cells are 5 to 10 times the size of normal astrocytes.[158] The relationship of the subependymal nodules to the germinal matrix also suggests disordered cell maturation.

In addition to the abnormalities described previously, small cystlike structures are present in the cerebral white matter in a significant number of TS complex patients.[176] These are isointense or isodense with cerebrospinal fluid and occur in periatrial white matter, corpus callosum, or elsewhere in the deep white matter. The cause is unknown (see Fig. 51–24).[176]

Subependymal giant cell astrocytomas are histologically benign neoplasms that for all practical purposes occur only in TS.[126, 177–179] Microscopic features of these tumors are the same as subependymal nodules, that is, giant cells with features of both astrocytes and neurons.[158] They do not seed the cerebrospinal fluid or spread hematogenously. The location of giant cell astrocytomas is characteristically adjacent to the foramen of Monro.[83, 180] Despite the benign histology and slow growth, these neoplasms often cause obstruction of the ventricular system because of their location. They are a cause of significant morbidity in TS (about 25% of deaths).[157] Age at presentation is usually between 8 and 18 years, but the tumors have been found as early as in neonates and as late as age 40.[181, 182] Incidence of subependymal giant cell

ependymomas in TS is 5% to 15%.[83, 150] Recurrence is uncommon after complete resection.[183]

Small subependymal giant cell astrocytomas may be difficult to differentiate from subependymal hamartomas. Enhancement is more common in subependymal giant cell astrocytomas, occurring in nearly all, than in subependymal nodules. Calcification is common in both. Signal intensity on MRI is often heterogeneous in subependymal giant cell astrocytomas, although in general the characteristics are parallel to tubers and hamartomas (Fig. 51–26). Prominent flow voids are sometimes seen, and intratumoral hemorrhage can also occasionally be identified.[83] The key imaging feature of subependymal giant cell astrocytomas is growth. An enhancing lesion near the foramen of Monro in TS complex should be followed with serial scans to evaluate for interval growth or obstruction of the lateral ventricle. One or both ventricles may be obstructed. Infrequently, degeneration into an infiltrating or more aggressive neoplasm can occur.[177, 180] Mild ventriculomegaly without evidence of obstruction is seen in about 25% of TS patients. Possible causes include atrophy, dysgenesis, or repeated transient hypoxia associated with seizures.[83]

There is a relationship between the amount of tissue abnormality detected on imaging studies of the brain and clinical manifestations.[184, 185] An evaluation of 34 children with TS found more abnormal electroencephalogram foci in those with more intermediate and large cortical tubers, although the overall number of lesions did not correlate.[186] In another, larger group of patients, early onset of seizures and mental impairment were both more likely in those with more lesions detected on MRI.[187] Other authors found no correlation between neurologic findings and tuber number, size, and location, but only five patients were studied.[166]

The cerebral lesions of TS consist of disordered collections of giant cells with features of both neurons and astrocytes, occurring in the periventricular region, especially near the origin of the germinal matrix, in the cortex, and in the white matter between. Subependymal tumors have the same histologic characteristics and cause symptoms by growth and obstruction of the ventricles. Imaging

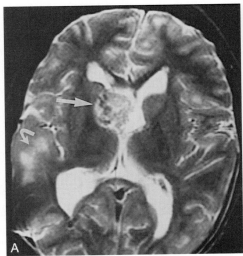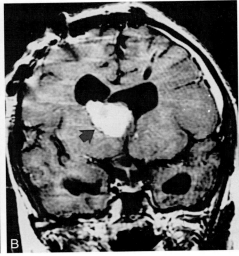

FIGURE 51–26 Subependymal giant cell astrocytoma in tuberous sclerosis complex. *A,* T2-weighted MRI study shows a heterogeneous mass (*straight arrow*) at the foramen of Monro. A cortical tuber is visible on the right (*curved arrow*), and there is signal void posterior to the tuber from a ventricular shunt catheter. *B,* Coronal contrast-enhanced T1-weighted MRI study shows intense contrast enhancement in the mass (*arrow*). (*A* and *B,* From Hart BL, Benzel EC, Ford CC. Fundamentals of Neuroimaging. Philadelphia, WB Saunders, 1997.)

characteristics of all of these lesions are similar but show some variation depending largely on the amount of calcification and enhancement present. Before the brain is myelinated, the hamartomatous areas are hyperintense on T1-weighted MRI and hypointense on T2-weighted MRI; the pattern tends to reverse after myelination of normal brain. Any of the lesions can calcify or show enhancement with MRI, but the subependymal nodules are especially prone to calcification.

Ocular Manifestations

The phakoma of TS complex was the source of the term *phakomatoses* in reference to neurocutaneous syndromes.[2, 28] It is an elevated lesion on or near the optic nerve, often described as *mulberry-like*. Histologically, this retinal hamartoma consists of fibrous astrocytes in a meshwork with large blood vessels, often with hyaline and calcium deposits.[117] Initially nearly flat and whitish, they become nodular and yellow or grayish in color. They consist of astrocytic proliferations. They are often multiple and bilateral. Calcified hamartomas are sometimes visible on CT.[149, 188, 189] Retinal hamartomas are usually asymptomatic unless they involve the macula or cause vitreous hemorrhage (Fig. 51–27).[190] They may produce leukocoria.[191]

Visceral Manifestations

Hamartomas characteristically occur in other organs in TS, some of which can also cause morbidity. Renal angio-

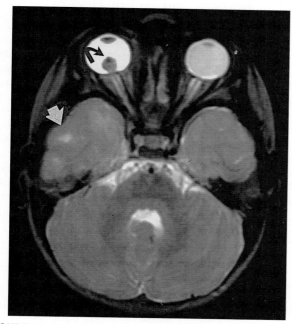

FIGURE 51–27 Retinal phakoma with hemorrhage. T2-weighted axial MRI study of a 2-year-old boy with a history of cardiac rhabdomyoma at birth, typical cortical tubers and subependymal nodules, and decreased vision. A retinal phakoma in the right globe has hemorrhaged (*black arrow*), an unusual complication of retinal hamartomas. High signal intensity of cortical tubers is visible in the anterior temporal lobe (*white arrow*).

myolipomas occur in 40% to 80% of patients with TS.[158, 192] These are not unique to TS complex. Sporadically occurring renal angiomyolipomas are seen most often in middle-aged women. Of all patients with angiomyolipomas, about half have TS. Renal angiomyolipomas are frequently bilateral and multiple in TS complex patients and usually solitary in sporadic cases. Clinical manifestations are quite variable. Many are asymptomatic, but they can cause bleeding, pain, or a palpable mass. Renal cysts are also common.[193, 194]

As the name suggests, renal angiomyolipomas typically contain vascular, smooth muscle, and fatty components. This heterogeneity is reflected on imaging studies. When fat is present, it causes a characteristic appearance on ultrasound, CT, or MRI studies. Sometimes there is minimal or no lipomatous component, however, in which case the lesions are much more nonspecific in appearance.

Renal cysts are common in TS complex. Severe cystic disease is more common in children than in adults and may lead to hypertension and renal failure. Rarely, renal cell cancer has occurred in TS complex, although it is not generally considered a cancer syndrome.[195–197]

Cardiac rhabdomyomas occur in up to two-thirds of patients with TS.[198] They can cause arrhythmias or obstruction, and they occur in all portions of the heart. They tend to regress with age.[158, 199] Embolization to the brain may rarely result.

Malformation of the lung, lymphangioleiomyomatosis, is uncommon in TS, occurring in fewer than 1% of patients.[158] The incidence is five times greater in females.[200] Histologically, there is hamartomatous proliferation of smooth muscle along the airways, resulting in parenchymal cystic changes and airway obliteration. Respiratory insufficiency, recurrent pneumothorax, and cor pulmonale can result. Lymphangioleiomyomatosis occurs sporadically in women of child-bearing age as well as in TS patients of both sexes, and progressive disease usually ends in respiratory failure.[201–204] Radiographically the disease appears as a coarse reticulonodular pattern early, with honeycombing a later manifestation. Therapeutic approaches have included hormonal treatment and lung transplantation.[205]

Bone findings in TS complex include sclerotic bone islands in the diploic space of the skull, flat bones of the pelvis, and spine. In the extremities, there are cystic changes in the phalanges, more often in the hands, and periosteal new bone formation, more often in the feet.[96, 158] Vascular disease has been reported in association with TS, including aortic aneurysm formation and occlusion resulting in a moyamoya pattern.[206, 207] Other visceral hamartomas in TS complex occur in the liver, pancreas, and spleen.

Recommendations for Screening Imaging Studies in Tuberous Sclerosis Complex

Imaging studies have a central role in the diagnosis of TS complex as discussed earlier. Screening examinations after diagnosis may be beneficial to detect subependymal giant cell astrocytomas before they cause serious complications. Screening with contrast-enhanced CT or MRI every 1 to

2 years during the peak ages of tumor presentation, from 8 to 18 years of age, has been suggested.[70, 208] MRI is more sensitive and has the advantage of avoiding repeated exposure to ionizing radiation.

VON HIPPEL–LINDAU DISEASE

von Hippel–Lindau disease is a condition of autosomal dominant inheritance that has as the most prominent features multiple CNS hemangioblastomas and a high risk of renal cell carcinoma. Retinal hemangioblastomas are also common in this disorder. von Hippel first described the retinal *angioma* that is a feature of this disease, and Lindau described the cerebellar tumor and recognized the association of eye and brain findings. von Hippel–Lindau disease was classified as one of the phakomatoses by Van der Hoeve.[3] Despite the CNS and ocular abnormalities, however, it differs from other phakomatoses in that it does not have cutaneous findings.[209] Another name for von Hippel–Lindau disease is *CNS angiomatosis*, referring to the multiple vascular tumors, hemangioblastomas, that occur.

Genetics

The von Hippel–Lindau disease gene on chromosome 3p (3p25-26) was cloned in 1993.[210] The function of the von Hippel–Lindau disease gene protein (pVHL) is hypothesized to relate, in part, to vasculogenesis.[209] von Hippel–Lindau disease follows an autosomal dominant pattern of inheritance, and von Hippel–Lindau disease gene mutations are identifiable in approximately in 80% of kindreds.[209] Commercial laboratories offer the gene test. A phenotype-genotype correlation exists for von Hippel–Lindau disease families, which may present with or without pheochromocytoma. Families with pheochromocytoma tend to have missense mutations, and those without tend to have deletions and protein-truncation mutations.[209] There is no racial or sexual predilection. The prevalence is approximately 1 per 35,000 to 40,000.[211, 212] About 1% to 3% of cases are thought to arise from new mutations.[210, 213] Despite the low overall rate of new mutations, a number of patients have no previously documented family history. It is likely that in many of these cases, there is an asymptomatic parent. Careful screening often discloses evidence of von Hippel–Lindau disease even in asymptomatic individuals.[211, 214, 215]

The von Hippel–Lindau disease gene is a tumor-suppressor gene. Absence or dysfunction of this gene predisposes to development of tumors. The *two-hit* hypothesis of cancer production postulates that both copies of a tumor-suppressor gene must be lost for cancer to develop in a tissue.[216] In diseases such as von Hippel–Lindau disease, one copy of the gene, the germ line mutation, is defective throughout the body. If the second copy becomes defective or lost in the somatic line in a target organ, that organ is susceptible to tumor formation. Target tissues in von Hippel–Lindau disease include those of the CNS, including cerebellum, retina, and spinal cord; those of neural crest origin; kidney; and pancreas.

Genetic analysis enables identification of some individuals with von Hippel–Lindau disease. If the specific mutation in a family is known, direct DNA analysis can be performed in a suspected individual. In other cases, linkage analysis for nearby flanking markers makes disease identification likely. Because at least two known family members must be used for linkage tests, in some cases this analysis is not possible.[217] Because DNA diagnosis may not be feasible in all cases, imaging plays an important role in diagnosis of the disease as well as monitoring disease in identified patients.

The National Cancer Institute has proposed a classification system that recognizes three distinct phenotypes, based on the various combinations of hemangioblastomas plus pheochromocytomas, renal cancers, and pancreatic disease (Table 51–4).[212, 214] Details are presented in following sections.

Diagnostic Criteria

Clinical criteria for diagnosis of the disease remain important. There are no strict criteria for diagnosis of the disease. It has been proposed by Maher and coworkers,[215] however, that more than one CNS hemangioblastoma, one hemangioblastoma plus visceral manifestations, or one CNS or visceral manifestation in a patient with a family member known to have von Hippel–Lindau disease are considered diagnostic. von Hippel–Lindau disease should be suspected in any individual with hemangioblastoma of the retina or CNS, familial or bilateral pheochromocytomas, bilateral endolymphatic sac tumors, or renal cell carcinoma of early onset.[207]

Clinical Findings and Natural History

Diagnosis of von Hippel–Lindau disease is uncommon in the first decade of life. Retinal hemangioblastomas are the most common initial manifestation, with a mean age in the 20s. Cerebellar hemangioblastomas usually present slightly later, and renal cell carcinoma is the most common initial manifestation in older patients. The risk of all of these tumors continues throughout life.[214] Careful screening of elderly asymptomatic known bearers of von Hippel–Lindau disease mutations can reveal unsuspected tumors and cysts in many.[211, 214] In a large population study from Great Britain, Maher and coworkers[215] studied 152 patients with von Hippel–Lindau disease. The initial manifestation was retinal hemangioblastoma in 43%, cere-

TABLE 51–4 National Cancer Institute Classification of von Hippel–Lindau Disease*

Type I.	von Hippel–Lindau disease without pheochromocytomas
Type II.	von Hippel–Lindau disease with pheochromocytomas
	A. Pheochromocytomas and retinal and CNS hemangioblastomas
	B. Pheochromocytomas, retinal and CNS hemangioblastomas, renal cancers, and pancreatic involvement

Abbreviation: CNS, central nervous system.
*The three phenotypes are listed in decreasing order of frequency.

bellar hemangioblastoma in 39%, and renal cell carcinoma in 10%. Many patients develop more than one complication. The cumulative risk of developing complications by age 60 was retinal hemangioblastoma, 0.7; cerebellar hemangioblastoma, 0.84; and renal cell carcinoma, 0.69. Overall frequency of major complications in this group plus 554 previously reported cases, a total of 706 patients, was retinal hemangioblastoma, 58%; cerebellar hemangioblastoma, 56%; spinal cord hemangioblastoma, 14%; renal cell carcinoma, 25%; and pheochromocytoma, 17%.[215, 217] The most common causes of death are complications of cerebellar hemangioblastoma and metastatic renal cell carcinoma.[218]

Clinical manifestations of hemangioblastomas include headache, vomiting, vertigo, and other posterior fossa symptoms. Often, there is sudden worsening of slowly progressive symptoms. Up to half of patients have hydrocephalus resulting from an obstructing tumor.[212] Solid tumors have been reported in one series to have more complications and a poorer prognosis than cystic tumors.[219]

Within individual families carrying the genetic mutation, disease patterns vary, especially with respect to the incidence of pheochromocytoma. Among all patients with von Hippel–Lindau disease, 7% to 18% have been reported to have pheochromocytoma.[214, 215, 220] The prevalence can be high (>50%) among certain families.[221, 222] The disease tends to present at an early age in these patients, but the overall morbidity is lower because of lower frequency of hemangioblastoma and renal cell carcinoma.[214] The National Cancer Institute classification phenotypes of von Hippel–Lindau disease is listed in Table 51–4. The two types of NF, NF-1 and NF-2, are actually entirely different diseases caused by mutations on different chromosomes, but the subtypes of von Hippel–Lindau disease, I, IIa, and IIb, are different phenotypes of the same disease, presumably resulting from different mutations within the same gene.

Considerably less morbidity is caused by other visceral manifestations of von Hippel–Lindau disease. Cysts within the pancreas are often found on screening studies and occasionally cause obstruction in critical locations. Nearly complete replacement of the pancreas or kidneys can cause organ failure. Endolymphatic sac tumors present with hearing loss, vertigo, or facial nerve paralysis. Islet cell tumors of the pancreas, although usually asymptomatic, can cause endocrinopathies or obstruction and can metastasize.[217]

Central Nervous System Hemangioblastoma

von Hippel–Lindau disease is manifested in the CNS by the occurrence of one or more hemangioblastomas, most commonly in the cerebellum. Hemangioblastomas are histologically benign neoplasms that contain prominent vascular components lined by cuboidal epithelial cells, amid lipid-laden stromal cells and pericytes. Mast cells are sometimes present and may be the source of erythropoietin.[223]

Cystic components are common. Microcysts are characteristic, and macroscopic collections of fluid are seen in roughly two-thirds of cases. In about one-third of cases, an intensely enhancing mural nodule is visible adjacent to or within a proteinaceous cyst (Fig. 51–28). About one-third of CNS hemangiomas appear solid on CT or MRI, and the remainder have combinations of solid and cystic components (Fig. 51–29).[95] The cyst wall in cases with a

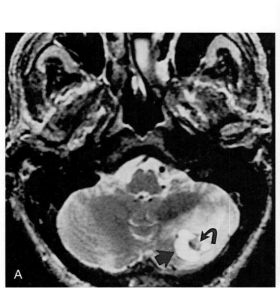 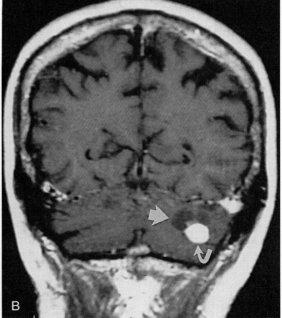

FIGURE 51–28 Hemangioblastoma, typical cystic appearance. *A,* Axial T2-weighted MRI study shows a left cerebellar hemisphere mass with cyst (*straight arrow*) and mural nodular mass (*curved arrow*). *B,* Coronal gadolinium-enhanced MRI study shows the cyst (*straight arrow*) and intense enhancement of the nodule (*curved arrow*).

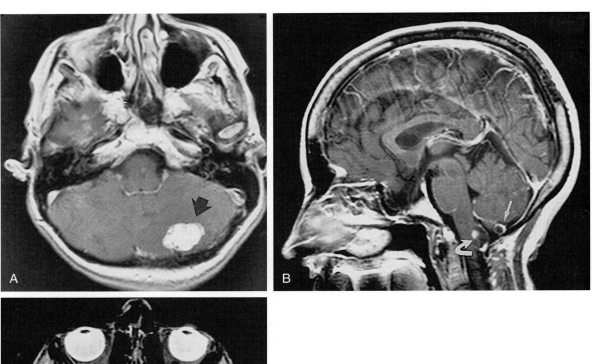

FIGURE 51–29 von Hippel–Lindau disease. *A* and *B*, Gadolinium-enhanced T1-weighted MRI studies demonstrate multiple enhancing well-defined masses in the cerebellar hemisphere, tonsil, and cervicomedullary junction (*arrows*) consistent with hemangioblastomas. The larger cerebellar lesions appear solid, whereas small cystic areas are seen in the tonsillar and cord lesions. *C*, T2-weighted MRI study demonstrates edema surrounding the larger left hemispheric lesion, which itself is hyperintense (*long arrow*), as well as an additional, smaller lesion of the right cerebellar hemisphere (*short arrow*).

single, large cyst is not neoplastic but consists of compressed tissue of the adjacent brain or reactive cells.[126, 224–226] Cysts or necrosis can also occur within the tumor, in which case the surrounding wall enhances. A mural nodule in a cyst cavity often lies adjacent to a pial surface. Completely solid tumors have been reported in 20% to 40% of tumors.[126, 212, 225, 227, 228] The hemangioblastoma cysts contain solute levels similar to blood, suggesting that they arise from diffusion from the vascular component of the tumor.[229]

A significant minority of hemangioblastomas (5% to 40%) secrete erythropoietin, which can cause polycythemia.[214, 225] Polycythemia has been reported more commonly to accompany solid tumors.[126, 225, 226, 230] The polycythemia resolves after surgical resection of the tumor. Erythrocytosis is apparently not a feature of solitary spinal hemangioblastomas.[223]

The characteristic vascularity of hemangioblastoma can be a helpful feature on both cross-sectional imaging and angiography (Fig. 51–30). Feeding or draining vessels can sometimes be identified on cross-sectional imaging. Low-signal-intensity foci on MRI can be due to flow void or hemosiderin deposition from prior internal hemorrhage. Earlier stages of hemorrhage may cause an appearance similar to cavernous angioma. Angiography can be helpful for preoperative planning, especially because of the highly vascular nature of the tumors. Hemangioblastomas typically cause a dense blush on angiography, often with early venous drainage.

The proteinaceous nature of the cyst fluid causes increased attenuation on CT and higher signal intensity on MRI than cerebrospinal fluid. The tumor nodule or solid tumor of hemangioblastoma is usually isodense to brain on CT and demonstrates intense contrast enhancement. The solid portion of the tumor also shows intense enhancement on MRI after gadolinium administration.

Hemangioblastomas are not unique to von Hippel–Lindau disease, and sporadically occurring hemangioblas-

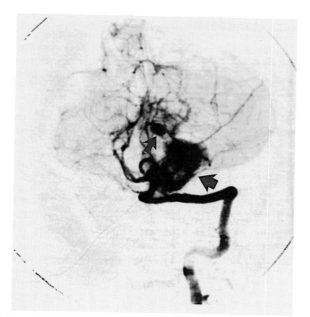

FIGURE 51–30 von Hippel–Lindau disease. Anteroposterior digital subtraction angiogram of left vertebral artery injection demonstrates intense vascularity of masses (*arrows*) during the early arterial phase, consistent with multiple hemangioblastomas.

TABLE 51–5 Suggested Clinical Diagnostic Criteria for von Hippel–Lindau Disease

>1 CNS hemangioblastoma *or*
1 hemangioblastoma plus 1 visceral manifestation° *or*
1 hemangioblastoma or 1 visceral manifestation° in a patient with a first-degree relative known to have von Hippel–Lindau disease

Abbreviation: CNS, central nervous system.
°Renal cysts, despite being especially prevalent in von Hippel–Lindau disease, are not considered without other visceral manifestations because they are so common in the general population.

tomas are histologically identical to those in von Hippel–Lindau disease. Approximately 10% to 20% of patients found to have one CNS hemangioblastoma have von Hippel–Lindau disease.[126, 212, 215, 226, 231] Careful evaluation of patients found to have hemangioblastoma may disclose an even higher proportion with other evidence of von Hippel–Lindau disease.[213] More than one hemangioblastoma has been considered diagnostic of von Hippel–Lindau disease (Table 51–5; Figs. 51–29 through 51–31). Evaluation of large numbers of cases of hemangioblastoma confirm this clinical criterion; multiple tumors were found in 42% of patients with known genetic carrier status and none of the patients without von Hippel–Lindau disease.[232] The mean age for diagnosis of CNS hemangioblastoma is younger in patients with von Hippel–Lindau disease (mean age in the 30s) than in sporadically occurring tumors (1 to 2 decades older).[212, 213, 228, 231] Prognosis of hemangioblastoma is also worse with von Hippel–Lindau disease.[215, 223]

The most common location for hemangioblastomas in von Hippel–Lindau disease is the cerebellum, followed by the spinal cord and brain stem. Approximately 75% to 80% of hemangioblastomas are detected in the cerebellum, where they constitute 7% to 12% of all posterior fossa tumors and 2% of all brain tumors.[126, 212, 214, 228] Brain

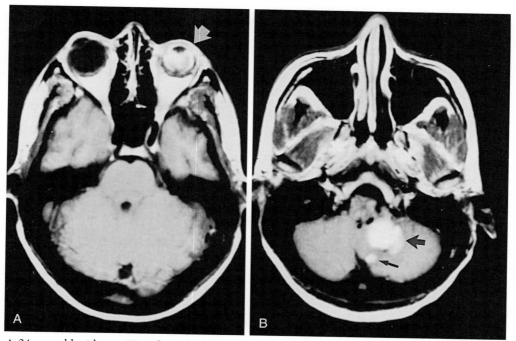

FIGURE 51–31 A 24-year-old with von Hippel–Lindau disease. *A*, T1-weighted MRI study demonstrates hyperintensity in the left globe (*arrow*) produced by subacute hemorrhage from a retinal hemangioblastoma. *B*, More inferiorly located MRI study with gadolinium demonstrates two enhancing solid hemangioblastomas (*arrows*).

stem hemangioblastomas are less common (about 5% of all cases). They occur in the area postrema on the dorsal medulla.[214] Supratentorial hemangioblastomas are rare.

Spinal cord hemangioblastomas are reported in 10% to 30% of cases, with more detected when extensive MRI screening is used.[214, 215, 232] The craniocervical junction and conus medullaris are especially common locations, but hemangioblastomas can occur throughout the spinal cord as well as nerve roots and cauda equina.[232] Severe involvement of the spinal cord and brain stem, essentially replacing the cord, has been reported in von Hippel–Lindau disease.[233] Spinal and medullary hemangioblastomas are associated with greater morbidity than cerebellar lesions.[212, 228] The association with von Hippel–Lindau disease is much higher (80%) in spinal hemangioblastomas than with cerebellar hemangioblastomas.[214] Cysts with enhancing mural nodules are a common appearance, and syringomyelia can also occur.

Endolymphatic Sac Tumors

Endolymphatic sac tumors are locally aggressive but slow-growing tumors thought to originate from the endolymphatic sac, in the posteromedial petrous temporal bone. There is a characteristic papillary adenomatous architecture. The tumors are often polypoid and may spread to the cerebellopontine angle and posterior fossa, to the middle ear and external auditory canal, into the middle cranial fossa, or to the clivus and adjacent structures.[234] The tumors are generally low grade and without metastatic potential but are locally invasive. More than 50% of endolymphatic sac tumors are sporadic, but 15% or more occur in patients with von Hippel–Lindau disease.[234-238] Among patients with von Hippel–Lindau disease, endolymphatic sac tumors are seen in 10% or more.[239] It is likely that some von Hippel–Lindau patients reported to have metastatic renal cell carcinoma to the temporal bone and extraventricular choroid plexus papilloma actually had endolymphatic sac tumors; similar papillary architecture may be confusing.[234, 237, 240, 241] There is histologic similarity to papillary cystadenoma of the epididymis, which is also a feature of von Hippel–Lindau disease.[214]

Clinical history in all patients with endolymphatic sac tumors includes hearing loss, often for more than 10 years before diagnosis of tumor.[234, 239] Facial nerve paralysis, vertigo, and lower cranial nerve deficits can also occur. Average age at presentation is about 50 years, with a range of 36 to 71 years.[234] Endolymphatic sac tumors should be included in the differential diagnosis of sudden hearing loss and in the differential diagnosis of cerebellopontine angle masses. Hearing loss also occurs in many patients with von Hippel–Lindau disease without radiographic evidence of endolymphatic sac tumors.[239]

The tumors can be seen on MRI as enhancing masses with an epicenter along the posterior margin of the petrous temporal bone (Fig. 51–32). Nonenhancing cystic or necrotic regions may be present, and hemorrhage or proteinaceous contents can result in high signal intensity on T1-weighted images.[242] Bone erosion can be seen on CT (Fig. 51–32).[238, 243] Extension can take place along any of the four directions described previously.

Ocular Manifestations

Retinal hemangioblastomas, the lesions that led to van der Hoeve's classifying von Hippel–Lindau disease with the phakomatoses, are histologically identical to hemangioblastomas elsewhere in the CNS. More than half of patients with von Hippel–Lindau disease have retinal hemangioblastomas, and many have bilateral tumors.[212, 215, 227, 231] Hemangioblastomas are raised masses with a dilated artery and draining vein.[92] They are most often peripheral in the retina but can involve the optic disk. Complications include visual loss from large lesions, exudation of fluid, hemorrhage, retinal detachment, glaucoma, uveitis, cataract, and sympathetic ophthalmitis (see Fig. 51–31).[214, 244] Laser photocoagulation is useful for preventing blindness, and screening is therefore advisable. Large lesions may be visible on contrast-enhanced MRI or CT, but ophthalmoscopy and fluorescein angiography are the best methods for detection of small hemangioblastomas.[245] Optic nerve hemangioblastomas have also been reported as a cause of blindness in von Hippel–Lindau disease.[245]

Visceral Manifestations

Visceral manifestations of von Hippel–Lindau disease include renal carcinoma, pheochromocytoma, renal and pancreatic cysts, islet cell tumors, and papillary cystadenoma of the epididymis and broad ligament. As previously discussed, identified subgroups of families with von Hippel–Lindau disease differ with respect to visceral manifestations (see Table 51–4).

Renal cell carcinoma is a significant risk in von Hippel–Lindau disease. It is reported in 24% to 45% of patients with the disease.[211, 215, 227] Although retinal and cerebellar hemangioblastomas usually present at an earlier age, renal cell carcinoma in von Hippel–Lindau disease presents about 20 years earlier on average than sporadic renal cell carcinoma.[213, 246] Renal cell carcinoma has been reported as early as 15 years of age, and the risk continues throughout life.[214] Multiple and bilateral tumors are common. Renal cell carcinoma has been reported as the cause of death of one-third or more of patients with von Hippel–Lindau disease.[215, 217, 220, 247] CT is highly sensitive and is the preferred test for screening, although ultrasound and MRI can have supplemental roles.[214]

Renal cysts occur in a large number of von Hippel–Lindau patients, from 60% to 80%.[228] These cysts are often complex, and the relationship with carcinoma is unclear. In some cases, tumors may arise from the cells lining the cyst wall, and all renal cysts in von Hippel–Lindau disease should be regarded with some suspicion and evaluated carefully.[214] Simple cysts carry little risk, but even small solid components can develop into tumors.[228]

Pheochromocytomas and pancreatic islet cell tumors are features of type II von Hippel–Lindau disease but not of type I. Within some families, pheochromocytoma has been found in more than half of the members.[221, 222] In comparison with sporadic pheochromocytomas, familial cases are more often multiple, bilateral, and ectopic to the adrenal gland.[213] Paragangliomas with the same histol-

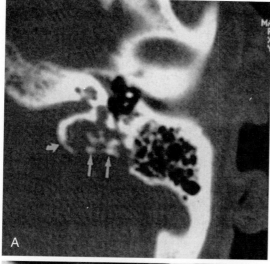

FIGURE 51–32 Endolymphatic sac tumor. *A,* Non–contrast-enhanced CT scan shows retrolabyrinthine bone destruction, intratumoral bone spicules (*straight arrows*), and a peripheral rim of calcification (*curved arrow*) from the expanded cortical margin of the petrous temporal bone. MRI studies of a different patient, before (*B*) and after (*C*) gadolinium administration, show multiple areas of increased signal intensity within the tumor (*B*). Flow void (*arrows*) demonstrates hypervascular nature of the tumor. *C,* Intense contrast enhancement is visible. (*A–C,* From Mukherji SK, Albernaz VS, Lo WWM, et al. Papillary endolymphatic sac tumors: CT, MR imaging, and angiographic findings in 20 patients. Radiology 1997;202:801–808.)

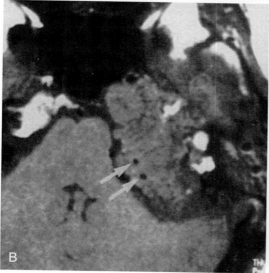 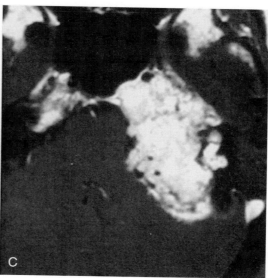

ogy as pheochromocytoma have been reported in the glomus jugulare, carotid body, organ of Zuckerkandl, spleen, kidney, and periaortic tissues.[214, 248] Metastasis can occur. Both adrenal and extra-adrenal tumors may be functional, producing catecholamines with associated signs and symptoms. Appropriate laboratory tests include serum and urinary levels of norepinephrine, epinephrine, and urinary vanillylmandelic acid. Because many pheochromocytomas in patients with von Hippel–Lindau disease are asymptomatic and do not have elevated catecholamine levels, imaging is important to detect these tumors.[214] CT, MRI, and radionuclide scintigraphy using metaiodobenzylguanidine can all be used. Nonionic iodinated contrast agents are preferred to ionic agents if CT is used because of the risk of catecholamine release.

Similar to pheochromocytomas, islet cell tumors are of neural crest origin. Symptoms arise from pancreatic obstruction or from hormone secretion. These tumors also can metastasize. Up to 20% of patients with type II von Hippel–Lindau disease develop islet cell tumors.[214]

Patients with von Hippel–Lindau disease are also prone to develop benign cysts and serous cystadenomas (microcystic adenomas) of the pancreas. Extensive cyst replacement can impair pancreatic exocrine function, and strategically located cysts can cause biliary obstruction. Adenocarcinomas of the pancreas and ampulla of Vater have been reported. Mucinous cystadenoma is not a feature of von Hippel–Lindau disease.[214]

Papillary cystadenomas of the epididymis are histologically similar to endolymphatic sac tumors. They occur in 10% to 26% of men with von Hippel–Lindau disease. The same tumor can rarely occur in the broad ligament in women, which is embryologically analogous to the epididymis.[214, 217, 220] Pulmonary and hepatic hemangioblastomas have rarely been reported in von Hippel–Lindau disease.[214]

Recommendations for Imaging in von Hippel–Lindau Disease

Recommendations have been made for screening patients with known or suspected von Hippel–Lindau disease (Table 51–6).[214] Although details of the scheduled examinations vary, regular tests should include MRI of the brain

TABLE 51–6 Screening Recommendations for von Hippel–Lindau Disease

Test	NIH	Cambridge, England	Hawaii
Urinary catecholamine	From age 2 yr: every 1–2 yr	Every year	At least once or if blood pressure is elevated
Ophthalmoscopy	From infancy: yearly	From age 5 yr: yearly	From age 6 yr: yearly
Fluorescein angioscopy	Not routine	Routine from age 10 yr: yearly	Not routine
Enhanced MRI of brain and spine	From age 11 yr: every 2 yr°; after age 60 yr: every 3–5 yr	From midteens: every 3 yr to age 50 yr then every 5 yr	Begin after age 20 yr, at least once per decade
Abdominal CT or ultrasound	From age 11 yr: yearly; from age 20 yr: CT yearly† or every other year‡ (ultrasound as needed to evaluate CT findings)	From midteens: ultrasound every year, CT every 3 yr	Begin age 15–20 yr, then ultrasound every year

From Choyke PL, Glenn GM, Wlather MM, et al. The natural history of renal lesions in von Hippel–Lindau disease: A serial CT study in 28 patients. AJR 1992;159:1229–1234.
°Examine middle ear for symptoms of hearing loss, tinnitus, or vertigo.
†After age 60 yr and still no evidence of von Hippel–Lindau disease, CT can be performed every 2 years with MRI of central nervous system.
‡Ultrasound annually at onset of puberty and during pregnancy.

and spine every 2 to 3 years, yearly ophthalmoscopy supplemented by fluorescein angiography in selected cases, and regular abdominal CT or ultrasound.

Neumann and colleagues[248] recommend screening all patients with pheochromocytomas for von Hippel–Lindau disease and multiple endocrine neoplasia type II. They found that a relatively high proportion of unselected patients with pheochromocytomas (19%) had von Hippel–Lindau disease. In addition, members of families with von Hippel–Lindau disease (and multiple endocrine neoplasia type II) should be screened for pheochromocytoma.[248] Because early diagnosis can lead to treatment that minimizes or avoids serious complications of the disease, it is important for radiologists to be familiar with the imaging findings of von Hippel–Lindau disease.

STURGE-WEBER SYNDROME AND RELATED CUTANEOUS CONDITIONS

Characterization of the phakomatoses that feature cutaneous vascular malformations is confounded by decades of confusion regarding the nomenclature used to describe them. Specifically, many authors have used the term *hemangiomas* to describe lesions that are actually vascular birthmarks and remain relatively static. In this chapter the nomenclature suggested by Mullikan and Young[249] is used whenever possible. A *hemangioma*, by definition, is a neoplasm of the vascular endothelium that typically proliferates then involutes. A *vascular malformation*, in contrast, is a congenital anomaly of the vascular system that does not proliferate or involute. The phakomatoses have a predominantly capillary vascular malformation component, but venous, arterial, or lymphatic vessels may also be involved.[250]

Sturge-Dimitri-Weber syndrome is an eponym for encephalotrigeminal angiomatosis, also known as *meningofacial angiomatosis*.[251] Principal features include a port wine stain capillary vascular malformation of the face and a leptomeningeal vascular anomaly that results in ischemia of the underlying cortex. Atrophy and calcification of the underlying cerebral cortex, hemiplegia, seizures, and glaucoma are common clinical features. Although there are not strict diagnostic criteria, it is generally agreed that the leptomeningeal venous malformation is the sine qua non of Sturge-Weber syndrome.

Embryology

In contrast to the previously discussed conditions, Sturge-Weber syndrome is almost always sporadic in occurrence. Although there have been a few reports of possible autosomal or autosomal recessive inheritance, most cases are not familial. The pathogenesis of Sturge-Weber syndrome is not completely understood. The defect most likely occurs at gestational weeks 4 to 8, when a primordial vascular mesenchyme lies adjacent to the neural tube and ectoderm that will overlie the head and face.[252] Abnormal development of the blood vessels at this time can thus ultimately affect both the skin and the brain and leptomeninges. A lack of differentiation of primitive vasculature into arteries, capillaries, and veins may result in a persistent, simple vascular pattern. Alternatively, others have hypothesized that the persistent primitive vascular plexus is a secondary result of impaired venous outflow caused by loss of normal connections between cortical veins and dural and calvarial circulation; that is, that the vascular plexus is a collateral channel.[28, 253, 254]

Practically speaking, regardless of the exact sequence of early embryologic defects, the consequences are clear and include the presence of a leptomeningeal angiomatous malformation that consists of simple vascular structures between the pia and arachnoid mater and a facial nevus. The venous drainage from the cerebral cortex is poor, and progressive cortical damage ensues.

Clinical Findings and Natural History

The port wine stain (*nevus flammeus*) of Sturge-Weber syndrome usually corresponds roughly to dermatomal distributions of the trigeminal nerve. Nearly all Sturge-Weber syndrome patients have involvement of the V1 distribution, especially the upper eyelid. Lower facial

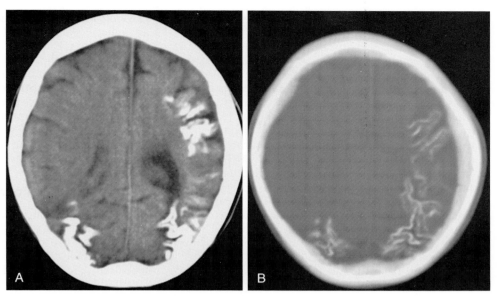

FIGURE 51–33 A 12-year-old boy with Sturge-Weber syndrome. Non–contrast-enhanced CT scan (A) demonstrates cortical calcification in the frontal and parietal lobes. The typical parallel, serpentine, *tram-track* appearance of the calcifications is best seen with bone window and level settings (B).

involvement is less common. Most cases have unilateral involvement, but bilateral facial nevi are not uncommon. Of all patients with facial port wine nevi, only 1% to 10% have Sturge-Weber syndrome with CNS involvement.[255–257] Those with upper eyelid involvement are much more likely to have eye and CNS disease as well. The nevus is typically a pink macule in infancy but darkens with age to a reddish purple. The dark color is attributed to deoxygenated blood within the telangiectatic vessels. The nevus often becomes raised by middle age as a result of progressive vascular ectasia. Laser therapy can be used effectively to treat the nevi.[224] The facial nevus can also extend into the mucosal surfaces and paranasal sinuses. Epistaxis has been linked to such mucosal involvement.[28]

Although classic Sturge-Weber syndrome involves only the face, cutaneous vascular malformations sometimes extend over the trunk and extremities as well. Some of these patients have Klippel-Trénaunay-Weber syndrome.

Up to 90% of patient with Sturge-Weber syndrome have generalized or partial seizures. The patients are usually neurologically intact at birth but develop seizure activity within the first year of life. Hypsarrhythmia is often found before generalized seizures. Developmental delay is common but not universal. Other patients may initially develop normally but lose milestones as ischemia or seizures become more significant. Hemiatrophy of the brain results in hemiparesis in about 30% of cases and, often, hemiatrophy of the contralateral extremities.[28, 258]

Central Nervous System Manifestations

The vascular malformation of Sturge-Weber syndrome is associated with impaired venous drainage and progressive ischemia of the underlying brain. The cortex gradually loses cells and calcifies, especially the middle layers 2 through 4.[95, 258] Calcification also occurs in subcortical white matter and in cerebral arterioles. Continued seizures may also contribute to metabolic damage. The result is progressive cortical atrophy and calcification.[28, 254]

The calcifications of the cortex can be identified early in life by CT but rarely at birth. The occipitoparietal region is most commonly involved, with more anterior involvement less common. Relative frequency of lobar involvement is a posterior-to-anterior pattern, occipital greater than parietal than temporal and frontal. Calcifications are usually unilateral, but bilateral involvement is seen in up 20% of cases (Fig. 51–33).[259] Skull radiographs show a tram-track appearance resulting from calcifications in apposing gyri separated by widened cerebrospinal fluid space (Fig. 51–34). Although tiny calcifications can occur in arterioles, these are far smaller than the cortical bands of calcification that are visualized by radiography and CT. CT can show some white matter calcification as well.[28, 254, 259–261] Calcifications appear as areas of low signal intensity

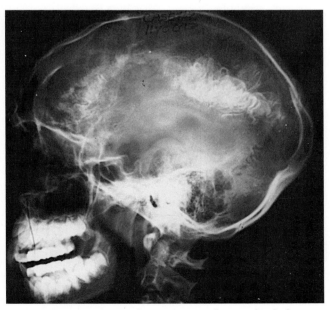

FIGURE 51–34 *Tram-track* appearance of cortical calcifications is apparent on lateral skull radiograph.

on MRI and are better detected with gradient-echo than spin-echo techniques.[262]

Despite less sensitivity for calcifications than CT, MRI has some advantages in evaluation of Sturge-Weber syndrome. Regional atrophy in Sturge-Weber syndrome is well demonstrated by MRI.[263, 264] White matter below the damaged cortex may show high signal intensity on long TR images as a result of ischemia and gliosis.[259, 265] Contrast-enhanced CT can show superficial meningeal enhancement, but subtle enhancement may be obscured near calcifications. Gadolinium-enhanced MRI is highly sensitive to meningeal enhancement, which often appears to fill the subarachnoid space (Fig. 51–35).[261, 266] The area of leptomeningeal angiomatosis shown by contrast-enhanced MRI can be larger than calcifications, which are a secondary phenomenon. Areas of thickened cortex with few sulci, presumed to represent migration abnormalities, have also been reported on MRI.[264]

The choroid plexus ipsilateral to the vascular malformation is often large, as a result of either hyperplasia or, less commonly, angiomatous involvement. Both CT and MRI demonstrate the enlarged choroid plexus (see Fig. 51–35). Enlarged deep perimedullary veins may also be seen on MRI.[267, 268]

With the availability of CT and MRI, angiography is not necessary now for diagnosis of Sturge-Weber syndrome. If used, angiography shows few or no cortical veins in the area of the malformation. There is poor transit and flow through the affected brain, with prominent but slow flow into the deep central veins.[267–270]

As with atrophy of other causes, Sturge-Weber syndrome can result in calvarial thickening and an enlarged diploic space on the side of atrophy, elevation of the petrous ridge and lesser wing of the sphenoid, and increased pneumatization of the paranasal sinuses. Dyke-Davidoff-Masson syndrome refers to these nonspecific, asymmetric skull findings that follow cerebral hemiatrophy.[271] Both CT and MRI demonstrate these changes. Enlargement of the skull on the side of the malformation resulting from a chronic subdural hematoma can be an unusual finding in Sturge-Weber syndrome.[272, 273] PET scanning usually shows the involved area in Sturge-Weber syndrome to be hypometabolic. Increased metabolism may be present in early stages, however, and there may a role for PET in planning surgery in cases unresponsive to medical management.[274]

Ocular Manifestations

Two different but important kinds of visual problems are strongly associated with Sturge-Weber syndrome, ocular and cortical. The cutaneous vascular malformation frequently includes the eye on the affected side of the face, specifically the sclera and choroid. Such involvement is seen in about one-third of Sturge-Weber syndrome patients. The retina is not usually involved, but glaucoma can result from the scleral and choroid involvement. Buphthalmos, a congenitally enlarged globe caused by congenital glaucoma, is seen in 10% to 30% of Sturge-Weber syndrome patients.[275] Retinal detachment can also occur.

Visual loss other than from glaucoma is commonly due to cortical blindness as the occipital lobe becomes ischemic and calcified. Unilateral occipital lobe involvement leads to homonymous hemianopsia.

Visceral Manifestations

Most cases of Sturge-Weber syndrome are not accompanied by significant visceral abnormalities. Some patients

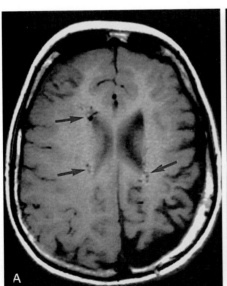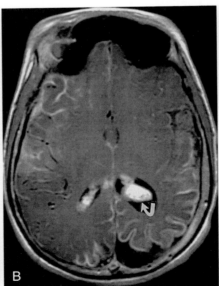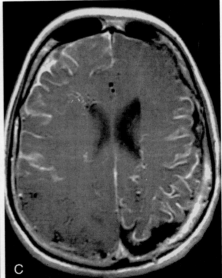

FIGURE 51–35 MRI of Sturge-Weber syndrome. *A,* Axial nonenhanced T1-weighted MRI study shows left cortical atrophy and small areas of flow around the lateral ventricles from enlarged deep veins (*arrows*). *B* and *C,* Axial postgadolinium T1-weighted MRI studies show prominent choroid plexus (*arrow in B*) and extensive superficial enhancement, some of which appears to fill the subarachnoid space. Calcification was limited to the areas of atrophy, much less than the areas of enhancement. (Compare with Fig. 51–33, CT of the same patient.)

have a more generalized vascular abnormality that involves, in addition to the cranial features of Sturge-Weber syndrome, angiomatous malformations in intestine, kidneys, spleen, ovaries, thyroid gland, lungs, or pancreas.[258]

Klippel-Trénaunay-Weber Syndrome

Klippel-Trénaunay syndrome also includes as a key feature cutaneous vascular capillary malformation. The port wine stain is usually unilateral and involves one or more extremities. Other features are venous varicosities and osseous and soft tissue hypertrophy of the affected body part.[276–278] Some patients have combined features of this and Sturge-Weber syndrome, termed *Klippel-Trénaunay-Weber syndrome.* CNS findings of Sturge-Weber syndrome, hemimegalencephaly, and deep white matter as well as subcortical calcifications have been reported in some of these patients (Fig. 51–36).[33, 276]

Cobb's Syndrome

Cobb's syndrome, also termed *cutaneomeningospinal angiomatosis,* is characterized by a port wine stain in the segmental dermatomal distribution of a vascular malformation of the spinal cord, with an associated medullary syndrome resulting from cord compression or ischemia.[279] The vascular malformation is present at birth, but the neurologic manifestations usually begin in childhood or adolescence. Symptoms of pain, paraplegia or monoplegia, incontinence, or sensory deficit may begin suddenly or gradually.[250]

OTHER NEUROCUTANEOUS SYNDROMES

A variety of other syndromes have been included in the category of neurocutaneous syndromes. Nearly all of

these are much less common than the conditions discussed earlier. Some syndromes that are notable for both CNS and cutaneous manifestations are presented subsequently.

Epidermal Nevus Syndrome and Linear Sebaceous Nevus Syndrome

The combination of an epidermoid or organoid nevus with congenital abnormalities elsewhere in the body has been referred to as epidermal nevus syndrome. Epidermal nevi arise from the basal layer of the epidermis and include elements of skin appendages, such as hair follicles and glands as well as keratinocytes. *Organoid nevus* is another term for these raised skin lesions that arise from more than one type of tissue. Different types of these nevi include linear nevus sebaceous, nevus verrucosus, nevus comedonicus, nevus syringocystadenosus papilliferus, nevus unius lateris, and ichthyosis hystrix. A wide variety of associated conditions have been described, including regional musculoskeletal hypertrophy or hyplasia; other cutaneous abnormalities, such as hypopigmented macules, café au lait spots, and capillary hemangiomas; various neurologic abnormalities; and infrequent cardiac and renal anomalies. Reported CNS abnormalities include hemimegalencephaly, gyral abnormalities and other neuronal migration abnormalities, callosal dysgenesis, porencephaly, vascular dysplasias, and partial absence of the dural venous sinuses and other venous anomalies.[280–282] Most cases are sporadic, although there are a few reports of familial cases.

One specific subtype of epidermal nevus is a linear sebaceous nevus, a waxy, roughly linear raised nevus that typically occurs on the head or neck. Other names are used for this nevus, including sebaceous nevus of Jadassohn. The clinical triad of linear sebaceous nevus, sei-

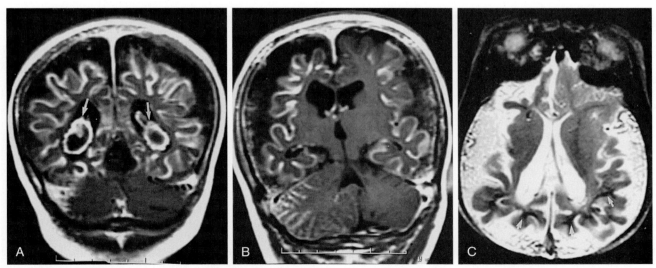

FIGURE 51–36 A 4-year-old with Klippel-Trénaunay-Weber syndrome. *A* and *B*, Gadolinium-enhanced MRI studies demonstrate extensive, avidly enhancing pial vascular malformations involving both cerebral hemispheres as well as the cerebellum. Also note enlarged, cystic, and avidly enhancing choroid plexus (*arrows* in *A*). *C*, Axial T2-weighted MRI study demonstrates extensive cerebral atrophy and focal serpentine areas of hypointensity (*arrows*) produced by calcification or possibly by deoxyhemoglobin in poorly perfused cortex beneath the pial angioma. The central nervous system imaging findings are similar to those of Sturge-Weber syndrome but are extensive in this patient.

zures, and mental retardation has been defined as the linear sebaceous nevus syndrome. Although some authors have used this term synonymously with epidermal nevus syndrome, the aforementioned triad appears to represent a more specific subset of epidermal nevus syndrome. There is a strong association of unilateral megalencephaly with this syndrome. A high incidence of unilateral megalencephaly has been noted by several authors.[283-285] Moreover, the imaging findings of unilateral megalencephaly are best revealed by MRI, and the radiographic features of this condition were defined in 1978. Careful review of older reports on linear sebaceous nevus syndrome suggest that unilateral megalencephaly was probably present in many of those cases as well. It is likely that in some cases ventricular enlargement noted on pneumoencephalography and early CT may well have been due to megalencephaly.[285]

Unilateral megalencephaly is a disorder of neuroblast migration that can involve all or part of one cerebral hemisphere.[272] Both the hemisphere and the lateral ventricle in the affected region are enlarged, and polymicrogyria is common. The enlargement can be seen with either CT or MRI. MRI can better demonstrate the findings of white matter gliosis and abnormal cortex in polymicrogyria as well as demonstrating other congenital anomalies (Fig. 51–37). Significantly, unilateral megalencephaly is often accompanied by developmental delay and seizures, often refractory. The CNS anomaly associated with linear sebaceous nevus syndrome, unilateral megalencephaly, thus explains the clinical features of that syndrome.[280, 282, 285, 286] Other neuronal migration anomalies are also reported with linear sebaceous nevus syndrome.

Ataxia Telangiectasia (Louis-Barr Syndrome)

Ataxia telangiectasia, also known as *Louis-Barr syndrome*, is an autosomal recessive condition in which multiple capillary telangiectasias occur in mucous membranes, conjunctivae, and elsewhere in skin. There is progressive cerebellar degeneration and significantly increased risk of lymphoma. The heterozygous carriers of ataxia telangiectasia are also at increased risk of malignancies, particularly breast cancer.[287] The skin manifestations may follow symptoms of cerebellar ataxia, which usually begin in childhood.[33, 272, 288] The ataxia telangiectasia gene (ATM) has been localized to chromosome 11q22-23 and was cloned in 1995.[289] The ATM gene appears to be related to a family of genes that are involved with cell cycle control and response of the cell to DNA damage.[290]

Patients with ataxia telangiectasia typically develop cellular and humoral immune deficiency. They have absence of the thymus and reduced lymphoid follicles in normal lymphoid locations, such as tonsils, lymph nodes, and spleen. There is also deficiency of IgA. Sinopulmonary infections are a major cause of morbidity and mortality. Chromosomal instability and sensitivity to ionizing radiation are characteristic. Lymphoid malignancies also occur with significant frequency, seen in 10% to 15% of patients with ataxia telangiectasia.[288, 291]

Imaging findings in the brain are best demonstrated with MRI. The cerebellum is small, especially the anterior vermis, and there is progressive degeneration over time (Figs. 51–38 and 51–39).[259, 272] Specific visceral manifestations are not present, but pulmonary infections are common, and the possibility of neoplasms, especially lymphoma, should be kept in mind.

Hereditary Hemorrhagic Telangiectasia

Hereditary hemorrhagic telangiectasia (HHT), also known as *Rendu-Osler-Weber disease*, is an autosomal dominant condition characterized by vascular abnormalities of skin and mucosal surfaces (telangiectasias) and arteriovenous malformations in multiple organs, including lungs and brain.[292, 293] The diagnostic criteria for HHT are not universally agreed on. Guttmacher and associates[292]

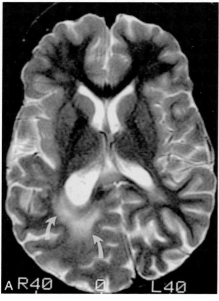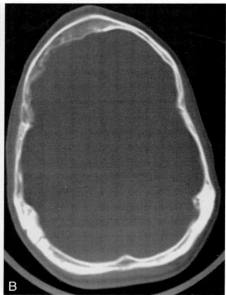

FIGURE 51–37 Linear sebaceous nevus syndrome and hemimegalencephaly. *A,* Axial T2-weighted MRI study of a teenage girl with seizures, mental retardation, and a waxy linear nevus over the scalp and forehead shows enlargement of the posterior right cerebral hemisphere and the atrium of the right lateral ventricle. There is gliosis in the white matter (*arrows*), also a common finding in hemimegalencephaly. Hemimegalencephaly can involve the entire hemisphere or, as in this case, a portion of the hemisphere. *B,* CT bone window scan of the same patient shows thickening of the left frontal calvaria and the overlying nevus. Skeletal asymmetry is common with linear sebaceous nevus syndrome.

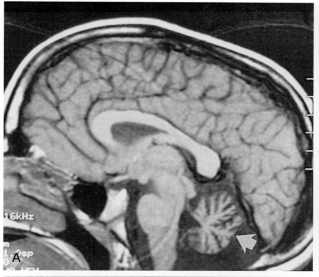

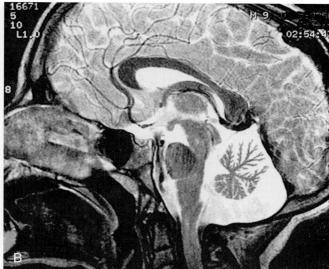

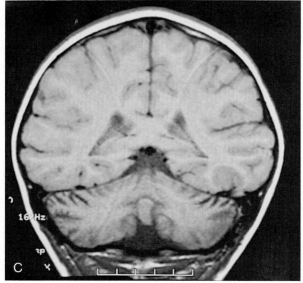

FIGURE 51–38 A 9-year-old with ataxia-telangiectasia. Sagittal T1-weighted (*A*), T2-weighted (*B*), and coronal T1 (*C*) MRI studies demonstrate atrophy of both the cerebellar vermis (*arrow* in *A*) and the hemispheres. The other cerebral structures are intact.

have suggested that the presence of any two of the following features is diagnostic: recurrent epistaxis, telangiectasias other than in the nasal mucosa, evidence of autosomal dominant inheritance, and visceral involvement. Haitjema and colleagues[293] have stated that the diagnosis should be based on a family history of HHT and the presence of multiple telangiectasias.

HHT has at least two genetic causes, with some families showing linkage to chromosome 9q3 and others to 12q. The first identified gene is endoglin (ENG) at 9q34.1, cloned in 1994.[294, 295] The ENG gene product encodes a glycoprotein found on endothelial cells that binds transforming growth factor-β. Linkage to chromosome 12q has been demonstrated in some families that did not show linkage to the ENG locus, and mutations in the activin receptor-like kinase-1 gene (ACVRLK1, or ALK1) at 12q11–q14 have been identified.[296–298]

Multiple vascular malformations occur in skin, mucous membranes, viscera, and CNS. The brain, lungs, and gastrointestinal tract, in particular, can be sources of mor-

tality or serious morbidity in HHT. Recurrent epistaxis, gastrointestinal bleeding, and hemoptysis occur frequently. Various vascular malformations have been described, but most involve abnormal arteriovenous connections. The skin telangiectasia consists of plexiform arteriovenous fistulas with arteriovenous shunting.[299] Arteriovenous malformations in the liver and especially the lungs may result in paradoxical embolization. Thus, significant CNS morbidity from brain abscess or infarction can result from the visceral arteriovenous malformations.[292, 300]

Within the brain itself, one or more vascular malformations are common in HHT. Most of these represent arteriovenous malformations (Fig. 51–40). In a clinic in which more than 100 patients with clinical evidence of HHT were screened by MRI, approximately 23% had MRI evidence of vascular malformations of the brain. Subsequent catheter angiography demonstrated evidence of additional small arteriovenous malformations not detected on MRI. Some small lesions have a nonspecific appear-

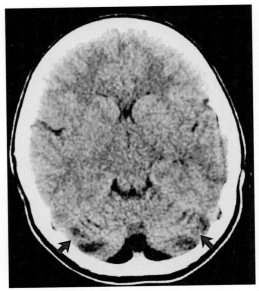

FIGURE 51–39 Ataxia-telangiectasia. Non–contrast-enhanced CT scan demonstrates diffuse cerebellar atrophy (*arrows*) with preservation of the cerebral cortex.

ance on MRI suggestive of cavernous malformations but often lacking some features, such as a complete hemosiderin rim, of typical cavernous malformations. Some of these nonspecific lesions on MRI can be shown on angiography to represent small arteriovenous malformations.[301, 302] The frequent multiplicity of arteriovenous malformations creates a challenge in management of these patients; the natural history of small lesions is uncertain, and surgical, endovascular, and radiation therapy may pose significant risks as well. Screening with MRI and supplementing with catheter angiography in selected cases may be a prudent approach.[301]

Wyburn-Mason Syndrome

Wyburn-Mason syndrome, also known as *Bonnet-Dechaume-Blanc syndrome, oculocephalic angiomatosis,* and *unilateral retinocephalic vascular malformation,* includes a retinal arteriovenous malformation and one or more ipsilateral arteriovenous malformations of the brain. A facial port wine stain is often present as well. The retinal malformation (cirsoid aneurysm) can produce minimal to severe visual impairment. The arteriovenous malformations in the brain involve midbrain and optic nerves in particular. Subcutaneous, mandibular, maxillary, or oral mucosal vascular malformations occur in up to half of patients.[250, 303, 304]

Other, Uncommon Neurocutaneous Syndromes

Nevoid Basal Cell Carcinoma Syndrome (Gorlin's Syndrome)

Basal cell nevus syndrome, more aptly termed the *nevoid basal cell carcinoma syndrome* (also Gorlin's syndrome) is an autosomal dominant disorder characterized by multiple basal cell carcinomas; odontogenic keratocysts of the jaw; palmar/plantar pits; and skeletal anomalies, including bifid ribs, short metacarpals, kyphoscoliosis, and segmentation anomalies of the vertebrae. Extensive dural calcifications in the falx and tentorium are characteristic features, observed in 65% and 20% of patients (Fig. 51–41).[305] There is an increased incidence of medulloblastoma in this syndrome, and meningioma, astrocytoma, and craniopharyngioma have also been reported.[306, 307] Because of the significantly increased risk of medulloblastoma up to age 7 years, individuals at risk for nevoid basal cell carcinoma syndrome should have neurologic evaluations at 6-month intervals in addition to annual MRI of the cerebellum until 7 years of age.[305]

The nevoid basal cell carcinoma syndrome has been

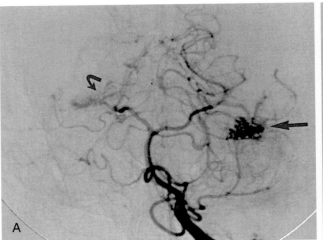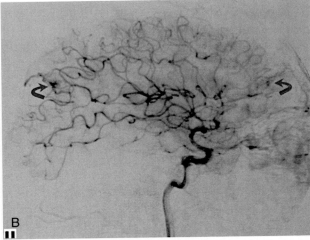

FIGURE 51–40 Hereditary hemorrhagic telangiectasia. *A* and *B*, Angiography of a man who presented with left cerebellar hematoma revealed at least four arteriovenous malformations. The largest, and source of the hemorrhage, is visible on the anteroposterior view after left vertebral injection (*straight arrow* in *A*). A smaller arteriovenous malformation is visible on the same injection (*curved arrow* in *A*), and two others are present on lateral view of right internal carotid injection (*arrows* in *B*).

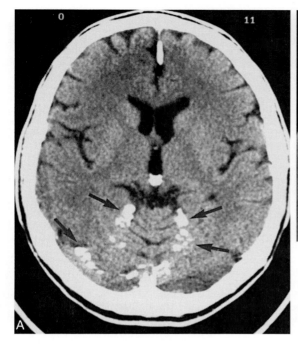
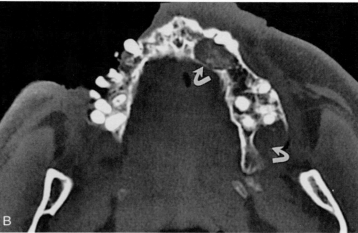

FIGURE 51–41 Gorlin's syndrome. *A,* Non–contrast-enhanced CT scan shows extensive dural calcifications (*arrows*). *B,* Axial non–contrast-enhanced CT scan of the face shows odontogenic cysts (*arrows*). A soft tissue defect over the right side of the face is from surgery for basal cell carcinoma.

mapped to 9q22.3–q31, and the causative gene (PTC) was cloned in 1996. The PTC gene is the human homologue of the *Drosophila* gene *patched* and appears to function as a tumor-suppressor gene.

Blue Rubber Bleb Nevus Syndrome

The nevi that give their name to this syndrome are multiple cutaneous venous malformations of rubbery consistency. Vascular malformations are found in the lungs, pleura, liver, gastrointestinal tract, peritoneum, and CNS. Venous angiomas and sinus pericranii are vascular anomalies reported in association with the CNS in this syndrome. The disorder is quite rare and is almost always a sporadic occurrence.[250]

Hypomelanosis of Ito (Incontinentia Pigmenti Achromians)

Hypomelanosis of Ito, or incontinentia pigmenti achromians, is a condition in which there are hypopigmented skin lesions with decreased size and number of melanosomes and melanocytes.[308] The cause is heterogeneous, and the finding most frequently indicates genetic or chromosomal mosaicism. A variety of CNS abnormalities have been reported, including migration anomalies, cerebral atrophy, and disordered cortical laminations with gliosis.[309–311]

Neurocutaneous Melanosis

Widespread lesions containing melanin-producing cells occur in this condition. There are multiple pigmented cutaneous nevi, sometimes hairy, and leptomeningeal melanotic proliferation. High signal intensity may be present in the thickened meninges, presumably as a result of T1-shortening effects of melanin. Intense contrast enhancement is also seen.[33, 312, 313] There is a high risk of malignant melanoma of the CNS (up to 40%).[33]

Cowden Disease

Cowden disease, also known as multiple hamartoma syndrome, is an autosomal dominant, multiple hamartoma-neoplasia syndrome characterized by verrucous skin lesions of the face and limbs, cobblestone-like papules of gingiva and buccal mucosa, multiple facial trichilemmomas, and tumors of the breast and thyroid. Multiple neoplasms occur of ectodermal, mesodermal, and endodermal origin. There is an association with Lhermitte-Duclos disease.[314–316] The PTEN gene responsible for Cowden disease was identified in 1997 and maps to 10q23.2.[317]

References

1. Van der Hoeve J. Augengeschwulate bei de tuberosen Hirnsklerose (Bourneville) Albrecht V. Graefes Arch Clin Exp Ophthalmol 1921;105:880.
2. Van der Hoeve J. Augengeschwulate bei de tuberosen Hirnsklerose (Bourneville) und verwandten Kunkheiten. Arch F Ophthalmol 1923;111:1.
3. Van der Hoeve J. Le phakomatoses de Bourneville, de Recklinhausen et de von Hippel Linda. J Belrge Neurol Psychiatr 1933;33:752–762.
4. Brower B, van der Hoeve J, Mahoney W, et al. Kon akada wet neerland. Tweede Sectie 1937;36:1.
5. Dorland's Illustrated Medical Dictionary, 28th ed., p. 1270. Philadelphia, WB Saunders, 1994.
6. Tilesius von Tilenau WG. Historia pathologica singularis entis turpitudinis. Jo Godofredi Rheinhardi viri 50 Annorum, Leipzig, SL Crusins, 1793.
7. Braffman B, Naidich T. The phakomatoses: Part I. Neuroimaging Clin North Am 1994;4:299–324.
8. Neurofibromatosis Conference Statement: National Institutes of Health Consensus Development Conference. Arch Neurol 1988;45:575–578.
9. Gutmann DH, Aylsworth A, Carey JC, et al. The diagnostic evaluation and multidisciplinary management of neurofibromatosis 1 and neurofibromatosis 2. JAMA 1997;278:51–57.
10. Von Recklinghausen FD. Uber die multiplen Fibrome der Haut und ihre Beziehung zu den multiplen neuromen. In Festschrift für Rudolf Virchow. Berlin, August Hirschwald, 1882.

11. Sorenson SA, Mulvihill JJ, Nielsen A. Long-term follow-up of von Recklinghausen neurofibromatosis. N Engl J Med 1986;314:1010–1015.
12. Cawthon RM, Weiss R, Xu G, et al. A major segment of the neurofibromatosis type 1 gene: cDNA sequence, genomic structure, and point mutations. Cell 1990;62:193–201.
13. Wallace MR, Marchuk DA, Anderson LB, et al. Type 1 neurofibromatosis gene: Identification of a larger transcript disrupted in three NF1 patients. Science 1990;249:181–186.
14. Rubinstein AE. Neurofibromatosis: A review of the clinical problem. Ann N Y Acad Sci 1986;486:1–13.
15. Berg BO. Current concepts of neurocutaneous disorders. Brain Dev 1991;13:9–20.
16. Huson SM, Harper PS, Compston DAS. Von Recklinghausen's neurofibromatosis: A clinical and population study in southeast Wales. Brain 1988;111:1355–1381.
17. Riccardi VM: Von Recklinghausen neurofibromatosis. N Engl J Med 1981;305:1617–1626.
18. Suh J-S, Abenoza P, Galloway HR, et al. Peripheral (extracranial) nerve tumors: Correlation of MR imaging and histologic findings. Radiology 1992;183:341–346.
19. Lubs M-LE, Bauer MS, Formas ME, Djokic B. Lisch nodules in neurofibromatosis type 1. N Engl J Med 1991;324:1264–1266.
20. Casselman ES, Mandell GA. Vertebral scalloping in neurofibromatosis. Radiology 1979;131:89–94.
21. Kumar AJ, Kahadja FP, Martinez CR, et al. CT of extracranial nerve sheath tumors with pathological correlation. J Comput Assist Tomogr 1983;9:1037–1041.
22. Coleman BG, Arger PH, Dalinka MA, et al. CT of sarcomatous degeneration of neurofibromatosis. AJR 1983;140:383–387.
23. Burk DL, Brunberg JA, Kanal E, et al. Spinal and paraspinal neurofibromatosis: Surface coil MR imaging at 1.5 T. Radiology 1987;162:797–801.
24. Listernick R, Charrow J, Greenwald M. Emergence of optic pathway gliomas in children with neurofibromatosis type 1 after normal imaging results. J Pediatr 1992;121:584–587.
25. Imes RK, Hoyt WF. Magnetic resonance imaging signs of optic nerve gliomas in neurofibromatosis 1. Am J Ophthalmol 1991;111:729–734.
26. Millar WS, Tartaglino LM, Sergott RC, et al. MR of malignant optic glioma of adulthood. AJNR 1995;16:1673–1676.
27. Lott IT, Richardson EP. Neuropathogenesis of neurofibromatosis. Adv Neurol 1981;29:23–31.
28. Smirniotopoulos JG, Murphy FM. The phakomatoses. AJNR 1992;13:725–746.
29. Brown EW, Riccardi VM, Mawad M, et al. MR imaging of optic pathways in patients with neurofibromatosis. AJNR 1987;8:1031–1036.
30. Alvord EC, Lufton S. Gliomas of the optic nerve or chiasm: Outcome by patient's age, tumor site, and treatment. J Neurosurg 1988;68:85–98.
31. Listernick R, Charrow J, Greenwald M, Mets M. Natural history of optic pathway tumors in children with neurofibromatosis type 1: A longitudinal study. J Pediatr 1994;125:63–66.
32. Brzowski AE, Bazan C III, Muma JV, Ryan SG. Spontaneous regression of optic glioma in a patient with neurofibromatosis. Neurology 1992;42:679–681.
33. Pont MS, Elster AD. Lesions of skin and brain: Modern imaging of the neurocutaneous syndromes. AJR 1992;158:1193–1203.
34. Menor F, Marti-Bonmati L, Mulas F, et al. Imaging considerations of central nervous system manifestations in pediatric patients with neurofibromatosis type 1. Pediatr Radiol 1991;21:389–394.
35. Fletcher WA, Imes RK, Hoyt WF. Chiasmal gliomas: Appearance and long-term changes demonstrated by computerized tomography. J Neurosurg 1986;65:154–159.
36. Imes RK, Hoyt WY. Childhood chiasmal gliomas: Update of the facts of patients in the 1969 San Francisco Study. Br J Ophthalmol 1986;70:179–182.
37. Mamelak AN, Prado MD, Obana WG, et al. Neurofibromatosis and multicentric gliomas: Response. J Neurosurg 82:151, 1995.
38. Listernick R, Louis DN, Packer RJ, Gutmann DH. Optic pathway gliomas in children with neurofibromatosis 1: Consensus statement from the NF1 optic pathway glioma task force. Ann Neurol 1997;41:143–149.
39. Jacoby C, Go R, Beren R. Cranial CT of neurofibromatosis. AJR 1980;135:553–557.
40. Pomeranz S, Shelton J, Tobias J, et al. MR of visual pathways in neurofibromatosis. AJNR 1987;8:831–836.
41. Holman RE, Grimson BS, Drayer BP, et al. Magnetic resonance imaging of optic gliomas. Am J Ophthalmol 1985;100:596–601.
42. Albert A, Lee BCP, Saint-Louis L, et al. MRI of optic chiasm and optic pathways. AJNR 1986;7:255.
43. Lovblad KO, Remonda L, Ozdoba C, et al. Dural ectasia of the optic nerve sheath in neurofibromatosis type 1: CT and MR features. J Comput Assist Tomogr 1994;18:728–730.
44. Berg BO. Neurocutaneous disorders. In Berg BO (ed). Neurologic Manifestations of Pediatrics, pp. 485–498. Boston, Butterworth-Heinemann, 1992.
45. Klatte EG, Franken EA, Smith JA. The radiographic spectrum in neurofibromatosis. Semin Roentgenol 1976;11:17–33.
46. Riccardi VM. Neurofibromatosis: Clinical heterogeneity. Curr Probl Cancer 1982;7:1–34.
47. Aoki S, Barkovich AJ, Nishimura K, et al. Neurofibromatosis types 1 and 2: Cranial MR findings. Radiology 1989;172:527–534.
48. Mulvihill JJ, Parry DM, Sherman JL, et al. Neurofibromatosis 1 (Recklinghausen disease) and neurofibromatosis 2 (bilateral acoustic neurofibromatosis). Ann Intern Med 1990;113:39–52.
49. Hochstrasser H, Boltshauser E, Valavanis A. Brain tumors in children with Recklinghausen neurofibromatosis. Neurofibromatosis 1989;1:233–239.
50. Barkovich AJ. The phakomatoses. In Pediatric Neuroimaging, 2nd ed., pp. 277–319. New York, Raven, 1995.
51. Raffel C, McComb JG, Bodner S, Gilles FE. Benign brain-stem lesions in pediatric patients with neurofibromatosis: Case reports. Neurosurgery 1989;25:959–964.
52. Parizel PM, Martin JJ, Van Vyre M, et al. Cerebral ganglioglioma and neurofibromatosis type 1. Neuroradiology 1991;33:357–359.
53. Bognanno J, Edwards M, Lee T, et al. Cranial MR imaging in neurofibromatosis. AJNR 1988;9:461–467.
54. Hurst R, Newman S, Cail W. Multifocal intracranial MR abnormalities in neurofibromatosis. AJNR 1988;9:293.
55. Braffman BH, Bilaniuk LT, Zimmerman RA. MR of CNS neoplasia of the phakomatoses. Semin Roentgenol 1990;25:198.
56. Braffman BH, Bilaniuk LT, Zimmerman RA. The central nervous manifestations of the phakomatoses on MR. Radiol Clin North Am 1988;26:773.
57. Ferner R, Chaudhuri R, Bingham J, Hughes R. MRI in neurofibromatosis 1: The nature and evolution of increased intensity T2 weighted lesions and their relationship to intellectual impairment. J Neurol Neurosurg Psychiatry 1993;56:492–495.
58. Mirowitz SA, Sarton K, Gado M. High-intensity basal ganglia lesions on T1-weighted MR images in neurofibromatosis. AJNR 1989;10:1159–1163.
59. Menor F, Marti-Bonmarti L. CT detection of basal ganglia lesions in neurofibromatosis type 1: Correlation with MRI. Neuroradiology 1992;34:305–307.
60. Sevick RJ, Barkovich AJ, Edwards MSB, et al. Evolution of white matter lesions in neurofibromatosis type 1: MR findings. AJR 1992;159:171–175.
61. Itoh T, Magnaldi S, White RM, et al. Neurofibromatosis type 1: The evolution of deep gray and white matter abnormalities. AJNR 1994;15:1513–1519.
62. Canale DJ, Bebin J. Von Recklinghausen disease of the nervous system. In Vinken PJ, Bruyn GW (eds). Handbook of Clinical Neurology: The Phakomatoses, pp. 132–162. Amsterdam, North-Holland, 1972.
63. Rubenstein LJ. The malformative central nervous system lesions in the central peripheral forms of neurofibromatosis: A neuropathological study of 22 cases. In Rubenstein AE, Bunge RP, Houseman DE (eds). Neurofibromatosis. Annals of the New York Academy of Sciences, Vol. 486, pp. 14–29. New York, Academy of Sciences, 1986.
64. Rosman NP, Pearce J. The brain in multiple neurofibromatosis (von Recklinghausen's disease): A suggested neuropathological basis for the associated mental defect. Brain 1967;90:829–837.
65. Rubinstein LJ. Tumors of the Central Nervous System. Washington, DC, Armed Forces Institute of Pathology, 1972.
66. DiPaolo DP, Zimmerman RA, Rorke LA, et al. Neurofibromatosis type 1: Pathologic substrate of high-signal-intensity foci in the brain. Radiology 1995;195:721–724.
67. North K, Joy P, Yuille D, et al. Specific learning disability in

children with neurofibromatosis type 1: Significance of MRI abnormalities. Neurology 1994;44:878–883.

68. Castillo M, Green C, Kwock L, et al. Proton MR spectroscopy in patients with neurofibromatosis type 1: Evaluation of hamartomas and clinical correlation. AJNR 1995;16:141–147.
69. Ferner R, Chaudhuri R, Bingham J, Hughes R. MRI in neurofibromatosis 1: The nature and evolution of increased intensity T2 weighted lesions and their relationship to intellectual impairment. J Neurol Neurosurg Psychiatry 1993;56:492–495.
70. Elster AD. Radiologic screening in the neurocutaneous syndromes: Strategies and controversies. AJNR 1992;13:1078–1082.
71. Bonawitz C, Castillo M, Chin CT, et al. Usefulness of contrast material in MR of patients with neurofibromatosis type 1. AJNR 1998;19:541–546.
72. Tomsick T, Lukin R, Chamber A, et al. Neurofibromatosis and intracranial arterial occlusive disease. Neuroradiology 1976;11:229–234.
73. Sobata E, Ohkuma H, Suzuki S. Cerebrovascular disorders associated with von Recklinghausen's neurofibromatosis. Neurosurgery 1988;22:544–549.
74. Woody RC, Perrot LJ, Beck SA. Neurofibromatosis cerebral vasculopathy in an infant: Clinical, neuroradiologic, and neuropathologic studies. Pediatr Pathol 1992;12:613–619.
75. Negoro M, Nakaya T, Terashima K, Sugita K. Exracranial vertebral artery aneurysm with neurofibromatosis. Neuroradiology 1990;31:533–536.
76. Gomori JM, Weinberger G, Shachar E, Freilich G. Multiple intracranial aneurysms and neurofibromatosis: A case report. Australas Radiol 1991;35:271–273.
77. Muhonen MG, Godersky JC, VanGilder JC. Cerebral aneurysms associated with neurofibromatosis. Surg Neurol 1992;36:470–475.
78. Schievink WI, Piepgras DG. Cervical vertebral artery aneurysms and arteriovenous fistulae in neurofibromatosis type 1: Case reports. Neurosurgery 1991;29:760–765.
79. Beyer R, Paden P, Sobel D, et al. Moya-moya pattern of vascular occlusion after radiotherapy for glioma of the optic chiasm. Neurology 1986;36:1173–1178.
80. Aizpuru RN, Quencer RM, Norenberg M, et al. Meningioangiomatosis: Clinical, radiologic, and histopathologic correlation. Radiology 1991;179:819–821.
81. Tien RD, Osumi A, Oakes JW, et al. Meningioangiomatosis: CT and MR findings. J Comput Assist Tomogr 1992;16:361–365.
82. Barnes PD, Korf BR. Neurocutaneous syndromes. In Wolpert SM, Barnes PD (eds). MRI in Pediatric Neuroradiology, pp. 299–315. St Louis, Mosby–Year Book, 1992.
83. Braffman BH, Bilaniuk LT, Naidich TP, et al. MR imaging of tuberous sclerosis: Pathogenesis of this phakomatosis, use of gadopentate dimeglumine, and literature review. Radiology 1992;183:227–238.
84. Holt J. Neurofibromatosis in children. AJR 1978;130:615.
85. Burrows EH. Bone changes in orbital neurofibromatosis. Br J Radiol 1963;36:549.
86. Sarwar M, Swischuk LE. Bilateral internal auditory canal enlargement due to dural ectasia in neurofibromatosis. AJR 1977;129:935–936.
87. Leeds NE, Jacobson HG. spinal neurofibromatosis. AJR 1976;126:617.
88. Zimmerman RA, Bilaniuk LT, Metzger RA, et al. Computed tomography of orbital facial neurofibromatosis. Radiology 1983;146:113–116.
89. Reed D, Robertson W, Rootman J, et al. Plexiform neurofibromatosis of the orbit: CT evaluation. AJNR 1986;7:259–263.
90. Rubenstein L. The malformative CNS lesions in central and peripheral forms of neurofibromatosis. Ann N Y Acad Sci 1986;486:14.
91. Duke-Elder S, Perkins ES. Diseases of the uveal tract. Syst Ophthalmol 1966;11:812.
92. Burk RR. Von Hippel-Lindau disease (angiomatosis of the retina and cerebellum). J Am Optom Assoc 1991;62:382–387.
93. Egelhoff JC, Bates DJ, Ross JS, et al. Spinal MR findings in neurofibromatosis types 1 and 2. AJNR 1990;13:1071–1077.
94. Halliday AL, Sobel RA, Martuza RL. Benign spinal nerve sheath tumors: Their occurrence sporadically and in neurofibromatosis types 1 and 2. J Neurosurg 1991;74:248–253.
95. DeRecondo J, Haguenau M. Neuropathologic survey of the phako-

matoses and allied disorders. In Vinken PJ, Bruyn GW (eds). Handbook of Clinical Neurology: The Phakomatoses, Vol. 14, pp. 19–72. Amsterdam, North Holland, 1972.
96. Feldman F. Tuberous sclerosis, neurofibromatosis, and fibrous dysplasia. In Resnick D (ed). Diagnosis of Bone and Joint Disorders, 3rd ed., pp. 4353–4395. Philadelphia, WB Saunders, 1995.
97. Bensaid AH, Dietermann JL, Kastler B, et al. Neurofibromatosis with dural ectasia and bilateral symmetrical pedicular clefts: Report of two cases. Neuroradiology 1992;34:107–109.
98. Nakasu Y, Minouchi K, Hatsuda N, et al. Thoracic meningocele in neurofibromatosis: CT and MR findings. J Comput Assist Tomogr 1991;15:1062–1064.
99. So CB, Li DKB. Anterolateral cervical meningocele in association with neurofibromatosis: MR and CT studies. J Comput Assist Tomogr 1992;13:692–695.
100. Miles J, Pennybacker J, Sheldon PH. Intrathoracic meningocele: Its development and association with neurofibromatosis. J Neurol Neurosurg Psychiatry 1969;32:99–110.
101. Hope DG, Mulvihill JJ: Malignancy in neurofibromatosis. In Riccardi VM, Mulvihill JJ (eds). Neurofibromatosis. Advances in Neurology, pp. 33–56. New York, Raven, 1981.
102. Evans DG, Huson SM, Donnai D, et al. A genetic study of type 2 neurofibromatosis in the United Kingdom: I. Prevalence, mutation rate, fitness and confirmation of maternal transmission effect on severity. J Med Genet 1992;29:841–846.
103. Evans DGR, Huson SM, Donnai D, et al. A clinical study of type 2 neurofibromatosis. Q J Med 1992;85:601–618.
104. Martuza R, Eldridge R. Neurofibromatosis 2 (bilateral acoustic neurofibromatosis). N Engl J Med 1988;318:684–688.
105. Rouleau GA, Merel P, Lutchman M, et al. Alteration in a new gene encoding a putative membrane-organizing protein causes neurofibromatosis type 2. Nature 1993;363:515–521.
106. Trofatter JA, MacCollin MM, Rutter JL, et al. A novel moesin-, ezrin-, radixin-like gene is a candidate for the neurofibromatosis 2 tumor suppressor. Cell 1993;72:791–800.
107. Pulst S, Rouleau G, Marineau C, et al. Familial meningioma is not allelic to neurofibromatosis 2. Neurology 1993;43:2096–2098.
108. Fontaine B, Hanson MP, VonSattel JP, et al. Loss of chromosome 22 alleles in human sporadic spinal schwannomas. Ann Neurol 1991;29:183–186.
109. Knudson AG Jr, Strong LC, Anderson DE. Heredity and cancer in man. Prog Med Genet 1973;9:113–158.
110. Merten DF, Goodlag CA, Newton TH, Malamud N. Meningiomas of childhood and adolescence. J Pediatr 1974;84:696–700.
111. Thomas PK, King RHM, Chiang TR, et al. Neurofibromatosis neuropathy. Muscle Nerve 1990;13:93–101.
112. Mori M, Morisaki S, Hazama R, et al. A family of von Recklinghausen's neurofibromatosis complicated by mononeuritis multiplex, bilateral acoustic neurinomas, and falx and spinal meningiomas. No To Shinkei 1985;37:403–408.
113. Kilpatrick TJ, Hjorth RJ, Gonzales MF. A case of neurofibromatosis 2 presenting with a mononeuritis multiplex. J Neurol Neurosurg Psychiatry 1992;52:391–393.
114. Pearson-Webb MA, Kaiser-Kupfer MI, Eldridge R. Eye findings in bilateral acoustic central neurofibromatosis: Association with presenile lens opacities and cataracts but absence of Lisch nodules [Letter]. N Engl J Med 1986;315:1553–1554.
115. Kaiser-Kupfer MI, Friedlin V, Datiles MB, et al. The association of posterior capsular lens opacities with bilateral acoustic neuromas in patients with neurofibromatosis type 2. Arch Ophthalmol 1989;107:541–544.
116. Kaye LD, Rothner AD, Beauchamp GR, et al. Ocular findings associated with neurofibromatosis type II. Ophthalmology 1992;99:1424–1429.
117. Bouzas EA, Friedlin V, Parry DM, et al. Lens opacities in neurofibromatosis 2: Further significant correlations. Br J Ophthalmol 1993;77:354–357.
118. Mautner V-F, Tatagiba M, Guthoff R, et al. Neurofibromatosis 2 in the pediatric age group. Neurosurgery 1993;33:92–96.
119. Silvingham A, Augsburger J, Perilongo G, et al. Combined hamartomas of the retina and retinal pigment epithelium in a patient with neurofibromatosis type 2. J Pediatr Ophthalmol Strabismus 1991;28:320–322.
120. Good WV, Brodsky MC, Edwards MS, Hoyt WF. Bilateral retinal hamartomas in neurofibromatosis type 2. Br J Ophthalmol 1991;75:190.

121. Landau K, Dossetor FM, Hoyt WF, Muci-Mendoza F. Retinal hamartomas in neurofibromatosis type 2. Arch Ophthalmol 1990;108:328–329.

122. Cotlier E. Cafe-au-lait spots of the fundus in neurofibromatosis. Arch Ophthalmol 1977;95:1990–1992.

123. Bouzas EA, Parry DM, Eldridge R, Kaiser-Kupfer MI. Familial occurrence of combined pigment epithelial and retinal hamartomas associated with neurofibromatosis 2. Retina 1992;12:103–107.

124. Harkin JC, Reed JR. Tumors of the Peripheral Nervous System. Washington, DC, The Armed Forces Institute of Pathology, 1969.

125. National Institutes of Health Consensus Development Conference Statement on Acoustic Neuroma, Dec 11–13, 1991. Arch Neurol 1994;51:201–207.

126. Rubenstein AR, Mytilinedau C, Yahr T, et al. Neurological aspects of neurofibromatosis. In Riccardi VM, Mulvihill JJ (eds). Neurofibromatosis, pp. 11–21. Advances in Neurology. New York, Raven, 1981.

127. Yamada K, Ohta T, Miyamoto T, et al. Bilateral trigeminal schwannomas associated with von Recklinghausen disease. AJNR 1992;13:299–300.

128. Baldwin D, King TT, Chevretton E, Morrison AW. Bilateral cerebellopontine angle tumors in neurofibromatosis type 2. J Neurosurg 1991;74:910–915.

129. Linskey ME, Lunsford LD, Flickinger JC. Tumor control after stereotactic radiosurgery in neurofibromatosis patients with bilateral acoustic tumors. Neurosurgery 1992;31:829–838.

130. Miyamoto RT, Campbell RL, Fritsch M, Lochmueller G. Preservation of hearing in neurofibromatosis 2. Otolaryngol Head Neck Surg 1990;103:619–624.

131. Kingsley DPE, Brooks GB, Leung AW-L, et al. Acoustic neuromas: Evaluation by magnetic resonance imaging. AJNR 1985;6:1–5.

132. Lhuillier FM, Doyon DL, Halami PhM, et al. Magnetic resonance imaging of acoustic neuromas: Pitfalls and differential diagnosis. Neuroradiology 1992;34:144–149.

133. Stack JP, Ramsden RT, Antoun NM, et al. Magnetic resonance imaging of acoustic neuromas: The role of gadolinium-DTPA. Br J Radiol 1988;61:800–805.

134. Allen RW, Harnsberger HR, Shelton C, et al. Low-cost high-resolution fast spin-echo MR of acoustic schwannoma: An alternative to enhanced conventional spin-echo MR? AJNR 1996;17:1205–1210.

135. Fukui MB, Weissman JL, Curtin HD, Kanal E. T2-weighted MR characteristics of internal auditory canal masses. AJNR 1996;17:1211–1218.

136. Stuckey SL, Harris AJ, Mannolini SM. Detection of acoustic schwannoma: Use of constructive interference in the steady state three-dimensional MR. AJNR 1996;17:1219–1225.

137. Beges C, Revel MP, Gaston A, et al. Trigeminal neuromas: Assessment of MRI and CT. Neuroradiology 1992;34:179–183.

138. Rodriguez HA, Berthrong M. Multiple primary intracranial tumors in von Recklinghausen's neurofibromatosis. Arch Neurol 1966;14:467–475.

139. Spagnoli MV, Goldberg HI, Grossman RI, et al. Intracranial meningiomas: High-field MR imaging. Radiology 1986;161:369–375.

140. Sze G, Abramson A, Krol G, et al. Gd-DTPA in the evaluation of intradural extramedullary spinal disease. AJNR 1989;9:153–163.

141. Valk J. Gd-DTPA in MR of spinal lesions. AJNR 1989;9:345–350.

142. Mautner V, Tatgiba M, Lindenau M, et al. Spinal tumors in patients with neurofibromatosis type 2: MR imaging study of frequency, multiplicity, and variety. AJR 1995;165:951–955.

143. Mayfrank L, Moyadjer M, Wullich B. Intracranial calcified deposits are part of the diagnostic spectrum of neurofibromatosis type 2. Neuroradiology 1991;33(Suppl):601–603.

144. Arts WFM, Van Dongen KJ. Intracranial calcified deposits in neurofibromatosis. J Neurol Neurosurg Psychiatry 1986;49:1317–1320.

145. Sadeh M, Martinovits G, Goldhammer Y. Occurrence of both neurofibromatosis 1 and 2 in the same individual with a rapidly progressive course. Neurology 1989;39:282–283.

146. Au K-S, Rodriguez JA, Finch JL, et al. Germ-line mutational analysis of the TSC2 gene in 90 tuberous-sclerosis patients. Am J Hum Genet 1998;62:286–294.

147. Roach ES, Smith M, Huttenlocher P, et al. Report of the Diagnostic Criteria Committee of the National Tuberous Sclerosis Association. J Child Neurol 1992;7:221–224.

148. Roach ES. Neurocutaneous syndromes. Pediatr Clin North Am 1992;39:591–619.

149. Hanno R, Beck R. Tuberous sclerosis. Neurol Clin 1987;5:351–360.

150. Kingsley DPE, Kendall BE, Fitz CR. Tuberous sclerosis: A clinicoradiological evaluation of 110 cases with particular reference to atypical presentation. Neurology 1986;28:171–190.

151. Lagos JC, Gomez MR. Tuberous sclerosis: Reappraisal of a clinical entity. Mayo Clin Proc 1967;42:26–49.

152. Curatolo P, Cusmai R, Cortesi F, et al. Neuropsychiatric aspects of tuberous sclerosis. Ann N Y Acad Sci 1991;615:8–16.

153. Hurwitz S, Braverman IM. White spots in tuberous sclerosis. J Pediatr 1970;77:587–594.

154. Chao DH. Congenital neurocutaneous syndromes in childhood. J Pediatr 1959;55:447–459.

155. Bell SD, MacDonald DM. The prevalence of café-au-lait patches in tuberous sclerosis. Clin Exp Dermatol 1985;10:562–565.

156. Gomez MR. Criteria for diagnosis in tuberous sclerosis. In Gomez MR (ed). Tuberous Sclerosis, 2nd ed., pp. 9–19. New York, Raven, 1988.

157. Shepherd CW, Gomez MR, Lie JT, Crowson CS. Causes of death in patients with tuberous sclerosis. Mayo Clin Proc 1991;66:792–796.

158. Bender BL, Yunis EJ. The pathology of tuberous sclerosis. Pathol Ann 1982;17:339–382.

159. Christophe C, Bartholome J, Blum D, et al. Neonatal tuberous sclerosis: US, CT, and MR diagnosis of brain and cardiac lesions. Pediatr Radiol 1989;19:446–448.

160. Altman NR, Purser RK, Post MJD. Tuberous sclerosis: Characteristics at CT and MR imaging. Radiology 1988;167:527–532.

161. Martin N, de Broker T, Cambier J, et al. MRI evaluation of tuberous sclerosis. Neuroradiology 1987;29:437–443.

162. Nixon JR, Houser OW, Gomez MR, Okazaki H. Cerebral tuberous sclerosis: MR imaging. Radiology 1989;170:869–873.

163. Wippold FJ II, Baber WW, Gado M, et al. Pre- and postcontrast MR studies in tuberous sclerosis. J Comput Assist Tomogr 1992;16:69–72.

164. Martin N, Debussche C, De Broucker T, et al. Gadolinium-DTPA enhanced MR imaging in tuberous sclerosis. Neuroradiology 1990;31:492–497.

165. Wilms G, van Wijck E, Demaerel PH, et al. Gyriform calcifications in tuberous sclerosis simulating the appearance of Sturge-Weber disease. AJNR 1992;13:295–297.

166. Takanashi J-I, Sugita K, Fujii K, Niimi H. MR evaluation of tuberous sclerosis: Increased sensitivity with fluid-attenuated inversion recovery and relation to severity of seizures and mental retardation. AJNR 1995;16:1923–1928.

167. Donegani G, Grattarola FR, Wildi E. Tuberous sclerosis: Bourneville disease—The phakomatoses. In Vinken PJ, Gruyn GW (eds). The Phakomatoses: Handbook of Clinical Neurology, p. 340. Amsterdam, Elsevier, 1972.

168. Castillo M, Whaley R. Gyriform enhancement in tuberous sclerosis simulating infarction. Radiology 1992;185:613–614.

169. Sieg KG, Harty JR, Simmons M, et al. Tc-99m HMPAO SPECT imaging of the central nervous system in tuberous sclerosis. Clin Nucl Med 1991;16:665–667.

170. Szelies B, Herholz K, Heiss WD, et al. Hypometabolic cortical lesions in tuberous sclerosis with epilepsy: Demonstration by positron emission tomography. J Comput Assist Tomogr 1983;7:946–953.

171. Inoue Y, Nakajima S, Fukuda P, et al. Magnetic resonance images of tuberous sclerosis: Further observations and clinical correlations. Neuroradiology 1988;30:379–384.

172. Iwasaki S, Nakagawa H, Kichikawa K, et al. MR and CT of tuberous sclerosis: Linear abnormalities in the cerebral white matter. AJNR 1990;11:1029–1034.

173. Barkovich AJ, Gressens P, Evrard P. Formation, maturation and disorders of brain neocortex. AJNR 1992;13:423–446.

174. Stefansson K, Wollmann RL, Huttenlocher PR. Lineages of cells in the central nervous system. In Gomez MR (ed). Tuberous Sclerosis, 2nd ed., pp. 75–87. New York, Raven, 1988.

175. Seidenwurm DJ, Barkovich AJ. Understanding tuberous sclerosis. Radiology 1992;183:23–24.

176. Van Tassel P, Cure JK, Holden KR. Cystlike white matter lesions in tuberous sclerosis. AJNR 1997;18:1367–1373.

177. Morimoto M, Mogami H. Sequential CT study of subependymal giant cell astrocytoma associated with tuberous sclerosis. J Neurosurg 1986;65:874–877.

178. Boesel CP, Paulson GW, Kisnik EJ, Earle KM. Brain hamartomas and tumors associated with tuberous sclerosis. Neurosurgery 1979;4:410–417.
179. Frerebeau PH, Penezech J, Segnarbieux F, et al. Intraventricular tumors in tuberous sclerosis. Childs Nerv Syst 1985;1:45–48.
180. Tsuchida T, Kamata K, Kwamata M, et al. Brain tumors in tuberous sclerosis. Childs Brain 1981;8:271–283.
181. Holanda FJCS, Holanda GMP. Tuberous sclerosis: Neurosurgical indications in intraventricular tumors. Neurosurg Rev 1980;3:139–150.
182. Tien RD, Hesselink JR, Duberg A. Rare subependymal giant-cell astrocytoma in a neonate with tuberous sclerosis. AJNR 1990;11:1251–1252.
183. Cooper JR. Brain tumors in hereditary multiple system hamartomatosis. J Neurosurg 1971;34:194–202.
184. Roach ES, Williams DP, Laster DW. Magnetic resonance imaging in tuberous sclerosis. Arch Neurol 1987;44:301–303.
185. Roach ES. Usefulness of magnetic resonance imaging in tuberous sclerosis. Arch Neurol 1988;45:830–831.
186. Cusmai R, Chiron C, Curatolo P, et al. Topographic comparative study of magnetic resonance imaging and electroencephalography in 34 children with tuberous sclerosis. Epilepsia 1990;31:747–755.
187. Shepherd CW, Houser OW, Gomez MR. MR findings in tuberous sclerosis complex and correlation with seizure development and mental impairment. AJNR 1995;16:149–155.
188. Nyboer JH, Robertson DM, Gomez MR. Retinal lesions in tuberous sclerosis. Arch Ophthalmol 1976;94:1277–1280.
189. Hedges TR III, Pozzi-Mucelli R, Char DH, Newton TH. CT demonstration of ocular calcification: Correlations with clinical and pathological findings. Neurology 1982;23:15–21.
190. Dotan SA, Trobe SD, Gebarski SS. Visual loss in tuberous sclerosis. Neuroradiology 1991;41:1915–1917.
191. Smirniotopoulos JG, Bargallo N, Mafee MF. Differential diagnosis of leukokoria: Radiologic-pathologic correlation. Radiographics 1994;14:1059–1079.
192. Chonko AM, Weiss SM, Stein JH, et al. Renal involvement in tuberous sclerosis. Am J Med 1974;56:124–132.
193. Bissada NK, White HJ, Sun CN, et al. Tuberous sclerosis complex and renal angiomyolipoma. Urology 1975;6:105–113.
194. Sherman JL, Hartman DS, Friedman AC, et al. Angiomyolipoma: Computed tomographic-pathologic correlation of 17 cases. AJR 1981;137:1221–1226.
195. Bernstein J, Robbins TO, Kissane JM. The renal lesions of tuberous sclerosis. Semin Diagn Pathol 1986;3:97–105.
196. Stefansson K. Tuberous sclerosis. Mayo Clin Proc 1991;66:868–872.
197. Weinblatt ME, Kahn E, Kochen J. Renal cell carcinoma in patients with tuberous sclerosis. Pediatrics 1987;80:898–903.
198. Gibbs JL. The heart and tuberous sclerosis—An echocardiographic and electrocardiographic study. Br Heart J 1985;54:596–599.
199. Smith HC, Watson GH, Patel RG, Super M. Cardiac rhabdomyomata in tuberous sclerosis: Their course and diagnostic value. Arch Dis Child 1989;64:196–200.
200. Dwyer JM, HIckie JB, Garvan J. Pulmonary tuberous sclerosis: Report of three patients and review of the literature. Q J Med 1971;40:115–125.
201. Corrin B, Leibow AA, Friedman PJ. Pulmonary lymphangiomyomatosis: A review. Am J Pathol 1975;79:348–382.
202. Bradley SL, Dines DE, Soule EH, Muhm JR. Pulmonary lymphangiomyomatosis. Lung 1980;158:69–80.
203. Kitaichi M, Nishimura K, Itho H, Izumi T. Pulmonary lymphangioleiomyomatosis: A report of 46 patients including a clinicopathologic study of prognostic factors. Am J Respir Crit Care Med 1995;151:527–533.
204. Taylor JR, Ryu J, Colby TV, Raffin TA. Lymphangioleiomyomatosis: Clinical course in 32 patients. N Engl J Med 1990;323:1254–1260.
205. Boehler A, Speich R, Russi EW, Weder W. Lung transplantation for lymphangioleiomyomatosis. N Engl J Med 1996;3335:1275–1280.
206. Ng S-H, Ng K-K, Pai S-C, Tsai C-C. Tuberous sclerosis with aortic aneurysm and rib changes: CT demonstration. J Comput Assist Tomogr 1988;12:666–668.
207. Imaizumi M, Nukada T, Yoneda S, et al. Tuberous sclerosis with moya-moya disease: Case report. Med J Osaka Univ 1978;28:345–353.
208. McLaurin RL, Towbin RB. Tuberous sclerosis: Diagnostic and surgical considerations. Pediatr Neurosci 1985–86;12:45–48.
209. Maher ER, Kaelin WG. von Hippel-Lindau disease. Medicine 1997;76:381–391.
210. Latif F, Tory K, Gnarra J, et al. Identification of the von Hippel-Lindau disease tumor suppressor gene. Science 1993;26:1317–1320.
211. Maher ER, Iselius L, Yates JRW, et al. von Hippel Lindau disease: a genetic study. J Med Genet 1991;28:443–447.
212. Neumann HPH, Wiestler OD. Clustering of features of von Hippel Lindau syndrome: Evidence for a complex genetic locus. Lancet 1991;337:1052–1054.
213. Richard S, Chavveau D, Chretien Y, et al. Renal lesions and pheochromocytoma in von Hippel Lindau disease. Adv Nephrol 1994;23:1–27.
214. Choyke PL, Glenn GM, Wlather MM, et al. The natural history of renal lesions in von Hippel–Lindau disease: A serial CT study in 28 patients. AJR 1992;159:1229–1234.
215. Maher ER, Yates JRW, Harries R, et al. Clinical features and natural history of von Hippel Lindau disease. Q J Med 1990;77:1151–1163.
216. Knudson AG. Genetics of human cancer. Annu Rev Genet 1986;29:231–251.
217. Glenn GM, Linehan WM, Hosoc S, et al. Screening for von Hippel Lindau disease by DNA polymorphism analysis. JAMA 1992;267:1226–1231.
218. Maddock IR, Maher ER, Teare MD, et al. A genetic register for von Hippel-Lindau disease. J Med Genet 1996;33:120–127.
219. Young S, Richardson AE. Solid hemangioblastomas of the posterior fossa: Radiological features and results of surgery. J Neurol Neurosurg Psychiatry 1987;50:155–158.
220. Horton WA, Wong V, Eldridge R. Von Hippel-Lindau disease: Clinical and pathologic manifestations in nine families with 50 affected members. Arch Intern Med 1976;136:769–777.
221. Green JS, Bowmer MI, Johnson GJ. von Hippel Lindau disease in a Newfoundland kindred. Can Med Assoc J 1986;134:133–146.
222. Glenn GM, Daniel LN, Choyke PL, et al. von Hippel Lindau disease: Distinct phenotypes suggest more than one mutant allele at the von Hippel–Lindau disease focus. Hum Genet 1991;87:207–211.
223. Lodrini S, Lasio G, Cimino C, Pluchino F. Hemangioblastomas: Clinical characteristics, surgical results and immunohistochemical studies. J Neurosci 1991;35:179–185.
224. Tan WS, Wilbur A, Spigus DG, et al. Cystic mural nodule in cerebellar hemangioblastoma: CT demonstration. J Comput Assist Tomogr 1984;8:1175–1178.
225. Silver ML, Hennigar G. Cerebellar hemangioma (hemangioblastoma): A clinicopathological review of 40 cases. J Neurosurg 1952;9:484–489.
226. Jeffreys R. Pathological and hematological aspects of posterior fossa hemangioblastoma. J Neurol Neurosurg Psychiatry 1975;38:112–119.
227. Fill WL, Lamiell J, Polk N. The radiographic manifestations of von Hippel-Lindau disease. Radiology 1979;133:289–295.
228. Ho VB, Smirniotopoulos JG, Murphy FM, Rushing EJ. Radiologic-pathologic correlation: Hemangioblastoma. AJNR 1992;13:1343–1352.
229. Cummings JN. The chemistry of cerebral cysts. Brain 1950;73:244–250.
230. Waldmann TA, Levin EH, Baldwin M. The association of polycythemia with a cerebellar hemangioblastoma: The production of an erythropoiesis stimulating factor by the tumor. Am J Med 1961;31:318–324.
231. Huson SM, Harper PS, Hourihan MD, et al. Cerebellar haemangioblastoma and von Hippel-Lindau disease. Brain 1986;109:1297–1310.
232. Filing-Kitz MR, Coyke PL, Oldfield E, et al. Central nervous system involvement in von Hippel-Lindau disease. Neurology 1991;41:41–46.
233. Rojiana AM, Elliott K, Dorovini-Zis K. Extensive replacement of spinal cord and brain stem by hemangioblastoma in a case of von Hippel-Lindau disease. Clin Neuropathol 1991;10:297–302.
234. Megerian CA, McKenna MJ, Nuss RC, et al. Endolymphatic sac tumors: Histopathologic confirmation, clinical characterization, and implication in von Hippel-Lindau disease. Laryngoscope 1995;105:801–808.

235. Gaffey MJ, Mills SE, Boyd JC. Aggressive papillary tumor of middle ear–temporal bone and adnexal papillary cystadenoma: Manifestations of von Hippel-Lindau disease. Am J Surg Pathol 1994;18:1254–1260.

236. Eby TL, Makek MS, Fisch U. Adenomas of the temporal bone. Ann Otol Rhinol Laryngol 1988;97:605–612.

237. Palmer JM, Coker NJ, Harper PL. Papillary adenoma of the temporal bone in von Hippel-Lindau disease. Otolaryngol Head Neck Surg 1989;100:64–68.

238. Poe DS, Tarlov EC, Thomas CB, et al. Aggressive papillary tumors of temporal bone. Otolaryngol Head Neck Surg 1993;108:80–86.

239. Manski TJ, Heffner DK, Glenn GM, et al. Endolymphatic sac tumors: A source of morbid hearing loss in von Hippel-Lindau disease. JAMA 1997;277:1461–1466.

240. Blamires TL, Friedmann I, Moffat DA. Von Hippel-Lindau disease associated with an invasive choroid plexus tumor presenting as a middle ear mass. J Laryngol Otol 1992;106:429–435.

241. Naguib MG, Chou SN, Mastri A. Radiation therapy of a choroid plexus papilloma of the cerebellopontine angle with bone involvement. J Neurosurg 1981;54:245–247.

242. Mukherji SK, Albernaz VS, Lo WWM, et al. Papillary endolymphatic sac tumors: CT, MR imaging, and angiographic findings in 20 patients. Radiology 1997;202:801–808.

243. Lo WWM, Applegate LJ, Carberry JN, et al. Endolymphatic sac tumors: Radiologic appearance. Radiology 1993;189:199–204.

244. Melmon KL, Rosen SW. Lindau's disease. Am J Med 1964;36:595–617.

245. Moore AT, Maher ER, Rosen P, et al. Ophthalmological screening for von Hippel–Lindau disease. Eye 1991;5:723–728.

246. Malek RS, Omess PJ, Benson RC, Zincke H. Renal carcinoma in von Hippel Lindau syndrome. Am J Med 1987;82:236–238.

247. Neumann H. Basic criteria for clinical diagnosis and genetic counselling in von Hippel-Lindau Syndrome. Vasa 1987;16:220–226.

248. Neumann HPH, Berger DP, Sigmund G, et al. Pheochromocytomas, multiple endocrine neoplasia type 2, and von Hippel-Lindau disease. N Engl J Med 1993;329:1531–1538.

249. Mullikan JB, Young AG. Vascular Birthmarks, Hemangiomas and Malformations. Philadelphia, WB Saunders, 1988.

250. Esterly NB. Cutaneous hemangiomas, vascular stains and malformations, and associated syndromes. Curr Probl Pediatr 1996;26:1–48.

251. Sturge WA. A case of partial epilepsy, apparently due to lesions of one of the vaso-motor centres of the brain. Trans Clin Soc Lond 1879;12:162–167.

252. Streeter GL. The developmental alterations in the vascular system of the brain of the human embryo. Contr Embryol Carneg Inst 1918;8:5–38.

253. Wohlwill FJ, Yakovlev PI. Histopathology of meningofacial angiomatosis (Sturge-Weber disease): Report of four cases. J Neuropathol Exp Neurol 1957;16:341–364.

254. Welch K, Naheedy MH, Abroms IF, Strand RD. Computed tomography of Sturge-Weber syndrome in infants. J Comput Assist Tomogr 1980;4:33–36.

255. Enjolras O, Rich MC, Merlan JJ. Facial port-wine stains and Sturge-Weber syndrome. Pediatrics 1985;756:48–51.

256. Tan OT, Sherwood K, Gilchrest BA. Treatment of children with port-wine stains using the flashlamp-pulsed tunable dye laser. N Engl J Med 1989;320:416–421.

257. Griffiths PD. Sturge-Weber syndrome revisited: The role of neuroradiology. Neuropediatrics 1996;27:284–294.

258. Alexander GL. Sturge-Weber syndrome. In Vinken PJ, Bruyn GWF (eds). Handbook of Clinical Neurology: The Phakomatoses, Vol. 14, pp. 223–240. Amsterdam, North Holland, 1972.

259. Gardeur D, Palmieri A, Mashaly R. Cranial computed tomography in the phakomatoses. Neuroradiology 1983;25:293–304.

260. Coulam CM, Brown LR, Reese DF. Sturge-Weber syndrome. Semin Roentgenol 1976;11:55–59.

261. Stimac GK, Solomon MA, Newton TH. CT and MR of angiomatous malformations of the choroid plexus in patients with Sturge-Weber disease. AJNR 1986;7:623–627.

262. Elster AD, Chen MYM. MR imaging of Sturge-Weber syndrome: Role of gadopentetate dimeglumine and gradient-echo techniques. AJNR 1990;11:685–689.

263. Wasenko JJ, Rosenbloom SA, Duchesneau PM, et al. The Sturge-Weber syndrome: Comparison of MR and CT characteristics. AJNR 1990;11:131–134.

264. Chamberlain MC, Press GA, Hesselink JR. MR imaging and CT in three cases of Sturge-Weber syndrome: Prospective comparison. AJNR 1989;10:491–496.

265. Bilaniuk LT, Zimmerman RA, Hochman M, et al. MR of the Sturge-Weber syndrome. AJNR 1987;8:945–950.

266. Lipski S, Brunell F, Aicardi J, et al. Gd-DOTA-enhanced MR imaging in two cases of Sturge-Weber syndrome. AJNR 1990;11:690–692.

267. Bentson JR, Wilson GH, Newton TH. Cerebral venous drainage pattern of the Sturge-Weber syndrome. Radiology 1971;101:111–118.

268. Probst FP. Vascular morphology and angiographic flow patterns in Sturge-Weber angiomatosis: Facts, thoughts and suggestions. Neuroradiology 1980;20:73–78.

269. Poser CM, Taveras JM. Cerebral angiography in encephalo-trigeminal angiomatosis. Radiology 1957;68:327–336.

270. Wagner EJ, Rao KCG, Knipp HC. CT-angiographic correlation in Sturge-Weber syndrome. J Comput Assist Tomogr 1981;5:324–326.

271. Dyke DG, Davidoff LM, Masson CB. Cerebral hemiatrophy with homolateral hypertrophy of the skull and sinuses. Surg Gynecol Obstet 1933;57:588–600.

272. Barkovich AJ, Chuang SH. Unilateral megalencephaly: Correlation of MR imaging and pathologic characteristics. AJNR 1990;11:523–531.

273. Enzmann DR, Hayward RW, Norman D, Dunn RP. Cranial computed tomographic scan appearance of Sturge-Weber disease: Unusual presentation. Radiology 1977;122:721–724.

274. Chugani HT, Mazziota JC, Phelps ME. Sturge-Weber syndrome: A study of cerebral glucose utilization with positron emission tomography. J Pediatr 1989;114:244–253.

275. Peterman AF, Hayles AB, Dockerty MB, Love JG. Encephalotrigeminal angiomatosis (Sturge-Weber disease). JAMA 1958;167:2169–2176.

276. Williams DW III, Elster AD. Cranial CT and MR in the Klippel-Trenaunay-Weber syndrome. AJNR 1992;13:291–294.

277. Murphey MD, Fairbairn KJ, Parman LM, et al. Musculoskeletal angiomatous lesions: Radiologic-pathologic correlation. Radiographics 1995;15:893–917.

278. Phillips GN, Gordon DH, Martin EC, et al. The Klippel-Trenaunay syndrome: Clinical and radiological aspects. Radiology 1978;128:429–434.

279. Cobb S. Haemangioma of the spinal cord, associated with skin naevi of the same metamere. Ann Surg 1915;62:641–649.

280. Rees JH, Smirniotopoulos JG, Matthews MS. Epidermal nevus syndrome. Int J Neuroradiol 1996;2:369–373.

281. Rogers M, McCrossin I, Commens C. Epidermal nevi and the epidermal nevus syndrome. J Am Acad Dermatol 1989;20:476–488.

282. Pavone L, Curatolo P, Rizzo R, et al. Epidermal nevus syndrome. Neurology 1991;41:266–271.

283. Clancy RR, Kurtz MB, Baker D, et al. Neurologic manifestations of the organoid nevus syndrome. Arch Neurol 1985;42:236–240.

284. Vles JS, Degraeuwe P, DeCock P, Casaer P. Neuroradiological findings in Jadassohn nevus phakomatosis: A report of four cases. Eur J Pediatr 1985;144:290–294.

285. Cavenagh EC, Hart BL, Rose D. Association of linear sebaceous nevus syndrome and unilateral megalencephaly. AJNR 1993;14:405–408.

286. Sarwar M, Schafer ME. Brain malformation in linear nevus sebaceous syndrome: An MR study. J Comput Assist Tomogr 1988;12:338–340.

287. Telatar M, Teraoka S, Wang Z, et al. Ataxia-telangiectasia: Identification and detection of founder-effect mutations in the ATM gene in ethnic populations. Am J Hum Genet 1998;62:86–97.

288. Hoskins G. Ataxia-telangiectasia. Dev Med Child Neurol 1982;24:77–80.

289. Savitsky K, Bar-Shira A, Gilad S, et al. A single ataxia telangiectasia gene with product similar to PI-3 kinase. Science 1995;268:1749–1753.

290. Lavin MF, Shiloh Y. The genetic defect in ataxia-telangiectasia. Annu Rev Immunol 1997;15:177–202.

291. Frizzera G, Rosai J, Dehner LP, et al. Lymphoreticular disorders in primary immunodeficiencies: New findings based on up-to-date histologic classification of 35 cases. Cancer 1980;46:692–699.

292. Guttmacher AE, Marchuk DA, White RI Jr. Current concepts:

Hereditary hemorrhagic telangiectasia. N Engl J Med 1995;333:913–924.

293. Haitjema T, Westermann CJ, Overtoom TT, et al. Hereditary hemorrhagic telangiectasia (Osler-Weber-Rendu disease): New insights in pathogenesis, complications, and treatment. Arch Intern Med 1996;156:714–719.

294. Shovlin CL, Huges JMB, Tuddenham EGD, et al. A gene for hereditary haemorrhagic telangiectasia maps to chromosome 9q33–34. Nat Genet 1994;6:197–204.

295. McDonald MT, Papenberg KA, Ghosh S, et al. A disease locus for hereditary haemorrhagic telangiectasia maps to chromosome 9q33–34. Nat Genet 1994;6:197–204.

296. Vincent P, Paluchu H, Hazan J, et al. A third locus for hereditary haemorrhagic telangiectasia maps to chromosome 12q. Hum Mol Genet 1995;4:945–950.

297. Johnson DW, Berg JN, Gallione CJ, et al. A second locus for hereditary hemorrhagic telangiectasia mapped to chromosome 12. Genome Res 1995;5:21–28.

298. Johnson DW, Berg JN, Gallione CJ, et al. Mutations in the activin receptor-like kinase 1 gene in hereditary haemorrhagic telangiectasia type 2. Nat Genet 1996;189–195.

299. Braverman IM, Keh A, Jacobson BS. Ultrastructure and three-dimensional organization of the telangiectases of hereditary hemorrhagic telangiectasia. J Invest Dermatol 1990;95:422–427.

300. Peery WH. Clinical spectrum of hereditary hemorrhagic telangiectasia (Osler-Weber-Rendu disease). Am J Med 1987;82:989–997.

301. Putnam CM, Chaloupka JC, Fulbright RK, et al. Exceptional multiplicity of cerebral arteriovenous malformations associated with hereditary hemorrhagic telangiectasia (Osler-Weber-Rendu syndrome). AJNR 1996;17:1733–1742.

302. Fulbright RK, Chaloupka JC, Putman CM, et al. MR of hereditary hemorrhagic telangiectasia: Prevalence and spectrum of cerebrovascular malformations. AJNR 1998;19:477–484.

303. Kikuchi K, Kowada M, Sakamoto T, et al. Wyburn-Mason syndrome: Report of a rare case with computed tomographic and angiographic evaluations. J Comput Assist Tomogr 1998;12:111–115.

304. Patel V, Gupta SC. Wyburn-Mason syndrome. Neuroradiology 1990;31:544–546.

305. Kimonis VE, Goldstein AM, Pastakia B, et al. Clinical manifestations in 105 persons with nevoid basal cell carcinomas syndrome. Am J Med Genet 1977;69:299–308.

306. Gorlin RJ, Rickers RA, Kellen F, et al. The multiple basal-cell nevi syndrome: An analysis of a syndrome consisting of multiple nevoid basal-cell anomalies, medulloblastoma, hyporesponsiveness to parathormone. Cancer 1965;18:89.

307. Lovin JD, Talarico CL, Wegert SL, et al. Gorlin's syndrome with associated odontogenic cysts. Pediatr Radiol 1991;21:584–587.

308. Ito M. Studies on melanin: XI. Incontinentia pigmenti achromians, a singular case of nevus dipigmentosus systematicus bilateris. Tohoku J Exp Med 1952;55:57–59.

309. Williams DW, Elster AD. Cranial MR imaging in hypomelanosis of Ito. J Comput Assist Tomogr 1991;14:981–983.

310. Moss C, Burn J. Genetic counseling in hypomelanosis of Ito: Case report and review. Clin Genet 1988;34:109–115.

311. Dunn V, Mock T, Bell WE, Smith W. Detection of heterotopic gray matter in children by magnetic resonance imaging. Magn Reson Imaging 1986;4:33–39.

312. Rhodes RE, Freidman HS, Halter HP Jr, et al. Contrast-enhanced MR imaging of neurocutaneous melanosis. AJNR 1991;12:380–382.

313. Sebag G, Dubois J, Pfister P, et al. Neurocutaneous melanosis and temporal lobe tumor in a child: MR study. AJNR 1991;12:699–700.

314. Lloyd KM, Dennis M. Cowden's disease: A possible new symptom complex with multiple system involvement. Ann Intern Med 1963;58:136–142.

315. Williams DW III, Elster AD, Ginsberg LE, Stanton C. Recurrent Lhermitte-Duclos disease: Report of two cases and association with Cowden's disease. AJNR 1992;13:287–290.

316. Padberg GW, Schot JDL, Vielvoye GJ, et al. Lhermitte-Duclos disease and Cowden disease: A single phakomatosis. Ann Neurol 1991;29:517–523.

317. Nelen MR, van Staveren WCG, Peeters EAJ, et al. Germline mutations in the PTEN/MMAC1 gene in patients with Cowden disease. Hum Mol Genet 1997;6:1383–1387.

52

Traumatic Brain Injury in Children

MARY K. EDWARDS-BROWN, M.D.
BLAINE L. HART, M.D.

INCIDENCE OF PEDIATRIC BRAIN INJURY

The significance of pediatric brain injury in the United States cannot be overstated. Trauma is the leading cause of death and disability in the pediatric population, and the incidence of traumatic brain injury is continuing to increase.[1, 2] Twice as many deaths are due to injuries and accidents than are caused by congenital malformations and childhood cancers combined.[3, 4] The causes of head trauma depend, in large part, on the age of the patient. The three major causes of brain injury are falls, motor vehicle accidents, and bicycle accidents.[1, 3, 5]

In the neonatal period, the major cause of brain injury is the trauma inflicted during the birth process.[6, 7] In the infantile period, up to 2 years of age, falls account for the majority of pediatric head injury, usually owing to the immaturity and curiosity of the toddler. Because the fall is usually not from a great height, toddlers rarely suffer severe accidental head injury. Even falls down stairways rarely cause significant injuries.[8] The exceptions to the rule of toddlers rarely suffering severe accidental head injury are injuries resulting from baby walkers and shopping carts.[9] Infant walkers have been called "a lethal form of transportation," in which a child can propel himself or herself down a flight of stairs with the head extended, vulnerable to head and cervical spine trauma.[9] Shopping-cart injuries are similar in incidence and in mechanism, with head and cervical spine injuries being most common.[9]

Child abuse and neglect, although much less common than accidental injury, still occur with an annual incidence of approximately 2.5% of children ages 0 to 17 years.[10] It is estimated that 30% of cases are physical abuse, 20% are sexual abuse, and 50% are neglect.[10] Physical abuse occurs less than one-tenth as often as accidental injury, but it is much more likely to be a cause of death.[11] Child abuse accounts for 80% of traumatic deaths in children less than 2 years of age.[12] Even though there is acknowledged underreporting of child abuse, at least 3000 deaths owing to abuse occur annually in the United States, the majority the result of head trauma. It has been estimated that child abuse is the cause of at least 10% of cases of mental retardation and cerebral palsy.[13–15] At least 10% of children under 5 years of age seen in the emergency room for trauma are actually victims of child abuse. Associated risk factors for abuse include poverty, unemployment, parental divorce, substance abuse, illegitimacy, previous social service intervention within the family, and a history of abuse to the perpetrator in childhood.[11] One-third of reported abuse is extrafamilial, and boys appear to be at greater risk than girls for extrafamilial abuse. Children with disabilities are also at greater risk for abuse.[12]

In later childhood, bicycle accidents are a more common cause of head injury than falls. Between 500 and 600 deaths owing to bicycle injuries are reported annually in the United States.[5] Bicycle-related injury rates are especially high in 10- to 14-year-old boys, who have an estimated rate of 13 emergency room–treated injuries/1000 population/yr.[5] Head injury is the most important determinant of bicycle-related mortality and permanent disability.[5] In spite of evidence that helmets can significantly reduce the risk of head injury, less than 10% of children routinely wear helmets while cycling.[5] In adolescents, there is a roughly equal incidence of falls, motor vehicle accidents, and bicycle accidents. In the 15- to 18-year-old age range, motor vehicle accidents are the most common cause of brain injury and the most common cause of death.[16] Athletic injury to the brain is an increasingly recognized problem in adolescents.[17] It has been estimated that 20% of high school football players suffer a closed head injury each season.[17] Although most are minor, injuries from high-risk sports (diving, gymnastics, horseback riding, ice hockey, trampolining, wrestling, and football) include arterial dissection, contusion, infarction, and intracranial hemorrhage.[17]

Recently, the incidence of violent trauma has increased in the older childhood and adolescent ages. Penetrating trauma is disproportionately higher in the urban setting, where firearm and stabbing injuries are responsible for three to four times more deaths compared with surrounding rural areas.[16, 18] In 1988, firearms were the cause of death in 4000 children.[18] A disproportionate number of young black males are victims of violent death, more than seven times that of white males of the same age. In fact, homicide is the leading cause of death in black males aged 15 to 24 years.[18]

MANAGEMENT OF BRAIN INJURY

The optimal management of brain trauma depends on timely diagnosis and treatment. A well-prepared rescue and transport team will assure that basic airway, cardiac, and respiratory resuscitation has been performed when necessary. Blood pressure must be maintained and bleeding stopped. Spinal immobilization is ensured to reduce further spinal cord injury. A common complication of nonaccidental brain injury is the delay in reporting the injury. When the child arrives at the emergency facility a neurologic assessment is performed. In adolescents, the Glasgow Coma Score is obtained.[1] In younger children, a modification of the Glasgow Coma Score is used.[1] A Glasgow Coma Score of 13 to 15 indicates a mild head injury, 9 to 12 indicates moderate injury, and less than 8 indicates severe head injury. It has been recommended that any patient with a score less than 15 should be observed and studied by computed tomography (CT) or magnetic resonance imaging (MRI) to evaluate the brain and help plan therapy.[19-22] Therapy for brain injury includes evacuation of hemorrhage and treatment of increased intracranial pressure. The role of CT is significant in that patients with a nonfocal neurologic examination and normal head CT scan are unlikely to develop neurologic defects and are usually discharged for observation at home, rather than admitted to the hospital.[22] In children with neurologic deterioration, reimaging is necessary. Delayed epidural, subdural, and even parenchymal hemorrhages are well-recognized complications of injury. As the blood pressure is restored in the hypotensive child, the increased cerebral perfussion increases the chance that hemorrhage will result from injured brain or blood vessels.

There is a significant difference in the response of children to brain trauma depending on age.[14] In infants, mild brain injury usually recovers without complication. In older children with mild injury, there is further deterioration in the Glasgow Coma Score in 10%, and 2% to 3% will require some form of neurosurgical intervention. In young children with moderate brain injury, there is a small risk of malignant brain edema with late deterioration and death (Fig. 52–1).[6] In children less than 2 years of age with severe brain injury, there is an increased mortality compared with older children and adults.[14] Child abuse is much more common in children under 2 years old and has a higher incidence of mortality than other forms of head trauma. For these reasons, it is likely that abuse accounts for the increased mortality in young children with severe brain injury.[14]

IMAGING CONSIDERATIONS

CT is commonly used for the acute evaluation of brain trauma.[23] Indications for CT include changing level of consciousness, seizures, focal neurologic deficits, de-

pressed or compound skull fracture, skull penetration, bulging fontanelle, and severe vomiting after injury. CT is usually easier to obtain, quicker, and less limited by life-support equipment than is MRI. CT scans will detect subarachnoid hemorrhages, which are rarely demonstrated on MRI. CT is also adequate for planning the acute neurosurgical treatment when necessary. A plain skull radiograph is a useful adjunct in the evaluation of suspected child abuse, and skull fractures are found in approximately 50% of children with intracranial injury resulting from abuse.[1, 10]

Although CT has been proved sufficient for the majority of acute brain injury, the use of MRI is increasing in the evaluation of subtle or complex brain trauma.[24, 25] The multiplanar capability, reduced artifacts, and increased resolution of MRI allow improved detection of hemorrhagic and nonhemorrhagic shear injuries, extra-axial hemorrhages, peripheral cortical contusions, and posterior fossa lesions. It has become common practice to perform a CT scan for acute brain injury and to perform the MRI examination of the brain later.[14] The most common reason for performing an MRI study is a neurologic presentation that is more severe than can be explained from the CT scan. Suspected child abuse may be better evaluated by MRI, given the increased detection of small injuries and the improved ability to detect hemorrhages of different ages (Fig. 52–2).

Several recent improvements in MRI pulse sequences result in superior imaging of brain trauma. The fast spin echo techniques, by shortening scan time, reduce the need for sedation and are less degraded by motion artifacts. The decreased sensitivity to hemorrhage with fast spin echo techniques can be compensated for by adding a gradient-echo image, which is more sensitive to hemorrhage than conventional spin-echo techniques.[14] MRI angiographic techniques are also quite helpful in evaluating dissection and other vascular injuries.[25] In general, MRI is a better method than CT for evaluating the extent and nature of injury, and it may help provide prognostic information (Fig. 52–3).

SPECIAL CONSIDERATIONS IN PEDIATRIC VERSUS ADULT BRAIN INJURY

As in all other disease considerations, children are not young adults. Compared with adults, there are significant differences in the response of the child's brain to the effects of trauma.[26] Even within the childhood years, there are significant differences. Not only is the response to injury different, the mechanisms of injury are also significantly different between children and adults and between children of different ages.

The child's head is relatively much larger and heavier compared with the body than in the adult and is supported by smaller, weaker neck musculature. For this reason, the head is frequently the contact point on impact. In addition, the facial skeleton is smaller and weaker and provides less protection for the brain. Because of the necessity for the skull to compensate for brain growth, the calvarium is also thinner and provides less protection.

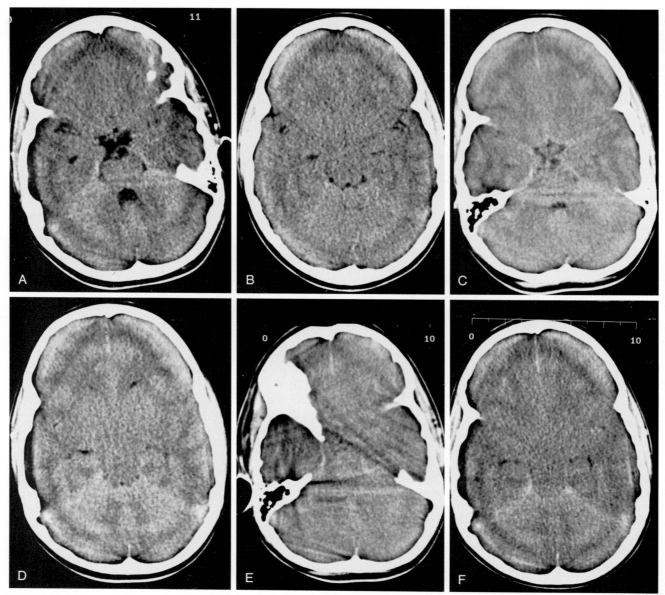

FIGURE 52–1 Sequential cranial computed tomography (CT) scans of a child who fell from a height of 12 to 13 feet. *A, C,* and *E* are at the level of the fourth ventricle and suprasellar cistern; *B, D,* and *F* are at the level of the quadrigeminal cistern. *A* and *B,* The initial scan, shortly after admission, was normal. A lucid interval was followed by clinical deterioration and coma. *C* and *D,* A scan about 20 hours later demonstrates diffuse edema. *E* and *F,* Despite aggressive therapy, on the final scan, 5 hours later, there is near-complete effacement of the cisterns and ventricles. The child died shortly thereafter. (Density over the frontal lobes is artifact.)

The calvarium is unilaminar until approximately 4 years, and it lacks a diploic space. Facial nerve injury is also more common in children, owing to the underdevelopment of the mastoid air cells and more lateral location of the stylomastoid foramen.[27] There is a propensity for compression of the nerve during the birth process.[27] Facial nerve injury is the most common manifestation of birth trauma, occurring in up to 6% of cases.[27]

Compared with adults, epidural hematomas are much less common in children and are more frequently caused by venous rather than arterial bleeding. Several reasons have been suggested: (1) there is a greater adherence of the dura to the inner table of the skull; (2) the pediatric skull is more malleable, allowing mild deformity without

fracture or dural tearing; (3) the middle meningeal artery is in a superficial location, allowing more displacement before tearing; and (4) there is a greater tendency toward venous thrombosis (Fig. 52–4).[1]

Shear, or axonal stretch, injuries are more common in children's brains than in adults'.[28, 29] This is due in large part to the different consistency of the pediatric brain. Because of the relative absence of myelination, the pediatric brain is much less firm, more like gelatin, and more likely to deform on impact.[1] Also, the weak neck musculature provides less protection against rapid movements such as are generated with shaking or motor vehicle accidents. Children under 1 year of age also have a greater subarachnoid space than do older children and

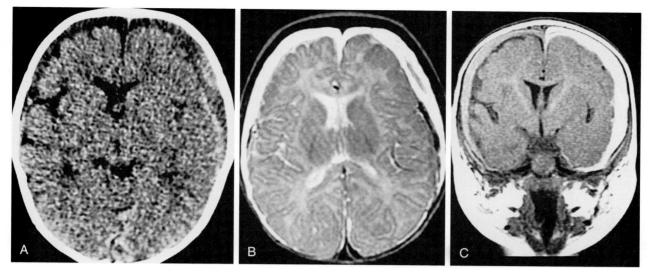

FIGURE 52–2 CT and magnetic resonance imaging (MRI) studies of a victim of child abuse (age 5 mo) with subdural blood of differing ages. *A*, CT scan shows low-density extra-axial fluid on the patient's right and mixed-density fluid on the patient's left. MRI was performed within 12 hours of the CT scan. *B*, Axial T2-weighted image confirms three distinct components on the patient's left, with low, intermediate, and high signal intensity. *C*, Coronal T1-weighted image shows very clearly the different signal intensities of the largest subdural hematomas.

FIGURE 52–3 CT and MRI studies of a victim of child abuse (age 2 mo). *A*, Initial CT scan shows only a very small area of mildly increased attenuation over the right frontal convexity. Most slices appeared normal. MRI was performed within 12 hours of the CT scan and demonstrates much more clearly the intracranial hemorrhage. *B*, Intermediate-weighted image shows an extra-axial fluid collection on the patient's right, with a small area of higher signal intensity within. *C*, Coronal T1-weighted image shows a small hematoma overlying the superomedial aspect of the right cerebral hemisphere, extending into the interhemispheric fissure. *D*, On coronal gradient-recalled image, the hematoma has very low signal intensity. Retinal hemorrhages were present on physical examination.

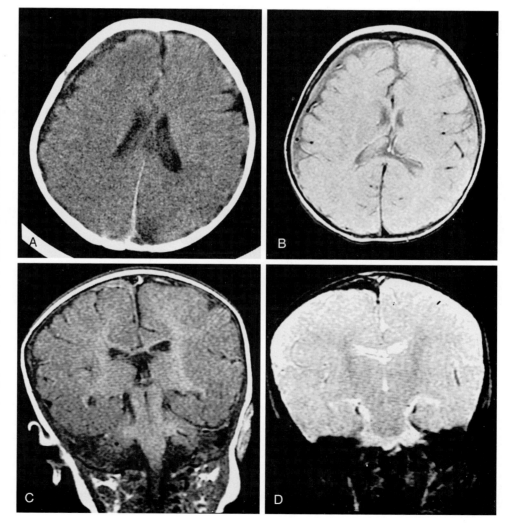

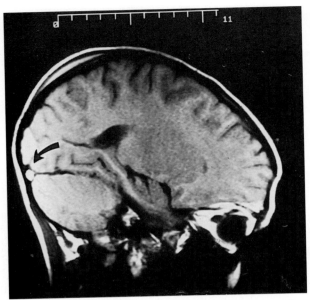

FIGURE 52–4 Four-year-old child, pedestrian, hit by an automobile. Brain injury is complicated by thrombosis of the transverse sinus *(curved arrow)*, demonstrated as a bright area on T1-weighted MRI, indicating the presence of methemoglobin.

young adults, permitting more motion of the brain within the skull and allowing more rotational and shearing forces.

Well-recognized lesions occur more commonly or even uniquely in children compared with adults, including cerebellar hemorrhages, brain stem injury, periventricular leukomalacia, status marmoratus (hypermyelination of the thalamus and basal ganglia owing to ischemia), and other less-common lesions.[30, 31]

The increased subarachnoid space and the open sutures of the young infant allow an increase in intracranial mass to occur without an associated increase in intracranial pressure until late.[32] This feature protects the child from suffering injury from small masses, but it may mask early signs of hemorrhage or swelling. Unlike adults, children may lose a considerable proportion of their blood volume in intracranial hemorrhage. This is due both to the small total blood volume of children and to the relatively large calvarium.

Injuries to the neck and the child's relatively large tongue cause an increase in the incidence of airway obstruction and secondary hypoxic brain injuries. Also, establishing and maintaining intubation in the small child carry increased risks. Injuries to the cervical spine and cord are relatively less common, however, due to the increased flexibility of the pediatric spine. Neither fractures nor spinal cord traumatic lesions are seen with any frequency in children compared with adults.[33] It has been recommended that children who are capable of verbal communication who do not report cervical discomfort do not need cervical spine x-rays.[33] When bony injury occurs in children, it is more common in the upper cervical region, compared with the more common injury to the lower cervical spine in adults. Where the spine is more fixed, in the lower cervical region, there is increased risk of cord injury, even though bony injury is more common in the upper cervical spine.

Posttraumatic seizures are a more common complication of brain injury in children than in adults.[34] As many as 10% of children under 5 years old develop posttraumatic seizures, twice the number occurring in older children and adults. Young children develop seizures within minutes to hours of the impact, much sooner than adults. Unlike in adults, posttraumatic seizures do not imply a poor prognostic outcome.[34] Children who suffer multiple posttraumatic seizures are more likely to develop epilepsy.

Malignant brain edema is more common in children than in adults, owing to an increase in cerebral blood flow.[35, 36] The immature pediatric brain is prone to loss of cerebral autoregulation resulting in hyperemic cerebral edema (Fig. 52–5).[35, 37] By contrast, in adults cerebral edema is usually associated with a decrease in cerebral blood flow.[38]

A continuum of development of the brain and myelination of the cerebral white matter in children from the fetal period until young adulthood alters the effects of brain trauma.[39] Those portions of the brain that are most metabolically active at a given period of time are most susceptible to ischemic injury.[7, 39, 40] The precentral gyrus, for example, is most susceptible in the neonatal period, accounting for the large numbers of children with cerebral palsy secondary to birth asphyxia. Myelination can be delayed by many factors that might accompany trauma, including malnutrition, asphyxia, and maternal drug abuse.

Although many factors contribute to the severity of pediatric brain injury, one positive factor is that children usually have a more complete neurologic recovery than adults with similar presenting injuries. This has been attributed to the plasticity of the developing undermyelinated brain or the ability of noninjured brain to assume the functions that would have been performed by the damaged brain.[41] The very young brain is also more likely to develop cavities in response to injury, related to the immature astrocytic response of the developing brain. This response is most marked in fetal or premature infantile injuries, in which porencephalic cavities may be smooth-walled, with no internal architecture, but it is well recognized that all young children have a greater tendency to cystic encephalomalacia than do adults.

SKULL INJURIES

Neonatal extracranial bleeding occurs in three compartments, the scalp or caput succedaneum, subgaleal space, and the subperiosteal space or cephalohematoma. Hemorrhage and edema in the scalp occur commonly after vaginal births, and although it may appear alarming to parents, it usually clears quickly in the first few days of life. Caput succedaneum is apparent clinically owing to the characteristic swelling, which is soft and superficial and may cross suture lines. Radiographic evaluation is not indicated. Subgaleal hemorrhages occur below the galea aponeurotica, a tendinous sheet that gives rise to the attachment of the frontalis and occipitalis scalp muscles (Fig. 52–6). Subgaleal hemorrhages also occur after vagi-

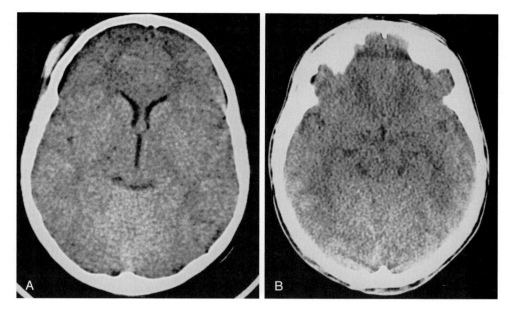

FIGURE 52–5 Progressive development of diffuse cerebral swelling. *A,* Brain appears normal on initial CT scan. *B,* The next day, complete effacement of the quadrigeminal cistern is seen, indicating an increase in intracranial pressure.

nal births, but they are less common than caput succedaneum. They may be clinically significant owing to a large volume of blood, but surgical intervention is rarely necessary and imaging is not indicated. The recent increase in use of "vacuum extraction" techniques for delivery has resulted in increased numbers of subgaleal hematomas. A cephalohematoma is caused by subperiosteal hemorrhage and is confined by the cranial sutures. Although cephalohematomas are uncommon, occurring in only 1% of births, the incidence is much higher with forceps deliveries (Fig. 52–7).[6] Cephalohematomas may increase in size after birth, presenting as a firm mass. If imaging is performed, calcification of the mass may be seen remarkably early, but resolution of the mass occurs as the skull grows and remodels (Fig. 52–8).

Imaging of skull fractures has become less common

since it was recognized that the presence or absence of skull fractures carries little or no prognostic value.[42] The major reasons for performing skull x-rays are to document the fracture in cases of nonaccidental injury (Fig. 52–9) and to characterize the more complex and depressed fractures (Fig. 52–10). When a skull fracture is accompanied by a tear of the dura, meninges and brain tissue may herniate into the fracture, preventing healing of the fracture and permitting cerebrospinal fluid pulsation to enlarge the fracture and extend into the subgaleal space.[43, 44] This entity is termed a *leptomeningeal cyst* or *growing fracture of childhood.* Although leptomeningeal cysts are rare, the fractures resulting in the cyst occur in children less than 3 years of age in 90% of cases.[43] The detection of leptomeningeal cyst is usually delayed. The average time of diagnosis is 14 months after the initial fracture.[43]

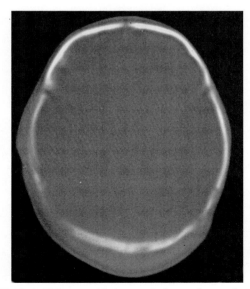

FIGURE 52–6 CT scan with bone windows of a newborn demonstrates a subgaleal hematoma in the occipital region.

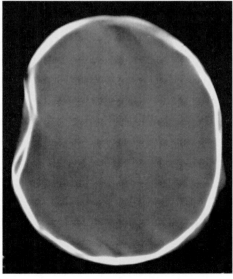

FIGURE 52–7 CT scan with bone windows of a newborn after forceps extraction shows a severe depressed skull fracture.

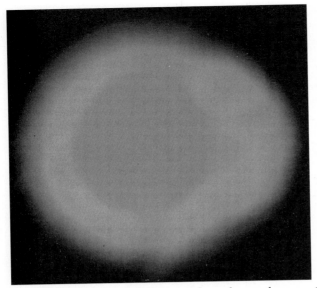

FIGURE 52–8 CT scan with bone windows shows a large, ossifying, left parietal cephalohematoma in a 10-day-old infant whose parents noticed an increase in the size of skull mass.

NEONATAL INJURIES

Hemorrhages within the tentorium, falx, and subdural space are not uncommon in infants after vaginal delivery. Posterior fossa subdural hematomas are especially common and do not require intervention unless they are massive. Massive hemorrhages may occur from tentorial or falx tears extending adjacent to the vein of Galen or other venous sinuses.[45] Epidural hematomas are frequent presenting findings in infants with venous sinus rupture.

Extra-Axial Hematomas

Epidural hematomas are uncommon in infants and increase in incidence with age. In the neonatal period, most

epidural hematomas are due to venous rupture.[1] In older children and adolescents, epidural hematomas are caused by the same mechanism as in adults, fractures across the middle meningeal artery. Unlike in adults, the child may adapt to the accumulation of blood by expansion of the pliable skull, and loss of consciousness is less common in children than in adults after epidural hematomas. Small epidural hematomas that do not result in loss of consciousness (and even some large epidurals) may be watched by frequent neurologic evaluation and imaging rather than evacuation. The findings of epidural hematomas on CT and MRI are a lentiform hyperdense collection that does not cross sutures, except in cases of rupture of the superior sagittal sinus (Fig. 52–11). Hematomas follow the same progression as seen in adults, and when they are acute, they are frequently bright on T1-weighted images and dark on T2-weighted images, reflecting the presence of intracellular methemoglobin.[29] A fluid-fluid level resulting from layering of clotted blood or blood products may be seen.[29]

Subdural hematomas are more common in young infants in whom widening of the subarachnoid spaces is normal (Fig. 52–12). As in elderly adults, subdural hemorrhaging results from ripping of cortical bridging veins crossing the subdural space.[46] Unlike in adults, bilateral subdural hematomas occur in more than 80% of infants. Many subdural hematomas result from birth trauma. As in all cases of brain injury, subdural hematomas in the absence of a history of significant trauma should alert the radiologist to the possibility of child abuse. Imaging of subdural hematomas in children is similar to adults, and contrast may reveal enhancement of the inner and outer membranes of the hematoma. MRI shows convexity subdural hematomas more clearly than CT because of the difference in the intensity of bone and the underlying hematoma (Fig. 52–13). As in adults, there is no hemosiderin seen within a chronic subdural hematoma because there are no macrophages in the subdural space to engulf

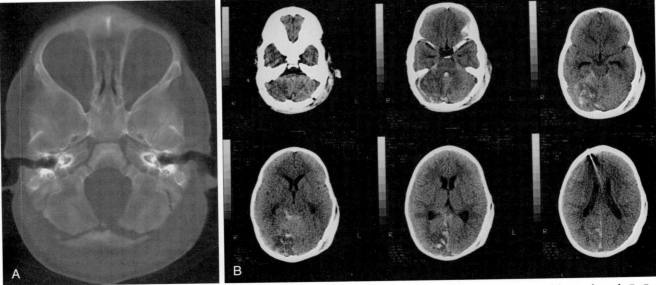

FIGURE 52–9 *A,* CT scan with bone windows shows a comminuted occipital skull fracture in a child who had been abused. *B,* Soft tissue windows show hemorrhagic contusion and subarachnoid hemorrhage.

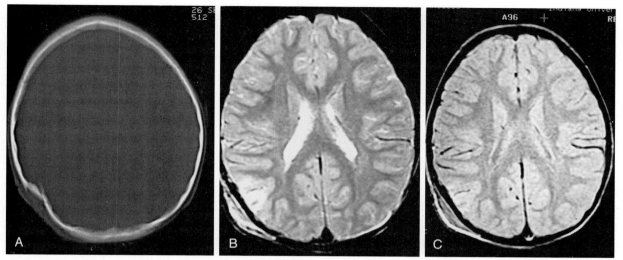

FIGURE 52–10 Five-year-old girl kicked in the head by a horse. *A,* Initial CT scan shows a depressed skull fracture. MRI with T2-weighting *(B)* and proton-density weighting *(C)* shows a nonhemorrhagic contusion subjacent to the fracture.

the blood, die, and remain as an indicator of prior hemorrhage. It is important to realize than unlike intraparenchymal hematomas, the absence of hemosiderin does not mean that a subdural hematoma is not chronic or that a prior subdural hematoma has not been present.

Subarachnoid hemorrhage is a frequent finding in children with parenchymal injuries. This may be a useful sign of more serious injury in a child in whom lesions are absent or subtle on CT (Fig. 52–14). MRI is rarely able to detect subarachnoid hemorrhage.[47] Subarachnoid hemorrhage is seen on CT scanning as increased density within the involved subarachnoid space, usually in the posterior interhemispheric fissure or along the tentorium (Fig. 52–15).

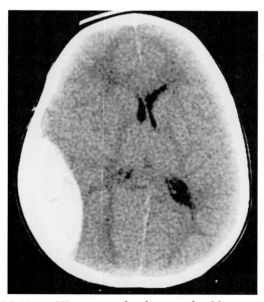

FIGURE 52–11 CT scan reveals a large epidural hematoma in a 9-month-old who fell from a highchair.

Intra-Axial Injuries

Acute parenchymal injuries include cerebral edema, contusions, and shear injuries. Both contusions and shear injuries may be hemorrhagic. Contusions are caused by the brain bouncing against the unyielding inner table of the skull, with bruising and edema resulting. Both coup and contrecoup contusions are common. Shear, or axonal stretch, injuries result from stretching or shear forces on the brain, usually from rotational injuries.[29] Shear injuries are most common at the gray-white junction, corpus callosum, internal capsule, basal ganglia, thalamus, and brain stem (Fig. 52–16).[1, 20, 29] Within the brain stem, the cerebral peduncles are especially prone to injury.[20] Shear injuries, contusions, and diffuse cerebral edema may contribute to cerebral swelling. Generalized cerebral swelling, as a result of brain injury, is more common in children than in adults (Fig. 52–17).[20, 30, 35, 36] The swelling probably results from edema as well as from a decrease in cerebrovascular resistance with vasodilatation and increased blood volume. Although cerebral swelling is rarely apparent within 18 hours after trauma, both CT and MRI will show decreased gray and white matter differentiation by 24 hours. Compression of cerebral sulci and effacement of the cisterns is also seen.[20] The quadrigeminal plate cistern is regarded as the most sensitive to the presence of swelling, and it should be observed for compression after head trauma. A focal decreased attenuation of the basal ganglia is common in brain-injured children.[20] If there is a unilateral mass effect, midline shift, transtentorial uncal herniation, and subfalcine herniation may also be evident.[20] Infarction may result from compression of the ipsilateral posterior cerebral arteries in the case of uncal herniation and the anterior cerebral arteries in the case of subfalcine herniation. In addition, distortion of the base of the brain owing to uncal herniation may cause stretching and occlusion of the thalamoperforator arteries and thalamic infarction. Poor prognostic signs include diffuse cerebral swelling and the "reversal sign" of increased density of the white

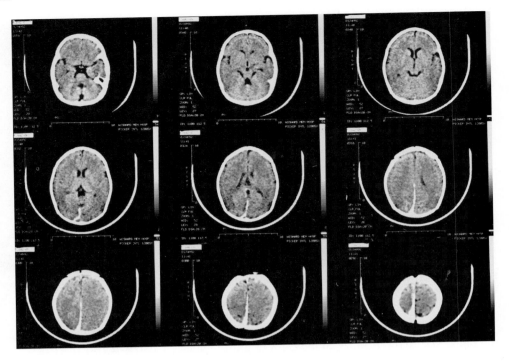

FIGURE 52–12 CT scans of a 10-month-old child with nonaccidental trauma, retinal hemorrhages, and seizures shows an interhemispheric subdural hematoma.

matter compared with the gray matter.[36] On CT scanning, axonal shear injuries are seen only as occasional punctate areas of hemorrhage.[29]

The use of MRI in the evaluation of brain injury is limited because of the extra care required to provide life support equipment, longer scan times, increased need for sedation, and high cost. MRI is superior to CT, however, in detecting non–life-threatening injuries and providing detailed anatomy of injuries.[20] MRI examination is much more sensitive to the presence of hemorrhagic shear injuries, which appear as dark lesions on gradient-echo

imaging, and of nonhemorrhagic shears, which appear as bright lesions on T2-weighted imaging (Fig. 52–18).[1, 24] Fluid attenuated inversion recovery imaging offers promise in the increased sensitivity to nonhemorrhagic shear injuries. In the subacute phase, hemorrhage appears bright on both T1- and T2-weighted sequences owing to the presence of methemoglobin. With time, the methemoglobin evolves to hemosiderin and appears dark on T2-weighted images. Areas of encephalomalacia appear bright on T2-weighted images, and cavitation appears dark on T1-weighted sequences. Both the MRI and the CT examinations may be misleading in the acute phase after trauma because reversible and profound cerebral

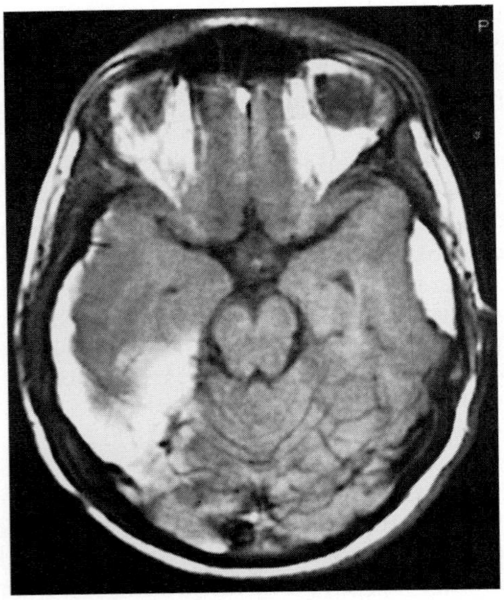

FIGURE 52–13 T1-weighted MRI study shows a large subdural hematoma on the right, layering on the tentorium as well as adjacent to the temporal bone, and a small left epidural hematoma.

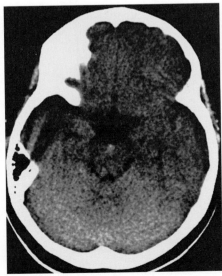

FIGURE 52–14 CT scan reveals a small subarachnoid hemorrhage within the interpeduncular cistern.

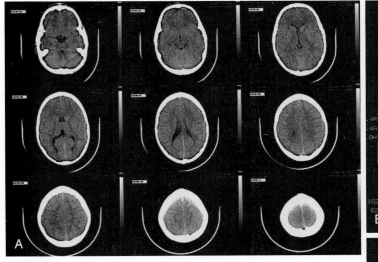
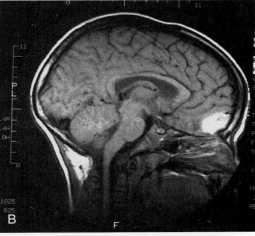
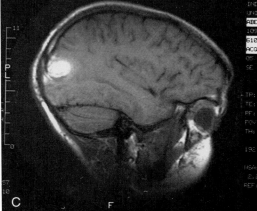

FIGURE 52–15 Motor vehicle accident in a 4-year-old. *A*, CT scans show a prominent posterior falx sign consistent with acute subarachnoid hemorrhage. *B* and *C*, Although the subarachnoid hemorrhage cannot be detected on the MRI study, coup-contrecoup hemorrhagic contusions are clearly seen.

injury may have a similar appearance. Follow-up examinations in children with severe injury will demonstrate atrophy, and the scans of children with mild injury will be normal by 3 months after injury. Parenchymal lesions are seen on MRI in 71% of children 3 months after moderate to severe closed head injury.[1] Another tool in the prosecution of suspected child abuse is the use of postmortem cranial MRI.[47] MRI is useful in directing the autopsy and brain cutting to focal areas of abnormality and may disclose abnormalities missed by autopsy (Fig. 52–19).[47]

Proton magnetic resonance spectroscopy shows some promise in differentiating cerebral swelling owing to shearing injury from the more benign increased blood volume.[48] Proton magnetic resonance spectroscopy shows decreased N-acetyl-aspartate and increased lactate in the face of severe brain injury, but it is normal in patients with mild injury.[48] Proton spectroscopy has not proved useful in detecting small injuries, such as seen with shear or axonal injury.[48] Positron emission tomography has been used to predict the outcome of children with traumatic brain injury, but it has not proved more useful than CT or MRI.[49]

Children with hemophilia present a special problem in the management and imaging of head trauma. Head trauma is the leading cause of mortality in hemophiliacs.[50] Hemorrhage may occur in the face of minor or "inconsequential" injury and can occur spontaneously. A history of

head trauma is recalled in only half of cases of intracranial hemorrhage in hemophiliacs.[50] Children with subdural hematomas typically have a symptom-free period of more than 24 hours. For these reasons, it is the typical practice to obtain a CT scan in most cases of head trauma in hemophiliacs, as well as repeat CT scans in all hemophiliacs with delayed symptoms.[50]

The most common late effects to the brain from trauma are infarctions, other vascular complications, and hydrocephalus. Infections and leptomeningeal cysts, although less common, are also seen (Fig. 52–20).[51] Infarctions and encephalomalacia are discussed in the previous section. Vascular brain lesions caused by trauma include carotid cavernous fistulas, arterial dissection, and venous thrombosis. Carotid cavernous fistulas are more common in adults than in children and are discussed elsewhere. Arterial dissections are caused by direct injury to the carotid or vertebral arteries. The trauma may be severe, such as a motor vehicle accident with whiplash injury to the vertebral artery in the bony foramen transversarium. The trauma may be almost inconsequential, such as occurs with "roughhousing" with parents or playmates. The neurologic presentation of arterial dissections reflects the portion of the brain with infarction. Paresis, dysphasia, and altered level of consciousness are common presenting signs.[1] The MRI appearance is characteristic. The infarction appears as a bright lesion on T2-weighted

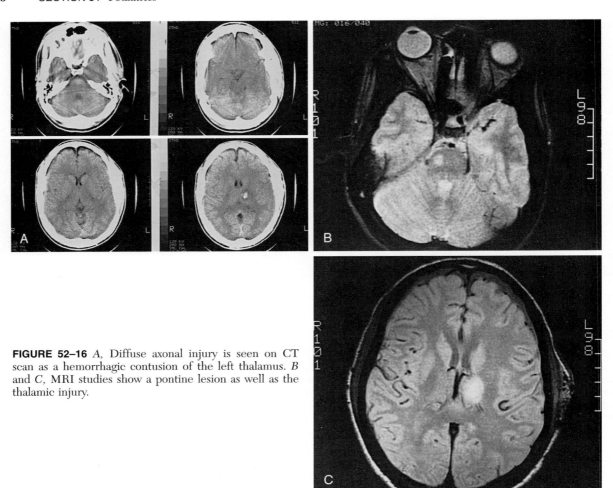

FIGURE 52–16 *A,* Diffuse axonal injury is seen on CT scan as a hemorrhagic contusion of the left thalamus. *B* and *C,* MRI studies show a pontine lesion as well as the thalamic injury.

sequences. The affected vessel appears narrowed on magnetic resonance angiography. A crescent of bright signal owing to methemoglobin is usually seen within the vessel wall on T1-weighted sequences. If a high-quality MRI and magnetic resonance angiography study shows arterial dissection clearly, there is usually no need for catheter angiography.[25] Hydrocephalus after head trauma is of the communicating type, resulting from subarachnoid hemorrhaging with subsequent occlusion of the arachnoid granulations. Although our focus is on brain injuries, it is important to recognize that the brain injury reflects the condition of the entire body. Cardiac injury, abdominal trauma, and even severe emotional trauma may affect the ability of the child to heal.[10] Pneumonia and sepsis may be a serious complication in children with head trauma.[51]

Venous thrombosis as a complication of trauma may occur because of direct injury to the sinus, infection, or dehydration, or a combination. Venous thromboses typically cause hemorrhagic infarctions in a distribution that cannot be explained by arterial occlusion. MRI, magnetic resonance venography, and catheter angiography may be used in the evaluation of venous thrombosis and are discussed elsewhere.

Brain injury rarely causes infection, unless there is a penetrating injury or basilar skull fracture. Bacterial seed-

ing through the dural laceration or through the penetrating injury may cause cerebritis or abscess.

Child Abuse

The most important clue in recognizing child abuse, also known as *nonaccidental injury,* is a discrepancy between the reported cause of injury and the severity of lesions observed on imaging studies.[1, 11] Retinal hemorrhages, especially when bilateral, are also strong indicators of child abuse.[52] Skull fractures are seen in 50% of children with known child abuse or neglect.[10, 11] A fracture caused by intentional trauma is more likely to be complex, multiple, and occipital or posterior parietal in location.[10, 11, 53] Symmetric cranial fractures in infants are most likely the result of bilateral compression of the head between two surfaces rather than the result of a localized impact.[54] The association of other fractures, such as those in long bones, should also increase the suspicion for abuse. Fractures caused by abuse include metaphyseal corner, posterior rib, and scapula fractures that are multiple or in different stages of healing, spinous process fractures, and spiral fractures in nonambulatory infants.[10, 53] A skeletal survey and bone scintigraphy should be performed in suspected child abuse, especially in children less than 2 years of age

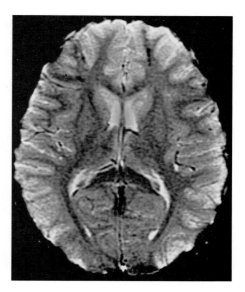

FIGURE 52–17 T2-weighted MRI study shows diffuse cortical swelling as a band of bright signal in the frontal regions in a 10-year-old after severe head trauma.

or older nonverbal children.[10, 53] Bone scintigraphy has been found to be a better initial screening tool for infants less than 1 year of age with suspected physical abuse.[10, 55] When physical abuse has occurred, CT has proved to be the best initial study for detecting the intracranial manifestations of injury.[12, 23, 24, 56] MRI is a useful additional tool in detecting blood of different ages and subtle areas of additional injury. Cerebral contusions, subdural hematomas, and rarely, epidural hematomas are found underlying skull fractures (Fig. 52–21).[12, 23, 24, 56] Fractures are caused by a direct blow to the child's head, usually owing to beating. As such, bruising is a common external sign.

A high-quality ophthalmologic examination is imperative in cases of suspected child abuse. The presence of retinal hemorrhages in a child with little external evidence of trauma, and without a history of significant external trauma, is considered pathognomonic for child abuse.[52, 57] The mechanism for retinal hemorrhages requires sudden deceleration after impact.[52, 57] In several series, the only nonaccidental injury capable of producing this type of hemorrhage was a side-impact automobile crash.[52] Causes of retinal hemorrhages other than injury include vaginal delivery, cardiopulmonary resuscitation, extracorporeal oxygenation, and massive increases in intrathoracic pressures such as caused by being run over.[52] This mechanism may also be a factor in the child who is shaken while the chest is compressed enough to cause rib fractures or the child who is strangled.[52] The use of MRI in the evaluation of orbital injuries is limited, because MRI cannot detect retinal hemorrhages. It is always useful to observe the orbits on MRI studies in cases of suspected abuse, however, because retinal detachment or gross hemorrhage may be seen (Fig. 52–22).

Shaken baby injury has become a well-recognized cause of severe head injury. The cause of the diffuse brain changes is a severe acceleration-deceleration injury best termed *shaken impact injury.* Skull fractures and

FIGURE 52–18 Hemorrhagic contusion in the right frontal region appears more conspicuous on the gradient-echo image *(A)* than on the routine spin-echo T2-weighted image *(B).*

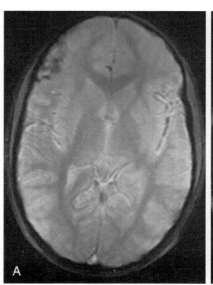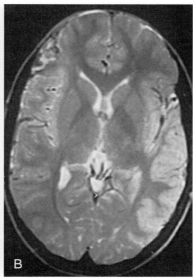

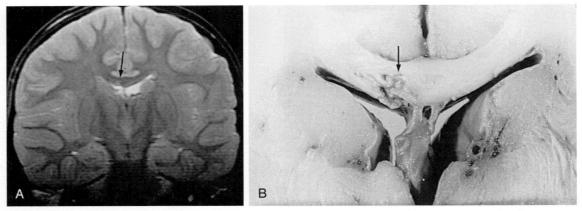

FIGURE 52–19 Coronal T2-weighted postmortem MRI study *(A)* and corresponding autopsy section *(B)* of a shearing injury of the corpus callosum *(arrows)* in a victim of child abuse. The autopsy photo is reversed to correspond with the radiographic convention. The pathologist had initially overlooked this as a presumed cutting artifact, but it is clearly present on the preautopsy MRI study and was called to the pathologist's attention by the radiologist. Careful microscopic examination showed a few red cells consistent with an acute injury.

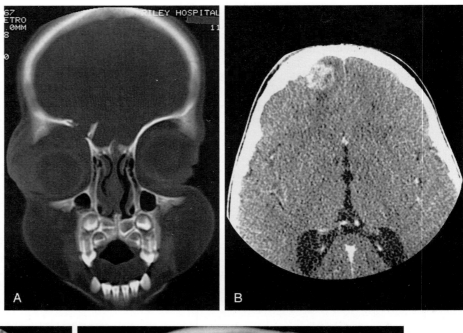

FIGURE 52–20 Penetrating injury secondary to a fall onto a twig. *A,* Coronal CT scan with bone windows shows an orbital roof fracture. *B,* Ten days after the injury, a frontal lobe abscess is seen.

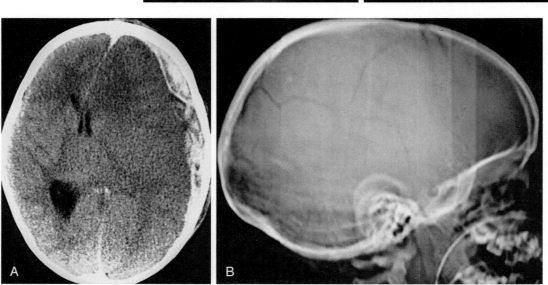

FIGURE 52–21 Nonenhanced axial CT scan *(A)* and scout image *(B)* of a victim of child abuse show a large left acute epidural hematoma with mixed attenuation and severe mass effect and shift. The scout image shows a large, stellate skull fracture.

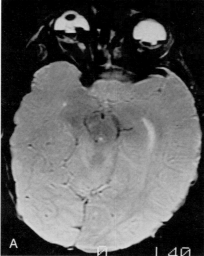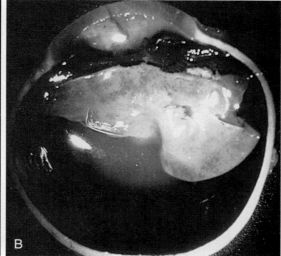

FIGURE 52–22 Axial MRI study (*A*) and postmortem section (*B*) of the eye of a victim of child abuse with bilateral retinal detachments.

bruises are not often seen. First described in 1946 by Caffey, shaken impact injury presented with subdural hematoma, retinal hemorrhages, and metaphyseal fractures of the long bones.[53] Rapid, violent shaking of the large infant head, with weak support from immature neck muscles, caused severe rotational shear injuries.[1, 53, 58] Posterior impact injuries such as hemorrhagic contusions are also seen with shaking injuries, indicating that shaking occurs against a surface such as a mattress.[1, 59] Ripping of the bridging veins causes subdural hematomas.[59] Shaking injuries may cause subdural and epidural hematomas in the spine as well as the brain (Fig. 52–23). Massive rotational forces generated from the shaking cause shearing injuries of the brain, most commonly at the gray-white junction (Fig. 52–24).[25] Brain stem injuries result

in respiratory depression; apnea and hypoxia are common complicating factors. It has been suggested that the perpetrator of the shaking impact injury shakes the crying child in frustration, and stops only when the child stops crying. The cessation of crying may be due to apnea or central brain injury with altered level of consciousness. In the most severe cases, cerebral swelling occurs causing increased intracranial pressure to exceed arterial pressure, and the child dies. The process is exacerbated by the usual delay in reporting the abuse and the delay in appropriate therapy. Subdural hematomas are the most frequent imaging finding in nonaccidental brain injury.[56, 59] On CT, 65% of child abuse victims were found to have subdural hematomas.[23] The subdural hematomas appear most obvious on CT in the interhemispheric fissure (Fig. 52–25), but they are best characterized on MRI, in which the convexity hematomas are better visualized (Fig. 52–

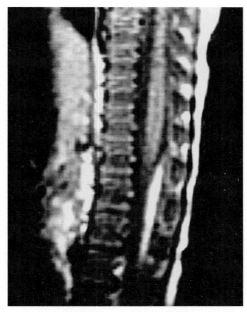

FIGURE 52–23 Sagittal T1-weighted MRI study of a shaken infant shows a high-signal-intensity dorsal extra-axial hematoma within the spinal canal just below the conus.

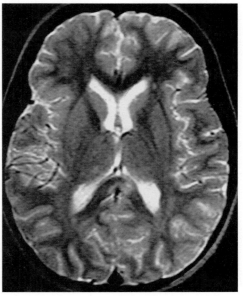

FIGURE 52–24 T2-weighted MRI study shows a corpus callosum shear injury in the splenium.

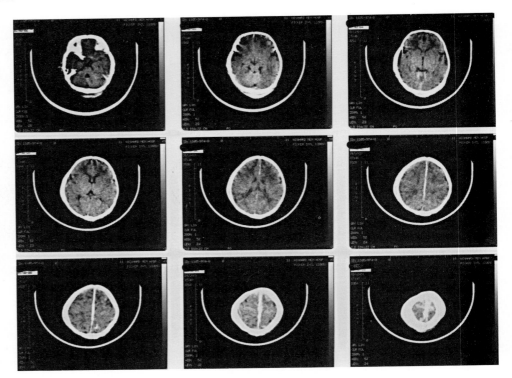

FIGURE 52–25 CT scan clearly shows a large interhemispheric subdural hematoma.

26).[24, 45] Subarachnoid hemorrhage is a common finding in abuse, occurring in approximately 50% of cases on CT. Cerebral swelling, as discussed previously, is a most frequent complication of shaken impact injury.[23] Because of the delay in reporting the injury, swelling is often present by the time the child is seen in the emergency room.[13] The child is usually put to bed after the shaking injury and taken to the hospital only when seizures or respiratory arrest is seen.

Strangulation and suffocation injuries are serious forms of nonaccidental injury that may be easily overlooked or misinterpreted as apnea or sudden death syndrome. The child may be in a coma with the imaging appearance of diffuse hypoxic injury or infarction, with no clear cause (Fig. 52–27). Strangulation will leave bruising on the neck, but suffocation may have no external signs.[1, 60] A typical mechanism for suffocation is smothering with a pillow. Nutritional deprivation is also a common form of abuse that is not suspected. Several forms of abuse may be present in the same child.

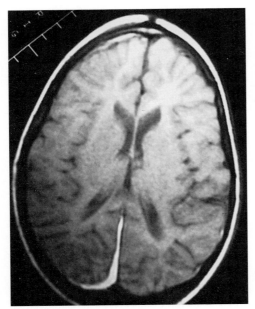

FIGURE 52–26 T1-weighted MRI study shows a right frontal as well as an interhemispheric subdural hematoma.

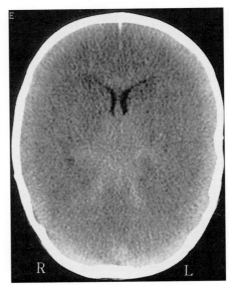

FIGURE 52–27 Complete loss of gray and white matter differentiation on CT scan in a child after an acute strangulation injury.

A child may present with late sequelae of abuse. Even though there is evidence of acute injury, evidence of old injury should be searched for, including cerebral atrophy, hemosiderin, infarction, healing fractures, and hydrocephalus.

References

1. Gean AD. Imaging of Head Trauma. New York, Raven, 1995.
2. Division of Injury Control, Centers for Disease Control. Childhood injuries in the United States. Am J Dis Child 1990;144:627–646.
3. Tepas JJ, DiSeala C, Ramenofsky ML, Barlo B. Mortality in head injury: The pediatric perspective. J Pediatr Surg 1990;25:92–96.
4. Dietrich AM, Bowman MJ, Ginn-Pease ME, et al. Pediatric head injuries: Can clinical factors reliably predict an abnormality on computed tomography? Ann Emerg Med 1993;22:1535–1540.
5. Li G, Baker SP, Fowler C, DiScala C. Factors related to the presence of head injury in bicycle-related pediatric trauma patients. J Trauma 1995;38:871–875.
6. Yancey MK, Herpolsheimer A, Jordan GD, et al. Maternal and neonatal effects of outlet forceps delivery compared with spontaneous vaginal delivery in term pregnancies. Obstet Gynecol 1991;78:646–650.
7. Rorke LB, Zimmerman RA. Prematurity, postmaturity, and destructive lesions in utero. AJNR 1992;13:517–536.
8. Chiaviello CT, Christoph RA, Bond GR. Stairway-related injuries in children. Pediatrics 1994;94:679–681.
9. Smith GA, Dietrich AM, Garcia CT, Shields BJ. Epidemiology of shopping cart–related injuries to children. Arch Pediatr Adolesc Med 1995;149:1207–1210.
10. Sirotnak AP, Krugman RD. Physical abuse of children: An update. Pediatr Rev 1994;15:394–399.
11. Goldstein B, Kelly MM, Bruton D, Cox C. Inflicted versus accidental head injury in critically injured children. Crit Care Med 1993;21:1328–1332.
12. Ball WS. Non-accidental craniocerebral trauma (child abuse). Radiology 1989;173:609.
13. Caffey J. On the theory and practice of shaking infants: Its potential residual effects of permanent brain damage and mental retardation. Am J Dis Child 1972;124:161–169.
14. Luerssen TG, Klauber MR, Marshall LF. Outcome from head injury related to patient's age. A longitudinal prospective study of adult and pediatric head injury. J Neurosurg 1988;68:409–416.
15. Bax M. Child abuse and cerebral palsy. Dev Med Child Neurol 1983;25:141–142.
16. Vane DW, Shackford SR. Epidemiology of rural traumatic death in children: A population-based study. J Trauma 1995;38:867–870.
17. Genuardi FJ, King WD. Inappropriate discharge instructions for youth athletes hospitalized for concussion. Pediatrics 1995;95:216–218.
18. Nance ML, Templeton JM, O'Neill JA Jr. Socioeconomic impact of gunshot wounds in an urban pediatric population. J Pediatr Surg 1994;29:39–43.
19. Davis RL, Hughes M, Gubler KD, et al. The use of cranial CT scans in the triage of pediatric patients with mild head injury. Pediatrics 1995;95:345–349.
20. Scherer LR. Diagnostic imaging in pediatric trauma. Semin Pediatr Surg 1995;4:100–108.
21. Mitchell KA, Fallat ME, Raque GH, et al. Evaluation of minor head injury in children. J Pediatr Surg 1994;29:851–854.
22. Dahl-Grove DL, Chande VT, Barnoski A. Closed head injuries in children: Is hospital admission always necessary? Pediatr Emerg Care 1995;11:86–88.
23. Cohen RA, Kaufman RA, Myers PA, Towbin RB. Cranial computed tomography in the abused child with head injury. AJR 1986;146:97–102.
24. Sato Y, Yuh WTC, Smith WL, etal. Head injury in child abuse: Evaluation with MR imaging. Radiology 1989;173:653–657.
25. Boyko OB. MR angiography of the central nervous system in pediatric patients: Clinical utility. In Proceedings of the Annual Meeting of the Radiological Society of North America, p. 246. Chicago, Radiological Society of North America, 1991.
26. Kissoon N, Dreyer J, Walia M. Pediatric trauma: Differences in pathophysiology, injury patterns, and treatment compared with adult trauma. Can Med Assoc J 1990;142:27–34.
27. Manning JJ, Adour KK. Facial paralysis in children. Pediatrics 1972;49:102–109.
28. Zimmerman RA, Bilaniuk LT. Pediatric head trauma. Neuroimaging Clin N Am 1994;4:349–366.
29. Zimmerman RA, Bilaniuk LT, Genneralli T. Computed tomography of shearing injuries of the cerebral white matter. Radiology 1978;127:393–396.
30. Steinlin M, Dirr R, Martin E, et al. MRI following severe perinatal asphyxia: Preliminary experience. Pediatr Neurol 1991;7:164–170.
31. Roland EH, Hill A, Norman MG, et al. Selective brain stem injury in an asphyxiated newborn: Correlation of clinical, radiological, and neuropathological features. Ann Neurol 1988;23:89–92.
32. Kleinman PK, Zito JL, Davidson RI, Raptopoulos V. The subarachnoid spaces in children: Normal variations in size. Radiology 1983;147:455–457.
33. Laham JL, Cotcamp DH, Gibbons PA, et al. Isolated head injuries versus multiple trauma in pediatric patients: Do the same indications for cervical spine evaluation apply? Pediatr Neurosurg 1994;21:221–226.
34. Zimmerman RA, Bilaniuk LT, Bruce D, et al. Computed tomography of pediatric head trauma: Acute general cerebral swelling. Radiology 1978;126:403–408.
35. Bruce DA, Alavi A, Bilaniuk L, et al. Diffuse cerebral swelling following head injuries in children: The syndrome of "malignant brain edema." J Neurosurg 1981;54:170–178.
36. Bird CR, Drayer BP, Gilles FH. Pathophysiology of "reverse" edema in global cerebral ischemia. AJNR 1989;10:95–98.
37. Han BK, Towbin RB, DeCourten-Myers G, et al. Reversal sign on CT: Effect of anoxic/ischemic cerebral injury in children. AJNR 1989;10:1191–1198.
38. Kjos BO, Brant-Zawadski M, Young RG. Early CT findings of global central nervous system hypoperfusion. AJNR 1983;4:1043–1048.
39. Valk J, van der Knaap MS. Myelination and retarded myelination. In Valk J, van der Knaap MS (eds). Magnetic Resonance of Myelin, Myelination, and Myelin Disorders. Berlin, Springer-Verlag, 1989.
40. Barkovich AJ, Truwit CL. MR of perinatal asphyxia: Correlation of gestational age with pattern of damage. AJNR 1990;11:1087–1095.
41. Goldman-Rakic PS. Development and plasticity of primate frontal association cortex. In Schmitt FO (ed). The Organization of the Cerebral Cortex, pp. 69–97. Cambridge, MA, MIT Press, 1981.
42. Harwood-Nash DC, Hendrick EB, Hudson AR. The significance of skull fracture in children: A study of 1187 patients. Radiology 1971;101:151–160.
43. Muhonen MG, Piper JG, Menezes AH. Pathogenesis and treatment of growing skull fractures. Surg Neurol 1995;43:367–373.
44. Tenner MS, Stein BM. Cerebral herniation in the growing fracture of the skull. Radiology 1970;94:351.
45. Osborn AG, Anderson RE, Wing SD. The false falx sign. Radiology 1980;134:421–425.
46. Orrison WW, Robertson WC, Sackett JF. Computerized tomography and chronic subdural hematomas (effusions) of infancy. Neuroradiology 1978;16:79–81.
47. Hart BL, Dudley MH, Zumwalt RE. Postmortem cranial MRI and autopsy correlation in suspected child abuse. Am J Forensic Med Pathol 1996;17:217–224.
48. Sutton LN, Wang Z, Duhaime AC, et al. Tissue lactate in pediatric head trauma: A clinical study using ¹H NMR spectroscopy. Pediatr Neurosurg 1995;22:81–87.
49. Worley G, Hoffman JM, Paine SS, et al. 18-Fluorodeoxyglucose positron emission tomography in children and adolescents with traumatic brain injury. Devel Med Child Neurol 1995;37:213–220.
50. Morgan LM, Kissoon N, deVebber BL. Experience with the hemophiliac child in a pediatric emergency department. J Emerg Med 1993;11:519–524.
51. Gooding AM, Bastian JF, Peterson BM, Wilson NW. Safety and efficacy of intravenous immunoglobulin prophylaxis in pediatric head trauma patients: A double-blind controlled trial. J Crit Care 1993;8:212–216.
52. Johnson DL, Braun D, Friendly D. Accidental head trauma and retinal hemorrhage. Neurosurgery 1993;33:231–235.
53. Caffey J. Multiple fractures in the long bones of infants suffering from chronic subdural hematoma. AJR 1946;56:163–173.

54. Hiss J, Kahana T. The medicolegal implications of bilateral cranial fractures in infants. J Trauma 1995;38:32–34.

55. Howard JL, Barron BJ, Smith GG. Bone scintigraphy in the evaluation of extra-skeletal injuries from child abuse. Radiographics 1990;10:67–81.

56. Kleinman PK. Diagnostic Imaging of Child Abuse, pp. 159–199. Baltimore, Williams & Wilkins, 1987.

57. Lambert SR, Johnson TE, Hoyt CS. Optic nerve sheath and retinal hemorrhages associated with the shaken baby syndrome. Arch Ophthalmol 1986;104:1509–1512.

58. Bruce DA, Zimmerman RA. Shaken impact syndrome. Ann Pediatr 1989;18:482–494.

59. Leestma JE. Neuropathology of child abuse. In Leestma JE (ed). Forensic Neuropathology, pp. 333–356. New York, Raven, 1988.

60. Bird CR, McMahan JR, Gilles GH, et al. Strangulation in child abuse: CT diagnosis. Radiology 1987;163:373–375.

Index

Note: Page numbers in *italics* refer to illustrations; page numbers followed by the letter t refer to tables.

Chondroid chordoma, 703, 704, 1003, 1344
Chondroma, of skull base, 993
Chondrosarcoma, 704–705
  fibrous dysplasia transformed to, 1114
  in masticator space, 1199–1200
  of larynx, 1450
  of petro-occipital synchondrosis, 703, 704, 705, *705*, 1003
  of skull base, 1002–1003, *1003*
  of spine, 1345
  petrous extension of, 969
  sinonasal, 1128–1129, *1130*
  vs. chondroid chordoma, 703
Chondrosis, intervertebral, 1303
Chordoma, 702–704, *704*
  chondroid, 703, 704, 1003, 1344
  of clivus, 703, *704,* 1003, *1004,* 1344, *1344*
    parapharyngeal extension of, 1192, *1194*
  of skull base, 1003–1005, *1004–1005*
    clival, 703, *704,* 1003, *1004,* 1192, *1194,* 1344, *1344*
  of spine, 1344
    cervical, 1344, *1345*
    sacral, 1337, *1340,* 1344
Choriocarcinoma, of pineal region, 660, 661, 1582
  of sellar region, 1596
Chorioretinitis, HIV infection causing, *1024*
Choristoma, 1244, *1245*
  of neurohypophysis, 693
Choroid, 1017, *1017*
  coloboma of, 1019
  detachment of, staphyloma with, 1020
  hamartoma of, in NF-2, 1728
  leukemic infiltration of, 1057, *1058*
  melanoma of, 1029, 1030t
  metastases to, 1030, *1030*
  staphyloma of, 1020
Choroid arch, of PICA, 238, *240*
Choroid plexus, adenoma of, 680
  calcifications in, 572, *572–573,* 670
    tumoral, 619
  carcinoma of (CPC), 669–671, *670*
    in children, 1609–1612, 1614, *1614*
  congenital tumors of, 315, 380, *381*
  CSF flow pattern and, 1711
  CSF overproduction by, 1706, *1706*
  CSF production by, 1704
  hemorrhage in, in preterm infant, 361
    in term infant, 361
  in infant, CT of, 1481, *1481*
    sonography of, *1486–1487*
  lipoma of, 679
  metastatic tumors in, 675
  papilloma of (CPP), 322–323, 669–671
    in children, 1609–1612, *1612–1613,* 1614, 1629, *1629,* 1630
    vs. central neurocytoma, 1617
    vs. endolymphatic sac tumor, 1744
    vs. meningioma, 638
  pseudocyst of, 303, *304*
  xanthogranulomas of, 572, *572–573,* 679, 1614
Choroid plexus cyst, 382, 677, 679, *681*

Choroid plexus cyst *(Continued)*
  fetal sonography of, 322–323, *323,* 679
  neonatal sonography of, 382, *384*
Choroidal artery(ies), anterior, 220–221, *221–223*
  posterior, 221, *222,* 235–236, *235–237*
Choroidal detachment, 1021, 1025, *1025–1026*
Choroidal fissure, cysts in, 567, *568*
Choroidal vein(s), 247, 248, *248–249*
Ciliary arteries, 218–219, 218t, *219*
Ciliary body, 1017, *1017*
  metastatic carcinoid to, *1030*
Ciliary muscle, 1017
Cine phase contrast, 39, 1708–1710
Cingulate gyrus, 536, *541*
  glucose consumption in, gender and, 92
  myelination in, 1510
Cingulate motor area, 523, 526, *527*
Circle of Willis, 61, 222, *224,* 226
  as collateral pathway, in ICA disease, 730
  Doppler sonography of, 411, *414,* 420
    in spinal headache, 435
    in vasospasm, 425, 426
    windows for, *421,* 422
  in young child, MRI of, 1490
    sonography of, 1484
  phase contrast MRA of, 731
  variations of, 222, 222t, *224–225,* 420, 730
Circumflex branches, of posterior cerebral artery, 235
Circumvallate papilla, 1149, 1151, 1164
Cirsoid aneurysm, 1752
Cisplatin, leukoencephalopathy caused by, 1654
  radiolabeled, PET studies of, 111
Cisterna magna, effacement of, in neural tube defects, 306, 307, 334
  fetal neurosonography of, 298–299, *299–300,* 300–301
  in young child, 1481, 1484
    MRI of, *1488,* 1489
  large, 567–570, 568–569, *569–570,* 1529, 1530, *1530*
    differential diagnosis of, 299
    fetal sonography of, 312, 313
    vs. arachnoid cyst, 1530
Cisternography. See also *CT cisternography.*
  in normal pressure hydrocephalus, 1706
  of CSF leaks, 1142–1143, *1143*
    with MRI, 1143
Cisterns, subarachnoid. See also specific cisterns.
  iophendylate residue in, 574, *574*
  large, 567–570, *569–570*
CIT (iodine-123–labeled), for SPECT, 128, 142, *143*
Citrullinemia, 1656
CJD (Creutzfeldt-Jakob disease), 770–771, 837t, 838t, 840–842, *842*
  PET studies of, 97
Clasp-knife deformity, *1316,* 1317
Claustrum, in normal 2-year-old, 1495, 1496

Claw osteophytes, 1319, *1319*
Clay-shoveler's fracture, 1422–1423, *1425*
Clear cell adenoma, salivary gland, 1256
Cleft palate, 1676–1677
Clinoid processes, 985, *987*
  pituitary gland and, 680
  pneumatization of, 1074, *1074–1075,* 1091
Clioquinol, necrotizing myelopathy caused by, 1375
Clival venous plexus, *243,* 245
Clivus, 985
  chondrosarcoma of, 704, *705*
  chordoma of, 703, *704,* 1003–1005, *1004–1005,* 1344, *1344*
    parapharyngeal extension of, 1192, *1194*
  dysplasia of, 991
  hypoglossal neoplasms and, 1001
  in nasopharyngeal atresia, 1679, *1680*
  petrous bone and, 947
Cloison sagittale, 1176
Clozapine, dopamine receptors and, 98
Cluster headache, Doppler sonography in, 435
Coagulation, hematoma imaging and, 858–859, 860–861, *866*
Coagulopathy, hematoma with, 859
  in amyloidosis, 857
  meningioma causing, 613
Coaptation, of frontal horn, 564, *564*
  of occipital horn, 564, *564*
Coats' disease, 1027
Cobb's syndrome, 1749
Cocaine abuse. See also *Drug abuse.*
  aneurysm and, 758
  Doppler sonography in, transcranial, 437
  hypopharyngeal burns in, 1467
  maternal, 321
    basal ganglia echolucency and, 375
  nasal granuloma caused by, 1100, *1100*
  PET studies of, 105
  septo-optic dysplasia and, 1526
  SPECT studies of, 146, *146*
  vasculitis in, 738
Coccidioidomycosis, 781, 783, 1386
  meningitis in, 788, *791*
Coccyx. See also *Sacrococcygeal teratoma.*
  agenesis of, 1545
Cochlea, 948, 949, *952–953*
  dysplasias of, 960–961, *961*
  schwannoma in, 963, *964*
Cochlear aqueduct, 948, 949
Cochlear duct, 948
Cochlear implants, MRI risk with, 492
  PET study of, 107
Cochlear nerve, 947, 949
  schwannoma of, 963
Cochlear otosclerosis, 964–965, *965*
Cochlear promontory, 949
Cochleosaccular dysplasia, 961
Cockayne's syndrome, 1645, *1646*
Cognitive systems. See also *Language; Memory; Mental activity.*